AF781343

FAO
FISHERIES
PROCEEDINGS

4

Regional Workshop on Preparedness and Response to Aquatic Animal Health Emergencies in Asia

21–23 September 2004
Jakarta, Indonesia

Edited by
Rohana P. Subasinghe
Inland Water Resources and Aquaculture Service
FAO Fisheries Department
Rome, Italy

and

J. Richard Arthur
Barriere
British Colombia, Canada

FOOD AND AGRICULTURE ORGANIZATION OF THE UNITED NATIONS
Rome, 2005

The designations employed and the presentation of material in this information product do not imply the expression of any opinion whatsoever on the part of the Food and Agriculture Organization of the United Nations concerning the legal or development status of any country, territory, city or area or of its authorities, or concerning the delimitation of its frontiers or boundaries.
The views expressed in this publication are those of the authors and do not necessarily reflect the views of the Food and Agriculture Organization of the United Nations.
The mention or omission of specific companies, their products or brand names does not imply any endorsement or judgement by the Food and Agriculture Organization of the United Nations.

ISBN 92-5-105395-2

All rights reserved. Reproduction and dissemination of material in this information product for educational or other non-commercial purposes are authorized without any prior written permission from the copyright holders provided the source is fully acknowledged. Reproduction of material in this information product for resale or other commercial purposes is prohibited without written permission of the copyright holders. Applications for such permission should be addressed to:

Chief
Publishing Management Service
Information Division
FAO
Viale delle Terme di Caracalla, 00100 Rome, Italy
or by e-mail to:
copyright@fao.org

© FAO 2005

Preparation of this document

This document contains the proceedings, including the texts of 14 papers presented, the Working Group reports and the recommendations resulting from the Regional Workshop on Preparedness and Response to Aquatic Animal Health Emergencies, held in Jakarta, Indonesia from 21-23 September 2004.

The workshop was jointly organized by the Food and Agriculture Organization of the United Nations (FAO) Inland Water Resources and Aquaculture Service (FIRI), the Network of Aquaculture Centres in Asia-Pacific (NACA) and the WorldFish Center (WFC), and was hosted by the Government of Indonesia, Ministry of Marine Affairs and Fisheries (MMAF). The editing, publishing and distribution of the document were undertaken by FAO, Rome.

The workshop was made possible with financial assistance through FAO/TCP/INS/2905 – Health Management in Freshwater Aquaculture and the FishCode Programme of the FAO Fisheries Department.

Abstract

This document contains the proceedings, including the texts of 14 papers presented, the Working Group reports and resulting recommendations of the Regional Workshop on Preparedness and Response to Aquatic Animal Health Emergencies, held in Jakarta, Indonesia, from 21-23 September 2004. The workshop was jointly organized by the Food and Agriculture Organization of the United Nations (FAO) Inland Water Resources and Aquaculture Service (FIRI), the Network of Aquaculture Centres in Asia-Pacific (NACA) and the WorldFish Center (WFC), and was hosted by the Government of Indonesia, Ministry of Marine Affairs and Fisheries (MMAF). The workshop was attended by 51 participants, including national policy-makers and scientists from the Asian region, and international experts and resource persons from both the region and elsewhere.

The papers contained herein cover a wide range of topics related to emergency planning and response to serious outbreaks of aquatic animal diseases, including a review of the history, current status and socio-economic impacts (including implications for international trade) of transboundary aquatic animal diseases (TAADs) in Asia; impacts of exotic diseases on aquatic biodiversity; experiences in the aquaculture and livestock sectors in developing and developed countries in the Asia-Pacific region and elsewhere (e.g. Canada, Norway) in dealing with major disease epizootics (including reviews of recent efforts in Indonesia and Japan to deal the serious outbreaks of Koi herpes virus disease); the role of national governments and the private sector; and analyses of regional needs in areas such as contingency planning, legislation (institutional and regulatory frameworks) and capacity building (training, infrastructure, disease diagnostics, surveillance, monitoring and reporting).

The major recommendations of the workshop are:
(i) at the national level, the capacity and awareness of personnel at producer, disease support and decision-making levels, should be strengthened and adequate resources allocated to support implementation of emergency preparedness strategies; (ii) at the regional level, existing disease reporting systems (e.g. NACA/FAO/OIE Quarterly Aquatic Animal Disease Reports) should be further strengthened to ensure increased sharing of information on national aquatic animal disease status and emerging aquatic animal diseases of significance to Asia; (iii) regional technical support mechanisms (e.g. the NACA Regional Advisory Group) should be used to provide expert teams and information to countries in order to assist in early response to disease problems; (iv) research to support early warning and early response should be targeted to rapid diagnostics (e.g. assessment of the accuracy of Level I diagnosis), epidemiology, risk assessments and biosecurity; (v) detailed post-mortem analyses of the outbreaks of Koi herpes virus (KHV) in Japan and Indonesia should be conducted to understand the actions taken by the government and private sector, the extent of their success and the lessons learned; and (vi) core funding should be allocated at national and regional levels to provide ready resources to respond rapidly to emergencies.

Subasinghe, R.P.; Arthur, J.R. (eds.)
Regional Workshop on Preparedness and Response to Aquatic Animal Health Emergencies in Asia. Jakarta, Indonesia, 21–23 September 2004.
FAO Fisheries Proceedings. No. 4. Rome, FAO. 2005. 178p.

Contents

Foreword

The epidemic spread of aquatic animal diseases is an increasing event in many parts of the world and many countries in the Asia-Pacific region have, to various degrees, suffered the consequences of such serious disease outbreaks. We have witnessed the devastating impacts of epizootic ulcerative syndrome (EUS) in freshwater fish during the 1980s and the 1990s, viral encephalopathy and retinopathy (VER) in marine fish since the 1990s, whitespot syndrome virus (WSSV) in penaeid shrimps from the early 1990s, and the emerging Taura syndrome virus (TSV) in *Penaeus vannamei*. There are still a number of unresolved diseases such as Akoya oyster disease in Japan and abalone mortalities in the People's Republic of China. Since 2002, Indonesia has faced a serious epizootic of Koi herpes virus (KHV), causing large-scale mortalities with significant economic losses among cultured common and koi carp (*Cyprinus carpio*) populations. More recently, during the last quarter of 2003, an outbreak of KHV also occurred in common and koi carp in Japan.

The above examples demonstrate the vulnerability of aquaculture and wild resource production to wide-scale infectious disease emergencies and the significant impacts that new diseases can have on local economies. Unless appropriate health management and biosecurity measures are continuously put in place and effectively implemented, the risk of major disease incursions and newly emerging diseases will continue to threaten the sector. Past experiences in dealing with disease epizootics can provide useful lessons towards better preparedness for and improved responses to similar events when they occur in the future.

In the case of KHV, the affected species is widely traded within and among countries inside and outside the region creating a considerable risk of spreading KHV with the movements of common and koi carp, a situation that can lead to transboundary epizootics. Common and koi carp are important commodities, as food fish and high-value ornamental fish, respectively. Many rural communities depend on koi and common carp to support their livelihoods, both in Indonesia and in several neighboring countries. Effective prevention and control measures, complemented by improved extension services, educational programmes and capacity building for farmers and producers are essential to reduce the risk of transboundary epizootics. A strong national approach, along with a well-planned regional strategy, is required to ensure that the operational capability is in place to respond effectively to disease emergencies. Equally important is a clear understanding by both government and the private sector of the benefits to be gained from investing and participating in emergency response systems.

It is clear from our knowledge and recent experience that the capacity for early detection and effective response to disease emergencies is inadequate in many countries in Asia due to several factors, such as limited diagnostic capacities, lack of information, insufficient human resources and infrastructure and lack of financial resources. Limited understanding of the gravity of the problem often results in failure to provide priority action at national and regional levels. This urgently needs rectifying in order to avoid further introduction of exotic pathogens and spreading of emerging diseases. KHV is a prime example, requiring immediate attention from relevant international research and development agencies, as well as the private sector. Concerted action is essential for controlling this serious epizootic and to regain both consumer and producer confidence.

In order to review and evaluate the national and regional status of emergency preparedness and response to infectious diseases in aquatic animals and to find avenues for providing guidance and assistance for national and regional improvements, the Food and Agriculture Organization of the United Nations (FAO) in partnership with the Government of Indonesia, the Network of Aquaculture Centres in Asia-Pacific (NACA) and the WorldFish Center (WFC) organized a workshop entitled "Emergency Preparedness and Response to Aquatic Animal Diseases". The purpose of the Workshop was to review the regional experiences in responding to disease emergencies, including the work accomplished through an FAO Technical Cooperation Programme project in Indonesia aimed at providing technical assistance to improve national capacity to respond to the ongoing carp disease epizootic. The Workshop was intended to assist Indonesia and other countries in the Asian region to: (i) identify actions to reduce the impacts of KHV on aquaculture and small-scale fisheries; and (ii) strengthen preparedness and response to serious aquatic animal disease emergencies.

The Regional Workshop on Emergency Preparedness and Response to Aquatic Animal Diseases was held from 21-23 September 2004 at the Santika Jakarta Hotel, Jakarta, Indonesia. The Workshop was hosted by the Government of Indonesia, under the patronage of the Hon. Minister of Fisheries. Assistance and support for the workshop was provided by the Office International des Épizooties (OIE) Regional Representation for Asia-Pacific (Tokyo), the Southeast Asian Fisheries Development Center (SEAFDEC), the Norwegian Agency for Development (NORAD), the Danish International Development Agency (DANIDA), the Australian Centre for International Agriculture Research (ACIAR), the Australian Agency for International Devlopment (AusAID) and the United Kingdom Department for International Development (DFID). The 51 participants included experts and policy personnel from the region who are responsible for handling health and disease situations in aquatic and terrestrial environments. It is hoped that the Workshop will prime the concept of emergency preparedness and response among aquatic animal health managers so that future national and regional aquatic production and conservation policy and programme development will take such preparedness plans into consideration.

This document presents the proceedings of the Workshop, including the papers presented, a summary of the Working Group discussions and the resulting recommendations. A separate set of guidelines outlining the procedures for contingency planning, emergency preparedness and response for aquatic animal diseases in developing countries will be published as *FAO Fisheries Technical Paper.* No. 486, Preparedness and response to aquatic animal health emergencies in Asia: guidelines.

Recommendations of the workshop

The recommendations presented below are drawn from the Working Group discussions and the final discussion session of the workshop.

Regional cooperation

National agencies have the primary responsibility for responding to disease emergencies, regional cooperation can provide essential support. Existing regional cooperation in aquatic animal disease control in Asia should be further strengthened to support national efforts to control serious aquatic animal disease outbreaks in the region.

Regional reporting and communications, the NACA/FAO/OIE Regional Quarterly Aquatic Animal Disease Reporting System, should be further strengthened to ensure increased sharing of information on national aquatic animal disease status and emerging aquatic animal diseases of significance to Asia. The regional list of aquatic animal diseases should continue to be used as a basis for supporting emergency disease response and preparedness for disease emergencies in the region. Communication between fishery and veterinary authorities should be strengthened so that Asia's regional concerns can be more effectively communicated to OIE. Collaboration and communication among countries should be promoted to influence international standard setting and disease notification.

Regional technical support and existing technical support mechanisms (e.g. the Regional Advisory Group, regional resource centres) should be used to provide expert teams and information to countries to assist in responding quickly to disease problems. Further development of the regional technical support mechanisms under the NACA umbrella is recommended to support harmonization in diagnostics among countries and the upgrading of skills. Collaborative research should be encouraged to understand and respond to significant and emerging diseases in the region.

Early warning and early response

Effective implementation of early warning and early response system at the national level requires participation of personnel at three levels: the producers, the disease support center and the decision-making level. Important recommendations for each of thse levels include:

- At the producer level, (i) disseminating information on disease diagnosis (Level 1); (ii) developing mechanisms for accessing and distributing disease information (including field guides in local languages) and having access to rapid field diagnostic tests, (iii) educating producers on methods of animal examination; (iv) developing a reporting culture among producers; (v) providing support for record keeping; (vi) supporting the development of farmer groups; (vii) providing increased advice on farm biosecurity, safe movement of live aquatic animals and their products; and (viii) providing guidance on methods for safe disposal and sanitation.
- At the disease support level, (i) increasing training and capacity building in diagnostics (Levels 2 & 3); (ii) increased epidemiological training; (iii) improving access to information; (iv) providing support for the establishment of laboratory information management systems; (v) encouraging a culture of disease investigation; and (vi) providing support for coordination between laboratories.

- At the decision-making level, (i) to continuously build awareness; (ii) to support development of practical surveillance systems with the flexibility to use different existing resources (e.g. those of the private sector and the livestock sector); (iii) conducting risk assessments on likely problems; (iv) to provide better description of emergency situations and "triggering" events; (v) to use systems analysis to provide clear descriptions of lines of authority, mandates and activities tuned to local conditions; and (vi) to develop mechanisms for financing.

Training
More work on human resource development is needed. Many training courses have been conducted in the region; however, technical training alone is not seen as sufficient. For example, specific training is needed on how to report scientific information for the purpose of early warning and early response.

Research
The region needs more needs-based, applied research. Research to support early warning should especially be targeted to three areas: pathology, microbiology (parasitology, virology, bacteriology, mycology) and epidemiology (including forecasting, risk assessment and assessment of the accuracy of Level 1 diagnosis). Collaborative research should be encouraged to understand and respond to significant and emerging diseases in the region.

Resources
The region needs resources to draw on in emergencies. Core funding should be allocated to regional organizations (e.g. NACA) to provide ready resources to respond rapidly to emergencies. For the less developed countries in the region (e.g. Cambodia, Laos, Bangladesh), lack of adequate human, institutional and financial resources is still the major constraint and thus training, capacity building and better infrastructure are urgently needed.

Communications
The profile of fish health and emergency preparedness needs to be raised to both the public and private sectors, highlighting the importance of emergencies from a socio-economic point of view. The role of "larger players" (geopolitical and supranational organizations and donor agencies) in addressing these issues needs to be strengthened.

Information transfer
Although there is a lot of knowledge about aquatic animal health in the world, the transfer of this knowledge to the Asian Region requires financial resources. Developed countries should invest on this issue because such knowledge is essential for the development of emergency preparedness systems.

Field exercises
Once countries have developed disease emergency contingency plans, staging field exercises for a simulated national disease emergency should be undertaken, as this will allow countries to test their contingency plans and see how their communication system works. Mock outbreaks (simulations) should be done at both the national and regional levels. These should involve various stakeholders such as the military, justice, finance, environment, agriculture etc.

Socio-economic impacts of disease epizootics
The investment of governments and the private sector in emergency preparedness and in aquatic animal health, in general, does not reflect the importance and value of the

aquaculture and fisheries resource. A desk study of the value of the aquatic resources in the different countries should be conducted, including an assessment of the magnitude of investment in the sector and the impact of disease. Such a study could be funded and undertaken by FAO and NACA.

Koi herpes virus outbreaks

Recent experience has shown that the systems in place in Indonesia and Japan to cope with disease emergencies were not effective against KHV infection. Detailed post-mortem analyses of the outbreaks of KHV in both countries should be conducted to determine why the respective governments were unable to contain the disease, the actions taken by government and private sector, the extent of their success. and the lessons learned.

It may be useful to have another workshop in a few years time to assess the progress made in Japan in establishing a system for early warning and preparedness.

Pilot projects on emerging diseases

Several emerging diseases are present in the region, and countries whose industries culture susceptible species should put in place some practical approaches. Pilot activities for key diseases such as abalone mortality, white tail disease etc. could be initiated by selecting a country to pilot a system for each disease. Each pilot system could involve people from the various countries most likely to be impacted by the disease and maybe also have people to visit different countries.

ANNEX 1

List of participants

Dr Juan D. Albaladejo	Supervising Aquaculturist Bureau of Fisheries and Aquatic Resources 860 Quezon Avenue Quezon City, Philippines 1103	E-mail: jalbaladejo@bfar.da.gov.ph
Dr J. Richard Arthur	Box 1216, Barriere, B.C. Canada V0E 1E0	E-mail: jrarthur@telus.net
Dr Francis Christian Baldock	Director, AusVet Animal Health Services PO Box 3180, South Brisbane Qld 4101 Australia	E-mail: chris@ausvet.com.au
Dr Peter Beers	Manager, Aquatic Animal Biosecurity Biosecurity Australia, Department of Agriculture, Fisheries and Forestry Edmund Barton Building, King Avenue Barton, ACT 2600, Australia	E-mail: peter.beers@daff.gov.au
Dr Supranee Chinabut	Senior Advisor on Fish Diseases Department of Fisheries Bangkok 10900 Bangkok, Thailand	E-mail: Supranee@fisheries.go.th
Mr Flavio Corsin	Aquatic Animal Health Specialist SUMA Office, Ministry of Fisheries 10 Nguyen Cong Hoan Street Ba Dinh District Hanoi, Viet Nam	E-mail: Flavio.corsin@enaca.org
Dr Sena S. De Silva	School of Ecology & Environment Deakin University PO Box 423, Warrnambool Victoria, Australia	E-mail: sena@deakin.edu.au
Mr Daniel Fegan	Regional Technical Manager Aquaculture Thailand 5th Floor, Preecha Building 2533 Sukhumvit Road Bangchack, Prakhanong Bangkok 10260, Thailand	E-mail: dfegan@alltech.com

Dr Simon Funge-Smith	Aquaculture Officer Food and Agriculture Organization of the United Nations Regional Office for Asia and the Pacific 39 Phra Atit Road Bangkok 10200, Thailand	E-mail: simon.fungesmith@fao.org
Dr Roar Gudding	Director General National Veterinary Institute PO Box 8156 DEP 0033 Oslo, Norway	E-mail: roar.gudding@vetinst.no
Dr A.N. Hasna Banu	Senior Scientific Officer Bangladesh Fisheries Research Institute Fish Disease Division Freshwater Station Mymensingh – 2201, Bangladesh	E-mail: fsbfri@bdonline.com; ismail@royalten.net
Mr Pedro Bueno	Director General Network of Aquaculture Centres in Asia-Pacific Kasetsart University Campus Ladyao, Jatujak, Bangkok 10900, Thailand	E-mail: pedro.bueno@enaca.org
Mr Nguyen Tu Cuong	Director, NAFIQAVED Ministry of Fisheries 10 Ngunyen Corg Hoan Street Ba Dinh District Hanoi, Viet Nam	E-mail: NAFIQAVED@mofi.gov.vn
Dr Doan Van Dai	Aquaculture Specialist Aquaculture Department Ministry of Fisheries 10 Ngunyen Corg Hoan Street Ba Dinh District Hanoi, Viet Nam	
Dr Darnas Dana	Directorate of Fish Health and Environment Directorate General of Aquaculture Ministry of Marine Affairs and Fisheries Jl. Harsono RM No.3 Gd. B lt. IV Ragunan-Jakarta Selatan, Indonesia	E-mail: dfhe@ditkeskanling.go.id
Ir Rubiyanto Haliman	PT. Tirta Mutiara Makmur PO Box 14 Besuki-Situbondo, Indonesia	E-mail: rhaliman@yahoo.com
Dr Hardjono	Center for Fish Quarantine Jl. MT Haryono Kav. 52-53 Jakarta Selatan, Indonesia	

Dr Tore Håstein	Senior Advisor National Veterinary Institute PO Box 8156 DEP 0033 Oslo, Norway	E-mail: tore.hastein@vetinst.no
Ir Dwika Herdikiawan	Directorate of Fish Health and Environment Directorate General of Aquaculture Ministry of Marine Affairs and Fisheries Jl. Harsono RM No.3 Gd. B lt. IV Ragunan-Jakarta Selatan, Indonesia	E-mail: dfhe@ditkeskanling.go.id; dwikahdk@indosat.net.id
Mrs Le Thi Hue	NAFIQAVED Ministry of Fisheries 10 Ngunyen Corg Hoan Street Ba Dinh District Hanoi, Viet Nam	E-mail: hue.nafi@mofi.gov.vn
Dr Takaji Iida	Aquatic Animal Health Division National Research Institute of Aquaculture Fisheries Research Agency Nansei Mei 516-0193 Japan	E-mail: takaji@fra.affrc.go.jp
Prof Dr Kamiso	University of Gadjah Mada Jurusan Perikanan, Fakultas Pertanian Yogyakarta, Indonesia	
Dr Celia R. Lavilla-Pitogo	Fish Health Specialist Southeast Asian Fisheries Development Center – Aquaculture Department Tigbauan 5021, Iloilo, Philippines	E-mail: celiap@aqd.seafdec.org.ph
Dr Juan Lubroth	Animal Production and Health Service Food and Agriculture Organization of the United Nations Vialle delle Terme di Caracalla 00100 Rome, Italy	E-mail: juan.lubroth@fao.org
Dr Nguyen Xuan Ly	Head, Science & Technology Department Ministry of Fisheries Hanoi, Viet Nam	E-mail: nguyenxuangly@mofi.gov.vn; khcn1@hn.vnn.vn
Dr C.V. Mohan	Aquatic Animal Health Specialist Network of Aquaculture Centres in Asia-Pacific Suraswadi Building, DOF Complex Kasetsart University Campus Ladyao, Jatujak, Bangkok 10900, Thailand	E-mail: mohan@enaca.org

Ir Endang Mudjiutami	Center for Freshwater Aquaculture Development Jl. Salabintana No. 17 Sukabumi, Indonesia	E-mail: bbat@sukabumi.wasantara.net.id
Dr M. Murdjani	Main Center for Brackishwater Aquaculture Development Jl. Pemandian Kartini PO Box 1 Jepara, Indonesia	E-mail: bbap@idola.net.id
Dr Kazuya Nagasawa	Fish Disease Expert Southeast Asian Fisheries Development Center – Aquaculture Department Tigbauan 5021, Iloilo, Philippines	E-mail: nagasawa@aqd.seafdec.org.ph
Dr Yoshiyuki Oketani	Deputy Regional Representative Office International des Épizooties Regional Representation for Asia and the Pacific East 311, Shin-Aoyama Bldg 1-1-1 Minami-Aoyama, Minato-ku Tokyo 107-0062, Japan	E-mail: oietokyo@tky.3web.ne.jp
Risza Oktavia S	Directorate of Fish Health and Environment Directorate General of Aquaculture Ministry of Marine Affairs and Fisheries Jl. Harsono RM No.3 Gd. B lt. IV Ragunan-Jakarta Selatan, Indonesia	E-mail: dfhe@ditkeskanling.go.id
Dr Fachriyan Hasmi Pasaribu	Institute Pertanian Bogor Jl. Agatis Kampus IPB Darmaga Bogor, Indonesia	E-mail: Fkh-ipb@bogor.wasantara.net.id
Dr Michael Phillips	Environment Specialist Network of Aquaculture Centres in Asia-Pacific Suraswadi Building, DOF Complex Kasetsart University Campus Ladyao, Jatujak, Bangkok 10900, Thailand	E-mail: Michael.Phillips@enaca.org
Prof. Dr Budi Prayitno	Fisheries Office Province of Central Java Jl. Imam Bonjol No. 134 Semarang, Indonesia	E-mail: budipr@indosat.net.id
Andi Rahman	Directorate of Fish Health and Environment Directorate General of Aquaculture Ministry of Marine Affairs and Fisheries Jl. Harsono RM No.3 Gd. B lt. IV Ragunan-Jakarta Selatan, Indonesia	E-mail: dfhe@ditkeskanling.go.id

M. Rifqi	Directorate of Fish Health and Environment Directorate General of Aquaculture Ministry of Marine Affairs and Fisheries Jl. Harsono RM No.3 Gd. B lt. IV Ragunan-Jakarta Selatan, Indonesia	E-mail: dfhe@ditkeskanling.go.id
Dr Djumbuh Rukmono	Directorate of Fish Health and Environment Directorate General of Aquaculture Ministry of Marine Affairs and Fisheries Jl. Harsono RM No.3 Gd. B lt. IV Ragunan-Jakarta Selatan, Indonesia	E-mail: dfhe@ditkeskanling.go.id
Dr S.D. Athula Senevirathne	Project Director Jaysons Aqua Products (Pvt) Ltd. Ferry Road Thoduwawa, Sri Lanka	E-mail: Jay.son@sltnet.lk
Prof Mohamed Shariff	Faculty of Veterinary Medicine Universiti Putra Malaysia 43400 Serdang Selangor, Malaysia	E-mail: shariff@vet.upm.edu.my
Dr Rohana P. Subasinghe	Fisheries Department Food and Agriculture Organization of the United Nations Viale delle Terme di Caracalla 00100 Rome, Italy	E-mail: Rohana.Subasinghe@fao.org
Dr Agus Sunarto	Fish Health Research Laboratory Jl. Ragunan 20, Pasar Minggu Jakarta Selatan, Indonesia	E-mail: agussunarto@hotmail.com; lariki@cbn.net.id
Dr Hambali Supriyadi	Fish Health Research Laboratory Jl. Ragunan 20, Pasar Minggu Jakarta Selatan, Indonesia	E-mail: lariki@cbn.net.id
Dr Arief Taslihan	Main Center for Brackishwater Aquaculture Development Jl. Pemandian Kartini PO Box 1 Jepara, Indonesia	E-mail: bbap@idola.net.id
Ir. Taukhid	Fish Health Research Laboratory Jl. Ragunan 20, Pasar Minggu Jakarta Selatan, Indonesia	E-mail: lariki@cbn.net.id
Mrs Thongphoun Theungphachanh	Head of Animal Production and Quality Control Unit Department of Livestock and Fisheries National Animal Health Centre PO Box 811 Vientiane, Lao, PDR	E-mail: theungphachanh@yahoo.com; laonachc@laotel.com

Mrs Phan Thi Van	Research Institute for Aquaculture No. 1 Dinh Bang, Tien Son Bac Ninh, Hanoi, Viet Nam	E-mail: phanvan@hn.vnn.vn
Ms Annick Van Houtte	Legal Officer Legal Office Food and Agriculture Organization of the United Nations Viale delle Terme di Caracalla 00100 Rome, Italy	E-mail: VanHoutte.Annick@fao.org
Mr Hav Viseth	Chief, Aquaculture Division Department of Fisheries No. 186, Norodom Blvd, PO Box 835 Phnom Penh, Cambodia	E-mail: aqua@online.com.kh
Mr D.E.M. Weerakoon	Director General National Aquaculture Development Authority Colombo, Sri Lanka	E-mail: aqua1@eureka.lk aqua2@eureka.lk
Drh Nila Widodari	Directorate Fish Health and Environment Directorate General of Aquaculture Ministry of Marine Affairs and Fisheries Jl. Harsono RM No.3 Gd. B lt. IV Ragunan-Jakarta Selatan, Indonesia	E-mail: dfhe@ditkeskanling.go.id

ANNEX 2

Reports of the working groups

The following section briefly summarizes the discussions and conclusions arising from the three Working Group Meetings.

WORKING GROUP 1 – REGIONAL COOPERATION

Members: Elmo Weerakorn, Simon Funge-Smith, Michael Phillips, Hardjono, Nguyen Tu Cuong, Nguyen Xuan Ly, Doan van Dai, Kazuya Nagasawa, Rubiyanto Haliman, Fachriyan H. Pasarien, Darnas Dana, Supranee Chinabut, Athula Seneviratna, Sena De Silva and Yoshiyuki Oketani

Objective – The objective of Working Group 1 was to identify needs and possible solutions related to improving regional cooperation to assist national efforts at emergency preparedness and response to outbreaks of serious aquatic animal diseases.

The Working Group recognized that while national agencies have the primary responsibility for responding to disease emergencies, regional cooperation can provide essential support. There is already collaboration in aquatic animal disease control in Asia that has helped in responding to emergency aquatic animal disease outbreaks. We should therefore build on these existing structures to strengthen cooperation to support national efforts to control serious aquatic animal disease outbreaks.

The Working Group then discussed the specific needs of the region with regards to improving international cooperation to address aquatic animal heath emergencies more effectively.

Regional reporting and communications – The Working Group noted that increased sharing of information on national aquatic animal disease status and emerging aquatic animal diseases of significance to Asia is required, and that the openness and accuracy of with which Asian nations provide this information needs to be improved. Awareness on methods for the control of aquatic animal diseases and emergency response should be increased. The Working Group noted that the NACA/FAO/OIE Regional Aquatic Animal Disease Reporting System is an important regional resource, and that the reporting system and the communication networks that support it at the national and regional levels should be further strengthened.

The Working Group noted the importance of the OIE in the setting of aquatic animal health reference standards for international trade, disease reporting and the disease control process. It also noted and that, for most Asian countries, the reporting of aquatic animal diseases to the OIE involves both the national fisheries and veterinary authorities. However, communication between Chief Veterinary Officers (CVOs) and senior fisheries officers within the OIE system is limited, and there are limited inputs from Asian countries to the standard setting process. Although the veterinary authorities have responsibility for official communication to OIE on livestock and aquatic animal diseases important for international trade, most veterinary authorities in Asia have limited experience with aquatic animal diseases. Thus communication between fishery and veterinary authorities should be strengthened so that Asia's regional concerns can be more effectively communicated to OIE. In this regard, national fisheries agencies need to be more proactive in developing the necessary linkages with their veterinary counterparts. Regional disease reporting is presently based on official quarterly reports. Countries should report more frequently on emergency diseases, to support rational decisions on emergency response measures.

The Working Group noted that the regional list of aquatic animal diseases – reviewed and developed annually by the Regional Advisory Group – includes both OIE-listed diseases and other diseases of emerging importance to the region. Such a list is useful and should continue to be used as a basis for supporting emergency disease response and preparedness for disease emergencies. The Regional Advisory Group should be strengthened through making formal recommendations to be passed through the veterinary channels to OIE.

Regional technical support – The Working Group considered that primary responsibility for prevention, preparedness and response to disease emergencies lies within each country. However, regional cooperation should be used to provide expert teams and information to countries to assist in responding quickly to disease problems. The Regional Advisory Group is a useful mechanism that can be more active in providing coordination and advice on recognizing emergencies and identifying the resources needed to respond effectively. Several competent regional institutions and resource centers exist to provide technical assistance (e.g. SEAFDEC-AQD, AAHRI) in disease emergencies. Collaboration between countries, particularly those countries sharing common borders and watersheds such as the Mekong Basin, on preventing the spread of aquatic animal diseases is also recommended for emergencies.

Diagnostic harmonization – The Working Work recognized that the sharing of information on significant aquatic animal diseases needs to be supported by better harmonization of disease diagnostic tests and techniques. Resource centers with specialist diagnostic skills are required to provide technical support to assist countries in dealing with aquatic animal disease problems. The further development of the resource centers and expert network under the NACA umbrella is recommended to support harmonization in diagnostics among countries and the upgrading of skills.

The Working Group recognized that the OIE code and diagnostic manual should be used as a reference in harmonizing diagnostic standards, and that care must be taken to ensure consistency with international standards. Collaboration and communication among countries should be promoted to influence international standard setting and disease notification. It is important for the region to be more active in getting information on aquatic animal diseases in the region into the OIE standards.

Research – Collaborative research should be encouraged to understand and respond to significant and emerging diseases in the region. The private sector must be involved, since they are also part of networks.

Resources – The Working Group agreed that the region needs resources to draw on in emergencies. Core funding should be allocated to NACA to provide ready resources to respond rapidly to emergencies; donor support should be sought.

Further regional cooperation – The Working Group recommended that joint activities between countries for testing of emergency response should be undertaken, and that regular meetings between countries and the exchange of expertise should be encouraged. Regional training on emergency preparedness is recommended. Regional centers to provide technical support to address emerging disease problems should be further developed.

WORKING GROUP 2 – EARLY WARNING

Members: Chris Baldock (Chairman), Agus Sunarto (Vice-chairperson), Flavio Corsin and C.V. Mohan (Rapporteurs), Celia R Lavilla-Pitogo, Phan Thi Van, Takaji Iida, Murdjani, Taukhid, Hambali Supriyadi , Ly Thi Thanh Loan, Viseth Hav, Thongphoun and Roar Gudding

Objective – The objective of Working Group 2 was to develop recommendations on what activities have to be carried out to implement early warning and detection of aquatic animal health problems and to identify the future steps to be taken at the national level.

Definition of emergency – The Working Group discussed the criteria that can be used to define an aquatic animal health emergency. The group agreed that the definition of emergency for producers and government may be different. For producers, an emergency would be a disease/syndrome (e.g. exotic disease, new disease) observed for the first time and/or any significant mortality/morbidity occurring in their system, including outbreaks of known diseases (e.g. EUS). From the perspective of a government, in addition to the above, emergencies would also include diseases having an impact on trade, human health or affecting the livelihood of poor communities. The Working Group recognized that although some diseases may not yet be considered emergencies, and thus might be ignored by decision makers, they may be recognized as emergencies in the future (e.g. white tail disease).

List of diseases for surveillance system – All the countries in the region have adopted the NACA/FAO/OIE regional disease list, which includes all diseases listed by OIE plus additional diseases of concern to the region. In addition, some countries have more comprehensive national disease lists that include pathogens/diseases of national concern.

Capacity requirements and delivery – A key point in the implementation of early warning systems is assessing the capacity requirements and how to deliver them. The following constraints were identified:

- Issues associated with the ability of field officers and other stakeholders to contribute to the flow of information (e.g. resources etc.); and
- Lack of staff, required skills, a system with the necessary flexibility, stakeholder motivation, and ability to confirm suspect outbreaks and their associated causes.

To alleviate the lack of field officers, farmer-group leaders and volunteer extension workers could be involved in the flow of information.

The Working Group identified three major levels at which capacity building is required: the producers, the disease support center and the decision-making level. Depending on the country, the latter two levels could be operating either at the provincial or national level. The responsibilities and the capacity required at the different levels for implementing an early warning system are identified in table 1.

Communication: warning system – The Working Group highlighted issues related to the slowness of information flow, which in some cases can take up to 1.5 months from emergency occurrence to response initiation. Of special concern is the fact that affected stock may be translocated in the time between emergency detection at the producer level and the initiation of a response, greatly increasing the risk of infectious disease spread. A potential solution to increase the speed of the warning system would be to limit the number of people/institutions involved in the information flow.

Web-based systems for disease reporting have been developed in some of the countries (e.g. Indofish), however, there are problems in populating databases. This is due to a number of constraints related to poor communication, including lack of lower level resources (e.g. at the level of producers, field officers etc.), internet culture, and strong leadership (people that can make it happen).

TABLE 1

Level	Responsibilities	Capacity Required
Producer	• recognize a disease emergency • report to the concerned authority	• ability to recognize an aquatic animal health problem • ability to recognize clinical signs (level 1 diagnosis) • ability to communicate the emergency to responsible authorities
Disease support center	• investigate emergencies • carry out targeted surveillance, when required • perform diagnostic tests (level 2 & 3) • ensure accuracy through a laboratory information management system • report to relevant authorities	• culture of disease investigation • capacity in diagnostics (Level 2&3) • expertise to establish lab information management systems • capacity to conduct surveillance
Decision making	• confirm disease emergencies & announce outbreaks • organize & coordinate surveillance systems & disease reporting for early warning • conduct risk analysis • develop national contingency plans for dealing with aquatic animal disease emergencies • communicate emergencies to relevant regional/international institutions	• awareness on significant health problems within the country & internationally • expertise in development of surveillance, risk analysis & other key areas

Encouraging producers to send information directly to the national level using modern communication tools (e.g. digital pictures, phone) is an approach that could be taken to overcome the slowness of the information flow and to make best use of the limited expertise available. The response from the national level could then be channeled to the producers through the local services (e.g. field officers, farmer groups). However, this approach may have limited application to the current Asian context.

The Working Group regarded the creation of regional awareness through the QAAD reporting system (e.g. for KHV) to be a part of an early warning system. This serves as an early warning for countries with susceptible species, so that they can take the necessary actions. It was recognized that regional awareness has the additional advantage of generating regional cooperation.

The Working Group identified possible tools for communicating emergencies at a wider level. These include Websites of regional organizations (e.g. NACA, SEAFDEC), aquafarmers' corner, on-line e-learning (which could involve a moderator), and mailing lists (e.g. Indonesian aquaculture mailing list for shrimp culture).

Motivation – The Working Group recognized that motivation at every level was a major concern. As the producers are normally the first to recognize an emergency, their motivation to report to the relevant authorities is essential to an early warning system. The Working Group discussed what would motivate producers to report and what can be done to promote motivation. The following issues were identified:

- building producers' trust in the field officers, who would need or have access to the knowledge required to help producers;
- creating awareness in producers on the risks faced when a disease emergency is not promptly reported;
- giving appropriate feedback on the problems reported and samples collected;
- providing solution to the problems – on this issue, the group expressed the concern that producers might stop reporting problems that cannot be solved;
- developing legislation to which the producers have to comply; and
- providing compensation (e.g. as in Japan).

Surveillance – The Working Group recognized that disease surveillance forms the basis for early warning and identified the following areas where improvements are necessary for the implementation of effective surveillance systems:

- better coordination at the national level;
- availability of adequate resources at every level;
- better problem definition and prioritization for using the often-limited resources;
- better management of laboratory information (e.g. sample tracking, validation); laboratory information management systems are well developed only in some countries;
- better diagnostic capability, with strong emphasis on better use of robust diagnostic techniques (e.g. pathology).

Enabling research – The Working Group recognized the importance of needs-based, applied research. Research to support early warning should especially be targeted to three areas: pathology, microbiology (parasitology, virology, bacteriology, mycology) and epidemiology (including forecasting, risk assessment and assessment of the accuracy of Level 1 diagnosis).

Legislation/notification-reporting – The Working Group recognized that legislation is an important support to the implementation of early warning (e.g. the Australian experience), although the existence of legislation, by itself, does not ensure the implementation of an effective system.

Regional/national planning and coordination – The Working Group recognized the need for awareness building at the national level on the importance of different levels of diagnosis (i.e. Levels 1, 2 and 3). This concern rises from the fact that Level 3 diagnosis is often perceived as sufficient. Another concern at the national level is the lack of awareness of diseases of aquatic animals by the livestock veterinary authority, which often hosts the OIE national delegate.

Interaction at the regional level was also recognized as essential to coordinate efforts, especially when countries share susceptible species. Issues such as the trade implications of reporting emergencies arise however, when a country considers whether or not to report an emergency associated with a non-OIE listed disease and ask for regional support.

PROBLEMS AND SOLUTIONS

For the purpose of identifying what needs to be done and the way forward, the group considered three disease emergency scenarios: (a) occurrence of an exotic disease, (b) outbreak of an unknown disease and (c) increased occurrence of a known endemic disease. Problems and solutions were identified at the producer, disease support and decision-making levels to support the implementation of an early warning system:

- **Producer level** – At the producer level, the major problems were identified as (i) poor ability to recognize the occurrence of a new or exotic disease, or to recognize a change in the magnitude of known disease; poor awareness of reporting protocol; and (iii) lack of motivation. Solutions suggested by the Working Group included (i) disseminating information on disease diagnosis (Level 1) and what to look at to identify problems; educating producers on methods of animal examination; (ii) developing a reporting culture among producers; (iii) providing support for record keeping; and (iv) supporting the development of farmer groups.
- **Disease support level** – At the disease support level, the Working Group identified problems due to (i) poor expertise in general pathology (inability to recognize new diseases) and disease diagnosis (Levels 2 & 3); (ii) inability of fish health workers to remain current with new diagnostic advancements; (iii) a general inadequacy in dedicated infrastructure and human resources in some countries (often with no obvious solution); (iv) poor awareness and/or motivation on the part of

fish health workers on the need to investigate all reports of disease outbreaks; (v) lack of active surveillance programmes; (vi) poor laboratory information management systems; and (vii) limited coordination between existing laboratories. The solutions identified included (i) increasing training and capacity building in diagnostics (Levels 2 & 3); (ii) improving access to information; (iii) providing support for the establishment of laboratory information management systems; (iv) encouraging a culture of disease investigation; and (v) providing support for coordination between laboratories.
- **Decision-making level** – At the decision-making level, the Working Group identified problems concerning (i) poor awareness of decision-makers on important issues (e.g. exotic disease), (ii) inadequate baseline data on diseases, (iii) lack of commitment in developing effective systems (e.g. quarantine, surveillance, risk analysis); (iv) slowness to report to the region and back to farmers; and (v) lack of motivation (in the case where a disease is already present). The solutions identified were (i) to continuously build awareness and (ii) to support development of practical surveillance systems with the flexibility to use different existing resources (e.g. those of the private sector and the livestock sector).

WORKING GROUP 3 – EARLY RESPONSE

Members: Dan Fegan (Chairman), Peter Beers (vice-chair), Mhd. Shariff and Richard Arthur (rapporteurs), Tore Hastein, Juan Albaladejo, Sarah Saleheen, Hasna Banu, Kamiso H. Nitimulyo, Arief Tasliihan, Doan Van Dai, Le Thi Hue Endang, Mudjintami and Dwika Herdikiawan .

Objective – The objective of Working Group 3 was to examine early response efforts both within and outside the region and develop recommendations on what activities have to be carried out to improve national capacity to mount timely and effective early responses to emergency disease situations.

After considerable discussion of individual country experiences, the Working Group considered the elements essential to mounting an effective early response to an emergency disease outbreak. These include:

- Authority to decide that an emergency response is required (may include pre-established criteria for identifying an emergency situation).
- Having a contingency plan in place. The plan should have been developed with the participation of all stakeholders, especially representatives from the farmers and industry. There is also a need to make new and/or emerging diseases reportable.
- Clear assignment/division of responsibilities. (For several countries, the issue of fisheries vs veterinary mandates and responsibilities has not been fully resolved. However, veterinarians have the authority to prescribe drugs in all countries.)
- Authority to place restrictions or enforce compliance on a farm or production facility (i.e. adequate legislation, enforcement and private-sector involvement).
- Access to adequate resources, including rapid access to funds needed to respond to an outbreak.
- Ability to develop an adequate case definition. (requires decisions on who is responsible for developing a national case definition and on how to access the necessary epidemiological expertise).
- Ability to define the extent of the problem and its pattern of spread.
- Ability to determine the costs vs benefits of potential interventions.
- Ability to implement movement restriction and determine the affected areas (feedback process).
- Capacity for adequate and effective communications, including publication of a case definition, internal communications, media relations, contacts with fish farmers etc.
- Presence of an established and effective disease reporting system.
- Access to adequate diagnostic capability
- Presence of an established education and extension system

The Working Group then considered in more detail some of the major requirements of effective early response to disease emergencies, the essential components and issues, the constraints, and the possible solutions.

Authority/responsibility – The essential components/issues for this major requirement were identified as (i) having defined responsibilities and lines of reporting, (ii) having an adequate case definition, (iii) being able to recognize an emergency situation (emergency recognition) and (iv) having adequate contingency planning to respond effectively to the emergency. The Working Group identified the following constraints: inadequate knowledge and training, unclear responsibilities, unclear chain of reporting, inadequate legislation and/or policy, inadequate private-sector cooperation, inadequate compensation and lack of donor support. The solutions were considered to be (i) better description of emergency situations and "triggering" events; (ii) use of systems analysis to provide clear descriptions of lines of authority, mandates and activities tuned to local conditions; (iii) effective implementation and coordination among agencies; and (v) assistance with contingency planning.

On-site investigation – The Working Group identified the essential components/issues for this major requirement as (i) trained local officers, (ii) expert backup, (iii) sample collection and (iv) farmer consultation. The main constraint noted was lack of resources. The solutions included increased epidemiological training, development of mechanisms for financing (local and international), development of effective animal health links (e.g. between fisheries departments and veterinary services), conducting risk assessments on likely problems; developing mechanisms for accessing and distributing disease information (including field guides in local languages) and having access to rapid field diagnostic tests.

Laboratory support – The Working Group identified the essential components/issues for this major requirement as (i) access to adequate resources, (ii) presence of an effective sample submission system, and (iii) the presence of adequate regional and national support. Lack of resources (human, infrastructure, financial etc.) was considered the main impediment, while potential solutions included increasing the availability of tests, developing rapid field diagnostic tests, developing collection and handling protocols, and developing laboratory accession and reporting systems.

Quarantine/movement restrictions – The Working Group identified the essential components/issues for this major requirement as (i) adequate biosecurity (water, vectors, stock); (ii) adequate and safe sanitation and disposal; (iii) appropriate and safe chemical usage; and (v) adequate supporting legislation. The primary constraints were seen as a lack of expertise and resources. Solutions included providing increased advice on farm biosecurity; developing local procedures; providing practical advice on safe movement of live aquatic animals and their products, on chemical usage, and on methods for safe disposal and sanitation; and developing GIS support systems for farm, geographical and trade mapping.

Epidemiological investigations – The Working Group identified the essential components/issues for this major requirement as (i) need to be able to trace disease outbreaks both forward and backward; (ii) to determine the extent of problem and its spread; and (iii) to have adequate record-keeping (both on and off site), coordination and data analysis. Lack of expertise and resources were identified as main constraints, while providing training in epidemiology and emergency management, and developing information management systems were seen as potential solutions.

Communications – The Working Group identified the essential components/issues for this major requirement as (i) having adequate local communication, including feed back; (ii) having adequate communication at the national level; (iii) dealing effectively with the media; (iv) developing effective reporting systems for communicating with stakeholders and (v) having mechanisms to provide regular updates of the disease emergency situation. The major constraint identified was a lack of experienced people to deal with media, while increasing the availability of information on biosecurity practices, providing media training and developing information reporting systems were seen as possible solutions.

Moving on (post-emergency actions) – The working group identified the essential components/issues for this major requirement as (i) making good decisions on control of movements of aquatic animals and/or zoning; (ii) conducting enabling research (including developing vaccines for major pathogens); and (iv) providing advice. The major constraints were identified as lack of expertise and resources, while the possible solutions included improving research infrastructure, developing and improving information dissemination systems, and developing zoning plans (including monitoring and surveillance programmes).

Post-mortem/cost-benefit analysis – The Working Group identified the essential components/issues for this major requirement as (i) learning from the experience, and (ii) providing feedback and improvement to stakeholders. The major constraints were identified as lack of expertise and resources, while obtaining access to cost/benefits expertise was seen as a solution.

Contributed papers

A historical overview of pathogen introductions and their transboundary spread in Asia

J. Richard Arthur
Barriere, British Colombia, Canada

Arthur, J.R.. A historical overview of pathogen introductions and their transboundary spread in Asia. p. 21–39. In: Subasinghe, R.P.; Arthur, J.R. (eds.). Regional workshop on preparedness and response to aquatic animal health emergencies in Asia. Jakarta, Indonesia, 21–23 September 2004. *FAO Fisheries Proceedings*. No. 4. Rome, FAO. 2005. 178p.

ABSTRACT

This paper briefly reviews the history of some of the major transboundary aquatic animal diseases in the Asia-Pacific Region and summarizes the status of some of the major diseases currently affecting the region (primarily those diseases listed by the Office International des Épizooties (OIE) or included in the Network of Aquaculture Centres in Asia-Pacific (NACA)/Food and Agriculture Organization of the United Nations (FAO)/OIE Quarterly Aquatic Animal Disease Reporting System). Emphasis is placed on those diseases having wide distributions and impacts in the region, with less attention paid to diseases of cold-water species such as salmonids, and those of very limited distribution. Some emerging diseases that could have significant impacts on aquaculture in the region in the near future are also discussed.

INTRODUCTION

Although parasites and pathogens are common in wild populations of aquatic animals, reports of serious disease outbreaks and associated mass mortalities in wild stocks due to their normal pathogen fauna are rare. This is because in natural systems the pathogen and the host have generally had a long period of time to adapt to each other, the pathogen often becoming less pathogenic and the host more tolerant of, or resistant to infection.

Serious epizootics of fish, shellfish and molluscs appear to be primarily a modern phenomenon, and are often associated with the intensification of aquaculture, where many animals are confined at high density and under conditions that are often stressful. Such conditions are often optimal for disease transmission, and organisms that are not a serious problem to the host species in the wild may become highly pathogenic. The international movement of aquatic animals for aquaculture purposes, while not entirely a recent development, has accelerated considerably during the past 50 years (see Arthur, 2004; Subasinghe and Bartley, 2004). As a result, exotic pathogens have been moved far outside their natural ranges, where they have gained exposure to new and naive host populations. Thus the vast majority of serious disease outbreaks that have occurred in the past 50 years are either known or believed to have been caused by transboundary aquatic animal pathogens (TAAPs) – exotic pathogens that have been transported between countries and regions into new geographic areas where they have flourished. Their economic impacts on aquaculture are well documented and include

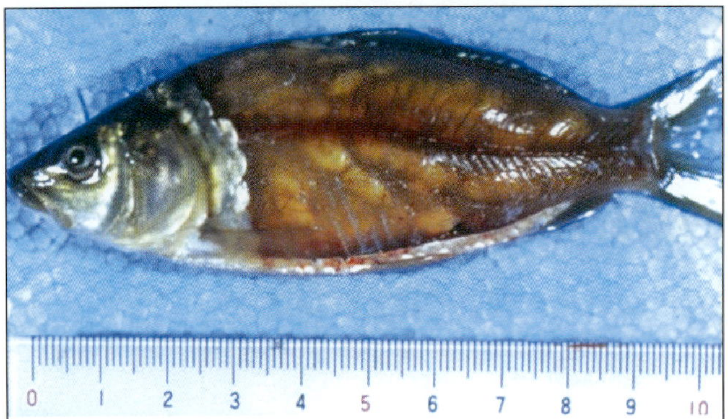

H. YOKOYAMA

Myxobolus artus *infection in the skeletal muscle of 0+ carp*

direct losses to production and secondary industries, as well as socio-economic hardships on communities (see Bondad-Reantaso, 2004). Impacts of TAAPs on wild populations of aquatic animals are less well-documented; but in at least one case, epizootic ulcerative syndrome (EUS) of freshwater fish, are thought to be considerable (Lilley, Callinan and Khan, 2002; Das, 2002).

This paper briefly reviews the history of some of the major transboundary aquatic animal diseases in the Asia-Pacific Region and summarizes the status of some of the major diseases currently affecting the region (primarily those diseases listed by the Organisation mondiale de la santé animale (OIE) or included in the Network of Aquaculture Centres in Asia-Pacific (NACA)/Food and Agriculture Organization of the United Nations (FAO)/OIE Quarterly Aquatic Animal Disease Reporting System). Emphasis is placed on those diseases having wide distributions and impacts in the region, with less attention paid to diseases of cold-water species such as salmonids, and those of very limited distribution. Some emerging diseases that could have significant impacts on aquaculture in the region in the near future are also discussed.

HISTORICAL ACCOUNTS

Ichthyophthiriasis hits Java

The first recorded disease epizootic in Asia thought to be due to an introduced pathogen was an outbreak of ichthyophthiriasis or "white spot disease" of freshwater fish that occurred on the island of Java, Indonesia in 1932 (see Buschkiel, 1935; Sachlan, 1952; Djajadiredja *et al.*, 1983; Arthur, 1996). The outbreak was reported by Alfred L. Buschkiel (Buschkiel 1935), a German scientist who worked at the Laboratorium voor de Binnenvisscherij in Buitenzorg (now Bogor) during the early 1930s. He reported that ichthyophthiriasis, due to the pathogenic ciliate *Ichthyophthirius multifiliis*, was particularly prevalent at the eastern border of West Java and that it spread rapidly eastward to Central Java with the transport of infected fish. Java barb (*Barbonymus gonionotus*), kissing gourami (*Helostoma temmincki*), common carp (*Cyprinus carpio*) and giant gourami (*Osphronemus goramy*) were the species most severely affected. The outbreak was associated with a very long drought that allowed the parasite to develop unchecked in the rather heavily stocked ponds. Although Sachlan (1952) noted that the parasite was first encountered in an aquarium at Bogor in 1928 and was probably introduced with ornamental fish from the United States and Europe, he also stated that many cases had been previously reported from Java and Sumatra. Measures taken to prevent the spread of the disease, which included ordering pond owners to drain infected ponds immediately and prohibiting the sale of infected fish, were ineffective. Losses due to the white spot epidemic in Indonesia were estimated at some 10 000 Dutch guilders, an amount that exceeded losses of salmonids in European countries caused by similar outbreaks between 1919-1928 (see Buschkiel, 1935; Sachlan, 1952).

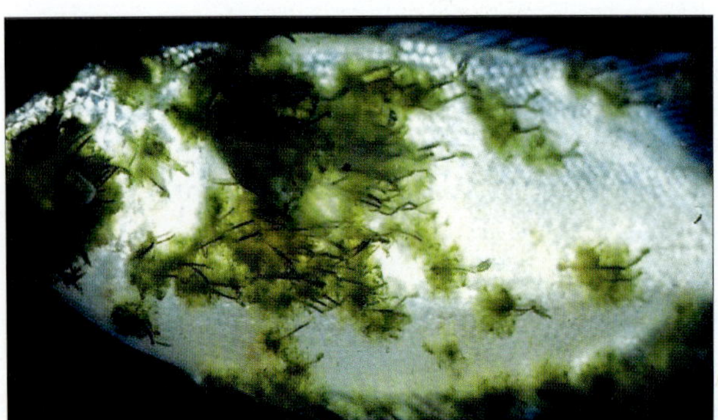

J.R. ARTHUR

Surface parasites, Lerneae cyprinacea *infection of giant gouramy*

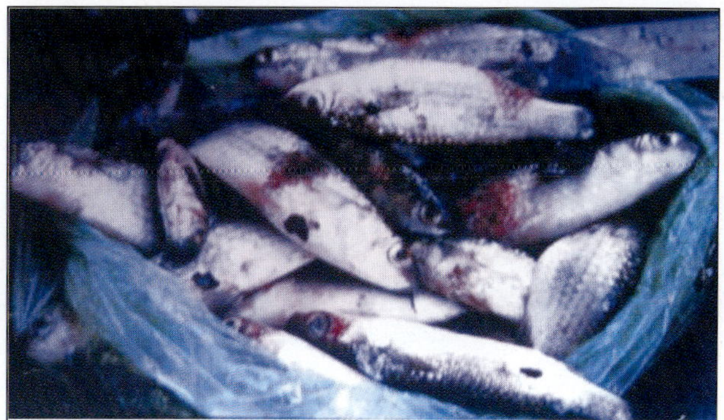

Wild mullet in Philippines (1989) with EUS

M.G. BONDAD-REANTASO

Myobolus and Lernaea problems in Indonesia

In 1951, another pathogen, tentatively identified as *Myxobolus pyriformis*, was reported to have killed thousands of Java barb fry in a government hatchery in Central Java (Sachlan 1952). Djajadiredja *et al.* (1983), who considered this myxosporean to have probably been introduced to Indonesia, reported in 1982 that this gill parasite had caused serious losses annually. These authors also noted that two other unidentified species of *Myxobolus*, suspected to have been introduced to Indonesia from Japan, have caused considerable losses (mortalities of 60-90 percent) of common carp fingerlings in Java since 1974.

Anchor worm (*Lernaea cyprinacea*) is a parasitic copepod that was introduced into Indonesia from Japan 1953 (Djajadiredja *et al.*, 1983). The parasite caused a serious epizootic in economically important species such as common carp, Java barb, kissing gourami and giant gourami, and quickly spread to other regions of the country. Losses were quite significant, with about 30 percent of hatchery production in the main hatchery centers of Java, northern Sumatra and northern Sulawesi affected. In Java, it was estimated that some 1.48 billion fry were lost, worth some 7.4 billion rupiahs (approximately US$11.4 million).

Epizootic ulcerative syndrome – a disease impacts wild fish stocks

Epizootic ulcerative syndrome (EUS) is a fungal-caused disease that has affected cultured and wild fresh and brackish-water fish species throughout much of the Asia-Pacific. It is now endemic in Southeast and South Asia and has recently expanded its range into West Asia (see FAO, 2001).

EUS is indistinguishable from mycotic granulomatosis of Japan, which was first recorded in 1971, red spot disease of eastern Australia, reported in 1972, and the ulcerative mycosis disease affecting Atlantic menhaden in the United States since 1978. Although more than 100 species of fish have been reported to be affected (see Chinabut & Roberts, 1999; Lilley, Phillips and Tonguthai, 1992), populations of some species are much more severely impacted than others.

Some idea of the impacts of EUS on the relative abundances of wild fish is given by Das (1994), who studied the landings at the Jorhat Fish Assembly Centre in Assam for species of EUS-affected fish from the capture fishery in the Brahmaputra River system before (1987–1988) and during the initial (1988–1991) three years in which outbreaks

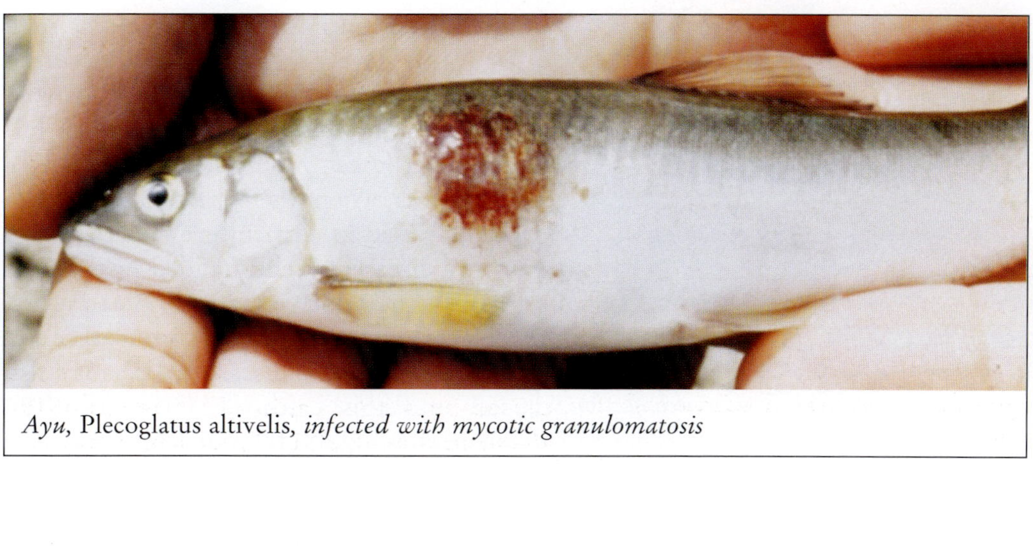

Ayu, Plecoglatus altivelis, *infected with mycotic granulomatosis*

K. HATAI

occurred in India (see Table 1). His data showed declines in catches of highly susceptible species by as much as 97 percent. Among the species most severely affected were snakeheads (Channidae – *Channa punctata*, *C. striata*) and native cyprinids (*Puntius* spp., *Labeo rohita*, *L. bata* and *Cirrhinus cirrhosus*).

TABLE 1
Impact of EUS on local abundance of highly susceptible species (modified from Das 1994)

Species	Decline in Landings (%)
Channa punctata	85–94%
C. striata	82–88%
Nandus nandus	82–97%
Puntius spp.	64–90%
Amblypharyngodon mola	37–71%
Labeo rohita	49–63%
L. bata	54–87%
Cirrhinus cirrhosus	28–66%

THE DISTRIBUTION OF SERIOUS TRANSBOUNDARY DISEASES IN THE ASIA-PACIFIC REGION

The geographic distributions of the major serious transboundary diseases affecting finfish, crustaceans and molluscs in the Asia-Pacific Region (excluding West Asia) are presented in Tables 2–4. The information given in these tables is drawn mainly from the International Database on Aquatic Animal Diseases (www.collabcen.net/toWeb/aq2.asp) and the NACA/FAO Quarterly Aquatic Animal Disease Reports (Asia and Pacific Region) (www.enaca.org/Health/QAAD), which summarize data submitted by the national authorities of participating countries to the NACA/FAO/OIE Quarterly Aquatic Animal Disease (QAAD) Reporting System. These tables represent a "best guess" as to the distribution of the various pathogens, and do not include a number of reports for countries such as India, Laos, Malaysia and Myanmar that are considered to be erroneous or highly suspect.

A number of the diseases of finfish listed by the OIE affect only Salmonidae or other cold or temperate-water fishes and thus have existing or potential ranges in the Asia-Pacific that are limited to countries having temperate climates, such as Japan, the Republic of Korea, northern China, southern Australia and New Zealand. These include infectious haematopoietic necrosis (IHN), viral haemorrhagic septicaemia (VHS), *Oncorhynchus masou* virus disease (OMVD), infectious pancreatic necrosis (IPN), bacterial kidney disease (BKD), epizootic haematopoietic necrosis (EHN) and red seabream iridoviral disease (RSBID). Although not reported from South Asia, those diseases affecting salmonids could potentially occur in a few mountainous regions of India, Sri Lanka and Nepal where trout (primarily rainbow trout, *Oncorhynchus mykiss*) have been introduced to support limited sport fisheries. However, any impacts in these areas would be quite localized.

Several of the OIE-listed diseases that are widespread across the Asia-Pacific Region have been present in the region for more than a decade. These include EUS of fresh and brackish-water fishes, viral encephalopathy and retinopathy (VER) of marine fishes, and white spot disease (WSD), yellowhead disease (YHD) and Penaeus monodon baculovirosis (PMV) of marine shrimp. Some diseases, such as VER, have probably always occurred throughout much on the region in wild populations of aquatic organisms but have only been reported to cause disease problems when their hosts have begun to be raised in aquaculture facilities. Two other diseases recently added to the OIE list that are poorly studied in Asia-Pacific, enteric septicaemia of catfish (ESC) and grouper iridoviral disease (GID), may also fall into this category. Other diseases, such as WSD, YHD and PMV probably

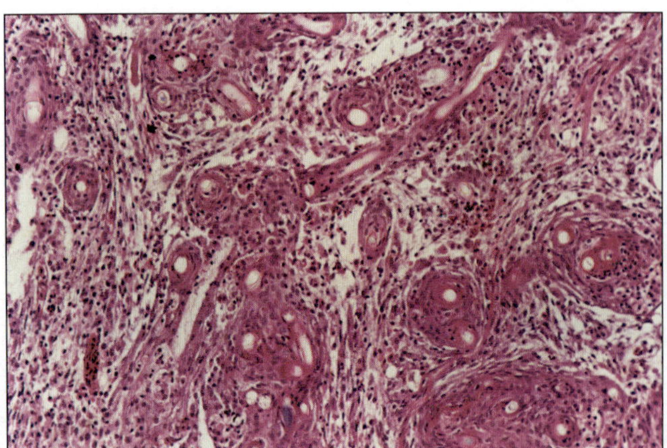
M.G. BONDAD-REANTASO

Typical severe mycotic granulomas from muscle section of EUS fish (H & E)

TABLE 2

Historical data on the occurrence of serious transboundary diseases of finfish in the Asia-Pacific Region.[1] (+=reported,?=suspected, [?]=report of uncertain status (primary sources: www.colabcen.net/toWeb/aq2.asp; www.oie-jp.org); www.enaca.org/Health/QAAD; FAO 2001

	OIE-listed Diseases[1]											Other Diseases Monitored		
Country	EHN	IHN	SVC	OMVD	VHS	VER	IPN	EUS	BKD	RSBID	ESC	KHV	Epi	GID
East Asia														
China P.R.		+	+			+	+			?		+		?
Japan		+		+	+	+	+	+	+	+		+		
Taipei China		+				+	+			?		+		+
Hong Kong China						+				+		+	+	+
Korea Rep.		+	?		+	+	+			+		?		
Southeast Asia														
Cambodia								+						
Indonesia						+		+			+	+		+
Laos[2]								+						
Malaysia[2]						+		+		+		+		+
Myanmar[2]								+						
Philippines						+		+						
Singapore						+		+						+
Thailand						+	[?]	+		+[?]	+		+	+
Viet Nam						+		+			+			+
South Asia														
Bangladesh								+						
India[2]								+						
Nepal								+						
Sri Lanka								+						
Australia/South Pacific														
Australia	+					+		+			+			
French Polynesia						+								
New Caledonia														
New Zealand							+							

[1] EHN=epizootic haematopoietic necrosis, IHN=infectious haematopoietic necrosis, SVC=spring viraemia of carp, OMVD=Oncorhynchus masou virus disease, VHS=viral haemorrhagic septicaemia, VER=viral encephalopathy and retinopathy, IPN=infectious pancreatic necrosis, EUS=epizootic ulcerative syndrome, BKD=bacterial kidney disease, RSBID=red sea bream iridoviral disease, ESC=enteric septicaemia of catfish, KHV=koi herpesvirus, Epi=eptheliocystis, GID= grouper iridoviral disease.

[2] A number of positive or suspected disease reports for these countries were corrected in subsequent country reports to OIE.

TABLE 3

Historical data on the occurrence of serious transboundary diseases of crustaceans in the Asia-Pacific Region.[1] (+=reported, ?=suspected, [?]=report of uncertain status) (primary sources: www.colabcen.net/toWeb/aq2.asp; www.oie-jp.org; www.enaca.org/Health/QAAD; FAO 2001

	OIE-listed Diseases								Other Diseases Monitored
Country	**IHHN**	**TS**	**WSD**	**SB (PMB)**	**TB (BP)**	**YHD/GAV**	**SMVD**	**NHP**	**BVMGN**
East Asia									
China PR		+	+			+			
Japan			+						+
Taipei China	+	+	+	+		+			
Hong Kong China			+						
Korea Rep			+						[?]
Southeast Asia									
Cambodia									
Indonesia	+	+	+			+			?
Laos									
Malaysia	+	?	+	+	[?]	+			
Myanmar	+		+						
Philippines	+		+	+		+	+		[?]
Singapore	+		+	+					
Thailand	+	+	+	+		+			
Viet Nam	?	+	+	+		+			
South Asia									
Bangladesh			+			+			
India	+		+	+		+	[?]		
Nepal									
Sri Lanka			+			+	+		
Australia/South Pacific									
Australia	+			+		+(GAV)	+		?
French Polynesia	+								
New Caledonia	+								
New Zealand									

[1] IHHNV-infectious hypodermal and haematopoietic necrosis, TS=Taura syndrome, WSD=whitespot disease, SB (PMB)=spherical baculovirosis (Penaeus monodon-type baculovirus), TB(BP)=tetrahedral baculovirosis (Baculovirus penaei), YHD/GAV=yellow head disease/gill- associated virus, SMVD=spawner-isolated mortality virus disease, NHP=necrotising hepatopancreatitis, BVMGN=baculoviral midgut gland necrosis.

TABLE 4
Historical data on the occurrence of serious transboundary diseases of molluscs in the Asia-Pacific Region. (+=reported) (primary sources: www.colabcen.net/toWeb/aq2.asp; www.oie-jp.org; www.enaca.org/Health/QAAD; FAO 2001)

Country	OIE-listed Diseases					Other Diseases Monitored		
	Bonamia exitiosa	*Marteilia sydneyi*	*Mikrocytos roughleyi*	*Perkinsis olseni/atlanticus*	*Haplosporidium nelsoni*	*Marteilioides chungmuensis*	Akoya Oyster Disease	Abalone Mortality Virus
East Asia								
China PR								
Japan					+	+	+	
Taipei China								
Hong Kong China								
Korea Rep.				+	+	+		
Southeast Asia								
Cambodia								
Indonesia								
Laos								
Malaysia								
Myanmar								
Philippines								
Singapore								
Thailand								
Viet Nam								
South Asia								
Bangladesh								
India								
Nepal								
Sri Lanka								
Australia/South Pacific								
Australia		+	+	+				
French Polynesia								
New Caledonia								
New Zealand	+			+				

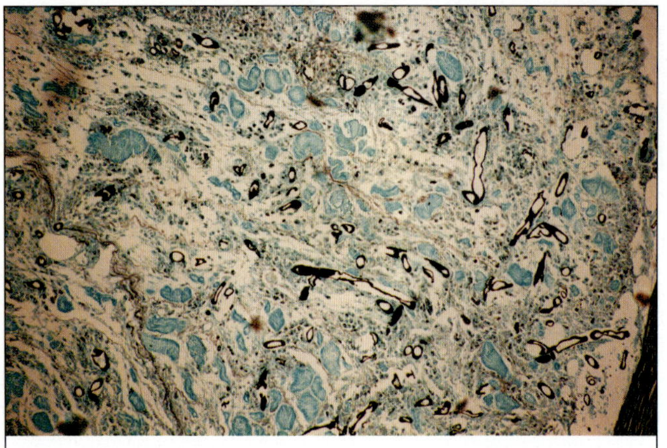
M.G. BONDAD-REANTASO

Mycotic granulomas showing fungal hyphae (stained black) using Grocotts stain

originated within the Asia-Pacific and were thus initially of very limited geographic distribution. However, they have now become widely distributed through the movement of infected hosts for aquaculture development. These diseases are now probably endemic in wild populations of aquatic animals throughout much of the region. In many cases, the problem that governments now face is not "How do we prevent the entry of these pathogens into our national territory?", but rather "How do we prevent their spread to those areas of the country that are still uninfected?", and "What can we do to prevent their introduction into individual aquaculture facilities, or to manage or eradicate these diseases in infected facilities?"

A few diseases, particularly some of those affecting marine shrimp (Penaeidae) are truly exotic to the Asia-Pacific, having recently been translocated into the region along with the introduction of infected exotic shrimp species, primarily white shrimp (*Litopenaeus vannamei*) and blue shrimp (*L. stylirostris*). These include infectious hypodermal and haematopoietic necrosis (IHHN), which has now widely distributed in Southeast Asia and the South Pacific, but apparently not in South Asia, and Taura syndrome (TS), which has recently been recorded from several East and Southeast Asian countries.

Unfortunately, the distribution of serious transboundary diseases in some countries in some parts of the Asia-Pacific Region remains unclear due to limited capacity for disease diagnosis, an absence of disease surveillance and monitoring programmes, and/or problems with accurate disease reporting. This is particularly true for diseases of molluscs throughout much of Asia, and for diseases of finfishes in developing countries such as Cambodia, Laos, Myanmar, Bangladesh, Nepal etc. In some countries, an additional problem is the apparent lack of awareness by the veterinary and/or fisheries authorities as to their country's national disease status. Thus in some cases, recent reports to NACA/FAO/OIE for some countries indicate that a given disease is either "never reported" or that there is "no information available" when reports of disease occurrence exist, either in the official reports to OIE, or elsewhere in the scientific literature.

THE CURRENT TRANSBOUNDARY DISEASE SITUATION IN THE ASIA-PACIFIC REGION

Tables 5–7 present summaries of the diseases listed or monitored by the NACA/FAO/OIE QAAD Reporting System for Asia-Pacific for the period 1 July 2003 – 31 June 2004, and include the most recent data available. It should be noted that these tables list only the reports of disease occurrence, and typically do not provide any indication of the seriousness or magnitude of the outbreaks. Nevertheless, the fact that a disease has recently been reported to occur in many countries gives some indication that the disease may still be a major problem in the region.

A number of serious diseases of finfish that are widely distributed in the Asia-Pacific were reported during the 12 months for which data are available. Viral encephalopathy and retinopathy (VER) of marine fish (groupers, seabass etc.) was reported from East Asia (Japan, Hong Kong and Taipei), Southeast Asia (Indonesia (?), Philippines, Thailand and Viet Nam), Australia and the South Pacific (French Polynesia), while epizootic ulcerative syndrome (EUS) was recorded from Southeast Asia (Cambodia,

TABLE 5

Summary of reports of the occurrence of serious transboundary diseases of finfish in the Asia-Pacific Region, July 2003–June 2004. (+ = reported or known to be present during period; +? = serological evidence and/or isolation of causative agent but not clinical disease; ? = suspected but presence not confirmed; +( ) = occurrence limited to certain zones; * = no information available; 0000 = never reported; - = not reported during period but disease is known to occur (Data for countries reporting to the NACA/FAO/OIE Regional Quarterly Aquatic Animal Disease (QAAD) Reporting System are taken from the FAO/NACA Quarterly Aquatic Animal Disease Reports (www.enaca.org/Health/QAAD); that for other countries (Taipei China, French Polynesia, New Caledonia and New Zealand) are taken from OIE (www.oie-jp.org)**

	OIE-listed Diseases[1]											Other Diseases Monitored		
Country	EHN	IHN	SVC	OMVD	VHS	VER	IPN	EUS	BKD	RSBID	ESC	KHV	Epi	GID
East Asia														
China PR	0000	-	***	0000	0000	0000	0000	0000	0000	0000	0000	0000	0000	0000
Japan	0000	+	0000	+	+	+	+	-	+	+	0000	+	+	0000
Taipei China	***	***	***	***	***	+	***	0000	***	0000	0000	-	***	-
Hong Kong China	0000	0000	0000	0000	000	+	0000	0000	0000	+	0000	0000	+? [-]	+
Korea, Rep	0000	-	?	0000	-	-	-	0000	0000	+		-		
Southeast Asia														
Cambodia	***	***	***	***	***	***	***	+	***	***	***	***	***	***
Indonesia	***	***	***	***	***	0000 [?][2]	0000	***	0000	0000	0000	+	0000	+( )
Laos	***	***	***	***	***	***	***	***	***	***	***	***	***	***
Malaysia	0000	0000	0000	***	0000	-	***	-	0000	0000	***	0000	***	-
Myanmar	0000	0000	0000	0000	0000	0000	0000	-	0000	0000	0000			
Philippines	0000	0000	0000	0000	0000	+	0000	-	0000	0000	***	0000	***	***
Singapore	0000	0000	0000	0000	0000	-	0000	0000	0000	0000	0000	0000	-	-
Thailand	0000	0000	0000	0000	0000	+	-	+	***	0000	***	0000	0000	0000
Viet Nam	0000	0000	0000	0000	0000	+	0000	+( )	0000	0000	0000			+
South Asia														
Bangladesh	***	***	***	***	***	***	***	+	***	***	***	***	***	***
India	0000	0000		0000	0000		0000	-	0000	0000				
Nepal	***	***	***	***	***	***	***	+	***	***	***	***	***	***
Sri Lanka	0000	0000	0000	0000	0000	0000	0000	?	0000	0000	0000	0000	0000	0000
Australia/South Pacific														
Australia	+	0000	0000	0000	0000	+	0000	+	0000	0000	-	***	***	***
French Polynesia	***	***	***	***	***	+( )	***	***	***	***	***			
New Caledonia	***	***	***	***	***	***	***	***	***	***	***	***	***	***
New Zealand	0000	0000	0000	0000	0000	0000	+?	0000	0000	0000	0000	0000	+	0000

[1] EHN=epizootic haematopoietic necrosis, IHN=infectious haematopoietic necrosis, SVC=spring viraemia of carp, OMVD=Oncorhynchus masou virus disease, VHS=viral haemorrhagic septicaemia, VER=viral encephalopathy and retinopathy, IPN=infectious pancreatic necrosis, EUS=epizootic ulcerative syndrome, BKD=bacterial kidney disease, RSBID=red sea bream iridoviral disease, ESC=enteric septicaemia of catfish, KHV=koi herpesvirus, Epi=eptheliocystis, GIV= grouper iridoviral disease.

[2] Disease was reported as present in reports for July-Sept, Oct.-Dec. 2003, but indicated as "never reported" in subsequent reports.

TABLE 6

Summary of reports of the occurrence of serious transboundary diseases of crustaceans in the Asia-Pacific Region, July 2003–June 2004. (+ = reported or known to be present during period; +? = serological evidence and/or isolation of causative agent but not clinical diseases; ? = suspected but presence not confirmed; +( ) = occurrence limited to certain zones; * = no information available; 0000 = never reported; - = not reported during period but disease is known to occur (Data for countries reporting to the NACA/FAO/OIE Regional Quarterly Aquatic Animal Disease (QAAD) Reporting System are taken from the FAO/NACA Quarterly Aquatic Animal Disease Reports (www.enaca.org/Health/QAAD), that for other countries (Taipei China, French Polynesia, New Caledonia and New Zealand) is taken from OIE (www.oie-jp.org)**

	OIE-listed Diseases[1]								Other Diseases Monitored
Country	TS	WSD	YHD/GAV	SB (PMB)	IHHN	SMVD	TB (BP)	NHP	BVMGN
East Asia									
China PR	+( )	+	0000	0000	0000	0000	0000	0000	0000
Japan	0000	+	0000	0000	0000	0000	0000	0000	0000
Taipei China	-	-	***	***	0000	***	***	***	***
Hong Kong China	0000	+?	0000	0000	0000	0000	0000	0000	0000
Korea Rep.	0000	-	0000		0000	0000			
Southeast Asia									
Cambodia	***	***	***	***	***	***	***	***	***
Indonesia	+	+	0000	0000	0000	0000	0000	0000	0000
Laos	***	***	***	***	***	***	***	***	***
Malaysia	?	+( )	-	-	-	0000	- [?]	0000	
Myanmar	0000	+( )	0000	0000	+( )	0000	0000	0000	
Philippines	0000	+	***	***	***	-	***	***	***
Singapore	***	-	***	-	***	***	***	***	***
Thailand	+	+	+	?	+	***	***	***	***
Viet Nam	+( )	+	+	+	?	0000	0000	0000	
South Asia									
Bangladesh	***	+	***	***	***	***	***	***	***
India	***	+( )	***		***	0000			
Nepal	***	***	***	***	***	***	***	***	***
Sri Lanka	0000	+	?	0000	0000	0000	0000	0000	0000
Australia/South Pacific									
Australia	0000	0000	+	-	+?	-(?)	0000	0000	0000
French Polynesia	***	***	***	***	***	***	***	***	
New Caledonia	0000	0000	0000	0000	+	0000	0000	0000	0000
New Zealand	0000	0000	0000	0000	0000	0000	0000	0000	0000

[1] TS=Taura syndrome, WSD=whitespot disease, YHD/GAV=yellow head disease/gill-associated virus, SB (PMB)=spherical baculovirosis (Penaeus monodon-type baculovirus), IHHN=infectious hypodermal and haematopoietic necrosis, SMVD=spawner-isolated mortality virus disease, TB (BP)=tetrahedral baculovirosis (Baculovirus penaei), NHP=necrotising hepatopancreatitis, BVMGN=baculoviral midgut gland necrosis.

TABLE 7.

Summary of reports of the occurrence of serious transboundary diseases of finfish in the Asia-Pacific Region, July 2003–June 2004. (+ = reported or known to be present during period; +? = serological evidence and/or isolation of causative agent but not clinical diseases; ? = suspected but presence not confirmed; +( ) = occurrence limited to certain zones; * = no information available; 0000 = never reported; - = not reported during period but disease is known to occur (Data for countries reporting to the NACA/FAO/OIE Regional Quarterly Aquatic Animal Disease (QAAD) Reporting System are taken from the FAO/NACA Quarterly Aquatic Animal Disease Reports (www.enaca.org/Health/QAAD), that for other countries (Taipei China, French Polynesia, New Caledonia and New Zealand) is taken from OIE (www.oie-jp.org)**

	OIE-listed Diseases					Other Diseases Monitored		
Country	**Bonamia exitiosa**	**Marteilia sydneyi**	**Mikrocytos roughleyi**	**Perkinsis olseni/ atlanticus**	**Haplosporidium nelsoni**	**Marteilioides chungmuensis**	**Akoya Oyster Disease**	**Abalone Mortality Virus**
East Asia								
China PR	0000	0000	0000	0000	0000	0000	0000	0000
Japan	0000	0000	0000	0000	-	+	+	0000
Taipei China	***	***	***	***	***	***	***	***
Hong Kong China	0000	0000	0000	0000	0000	0000	0000	0000
Korea Rep.	0000	0000	0000	+	0000	+	0000	
Southeast Asia								
Cambodia	***	***	***	***	***	***	***	***
Indonesia	0000	0000	0000	0000	0000	0000	0000	0000
Laos	***	***	***	***	***	***	***	***
Malaysia	0000	0000	0000	0000	0000	0000	0000	0000
Myanmar	***	***	***	***	***	***	***	***
Philippines	0000	0000	0000	0000	0000	0000	0000	0000
Singapore	***	***	***	***	***	***	***	***
Thailand	***	***	***	***	***	***	***	***
Viet Nam	0000	0000	0000	0000	0000	0000	0000	0000
South Asia								
Bangladesh	***	***	***	***	***	***	***	***
India	0000	0000	0000	0000	0000			
Nepal	0000	0000	0000	0000	0000	0000	0000	0000
Sri Lanka	0000	0000	0000	0000	0000	0000	0000	0000
Australia/South Pacific								
Australia	0000	+	+	+	0000	***	0000	***
French Polynesia	0000	0000	0000	0000	0000	0000	0000	***
New Caledonia	0000	0000	0000	0000	0000	0000	***	***
New Zealand	+( )	0000	0000	+( )	0000	0000	0000	0000

Thailand and Viet Nam), South Asia (Bangladesh, Nepal and Sri Lanka) and Australia. Red seabream iridovirus disease (RSBID) was reported from three countries in East Asia (Japan, Hong Kong and the Republic of Korea). Several diseases of salmonids continue to be reported from East Asia (primarily Japan). These include IHN, OMVD, VHS, IPN and BKD. Epitheliocystis was reported from East Asia (Japan and Republic of Korea) and New Zealand, while epizootic haematopoietic necrosis (EHN) was detected in redfin perch (*Perca fluviatilis*) following a fish kill in Australia. Two finfish diseases, Koi herpes virus (KHV) and grouper iridoviral disease (GID), appear to be spreading in the Asia-Pacific Region and thus will be discussed in detail later. Although the occurrence of spring viraemia of carp (SVC) in the Asia-Pacific Region has not yet been officially reported to the NACA/FAO/OIE Quarterly Aquatic Animal Disease Reporting System, the virus has recently been isolated from koi and common carp in China P.R (see the International Database on Aquatic Animal Diseases, www.collabcen.net/toWeb/aq2.asp). One other disease, enteric septicaemia of catfish (ESC), was not reported during the period in question

Several diseases of Crustacea were widely reported from the Asia-Pacific during the most recent 12 months of reporting to NACA/FAO/OIE. Whitespot disease (WSD) continues to plague shrimp production in much of East Asia (China P.R., Japan and Hong Kong), Southeast Asia (Indonesia, Malaysia, Myanmar, Philippines, Thailand and Viet Nam) and South Asia (Bangladesh, India and Sri Lanka). Yellowhead disease (YHD) was recorded from Southeast Asia (Thailand and Viet Nam) and South Asia (Sri Lanka), while the closely related gill-associated virus (GAV) was reported from Australia. Infectious hypodermal and haematopoietic necrosis (IHHN) was reported from Southeast Asia (Myanmar, Thailand and Viet Nam), Australia and the South Pacific (New Caledonia), while spherical baculovirosis (SB) was recorded from Southeast Asia (Thailand and Viet Nam). One exotic viral disease of penaeid shrimp (Taura syndrome, TS) is an emerging disease in Asia, and will be discussed in more detail later. Other diseases listed by NACA/FAO/OIE were either not reported during the period in question (spawner-isolated mortality virus disease, SMVD) and baculoviral midgut gland necrosis, BVMGN) or have never been confirmed or reported from the region (tetrahedral baculovirosis, TB, and necrotising hepatopancreatitis, NHP).

As previously mentioned, the ability of the majority of countries reporting to NACA/FAO/OIE to diagnose diseases of molluscs is very limited and thus the occurrence of outbreaks of disease may go unreported, particularly in South and Southeast Asia. During the 12-month period under consideration, Japan reported cases of *Marteilioides* and Akoya oyster disease, while the Republic of Korea reported cases of *Marteilioides* and *Perkinsis*. Australia reported cases of *Marteilia*, *Mikrocytos* and *Perkinsis*, and New Zealand reported cases of *Bonamia* and *Perkinsis*. Two molluscan diseases may be emerging in the region (Akoya oyster disease and abalone mortality virus) and thus will be discussed in more detail below.

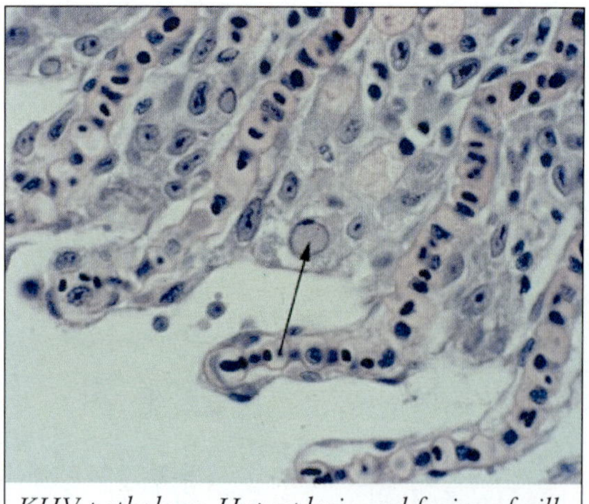
R. HEDRICK, UC DAVIS

KHV pathology. Hyperplasia and fusion of gill lamellae; intranuclear inclusion (arrow) in the branchial epithelium (gill section with H & E).

Information on the seriousness of the disease outbreaks that occurred in the Asia-Pacific Region during the past 12 months and their social and economic impacts is generally lacking. The impacts of Koi herpes virus on koi and common carp culture in Indonesia and Japan are briefly mentioned below, and are presented in more detail elsewhere (Iida *et al.*, 2004; Sano *et al.*, 2004; Sunarto *et al.*, 2004).

SOME CURRENT AND POTENTIAL EMERGING DISEASE PROBLEMS

The following section discusses several serious diseases of aquatic animals that are currently expanding their range in the Asia-Pacific or, although of limited distribution in the region, have the potential to expand their ranges and cause significant losses. Of these, white tail disease (WTD) has not been monitored by NACA/FAO/OIE and thus has received little attention. It will thus be discussed in more detail than the other, better known diseases.

White tail disease

White tail disease (WTD) (also reported as "whitish muscle disease" by Chinese workers) has caused epizootic losses of postlarval giant river prawns (*Macrobrachium rosenbergii*) in southern Taiwan Province of China (Taiwan POC) since 1992. The disease, which can cause mortalities of up to 100 percent of postlarvae (PL) in hatcheries, has also been reported from *M. rosenbergii* from mainland China, the French West Indies and India (see Arcier *et al.*, 1999; Sri Widada *et al.*, 2003; Qian *et al.*, 2003; Sahul Hameed, 2004). In India, it was first reported in 2003 as affecting many hatcheries at Nellore, Andra Pradesh and Chennai, and has also been seen in farms in Nellore, Andhra Pradesh (Hameed, 2004; NACA, 2004). WTD appears to spread rapidly, causing heavy economic losses due to high mortalities.

The probable cause of WTD is the *Macrobrachium rosenbergii* nodavirus (MrNV), also reported as *Macrobrachium* muscle virus (MMV) by Tung, Wang and Chen (1999). However, as noted by Sri Widada *et al.* (2003), the virus-host interactions and modes of transmission of this disease are still unknown.

The clinical signs of the disease in severely affected postlarvae (PL), which are similar to those of idiopathic muscle necrosis (IMN) syndrome (see Nash *et al.*, 1987) and thus not sufficient for presumptive diagnosis, include white opaque areas in the abdominal segments, commonly accompanied by lethargy and anorexia (see Tung, Wang and Chen, 1999; Arcier *et al.*, 1999; Sahul Hameed, 2004; NACA, 2004). Severe cases may show degeneration of the telson and uropods. Mortalities of 100 percent may occur within two or three days of the appearance of muscle opacity. Experimental infections indicate that infections may be responsible for branchostegite blister disease (BBD) or "swollen head syndrome" in adults (see Sahul Hameed, 2004; NACA, 2004).

The histopathological changes seen are similar to those described for IMN and include progressive segmental myofibre degeneration of muscle fibres and necrobiotic myopathy with numerous single, rows, aggregations and sheets of hyperchromatic myonuclei. Centrally or eccentrically placed (nuclear internalization) pyknotic nuclei were also frequently observed. However, unlike IMN, cytoplasmic inclusion bodies have been detected in the necrotic muscle of diseased prawns (see Tung, Wang and Chen, 1999). Transmission electron microscopy (TEM) of tissue homogenates from diseased prawns has revealed the presence of numerous non-enveloped virus-like particles of about 30 nm in diameter (Arcier *et al.*, 1999).

Initially, the use of pryonin methyl green was recommended (see Tung, Wang and Chen, 1999) to distinguish the characteristically green-stained MrNV viral inclusions from hemocyte nuclei. More recently Sri Widada *et al.* (2003) have developed three complimentary genome-based detection methods (dot-blot hybridization, *in situ* hybridization and reverse transcriptase-polymerase chain reaction (RT-PCR)) for detection of MrNV, dot-blot hybridization being considered the easiest to perform. In addition, Romestand and Bonami (2003) have developed a sandwich enzyme linked immmunosorbent assay (S-ELISA) for detection of this virus.

A second virus, extra small virus (XSV), whose role, if any, in producing WTD is unclear, was first reported in *M. rosenbergii* postlarvae from mainland China having concurrent infections with MrNV (Qian *et al.*, 2003). Qian *et al.* (2003) suggested that XSV, which is located in the muscle and connective cells of diseased animals, could be a helper virus for MrNV or a satellite-like virus, possibly acting as a disease modulator. It has also been considered a satellite virus by Widada and Bonami (2004). Although Qian *et al.* (2003) believed that XSV was always associated with MrNV, results presented by Sri Widada *et al.* (2004) suggest that this is not always the case. These authors concluded that the cause of WTD may be more complex than previously thought and thus further investigation is required.

Transmission electron microscopy (TEM) has revealed that the XSV viral particle is isocohedral and about 15 nm in diameter. Genome-based diagnostic techniques (dot-blot hybridization and RT-PCR) for XSV have been developed by Sri Widada *et al.* (2004).

Taura syndrome

Taura syndrome (TS) was first detected in shrimp farms near the Taura River, Ecuador (hence the name of the disease) in 1992. It then spread throughout most shrimp-growing regions of Latin America and the Pacific coasts of Colombia, Costa Rica, Ecuador, El Salvador, Guatemala, Honduras, Mexico, Nicaragua, Panama and Peru. It was also introduced to Hawaii but was successfully eradicated.

Erickson *et al.* (2002) reported that anecdotal evidence of occurrences of TS epizootics in *L. stylirostris* since 1999 in Mexico suggests that a closely related virus might have evolved from the original Ecuadorian/Hawaiian isolate characterized by Bonami *et al.* (1997) and Mari *et al.* (2002). They noted the possibility that since 1994 a change in Taura syndrome virus (TSV) structural protein may have occurred and that this change is now responsible for the emergence of TS in *L. stylirostris*, a previously refractive species (Brock *et al.*, 1997).

Survivors of acute TSV infection pass through a brief transitional phase and enter the chronic phase, which may persist for the rest of their lives. This subclinical phase of infection is believed to have contributed to the spread of the disease via carriage of viable virus.

TS has recently spread to Asia through the introduction of *Litopenaeus vannamei* and has now been reported from Taiwan POC, Indonesia, Malaysia (suspected), Thailand and Viet Nam (Palanisamy, 2004; Sunarto *et al.*, 2004; de la Peña, 2004; Van, 2004).

In Indonesia, TSV was first discovered in shrimp culture in November 2002 in *L. vannamei* from East Java (see Sunarto *et al.*, 2004). It is suspected that TSV first occurred in Banyuwangi and Situbono before spreading to other districts of East Java through the movement of infected PL. Samples testing positive by PCR have also been detected from Brebes (central Java), Situbondo (East Java) and the islands of Bali, Sulawesi and Sumbawa. It thus appears that the virus is now widespread in Indonesian shrimp culture where it causes mortalities in 1-2 month old *L. vannamei* reared in intensive culture systems.

Koi herpes virus (=carp nephritis and gill necrosis virus)

Koi herpes virus disease first appeared in the Asia-Pacific Region in March 2002 in Indonesia and in Taiwan POC in December of the same year, with subsequent outbreaks in Japan beginning in October 2003 (see Lio-Po, 2004; Tu *et al.*, 2004, Sano *et al.*, 2004; Sunarto *et al.*, 2004). Earlier reports of infections with Koi herpes virus (KHV) are recorded for the Republic of Korea (1998, suspected –reported as viral infection causing mass mortality of koi and common carp), Malaysia (2000) and Japan (2000).

An interesting characteristic of the disease has been its rapid spread across Indonesia and Japan through the trade in live koi for the ornamental fish trade and common carp for foodfish production. In both cases this has been due to the disease appearing rapidly in major production areas, and its rapid dissemination through the live fish trade. By the end of May 2004, KHV had been reported from 24 of Japan's 47 prefectures (Sano *et al.*, 2004), while in Indonesia, the disease has now spread throughout much of Java and into South Sumatra (see Sunarto *et al.*, 2004).

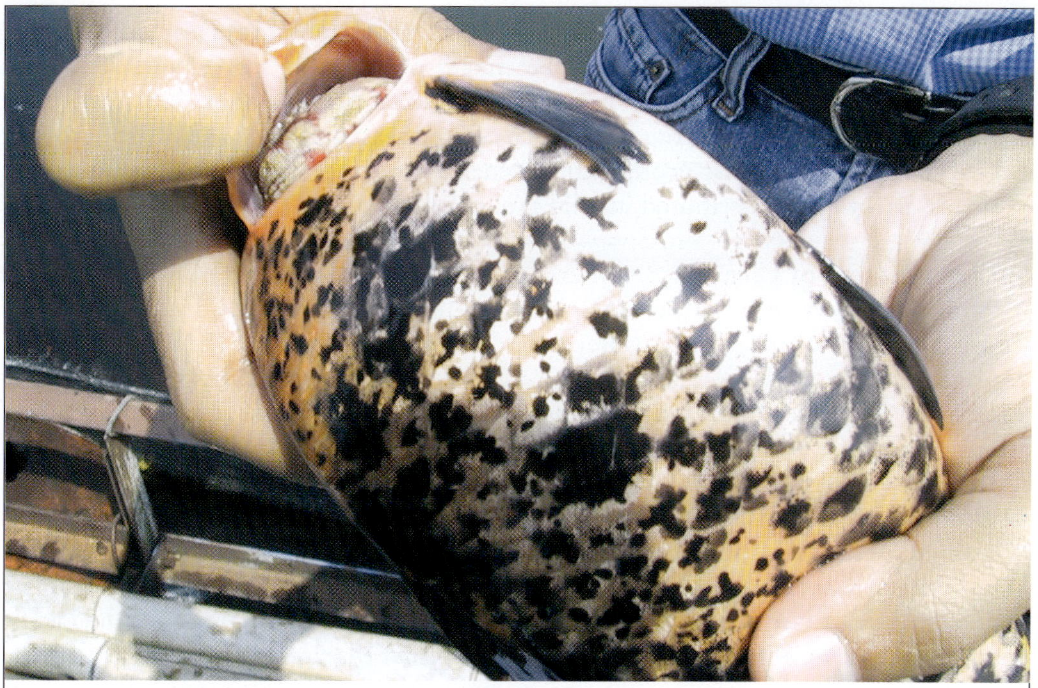

STUART MILLAR

Koi carp infected with Koi herpesvirus (KHV)

In both Indonesia and Japan, losses have been significant. In Lake Kasumigaura, Japan, mortalities of almost 100 percent occurred in netpen culture, with a total loss of almost 25 percent of the lake's annual production. In Indonesia, the first occurrence of mass mortalities due to KHV occurred in cultured koi in March 2002 in Blitar, East Java. Mortalities of up to 80-95 percent were seen in koi carp of all ages. As Blitar is the center of koi production for Indonesia, diseased fish were rapidly transported throughout the country, with Central Java, West Java and Jakarta being the main markets. Common carp is an important foodfish in Indonesia, and KHV rapidly impacted carp aquaculture production. Epizootics subsequently occurred in Subang Regency (West Java) in April 2002 and then in neighbouring areas. The disease has continued to spread through the transfer of live infected carp, with outbreaks occurring in May-June in carp cultured in netcages in the Citarum River system and by February 2003, it had been translocated to Lubuk Lingau Regency, South Sumatra along with carp moved from West Java by fish traders. It has since continued its spread to neighbouring provinces.

The origins of KHV remain obscure. In Indonesia, the disease is thought to have been introduced with the importation of koi from mainland China (via Hong Kong) in December 2001 and January 2002. Earlier, KHV had been reported from Israel, the United States and the United Kingdom in 1998, with subsequent cases in nine other European countries and in South Africa (see Crane, Sano and Komar, 2004).

The social and economic impacts of KHV in Indonesia are still being felt. In Blitar alone, the disease has affected more than 5 000 carp culturists with economic losses exceeding Rp 5 billion during the first three months of the outbreak. As of December 2003, the total losses due to KHV due to revenue lost to the carp culture sector and the accompanying impact on rural farming communities was estimated at some US$15 million (Sunarto *et al.*, 2004).

Grouper iridoviral disease

Grouper iridoviral disease, also known as "sleepy grouper disease", is caused by grouper irodovirus (GIV). It affects groupers (*Epinephelus* spp.) in South and East Asia, having been reported from Taipei, Hong Kong and PR China (suspected), Singapore and Viet Nam (see Nakajima, 2003; Table 2). It is a problem in grouper culture, where it causes losses of fry, juveniles and market-size fish. As "sleeper grouper disease" has also been reported from Malaysia and Thailand (see Kasornchandra, 2002), the virus probably naturally occurs throughout much of Southeast and East Asia where grouper are cultured. Because most grouper fry used for stocking are still wild-caught, it is probably also widely distributed in wild grouper populations.

Spring viraemia of carp

Although spring viraemia of carp (SVC) has traditionally been considered a disease of European countries having low water temperatures during winter (FAO, 2001), SVC virus has recently been isolated from China P.R. As Chinese carps, the principal species affected by SVC, are widely cultured throughout Asia, the disease has the potential to affect carp culture wherever suitably low temperatures (11-17 °C) occur.

Withering syndrome of abalone

Withering syndrome of abalone is caused by an intracellular prokaryote, the rickettsia-like organism *Candidatus Xenohaliotis californiensis*, which infects the epithelium of the digestive tract (see Bower, 2004). Although its confirmed distribution is the Pacific coast of southern California to Baja, Mexico, a similar disease has been reported from northern China, and rickettsia-like organisms have also been reported from abalone cultured in South Africa. Although the presence of this pathogen in the Asia-Pacific has not yet been confirmed, the disease was recently added to the NACA/ FAO/OIE Quarterly Aquatic Animal Disease (QAAD) Reporting System.

The disease is lethal to all sizes of abalone (genus *Haliotis*), in which it causes lethargy, retracted visceral tissues and atrophy of the foot muscle, affecting the abalone's ability to adhere to the substrate.

Akoya oyster disease

Akoya oyster disease is as yet known only from Japan, where it first appeared in 1994. It affects Japanese pearl oyster, *Pinctata fucata martensii*, of at least one year old or older, causing stunting, tissue atrophy and cytopathological changes (see Wada, 2003). It causes significant economic losses to the pearl culture industry in southern Japan, disease outbreaks occurring at high water temperatures (above 20 °C). Although a virus has been isolated from diseased oysters, its role in the disease has not been shown, and thus the causative agent is still considered to be unknown. Because the disease is believed to be caused by a biological agent, and causes significant mortalities of pearl oysters, which are widely cultured and have significant economic value in many countries of the Asia-Pacific Region, Akoya oyster disease was recently added to the NACA/FAO/OIE QAAD Reporting System.

CONCLUSIONS

Countries in the Asia-Pacific remain highly vulnerable to transboundary aquatic animal diseases. As the recent introduction and spread of KHV throughout most of Japan and in Indonesia has shown, governments can be easily caught unawares by new diseases. To better protect themselves from exotic diseases, countries in the Asia-Pacific Region should undertake risk analyses to determine which transboundary diseases are most likely to gain entry via their current trading practices, and of these, which are most likely to cause serious damage to their aquaculture industries and capture fisheries. Based on this knowledge, national governments should take steps to reduce the risk of pathogen entry through health certification, quarantine and/or other appropriate risk mitigation measures. They should also initiate contingency planning to develop emergency response plans that will limit the spread and impacts of such diseases. Along with this, the other components of a National Aquatic Animal Health Strategy should be given high priority, so that the necessary legislation, expertise and capacity to deal with a disease emergency is in place before a serious disease outbreak due to an exotic pathogen occurs.

LITERATURE CITED

Arcier J.-M., Herman, F., Lightner, D.V., Redman, R.M., Mari, J. & Bonami, J.-R. 1999. A viral disease associated with mortalities in hatchery-reared postlarvae of the giant freshwater prawn *Macrobrachium rosenbergii. Dis. Aquat. Org.*, 38: 177-181.

Arthur, J.R. 1996. A history of fisheries parasitology in Southeast Asia. In: S.S. De Silva, ed. *Perspectives in Asian fisheries – a volume to commemorate the 10th anniversary of the Asian Fisheries Society.* pp. 383-407. Manila, Asian Fisheries Society.

Arthur, J.R. 2004. A brief review of international trade in live aquatic animals. In: J.R. Arthur & M.B. Reantaso, eds. *Capacity and awareness building on import risk analysis for aquatic animals.* Report of the Joint APEC/FAO/NACA/OIE/DoF-Thailand/INP/CONPESCA/SAGARPA Workshops, Bangkok, Thailand, 1-6 April 2002 and Mazatlan, Sinaloa, Mexico, 12-17 August 2002. pp. 1-7. Asia-Pacific Economic Cooperation, APEC Fisheries Working Group.

Bonami, J.R., Hasson, K.W., Mari, J., Poulos, B.T. & Lightner, D.V. 1997. Taura syndrome of marine penaeid shrimp: characterization of the viral agent. *J. Gen. Virol.*, 78: 313-319.

Bondad-Reantaso, M.G. 2004. Trans-boundary aquatic animal diseases/pathogens. In: J.R. Arthur & M.B. Reantaso, eds.. *Capacity and awareness building on import risk analysis for aquatic animals.* Report of the Joint APEC/FAO/NACA/OIE/DoF-Thailand/INP/CONPESCA/SAGARPA Workshops, Bangkok, Thailand 1-6 April 2002 and Mazatlan, Sinaloa, Mexico, 12-17 August 2002. pp. 9-22. Asia-Pacific Economic Cooperation, APEC Fisheries Working Group.

Bower, S.M. 2004. Synopsis of infectious diseases and parasites of commercially exploited shellfish: withering syndrome of abalone. (www-sci.pac.dfo-mpo.gc.ca/shelldis/pages/fwsab_e.htm)

Brock, J.A., Gose, R.B., Lightner, D.V. & Hasson, K. 1997. Recent developments and an overview of Taura syndrome of farmed shrimp in the Americas, In: T.W. Flegel & I.H. MacRae, eds. *Diseases in Asian aquaculture III.* pp. 275-283. Manila, Fish Health Section, Asian Fisheries Society.

Buschkiel, A.L. 1935. Neue Beiträge zur Kenntnis des *Ichthyophthirius multifiliis* Fouquet. *Arch. Néerland. Zool.*, 2: 178-224

Crane, M., Sano, M. & Komar, C. 2004. Infection with koi herpesvirus – disease card. In: NACA/FAO. *Quarterly aquatic animal disease report (Asia and Pacific Region).* April-June 2004, 2004/2. pp. 43-47. Bangkok, NACA.

Chinabut, S. & Roberts, R.J. 1999. *Pathology and histopathology of epizootic ulcerative syndrome (EUS).* Bangkok, Aquatic Animal Health Research Institute, Department of Fisheries, 33 pp.

Das, M.K. 1994. Outbreak of the fish disease epizootic ulcerative syndrome in India – an overview. In: R.J. Roberts, B. Campbell & I.H. MacRae, eds. *ODA Regional Seminar on Epizootic Ulcerative Syndrome at the Aquatic Animal Health Research Institute, Bangkok, Thailand, 25-27 January 1994.* pp. 21-38.

Das, M.K. 2002. Social and economic impacts of disease in inland open-water and culture-based fisheries in India. In: J.R. Arthur, M.J. Phillips R.P. Subasinghe, M.B. Reantaso, & I.H. MacRae, eds. *Primary aquatic animal health care in rural, small-scale, aquaculture development.* pp. 333-344. FAO Fisheries Technical Paper No. 406, Rome.

de la Peña, L. 2004. Transboundary shrimp viral diseases with emphasis on white spot syndrome virus (WSSV) and Taura syndrome virus (TSV). *In* C.R. Lavilla-Pitogo & K. Nagasawa. *Transboundary fish diseases in Southeast Asia: occurrence, surveillance, research and training.* pp. 67-69. Tigbauan, Iloilo, Philippines. SEAFDEC Aquaculture Department.

Djajadiredja, R., Panjaitan, T.H., Rukyani, A., Sarono, A., Satyani, D. & Supriyadi, H. 1983 Country Reports: Indonesia. In: F.B. Davy & A. Chouinard, eds. *Fish quarantine and fish diseases in Southeast Asia.* pp. 19-30. Report of a workshop held in Jakarta, Indonesia, 7–10 December 1982. International Development Research Centre Publication IDRC-210e, Ottawa.

Erickson, H.S., Zarain-Herzberg, M. & Lightner, D.V. 2002. Detection of Taura syndrome virus (TSV) strain differences using selected diagnostic methods: diagnostic implications in penaeid shrimp. *Dis. Aquat. Org*., 52: 1-10.

FAO. 2001. *Asia diagnostic guide to aquatic animal diseases.* M.G. Bondad-Reantaso, S.E. McGladdery, I. East & R.P. Subasinghe, eds. FAO Fisheries Technical Paper No. 402, Suppl. 2, 240 pp, Rome.

Iida, T., Sano, M., Ito, T., Kurita, J., Yuasa, K. & Miwa, S. 2005. Responses to koi herpesvirus (KHV) outbreaks in Japan In: R.P. Subasinghe & J.R. Arthur, eds. *Preparedness and response to aquatic animal health emergencies in Asia.* pp. xx-xx. FAO Fisheries Technical Paper No. xxx.

Kasornchandra, J. 2002. Major viral and bacterial diseases of cultured seabass and groupers in Southeast Asia. In: C.R. Lavilla-Pitogo & E.R.. Cruz-Lacierda, eds. *Diseases in Asian aquaculture IV*. pp. 205-212. Manila, Fish Health Section, Asian Fisheries Society.

Lilley, J.H, Callinan, R.B. & Khan, M.H. 2002. Social, economic and biodiversity impacts of epizootic ulcerative syndrome (EUS). In: J.R. Arthur, M.J. Phillips, R.P. Subasinghe, M.B. Reantaso & I.H. MacRae, eds. *Primary aquatic animal health care in rural, small-scale, aquaculture development*. pp. 127-139. FAO Fisheries Technical Paper No. 406, Rome.

Lilley, J.H., Phillips, M.J. & Tonguthai, K. 1992. *A review of epizootic ulcerative syndrome (EUS) in Asia.* Bangkok, Aquatic Animal Health Research Institute and Network of Aquaculture Centres in Asia-Pacific, 73 pp.

Lio-Po, G.D. 2004. Summary brief: International Symposium on Koi Herpesvirus Disease. *In* C.R. Lavilla-Pitogo and K. Nagasawa. *Transboundary fish diseases in Southeast Asia: occurrence, surveillance, research and training*. pp. 71-73. Tigbauan, Iloilo, Philippines. SEAFDEC Aquaculture Department.

Mari, J., Poulos, B.T., Lightner, D.V. & Bonami, J.R. 2002. Shrimp Taura syndrome virus: genomic characterization and similarity with members of the genus cricket paralysis-like viruses. *J. Gen. Virol*., 83: 917-928.

NACA. 2004. White tail disease (WTD) of *Macrobrachium rosenbergii* in India. (www.enaca.org/modules/news/articlephp.storyid=50 (posted 20/11/32003).

Nakajima, K. 2003. Grouper iridoviral disease – disease card. Developed to support the NACA/FAO/OIE Regional Quarterly Aquatic Animal Disease (QAAD) Reporting System in the Asia-Pacific. Bangkok, NACA, 4 pp. (www.enaca.org/Health/DiseaseLibrary/Disease_card_GIV_Nakajima.pdf)

Nash G., Chinabut, S. & Limsuwan, C. 1987. Idiopathic muscle necrosis in the freshwater prawn, *Macrobrachium rosenbergii* de Man, cultured in Thailand. *J. Fish Dis.,* 10: 109-120.

Palanisamy, V. 2004. Part II: Associated transboundary aquatic animal pathogens. Paper presented at the Workshop On "Building Capacity to Combat Impacts of Aquatic Invasive Alien Species and Associated Trans-boundary Pathogens", 12-16 July 2004, Penang, Malaysia, 14 pp.

Qian D., Shi, Z., Zhang, S., Cao, Z., Liu, W., Li, L., Xie, Y., Cambournac, I. & Bonami, J.R. 2003. Extra small virus-like particles (XSV) and nodavirus associated with whitish muscle disease in the giant freshwater prawn, *Macrobrachium rosenbergii*. *J. Fish Dis.,* 26: 521-527.

Romestand B. & Bonami, J.R.. 2003. A sandwich enzyme linked immunosorbent assay (S-ELISA) for detection of MrNV in the giant freshwater prawn, *Macrobrachium rosenbergii* (de Man). *J Fish Dis.,* 26: 71-75.

Sachlan, M. 1952. Notes on parasites of fresh-water fishes in Indonesia. *Contributions of the Inland Fisheries Research Stations,* 2: 1-60.

Sahul Hameed, A.S. 2004. White tail disease of *Macrobrachium rosenbergii.* (www.enaca.org).

Sano, M., Ito, T., Kurita, J., Yuasa, K., Miwa, S. & Iida, T. 2004. Experience on common carp mass mortality in Japan. *In* C.R. Lavilla-Pitogo & K. Nagasawa. *Transboundary fish diseases in Southeast Asia: occurrence, surveillance, research and training.* pp. 13-19. Tigbauan, Iloilo, Philippines. SEAFDEC Aquaculture Department.

Sri Widada, J., Durand, S., Cambournac, I., Qian, D., Shi, Z., Dejonghe, E., Richard V. & Bonami, J.R. 2003. Genome-based detection methods of *Macrobrachium rosenbergii* nodavirus, a pathogen of the giant freshwater prawn, *Macrobrachium rosenbergii*: dot-blot, *in situ* hybridization and RT-PCR. *J. Fish Dis.,* 26: 583-590.

Sri Widada J., Richard, V., Shi, Z., Qian, D. & Bonami. J.R. 2004. Dot-blot hybridization and RT-PCR detection of extra small virus (XSV) associated with white tail disease of prawn *Macrobrachium rosenbergii. Dis Aquat Org.,* 58: 83-87.

Subasinghe, R.P. & Bartley, D. 2004. Risks of species introduction. In: J.R. Arthur, & M.B. Reantaso, eds. *Capacity and awareness building on import risk analysis for aquatic animals.* Report of the Joint APEC/FAO/NACA/OIE/DoF-Thailand/INP/CONPESCA/SAGARPA Workshops, Bangkok, Thailand 1-6 April 2002 and Mazatlan, Sinaloa, Mexico, 12-17 August 2002. pp.23-31. Asia-Pacific Economic Cooperation, APEC Fisheries Working Group.

Sunarto, A., Widodo, Taukhid, Koesharyani, I., Supriyadi, H., Gardenia, L., Sugianti, B. & Rukmono, D. 2004. *In* C.R. Lavilla-Pitogo and K. Nagasawa. *Transboundary fish diseases in Southeast Asia: occurrence, surveillance, research and training.* pp. 91-121. Tigbauan, Iloilo, Philippines. SEAFDEC Aquaculture Department.

Tu, C., Lin, S.-Y. & Sung, H.-T. 2004. Current status of koi herpesvirus in Taiwan. *In* C.R. Lavilla-Pitogo and K. Nagasawa. *Transboundary fish diseases in Southeast Asia: occurrence, surveillance, research and training.* pp. 21-24. Tigbauan, Iloilo, Philippines. SEAFDEC Aquaculture Department.

Tung, C.W., Wang, C.S. & Chen, S.N. 1999. Histological and electron microscopic study on *Macrobrachium* muscle virus (MMV) infection in the giant freshwater prawn, *Macrobrachium rosenbergii* (de Man), cultured in Taiwan. *J. Fish Dis.,* 22: 319-324.

Van, V.K. 2004. Current status of transboundary fish diseases in Vietnam: occurrence, surveillance, research and training. *In* C.R. Lavilla-Pitogo and K. Nagasawa. *Transboundary fish diseases in Southeast Asia: occurrence, surveillance, research and training.* pp. 221-227. Tigbauan, Iloilo, Philippines. SEAFDEC Aquaculture Department.

Wada, K.T. 2003. Akoya oyster disease – disease card. Developed to support the NACA/FAO/OIE Regional Quarterly Aquatic Animal Disease (QAAD) Reporting System in the Asia-Pacific. Bangkok, NACA, 3 pp. (www.enaca.org/Health/DiseaseLibrary/AkoyaDisease.pdf)

Widada, J.S. & J.R. Bonami. 2004. Characteristics of the monocistronic genome of extra small virus, a virus-like particle associated with *Macrobrachium rosenbergii* nodavirus: possible candidate for a new species of satellite virus. *J. Gen. Virol.,* 85: 643-646.

Aquatic disease emergencies and implications to international trade

Peter Beers
Biosecurity Australia, Department of Agriculture Fisheries and Forestry
Edmund Barton Building, Kings Avenue
Canberra, Australia
peter.beers@daff.gov.au

Beers, P. 2005. Aquatic disease emergencies and implications to international trade. p. 41–45. In: Subasinghe, R.P.; Arthur, J.R. (eds.). Regional workshop on preparedness and response to aquatic animal health emergencies in Asia. Jakarta, Indonesia, 21–23 September 2004. *FAO Fisheries Proceedings*. No. 4. Rome, FAO. 2005. 178p.

ABSTRACT

The threat to international trade as a result of aquatic animal disease emergencies is growing. Increasingly, the response to health emergencies is to guard aquatic animal resources from disease in order to protect environmental values, investment, production, market access and consumer confidence. The Sanitary and Phytosanitary Agreement (SPS Agreement) of the World Trade Organization (WTO) provides the international framework within which governments respond to disease emergencies. The SPS Agreement provides special status to the recommendations of the World Organisation for Animal Health (OIE) that deal with trade in aquatic animal commodities and related matters. The effectiveness of emergency response procedures will inevitably impact on the response of trading partners to disease threats.

INTRODUCTION

The sources of aquatic animal products and the patterns of international trade in them are changing. Aquaculture production is growing rapidly, at a higher rate than for the terrestrial farmed meat production sectors (since 1970, at 9.2 percent *per annum* compared to 2.8 percent). In the same period, the capture fisheries sector has only grown at 1.4 percent *per annum*. About 27 percent of aquatic animal production (by weight) is now from aquaculture. The pattern of international trade in aquatic animal products is also changing, and 37 percent of aquatic animal production is traded internationally, with significant shifts in the source and destination of the product (FAO, 2002).

Aquaculture is an innovative industry; many species are being cultured, in many locations, under a variety of environmental and husbandry conditions. This has lead to new challenges, particularly when new disease syndromes emerge, often precipitated by high stocking densities, exposure to alien pathogens, stressful environmental conditions and inadequate husbandry.

Investment in aquaculture and the property values of capture fisheries bring new economic imperatives to derive a return and protect the investment from threats such as disease. Disease outbreaks are a common event in modern aquaculture, and concerns of spill-over into wild populations are regularly aired. In light of this, the response to dealing with and preventing aquatic animal disease emergencies is changing.

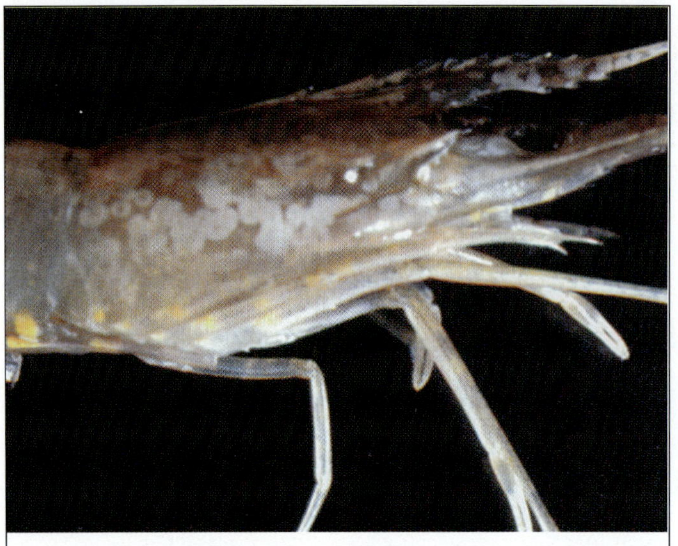

DV LIGHTNER

A juvenile P. monodon *with distinctive white spots of WSD*

EMERGENCIES

Emergency situations can arise for different reasons, such as environmental disasters, significant disease occurrences and residue findings. The common result is that sudden and urgent action is required to manage the situation to minimize losses. Disease emergencies can take several different forms – the recognition of a novel disease, the appearance of a disease in a new location or in a new host species (including humans), or a disease taking on a more virulent form. A rapid response is required to assess the situation, limit further biological losses, stop spread and provide reassurance to markets.

In recent times, there are many examples of disease emergencies affecting aquatic animals, such as whitespot, Taura syndrome, infectious salmon anaemia and Koi herpes virus. It is reasonable to expect that aquatic animal emergencies will continue to occur for the foreseeable future because of the widespread movement of genetic materials for aquaculture purposes, the movement and reswimming (re-immersion) of live product for human consumption, the movement of aquaculture species into environments where they encounter new pathogens, the adaptation of new aquaculture species to commercial production exposing them to hitherto unrecognized pathogens and so on.

With the terrestrial animal industries, disease emergencies are frequently associated with the disruption of markets for two reasons: firstly, from the loss of consumer confidence and their switching to alternative products and secondly, from loss of market due to technical impediments. The response to the emergency, especially the level of trust in the authorities undertaking the response, will be instrumental in determining how rapidly the market can be regained.

Historically, there have been few restrictions on the international movement of aquatic animals and their products. Thus the biological loss of production caused by the disease emergency has been in general greater than losses due to disruption of markets, though the loss of markets to competing traders may have a continuing longer-term impact.

This is changing as the economic, environmental and social values of aquatic animals are recognized and as the increased threat of disease spread is appreciated. In general, restrictions in response to emergencies are likely to be directed at the movement of live animals and their genetic materials. However, it should be expected that increased scrutiny will be paid to the movement of aquatic animal products during disease emergencies, especially to those from emergency harvest or those that are not highly processed.

WORLD ORGANISATION FOR ANIMAL HEALTH – OIE

International biosecurity standards for the movement of aquatic animals and their products have lagged behind those for terrestrial animals. As aquaculture has increased in importance, international standards have been developed by the World Organisation for Animal Health (the Office International des Épizooties, OIE). The diseases addressed by the OIE have reflected the species that are of importance to aquaculture and the state of knowledge. The movement of broodstock and genetic materials have been the focus of its activities, but more recently the movement of products is being increasingly considered.

The current OIE Aquatic Animal Health Code 2004 – the Aquatic Code (OIE, 2004) contains recommended measures for the movement of live aquatic animals and their genetic material susceptible to the listed diseases. The Aquatic Code also contains recommendations for dead, uneviscerated fish and dead crustaceans of species susceptible to the OIE-listed diseases. The Aquatic Animal Health Standards Commission will be redrafting the Aquatic Code to introduce the concept of "safe commodities". These are commodities that can be traded safely, regardless of the animal health status of the source. The Commission will also attempt to grade the level of risk for other commodities.

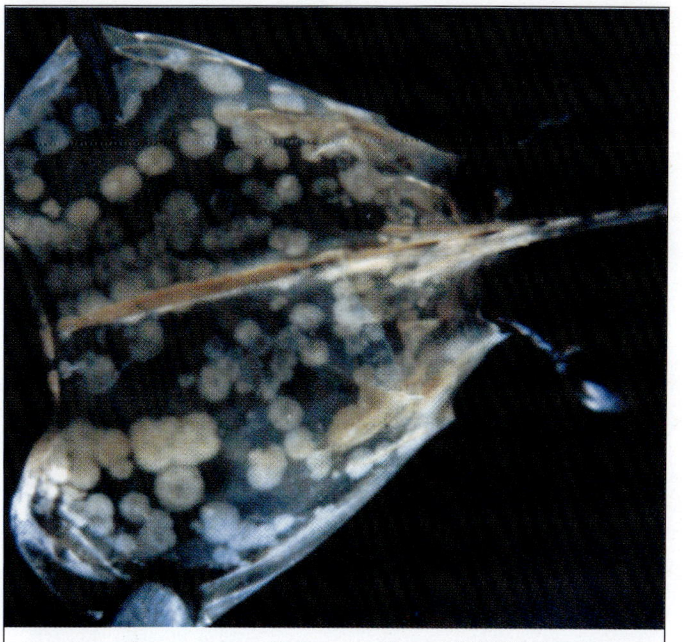

DV LIGHTNER/P. SAIBABA

Carapace from a juvenile P. monodon *with WSD. Calcareous deposits on the underside of the shell account for the white spots*

Member countries of the OIE also have obligations with regard to reporting particular disease occurrences through the OIE to the international community. Disease reporting is intended to assist in minimizing disease spread and aiding disease control. OIE members are obliged to report not only the occurrence of disease but also the presence of the causative agent in the absence of clinical disease.

In certain circumstances, such as a change in disease status or where information will be of epidemiological significance to trading partners, reports must be made within 24 hours. This is commonly referred to as emergency reporting. Situations covered by emergency reporting include the outbreak of a disease in countries or zones previously considered to be free, occurrence of a listed disease in a new host species, identification of a new strain or disease manifestation of a listed disease, situations where a listed disease has potential to spread internationally, newly recognized zoonotic potential for a listed disease and recognition of new emerging diseases and pathogens.

The Aquatic Code also provides rules by which a free status can be restored to a country or zone that has suffered a disease outbreak. In the case of "stamping out" (i.e. disease eradication), this relies on following the methods detailed in the appropriate chapters of the Aquatic Code, a surveillance scheme and no new infections being recognized.

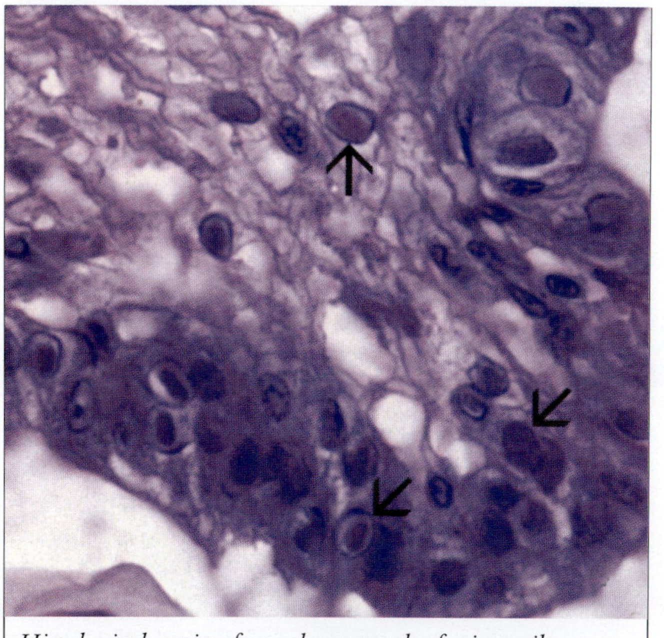

DV LIGHTNER

Histological section from the stomach of a juvenile P. chinensis *infected with WSD. Prominent intranuclear inclusion bodies are abundant in the cuticular epithelium and subcuticular*

Timely and accurate reporting to the OIE is usually an important consideration when assessing trading partners and responding to disease

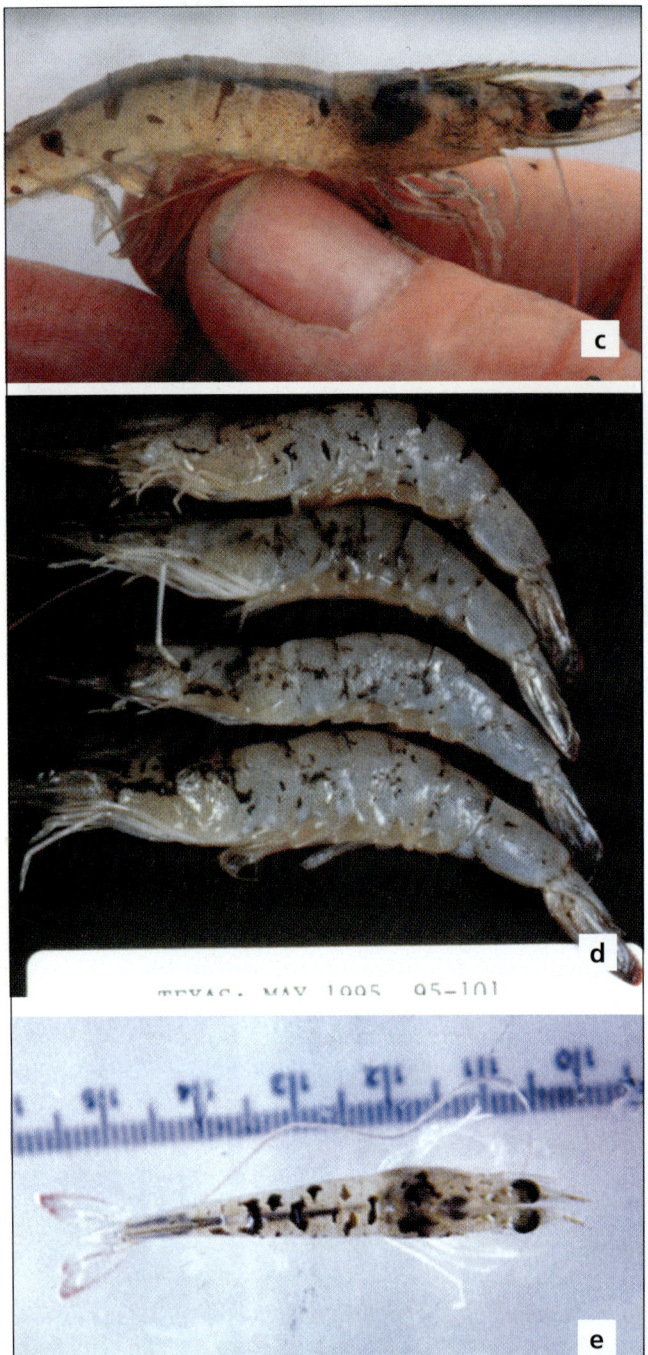

Juvenile, pond-reared P. vannamei *(c – from Ecuador; d – from Texas; e – from Mexico) showing melanized foci mark sites of resolving cuticular epithelium necrosis due to TSV infection.*

DV LIGHTNER/F. JIMENEZ

emergencies. Members are also to provide information on control measures taken to prevent spread, including on live animals, animal products and other things that could transmit disease.

Health certification is the basis of much international trade where measures are used to address sanitary and phytosanitary (SPS) concerns. Unreliable and inaccurate reporting of disease emergencies may have a broader effect on the trading relationship, spilling over into the acceptance of routine certification.

THE AGREEMENT ON THE APPLICATION OF SANITARY AND PHYTOSANITARY MEASURES

The World Trade Organization's (WTO) Agreement on the Application of Sanitary and Phytosanitary Measures (SPS Agreement) provides a basic right to WTO member countries to take necessary measures to protect human, animal or plant life or health. With this right come certain obligations, including that such protective measures must be based on a risk assessment or conform to an international standard. In the case of aquatic animal health, the measures in the Aquatic Code are the relevant international standards. If an aquatic disease emergency involved a disease listed by the OIE, a WTO member would be justified in restricting trade to the extent specified in the Aquatic Code.

WTO members are also able to take provisional measures in cases where relevant scientific evidence is insufficient for the risk assessment. This is often the situation in aquatic disease emergencies while the disease agent is being identified, the extent of its spread determined, the effectiveness of control measures assessed, and trace back and trace forward investigations are continuing. A WTO member adopting provisional measures must consider the available pertinent information, including international standards, seek further information to assess the risk and review the measure in a timely manner.

In practice, trading partners are becoming more likely to restrict trade in response to an aquatic disease emergency if they perceive a threat to their own aquatic resources. Such restrictions will be minimized by accurate international reporting and prompt action to control the outbreak. Previously prepared contingency plans effectively implemented increase the probability that disease outbreaks will be efficiently controlled. Obtaining cooperation from all of the participants in the midst of a response is likely to be difficult and may compromise the potential effectiveness of control and eradication. Trading partners need early and accurate advice, which is frequently updated, if they are to have confidence in the response and remove unnecessary trade restrictions.

Individual aquaculture producers can practice on-farm biosecurity to help minimize losses and facilitate a faster return to market. The OIE's Aquatic Animal Health Standards Commission is introducing the concept of "compartment" into the Code, which will help facilitate recognition of a higher health status on individual farms based on their health status, surveillance, control and biosecurity measures.

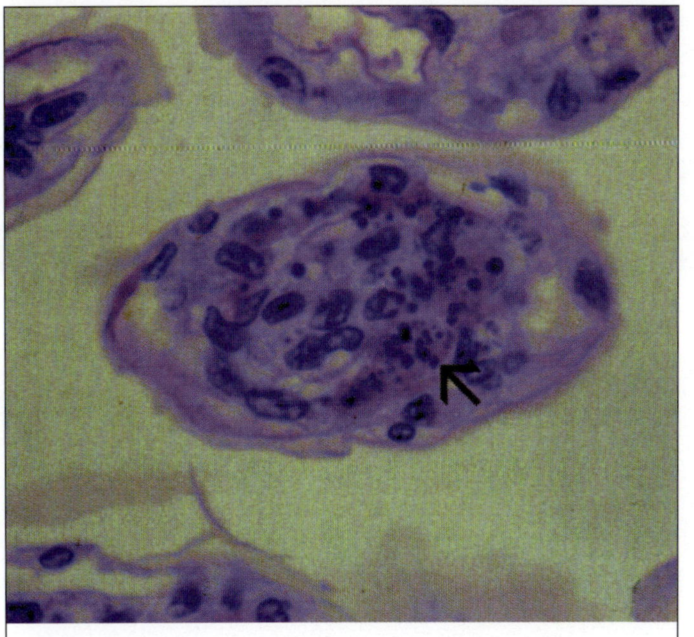

DV LIGHTNER

Focal TSV lesions in the gills (arrow). Nuclear pykinosis and karyorrhexis, increased cytoplasmic eosinophilia, and an abundance of variably staining generally spherical cytoplasmic inclusions are distinguishing characteristics of the lesions. 900x magnification.

CONCLUSIONS

At present, the impact on international trade resulting from aquatic disease emergencies is not great when compared to impacts that follow disease emergencies affecting terrestrial animals. This is not to diminish or understate the economic, social and environmental losses that occur in aquatic disease emergencies, particularly when there are severe biological losses in the affected species. However many countries have few biosecurity controls on the movement of aquatic animals and their products when compared to the terrestrial animal situation. This approach is changing with the recognition of the value of wild fisheries and the level of investment in aquaculture.

The SPS Agreement provides for the use of biosecurity measures to protect life and health. The OIE has disease-reporting obligations and recommendations for trade in aquatic animals and their products with regard to listed diseases. Although rapid and accurate reporting of aquatic disease emergencies may have consequences for trade, the building of trust will have longer-term benefits. Trust is the basis of trade, the international trading system and its certification system for SPS matters.

Early and accurate reporting of disease emergencies helps to build trust and facilitates the reinstatement of normal trading relations following a disease emergency. The longer access to a market is lost, the more difficult it becomes to regain market share taken by competitors and to rebuild commercial confidence as a reliable supplier.

For countries to meet their SPS obligations and international standards of the OIE Aquatic Code, a suitable infrastructure is required. The aquatic animal industries are growing globally at a rate faster than the development of the supporting infrastructure and expertise. SPS capacity can be strengthened in a number of ways, and this workshop will offer guidance and assistance to this end.

LITERATURE CITED

FAO. 2002. *The state of world fisheries and aquaculture 2002.* Food and Agriculture Organization of the United Nations, Rome. (available at www.fao.org)

OIE. 2004. *Aquatic animal health code*, 7th Edn, Office International des Épizooties, Paris. (available at www.oie.int)

The Food and Agriculture Organization of the United Nations' Emergency Prevention System (EMPRES-Livestock) and experiences in developing countries

Juan Lubroth[1], Peter Roeder[1], Moisés Vargas-Terán[2], William Amanfu[1], Vincent Martin[1], Wolfgang Boehle[3], George Chizuka[4], Carolyn Benigno[5], Akiko Kamata[1] and Fairouz Larfoui[1]

Lubroth, J., Roeder, P., Vargas-Terán, M., Amanfu, W., Martin, V., Boehle, W., Chizuka, G., Benigno, C., Kamata, A. & Larfoui, F. 2005. The Food and Agriculture Organization of the United Nations' Emergency Prevention System (EMPRES-Livestock) and experiences in developing countries. p. 47-65. In: Subasinghe, R.P.; Arthur, J.R. (eds.). Regional workshop on preparedness and response to aquatic animal health emergencies in Asia. Jakarta, Indonesia, 21–23 September 2004. *FAO Fisheries Proceedings*. No. 4. Rome, FAO. 2005. 178p.

ABSTRACT

FAO's Emergency Prevention System for Transboundary Animal and Plant Pests and Diseases (EMPRES), promotes the effective containment and control of the most serious epidemic livestock diseases, such as foot-and-mouth disease, rinderpest, contagious bovine pleuropneumonia, avian influenza, classical swine fever and Rift Valley fever, some which have public health implications. EMPRES also attends to newly emerging diseases and applies methods of progressive elimination on a regional and global basis through international cooperation involving (i) early warning, (ii) early reaction, (iii) enabling research and (iv) coordination. Major economic losses to livestock and producers the world over due to major outbreaks of transboundary animal diseases (TADs) such as foot-and-mouth disease (1997–2003), classical swine fever in the Caribbean and Europe (1996–2002), rinderpest in the Somali ecosystem (2001 and 2003), and Rift Valley fever into the Arabian Peninsula (2000) have been the main stimulus for the initiative to create a Global Framework for the Progressive Control of TADs with the Office International des Épizooties. Both organizations have examined the problem of TADs from the perspective of the complexity of the world food chain and human welfare, as well as the international public goods of equity, conservation of natural resources and public health

[1] Animal and Health Service
Animal Production and Health Service
FAO, Rome, Italy
Juan.lubroth@fao.org

[2] FAO, Santiago, Chile

[3] FAO, Harare, Zimbabwe

[4] FAO, Accra, Ghana

[5] FAO, Bangkok, Thailand

and propose that effective prevention and progressive control of the major transboundary animal diseases is an essential contribution to the achievement of the Millennium Development Goals. The objectives of the GF-TADs initiative are to: safeguard the livestock industry of developed as well as developing countries from repeated incursions of infectious disease epidemics, to improve food security and incomes of developing countries, and to promote safe trade in livestock and animal products at the national, regional and international levels. These goals can be best achieved if the major TADs are controlled at *source of infection*, which is mainly in the developing countries.

INTRODUCTION

The overall priority of the Food and Agriculture Organization of the United Nations (FAO) is the encouragement of sustainable agriculture and rural development. This priority is met by FAO's long-term strategy to increase food production and food security while conserving and managing natural resources and reducing poverty. According to its constitution and mandate, granted by the Member Countries, FAO provides independent advice to governments on agricultural policy and planning, as well as on the legal structures needed for development (including rural development, food security and the alleviation of poverty); development assistance through a wide range of technical assistance projects; the collection, analysis, interpretation and dissemination of information relating to food, agriculture, forestry and fisheries; and offers reference and educational material to farmers, scientists and non-governmental organizations (NGOs) so as to enable rational decisions on planning, investment, marketing, research and training. FAO provides a neutral forum where all nations can discuss, formulate and negotiate policy on major food and agriculture issues.

THE PRIORITIES OF THE FAO

The five corporate strategies expressed in FAO's Strategic Framework 2000–2015 are:

- contributing to the eradication of food insecurity and rural poverty;
- promoting, developing and reinforcing policy and regulatory frameworks for food, agriculture, fisheries and forestry;
- creating sustainable increases in the supply and availability of food and other products from the crop, livestock, fisheries and forestry sectors;
- supporting the conservation, improvement and sustainable use of natural resources for food and agriculture; and
- improving decision-making through the provision of information and assessments and fostering of knowledge management for food and agriculture.

In 1994, the Director-General of FAO established two priority programmes in support of such strategy, the Special Programme in Food Security (SPFS) and the EMPRES[1]. The two components of EMPRES are those of the desert locust in crops and the livestock component that focuses on epidemic animal diseases. The latter is placed within the Infectious Diseases Group, Animal Health Service (AGAH) within the Division of Animal Production and Health (AGA). The EMPRES concepts are encompassed in all five of the FAO priorities.

THE EMPRES VISION AND CONCEPT

FAO, within its global mandate related to animal health, has traditionally played an eminent role in the fight against epidemic diseases of livestock.[2] However, upon taking office, the Director-General decided to step up FAO's role in the control and prevention

---

[1] 106th FAO Council Session, May-June, 1994.

[2] Rinderpest (Pan African Rinderpest Campaign 1980 and Joint Programme 15 (1970); foot-and-mouth disease (European Commission for FMD since 1952); screwworm in Libya/North Africa (1988).

of emergencies, to respond to the need to develop more effective mechanisms that would alert Member Countries to impending transboundary disease problems, as well as to develop FAO's ability to monitor and forecast the spread of animal diseases. The EMPRES concept encompasses animal diseases of a transboundary nature, which have been defined as:

> *"... those that are of significant economic, trade and/or food security importance for a considerable number of countries; which can easily spread to other countries and reach epidemic proportions; and where control/management, including exclusion, requires co-operation between several countries".*

The EMPRES vision is to promote the effective containment and control of the most serious epidemic livestock diseases. EMPRES also attends to newly emerging diseases and applies methods of progressive elimination on a regional and global basis through international cooperation involving (i) early warning, (ii) early reaction, (iii) enabling research and (iv) coordination.. The EMPRES Programme has established itself as a major initiative of FAO, well acknowledged as fulfilling an important development role. The World Food Summit in 1996 under Commitment Number 3[3] and FAO conferences have emphasized its relevance and importance.

Funding for EMPRES activities is part of the FAO Regular Programme described under the Department of Agriculture. These activities are normative in nature and address aspects of disease spread and strategy development for containment, capacity building, awareness and technology transfer, as well as information in the form of manuals, booklets, CDs, videos etc. Included is the financial support to the World Reference Laboratory for Foot-and-Mouth Disease and the World Reference Laboratories for Rinderpest and other Morbilliviruses, located at Pirbright, United Kingdom, and Montpellier, France, and the extensive collaboration with the Joint Division of FAO/International Atomic Energy Agency (IAEA) in Vienna. There are some 30 FAO Collaborating Centres and Reference Laboratories that assist EMPRES in their speciality areas or competence in applied research for specific diseases of direct relevance to EMPRES needs. EMPRES also incorporates the Secretariat for the Global Rinderpest Eradication Programme, actively participates in Office International des Épizooties (OIE) standard setting upon request, and forms part of advisory or steering committees in several initiatives around the world (e.g. the Pan African Programme for the Control of Epizootics/African Union-Inter African Bureau for Animal Resources). Also within the Animal Health Service, the Secretariat of the European Commission for the Control of FMD resides, dedicating its efforts to prevent incursion of foot-and-mouth disease (FMD) into Europe, promoting applied research and technology exchange, and supporting countries neighbouring Europe in FMD surveillance activities. This commission, financed through a European Community (EC) Trust Fund, extends well beyond the European Union, to include 33 countries.

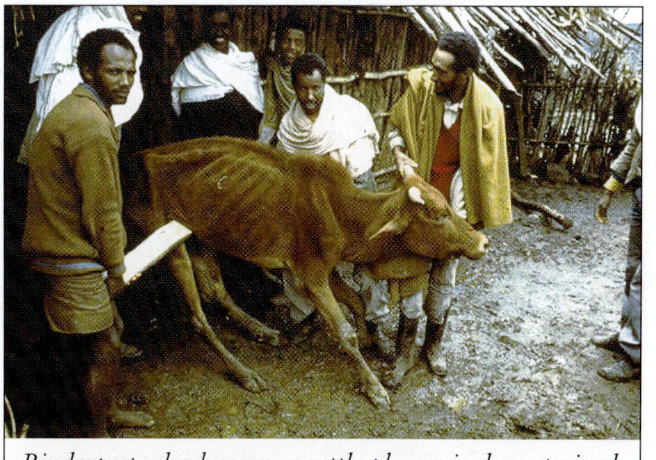

FAO

Rinderpest, also known as cattle plague, is characterized by fever, depression, dehydration, diarrhoea, and high mortality

FAO Member Countries requesting assistance can benefit from its Technical Cooperation Programme, which may provide funds (up to US$400 000 per project), training, equipment, vaccine

[3] Commitment Number 3: "Seek to ensure effective prevention and progressive control of plant and animal pests and diseases, including especially those which are of transboundary nature, such as rinderpest, cattle tick, foot and mouth disease and desert locust,...".

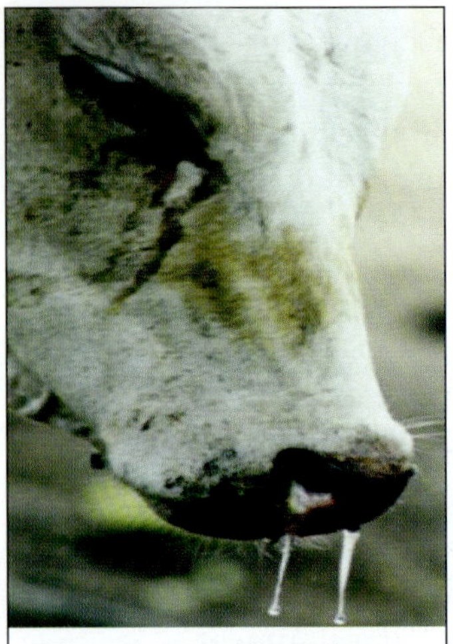

JUAN LUBROTH

Clinical signs of Rinderpest

and expertise to meet priority development needs. EMPRES operates numerous emergency or regular Technical Cooperation Projects (TCPs, Figure 1) for several of the most devastating animal diseases such as FDM, rinderpest, contagious bovine pleuropneumonia, *peste des petits ruminants,* Newcastle disease, Rift Valley fever, classical swine fever (CSF), African swine fever, sheep pox, brucellosis and haemorrhagic septicaemia. In addition, inputs from FAO include: surveillance systems (including global information systems (GIS) based field observation/abattoir data software) known as TAD*info*, emergency preparedness, contingency planning, veterinary vaccine technology transfer, participatory epidemiological approaches, enabling legislation and evaluation of veterinary services.

The diseases or needs addressed by EMPRES were: In **Asia**, FMD, Rift Valley fever, CSF, rinderpest, *peste des petits ruminants*, information systems, project evaluation and border control. In **Africa**, contagious bovine pleuropneumonia, African swine fever, FMD, Rift Valley fever, rinderpest, *peste des petits ruminants*, Newcastle disease, veterinary vaccines, laboratory training and equipment, molecular analysis of viral strains, surveillance systems, participatory approaches to epidemiology and participatory disease search, modeling of disease transmission, remote sensing and prediction, animal identification and evaluation of legislation. In the **Americas**, EMPRES inputs included molecular characterization of FMD viral strains, the promotion of the Hemispheric Plan for CSF eradication, public awareness, surveillance methods and information systems.

Other activities in which EMPRES (including others within the Animal Health Service and AGA) has been involved include:

- inputs for the livestock sector rehabilitation in post-war Iraq;
- livestock sector rehabilitation in Afghanistan, Kosovo and Rwanda;
- studies to identify possible animal reservoirs for the severe respiratory acute syndrome (SARS) coronavirus in China; and
- presentations at the Biological Weapons Convention meetings.

The EMPRES Projects depicted in Figure 1 (2002–2004) do not include trust-funded projects or specific extra-budgetary projects for agriculture or animal health where the Infectious Disease Group has held responsibility.

It is apparent to EMPRES itself that all its inputs are insufficient to curtail the devastation caused by transboundary animal diseases and their impacts on food security and the livelihoods of poor animal farmers, pastoral communities, and the viability of dairy cooperatives and commercial enterprises. The long-term vision of EMPRES is to have a large cadre of trained professionals and para-professionals that would curb disease incidence and implement the required control strategies through better surveillance, early warning, early detection and early reaction. As EMPRES works to meet these needs for individual countries, these inputs are often not sustainable for various reasons. These include such factors as: the poor animal health status of a neighbouring country; low efficiency in carrying out planned activities, inconsistent training; attrition of personnel (i.e. key individuals departing from public service for the acceptance of greater administrative responsibilities[4], succumbing to disease[5] or desiring to find a place within the private sector in

[4] Sometimes precisely because a postgraduate technical degree was obtained.

[5] Reference is made to the devastating effect of human immunodeficiency virus infection and the acute immunodeficiency syndrome (HIV/AIDS) on a village population, where mortality among adults in certain parts of Africa exceeds 30 percent. A capacity building course on community animal health and production would theoretically need to be repeated every two years or else the need to commence the process from the beginning every time. The same would be true for water management, soil conservation, fisheries or crop rotation initiatives etc.

clinical practice, pharmaceutical representation or consultancy). Recognizing that transboundary animal disease respects no political boundaries, EMPRES, has sought to work beyond individual country projects at the regional level in coordination with various countries and stakeholders. An initiative, in partnership with the Office International des Épizooties (OIE), to coordinate counter-epizootic measures and strengthen veterinary systems was therefore undertaken in 2002, under the working title: "The Global Framework for the Progressive Control of Transboundary Animal Diseases (GF-TADs)."

THE GLOBAL FRAMEWORK FOR THE PROGRESSIVE CONTROL OF TRANSBOUNDARY ANIMAL DISEASES (GF-TADS)[6]

Major economic losses to livestock and producers the world over due to major outbreaks of transboundary animal diseases (TADs) such as foot-and-mouth disease (1997–2003), classical swine fever in the Caribbean and Europe (1996–2002), rinderpest in the Somali ecosystem (2001 and 2003), and Rift Valley fever into the Arabian Peninsula (2000) have been the main stimulus for the initiative to create a Global Framework for the Progressive Control of TADs. The unprecedented epidemics, both in scope and geographical occurrence, of highly pathogenic avian influenza (HPAI) that came into international attention in Asia in 2004 are symptomatic of the problems facing disease control, regional collaboration and understanding of disease ecology for better prevention. Other diseases remain unchecked – such as contagious bovine pleuropneumonia in Zambia, Angola, DR Congo and Namibia or *peste des petits ruminants* in India, Bangladesh, North Africa and the Middle East. African swine fever still causes hardship for swine production in rural and peri-urban areas in Central and West Africa.

Several international institutions have emphasized the need to control TADs due to their devastating impact on livestock agriculture, trade and food security:

- The World Food Summit (WFS), November 1996, recognized the pivotal, constraining role of TADs, and the Heads of State and Governments pledged to *"seek to ensure effective prevention and progressive control of plant and animal pests and diseases, including especially those which are of transboundary nature, such as rinderpest, cattle tick, foot and mouth disease and desert locust,..... ".*

FIGURE 1

Technical Cooperation Projects 2002–2004; EMPRES (full circle) and those with EMPRES involvement or of notable mention (open circles)

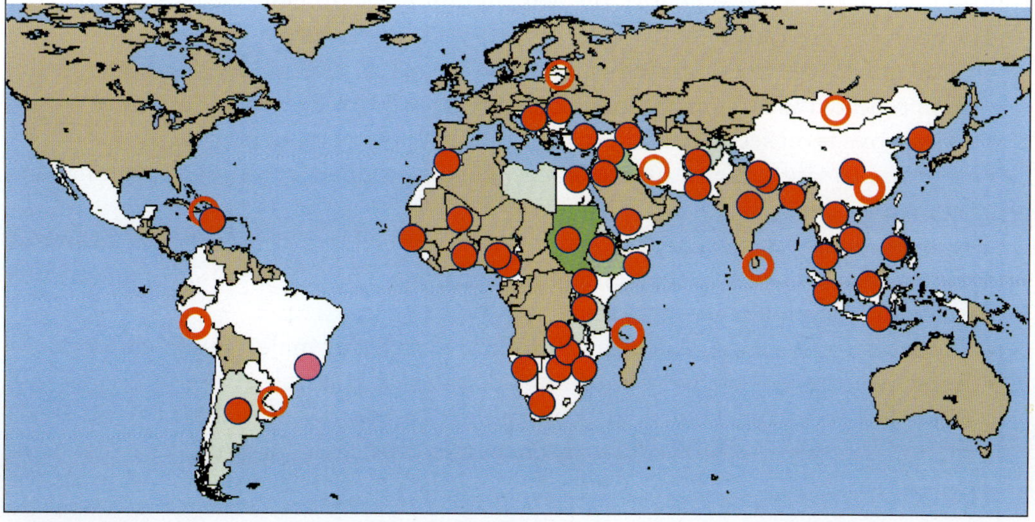

[6] GF-TADs was endorsed by Member Countries at FAO's 32nd Conference held in Rome in December 2003 and by the 72nd General Session of the OIE in Paris.

- The OIE's International Committee in 2002, called on the OIE and FAO to pursue an international concerted action against a number of diseases having significant effects on food security, poverty alleviation, food safety, public health and access to formal markets.
- The 31st Session of the FAO Conference (2001) also recognized the widespread and increasing impact of epidemic animal diseases, like FMD, and stressed the need to continue the work to combat the disease at the national, regional and international levels, involving all relevant stakeholders.
- The report of the Temporary Committee on Foot and Mouth Disease of the European Union Parliament (3 October, 2002)[7], concluded:

  "In view of the intensification of world trade and global warming, a thorough analysis of the existing and likely future threats arising from the introduction of animal diseases into the EU which could cause major economic damage is urgently needed at European level.

  Lasting success can be achieved in efforts to control FMD worldwide only if it proves possible, through close international cooperation, to curb the disease decisively in areas where it is still endemic. The Commission should therefore do more to assist the countries concerned in their efforts to control or eradicate FMD and seek to improve cooperation with regard to information (early warning systems)."
- The WFS, five years later (2002), reiterated the 1996 commitment and called for specific action and voluntary financial contribution to the FAO Global Trust Fund to facilitate food security programmes and combat TADs.

There is ample evidence from various studies that the risk of spread of TADs will increase unless concerted international actions are put into place for effective prevention and progressive control. This conclusion is predominantly based on predictions of an unprecedented growth of the livestock sector and of the consumption of livestock products, particularly in TAD-endemic developing countries. The predicted growth in livestock is expected to result in increased livestock farming in tropical/subtropical zones, with trends towards large farming units and increase in trade in livestock and livestock products through informal and formal markets regionally and internationally.

OIE and FAO have examined the problem of TADs from the perspective of the complexity of the world food chain and human welfare, as well as the international public goods of equity, conservation of natural resources and public health. Thus the GF-TADs that is being promoted by the two organizations proposes the effective prevention and progressive control of FMD and other major TADs as an essential contribution to the achievement of the Millennium Development Goals.

The goals of GF-TADs are:

- to safeguard the livestock industry of developed as well as developing countries from repeated incursions of infectious disease epidemics;
- to improve food security and incomes of developing countries; and
- to promote safe trade in livestock and animal products at national, regional and international levels.

The above goals can be best achieved if the major TADs are controlled at **source of infection**, which is mainly in the developing countries. The GF-TADs programme will be developed along four main thrusts:

- Global Early Warning, Alert and Response System for major animal diseases;
- Implementing knowledge gained after decades of research at the molecular and ecological level and how it may be applied to other TADs. FMD is the TAD that all regions of the world consulted identified as a priority, as it concerns

[7] European Parliament: Temporary Committee on Foot and Mouth Disease. Draft Report. Provisional 2002/2153(INI). 3 October 2002.
www.europarl.eu.int/meetdocs/committees/fiap/20021107/475314en.pdf

both developed and developing countries and it offers the best opportunity for developing good practices in disease management in all regions of the world;
- Completion of global rinderpest eradication[8]; and
- A flexible Regional Thrust to take account of the regional priorities in terms of target disease, epidemiology and strategy for progressive control of FMD and priority diseases agreed through regional collaboration.

The Outputs for the initial six-year (2004–2009) period are:
- establishing a robust FAO-OIE-WHO (World Health Organization) Global Early Warning System for TADs and versions for each of the major regions, in partnership with regional organizations;
- securing a global status of internationally verified freedom from rinderpest;
- defining primary endemic areas for FMD and the other selected TADs;
- developing disease control strategies based on sound epidemiological knowledge for participating countries coordinated through relevant regional organizations;
- establishing an international early response capacity for prompt and authoritative disease diagnosis and for targeted local disease control in order to limit the spread of new outbreaks of TADs;
- identifying new research programmes through advanced research institutes (ARIs), including Consultative Group on International Agricultural Research (CGIAR) centers; and
- strengthening of referral diagnostic and molecular biological capacity of FAO/OIE Reference Laboratories and a follow-up technology transfer to National Agricultural Research Systems (NARS), primarily through the established system of a network of national laboratories supported by the FAO/IAEA Joint Division and north-south/south-south partnerships.

The GF-TADs initiative is designed to provide strategic regional cooperation for the control of transboundary animal diseases by:
- Improving national knowledge and information/data retrieval systems on animal production, disease surveillance, land use, animal and product movement, and related factors that affect or threaten animal health, as do climate change, worker migration and refugee movements, and price differentials across borders;
- Strategic use of quality vaccines – where such vaccines exist, and enabling research where they do not;
- Improved diagnostic laboratory performance at the national level and support for reference laboratories for the region/world through technology transfer and internal and external quality control;
- Technical guidance in the establishment of regional initiatives ensuring collaboration across borders; and
- Implementation of Good Emergency Management Practices that include early detection, reporting and counter-epizootic measures. The epidemiologically based strategy advocated in the GF-TADs is founded on two notions: risk-based surveillance and risk-mitigation disease control.

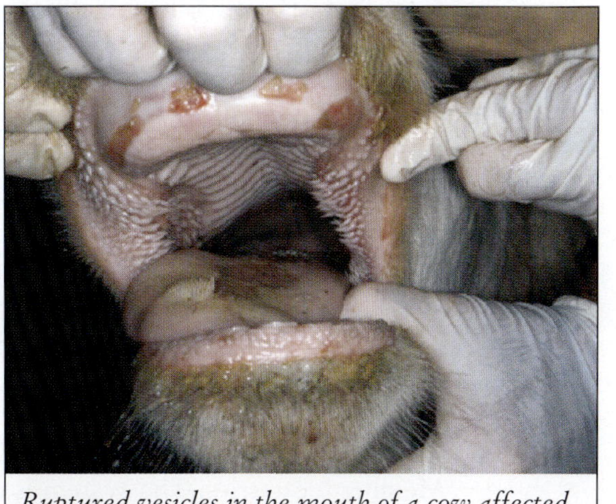

USDA

Ruptured vesicles in the mouth of a cow affected by FMD

[8] This thrust builds on the success of the on-going FAO Global Rinderpest Eradication Programme (GREP). Eradication is planned for 2010. Completing this major and unique undertaking of global eradication of an animal disease offers opportunity for good disease management practices through lessons learned through GREP.

It is expected that the GF-TADs programme will oversee a flexible progression in disease containment according to the various target regions, addressing features of risk reduction, evolved and strengthened national/regional control programmes, and the creation and maintenance of free zones or prescribed disease free zones. Verification of disease and infection-free status will be a reiterative process of national responsibility to ensure safe animal trade.

In addition, research into a new generation of vaccines their delivery, and diagnostic tests that will advance disease control programmes, early detection or prevention is being considered by several research centers with vast experience in FMD. Meetings with partners in the United States, the United Kingdom, Australia and Canada have already taken place to determine researchable priorities with the hope of obtaining promising advances in short periods of time, after which pilot projects could be carried out. This research programme is suggested to be coordinated with the Global Framework by an Inter-Agency Steering Committee.

It is expected that the Joint FAO/IAEA Division will continue to provide transfer of the new diagnostic technologies to developing countries as they become available, building on its 30-year experience of coordinated research and technical cooperation programmes. It is envisaged to include a financial subcontract arrangement with the FAO/OIE World and Regional Reference Laboratories in order to enhance their capacity for rapid and coordinated provision of authoritative diagnosis of epidemiologically important outbreaks, characterization and analysis of the genetic and antigenic make up of causal agents, monitoring of regional and global trends in pathogens and capacity building in national and regional laboratories. Other advanced research institutes will be contracted for specific expertise in the development of predictive methodologies and sensors, novel diagnostic techniques and more efficacious vaccines.

EARLY WARNING ACTIVITIES

Early warning concept

Early Warning was seen from the outset as a key component of EMPRES. The 1994–1995 Programme Review Report, Chapter V, observed thus:

> *"Early warning of T-PP/AD[9] situations is an important function of FAO, which has to rely largely on national systems for identifying and reporting outbreaks. Strengthening of national and regional capacities has thus been an important priority for FAO".*

Early warning has been defined as all disease initiatives, which predominantly would be based on epidemiological surveillance, that would lead to improved knowledge of the distribution of disease or infection and that might permit the forecasting or further evolution of an outbreak.

Capacity building in surveillance and early warning

This has been undertaken through a series of regional and national workshops, especially in Africa, North Africa and the Near East and in Asia. These training activities have been augmented by two specific manuals on surveillance and participatory epidemiology.

A development of greatest impact has been the development of a hierarchical software system aimed at assisting epidemiological surveillance, collection and analysis of GIS-based animal disease information at the national, regional and global levels. This unique system, called TADinfo, has been adopted or is being evaluated in several Member Countries. The system is described on the EMPRES website:
www.fao.org/ag/AGA/AGAH/EMPRES/tadinfo2/e_tadinf.htm

Regional TAD*info* is currently being field tested by the Southern African Development Community Regional Epidemiology Unit. A "global" TAD*info* system is expected to act as a major platform for the proposed FAO-OIE-WHO Global Early

[9] Transboundary plant pest or animal disease

Warning System for Transboundary Animal Diseases (GLEWS). The global aspects are under the incipient EMPRES-*i* (*i* for *information*, *intelligence* and *intervention*) database for disease tracking and references linked to the FAO Global Livestock Production and Health Atlas (GLIPHA).

Early warning projects

EMPRES-Livestock has been providing technical assistance to three major regional projects:

- ***The Pan African Programme for the Control of Epizootics (PACE)*** is conducted in collaboration with the Inter-African Bureau for Animal Resources of the African Union (AU-IBAR), with funding from the European Union. EMPRES-Livestock has provided the main epidemiologist for this five-year programme. The objective of the programme is to develop epidemio-surveillance networks for 34 countries in tropical Africa to assist with the surveillance and eventual early warning for transboundary animal diseases.
- ***Regional Animal Disease Surveillance and Control (RADISCON):*** This International Fund for Agricultural Development-funded project has been operating in 29 countries of North Africa, the Horn of Africa and the Middle East since 1997 and is expected to enter another phase of three years. This project has the objective of developing capacity in the region through (1) enhancing training in data management and analysis, (2) passive and active surveillance, and (3) outbreak investigation and risk analysis. The project has established national animal disease databases in a number of countries (Algeria, Egypt, Morocco, Sudan, Tunisia, Libya, Yemen, Saudi Arabia, Iraq, Kuwait) based on the TAD*info* system plus a regional reporting system, with standardized forms and an electronic information network linked to EMPRES-Livestock.
- ***Early Warning in SADC:*** A TCP regional project entitled Promotion of Transboundary Disease Early Warning Systems in the SADC Region covering 11 SADC countries (Angola, Botswana, Lesotho, Malawi, Mozambique, Namibia, South Africa, Swaziland, Tanzania, Zambia and Zimbabwe) has assisted in strengthening the SADC Livestock Disease Early Warning system through the procurement of equipment and installation of the TAD*info* system and the associated training of national epidemiologists. This has now formed the catalyst for a pipeline project by SADC seeking to institutionalize early warning for TADs in the region.

Pipeline projects

EMPRES-Livestock is developing three pipeline projects that are likely to have a long-term impact on early warning for transboundary animal diseases. The first involves capacity building and development of an early warning system for Central Asia, with ear-marked funding from the FAO Trust Fund; the second involves enhancing national uptake of the TAD*info* system – which is still largely unfunded; and the third is expected to be developed jointly with the OIE and WHO as the Global Early Warning System for Transboundary Animal Diseases (GLEWS). The FAO-OIE-WHO GLEWS is being designed along the principles shown in Figure 2.

FIGURE 2
Schematic representation of the FAO/OIE/WHO Global Early Warning System (GLEWS) and response

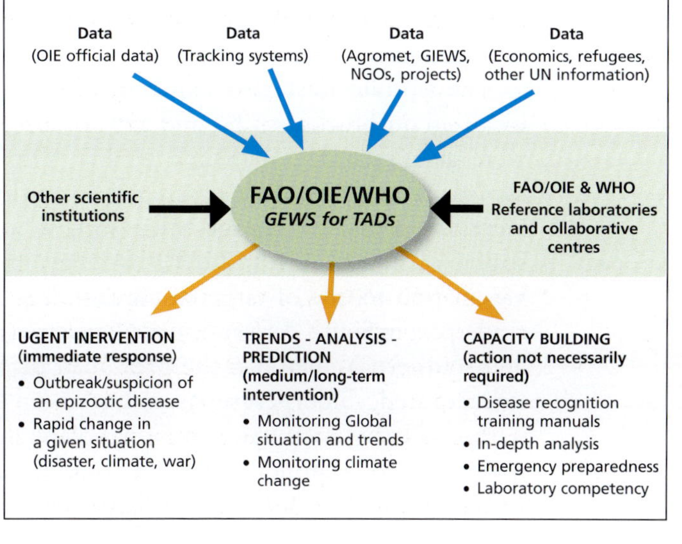

SPECIFIC EXAMPLES FOR COOPERATION AND LESSONS TO BE LEARNED

The Global Rinderpest Eradication Programme (GREP)

The immediate post-World War II period in Asia was followed by a major rinderpest epidemic in the 1950s affecting many countries in south and eastern Asia. National and regional programmes were set up to control rinderpest, the principal strategy for which was mass vaccination of the national herd. Once under control and with considerable investment, the disease likely persisted only in southern India and southern Pakistan. Nevertheless, the rinderpest control programmes initiated from 1987 were still based on the strategy of national mass vaccination, with relatively little impact on the perceived incidence of rinderpest in the region (Figure 3). The breakthrough happened once the region started to adopt an epidemiologically determined approach to disease eradication. In India, this led to recognizing that the disease was really endemic in the southern states (Tamil Nadu, Karnataka and Andra Pradesh) and that rinderpest elsewhere occurred by epidemic extension. Indian veterinary authorities concentrated their vaccination programme in the southern states and stopped vaccination in the north. No further outbreak of rinderpest has been reported in India since September 1995, and vaccination ceased in 2001. It is likely that the entire country will gain freedom of disease status by the end of 2004.

Similarly, by analysing the epidemiology of rinderpest in Pakistan and Afghanistan, it became obvious by 1996 that the 1994–1995 rinderpest epidemic in the Northern Areas of Pakistan and the 1995 and 1997 outbreaks in Afghanistan had merely represented a disease incursion from the endemic areas of southern Pakistan. On the three occasions, the outbreaks were controlled by targeted, peri-focal intensive vaccination without resorting to nation-wide blanket rinderpest vaccination.

During the regional workshop jointly organized by FAO/EMPRES and the Animal Production and Health Commission for Asia (and the Pacific [APHCA]) in 1998 in Sri Lanka, each country presented its rinderpest status. It became clear that in the entire South and East Asia, there was only a single endemic focus in southern Pakistan. As a consequence, there was no justification for countries to conceive expensive programmes involving national or regional mass vaccination campaigns against rinderpest, but rather to focus on the nidus of infection.

In Pakistan, the veterinary authorities were motivated since 1998 to pursue a strategy that would be epidemiologically determined rather than the 100-fold more costly generalized blanket vaccination campaign. In the following two years, Pakistan embarked on clinical and serological surveillance with targeted vaccination of buffalo herds in the presumed endemic areas encompassing the dairy colonies of Karachi in Sindh Province. The last recorded case of rinderpest in Pakistan was in 2000, with a status of provisional freedom from disease declared in 2003. This once-Asian disease may now have been eradicated from the continent; yet, active surveillance in the most remote villages must be exhaustive.

The Middle East also experienced an epidemic of rinderpest in the 1980s, and localized outbreaks in 1991 and 1994 occurred in Turkey and northern Iraq. Outbreaks were also recorded in Saudi Arabia, Oman and Yemen between 1994 and 1996. Molecular analysis of virus samples from the region showed that the causative strains were of the Asiatic lineage, suggesting a South Asian rather than an African link to source of infection. The GREP strategy in 1994–1996 shifted from advocating mass vaccination to one of targeted control. This concentrated on three fronts: controlling rinderpest in South Asia and surveillance plus targeted control in the Kurdish ecosystem and southern Yemen, i.e. the presumed primary endemicity. Although verification is still required, rinderpest seems to have been eliminated from the Middle Eastern region without further recourse to regional blanket vaccination. Only Syria still vaccinates its national herd, although there is a commitment to halt the practice at the end of 2004. In December 2003, GREP/EMPRES held a joint Technical Advisory Meeting with the

FIGURE 3

In the early 1980s (a), rinderpest was known to have been present in many countries, extending from Mauritania in the west to India in the east and as far south as Tanzania in Africa (years earlier, rinderpest extended to countries further east, including the Philippines). By the early 1990s (b), western and most of central Africa had been cleared of rinderpest, but it was still prevalent in eastern Africa. Many countries in South Asia, the Near East and the Arabian Peninsula continued to be affected. Even Europe was affected when rinderpest occurred in Georgia (and eastern Russia – not shown). In 2001 (c), there were suspicions of rinderpest persistence only in southern Sudan, the Somali ecosystem and Pakistan. The Pakistan reservoir was eliminated in 2002 (by virtue of Pakistan/EC/FAO joint effort), and this country declared provisional freedom in 2003 with subsequent recognition by the OIE. The first two maps (1980s and 1990s) show rinderpest infection status of countries by depicting whole countries as being infected, which epidemiologically is known not to be the case, even where disease occurrence was reported. The map for 2001 depicts livestock populations in which infection was suspected to be persisting and indicative of an improved epidemiological understanding. Currently, in 2004 (d), rinderpest virus is suspected to occur in the Somali ecosystem, crossing over several international borders

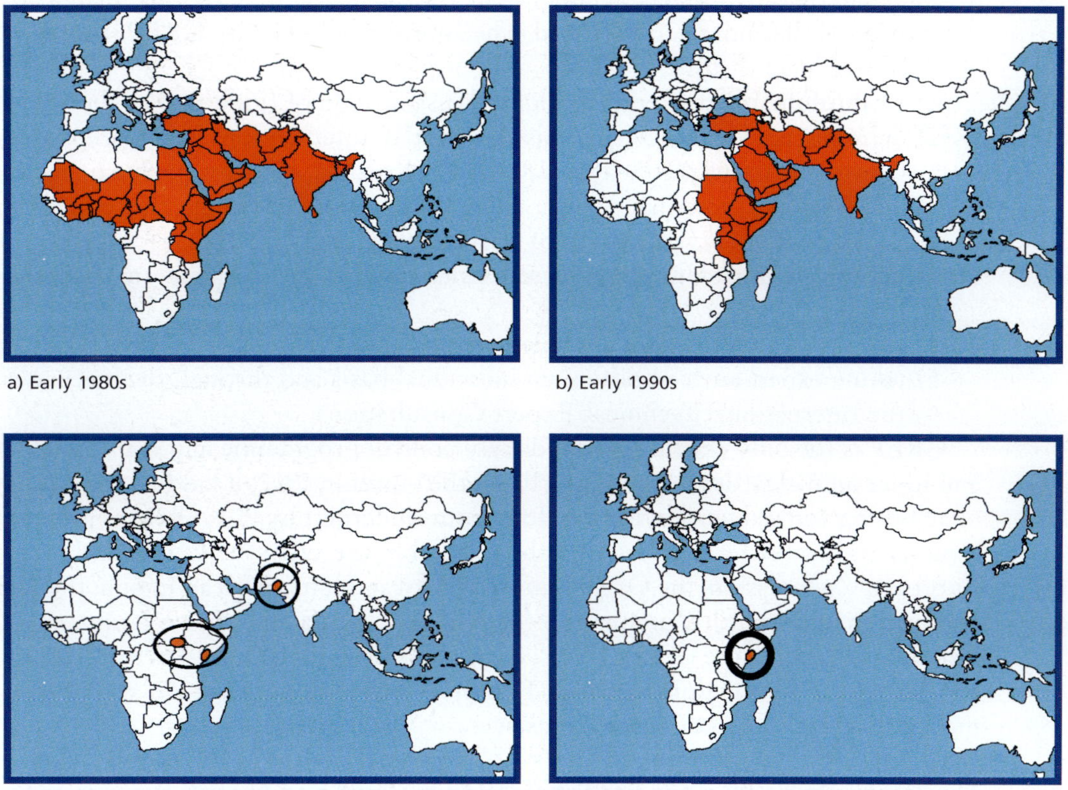

a) Early 1980s — b) Early 1990s — c) 2001 — d) 2004

OIE in Lebanon to provide the assistance required for countries in the Middle East and Arabian Peninsula (and Iran and Iraq) to meet the internationally recognized goals of freedom from disease and infection.

In Africa, the 10-year, multidonor programme coded JP-15 from 1964 to 1975 was based on blanket vaccination of the national herds throughout Tropical Africa. Although it was expected to have countries assume responsibilities, by 1982–1984 a pandemic of rinderpest had broken out in 20 countries of Tropical Africa stretching from Somalia in the east to Mauritania in the west. A new programme, the Pan African Rinderpest Campaign (PARC) was developed in 1986 with financial support primarily from the European Union. Initially, the approach was mass vaccination. It was not until the early 1990s that the approach of addressing the disease at source started to be vigorously pursued. Using community-based vaccination and disease search methodologies with several NGOs proved an extremely useful programme in remote areas and those under civil strife (e.g. southern Sudan, with its last confirmed case in 1998).

There is an urgent need to provide such a community-based animal health programme delivery system in the area that almost certainly constitutes the last rinderpest reservoir, situated in the Horn of Africa, and to institute specific actions aimed at eliminating foci of viral infection there. Fortunately, there exists a coordinated African programme with the work being undertaken predominantly through the Pan African Programme for the Control of Epizootics (PACE), implemented by the African Union/Inter-African Bureau for Animal Resources with financial support from the European Commission and the United Kingdom through its development agency. FAO and OIE, both on the advisory committee with PACE, assist in defining the actions required to define the rinderpest situation and bring about rapid elimination of the last reservoir of infection, with appropriate surveillance programmes to verify freedom.

One of the main lessons to be learnt from GREP is that the cost of a disease eradication programme can be reduced considerably by targeting disease control to epidemiologically defined endemic areas instead of undertaking blanket, mass vaccination of the entire national herd. The approach adopted by GREP since 1994 has involved five main thrusts:

1) establishing the true epidemiological distribution of rinderpest in the world;
2) defining epidemiologically based targeted interventions for the progressive control of rinderpest where disease is suspected, thereby persuading national and regional veterinary authorities away from pursuing the conventional, generalized mass vaccination of the entire national heard;
3) defining epidemiologically based strategies for the verification of rinderpest freedom;
4) establishing participatory involvement of key stakeholders in the GREP: and
5) taking expert advice both on an individual basis and through the mechanism of the International Technical/Expert Consultations.

GREP is the only existing global disease control programme and is the single most ambitious animal health programme. From the outset in 1992, it has had the stated goal of achieving verified worldwide freedom from rinderpest by 2010. Recognition for the achievements must be shared with others, notably the OIE; the European Union and European Commission; the Organisation of African Unity/African Union; the Animal Production and Health Commission for Asia and the Pacific; the governments of the Republic of Ireland, the United States, the United Kingdom, Australia, the Netherlands and Japan; the International Atomic Energy Agency's Joint Division with FAO; and most importantly, the countries themselves.

The Hemispheric Plan for the Eradication of Foot-and-Mouth Disease – Americas

Control of this relatively new disease to South Americas[10] has benefited from concerted action by the Pan American Health Organisation (PAHO) through the establishment of the Pan American Centre for Foot-and-Mouth Disease (Panaftosa), located in Rio de Janeiro, Brazil. In 1978, the Inter-American Meeting, at the Ministerial Level, on Health and Agriculture agreed on the Hemispheric Plan for Eradication of FMD in the Americas. The three subregional plans focussed on the level of endemicity of FMD (none, as in North America; endemic – South America; and a third sphere reflective of risk and proximity). The South American countries formed a commission *(Comisión Suramericana para la Lucha Contra la Fiebre Aftosa or COSALFA), which in its early years consisted* of the official veterinary service representatives or Ministers of Agriculture, but today incorporates the private sector, through representatives from dairy cooperatives, rancher syndicates or presidents of rural associations sitting side by side with the government to strategize methods for control and evaluate performance,

[10] First reported in Argentina in 1870; Colombia and Venezuela in 1950, for example.

accountability and conformity. The *Comisión* meets annually and more frequently if an emergency arises (as it did in 2001). This partnership between the public and private sectors was extremely successful in Colombia in 1985, when a new type of FMD virus appeared in the Sabana de Bogota, in central Colombia. This particular virus appears to have been extinguished from circulation. In Argentina, this partnership extended this model to the rural communities and livestock associations, with the involvement of schools, churches, universities and police, which rapidly led to the countries' recognition of freedom with vaccination in the late 1990s.[11]

Some of the major contributions of Panaftosa in the field of FMD control are a better understanding of FMD epidemiology, persistent infections of cattle and buffalo, and vaccine use. Epidemiologists at Panaftosa devised a structure to correlate "*ecosistemas*" – virus ecological systems, land use, farming and husbandry practices, and cattle movement to identify primary endemic areas (i.e. virus maintenance areas), secondary endemic areas (areas of virus propagation) and epidemic areas (i.e. areas of explosive outbreaks). They showed that the most cost-effective and sustainable strategy for FMD control was that which targeted first the primary endemic ecosystem, which is highly correlated with a calf:cow ratio of 1. If disease is first brought under control in this ecosystem, it becomes relatively easy to achieve sustained control in the other zones and diminishes risk to elsewhere.

Panaftosa also provides regional reference diagnostic support and training, and independent vaccine evaluation for manufacturers (private or governmental). This last activity is highly relevant for FMD vaccine use elsewhere around the world, where such quality assurance is lacking. Today, major efforts by Panaftosa include country collaboration along adjoining borders and robust rural integration for animal health development.

Avian influenza – Asia, poultry, livelihoods and human health[12]

Official reports to FAO, OIE and WHO suggested that avian influenza, more commonly know as bird flu, started to assume epidemic proportions towards the end of the year 2003. However, recent, retrospective analysis suggests that in most countries the disease may have been around for many more months. This would signify that a major veterinary public and animal health problem and a socio-economic disaster of subcontinental scale unfolded itself before causing any widespread alarm. This in turn illustrates that the current avian influenza crisis is not just an emergency but also a symptom, reflecting major institutional and policy-level deficiencies that also need addressing.

The FAO/OIE/WHO Technical Consultation on the Control of Avian Influenza, held 3–4 February 2004, concluded that the current epidemic is evolving and is anticipated to continue to expand both in geographic distribution and incidence. Given that the virus circulation in the region is not considered to be under control, there is need for a concerted emergency response. Without the implementation of appropriate methods of disease control, the risk of epidemic spread to further countries, including those in distant regions, is likely to remain high, and the disease may persist as a result of infection becoming endemic in the domestic poultry population. There will be a continuing threat to human health as long as the infection is present in the poultry production systems in Asia.

As an emergency measure, the above scientific panel recommended that control programmes be immediately intensified and monitored, and that public education

[11] In 2001, shortly after receiving declaration of freedom without vaccination from the OIE, Argentina was infected by FMD virus type A after the movement of animals from a neighbouring country. Interestingly, it was the private sector that demanded immediate action although they would be adversely affected as to the loss of their privileged status.

[12] Selected and updated text from "Halting the spread of avian influenza in Asia and promoting recovery" by FAO and OIE (original February 2004).

in veterinary training and national and regional capacity building, particularly for veterinary services, is an important part of the development of long-term surveillance and the control of highly pathogenic avian influenza (HPAI) and other priority diseases. National avian influenza task forces require major strengthening and improved surveillance. Transparent and timely reporting of infection to the OIE by the veterinary administration is required at the national, regional and international levels. Extensive international coordination should be established for short and long-term control of influenza viruses of human and animal health significance.

Preventing a similar emergency in the future makes it necessary to reflect on the factors in the Asian poultry subsectors that led to this problem. Of paramount importance is the human health risk posed by HPAI flare-ups and the threat emanating from the combination of wild bird reservoirs, backyard poultry and rapid intensification and industrialization. The meeting highlighted that the current spread of HPAI virus may be viewed as a consequence of failure of surveillance networks, early warning implementation, and control of movement of infection between domestic poultry. The HPAI crisis also serves to indicate the need for a veterinary surveillance framework for early warning of disease risk at the regional level, which should serve the needs of the agricultural and medical communities of the region and the wider international community. Regional networks for epidemiological surveillance, typing of influenza and other infectious pathogens, vaccine banks and contingency stocks of vaccines complying with OIE standards may all be necessary for timely national and international early warning and effective action. Novel approaches and thinking will almost certainly be required.

Rehabilitation and restructuring of the subsector should duly reflect the importance of the smallholder and the semicommercial sector. A sizeable segment of the poultry population remains within this sector. An estimated total of 200 million farmers, mostly keeping somewhere between 10 to 100 birds including chicken, ducks, geese, turkeys and quail, constitutes a vitally important contribution to the food and income security of the rural sector. FAO is especially concerned with the loss of livelihood for the proportion of dependent poor in the affected region. Not only poultry producers but also traders, processors, marketers and food vendors, as well as persons employed in the poultry sector, are at risk of losing their livelihood. Recovery of export capabilities for regional and international market access in compliance with OIE standards of the *Terrestrial Animal Health Code* is also crucial for the rural economy of some countries of the region.

While the present document seeks to categorize the support required today (Emergency Response), tomorrow (Emergency Prevention) and beyond (Rehabilitation and Restructuring), none of these components should be viewed in isolation. On the contrary, without integrating the immediate, medium and long-range responses required, there will be no effective containment of the current emergency.

The FAO Technical Cooperation Programme (TCP) has allocated US$5.5 million to assist countries in Asia with emergency/short-term support. Within this budget, US$2.7 million was approved by mid-February 2004 for one regional TCP covering Southeast Asia and six national TCPs (China, Pakistan, Viet Nam, Cambodia, Laos and Indonesia). At the time of this writing, September 2004, all six national TCPs are far in implementation and three subregional TCPs are underway, with two additional ones approved, with launching planned in the next four to six weeks (all regional TCPs cover 21 countries of the Region. See Table 1). Such TCP-mobilization for an animal health crisis was unprecedented in scope and nature. Some of these funds, however, have been used for advocacy channels to seek additional donor input successfully for countries or regional interventions. The emergency response cannot be viewed in isolation from the longer-term rehabilitation of the poultry sector, including supportive veterinary administrations and animal health services both in the public and private sectors.

TABLE 1
Regional support units identified for the avian influenza emergency.

East Asia	PR China, Japan, North Korea, South Korea, Taiwan Province of China
Southeast Asia/Oceania	Cambodia, Laos, Viet Nam, Thailand, Myanmar, Indonesia, Malaysia, Philippines, East Timor, Papua New Guinea
South Asia	India, Bangladesh, Sri Lanka, Nepal, Bhutan, Pakistan

The strategy decisions require early identification of the desired health status by production system, a timetable to achieve this, and surveillance systems and criteria required to permit re-opening of export markets in compliance with international standards. The inputs required for individual countries depend also on the level of risk of reintroduction of infection from sectors or regions that have not controlled or eliminated reservoirs of infection (and perhaps may never). For the moment, the situation in most of the Asia Region is far from clear, and the problem in some countries is still evolving.

In order to bring the diseases back in check, the affected countries are currently engaged in a number of the following disease emergency measures:

- establishment of central command structure;
- coordination by national disease emergency control centers in veterinary administrations;
- information, reporting and communication units;
- mapping and epidemio-surveillance office;
- establishment and running of local disease control centers;
- logistical support, administration and planning;
- training and capacity building;
- consultative technical committee and inter-ministerial representation;
- use of personal protection equipment and general safety precautions;
- in-field and laboratories: surveillance and diagnostics, particularly for any suspected outbreaks; tracing contacts; sampling; laboratory support for confirmation; and assisted delivery to OIE/FAO reference laboratories;
- design and carrying out of enhanced border inspection, quarantine measures, marketing control, movement restrictions and strategic stand-still for live animal transportation;
- stamping out or culling of the affected, suspected and (high) risk units using internationally recognized methods of killing;
- disposal of birds and contaminated materials, including products;
- cleaning out and disinfection of premises;
- implementation of targeted vaccination in compliance with international requirements;
- post-outbreak surveillance to monitor infection status;
- communication with stakeholders;
- compensation to farmers; and
- monitoring and resourcing of the entire control operation.

In terms of financial resources, the operations in the field are the most costly. The killing and disposal of birds demand large numbers of staff and involve high running costs for transport, earth moving equipment and various supplies. Round-the-clock deployment of staff resources is sometimes necessary in local and national centers. Considerable financial resources go to the compensation of the affected farmers.

On the basis of all the above considerations and taking into account the variable size of the country epidemics, a conservative estimate is possible. Preliminary figures suggest that the total campaign costs may amount to several million US dollars for each of the least affected countries and up to tens of millions of US dollars for the more seriously affected countries. However, the total costs for the control operations may continue to go up in the case of a prolonged campaign necessitated by the persistence of disease flare-ups in areas that were believed to have been freed from infection. This now brings the expenditure for the control of the avian influenza epidemic across the Asia Region, excluding China, to over US$250 million.

It is anticipated that more details on the total cost of the control of the disease; its economic impact; and the requirements for rehabilitation, restructuring and restocking will become available in the coming months. With more accurate information being collated, analyzed and synthesized, it also becomes more realistic to optimize control strategies in economic terms and base different scenarios on detailed and rigorous economic analysis.

Given the current deficiencies in disease reporting, there is an urgent need to enhance early and adequate risk assessment for use within the regions and to provide a wider warning to the international community.

The FAO/OIE proposal for strengthened surveillance and control of epizootic animal diseases – through support of disease surveillance units – is expected to operate at the regional level, placing emphasis on disease risk assessment and communication within each region. Through embedding epidemiologic expertise in regional specialized organizations whose mandate is to serve member states as well as to provide essential information for early detection of changing risk, benefits go to and ownership is with the countries in each region. Clearly, the avian influenza situation highlights the need for such a regionally focussed programme.

On a regional basis and under the guidance of the GF-TADs OIE/FAO steering committee, three Regional Support Units (RSU) (in East, South East and South Asia) have been identified to support regional needs on a range of animal diseases, working with and in support of the Association of Southeast Asian Nations (ASEAN); the Southeast Asia FMD, Animal Production and Health Commission of Asia and the Pacific; and the South Asian Association for Regional Cooperation (SAARC). The principal activities of the RSU are (in relation with national veterinary services) to:

- conduct needs assessments in epidemiology units and laboratories, assess gaps in legislation and compliance with trade regulations, and organize capacity building in priority subjects;
- advise and support national priority activities identified in the GF-TADs and assist in the preparation of bankable projects in the region to address priority requirements;
- assist in activities for disease surveillance and national and international reporting;
- report and liaise with Regional Specialised Organisations, regional FAO and OIE offices and Commissions, and the GF-TADs Secretariat; and
- arrange and participate in national and regional workshops.

Regional network for laboratory support

Networking of veterinary laboratories within regions, with support from international specialist (reference) laboratories has been of proven value in raising capacity and preparedness for diagnostic activities, and especially in introducing and establishing quality assurance. A support project for laboratories in the South, East and Southeast Asian region could play a very important role to network laboratories to raise cooperation within the region, with training and technical support from FAO/OIE Reference Laboratories (e.g. Weybridge, United Kingdom and Geelong, Australia). In addition to capacity building (e.g. to comply with OIE guidelines), quality control of laboratories and inter-laboratory proficiency testing will be promoted. Contract arrangement with OIE/FAO World and Regional Reference Laboratories should support authoritative diagnosis of epidemiologically important outbreaks, characterization and analysis of the genetic and antigenic make up of causal agents, and expert input into monitoring of regional and global trends in avian influenza circulation.

PARADIGM SHIFTS

It may appear as an insurmountable task: *the Global Control and Eradication of FMD*. However, understanding of where, how and when infections occur is key in defining strategies of intervention. Although the experience of the remarkable successes against rinderpest for some 50 years was based on widespread vaccinations with a vaccine unsurpassed in medicine that conferred life-long immunity (with concurrent circulation of a immunologic similar virus, *peste des petits ruminants*), today the strategy is on halting vaccination to identify areas of specific virus maintenance, and then targeting the specific population at risk with intensive vaccination with the object of immunosterilizing susceptible animals and banishing the virus from the particular ecosystem. Discovering where agents of disease are maintained is not an easy task and requires the participation of many sectors of society, perhaps the most important being at the local village level, and as such, participatory epidemiological approaches and the use of community animal health groups become essential. In contrast, FMD has several serotypes and the current vaccine does not confer long protection. But FMD viruses share with rinderpest virus, as with other disease-causing pathogens, primary endemic areas where the virus is maintained. The shift in strategy against FMD would be better served if FMD were thought of not as caused by one virus but by seven different viruses, with a plethora of variants, each of which can cause a similar clinical disease, but each with distinctive epidemiological parameters and varied biochemistry. It is then that we can begin to appreciate FMD dynamics and design strategies to tackle subtype to subtype, occurrence to occurrences in the field, and understand the behaviour of the virus within a particular ecosystem. Such focussed campaigns would become more rational and logistical, as well as scientific, than they are today. Likewise, the lessons learnt from the experience with rinderpest, which is approaching extinction, and international efforts required to maintain interest and momentum for active surveillance and verifiable freedom from disease and infection are most valuable. Thorough epidemiological understanding of host, environment and agent are to be applied – against FMD, rinderpest and other TADs.

Vaccines are tools that assist in protecting hosts from disease but may not eliminate infection. Intelligent use of these tools (i.e. targeted vaccination, information systems, animal movement management) is not widely applied. In the case of FMD where multivalent vaccines are applied, success may be better achieved with one serotype over another, or vaccines should be better tailored to select master seed vaccine strains that better protect against circulating strains. Cooperation and designing identical strategies across borders are essential in the attempt to decrease the load of agent circulation. With the exception of South America and perhaps part of Southeast Asia, this unification of strategies against FMD is not common. The Hemispheric Plan for the control of classical swine

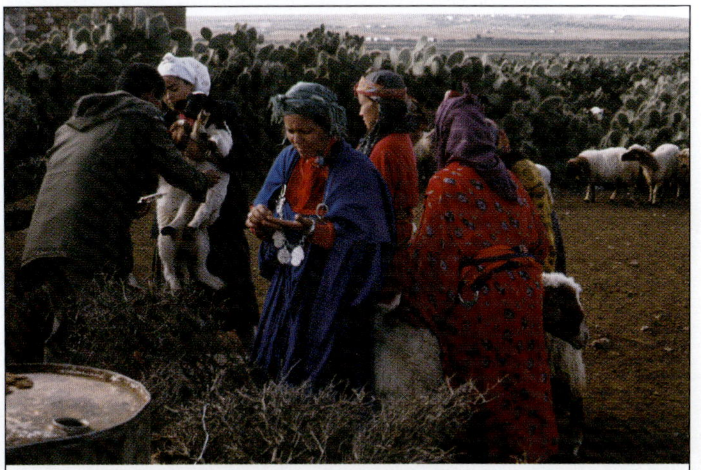

JUAN LUBROTH

Vaccination campaigns for the control of transboundary animal diseases, such as FMD, need to be coordinated at the central, regional and local level. Quality vaccines need to be approved by governments

fever addresses this issue, but it is the responsibility of the national programmes to implement such plans with realistic strategies, with membership of the public and private sectors and follow through using self-realized performance indicators.

To diminish the risk to the areas where a transboundary animal disease (or other) does not occur, engagement with countries and regional associations to assess out the environments where they do exist is essential, as proposed in the GF-TADs initiative. Paramount to the success of GF-TADs is the identification of primary endemic regions (i.e. hot zones). EMPRES and the GF-TADs initiative propose to address these issues to the interested investors.

CONCLUSIONS

This seminar on the emergency preparedness of transboundary animal disease in aquaculture, and fisheries in general, should ask: (1) *What can be done to reduce the vulnerability of individual countries* (vis-à-vis *risk analysis and threat mitigation)?*, (2) *What can be done to streamline resumption of trade after an occurrence of disease (recovery and rehabilitation)? and* (3) *What can be done to enhance the capacity of a developing country's trading partners in meeting SPS (sanitary and phytosanitary) requirements*?

From the perspective of transboundary animal diseases as dealt with by EMPRES, the reduction of the vulnerability of countries to disease exposure relies on their participation in ongoing regional and international efforts to curb disease incidence where such agents are known to occur naturally; on supporting efforts to identify ecological zones that are the origin of infection or where new pathogen subtypes emerge; and on undertaking prevention measures by applying risk mitigation, including networking with close and distant partners in an agreed development agenda. This latter point is essential, as it creates an understanding of risk assessment, risk management and risk communication among all involved. Thus it is to better to consider that a neighbour's situation (i.e. an incipient animal health problem) should be of concern to the region as a whole, and stimulate the preparation of contingency plans at that level prior to an emergency situation.

Among the tools required are: (1) good communication links between the field (production areas), the diagnostic and research laboratories, and the central command structures; (2) rapid and accurate diagnostic methods with epidemiologically sound response; and (3) efficacious and safe prophylactic or treatment options that can be deployed under emergency operations or programmed in progressive control campaigns.

The resumption of trade after the occurrence of a disease such as FMD, rinderpest, contagious bovine pleuropneumonia, highly pathogenic avian influenza or bovine spongiform encephalopathy, to name a few important livestock diseases,[13] would require a robust veterinary service with the necessary institutional framework to demonstrate all activities carried out in the field, the laboratory and abattoirs on the progressive control, and passive and active surveillance leading to the absence of the condition. These methods should be scientifically based and stand up to internal and external auditing. FAO has on several occasions provided assistance and inputs to strengthen such activities (notably, in the cases of rinderpest in Africa and Asia, bovine spongiform encephalopathy surveillance in South America, and the current avian influenza crisis in Asia). The OIE is the standard-setting body in its guidelines for trade in animals and commodities of animal origin (aquaculture is handled in a parallel manner but separate from terrestrial animals). Yet, trade is a relationship between

[13] The OIE only has specific declarations for freedom for the four mentioned diseases. Bovine spongiform encephalopathy is not considered a transboundary animal disease, as it is not explosive or highly contagious.

two consenting countries or partners and independent of OIE guidelines; but as an increasing number of countries become signatories to the World Trade Organization (and are members of the OIE), they should observe OIE guidelines and standards in their trade relationships, thus providing necessary transparency and expediency of action.

Enhancing the capacity of a developing country to meet international sanitary and phytosanitary requirements relies on investment in training in all aspects of administration, governance, regulation and legislation, technology, information and documentation. It should be based on equitable systems providing a level playing field (i.e. subsidies to agriculture in the developed world) and enhanced in a realistic, practical manner that allows the country to have the necessary depth with succession planning in human resources and self-assessed performance indicators. Capacity building is not a single occasion event; inputs are needed more often than is appreciated. Again, the OIE, FAO and numerous private consultancies are able to provide such guidance.

The priority within FAO is sustainable agriculture and rural development. The Global Framework for the Progressive Control of Transboundary Animal Diseases represents the collaboration of the two lead international institutions to curb the crippling effect of selected epidemic animal diseases on livestock production and trade. Under GF-TADs, developed countries would decrease the risk of introduction by reducing incidence in endemically affected areas. Developing countries, where these diseases are most often reported, would benefit from the Global Framework as the effort to strengthen veterinary services, build the necessary institutions and foment public/private partnership, which should lead to development of healthy animal production and allow rural economies to participate better in formal trade, whether local, regional or international.

ADDITIONAL RESOURCE INFORMATION

- FAO/WHO *Codex Alimetarius* (www.fao.org/docrep/w9114e/W9114e01.htm)
- EMPRES - Emergency Prevention System – Livestock Component (new URL coming soon) (www.fao.org/ag/AGA/AGAH/EMPRES/index.asp)
- FAO/IAEA Joint Division (www.iaea.org/programmes/nafa/d3/index.html)
- *FAO and Food Safety* – "Protecting the food chain" article in AG21 www.fao.org/ag/magazine
- World Health Organization (www.who.int)
- Office International des Épizooties www.oie.int)
- Pan African Programme for the Control of Epizootics (i.e. Uganda) (www.deluga.cec.eu.int/en/eu_and_uganda/pace.htm)
- Centro Panamericano para la Fiebre Aftosa (www.panaftosa.org.br/novo)

ACKNOWLEDGEMENTS

The authors are indebted to Samuel Jutzi, Director, Animal Production and Health Division, Joseph Domenech and Yves Cheneau, current and previous Chiefs of the FAO Animal Health Service, and Mark Rweyemamu (Tanzania) and Roger Paskin (Namibia) for their unwavering commitment, fine insight, commentary and development of the EMPRES-Livestock programme.

Experiences in dealing with aquatic animal disease emergencies in Asia

Rohana P. Subasinghe
Fishery Resources Division
Fisheries Department
Food and Agriculture Organization of the United Nations
Viale delle Terme di Caracalla
00100 Rome, Italy
E-mail: Rohana.Subasinghe@fao.org

Subasinghe, R.P. 2005. Experiences in dealing with aquatic animal disease emergencies in Asia. p. 67–72. In: Subasinghe, R.P.; Arthur, J.R. (eds.). Regional workshop on preparedness and response to aquatic animal health emergencies in Asia. Jakarta, Indonesia, 21–23 September 2004. *FAO Fisheries Proceedings*. No. 4. Rome, FAO. 2005. 178p.

ABSTRACT

This paper presents a brief introduction to the disease problems facing aquaculture in Asia and some current efforts to deal with epizootics caused by transboundary aquatic animal diseases (TAADs).

INTRODUCTION

Aquaculture is the fastest growing food-producing sector in the world. A great proportion (over 90 percent) of this production comes from the developing world. In contrast to terrestrial farming systems, where the bulk of global production is based on a limited number of animal and plant species, the aquaculture sector comprises of over 230 different species. This large number of species cultivated reflects the diversity of the sector, particularly the wide variety of candidate species cultivated and the different production systems used. According to the latest Food and Agriculture of the United Nations (FAO) statistics, the contribution of aquaculture to global supplies of fish, crustaceans and molluscs continues to grow, increasing from 3.9 percent of total production by weight in 1970 to 29.9 percent in 2002. Aquaculture continues to grow more rapidly than all other animal food-producing sectors. Worldwide, the sector has grown at an average rate of 8.9 percent per year since 1970, compared with only 1.2 percent for capture fisheries and 2.8 percent for terrestrial farmed meat production systems over the same period. Production from aquaculture has greatly outpaced population growth, with per capita supply from aquaculture increasing from 0.7 kg in 1970 to 6.4 kg in 2002, an average annual growth rate of 7.2 percent.

In 2002, total world aquaculture production (including aquatic plants) was reported to be 51.4 million tonnes by volume and US$60.0 billion by value. This represents an annual increase of 6.1 percent in volume and 2.9 percent in value, respectively, over reported figures for 2000. In 2002, countries in Asia accounted for 91.2 percent of the production and 82.0 percent of the value. Of the world total, the People's Republic of China produced 71.2 percent of the total volume and 54.7 percent of the total value of

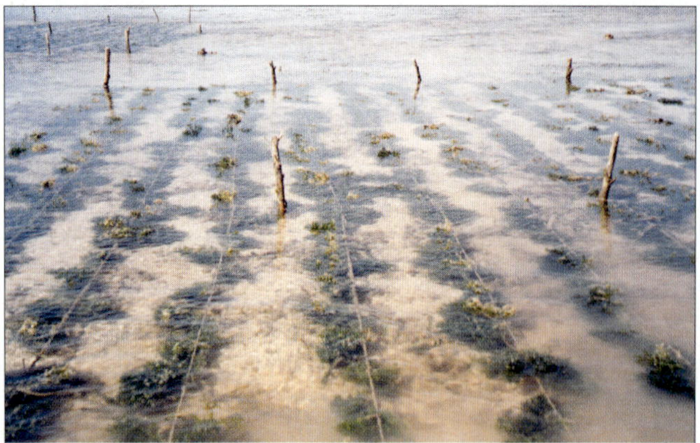

Cultured Kappaphycus alvarezii *in fixed, off-bottom lines in Batangas, Philippines*

M.G. BONDAD-REANTASO

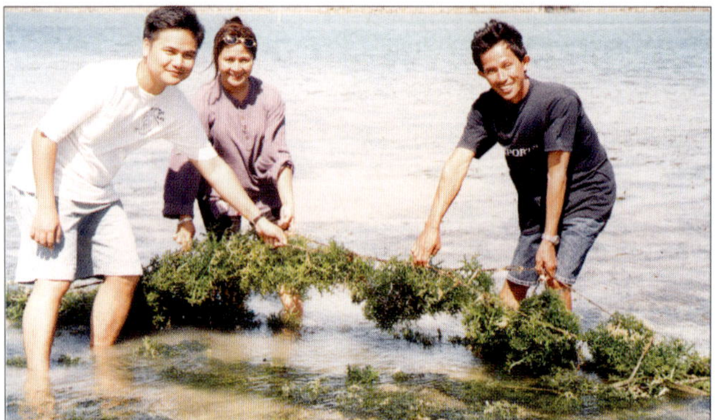

Seaweed farming (aquatic plant) in Batangas Province, Philippines

M.G. BONDAD-REANTASO

aquaculture production. The majority of aquaculture production of fish, crustaceans and molluscs continues to come from the freshwater environment (57.7 percent by volume and 48.4 percent by value). Mariculture contributes 36.5 percent of production and 35.7 percent of the total value. Although brackishwater production represented only 5.8 percent of production volume in 2002, it contributed 15.9 percent of the total value, reflecting the prominence of high-value crustaceans and finfish.

FISH AS NUTRITIOUS FOOD

Fish is an important part of the diet for a large proportion of the people living in the developing world. Many types and forms of fish and aquatic products are available at affordable prices in developing countries. Economic affordability is a key factor as to why aquaculture is making an essential contribution to human health in the developing world. More "foodfish" is consumed globally on a per capita basis than any other type of meat or animal protein. The main reason for the high demand for staple foodfish within most developing countries is its greater affordability to the poorer segments of the community. At present, foodfish represents the primary source of animal protein (contributing more than 25 percent of the total animal protein supply) for about one billion people within 58 countries worldwide, including many developing countries and low-income food-deficit countries (LIFDCs) (value excludes China).

Fish are important sources for many nutrients, including protein of very high quality, retinol (vitamin A), vitamin D, vitamin E, iodine and selenium. Evidence is increasing that the consumption of fish enhances brain development and learning in children, protects vision and eye health, and offers protection from cardiovascular disease and some cancers. The fats and fatty acids in fish, particularly the long-chain n-3 fatty acids (n-3 PUFA), are highly beneficial and difficult to obtain from other food sources.

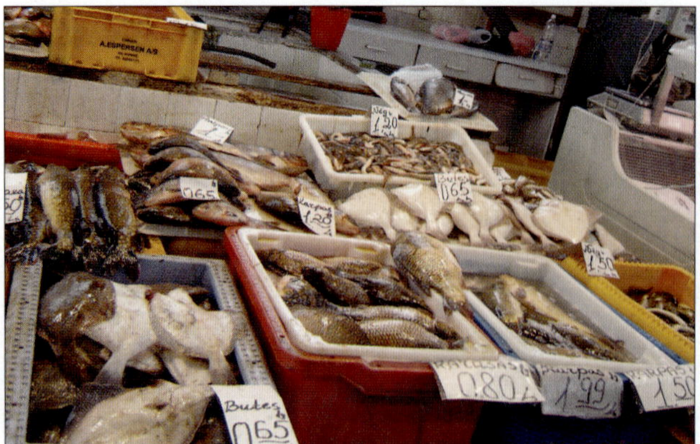

Various species of aquacultured fresh and marine food fish sold in a wet market in Riga, Latvia

M.G. BONDAD-REANTASO

DISEASES AND HEALTH AS A CONSTRAINT TO AQUACULTURE PRODUCTION

Although aquaculture is the fastest growing food-production sector in the world, diseases are a primary constraint to the growth of the aquaculture sector in many parts of the world. A multitude of factors has contributed to the health problems currently faced by aquaculture. Over the past three decades, aquaculture has expanded, intensified and diversified, based heavily on movements of live aquatic animals and their products (broodstock, seed and feed). This trend has been triggered by changing circumstances and perspectives, especially the liberalization of world trade. New outlooks and directions have accelerated the accidental spread of diseases into new populations and geographic regions, for example, through movements of hatchery-produced stocks and new species for culture, enhancement and development of the ornamental fish trade.

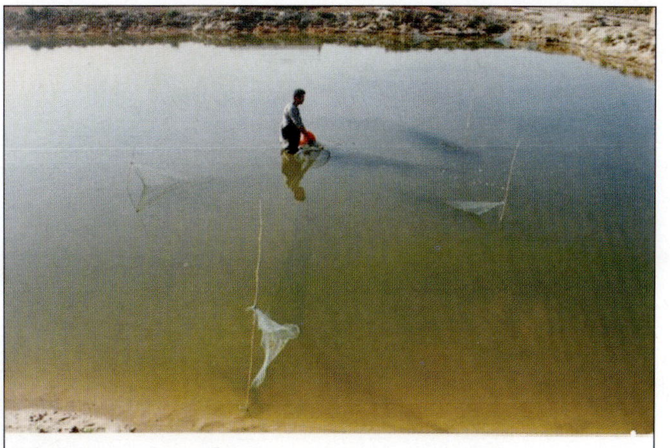

Shrimp pond in China

There is now convincing evidence of the serious socio-economic, environmental and international trade consequences arising from transboundary aquatic animal diseases (TAADs). These impacts occur on top of the routine needs of managing the opportunistic disease challenges mentioned in the Introduction. Bearing this in mind, and taking Asia-Pacific as an example of a region highly dependent upon aquaculture production and capture fisheries, we need to look at exactly what these impacts are.

Although translocation of pathogens and diseases with movements of their hosts is by no means a new phenomenon, it has only recently gained focussed attention in many regions. Advances in live aquatic animal trade, facilitated by improved transportation efficiency, are now recognized as having played a pivotal role in the introduction and spread of pathogens and diseases into many aquaculture systems. There is now convincing evidence of the serious socio-economic, environmental and international trade consequences arising from transboundary aquatic animal diseases. For instance, combined losses from shrimp diseases at the global level from 11 countries for the period 1987 to 1994 were estimated at US$3 019 million. More recent examples of major losses due to the spread of aquatic animal diseases include that of carp mortalities (losses estimated at 50 billion Indonesian rupiah, approximately US$5.5 million) in Indonesia; Koi herpes virus (KHV) (losses estimated at 150 million yen, approximately US$1.4 million) in Japan; and abalone mortalities (losses estimated at 400 million TWD, approximately US$11.4 million) in Taiwan, Province of China.

In addition to the obvious effects of large-scale aquaculture losses on rural communities, diseases also cause considerable financial impact on investor confidence. These losses are even more alarming where the success or failure of a harvest will determine the raising of families above or below the United Nations (UN) poverty threshold. In southern Viet Nam, approximately 1 200 families dependent on rice-shrimp culture have experienced annual losses of more than US$300 000 due to shrimp diseases. Between 1995 and 1997, the "red spot disease" of grass carp affected 4 000 of 5 000 cages in operation, with losses estimated at US$0.5 million. Such losses in these situations directly threaten the livelihoods of the communities they occur in through reduced food availability and loss of income and employment, as well as other associated social consequences.

Besides recent outbreaks of Taura syndrome virus (TSV) and KHV, which will be dealt with in detail in other presentations, some other examples of transboundary aquatic animal diseases in the Asia-Pacific and their impacts are briefly discussed below:

Epizootic ulcerative syndrome (EUS)

This serious epizootic, first reported in Japan as mycotic granulomatosis (MG) of freshwater ayu (*Plectoglossus altivelis*) in 1971 and observed in eastern Australia in 1972, is now reported to occur in most Southeast and South Asian countries, affecting

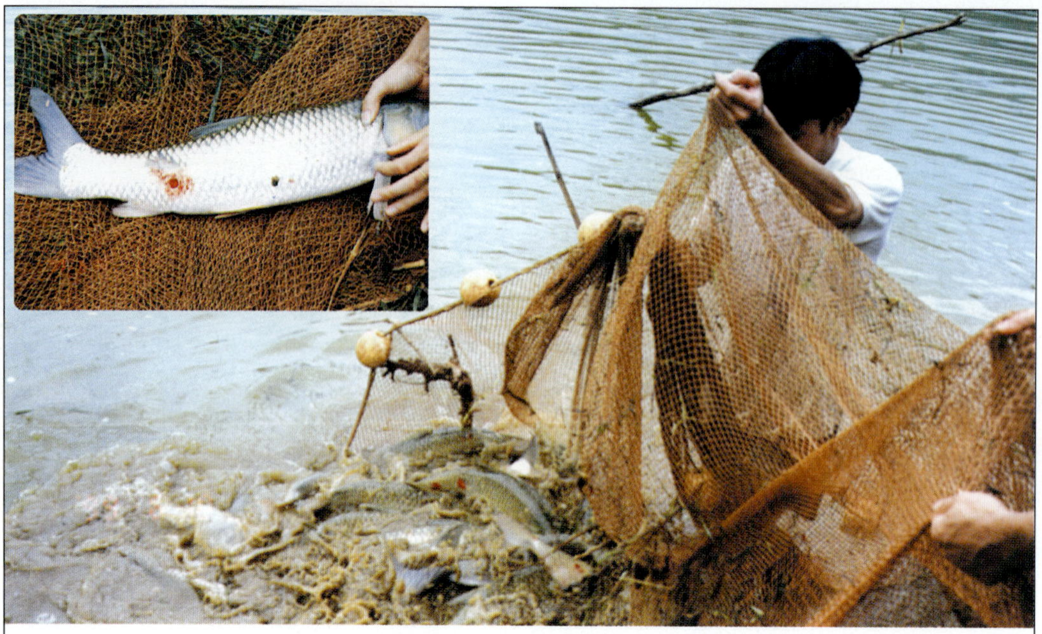

M.G. BONDAD-REANTASO

Red spot disease of grass carp in Viet Nam

over 100 species of wild and cultured fresh and to a lesser extent brackishwater fish. The primary causative agent of this disease has been confirmed as a fungus of the genus *Aphanomyces*. Combined losses from EUS in several Asian countries before 1990 were more than US$10 million; losses in Thailand alone from 1983–1993 were US$100 million. EUS continues to expand its range, the latest extension being into the rivers of the Indus in the Punjab of Pakistan. Outbreaks of ulcerative disease in *Brevoortia tyrannus* in the United States are very similar to EUS in Asia.

White spot syndrome virus (WSSV)

First reported in Taiwan Province of China and PR China between 1991-1992, then in Japan in 1993 from shrimp imported from China, this major viral disease of shrimp is now affecting almost all shrimp-producing countries in Asia and the Americas. WSSV has been officially reported from 10 countries in the Asia-Pacific Region including Bangladesh, PR China., Republic of Korea, India, Indonesia, Malaysia, Philippines, Sri Lanka, Thailand and Viet Nam. As of 1999, WSSV has also been officially confirmed in at least nine countries in the Americas: Columbia, Ecuador, Guatemala, Honduras, Mexico, Nicaragua, Panama, Peru and the United States. Losses were in the range of more than US$400 million in China in 1993, US$17.6 million in India in 1994, US$600 million in 1997 in Thailand, and to a global estimate of US$3 000 million.

Viral encephalopathy and retinopathy (VER)

Among many other viral diseases, VER causes serious problems to grouper culture in the Asia-Pacific. VER was first reported in Japan in 1991 and has since been reported in Indonesia, Republic of Korea, Singapore and Thailand. The expanding trend in grouper aquaculture and related trade, without appropriate health management, increases the risk of introducing the pathogen into new localities and environments.

Neobenedenia girellae

One of the most commonly reported monogenean parasites of grouper and other marine fishes, this parasite was introduced to Japan along with importation of amberjack fry from Hainan, China and China, Hong Kong Special Administrative

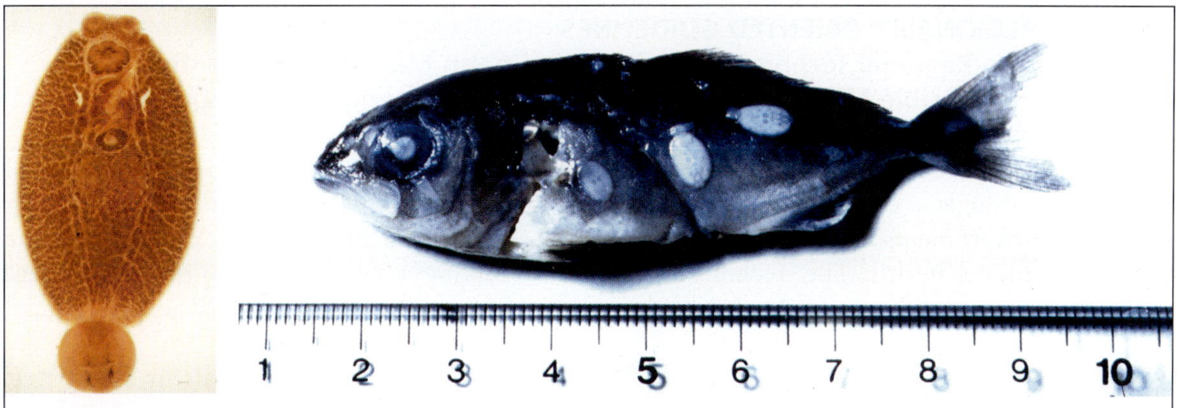

K. OGAWA

Right: Amberjack fry (Seriola dumerili) *infected with adult* Neobenedenia girellae, *on the day of arrival in Japan from China. Left: Stained whole mount of* Neobenedenia girellae.

Region. This parasite caused heavy infection and mortalities among flounder cultured in floating netcages in 1991 and of one-year-old amberjack in 1992 in Japan, where a total of 15 cultured marine fishes (e.g. groupers and flounders) and brackishwater cultured tilapia are susceptible. *Neobenedenia girellae* now causes serious problems in grouper culture in most countries of Southeast Asia.

Control measures

Measures to combat diseases of fish and shellfish have only recently assumed a high priority in many aquaculture-producing regions of the world. Development of such measures was stimulated by the serious socio-economic losses and environmental impacts caused by aquatic animal diseases, as well as by threats to food security and the livelihoods of vulnerable sectors of society. Many countries have improved their laboratory facilities, diagnostic expertise, control protocols and therapeutic strategies in order to better handle disease outbreaks. In addition, many farmers, especially in developed countries, have improved their capacity to respond quickly and effectively to emergent disease situations. They have also greatly enhanced their disease prevention awareness. Similar efforts towards strengthening aquatic animal health capacities in many developing countries are also being actively pursued, although the capabilities of many countries are still marginal.

INTERNATIONAL CODES

A number of international codes of practice, agreements and technical guidelines exist and are aimed, at least in part, at providing a degree of standardization for the protocols used to minimize the risks of disease associated with movements of aquatic animals.

These include:

- the World Organisation for Animal Health (OIE) Aquatic Animal Health Code and Manual of Diagnostic Tests for Aquatic Animals;
- the International Council for the Exploration of the Sea (ICES) Code of Practice on the Introductions and Transfers of Marine Organisms;
- the European Inland Fishery Advisory Council (EIFAC) Codes of Practice and Manual of Procedures for Consideration of Introductions and Transfers of Marine and Freshwater Organisms;
- the FAO's Code of Conduct for Responsible Fisheries (CCRF);
- the Convention on Biological Diversity; and
- the World Trade Organization's (WTO) Sanitary and Phytosanitary (SPS) Agreement.

REGIONALLY ORIENTED GUIDELINES

Asia Regional Technical Guidelines on Health Management for the Responsible Movement of Live Aquatic Animals and the Beijing Consensus and Implementation Strategy

The "Technical Guidelines" were based on a set of guiding principles developed through a consultative process that involved representatives from 21 participating governments and technical assistance from regional and international experts on aquatic animal health. The Technical Guidelines describe a number of health management considerations aimed at minimizing the risk of disease spread via aquatic animal movements and were developed to:

- assist countries in the Asia-Pacific to move live aquatic animals in a way that minimizes the disease risks associated with pathogen transfer and disease spread, both within and across boundaries;
- enhance protection of the aquatic environment and biodiversity, as well as the interests of aquaculture and capture fisheries;
- provide a mechanism to facilitate trade in live aquatic species and avoid unjustifiable trade barriers based on aquatic animal health issues; and
- implement relevant provisions of FAO's CCRF and other international treaties and agreements (e.g. WTO's SPS agreement) applicable to the Asian Region.

The development of the Technical Guidelines took into account the different socio-economic and environmental circumstances of the participating countries in the Asia-Pacific Region, the diversity of infrastructures (in terms of trained expertise and institutional capability), the wide range of aquatic species being moved, the different reasons for such movements and the diversity of pathogens currently known.

DISEASE EMERGENCIES

With all efforts in place, disease emergencies still occur. They either result from the movement of exotics or introduced species, from simple trade-related movements or from an outbreak of an existing disease. In all cases, preparedness appears to be inadequate and the response to control is thus slow.

The present workshop attempts to address this issue with the view to develop an Asia Regional Strategy to deal with disease emergencies in aquatic animals.

OIE Asia-Pacific's experience in dealing with livestock disease emergencies in the Asia-Pacific

Yoshiyuki Oketani
OIE Deputy Regional Representative for Asia and the Pacific
East 311, Shin Aoyama Building
1-1-1 Minami Aoyama
Minato-ku, Tokyo 107-0062, Japan
oietokyo@tky.3web.ne.jp

Oketani, Y. 2005. OIE Asia-Pacific's experience in dealing with livestock disease emergencies in the Asia-Pacific. p. 73–78. In: Subasinghe, R.P.; Arthur, J.R. (eds.). Regional workshop on preparedness and response to aquatic animal health emergencies in Asia. Jakarta, Indonesia, 21–23 September 2004. *FAO Fisheries Proceedings*. No. 4. Rome, FAO. 2005. 178p.

ABSTRACT

Since 1924, the World Organisation for Animal Health (OIE) has worked to promote world animal health. The Regional Representation for Asia and the Pacific (OIE Tokyo) has worked to help the Member Countries deal with animal health improvement, including disease emergencies. The OIE Tokyo's experiences of emergency measures against terrestrial animal diseases serve as a good reference in order to prepare for aquatic animal disease emergencies. Three infectious animal diseases, foot and mouth disease (FMD), bovine spongiform encephalopathy (BSE) and highly pathogenic avian influenza (HPAI), have recently become a serious problem in the Asian Region. The lesson learned from these emergencies is the necessity to fight against the disease itself and, at the same time, to protect the livestock industry from international trade disputes. To fight against serious infectious diseases, it is important to establish cooperation systems between veterinary administrations and related ministries, departments and local governments. The OIE calls on the fishery authorities to make steadfast linkages with veterinary administrations to deal with aquatic animal disease emergencies. To protect the livestock industry from international trade disputes, it is indispensable to recover the disease-free status in accordance with international standards. The OIE has played important roles for aquatic animal health as well. The OIE Aquatic Animal Health Standards Commission develops the Aquatic Animal Health Code in line with the terminology of the Sanitary and Phytosanitary Agreement (SPS Agreement) of the World Trade Organization (WTO) to assure sanitary safety and international trade in aquatic animals and their products.

INTRODUCTION

The World Organisation for Animal Health (Office International des Épizooties, OIE) is an intergovernmental organization established in Paris, France in 1924 in order to promote world animal health. Since then OIE has worked as an informative and normative organization for animal diseases.

At the General Agreement on Tariffs and Trade (GATT) Uruguay Round trade negotiations, it was concluded that OIE be approved as one of the international standards-setting organizations by the World Trade Organization (WTO). Now, the OIE standards are used as judgment criteria in the WTO dispute settlement procedures.

In 1991, the OIE General Session decided to create the OIE Regional Representation for Asia and the Pacific in Tokyo, Japan (OIE Tokyo), aiming at providing its Member Countries with services adapted to the regional characteristics and more especially, to help them strengthen, in a coordinated manner and through the setting up of regional programmes, the surveillance and control of major diseases. Since then the OIE Tokyo Office has worked for the Member Countries in dealing with animal health improvement, including disease emergencies in this region. Some experiences with the diseases are given below as examples.

FOOT AND MOUTH DISEASE (FMD)

FMD is a typical OIE List A disease. OIE List A means transmissible diseases that have the potential for very serious and rapid spread, irrespective of national borders, that are of serious socio-economic or public health consequence and that are of major importance in the international trade of animals and animal products.

Reports are submitted to the OIE as often as necessary to comply with the OIE Terrestrial Animal Health Code (OIE, 2004a). The veterinary administration of an OIE Member Country has to send notification by telegram, fax or e-mail, within 24 hours, of any of the suspected or confirmed first occurrences or reoccurrence of a List A disease, if the country or zone of the country was previously considered to be free from that particular disease.

The OIE has been publishing the "Disease Free Country Lists" for specific diseases, namely FMD, rinderpest, contagious bovine pleuropneumonia and bovine spongiform encephalopathy (BSE).

In 1997, the OIE received the official notification of FMD outbreaks from Taiwan Province of China (Taiwan POC). The OIE immediately sent alert messages to all Member Countries and deleted the name of Taiwan POC from the list of FMD-free countries or zones, which was published through the Internet.

As a result of this change in the list of FMD-free countries or zones, trade partner countries, including surrounding countries, took necessary quarantine measures, including the import ban on animals and animal products from Taiwan POC and disinfection of tourists' shoes at airports and seaports. Importing countries that took the import ban notified their measures to the WTO. Veterinary administrations also instructed their police and coast guard departments to check the smuggling of animals and animal products more strictly.

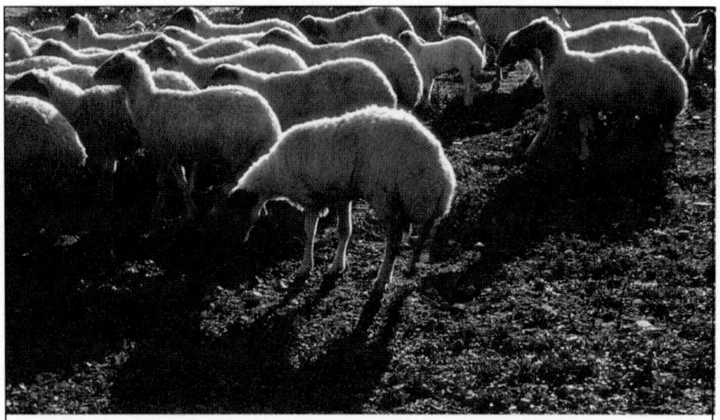

USDA

Lameness in small ruminants, such as sheep and goats, can be quite difficult to see in FMD

Throughout the history of FMD accidents in the world, there are many cases where the FMD virus was transferred by wind, and sometimes it invaded into neighboring countries beyond channels. In the case of FMD in Taiwan POC, an island country surrounded by the sea, it was not demonstrated that the virus was transferred by wind. As a precautionary measure, the Japanese Government decided to kill all the pigs being raised in its small islands located just like steppingstones between Japan and Taiwan POC.

Between 1998 and 1999, there were no significant changes in the FMD situation of this region. But in 2000, the OIE received official notifications of FMD outbreaks from Kazakhstan, the Republic of Korea, Japan and Mongolia. The disease had been absent in the Republic of Korea since 1934, while in Japan the previous FMD outbreak dated back to 1908. OIE dispatched alert messages to all Member Countries again and deleted the names of the Republic of Korea and Japan from the list of FMD-free countries.

In May 2000, OIE Headquarters and OIE Tokyo sent experts to the Republic of Korea to investigate the origin of the FMD outbreak and to advise the government on the control measures to be taken.

In April 2001, OIE and FAO held the joint International Scientific Conference on Foot and Mouth Disease in Paris.

In the cases of Taiwan POC, the Republic of Korea and Japan, veterinary administrations set up infected zones and protection zones surrounding infected farms, and supervised and restricted the movement of animals in cooperation with local police departments. At first these three countries adopted the stamping-out policy, and then Taiwan POC and the Republic of Korea secondly adopted emergency vaccination.

In general, stamping-out is carried out under the authority of the veterinary administration, on confirmation of a disease. It involves the killing of the animals that are affected and those suspected of being affected in the herd and, where appropriate, those in other herds that have been exposed to infection by direct animal to animal contact or indirect contact likely to cause the transmission of the causal pathogen. All susceptible animals on an infected premise should be killed and their carcasses destroyed by burning, burial or any other method that will eliminate the spread of infection through the carcasses or products of the animals killed.

In those countries, carcass disposal work was undertaken by veterinary administrations assisted by local government officers and sometimes by national army soldiers. However, it was very difficult to find appropriate places to bury carcasses, and veterinary administrations faced hard negotiations with mayors and governors.

The OIE strongly recommends that veterinary administrations exercise the simulation of disease prevention, including establishment of cooperation systems with other related ministries, departments and local governments, and the secured plan of carcass disposal.

When a country or a zone in the country was previously considered to be free from FMD, the Chief Veterinary Officer would, with necessary documents including results of monitoring and surveillance, apply to the OIE to declare freedom from the disease.

Japan began its effort to recover the FMD-free status. In September 2000, when more than three months had elapsed since the last case was observed, stamping out without vaccination had been implemented, and serological surveillance had detected no signs of existing FMD virus, Japan submitted its formal application for FMD-free status to the Director General of the OIE. Its application was evaluated by the OIE FMD and Other Epizootics Commission. By the end of the month, Japan regained its status as a FMD-free country.

In the Republic of Korea, stamping out was applied in the affected farms and farms in the vicinity. Given the severity of the clinical signs observed in cattle, emergency vaccination was applied to cattle in the protection zones around the outbreaks. As no other outbreaks occurred, the movement restrictions that had been imposed were lifted in May 2000. However, the emergency vaccination (given to nearly 600 000 animals in over 11 052 farms) delayed recovery of its disease-free status. Finally, in May 2004, the Republic of Korea regained its status as a FMD-free country.

Taiwan POC has to date not recovered disease-free status because of its nationwide vaccination practices.

For other FMD-infected countries in the region, the OIE carries out the South-East Asia FMD Control Campaign (so-called SEAFMD), which has been successfully progressing. SEAFMD aims at establishing the status of a FMD-free area to be accepted internationally, and the participating countries are using the OIE Code and Manual (OIE, 2004a, 2004b) as their guidelines.

The SEAFMD Campaign serves as a good model for the future establishment of the Global Framework for Progressive Control of Trans-boundary Animal Diseases (GF-TADs). The joint OIE/FAO initiative of the GF-TADs project will strongly assist Member Countries in establishing control programmes against specific animal diseases on a regional basis.

BOVINE SPONGIFORM ENCEPHALOPATHY (BSE)

BSE is considered as a kind of zoonosis (in human cases, it is known as variant Creutzfeld-Jakob disease) and classified as an OIE List B disease. OIE List B means transmissible diseases that are considered to be of socio-economic and/or public health importance within countries and that are significant in the international trade of animals and animal products. Reports are normally submitted to the OIE once a year, although more frequent reporting may in some cases be necessary to comply with the OIE Terrestrial Animal Health Code. So far, to meet the demand of Member Countries, the OIE decided to publish the "Disease Free Country List" for BSE.

In recent years, many Member Countries submitted formal applications for BSE-free status to the Director General of the OIE. These applications were evaluated by an ad hoc group of experts on BSE that had been set up, and also by the Scientific Commission. However, the conclusions did not come out easily, because the OIE cannot take responsibility for publication of a country's inaccurate disease status based on inaccurate information or change in epidemiological status or other significant events that were not promptly reported to the Central Bureau. After accurate and complete data were received, during the 72nd OIE General Session held in May 2004, the Director General established a list of BSE provisionally free countries or zones in accordance with the chapters of the Terrestrial Animal Health Code. The first list of provisionally free countries included Argentina, Uruguay, Iceland and Singapore.

In Asia and the Pacific, so far the OIE has received official notifications of BSE outbreaks only from Japan. In 2001, Japan reported three cases of BSE for the first time; two cases were reported in 2002 and one atypical BSE case in 2003.

In Japan, repeated reporting of BSE cases in various ways by mass media contributed to drastic reduction in consumption of not only domestically produced beef but also of imported beef. When a serious infectious disease occurs, sometimes various rumors circulate and unconfirmed reports are accepted as facts. Producers, government officials, policy-makers, exporters, importers, consumers etc. ask for official information provided by a responsible source.

The OIE Regional Representation for Asia and the Pacific based in Tokyo held the Consultation Meeting on BSE Public Awareness in Chiang Mai, Thailand in October 2003, in collaboration with the FAO-Animal Production and Health Commission for Asia and the Pacific (FAO-APHCA) and the Department of Livestock Development, Thailand (DLD). The Consultation Meeting drafted three different types of model information papers for public awareness. The pamphlet for policy-makers aims at facilitating legislation and funding of measures, that for veterinary services is aimed at understanding the basis for implementation of various BSE programmes, and that for consumers, at understanding what BSE is and what is safe. The model information papers will be modified and translated into local languages in the respective countries in the region, where appropriate.

OIE Tokyo has also held the Regional Workshop on BSE Diagnosis and Surveillance in collaboration with FAO-APHCA and DLD since 2001. The purpose of the Hands-on Training Workshop was to train laboratory staff from selected countries in Asia and the Pacific.

HIGHLY PATHOGENIC AVIAN INFLUENZA (HPAI)

HPAI is a typical zoonosis and classified as an OIE List A disease. Since the end of 2003, the OIE has received notifications of HPAI outbreaks from many Asian countries and areas.

In the Republic of Korea, HPAI virus subtype H5N1 was isolated from samples collected from broilers and ducks in December 2003.

In 2004, the OIE received official notifications of HPAI confirmation from Viet Nam, Japan, Taiwan POC, Thailand, Cambodia, Hong Kong Special Administrative Region and Laos in January, and from Indonesia and the People's Republic of China in February. Viet Nam reported outbreaks in three parent-stock farms for broilers that had started in December 2003. This was the first occurrence of HPAI reported in Viet Nam. Indonesia reported several outbreaks of HPAI initially confirmed in December 2003. The OIE immediately dispatched alert messages to all Member Countries.

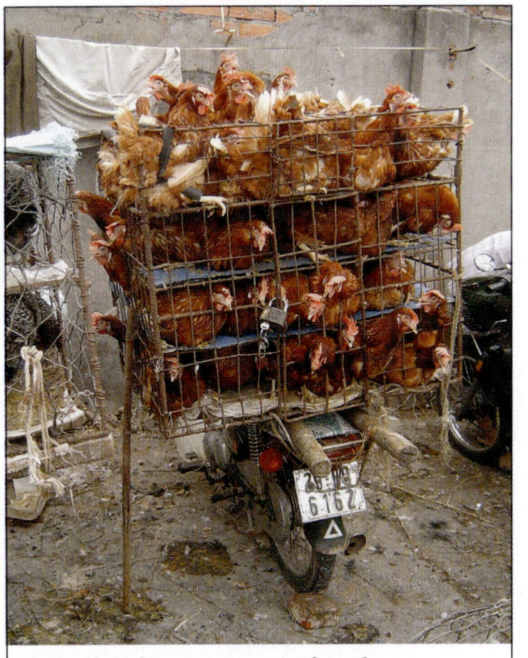

FAO

Control and management of poultry movement is key in the fight of transboundary animal diseases such as avian influenza

Before the OIE received official notifications from the governments of the Member Countries, various rumors had already circulated in the mass media. Therefore, people asked for official information provided by a responsible source as quickly as possible.

The OIE receives official disease notification with the signature of the Chief Veterinary Officer directly from a relevant Member Country. Furthermore, the OIE collects animal health information based on the active search policy. The information thus collected, including nonofficial information from scientific journals, local newspapers, TV news etc., is systematically evaluated before deciding whether to verify it with the Chief Veterinary Officer of the relevant Member Country.

OIE information is recognized and used as official information around the world. Therefore, during the avian influenza crisis, more than 40 000 people visited the OIE Web site during only one week. OIE information is commonly used as official information by the Food and Agriculture Organization of the United Nations (FAO) and the World Health Organization (WHO) in their Web sites

In February 2004, in Bangkok, OIE and FAO jointly organized the Emergency Regional Meeting on Avian Influenza Control in Animals in Asia in collaboration with WHO. The meeting discussed various areas and recommended important activities to be undertaken for short- and long-term disease control strategies, including networking of the countries and a future Global Framework for Progressive Control of Trans-boundary Animal Diseases (GF-TADs) project. HPAI will be selected as one of serious transboundary animal diseases to be targeted by GF-TADs.

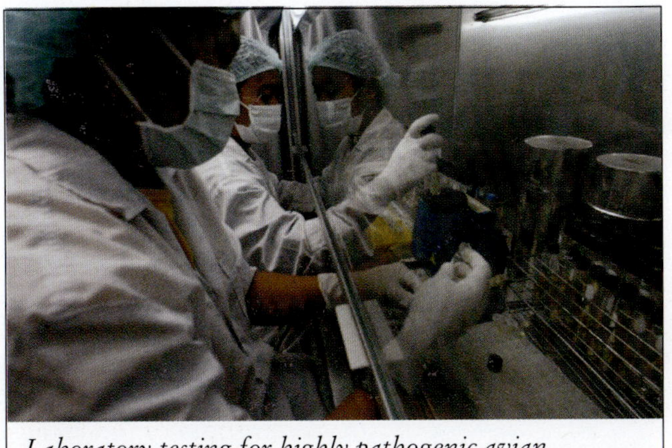

FAO

Laboratory testing for highly pathogenic avian influenza in Southeast Asia

CONCLUSIONS

The lessons learned from the above-mentioned emergency experiences are as follows:

- In order to perform an official notification, and in order to carry out stamping-out measures accompanied by compensation, implementation of diagnosis in accordance with international standards is indispensable; and
- In order to recover the disease-free status, implementation of surveillance and monitoring in accordance with international standards is indispensable.

OIE has been widely considered as an international and intergovernmental organization for terrestrial animal health, but has played important roles for aquatic animal health as well. The OIE Headquarters and the Regional Representation for Asia and the Pacific based in Tokyo are working with Member Countries to collect and disseminate aquatic animal health information and to organize meetings such as the International Conference on Risk Analysis in Aquatic Animals, the International Symposium on Koi herpes virus Disease and Regional Hands-on Workshop on Diagnosis and Surveillance of Aquatic Animal Diseases.

One of the OIE Specialist Commissions, namely the OIE Aquatic Animal Health Standards Commission, develops the Aquatic Animal Health Code (OIE, 2004c) in line with the terminology of the Sanitary and Phytosanitary Agreement (SPS Agreement) of the WTO to assure the sanitary safety and international trade in aquatic animals and their products. Fortunately no serious arguments on international trade of aquaculture products have so far been brought for WTO dispute settlement as SPS issues.

The aquaculture sector has been growing rapidly in Asia and Pacific and now this region is producing approximately 79 percent in value and 88 percent in volume of aquaculture products worldwide. However, we are now confronting the threat of transboundary aquatic animal diseases such as Koi herpes virus (KHV). To protect aquaculturists in this region not only from serious infectious diseases but also from future international trade disputes, the OIE Regional Representation for Asia and the Pacific calls on the fishery authorities in Member Countries to make steadfast linkages with veterinary administrations and to take advantage of OIE information and standards to deal with of aquatic animal disease emergencies.

LITERATURE CITED

OIE. 2004a. *Terrestrial animal health code*. 13th Edn, Paris.

OIE. 2004b. *Manual of diagnostic tests and vaccines for terrestrial animals*. Parts 1 and 2, 5th Edn, Paris.

OIE. 2004c. *Aquatic animal health code*. 7th Edn. Paris.

Emergency preparedness of aquatic animal diseases: Norwegian experiences

Tore Håstein and Roar Gudding
National Veterinary Institute
Oslo, Norway
tore.hastein@vetinst.no
roar.gudding@vetinst.no

Håstein, T. & Gudding, R. 2005. Emergency preparedness of aquatic animal diseases: Norwegian experiences. p. 79–85. In: Subasinghe, R.P.; Arthur, J.R. (eds.). Regional workshop on preparedness and response to aquatic animal health emergencies in Asia. Jakarta, Indonesia, 21–23 September 2004. *FAO Fisheries Proceedings*. No. 4. Rome, FAO. 2005. 178p.

ABSTRACT

Outbreaks of disease may have large consequences for aquaculture production and thus significant impact on the economy at the local, regional and national levels. This paper describes the key elements in emergency preparedness based on Norwegian experiences. Norway has had fish disease legislation since 1968. Management of disease emergencies is a core responsibility of governmental authorities based on appropriate legislation. Regulations on notification, diagnosis, epidemiology and restrictions on trade as well as fallowing and disinfection are important tools in disease management. An effective organization and adequate personnel resources, as well as competent diagnostic laboratories, are also key elements. Furthermore, emergency preparedness includes disease prevention and control through implementation of factors such as movement control, sanitary slaughter and zoning. With the tools described, it is possible to handle emergencies in aquaculture optimally.

INTRODUCTION

Over the last decades, emerging or serious diseases such as viral haemorrhagic septicaemia (VHS), infectious haematopoietic necrosis (IHN), infectious pancreatic necrosis (IPN), viral nervous necrosis (VNN), epizootic ulcerative syndrome (EUS) and many others have been diagnosed in feral and farmed fish populations in different parts of the world where they were previously unknown to occur.

Outbreaks of severe disease may have dramatic consequences for aquaculture production and thus have significant impact on the economy at the local, regional and national levels. The losses may be due to reduced production, increased labour costs and increased expenses due to medication. In addition, restrictions on trade are becoming increasingly important as an economic consequence. Furthermore, diseases in farmed aquatic animals may affect the environment in different ways, for instance by transmission of infectious disease to the wild fish population, which may have a negative impact on the wild stock, e.g. infection of *Gyrodactylus salaris* in Norwegian rivers.

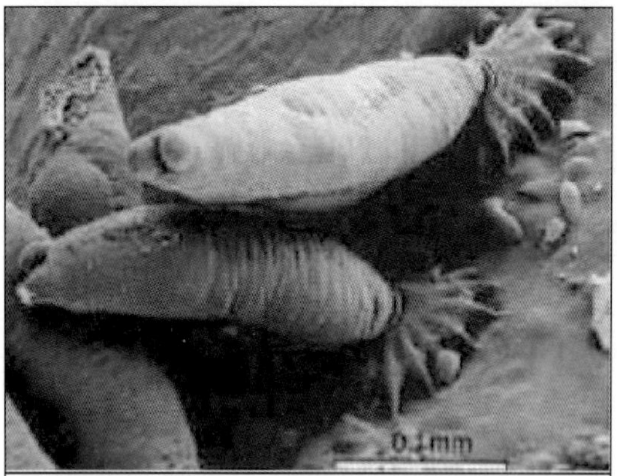

Gyrodactylus salaris *of salmon*

The food safety aspect of diseases of aquatic animals is less important than for diseases in terrestrial animals, as few aquatic animal diseases have true zoonotic potential. However, as microbial diseases in farmed fish are often treated with antibiotics, both residues and microbial resistance against antibiotics may be undesired effects of fish disease.

Effective emergency management is therefore crucial in order to reduce the economic, social and environmental impacts of serious diseases in aquaculture, and many countries, including Norway, have thus initiated emergency programmes for the control and/or eradication of such diseases (Folkestad and Torgersen 1999, Håstein, Hill and Winton 1999). The efficiency and success of such programmes are dependent on rapid initiation of the necessary measures/actions.

DISEASE AETIOLOGY

The most serious diseases in aquatic animals are caused by micro-organisms (bacteria, fungi, viruses, parasites). Such diseases may be introduced to a region/country, while others may already exist, but show a rapid increase in incidence due to predisposing factors such as high population density, bad water quality etc. The nature of the diseases, including their contagiousness and severity, may, however, vary significantly. Non-infectious diseases due to toxic components or nutritional factors may also have severe impact in aquaculture. Diseases with complex aetiology, involving both microorganisms as well as various predisposing factors, are becoming more common in some countries with a developed aquaculture.

RESPONSIBILITY

The management of disease emergencies remains a core responsibility for governmental authorities. The government should provide the necessary legislation and should also have an important role in leadership and intellectual input in such work. However, cooperation with the private sector, for example industrial organizations, local enterprises and farmers, is also an important element in the management of emergencies.

In Norway, the Ministry of Agriculture has had responsibility for aquatic animal diseases since 1968. As of 2004, the Ministry of Fisheries took over this responsibility as part of the reorganization of legislation related to food safety and the health of animals, aquatic animals and plants. A new agency, the Norwegian Food Safety Authority, has responsibility for implementing the Act and regulations given in pursuance of the Act.

LEGISLATION

Appropriate legislation is a fundamental instrument in emergency management. All biosecurity measures must have a legal basis. This includes disease notification, disease diagnosis or suspicion of disease, collection of specimens or epidemiological information, restrictions on trade or movement, disposal and decontamination of material, and cleaning and disinfection of premises.

The statutory definition of action to be taken is one of the most significant legal steps for disease control in aquatic animals and may have tremendous implications for on-farm management practices aimed at disease control. Depending upon the classification and importance of a notifiable disease, different management practises may be laid down by law to achieve sufficient disease control.

In Norway, fish disease legislation was established in 1968 due to the introduction of serious diseases such as viral haemorrhagic septicaemia (VHS) and furunculosis into Norway by imports of live rainbow trout (*Oncorhynchus mykiss*) from Denmark (Håstein, Holt and Krogsrud 1968, Holt and Håstein 1970).

The first "Fish Disease Act" covered only diseases of freshwater fish, including anadromous and catadromous fish species as well as freshwater crayfish. The reason for this was that diseases in salmonid species and freshwater crayfish were of major importance, and farming of other species had not been considered at that time.

In 1990, an interim Act covering all aquatic organisms, including marine species, was adopted. However, as regards marine aquatic organisms, only those kept under culture conditions were covered. The intention was to replace this interim Act by a permanent Act in 1992, but this permanent Act did not come into force until 1997.

As of January 2004, a new legislation, the so-called "Food Act", covering all aspects of animals and aquatic animals from fiord and pasture to the table was introduced (Anon., 2004a).

Several regulations have been introduced in pursuance of the acts referred to above, and these regulations have been improved over the years since 1968 until today. Some 36 regulations are now in force in pursuance of the current Act.

The "Food Act" is an enabling act as regards control of animal health and gives wide authority to prevent, eradicate and keep diseases and infective agents in aquatic animals under surveillance. The Act also includes particular powers to ensure eradication of exotic diseases.

ORGANIZATION

An effective organization with functional responsibilities for preparedness is the basis for the work of the governmental authority. In addition to a central unit with direct link to the policy decision-makers within the political system, including those at the ministerial level, there should be a regional and a local organization with professional and paraprofessional personnel. The command principles between the levels of the organization, as well as the relationship to institutions providing scientific and technical support, should be well defined. As cooperation with the industry and information to the public are important for the success of any emergency management, a well-organized communications system should be integrated into the organization.

In Norway, the Norwegian Food Safety Authority consists of three levels: a Central Unit, eight Regional Offices and 64 District Offices covering the entire country. In emergency situations, the District Offices have the main responsibility for immediate implementation of measures such as:

- restrictions on a farm on suspicion;
- confirmation of diagnosis of the notifiable disease in question;
- provision of any supplementary information/changes in earlier information; and
- repeal of restrictions.

The tasks of the District Offices include reporting to the regional and central authorities.

PERSONNEL RESOURCES

Depending on the infrastructure within a country, a national and/or a regional (local) emergency team (disease experts, operational team, administrative personnel) should be established in order to cope with outbreaks of serious diseases.

In Norway, we have a network of veterinarians, fish health biologists and diagnostic laboratories that may be involved in implementation of actions necessitated by an emergency disease outbreak. With such a good infrastructure, it has been relatively easy to implement any information and measures to be taken in case of an outbreak of an unknown disease.

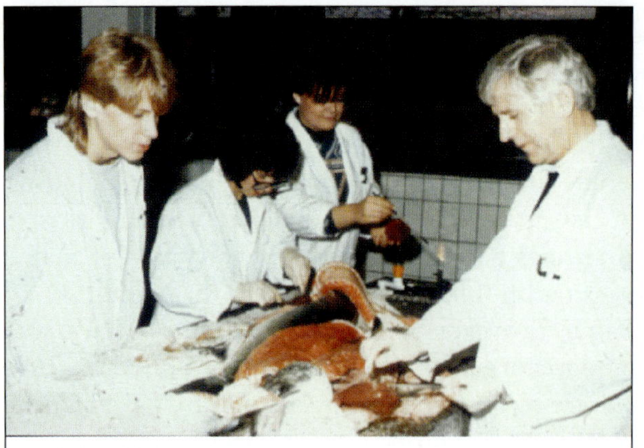

TORE HÅSTEIN

Fish health training

TRAINING PROGRAMMES

In order to maintain the state of readiness, announced and unannounced exercises in handling exotic diseases or any serious disease should be carried out for personnel at all levels that will become involved in the different aspects of control of aquatic animal diseases. For fish health personnel, this must include updated information on the disease in question, epidemiology of the disease, sampling and diagnostic methods, new disinfection procedures etc. Specific training programmes should also involve people from the fish farming industry. The responsibility for these training programmes should involve the responsible authorities at the central, regional and local levels. Norway has good experience with such types of training programmes.

EQUIPMENT AND FACILITIES

Handling of emergency situations requires necessary equipment and supplies. These include communication equipment and maps covering coastal and continental areas of the country, as well as equipment for necropsy and the introduction of sanitary measures. Furthermore, routines for how to issue warning notices to inform the public relating to restricted access to the premises in question, as well as access to transportation units (boats, vehicles) are needed and whether sanitary slaughtering, etc. is required. All this will have to be a part of a contingency plan.

MANUAL

Preparation for emergency situations is crucial for success during a disease crisis. A simple but thoroughly written plan describing responsibilities and activities in case of a disease outbreak is a major element in the emergency management. Professional and paraprofessional personnel with theoretical and practical training must be available in order to carry out the activities at the central and regional units, as well as on the local level.

Although Norway, presently has in force only a contingency plan for infectious salmon anaemia (ISA) (Anon., 2004b), the principles laid down in this plan have also been used to bring other serious diseases under control.

DIAGNOSTIC LABORATORIES

Rapid, reliable and effective diagnostic work should be carried out by national or provincial laboratories designated for such purposes by the competent authority, as this may be essential for a successful outcome of a crisis. Diagnoses of serious disease should, if necessary, be confirmed by an international reference laboratory for the disease in question.

Each country should thus establish a national fish disease reference laboratory that should have a key responsibility for aquatic animal diseases and with well-qualified personnel, facilities and equipment in order to handle a crisis. This responsibility

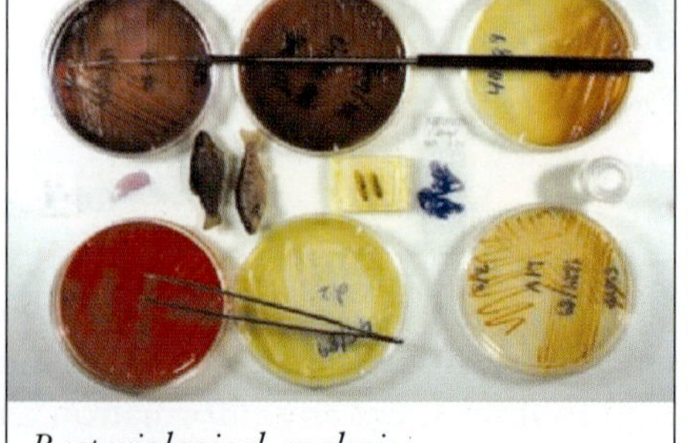

TORE HÅSTEIN

Bacteriological analysis

should include reference functions for regional and local laboratories with official or private funding. A decentralized laboratory structure is especially essential in countries with large fish populations that are distributed over large geographical areas.

The expertise of the laboratories should include scientifically based diagnostic procedures in addition to research, but also competence in preventive medicine and emergency management is needed. Descriptive and analytical epidemiology and risk assessment are areas with increasing significance in emergency situations in aquaculture and should be part of the scientific advice given to the authorities by the laboratories.

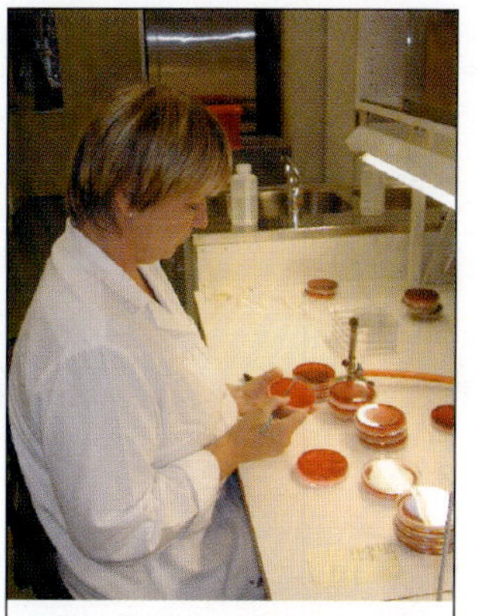

TORE HÅSTEIN

Microbiology laboratory

New methods for diagnostic work and surveillance are under continuous development, and the laboratory should have the competence and capacity to be updated on the international progress in diagnostic procedures.

Pathology is considered as the most essential area of competence for an aquatic animal health laboratory with diagnostic responsibilities. The clinical signs in diseased aquatic animals are often vague and non-specific, and necropsy is the major method for diagnosing diseases. The post-mortem lesions should be supported by histological examinations. Techniques based on histochemistry and immunological methods may contribute to a more precise diagnosis, including the aetiology of a given disease.

Necropsy should be performed in an equipped laboratory with good technical support. However, if transport to a pathological laboratory is long and costly, necropsy in the field may be an alternative. If performed by skilled personnel, a preliminary diagnosis may be obtained, creating a basis for control measures. Furthermore, samples may be taken, preserved and shipped to regional or central laboratories for further examination and confirmation.

Bacteriological examinations should be available in any diagnostic laboratory. Diagnostics for viral diseases requires cell or tissue cultures and personnel with special expertise. Viral isolation should consequently be performed in the central and most specialized laboratories.

Methods based on molecular biology are becoming more and more used as part of the diagnostic work in bacteriology, virology, mycology and parasitology. These techniques offer great advantages in sensitivity and speed, but the analyses should take place in well-equipped laboratories due to the risk of false positive and negative reactions.

Over the years, the National Veterinary Institute has built up its expertise in all the fields mentioned above and functions as a national reference laboratory for Norway, giving scientific advice to the authorities based upon research, surveillance programmes and the results of diagnostic investigations.

COMMUNICATION

Since most aquatic animal diseases constitute no human health hazard, it may not be necessary to direct special efforts towards public education. Nevertheless, it may be worth while to prepare some press releases giving definite information on the disease in question to avoid rumours and incorrect information. Such information should clearly state that the disease does not represent any health risks to humans.

However, from an aquatic animal disease aspect, there is a need for emergency information between the field and the international society when a listed disease has been diagnosed. Thus, neighbouring countries should be informed, in addition to international organizations (i.e. the European Union (EU), the Network of Aquaculture Centres in Asia-Pacific (NACA), the Office International des Épizooties (OIE) etc.).

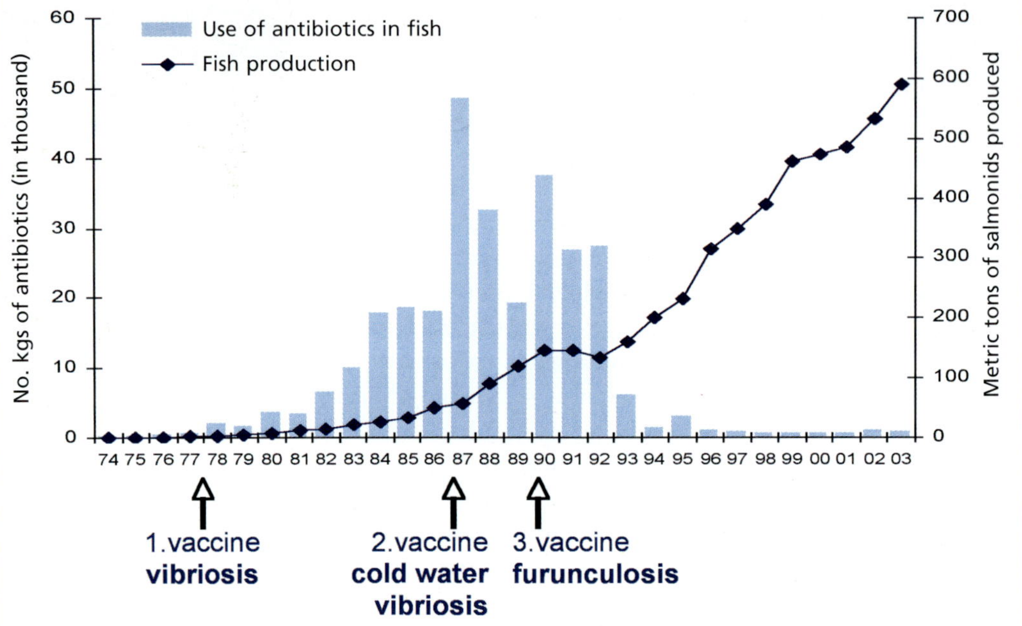

Effect of vaccination on the use of antibacterials in Norway 1974 - 2003

DISEASE PREVENTION AND CONTROL

Emergency preparedness for aquatic animal diseases also includes establishment of disease prevention and control measures. Since production of animal protein has to be sustainable, the preventive measures to be used have to be acceptable from a biological and environmental point of view. Vaccination is now the single most important measure for prevention of bacterial diseases in farmed fish, especially in salmonid fish (Håstein, Gudding and Evensen, 2005).

In Norway, the use of vaccination as a preventive measure started as early as 1977, and regulations regarding vaccination of fish were established in 1983. These regulations were updated in 1999 (Anon., 1999). Only vaccines authorized by the Norwegian Medicinal Authority are allowed to be used. The vaccination policy in Norway has had a large influence on the use of antibacterials.

Effective control of an emerging disease may be obtained through implementation of measures such as movement restriction, stamping out, sanitary slaughter and establishment of control and surveillance zones.

CONCLUSIONS

Based on the experiences gained in Norway after some 35 years of disease control in aquatic animals, we still have to live with certain diseases, but the legislation and regulations have given us the necessary tools to handle emergency crises in an optimal way. Since the infrastructure and disease situation may vary from country to country and between regions, it is important that the regulations are as flexible as possible in order to retain sufficient precautions should an emergency situation occur.

LITERATURE CITED

Anon. 1999. Regulations of 20th December 1999 No. 1310 relating to vaccination of domestic animals, wildlife, fish and other aquatic animals (The regulations of vaccination).

Anon. 2004a. Lov 2003-12-19 nr 124: Lov om matproduksjon og mattrygghet mv. (matloven). [Act of 19th December 2003 No. 124 relating to food production and food safety ("The Food Act")] (In Norwegian).

Anon. 2004b. Contingency plan for control of infectious salmon anaemia (ISA) in Norway.

Folkestad, P. & Torgersen, Y. 1999. Disease prevention and control in aquatic animals from a legislative point of view with special reference to Norwegian experiences. 9 pp. Presentation at the Second Workshop of the National Coordinators. FAO/NACA/OIE Regional Programme for the Development of Technical Guidelines on Quarantine and Health Certification and Establishment of Information Systems for the Responsible Movement of Live Aquatic Animals in Asia. Bangkok, 1–5 February 1999.

Håstein, T., Gudding, R. & Evensen, Ø. 2005. Bacterial vaccines for fish; an update of the current situation world wide. In: *Fish Vaccinology. Developments in Biological Standardisation.* (In press).

Håstein, T., Hill, B.J. & Winton, J.R. 1999. Successful aquatic animal disease emergency programmes. *Rev. Sci. Tech. Off. Int. Epiz.*, 18: 214-227.

Håstein, T., Holt, G. & Krogsrud, J. 1968. Hemorrhagisk virusseptikemi (Egtvedsyke) hos regnbueørret i Norge. [Haemorrhagic viral septicaemia in rainbow trout in Norway.] *Nord. Vet.*, 20: 708-711. (In Norwegian, English summary).

Holt, G. & Håstein, T. 1970. Furunkulose hos fisk i Norge [Furunculosis in fish in Norway.] *Nord. Vet.*, 22: 505-509. (In Norwegian, English summary).

Response to mass mortality of carp: an Indonesian experience[1]

Agus Sunarto
Fish Health Research Laboratory
Jl. Ragunan No. 20
Jakarta 12540, Indonesia
agus.sunarto@gmail.com
Angus Cameron
AusVet Animal Health Services
140 Falls Road
Wentworth Falls NSW 2782, Australia
angus@ausbet.com.au

Sunarto, A. & Cameron, A. 2005. Response to mass mortality of carp: an Indonesian experience. p. 87–105. In: Subasinghe, R.P.; Arthur, J.R. (eds.). Regional workshop on preparedness and response to aquatic animal health emergencies in Asia. Jakarta, Indonesia, 21–23 September 2004. *FAO Fisheries Proceedings*. No. 4. Rome, FAO. 2005. 178p.

ABSTRACT

Since March 2002, Indonesian carp culture has faced a serious epizootic that has caused severe economic loss and significant social impact. As of December 2003, losses were estimated at US$15 million, with total fish mortality of up to 80-95 percent. The disease outbreaks affected koi and common carp (*Cyprinus carpio*) populations of all ages and sizes cultured in different grow-out facilities (ponds, lakes, cages etc.), regardless of stocking density. Epidemiological observations indicated that the first outbreak occurred in imported koi carp that had just been transported from Surabaya to Blitar, both in East Java. The heavy rain prior to the initial outbreak indicated the possibility of an environmental triggering factor, such as temperature. Based on the history, clinical signs, epidemiological features, histopathological changes, results of experimental infection, PCR detection of naturally and experimentally diseased fish, and analysis of DNA sequence, it is confirmed that Koi herpes virus (KHV) was involved in this serious outbreak. To prevent the spread of the disease to other islands, the Government of Indonesia declared the islands of Java and Bali as isolated areas infected with the disease, and movement of koi and common carps from Java to other islands has been restricted to quarantined animals. The government has also taken measures to reduce the possible re-introduction of the disease through importation of koi and common carps into the country. This paper includes information collected in July 2002 during the initial investigation conducted by the Emergency Disease Control Task Force on a Serious Disease of Koi and Common

[1] Initially, many factors were speculated to be responsible for this new outbreak, including water pollution, contaminated feed and bacterial infection. NACA's Task Force found that koi herpesvirus (KHV) might have played a role in the mass mortalities, and since then, Indonesian scientists have used the term KHV. However, the Task Force recommended that this serious outbreak be called "mass mortality of koi and common carp" until a clear association with KHV could be established (NACA, 2002). During the International Workshop on Koi Herpesvirus held in London in February 2004, it was agreed that the cause of the Indonesian outbreak was KHV (see Crane, Sano and Komar, 2004).

Carps in Indonesia organized by the Network of Aquaculture Centres in Asia-Pacific (NACA) and partners, results of the on-going work undertaken by the National Disease Task Force, and the Food and Agriculture Organization of the United Nations' (FAO) follow-up assistance through a Technical Cooperation Project.

INTRODUCTION

Aquaculture plays an important role in rural development, provides a source for export earning and has proved to be a leading sector in economic growth in Indonesia. Freshwater, brackishwater, and marine cage culture still have an opportunity to be expanded and developed. However, since March 2002, Indonesian carp culture has faced a serious epizootic that has caused severe economic loss and significant social impact. The epizootic nature of the disease and its potential for spread to neighbouring Asian countries, the current economic impact and the potential threat to the production of this important foodfish, and the potential trade and economic implications are significant and require urgent implementation of containment and control procedures.

Responding to an official request from the Government of Indonesia, immediate assistance was provided by the Network of Aquaculture Centres in Asia-Pacific (NACA) and partners, by fielding an Emergency Disease Control Task Force on a Serious Disease of Koi and Common Carps in Indonesia consisting of three fish health experts in July 2002. The Task Force provided several key recommendations to improve the fish health status of Indonesia and to reduce possible disease outbreaks. The Task Force report provides supportive evidence of possible Koi herpes virus (KHV) infection, the confirmed aetiology of which is yet to be found. To further assist Indonesia in finding a resolution to this emergency situation, the Food and Agriculture Organization of the United Nations (FAO) approved emergency assistance to the Government of Indonesia through a Technical Cooperation Project – TCP/INS/2905(A) entitled "Health Management in Freshwater Aquaculture", which commenced on 10 January 2003.

This paper includes vital information collected in July 2002 during the initial investigation conducted by the Emergency Task Force organized by NACA and partners, results of the on-going work undertaken by the National Disease Task Force, and FAO's follow-up assistance through a Technical Cooperation Project.

EMERGENCY RESPONSE

The Government of Indonesia immediately responded to the outbreak of mass mortality of koi and common carp. Initial actions taken included announcing the occurrence of the disease outbreak to stakeholders, issuing a regulation restricting the movement of diseased fish, organizing the National Disease Task Force, reporting the outbreak to the Office International des Épizooties (OIE) (Rukyani, 2002), and seeking assistance from international agencies that lead to the formation of NACA's Task Force and an FAO Technical Cooperation Project. In addition, the government also provided various assistances to affected carp farmers.

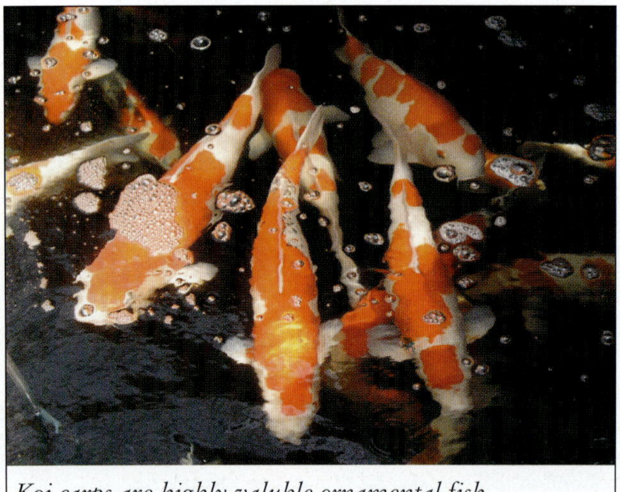

AGUS SUNARTO

Koi carps are highly valuble ornamental fish

Rules and regulations

The first episode of the outbreak in koi occurred in March 2002 in Blitar, East Java. On 17 May 2002, the Director General of Aquaculture (DGA) issued Circulation

Letter No. 1874 pertaining to the disease outbreak in koi and common carp. The announcement letter was circulated to provincial governments, fisheries offices and other stakeholders. As the outbreak was escalating and spreading to new areas, the government organized a National Disease Task Force (DGA's Letter No. 2101 dated 4 June 2002). The main mandate of the National Task Force is to control the outbreak and to minimize the economic losses.

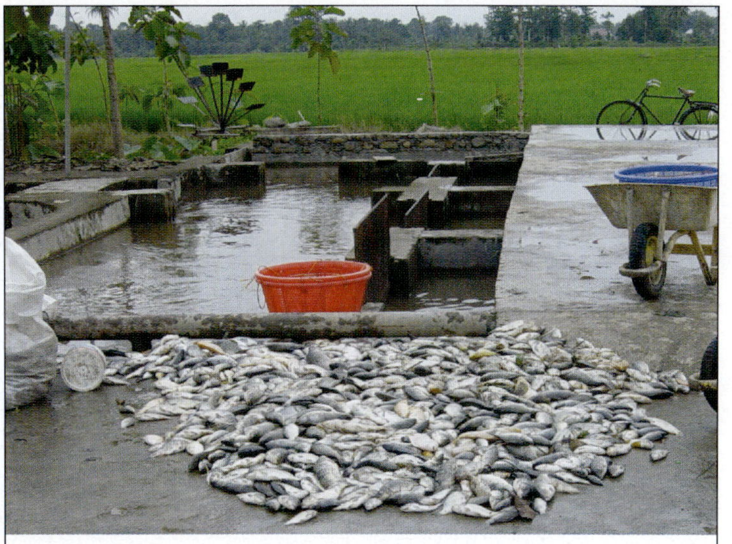

AGUS SUNARTO

Common carps are important food fish

Based on the recommendation of the National Task Force, the government declared Java Island as an isolated area of the disease, strictly prohibited the movement of koi and common carp from Java to other islands, and permitted the importation of koi and common carp only from KHV-free countries (DGA's Letter No. 2317 dated 14 June 2002 and Ministerial Decree No. 28 dated 2 July 2002). The regulations were issued in order to protect the country from re- introduction of the disease, to prevent wider spread of KHV and to minimize losses in common carp and koi culture. However, due to the restriction on movement of koi and common carp, there was an over-supply of common carp on Java Island.

To solve this problem and due to social pressure, the government issued Ministerial Decree no 40 dated 3 October 2002. The degree declared Java and Bali islands as an isolated area of Koi herpes virus (KHV) and specified that the movement of koi and common carp from Java and Bali to other islands should follow a quarantine check for KHV. However, because trucks with live fish often cross the strait without reporting to the checkpoint office, the application of Decree No. 40 has not been effective. Such trucks are usually without documents or certificates of fish health. At Merak, the checkpoint for the movement of live fish from Java into Sumatera Island is not equipped with simple laboratory equipment. Live fish traffic, especially carp, destined to Sumatera, involves around 5-10 trucks per day. The live carp transported to Sumatera originate from KHV-infected areas, i.e. Cirata Reservoir, Sukabumi, Subang, Pandeglang and Jatiluhur. Thus, Merak is a strategic point for the spread of fish disease from Java to Sumatra, since it is the most convenient entry point for inter-island live fish movement between the islands. The spread of KHV disease to the whole of Sumatera through the Merak Check Point is just a matter of time unless there is other policy to stop the infected live fish movement to Sumatera. If Decree No. 40 is to be effective, officers at key checkpoints must be given the necessary infrastructure, authority and manpower to fully enforce regulations (Arthur, 2003). The provincial and district authorities of uninfected regions should be encouraged to regulate the movement of live carp from Java to their regions (Prayitno, 2003). However, the disease spread to Sumatera Island in January 2003 (Yuasa *et al.*, 2004).

Governmental assistance

Besides issuing rules and regulations soon after the outbreak, the government also provided assistance to affected carp farmers. This included new broodstock, disinfectants, diagnostic services, training and consultancies. A website (www. ditkeskanling.go.id) was also established to provide information on the outbreak and fish health management in general. Intensive information dissemination was also undertaken to raise awareness and inform the public sector about KHV and the relevant information available at that time.

Fulfilling international obligations

As a member of the international community, the Government of Indonesia has fulfilled its obligation to report important diseases to the Office International des Épizooties (OIE). A report of the KHV epidemic was sent to OIE on 26 June 2002 (Rukyani, 2002). Since then, a regular report on the KHV outbreak has also been sent to OIE through the NACA/OIE/FAO Asia-Pacific Quarterly Aquatic Animal Disease Reporting System.

NACA's Task Force

In 20 June 2002, Dr. Fatuchri Sukadi, Director General of Aquaculture, Ministry of Marine Affairs and Fisheries, requested assistance for the solution to the outbreak to NACA. NACA's response was to organize the Emergency Disease Control Task Force on a Serious Disease of Koi and Common Carps in Indonesia, subsequently referred to as NACA's "Task Force", in cooperation with the Australian Centre for International Agricultural Research (ACIAR) and the Aquatic Animal Health Research Institute (AAHRI). The Task Force, which consisted of international and national experts and a number of participating laboratories and organizations, conducted an emergency assessment of the disease situation in July 2002 through field observations (i.e. field visits, interviews with local/district officials and farmers) and laboratory examinations (e.g. histopathology and virology, including use of polymerase chain reaction (PCR), and electron microscopy (EM)) of collected samples).

The Task Force collected vital information about the disease occurrence, epidemiological perspective and provided supportive evidence of a possible KHV infection, the confirmed aetiology of which is yet to be found. The Task Force findings recommended that this serious outbreak of koi and common carp be called "Mass mortality of koi and common carp (MMKC)" until a clear association with KHV or another specific disease can be established. The Task Force also provided several key recommendations for improving the fish health status of Indonesia and reducing possible disease outbreaks (NACA, 2002).

FAO's Technical Cooperation Programme

As follow-up to the recommendations of NACA's Task Force and in response to a request from the Government of Indonesia, FAO immediately provided emergency assistance through a Technical Cooperation Project "Health Management in Freshwater Aquaculture" (TCP/INS/2905(A)), to find resolution to this disease emergency. The project was set up to:

- strengthen diagnostic and control capabilities within the responsible state agencies for major diseases of cultured freshwater fish, including koi and common carp;
- improve capacity for vulnerable rural aqua-farmers to face future outbreaks in their culture systems;
- enhance national regulatory frameworks and legislation, improve biosecurity measures and strengthen national disease surveillance and reporting to reduce the risk of movement of pathogens, both nationally and internationally, through movement of live animals; and
- develop and implement Indonesia's National Strategy on Aquatic Animal Health Management.

Under the project, various issues on fish health management in Indonesia were addressed. These included review of policy and legislation, enhancement of the national regulatory framework and development of a national strategy on fish health management. Other related issues on fish health management such as strengthening diagnostic and control capability; improving surveillance, monitoring and disease reporting systems; human resource development and public awareness are being addressed. The project is also concerned with the identification and confirmation of the aetiological agent of the disease and is looking for assistance from international laboratories.

Legislation: The major accomplishments arising from the consultancy on fish health legislation include:

- a one-day national workshop on import risk analysis (IRA);
- a workshop on legislation on fish health management;
- review and revision of the National Strategy on Fish Health Management;
- identification and brief summary of the contents of national legislation dealing with fish health management and;
- recommendations with regard to future activities.

It should be noted that the short duration of the consultancy, combined with the complicated and extensive nature of the Indonesian legislation on fish health and the complicated structure of the Indonesian fish quarantine service made it impossible to undertake anything more than an initial and incomplete examination of the issues surrounding these sectors. Recommendations are made for more detailed future reviews in these two important areas (Arthur, 2003; Prayitno, 2003).

Fish health management: A consultancy was undertaken to understand the fish health management practices by stakeholders. Below is summary of the findings based on the report of the consultants (Shariff, 2004; Pasaribu, 2004). Investigations revealed that disease outbreaks were a common phenomenon due to the following:

- lack of appropriate infrastructure and trained personnel;
- lack of stakeholder knowledge regarding good fish health management practices;
- lack of stakeholder understanding of the complexity of fish health management due to an array of potential sources of disease outbreak;
- farming communities spreading diseases through movement of apparently healthy fish that are carriers of disease;
- lack of manpower and funds for extension services to reach the fish farming community;
- lack of understanding on the part of officers providing extension service of the complex issues related to fish disease outbreaks and their inability to communicate effectively with the fish farming community;
- in some cases, lost faith by the farming community in the extension services, as the information provided is considered unreliable;
- poor infrastructure at fish breeding centers and live fish markets, which are centers for distribution of disease;
- even when KHV had caused severe economic losses to farmers, movement of fish suspected to be infected with KHV still continues freely, spreading it to new localities;
- poor networking among the various agencies related to the aquaculture industry; and
- insufficient collaboration among the various institutions for research in fish health.

The major accomplishments arising from the consultancy include:

- identification of fish health management problems faced by farmers and their needs to overcome these problems;
- development of a module for fish health management practices that can be used as standard teaching material for fisheries officers and fish farmers;
- conducting national training programmes on fish health management for fisheries officers and fish farmers respectively; and
- recommendations with regard to future activities on fish health management.

Epidemiology: The major accomplishments arising from the consultancy are as follows:

- field investigation to affected and unaffected common carp production areas to formulate prevention strategy;
- assessments of the disease reporting capabilities and communication infrastructure;
- description the general characteristics and components of an aquatic animal disease surveillance system;
- national survey on the geographic distribution and progression of KHV in the country;
- construction of a web-based information system on fish health management with special emphasis on a disease reporting system (www.ausvet.com.au/indofish); and
- recommendations with regards to future activities on research, information system, epidemiology and control of KHV (Cameron, 2003; Rukyani, 2003).

Virology: Equipment, facilities and human resources were reviewed at major laboratories involved in fish health management, and fish disease diagnostics laboratories were visited in order to evaluate current diagnostic capabilities, with particular reference to fish virology. The major accomplishments arising from the consultancy are as follows:

- a total of 13 major laboratories were visited, with a view to setting up a national center for virology;
- assistance was given to a number of laboratories visited in terms of advice on laboratory design, equipment use and requirements for fish disease diagnostics and research;
- a National Virology Unit was established at the Fish Health Research Laboratory (FHRL), which is the first of its kind in the country;
- a laboratory manual was developed for the operation of the virology unit that can be used as standard operating procedures (SOP) for other virology laboratories;
- a three-day training workshop on fish virology was conducted for staff from 17 major laboratories in Indonesia;
- an Inter-laboratory Network (ILAN) was established in order to facilitate information exchange among laboratory workers; and
- recommendations were made with regard to the future development and activities to sustain the function and operation of the National Virology Unit (Millar, 2003; 2004; Sunarto, 2004).

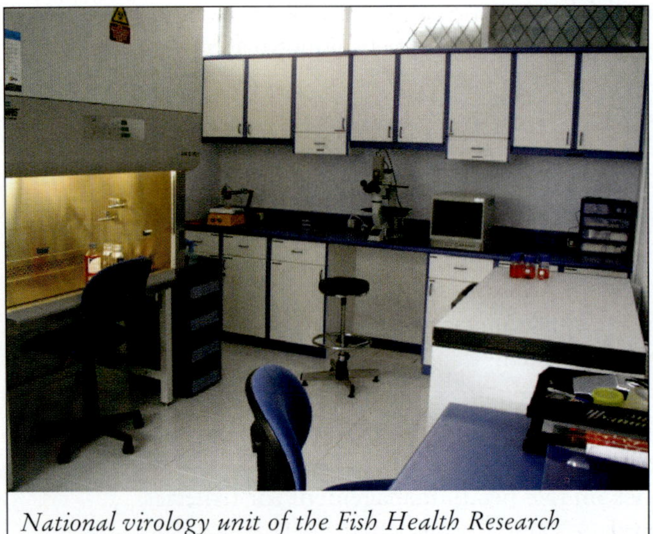

AGUS SUNARTO

National virology unit of the Fish Health Research Laboratory of Indonesia

Surveillance and information system: These issued were addressed mostly by the consultant in epidemiology. The major accomplishments arising from the consultancy are as follows:

- description of the general characteristics and components of an aquatic animal disease surveillance system; and
- construction of a pilot web-based information system on fish health management in Indonesia, with special emphasis on disease reporting system by Dr. Angus Cameron (www.ausvet.com.au/indofish).

A website of the Directorate for Fish Health and Environment (www.ditkeskanling.go.id) was also set up to provide general information on fish health management. Indofish is being placed in the directorate's website.

Human resource development: Under the project, five training workshops on legislation, epidemiology, virology and fish health management for fisheries officers and key farmers were completed. Four persons attended two-week overseas training at the Aquatic Animal Health Research Institute (AAHRI) in Bangkok, Thailand. The project termination workshop was expanded to an FAO regional workshop conducted on 21-23 September 2004. Dissemination of information regarding fish health management including technical guidelines for KHV and whitespot syndrome virus (WSSV) and a poster for import risk analysis (IRA) were produced and distributed to stakeholders.

HISTORY OF THE OUTBREAK

The history of the outbreak including the first three episodes was chronologically described by Sunarto *et al.* (2002). The first episode of mass mortalities of cultured koi carp was recorded in March 2002 in Blitar, East Java. It occurred after heavy rains among new fish introduced from Surabaya, the capital city of East Java. The fish were imported from PR China through Hong Kong in December 2001 and January 2002. Blitar is well known as the center for koi production in the country. The koi, including the infected animals, were distributed to the provinces of Central Java, West Java and Jakarta as the main market. The second disease outbreak occurred in cultured common carp during the end of April 2002 in Subang Regency, West Java. The gross signs shown by the diseased fish were extremely similar with that observed previously in koi carp. Subang is one of the production centers of common carp in West Java. Since then the outbreaks spread to neighbouring regencies, mainly through the movement of infected fish. The third episode of the outbreak occurred in the end of May to early June 2002 in cultured common carp in floating netcages at Cirata Reservoir, West Java. Weeks before the outbreak, farmers introduced common carp from the Subang region, due to the low price of these fish.

The fourth episode of the outbreak occurred in January 2003, affecting cultured common carp in Lubuk Lingau Regency, South Sumatera. The gross signs of the diseased common carp were extremely similar to those observed previously in koi and common carp in Java. Mass mortality of more than 90 percent was observed during the outbreak. Common carp farms at Lubuk Lingau were infected with the disease coming from Cirata Reservoir, West Java through fish transfer by traders. In January, the outbreak spread to neighbouring Provinces, including Bengkulu in the south and Jambi in the west (Sunarto, Rukyani and Itami, 2004; Yuasa *et al.,* 2004).

In this paper, two new outbreaks are reported. Although a public awareness campaign conducted by the central and local governments delayed the spread of the disease from southern Sumatera to West Sumatera, in August 2004, an outbreak that killed more than 200 tonnes of cultured common carp occurred in Singkarak Lake and Maninjau Lake, West Sumatera. The gross signs of the diseased fish were extremely similar with those observed previously in koi and carp in Java and southern Sumatera. Common carp farms on West Sumatera were infected with the disease via contaminated seed that is believed to have been transferred from Jambi Province, where KHV disease has occurred since 2003.

The sixth episode of KHV outbreak occurred in carp culture in Banjar Baru, South Kalimantan. The outbreak killed 600 tonnes of common carp in the running water culture system in September 2004. However, the mortality rate was quite low (30-50 percent) as compared with the outbreaks on Java and Sumatera islands. It is speculated that the polyculture of common carp with tilapia and high water temperate (29°C) may reduce mortality rate due to KHV. The spread of KHV into Kalimantan was thought to be due to the irresponsible movement of infected carp broodstock from Malang, East Java, where KHV is endemic.

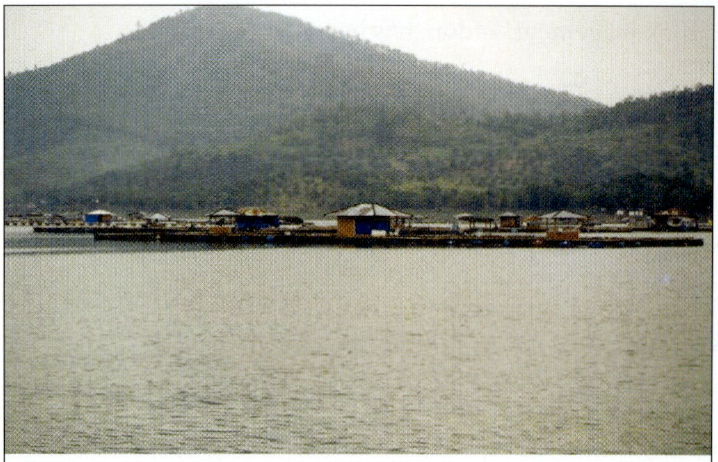
AGUS SUNARTO

Double cage culture system with first level using common carp and second level using tilapia

EPIDEMIOLOGY

The epidemiological investigation was conducted by NACA's Task Force in July 2002. The information presented below is based on the report of Dr. Angus Cameron (Cameron, 2002).

Methodology

Investigations were conducted in the east of Java, with visits to Surabaya, Malang and Blitar. The approach used to investigate the disease was as follows:

- initial discussions with central staff in Java, and collection of existing information on the nature and distribution of the disease;
- discussions with local Kabupaten and Kotamadya officers in Blitar to collect information on the distribution of the disease in the local area;
- field visits to two farms to the northwest of Blitar and three farms to the southeast and east. At each visit, farmers were questioned about the origin, progression and behaviour of the disease;
- one visit to the Surabaya fish quarantine offices and laboratory for examination of import documents and discussion with staff relating to the importers premises; and
- in conducting the epidemiological investigations, analyzing the findings, and formulating conclusions, the team maintained contact with the laboratory investigation team to assess findings from the west of the island.

Results

The following section presents the results of epidemiological observations gathered during the investigation:

Confirmation of a disease outbreak: The 50-100 percent mortality rates reported by farmers far exceed what is considered normal and therefore a disease outbreak is confirmed.

Pattern of spread of disease: The pattern is typical of a propagating infectious disease, starting in one location and subsequently spreading both locally and over long distances. From each new disease location, further local spread has occurred. The evidence of spread of disease within farms after the introduction of fish is also consistent with the disease being caused by an infectious agent. Disease is spread downstream, with the second case-farm being located about 500 m downstream from the index farm, with a delay of about 20 days between the onset of disease in the two farms. It is still unclear what the main mechanism of water-borne between-farm spread is (whether it is through direct carriage of the virus or through either mechanical or biological vectors). It is suspected that vectors may play a role, as the relatively fragile herpes virus is unlikely to survive for long periods exposed to sunlight in the shallow streams of the region.

Nature of the pathogen: Based on available epidemiological evidence, it can be reported with extreme confidence that the disease is caused by a directly transmitted infectious agent. The rapid transmission of the disease (about seven days between introduction of infected fish and the onset of clinical signs in contact fish) and the observation that transmission has occurred in clean cement tanks with very few potential intermediate hosts present both strongly indicate that the disease is directly transmitted.

Spread of disease: Several mechanisms for spread of disease have been identified. These are:

- spread between enclosures in a farm through fish to fish contact, through water and possibly through movement of dead fish or tissues;
- local spread between farms through water and possibly non-water mechanisms such as transport of live fish or the transport of the pathogen via humans, other animals or inanimate objects (fomites) such as aquaculture equipment, and feed; and
- long distance spread – mainly through fish movements.

Incubation period: The incubation period is about seven days, and the contact rate is very high, allowing a large number of fish to become infected from a single shedding fish.

Cause of the current outbreak: There are a number of pieces of evidence that strongly suggest that the cause is viral, and is most likely to be KHV. The host specificity and pattern of mortality is the same as that described for KHV (Hedrick *et al.*, 2000) in earlier outbreaks (*analogy*). The observation in one experiment that the disease recurred in recovered fish once they were stressed is typical of latent herpes virus behaviour, and unlikely in any of the other pathogens under consideration (*experimental*). The failure of response to treatment with antibiotics reported in a number of cases probably provides a weak evidence that the cause may not be bacterial (*response to treatment*). The finding of positive PCR results from affected fish (and the negative finding from unaffected fish) confirms these epidemiological assessments.

Risk factors: A number of risk factors may play a role in disease development, based on direct field observations and anecdotal evidence. These include the following:

- size of fish (large fish are sometimes reported to be more susceptible, but this may well be due to the fact that gill damage is one of the first signs of disease, and their increased requirements for oxygen);
- water oxygen levels (increasing water oxygen levels may minimize mortality in less severely affected fish);
- water flow;
- rapid collection of affected fish (to decrease the level of virus transmission);
- temperature (previous reports indicate that the virus is only active within a relatively narrow temperature range); and
- water quality, management factors, feed and treatments.

GEOGRAPHICAL DISTRIBUTION

A survey of KHV was conducted in April 2003 under FAO's Technical Cooperation Programme. The information presented below is based on the reports of Dr. Angus Cameron and Dr. Akhmad Rukyani (Cameron, 2003; Rukyani, 2003).

Objective

The main objectives of the survey were to determine the extent and the distribution of the population at risk against KHV, the current distribution of the disease and extent of the disease.

Methods

In order to achieve these objectives and meet the criteria listed above, a rapid survey at the district (kabupaten) level as a unit of interest was conducted. The survey was conducted in all of the country's 353 districts. A printed questionnaire was used to collect data. The questionnaire was pre-printed with the name of each district and province, as well as the district code, to simplify the data entry. The questionnaire was designed to be as simple and as rapid as possible to be completed, consisting of only seven questions. These related to:

- presence of at-risk species (common and koi carp);
- extent of the population at risk, measured both in terms of hectares under culture and the number of farms;
- presence of KHV disease in the district;
- date of the first report of KHV; and
- an estimate of the number of farms affected by KHV.

The questionnaire was delivered by mail to each district office. It was accompanied by an official covering letter explaining the survey and giving instructions on how to fill out the questionnaire, and an information sheet on KHV (with case definition) to enable district fisheries staff that were not familiar with the disease to determine if outbreaks in their area met the case definition.

Results

This survey is the first epidemiological survey that has been conducted in the field of fish health in Indonesia. The survey was very successful, not only in terms of the high response (90 percent of questionnaires returned), but also in terms of developing better communication and networking between the central and district levels.

Population at risk: Based on the survey results, the distribution of the population at risk (i.e. koi and common carp) is shown on the map given in Figure 1.

Progression and geographic distribution of the disease: There are arguments among scientists on when the first KHV outbreak occurred in Indonesia. This survey was designed to address this issue. The results show that the outbreak first occurred at Blitar, East Java in March 2003 and then spread to Subang, West Java (Figure 2.). The geographic distribution of KHV in Indonesia as of February 2003 is illustrated in Figure 3. The red colour indicates the districts affected by disease.

SURVEY CONCLUSIONS

This is the first epidemiological survey that has been conducted in the field of fish health in Indonesia. The communication established during the survey should lead to better communication and cooperation among institutions in the central and district level in the future. Networking with key districts should be maintained and further developed through regular communication and sharing of information on fish health matters. Finally, 90 percent (315 out of 353) of the survey questionnaires were returned. From the survey, it was found that the disease has infected most of Java, Bali, Lampung, Bengkulu and South Sumatra, as well as making incursions into Kalimantan and Sulawesi. Nationally, 31 percent of the districts culturing susceptible species (common and koi carps) reported the presence of KHV.

Patterns of local and long-distance spread were further assessed by a district (kabupaten) level national survey. The survey found that there was gradual local spread from numerous foci of infection, as well as occasional long-distance spread, initially within Java, but also to other islands. It is hypothesised that the long-distance spread is mainly associated with the transport of the high-value ornamental koi carp, while local spread is through water and local transport of common carp for human consumption.

CLINICAL ASPECTS

Infected fish were lethargic, showed loss of balance and gasped for air. Some dead fish had sloughing off the epithelium with loss of mucus and rough appearance of the skin, darkened skin or showed blister-like lesions on the skin and haemorrhages of the operculae, fins and abdomen. However, the most common clinical sign was gill damage seen as whitish coloration, white patches or severe necrosis (Figure 4).

FIGURE 1
Map showiing the distribution of common (red) and koi (blue) carp production areas in Indonesia. Pale grey areas indicate no data, dark grey indicates no production (source: Cameron, 2003; Rukyani, 2003).

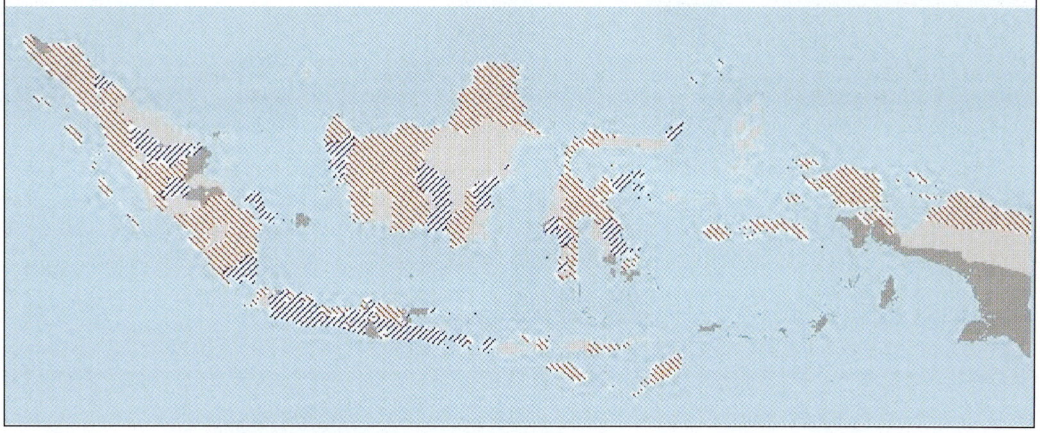

FIGURE 2
Map of the KHV outbreak during its first occurrence at Blitar (koi) and Subang (common carp) in March 2002. Pale grey areas indicate no data, green areas indicate no reported KHV, red areas have reported KHV in either common or koi carp (source: Cameron, 2003; Rukyani, 2003)

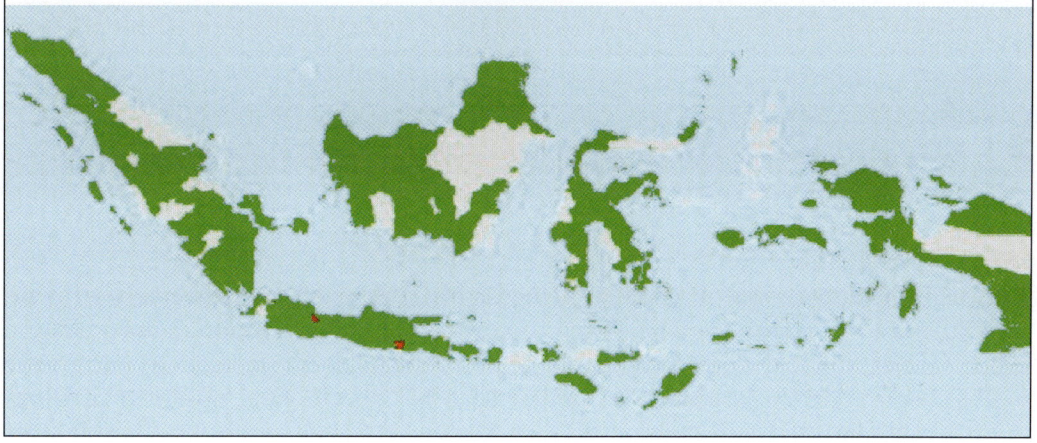

FIGURE 3
Map showing the geographic distribution of reported KHV in Indonesia as of February 2003. Pale grey areas indicate no data, green areas indicate no reported KHV, red areas have reported KHV in either common or koi carp (source: Cameron, 2003; Rukyani, 2003)

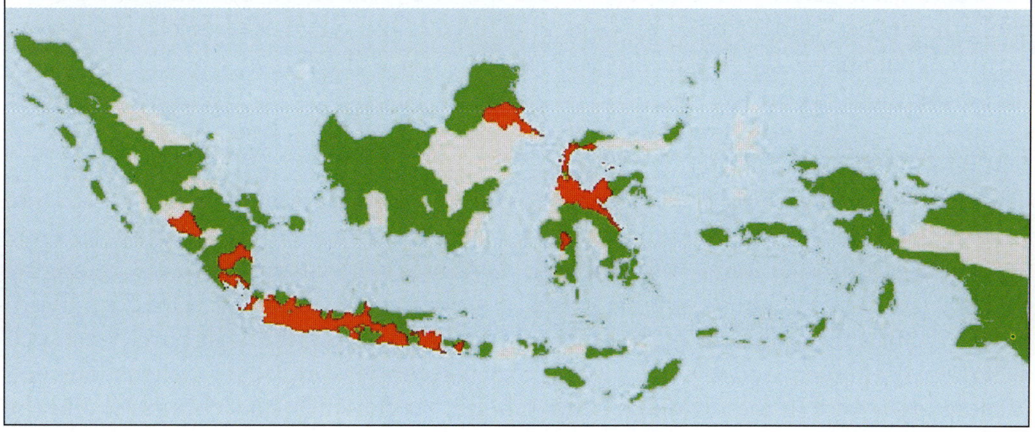

FIGURE 4
Diseased fish showing typical clinical signs – gill damage such as whitish gills (A) and severe gill necrosis (B). Some fish also showed blister-like lesions on the skin and white patches on the gills (C).

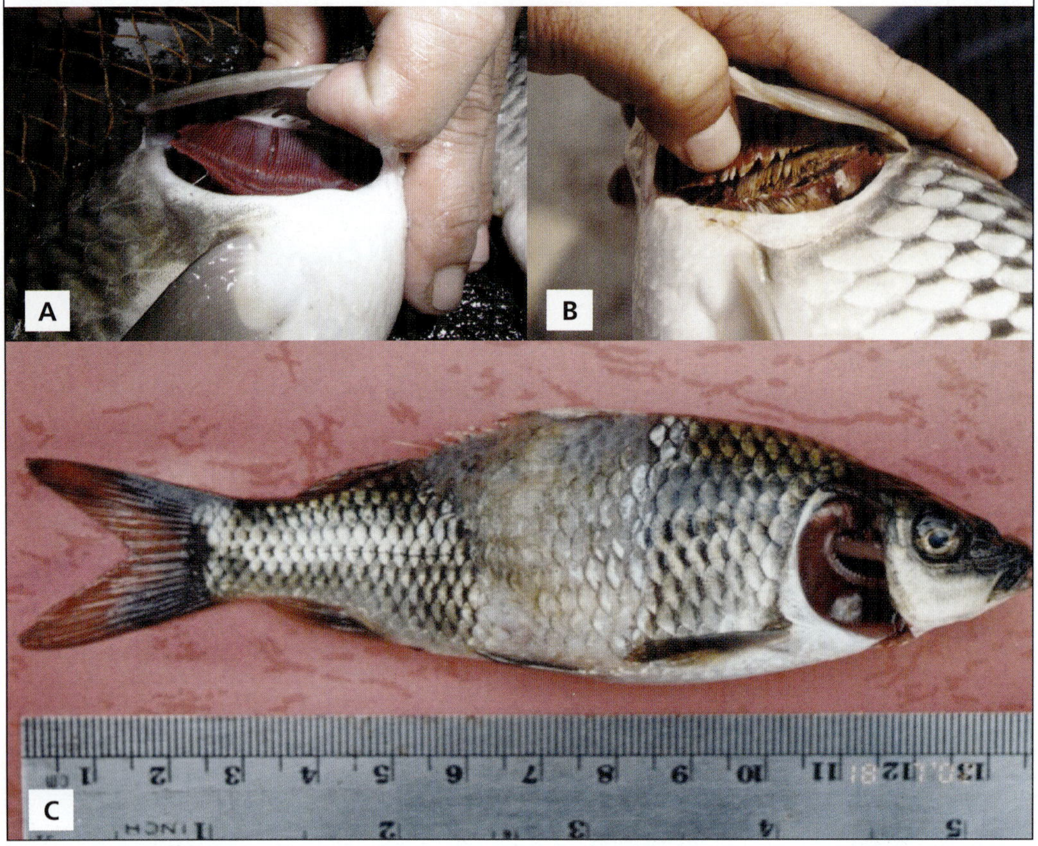

SPECIES AFFECTED

Although the disease was observed as being highly contagious and extremely virulent, morbidity and mortality were restricted to koi and common carp populations. Several other species stocked within the same ponds remained completely asymptomatic to the disease. Co-culture with a number of other species was observed in Blitar (with tilapia and gouramy) and in Cirata Reservoir (which utilizes a double cage system using carp and tilapia), and in all cases only carp were affected by the disease. However, it is not known yet whether the fish harbour the virus and act as carriers. Screening of other cultured and wild fishes such as tilapia, giant gouramy, catfish and Siam catfish, collected from the same cage, pond or canal of surrounding farms showed PCR negative results against KHV. The fish were tested with single step PCR using the primer set developed by Gray *et al.* (2002) and Gilad *et al.* (2002). However, further screening of the fish using double step PCR will confirm whether the fish is harboring the virus or not.

SOCIO-ECONOMIC IMPACT

The first report regarding the economic losses due to the outbreak was made by the head of the Association of Ornamental Fish Culture of Blitar Regency, East Java. They reported that in Blitar alone, the outbreak destroyed high quality koi carp belonging to 5 000 fish farmers with economic losses of more than Rp. 5 billion (US$0.5 million) within the first three months of the outbreak. As of July 2002, the Task Force estimated that the loss of revenue to the sector and the socio-economic impact to the rural farming communities were in the region of US$5 million. As the outbreaks continued and the disease spread to new areas, the socio-economic impact escalated. The Directorate of Fish Health and Environment (DFHE) estimated that as of December 2002 and 2003, losses due to KHV were US$ 10 million and US$15 million, respectively (Sunarto *et al.*, 2004).

PUBLIC HEALTH

There has been a great deal of local apprehension as to the consequences of consuming diseased fish. This is particularly affected by the fact that the some of the diseased fish showed blister-like lesions (Figure 4) and the word "herpes", which is associated with herpes virus in humans. There is however, no scientific evidence that the disease causes any human illness. In some outbreaks, large volumes of affected fish were sold or given away to people living in the local area for consumption, and there have so far been no reports of ill effects as a result of this. The government has conducted campaigns to eat carp. Fortunately, the Indonesian community has the habit of eating cooked fish, either fried or steamed.

AETIOLOGY

Screening for parasites, fungi and bacteria showed multiple infections on affected fish. *Dactylogyrus* sp., *Trichodina* sp., *Ichthyophthyrius multifiliis* and *Argulus* sp. were found on some debilitated fish. *Flexibacter columnaris* and *Aeromonas hydrophila* were isolated from necrotic gill filaments and skin ulcers of affected fish, respectively. *Saprolegnia* sp. and *Achyla* sp. were found in some fish showing blister-like lesions. All these species are suspected to be endemic in Indonesia and can be found in unaffected fish, so are unlikely to play a central role in the development of the disease. Attempts have been made to treat the infected fish with potassium permanganate and antibiotics (enrofloxacin, erythromycin, amoxicylin and oxytetracycline), but with no success.

At the beginning of these outbreaks, many causative factors were proposed, including water pollution, contaminated feed and bacterial infection. An infectivity trial was then conducted to elucidate the causative agent of the outbreak. Cohabitation of diseased fish with healthy common carp resulted in 100 percent mortality within an 8-day period. Experimental infections with 0.45 m-filtered homogenates resulted in 70 percent mortality during a 14-day period. Similar clinical signs (i.e. gill necrosis) were observed in both groups in the cohabitation test and injection of filtrate homogenate test.

PCR detection of KHV naturally diseased fish showed that some affected common carp produced a single band 290 base pair (bp) (Gray *et al.*, 2002) or 484 bp (Gilad *et al.*, 2003) in size, that would be expected if KHV DNA was present. However, other common carp collected from the same pond gave negative results. Partial DNA sequencing of the 484 bp amplicon revealed that the DNA sequence of KHV from Indonesia has high similarity (99.65 percent) with the DNA sequence of KHV from the United States. Nucleotide sequences of the three regions (KHV9/5 primer set amplicon, SphI-5 primer set amplicon, and thymidine kinase) of KHV DNA from Indonesia, Japan and Taiwan were identical (Ito *et al.*, 2004).

Virus isolation was attempted onto the KF-1 cell line, the cell line most appropriate for the isolation of KHV, as well as onto GP, EPC, BB, BF-2, DT and SSN-1, but did not result in any observable cytopathic effects (CPE). However, these negative results may be caused by inappropriate sample preparation. The samples were collected in various infected farms, brought to the laboratory and processed prior sending to Intervet Singapore, AAHRI (Thailand) and the University of California at Davis (United States). These extracts had arrived in the laboratories after several days of shipping and no refrigeration. Thus, it would not be surprising that no viral agents could be isolated.

However, based on the history, clinical signs, epidemiological features, histopathological changes, results of experimental infection, PCR detection of naturally and experimentally diseased fish, and analysis of DNA sequence, it is confirmed that KHV involved in this serious outbreak.

ENVIRONMENTAL FACTORS

Most of the outbreaks occurred when infected fish were introduced to non-infected fish, farms or areas. The heavy rain prior to the initial outbreak indicated the possibility of an environmental triggering factor, such as water temperature. Another environmental factor that may trigger outbreaks is stress caused by, for example, high stocking density and low water quality. However, research is needed to elucidate the environmental and other factors that trigger outbreaks.

DIAGNOSTIC METHODS

Appropriate diagnosis of KHV is important to avoid confusion with other diseases in carp. The haemorrhage and blister-like lesions seen in diseased fish may lead to a misdiagnosis as *Aeromonas hydrophila* infection. *Flexibacter columnaris* also causes gill necrosis. In fact these two bacteria were also found in the infected carp during the episode of mass mortality. Therefore, a case definition was established as an important step in the disease investigation in order to determine whether or not an individual fish, pond or tank is suffering from the disease. The case definition was used to minimize misdiagnosis. In the case of KHV, the case definition used was high mortality in koi or common carp, in which the fish shows gill damage, with or without other clinical signs.

Clinical signs and gross pathology

Infected fish were lethargic, showed loss of balance and gasped for air. Common gross signs included sloughing off the epithelium with loss of mucus and a rough appearance of the skin, haemorrhages of operculae, fins and abdomen, and severe gill damage. Some diseased fish showed a blister-like lesion on the skin, so called "penyakit melepuh" in the Indonesian language. As the outbreak continued, various clinical signs were observed or reported; however, the only consistent clinical sign was severe gill necrosis. Therefore, this pathognomonic clinical sign was used to establish a presumptive diagnosis against KHV (diagnosis level 1).

Histopathology

Although histopathological changes due to KHV were not obvious in most of the diseased fish, some diseased fish showed consistent findings with various lesions. Acute dermatitis with bacterial colonies occurred on the skin. Branchitis and numerous parasites including protozoans and metazoans, and bacterial colonies were present on the gills. Occasionally, intranuclear amphophilic inclusion bodies with peripheral chromatin margination were observed within the gill's epithelium. Similar inclusions were also observed within the kidney tubular epithelium accompanied by nephrocalcinosis. The interrenal extramedullary hematopoetic tissue showed haemorrhage or haemosiderosis. Epicarditis, myocarditis and endocarditis were demonstrated in the heart. Multifoci of chronic pancreatitis with acinar cell necrosis were present in the pancreas. The liver displayed various types of degeneration such as hydrophic degeneration and fatty change. Occasionally, vasculitis and bile stases were observed within the sinusoid of the liver. The spleen was congested and displayed the occurrence of perivascular amyloidosis (diagnosis level 2).

PCR detection

PCR detection of KHV was carried out using specific primers set developed by Gray *et al.* (2002) and Gilad *et al.* (2002). Nine laboratories in Sumatera, Java and Sulawesi have routinely used PCR assay for confirmative diagnosis against KHV (diagnosis level 3). However, mixed results were occasionally found by using this molecular-based method. As the detection of fish pathogens in Indonesia using PCR assay is still in its early development, standardized methods and harmonization of PCR application is urgently needed to ensure high quality results.

CONTROL MEASURES

The recent increase in live-fish traffic is increasing the risk of introduction and spread of fish pathogens throughout the country. Past and recent disease outbreaks among cultured and wild fish have prompted the government to carry out a programme to control disease and protect fishery resources.

Attempts to control the outbreak at the farm level have also been made. These efforts include curative approach (treatment by using of antibiotics, disinfectants and other pharmaceuticals) and a preventive approach (by quarantine measures, biosecurity, vaccination and good management practices (GMPs)).

Treatment

No drugs or other pharmaceuticals have been found to be effective in combating the disease. Attempts have been made to treat the infected fish with antibiotics, but without success. Some fish farmers have tried to use potassium permanganate (PK) for treatment. However, PK tends to irritate the gills, leading to a surging mortality up to 80-95 percent of affected fish. Since other pathogens such as parasites, fungi and bacteria were also found in the diseased fish, antibiotics and disinfectants were used to treat these secondary infections. Enrofloxacine (5-10 ppm) was used to treat secondary bacterial infection. Dyvon (dichlorphos) at 1-5 ppm and benzalkonium chloride (BKC) at one drop/100 L were used to treat *Argulus* and other parasitic infections.

Quarantine

Since most outbreaks occur after the introduction of new infected fish, it is obvious that the disease is spread by direct contact. Therefore, the effective way to protect a non-infected area from being infected with the disease is by preventing the introduction of infected fish. It is recommended that all new fish be quarantined for at least two weeks, together with sentinel fish at a permissive water temperature between 18-28 °C.

Biosecurity

Most outbreaks occurred after the introduction of new fish from an infected area or through infection via contaminated equipment or water source. Therefore, the biosecurity concept may be applied to prevent or reduce the possibility of KHV infection. For areas where KHV is presently endemic, a prevention programme should include eradication and exclusion activities. Given that KHV also occurs in wild carp stocks, it can be difficult to control outbreaks in common waterbodies such as in floating netcages in lakes and in raceways in rivers. Although little is known about how the virus survives between the outbreaks, available evidence suggested that infections may persist in the susceptible fish population remaining at the site between crops. Accordingly, measures to eradicate the virus should include: removal of all fish (particularly all susceptible fish species) from ponds, reservoirs, and water canals prior to restocking, drying out and liming the ponds and disinfecting of contaminated equipment. Potassium permanganate (10 ppm), chlorine (200 ppm) and formalin (500–1 000 ppm) were commonly used as disinfectants. Once the virus has been eradicated from a site, it is important to prevent re-introduction. It is likely that infection is spread by affected fish, as well as by contaminated water and equipment. Ronen *et al.* (2003) reported that KHV remains active in the water for at least four hours. Accordingly, the following measures should be considered for the exclusion of the virus from fish farms: seed and broodstock should be KHV-free or be obtained from KHV-free areas, all wild carps must be rigorously excluded from farms in endemic areas, use only KHV-free water, either decontaminated or originating from KHV-free water sources, and equipment which may have been used at infected sites must be disinfected. These practices have been adopted and proved to be effective to prevent the outbreak in an isolated koi farm. However, they may not applicable for culture systems in open waters such as cage culture in lakes and raceway culture in rivers. In these systems, GMPs may be applied to reduce mass mortality due to KHV infection.

Good management practices

KHV now appears to be endemic in most areas of Indonesia where carp and koi are cultured including Java, Bali, Sumatera and Kalimantan. Emphasis should now be placed on learning how to manage the disease so that carp production in infected areas can be maintained (Arthur, 2003). There are scattered reports from fish farmers that GMPs can reduce the incidence of and mortality due to KHV infection in koi and carp culture. However, these reports need to be backed up with scientific data. The koi farmer association of Blitar Regency reported that although KHV is still found in their koi, the mortality due to KHV is very low. There is an area in Cirata Reservoir that managed to get free from the outbreak, even though sharing the same waterbody with other infected areas. Blitar and Cirata are the centers of production of koi and common carp, respectively. These two areas were badly affected by the outbreak in 2002. There are reports that transferring diseased fish from raceways to earthen ponds will decrease mortality and prevent further losses. It seems that this practice reduces the stocking density and provides stable water temperature, hence providing a better environment for the fish. Other farmers have reported that polyculture of common carp with other fish species such as tilapia and gouramy, also reduces the severity and frequency of KHV outbreak.

It is important that the general health, as well as the KHV status, of a susceptible fish population is monitored regularly during the grow-out period. High doses of vitamin C (500 mg/kg feed) were used to enhance fish immunity against infection. It is hypothesized that the disease outbreaks do not occur if the fish's defence mechanisms manage to contain low-intensity of KHV infection under low-stress culture conditions. Conversely, outbreaks may occur under stressful conditions. Therefore, avoiding stress factors such as high stocking density, fluctuating water temperature, low dissolved oxygen and improper handling of fish are essential to reduce the risk of outbreak. It is recommended to remove dead and moribund fish from the pond, as they are a good reservoir for the virus. Record keeping, epidemiological analysis and accurate diagnostic tools are essential for pond monitoring. To break the life cycle of KHV and to avoid re-occurrence of outbreaks in endemic areas, it is recommended to farm species that are resistant to KHV, such as tilapia, gouramy and catfish.

Vaccination

Attempts have been made to control outbreaks by using antibiotics and other drugs, but this has had no success. As KHV is an immunogenic virus, preventive measures a using vaccination programme would be effective to control the disease (Ronen *et al.*, 2003). A preliminary "vaccination trial" by temperature manipulation has been conducted in the Fish Health Research Laboratory (Gardenia *et al.*, 2004). The trial methods involved the cohabitation of healthy fish with sick fish at permissive temperature (26-28 °C) and their subsequent transfer to non-permissive temperature (32-35 °C). At thirty days post-exposure, the vaccinated fish were then challenged by cohabitation with sick fish. The results show that the vaccinated group has lower mortality (33 percent) compared with the control group (86 percent). Although beneficial to reduce the mortality of fish, this vaccination method involves a serious risk due to the use of live virus. Research on the development of inactivated vaccine is being conducted.

CONCLUSIONS

The NACA's Task Force findings revealed that an infectious agent is involved in the current outbreak. Epidemiological evidence and positive PCR findings from 82.5 percent (33/40) of the case samples indicated that the outbreak was most probably caused by KHV, despite the failure to isolate the virus, to observe the virus with electron microscopy and to find typical histopathological changes described in other cases of KHV. The disease was introduced into Indonesia through fish importation and spread to other areas within the country through fish movements. Since most of the episodes of mass mortality in koi and common carp occurred within a few weeks after the introduction of infected fish into disease-free areas, the responsible movement of live fish and quarantine of incoming fish seem to be a logical way to prevent the introduction and spread of the disease to new areas.

Although KHV is strongly suspected to be the cause of the outbreak, this has yet to be confirmed. Further research on the identification and confirmation of the disease is urgently needed. Other areas of research that need to be pursued include the development of standardized procedures for the detection of the virus, with emphasis on the detection of subclinical fish and potential carriers, if any. Research is also needed to identify environmental and predisposing factors and to analyze risk factors that trigger the outbreaks. Control strategy through the development of vaccines is another area of research that should be considered.

Despite the difficulties in the control of outbreaks in common waterbodies such as raceway culture in rivers and netcages in reservoirs and lakes, a vaccination programme, biosecurity measures and GMPs seem to provide alternative control strategies at the farm level. However, further research is needed to analyse the cost effectiveness of a vaccination programme in common carp and to identify the key components of biosecurity and GMPs that are effective to control KHV outbreaks. Although, the government has attempted to restrict the spread of the disease to new areas by issuing rules, regulations and technical guidelines, the disease is still spreading to new areas. Better law enforcement and improved public awareness are essential to ensure the proper implementation of the regulations and guidelines.

The Government of Indonesia still faces significant challenges in the implementation of emergency response to disease outbreak. Capacity building on emergency preparedness and response is needed to properly manage disease emergencies. The general approach would be the proper development and implementation of the National Strategy for Fish Health Management.

ACKNOWLEDGEMENTS

The authors wishes to thank NACA Task Force members Dr Somkiat Kanchanakhan and Dr Melba Bondad-Reantaso and FAO's national and international consultants Prof Mohamed Shariff, Dr Richard Arthur Mr Stuart Millar, Prof S.B. Prayitno, Dr Fachriyan H. Pasaribu and the late Dr Akhmad Rukyani for sharing their reports and findings before publication.

LITERATURE CITED

Arthur, J.R. 2003. *Fish health management for Indonesia.* Report of international consultant on legislation. Project TCP/INS/2905(A). Health Management in Freshwater Aquaculture 55 pp. FAO, Rome.

Cameron, A. 2002. *Report of an epidemiological investigation of a serious outbreak of disease amongst koi and common carp in Indonesia.* Report prepared for the Emergency Disease Control Task Force on a Serious Disease of Koi and Common Carps in Indonesia. 72 pp. NACA, Bangkok.

Cameron, A. 2003. *Report of international consultant in epidemiology.* Project TCP/INS/2905(A). Health Management in Freshwater Aquaculture 62 pp. FAO, Rome.

Crane, M., Sano, M. & Komar, C. 2004. Infection with koi herpesvirus – disease card. In: NACA/FAO. *Quarterly aquatic animal disease report (Asia and Pacific Region).* April-June 2004, 2004/2. pp. 43-47. Bangkok, NACA.

Gardenia, L., Sunarto, A., Koesharyani, I., Taukhid & Novita, H. 2004. *Immunogenic potency of koi herpesvirus in common carp*. Technical Report submitted to the Research Institute for Freshwater Fisheries. Bogor. 12 pp. (in Bahasa Indonesia)

Gilad, O., Yun, S., Adkison, M.A., Way, K., Willits, N.H., Bercovier, H. & Hedrick, R.P. 2003. Molecular comparison of isolates of an emerging fish pathogen, koi herpesvirus, and the effect of water temperature on mortality of experimentally infected koi. *J. Gen. Virol.*, 84: 2661-2668.

Gray, W.L., Mullis, L., LaPatra, S.E., Groff, J.M. & Goodwin, A. 2002. Detection of koi herpesvirus DNA in tissue of infected fish. *J. Fish Dis.*, 25: 171-178.

Hedrick, R.P., Gilad, O., Yun, S., Spangenberg, J.V., Marty, G.D., Nordhausen, R.W., Kebus, M.J., Bercovier, H. & Eldar, A. 2000. A herpesvirus associated with mass mortality of juvenile and adult koi, a strain of common carp. *J. Aquat. Anim. Health,* 12: 44-57.

Ito, T., Kurita, J., Miwa S., Yuasa, K., Hedrick, R.P., Engelsma, M., Haene, O., Chou, H.Y., Tung, M.C., Sunarto, A., Sano M. & Iida, T. 2004. *Outbreak of the koi herpesvirus infection in Japan*. Book of Abstracts, the 7th Asian Fisheries Forum, Penang, Malaysia, 30 November – 4 December 2004. p. 409.

Millar, S.D. 2003. *Report of international consultant in virology: first mission*. Project TCP/INS/2905(A). Health Management in Freshwater Aquaculture. 44 pp.FAO, Rome.

Millar, S.D. 2004. *Report of international consultant in virology: second mission*. Project TCP/INS/2905(A). Health Management in Freshwater Aquaculture. 45 pp. FAO, Rome.

NACA. 2002. *Report of Emergency disease control task force on a serious disease of koi and common carps in Indonesia*. 24 pp.NACA, Bangkok.

Pasaribu, F.H. 2004. *Report of national consultant in fish health management*. Project TCP/INS/2905(A). Health Management in Freshwater Aquaculture. 38 pp. FAO, Rome.

Prayitno, S.B. 2003. *Legislation on fish health management: report of national consultant in legislation*. TCP/INS/2905(A). Health Management in Freshwater Aquaculture. 38 pp. FAO, Rome.

Ronen, A., Perelberg, A., Abramowitz, J., Hutoran, M., Tinman, S., Bejerano, I., Steinitz, M. & Kotler, M. 2003. Efficient vaccine against the virus causing a lethal disease in cultured *Cyprinus carpio. Vaccine*, 21: 4677-4684.

Rukyani, A. 2002. *Koi herpesvirus in Indonesia: suspicion*. Report of KHV epidemic to OIE (available at www.oie.int).

Rukyani, A. 2003. *Report of national consultant in epidemiology*. Project TCP/INS/2905(A). Health Management in Freshwater Aquaculture. 54 pp. FAO, Rome.

Shariff, M. 2004. *Fish health management for Indonesia: report of international consultant in fish health management*. Project TCP/INS/2905(A). Health Management in Freshwater Aquaculture. 47 pp. FAO, Rome.

Sunarto, A. 2004. *Report of national consultant in virology*. Project TCP/INS/2905(A). Health Management in Freshwater Aquaculture 72 pp. FAO, Rome.

Sunarto, A., Rukyani, A., Cameron, A., Bondad-Reantaso, M. & Subasinghe, R. 2004. *Outbreak of disease causing mass mortality in koi and common carp* (Cyprinus carpio*) in Indonesia*. Book of Abstracts, the International Workshop on Koi Herpesvirus, London, England, 12-13 February 2004. p. 12.

Sunarto, A., Rukyani A. & Itami, T. 2004. *Indonesian experience on the outbreak of koi herpesvirus in koi and carp* (Cyprinus carpio*)*. Bull. Japan Fish. Res. Agency, Supp. 2: 12-19. (in press)

Sunarto, A., Taukhid, Rukyani, A., Koesharyani, I., Supriyadi, H., Gardenia, L., Huminto, H., Agungpriyono, D.R., Pasaribu, F.H., Widodo, Herdikiawan, D., Rukmono, D. & Prayitno, S.B. 2002. *Field investigations on a serious disease outbreak among koi and common carp* (Cyprinus carpio) *in Indonesia*. Diseases in Asian Aquaculture V. (in press).

Yuasa, K., Panigoro, N., Bahnan, M., Kholidin, E.B., Koesharyani, I. & Hatai, K. 2004. *Outbreak of KHV infection in common carp in Sumatera, Indonesia*. Book of Abstracts, 7th Asian Fisheries Forum, 30 November – 4 December 2004, Penang, Malaysia. p. 133.

Responses to Koi Herpes Virus (KHV) outbreaks in Japan

Takaji Iida, Motohiko Sano, Takafumi Ito, Jun Kurita, Kei Yuasa and Satoshi Miwa
Aquatic Animal Health Division
National Research Institute of Aquaculture (NRIA)
Fisheries Research Agency
Nansei, Mie 516-0193, Japan

Iida, T., Sano, M., Ito, T., Kurita, J., Yuasa, K. & Miwa, S. 2005. Responses to Koi herpes virus (KHV) outbreaks in Japan. 107–111. In: Subasinghe, R.P.; Arthur, J.R. (eds.). Regional workshop on preparedness and response to aquatic animal health emergencies in Asia. Jakarta, Indonesia, 21–23 September 2004. *FAO Fisheries Proceedings*. No. 4. Rome, FAO. 2005. 178p.

ABSTRACT

The mass mortality among common carp (*Cyprinus carpio*) caused by Koi herpes virus (KHV) infection occurred in early October 2003 in Japan. KHV infection has been diagnosed in accordance with a guideline for the disease, and confirmation is based on the results of the polymerase cahin reaction (PCR) examinations. The local authorities have officially declared that the movement of KHV-affected common carp and koi is prohibited and have ordered the destruction of KHV-affected common carp and koi under the Law to Ensure Sustainable Aquaculture Production.

INTRODUCTION

Koi herpes virus (KHV) is highly contagious and virulent in common carp and koi (*Cyprinus carpio*). KHV infection first occurred in 2003 in Japan, and has caused heavy damage to common carp culture. In this report, we present responses to the KHV outbreak and the current status of the disease in Japan.

DIAGNOSTIC SYSTEM FOR EXOTIC DISEASES AND KOI HERPES VIRUS DISEASE

In Japan, some exotic diseases are designated as "Specific Diseases" in the Law to Ensure Sustainable Aquaculture Production (Law No. 51, 1999). This designation is used for exotic diseases such as spring viraemia of carp (SVC) and viral haemorrhagic septicemia (VHS) of salmonid fish that have the potential to devastate the aquaculture industry in Japan. For such diseases, protective guidelines are established. The guidelines provide etiological information, diagnostic procedures, and description of the clinical signs and other important characteristics of the disease. Laboratory diagnoses of the diseases should be conducted in accordance with these guidelines.

A newly isolated herpes virus, Koi herpes virus (KHV), was first reported as a pathogen causing of mass mortality of common and ornamental (koi) carp cultured in Israel and the United States in 1998 (Hedrick *et al.*, 2000). In Japan, no such mass mortality of cultured carp had been reported, and KHV had not been detected by a survey conducted in Niigata Prefecture (Amita *et al.*, 2002). It has been shown that

FIGURE 1
Inspection chart for KHV infection according to the Japanese guidelines

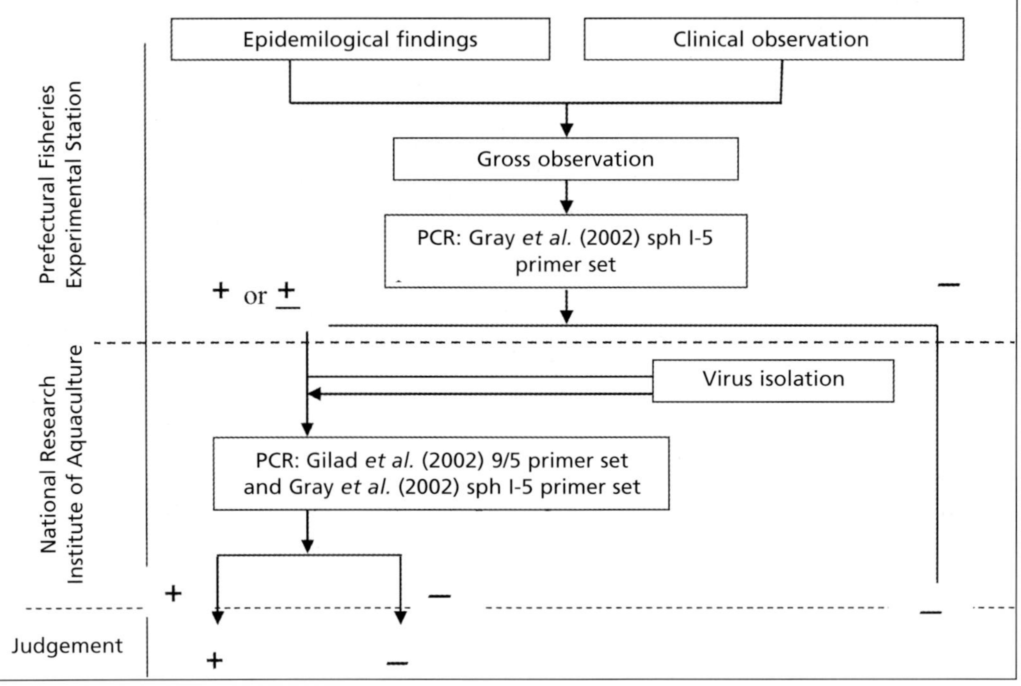

KHV is highly contagious and virulent in juvenile and adult carp (Hedrick *et al.*, 2000, Perelberg *et al.*, 2003). Therefore, on 30 June 2003 KHV infection was added to "Specific Diseases" in the Law, and an inspection chart was established in the guidelines (Fig. 1).

According to the chart, the Prefectural Fisheries Experimental Stations first conduct epizootic and routine clinical examination on diseased fish. The most important epizootilogical aspects of KHV disease are that it only affects common and koi carp (*C. carpio*) and it occurs, remarkably, at temperatures from 18 to 28 °C (Hedrick *et al.*, 2000; Gilad *et al.*, 2003). Therefore, the water temperature and affected species of fish should be determined during a field examination. Few external signs are usually visible, but pale and necrotic gills are frequently evident. Infections by *Flavobacterium columnare* (=*Flexibacter columnaris*) and some protozoan parasites such as *Chilodonella* and *Trichodina* are sometimes found on necrotic gill lesions, easily leading to misdiagnoses.

If any doubt remains as to the presence of KHV infection, a polymerase chain reaction (PCR) test can be used to detect KHV DNA in the tissues of fish, usually gills. The PCR method described by Gray *et al.* (2002) was adopted in the inspection chart as the primary examination to be conducted by the Prefectural Fisheries Experimental Stations. When there is some evidence of a positive reaction in the PCR test for KHV, the sample is sent to the National Research Institute of Aquaculture (NRIA) for further examination by the PCR methods of both Gilad *et al.* (2002) and Gray *et al.* (2002) for confirmation. Viral isolation is also attempted using KF-1 cell line (Hedrick *et al.*, 2000). Because of the difficulty of isolating the virus in the cell line, the results of the isolation trial are considered supplementary data. Confirmation is based on the results of the PCR examinations.

OCCURRENCE OF KHV INFECTION IN JAPAN AND PRACTICAL DIAGNOSIS OF THE DISEASE

The mass mortality among common carp cultured in net-pens at Lake Kasumigaura, Ibaraki Prefecture, central Japan, began in early October 2003 (Fig. 2). At the time, the water temperature of the lake was 16-18 °C. The fish swam lethargically near the water surface. No marked external signs were observed in the most affected fish, but a whitish mucous-like substance on the body surface, redness of the fins and body, fin rot, and discoloration of the gills with some necrosis were sometimes noticed. The mortality was over 60 percent in the most severe cases, especially in larger carp (those in older than 2-years-old). The losses of the cultured carp were estimated to be 660 metric tonnes in early November and reached approximately 1 200 tonnes by mid-November, which is approximately one quarter of the annual production of the lake.

FIGURE 2

Mass mortality of common carp caused by KHV at Lake Kasumigaura

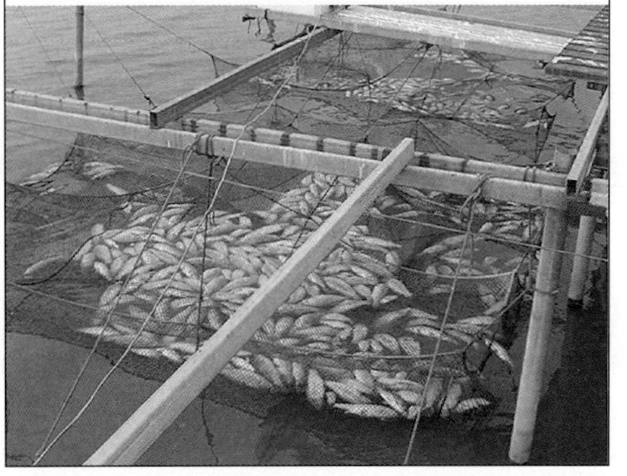

External parasites, such as *Chilodonella*, *Trichodina* and *Gyrodactylus*, were sometimes seen on the necrotic gill tissues of the affected fish. Marked histopathological changes were observed in the gill of the diseased carp (Fig. 3). The secondary lamellae were often fused with hyperplastic branchial epithelium where cell necrosis or the infiltration of lymphocytes was often observed. Congestion and hemorrhage were sometimes observed. In some cases, the branchial tissues were severely degraded and numerous bacteria were seen in the lesions. These histopathological changes are similar to those seen in the previous reports of KHV infection (Hedrick *et al.*, 2000; Tu *et al.*, 2004). Unlike with the previous report of Hedrick *et al.* (2000), nuclear changes characterized by hypertrophy and margination of chromatin were rarely observed. No bacteria dominantly isolated from the kidney of affected fish were observed on trypticase soy agar (TSA). The PCR for KHV amplified specific bands by the methods of Gray *et al.* (2002) and Gilad *et al.* (2002) (Fig. 4). Direct sequence of the amplicon by the primer set of Gray *et al.* (2002) corresponded completely with the GenBank accession no. AY568951, and that by the primer set of Gilad *et al.* (2002) showed 99 percent matching to AF411803.

FIGURE 3

A tissue section of the gill from affected common carp cultured at Lake Kasumigaura. Arrowheads indicate secondary lamellae. H&E stain

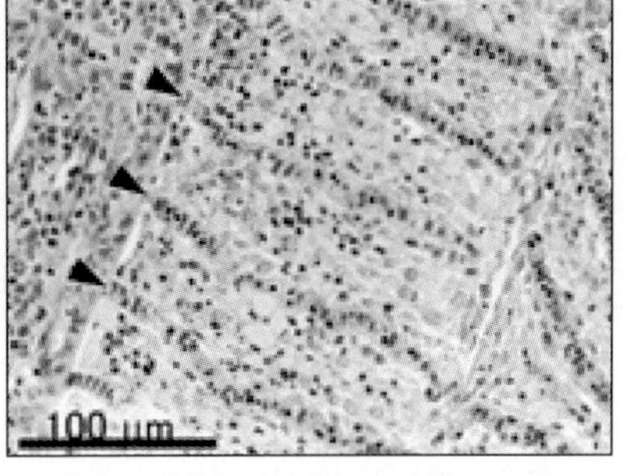

FIGURE 4

Gel electrophoresis of the products (292bp) amplified with the primer set sph I-5 of Gray et al. (2002) from the extracted sample of gill and kidney of affected fish cultured in Lake Kasumigaura. Pc: positive control, Nc: negative control. 1 percent agarose gel stained with ethidium bromide

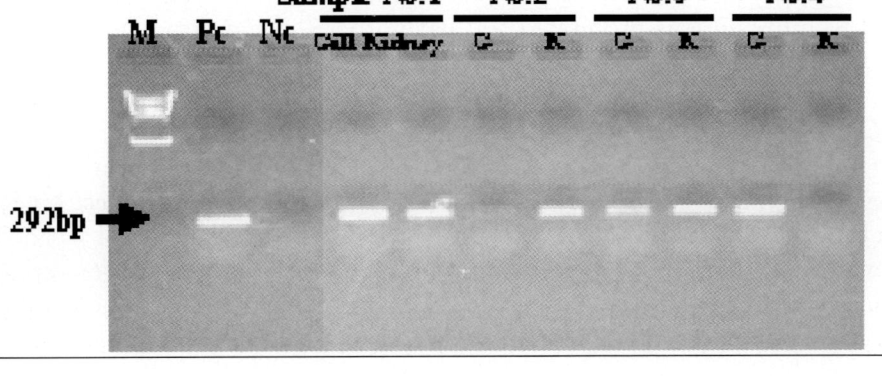

Properly, on 2 November 2003, the Ministry of Agriculture, Forestry and Fisheries of Japan officially announced the first occurrence of the disease in Japan. It was also reported to the Office International des Épizooties (OIE). According to the Law, the Governor of Ibaraki Prefecture officially prohibited the movement of cultured carp from the lake, and ultimately ordered that all carp cultured in the lake were to be destroyed by the end of March 2004.

OTHER EVIDENCE OF KHV BEFORE THE OUTBREAK AT LAKE KASUMIGAURA

Independently of the KHV outbreak at Lake Kasumigaura, a massive loss in excess of 10 000 carp occurred in the rivers and a lake in Okayama Prefecture, western part of Japan, in late May to mid-July 2003. In November 2003, the NRIA detected KHV DNA by PCR in the samples of the diseased fish stored in a freezer. This demonstrates that KHV had been introduced into Japan by May before the Lake Kasumigaura outbreak.

THE SPREAD OF KHV IN JAPAN

The KHV-infected common carp cultured in Lake Kasumigaura had been transferred to other areas in Japan before the first detection of the KHV DNA by PCR, and therefore, the virus had spread as a result. In warm-water facilities such as those used for indoor game fishing, some mortality of carp was recorded. However, in many cases KHV was detected in carp with no mortality; this was attributed to the fact that the water temperature was gradually decreasing at the time. By the end of 2003, the NRIA has accepted 529 individuals of 87 cases to be diagnosed, and KHV-infected carp were found in 23 out of 47 prefectures in Japan.

No occurrence of the disease was reported during the winter period. However, as the water temperature increased in the spring of 2004, KHV reappeared in the area where the disease had been recorded and also in new places. In many of the facilities that experienced outbreaks of KHV infection during the previous season, the disease has not been observed so far this year. In these places, all the carp, as well as other fish species, were removed and the facilities were properly treated with disinfectants after the outbreaks. By the end of July 2004, KHV infections have been reported in 39 prefectures in Japan.

OFFICIAL CONTROL MEASURES IN JAPAN

The Government of Japan has conducted surveillance throughout the country and has controlled the movement of common and koi carp through local governments in accordance with the advice issued by the Technical Commission for KHV Disease. The commission is comprised of experts in fish pathology and representatives from the Prefectural Fisheries Experimental Stations.

Each local government has inspected common and koi carp within its territory for signs of infection and has checked for the presence or absence of KHV infection using a PCR test. The local authorities of the KHV-affected area have officially declared that the movement of common carp and koi carp from the area where KHV has been confirmed to other areas is prohibited and have ordered the destruction of common and koi carp in the area under the Law.

RESEARCH ACTIVITIES ON KHV AT NRIA

The NRIA and other research groups, including universities and the Southeast Asian Fisheries Development Center (SEAFDEC) have begun a research project on KHV infection funded by the Ministry of Agriculture, Forestry and Fisheries of Japan. This project, which will have a duration of three years, consists of three major activities: 1) molecular virology and histopathology of KHV infection, including viral behavior in infected fish at different temperatures and a carrier state; 2) development and evaluation of diagnostic tools such as a loop-mediated isothermal amplification (LAMP) method and immunocytochemistry; and 3) measures to control infection, including the efficacy of disinfectants, vaccination and elevation of the rearing water temperature. The results could contribute for controlling KHV infections in both wild and cultured populations of carp.

ACKNOWLEDGEMENTS

We are grateful to Prof. Ronald P. Hedrick of the University of California, Davis, the United States, for his invaluable suggestions and for providing the KF-1 cell line and a KHV isolate. We thank the Ibaraki Prefectural Experimental Station and Okayama Prefectural Experimental Station for providing the sample fish, and the staff of the Aquatic Animal Health Division, National Research Institute of Aquaculture for running diagnoses of KHV infection.

LITERATURE CITED

Amita K., Oe, M., Matoyama, H., Yamaguchi, N. & Fukuda, H. 2002. A survey of Koi herpes virus and carp edema virus in colorcarp cultured in Niigata Prefecture, Japan. *Fish Pathol.*, 37: 197-198.

Gilad O., Yun, S., Andree, K.B., Adkison, M.A., Way, K., Willits, N.H., Bercovier, H. & Hedrick, R.P. 2003. Molecular comparison of isolates of an emerging fish pathogen, Koi herpes virus, and the effect of water temperature on mortality of experimentally infected koi. *J. Gen. Virol.*, 84: 2661-2668.

Gilad O., Yun, S., Andree, K.B., Adkison, M.A., Zlotkin, A., Bercovier, H., Eldar, A. & Hedrick, R.P. 2002. Initial characteristics of Koi herpes virus and development of a polymerase chain reaction assay to detect the virus in koi, *Cyprinus carpio koi. Dis. Aquat. Org.*, 48: 101-108.

Gray, W.L., Mullis, L., LaPatra, S.E., Groff, J.M. & Goodwin, A. 2002. Detection of Koi herpes virus DNA in tissues of infected fish. *J. Fish Dis.*, 25: 171-178.

Hedrick, R.P., Gilad, O., Yun, S., Spangenberg, J.V., Marty, G.D., Nordhausen, R.W., Kebus, M.J., Bercovier, H. & Eldar, A. 2000. A herpes virus associated with mass mortality of juvenile and adult koi, a strain of common carp. *J. Aquat. Anim. Health*, 12: 44-57.

Perelberg, A., Smirnov, M., Hutoran, M., Diamant, A., Bejerano, Y. & Kotler, M. 2003. Epidemiological description of a new viral disease afflicting cultured *Cyprinus carpio* in Israel. *Israeli J. Aquacult. – Bamidgeh*, 55: 5-12.

Tu, C., Weng, M.-C., Shiau, J.-R. & Lin, S.-Y. 2004. Detection of Koi herpes virus in koi *Cyprinus carpio* in Taiwan. *Fish Pathol.*, 39: 109-110.

Preparedness and response to aquatic disease emergencies: the relevance and role of the private sector

Daniel F. Fegan
Alltech Inc.
Bangkok, Thailand
dfegan@alltech.com

Fegan, D.F. 2005. Preparedness and response to aquatic disease emergencies: the relevance and role of the private sector. 113–121. In: Subasinghe, R.P.; Arthur, J.R. (eds.). Regional workshop on preparedness and response to aquatic animal health emergencies in Asia. Jakarta, Indonesia, 21–23 September 2004. *FAO Fisheries Proceedings*. No. 4. Rome, FAO. 2005. 178p.

ABSTRACT

The private sector is often the most seriously impacted in disease emergencies and yet, paradoxically, is frequently overlooked in the planning and development of contingency plans and responses to aquatic disease emergencies. While it is true that some disease problems can be self-inflicted, this is most often due to lack of an adequate knowledge or appreciation of the disease risks associated with a particular activity. This is exacerbated by the multi-functional structure of the private sector, where different stakeholders may have drastically different motivations and attitudes to risk. Preparation of contingency plans and disease responses without adequate consideration and communication with the different private-sector stakeholders will usually result in severe problems in their implementation. This paper looks at the structure and role of the various private-sector stakeholders in the aquaculture industry and uses two shrimp disease case studies – yellowhead and white spot diseases in Thailand and “loose shell syndrome” in India – to illustrate how the public and private sectors can effectively collaborate in a structured approach to aquatic animal disease emergencies.

INTRODUCTION

Most aquaculture activities in Asia, and around the world, are conducted by the private (i.e. non-governmental) sector. These range in size and complexity from the growth of trapped fish in small ponds for household or local consumption to large conglomerates breeding and growing expensive seafood items for export, and everything in between. Governments, in general, tend to play a facilitating role (through technology transfer and extension), a regulatory role or some combination of the two. There is also a tendency of governments in Asia to adopt a largely “laissez faire” attitude, either due to the importance of private-sector aquaculture in local and national economies (including as a source of food security), or as a result of a lack of sufficient resources to manage private-sector aquaculture activities. Only recently have some governments begun to regulate more closely private-sector aquaculture, often as a result of external pressures such as disease, market pressure and/or food safety concerns. In general, however, private-sector aquaculture is generally left to develop on its own, except where obvious resource conflicts lead to the need for regulatory agencies to take action. By the same token, it is the same private sector that suffers in the event of aquatic disease emergencies through loss of stock, food, income and livelihood.

Although there are some examples of large conglomerates involved in aquaculture, usually for high-value species, this is far from common. Asian aquaculture is largely "small-scale", even in high-value species such as shrimp, individual farmers owning a few small ponds or cages. Thus, the typical scenario in most countries is of large numbers of small farms, each owned and operated independently. This type of development also leads to constraints in effective government regulation, since the resources and logistics required to contend with large numbers of small farms, many of which may be geographically remote, are often beyond the capacity of state agencies.

THE STAKEHOLDERS

However, the farming sector represents only one group in the complex web of interconnected activities that comprise the private sector in aquaculture. If we consider the various stakeholders that have a direct stake in aquaculture production (i.e. where the aquaculture product is handled), the picture becomes more complex (Figure 1). In the direct production chain for example, we may have a differentiation between breeders, hatcheries, nurseries or fry producers and farmers. Then there are numerous trading links. Any or all of these producers may sell their products through wholesalers, brokers, shippers or exporters to other producers, distributors, processors, retailers or end users. This may involve purely local movements, or there may be a large geographic distribution. Live fish may be transported between different islands as fry or fingerlings, shrimp postlarvae are typically transported large distances and live fish may be shipped to distant markets. The latter is especially important in Asia given the traditional preference for buying live, or at least fresh, seafood.

Added to this network of direct stakeholders, are a few indirect stakeholders. The most important of these are feed manufacturers, feed suppliers and suppliers of various goods and equipment used by producers. In some countries, there is also a network of private advisors or consultants and laboratories offering services and advice to producers. Although not involved in the day-to-day running of aquaculture operations, such advisory service providers can play an important and influential role in the producers' decision-making.

FIGURE 1
Typical network of direct stakeholders in aquaculture

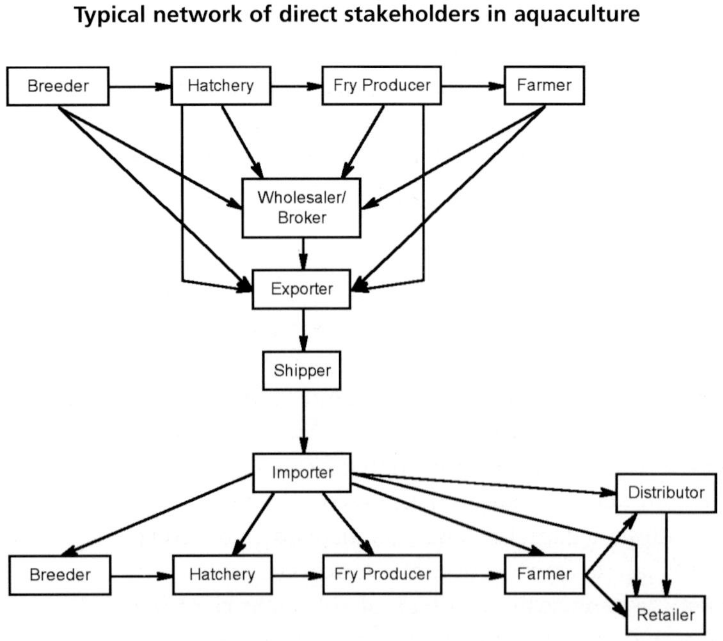

With such a complex network of stakeholders, it is interesting to consider what factors drive the decision-making process. Obviously, with such a large number of players and a diverse range of interests, there is seldom any hierarchical management structure that will influence the entire process. Rather, the development of private-sector aquaculture (i.e. what the private sector "does") is the net result of decisions made in the self-interest of all of the stakeholders involved – both direct (farmers and producers) and indirect (suppliers and consultants). In each of these groups, self-interest may result in some contradictions. Feed companies want to sell more feed, and thus there is a pressure to intensify production and increase the dependence on formulated feeds. Farmers want to increase profit and reduce costs, one of the largest of which is feed. Greater intensity of production has the potential to result in more disease outbreaks but also the potential for higher profits and so on.

Much of the decision-making at farm level is based on the familiar risk:reward scenario and is largely driven by economic considerations. Even in small-scale, so-called "subsistence" farms, decisions are often made on what will provide the highest return. Higher intensity farming may carry greater risk, but the potential reward is also attractive. This can be seen particularly in the case of the rice vs shrimp farming debate. Many rice farmers who switched to shrimp saw it as a worthwhile risk given the poverty associated with rice farming and the comparatively high return from a single successful crop of shrimp. This enabled many poor rice-farming families in coastal areas to escape the poverty trap but unfortunately, outbreaks of yellowhead virus (YHV) and white spot syndrome virus (WSSV) meant that others lost more than they could afford due to the higher costs of shrimp production. Only when the perceived risk of losses due to disease was higher than the potential reward did attitudes change.

Attitude to risk, however, is also an important aspect of decision-making within private-sector aquaculture, especially with respect to disease. The acceptance of risk varies between individuals and also with the distance from the direct impact (particularly economic impact) of a given risk on an individual business. Different individuals vary in their aversion to risk, and it is clear that some farmers accept a higher level of risk than others. For example, some farmers are willing to pay extra for shrimp postlarvae that test negative for serious viral diseases such as WSSV, whereas others prefer to pay less for postlarvae that have not been tested, despite the experience of many farmers and the results of epidemiological investigations that show the probability of disease outbreaks is much lower with negative-tested postlarvae. In the case of catastrophic, easily transmitted, epidemic diseases, individuals may accept a level of risk that exposes not just themselves, but all of their neighbours, to a high risk of disease outbreak. Disease is often considered as an "external" risk factor outside the control of the producer until such time as it becomes widespread and endemic, by which time it is often too late to impose any form of control.

Similarly, the impact of disease on a single farm may be devastating for that farmer but has less effect on, for example, a hatchery or feed supplier, since their business is not dependent on a single farm and they are less exposed to the disease risk until it becomes widespread. For example, poor hatchery biosecurity and hygiene may result in problems that manifest themselves long after the animals have been stocked in ponds, resulting in losses to the farmer that may or may not be clearly attributable to the hatchery practices.

The private sector is generally concerned with its local situation and direct threats to livelihood such as disease, market demands and even government regulation (e.g. in the case of bans, moratoria and restrictions on business activities). By comparison, the public or government sector has to take account of the total picture and balance the needs of all stakeholders on a national, and sometimes international, basis. The key is how to take both of these concerns into account and balance the reduction of disease risk through means that do not excessively affect livelihoods in the private sector.

The private sector response to a disease threat or outbreak depends on several factors, and not all of the stakeholders have the same resources or access to resources that may be required. If the impact on business, real or perceived, is great, there will be a greater likelihood that the private sector will act quickly and comprehensively, especially if there is a short-term impact. This is not to say that such efforts will be concerted or well coordinated. An emergency on a single farm may result in a greater level of precaution on nearby farms but will not translate into concerted action to respond to the emergency until a disease affects a greater number of farms or appears to be spreading. This may not engender a response by suppliers until enough farms are affected that their business suffers. Similarly, processors and exporters may not be motivated until they are unable to source sufficient raw materials for their needs and so on. Only rarely, and under specific, usually epidemic, situations will the entire industry work together to resolve the problem. This is not so different from government agencies that may be unaware of the importance of a developing disease situation until a sufficiently large number of farms are affected.

Farmers

At the farm level, farmers may have access to their own, usually limited, financial resources as well as their staff and on-farm equipment. Although this would generally be used to deal with problems at their own farm, in the case of a serious epidemic, they may be pooled among a number of farms. The level of effectiveness will depend upon the level of training and education of the farmers and their staff, as well as their level of preparedness. Few farms have a contingency plan in place for catastrophic disease and thus depend on the experience of the staff on site. Training and assistance in developing on-farm contingency plans, ability to identify problems early and a well-defined system of communication can all be used to improve the level of preparedness and response to disease emergencies. This is especially true when there are well-organized farmers' groups or associations that can assist in organizing training and disseminating information. The farmers' motivation to assist in such planning is clearly linked to their suppliers.

Suppliers

Farm suppliers have the advantage of a network of sales and technical advisory staff who can support extension activities to the farms. Although often viewed as being in competition with government services or as being unreliable technically, they are generally able to provide a more frequent and better level of service and support, since their funding is derived from profits, and can usefully complement government services in some cases. For example, feed company support was elicited in the cases of WSSV and YHV outbreaks in Thailand to disseminate information (brochures, newsletters, posters etc.) prepared by the Thai Department of Fisheries to the farm level, as well as providing some additional funds for printing etc. This was justified as a way of supporting their customers to prevent disease transmission and thus protecting their market.

The major issue with private-sector technical support is the quality of services provided, especially in the event of a disease outbreak. Under such situations, opportunistic suppliers can exacerbate the problem by providing ineffective "cures". This causes confusion and can actually delay or reduce the effectiveness of prevention and eradication programmes. Nor are such situations necessarily simply the result of unscrupulous individuals taking advantage of farmers. During an epidemic, farmers desperately search for solutions, and when they find an apparent solution, they will spread the information by word-of-mouth. Such opinions are seldom, if ever, supported by other than anecdotal evidence but often find widespread adoption. If this involves a particular product, salespeople of the product will actively promote the solution to others, especially when many farmers insist that they have seen results. Indeed, sometimes the weight of popular belief is such that government technical support services also spread the information in an attempt to assist as many farmers as possible. This is not due to a conscious attempt to take advantage of farmers but a sincere desire to help and a belief that, in the absence of scientific evidence to evaluate the claims, popular opinion carries considerable weight as evidence of efficacy.

Ensuring quality of technical support services is complex and requires considerable effort and communication between the support providers. Preparedness plans need to recognize and take account of the varied roles played by different stakeholders, their ability and willingness to assist and ensure regular communication and update between them and the relevant authorities.

In many cases, suppliers can also provide a significant source of assistance and access to finances, usually through marketing and technical support funding. Many feed companies and other suppliers provide newsletters and seminars to farmers, for example. Although primarily aimed at product support, they frequently invite third parties to contribute in key areas of expertise and interest to their customers. Prevention and control of aquatic animal diseases are usually of interest to farmers, and company-sponsored communications can be used to provide information to farmers on what to do and who to contact in the event of an emergency. Some suppliers also provide laboratory services and analyses to customers. These can be integrated so that they complement, rather than compete with, existing government services.

Buyers

Buyers may be the last group to be significantly affected by outbreaks of disease, especially if these are confined to a limited area, since they may be able to compensate for local shortfalls by sourcing raw materials from other areas. However, as businesses they are often aware of the potential impact of catastrophic disease on their profitability and ability to fulfil forward contracts and can be a significant source of support for preventative activities.

Apart from financial support, they can play an effective role in planning, since they usually have good connections directly to farms, especially with respect to harvesting. Information on harvest yields, emergency harvests and presence of unusual clinical signs in harvested animals can be gathered. They can also be an invaluable source of information on trading networks, both formal and informal. These networks need to be taken into account in preparation of contingency and preparedness plans for disease outbreaks, since they may play an important role in transmission of disease.

Multinationals

Some aquaculture industries, especially the high value ones, may involve companies that have a multinational presence. Their business may be related to feed or other supplies, or to other areas, such as animal health. Such groups may have access to international expertise, either in-house or in their network of contacts and in some cases, may be willing to use these to deal with disease outbreaks. Some companies also have access to sophisticated laboratory facilities that can complement those available to local or regional organizations. A good example of this is the assistance provided by the Intervet company in dealing with the outbreak of disease in koi carp in Indonesia in 2003.

Others

Some countries (e.g. India) have extensive private consulting networks supporting farmers. These operate as quasi-independent extension services and usually service clients in a limited local area. Many of the comments related to suppliers are also relevant here, especially when a significant portion of their income is derived from product sales or distribution.

Stakeholder motivation

Clearly, the different stakeholders need to have some motivation. This will vary depending on their involvement and role in the industry (Table 1).

TABLE 1.
Possible roles and motivations for different private-sector stakeholders.

Stakeholder	Role	Motivation
Farmers/farmer groups	Development of contingency plans (farm and local), implementation	Livelihood
Suppliers	Reporting, advisory, dissemination of information, laboratory services	Customer support, market reputation, competitiveness
Buyers	Reporting, provision of incentives(?)	Maintain supply, cost-competitiveness
Multinationals	Technical support, information dissemination, development assistance	Investment, market development, political influence

CASE STUDIES

The following two case studies can serve to demonstrate how the private sector can play an effective role in the development of a response to disease outbreaks – WSD and YHD of shrimp in Thailand and "loose shell syndrome (LSS)" of shrimp in India. Both of these case studies involve shrimp, mainly due to the author's experience but also due to the fact that the shrimp private sector is among the best developed in Asian aquaculture.

Case study 1: Yellowhead Disease (YHD) and White Spot Disease (WSD) in Thailand

The Thai response to the initial outbreak of WSD in shrimp benefited considerably from the experience of the industry and government agencies involved with the outbreak of YHD that had occurred a year earlier. In the YHD outbreak, a multidisciplinary task force was established which comprised members from the public and private sectors. Two government agencies were involved - The Royal Thai Department of Fisheries (DOF) and the National Center for Genetic Engineering and Biotechnology (BIOTEC), as well as researchers from several key universities such as Chulalongkorn University, Kasetsart University, Mahidol University and Prince of Songkhla University, and key groups in the aquaculture industry, mainly farmers' associations and some feed companies, such as Aquastar and Charoen Pokphand.

Following initial meetings to discuss what was known about the disease, a committee was established to determine what information was required, what steps should be taken and, more importantly, what funding was available. Based on this, several short-term research projects were established to answer specific questions aimed at managing the outbreak, such as how the disease was transmitted and, once it was established that a virus was involved, whether it could be transmitted through the feed, a major concern of farmers and feed companies alike. These projects were funded through a combination of public and private-sector funds, since government budgets did not include contingency funds for emergencies and private-sector collaboration in research was a key component of most of these projects. At the same time, it was clear that information had to be widely disseminated to farmers to allow them to identify the problem and what steps to take. The DOF oversaw the preparation of a series of brochures and posters that were partly funded by the private sector and were widely distributed through the DOF's fisheries stations and by feed companies and other farm suppliers.

These steps did not completely halt the outbreak of YHD, but it was widely agreed that they served to limit the extent of the damage, allowing the industry to recover more rapidly than would otherwise have been the case. It also provided a good model of public and private-sector collaboration to deal with a disease emergency.

In the case of WSD outbreaks (and as is the case in most disease outbreaks), the initial reports of disease came from farmers. News of unusually high mortalities was spread by word of mouth between farmers and through feed salespeople, suppliers and government agencies. The most obvious clinical signs, white spots on the carapace, led to the naming of the problem "white spot disease" and allowed easy diagnosis of affected ponds.

Initially, management and treatment efforts were based on earlier experience with YHD. Farmers' efforts were supported with advice by the DOF and the technical support teams of various suppliers. When these were unsuccessful, some of the major private-sector organizations (large farms and feed companies) requested the government agencies to reactivate the Yellowhead Task Force to plan a nationwide response. Information and experience with the problem were freely shared in order to establish an appropriate picture of the progress of the disease. Through careful examination of the available data submitted by the private sector, it was clear that mortalities were associated with postlarvae, even though at this point no pathogen had been identified. This resulted in a focus on broodstock, hatcheries and postlarvae as a principal route of transmission.

Many samples of infected shrimp were sent for histopathology, much of it paid for by the private sector. Eventually, a virus was found and transmission studies showed that it was indeed responsible for the disease. Under the guidance of the task force, the next priority was to develop a rapid diagnostic test to detect subclinical infection with a view to screening postlarvae. Researchers at Mahidol University had experience with polymerase chain reaction (PCR) technology as a diagnostic tool and quickly developed primers that could be used as a rapid test for screening. The primers were shared with other laboratories, and testing was widely implemented both for screening broodstock and postlarvae, and for searching for potential carriers or reservoir hosts.

Once again, the private sector collaborated in the preparation, funding and dissemination of information on the disease and possible control measures to mitigate the situation. In some cases, affected farmers were given additional credit by suppliers, allowing them to restock and get back into production quickly. Unfortunately, subsequent disease outbreaks and stock losses often meant that farmers were unable to meet their obligations, causing major debt problems. This, together with problems in managing debt and revenue collection, resulted in the collapse of the Aquastar contract farming system in the south of the country.

As in the YHD outbreak, it is difficult to assess how effective these efforts were in reducing losses due to the disease. However, the relatively rapid recovery of the Thai shrimp industry following the WSD outbreaks compared to that of other countries does give some idea of the effectiveness of the public/private-sector collaboration in dealing with disease emergencies. In addition, the legacy of this experience can be seen in the involvement of the industry itself in preparing its own preparedness plans. Privately operated PCR laboratories, some owned by the farmers' associations themselves, now screen broodstock and postlarvae for a range of viruses, and farmers' organizations provide regular updates to members on the disease situation in the country. Some are even developing their own preparedness plans for new diseases (e.g. Taura syndrome) before they become significant problems. Feed companies and other suppliers organize

FIGURE 2.
Estimated prevalence of LSS in India in 1996–2003 (courtesy Indian Society of Aquaculture Professionals)

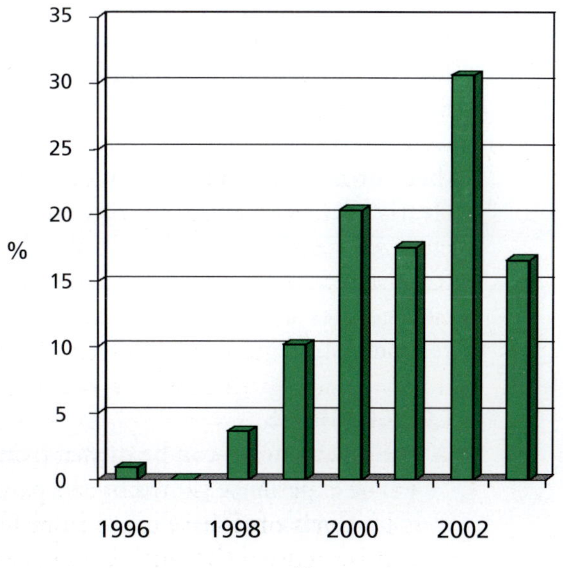

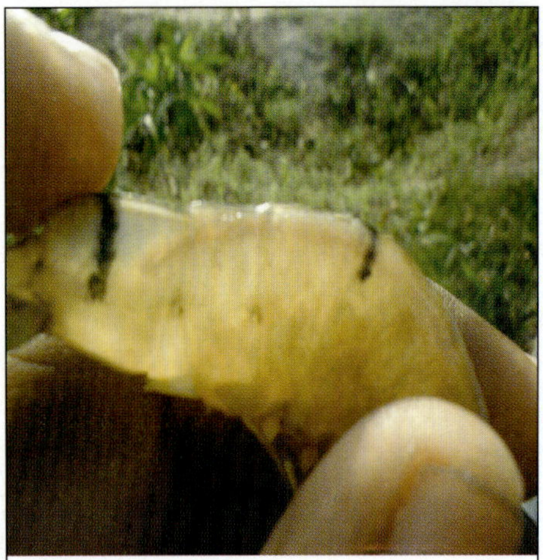
DANIEL FEGAN

Loose shell syndrome of P. monodon *in India*

regular seminars/workshops to update on important issues facing the industry, including disease threats, and the private sector is collaborating with the DOF in the development and implementation of Codes of Conduct and Good Management Practices for quality shrimp.

Case study 2: Loose Shell Syndrome (LSS) in India

Loose shell syndrome (LSS) of shrimp, in which the meat in the tail portion of the shrimp appears shrunken inside the carapace, was first noted in 1996 but significant losses were not experienced until 1998 (Figure 2). The number of farms affected has increased over the past five years, and it is now regarded as a major factor affecting shrimp farm profitability.

Studies into the syndrome have been hampered due to the lack of a clear, consistent case definition and conflicting information as to cause. No pathogen has been identified and so transmission studies have been impossible. This made research into the problem very difficult and few studies have been reported on the disease, its development and control strategies.

As a result of industry concerns and to coordinate efforts between the public and private sectors, the newly formed Society of Aquaculture Professionals (SAP) conducted a survey in early 2004 to investigate LSS. The survey objectives were to:

- understand the occurrence and severity of LSS in shrimp farms;
- identify biological and environmental factors and conditions that are associated with LSS; and
- understand the views of farmers, farm technicians, farm consultants and technical support staff from farm suppliers on possible causative factors.

Although the conduct of the survey suffered from some constraints, the survey was able to identify to some extent, the scale of the problem and some potential factors associated with the syndrome. The survey results, as well as the results of some research projects supported by the SAP, were presented and summarized in a specially convened workshop, again funded and organized by the SAP. The workshop participants discussed and prioritized possible causes of the syndrome and established a clearer working case definition. The SAP then agreed on an investigative strategy and arranged for samples to be collected and submitted to pathology laboratories in India and other countries such as Thailand and the United States for more detailed analysis. In order to coordinate the investigations, the SAP also established a smaller "Task Force" of farmers, consultants and private laboratories whose responsibility was to follow up on the investigation and report to the SAP and its members.

The efforts of the SAP in dealing with LSS have been undertaken largely using their own funds and resources. However, as in the Thai case study, this example clearly demonstrates the role that the private sector can play in dealing with emergencies. Experience gained in such situations provides an invaluable resource for the development of contingency and preparedness plans for subsequent disease emergencies and represents an important resource for the development of official response strategies.

CONCLUSIONS

A few observations can be drawn from these case studies:

- The experience gained by the private sector in dealing with disease outbreaks is an invaluable resource in contingency planning and response to disease emergencies. It is essential that such experience is utilized if an efficient and effective response is to be developed.

- If an emergency response plan is to be effective, it must be prepared in consultation with the private sector. Greater involvement of the private sector in the development of preparedness plans and the control measures to be implemented will increase the likelihood that it will understand the need for such plans and its role and responsibilities within the emergency response.
- Effective involvement of the private sector requires its role be clear and that it understand the objectives and activities within the plan and how they relate to those of other agencies.
- Where the private sector is well-organized, it is capable of developing strategic plans, either on its own or in collaboration with government agencies.
- Although the lead role in such organizations is usually taken by wealthier, better-educated players, smaller farmers usually benefit from the knowledge gained and implementation of better health management strategies.
- Different stakeholders in the private sector will work together to solve common problems where these are perceived to be a threat to the entire industry rather than a threat to a limited number of players or sectors.
- In higher value species, more financial resources are available from within the industry itself, and these can be committed under circumstances where the industry is under threat. Even where money is not available, "in-kind" support can provide a significant resource in emergency response.
- Effective collaboration between the public and private sectors requires good communication between the two. With appropriate guidance and training, the private sector can play a significant role and provide a valuable partner for government agencies.
- Private-sector training in disease emergency preparedness and response is an essential part of the risk communication and risk management processes. Such training should be included in any development plan and should involve the public and private sectors, both individually and jointly.

Protecting aquatic biodiversity through health management and risk analysis: on-going initiatives and future prospects

J. Richard Arthur
PO Box 1216
Barriere, B.C., Canada V0E 1E0
jrarthur@telus.net
Rohana P. Subasinghe
Fishery Resources Division, Fisheries Department
Food and Agriculture Organization of the United Nations
Viale delle Terme di Caracalla, 00100 Rome, Italy
Rohana.Subasinghe@fao.org

Arthur, J.R. & Subasinghe, R.P. 2005. Protecting aquatic biodiversity through health management and risk analysis: on-going initiatives and future prospects. p. 123–131. In: Subasinghe, R.P.; Arthur, J.R. (eds.). Regional workshop on preparedness and response to aquatic animal health emergencies in Asia. Jakarta, Indonesia, 21–23 September 2004. *FAO Fisheries Proceedings*. No. 4. Rome, FAO. 2005. 178p.

ABSTRACT

This discussion paper reviews some of the activities related to protecting aquaculture and aquatic biodiversity from transboundary aquatic animal pathogens (TAAPs) that have recently occurred or are being planned for the Asia-Pacific Region. It also speculates on where aquatic animal health in the region is headed in the next few years.

INTRODUCTION

The impacts of transboundary diseases on cultured stocks of aquatic animals are often well documented, due to the fact that in semi-intensive and intensive aquaculture production outbreaks of disease and associated mortalities are readily observed and the losses, in terms of numbers of dead animals and their monetary value, are easily quantified when ponds or cages are harvested. In contrast, the impacts of exotic diseases on wild populations of aquatic animals are less easily seen, as moribund animals are easy prey and may be quickly taken by piscivorous fish, birds and mammals. Additionally, accurate quantification of losses is usually impossible, as estimates of original population size are often not available, and any impacts on host population structure and aquatic biodiversity are difficult to measure, due to the problems inherent in working with natural ecosystems. Nonetheless, aquatic animal health workers are beginning to realize that the impacts of exotic diseases on wild populations of fish, shellfish and molluscs may be more significant, in terms of economic and social losses and long-term ecological impacts, than diseases confined to aquaculture systems (see, for example, Arthur and Subasinghe, 2002). This discussion paper will review some of the activities related to protecting aquaculture and aquatic biodiversity from transboundary aquatic animal pathogens (TAAPs) that have recently occurred or are being planned for the Asia-Pacific Region. It will also speculate briefly on where aquatic animal health in the region is headed in the next few years.

RECENT INITIATIVES

Aquatic animal health has recently become a rather dynamic field, thanks to outbreaks of serious transboundary diseases affecting the aquaculture industry, and to international efforts by the World Trade Organization (WTO) to remove barriers to free trade, while also providing the mechanisms for member countries to protect national human, animal and plant health (the Sanitary and Phytosanitary Agreement). These events have led to a large number of recent initiatives on reducing the risks due to transboundary aquatic animal pathogens, including the use of risk analysis as a decision-making tool, and to efforts to link concerns related to transboundary aquatic animal pathogens (TAAPs) to the larger concerns associated with aquatic invasive alien species (aquatic IAS) in the Asia-Pacific Region. This section highlights some of these activities.

Risk analysis initiatives

Good risk analysis is fundamental to protecting national aquaculture, capture fisheries and biodiversity from the adverse impacts of aquatic IAS and TAAPs. However, while most Asia-Pacific countries now recognize this fact, many are still struggling with how to move beyond theory to actual practice. Thanks to a number of recent regional meetings and activities, risk analysis procedures are becoming widely understood in the Asia-Pacific Region and are increasingly being adopted by countries as a way to reduce possible ecological, pathogen and genetic risks associated with international trade in live aquatic animals and their products.

A major step forward in this direction was the Asia Pacific Economic Cooperation (APEC) Fishery Working Group (FWG) Project on Capacity and Awareness Building on Import Risk Analysis for Aquatic Animals (FWG/01/2002), which included Asian and Latin American regional meetings on risk analysis that were held in Bangkok, Thailand and Mazatlan, Mexico. The primary outputs of this project were a volume containing the proceedings of the two meetings (Arthur and Reantaso, 2004) and a risk analysis manual designed for use by developing countries (Arthur *et al.*, 2004), documents that will prove useful to developing countries when starting risk analyses.

The World Organisation for Animal Health (OIE) has also recently published a two-volume set on qualitative and quantitative import risk analysis for animals and animal products (see Murray *et al.*, 2004; Murray, 2004).

Another extremely useful document for those attempting a first risk analysis is the Government of Australia's "Draft Import Risk Analysis Guidelines" (AFFA, 2001).

Most encouragingly, several risk analyses have recently be undertaken by countries in the Asia-Pacific:

- In April 2004, the Secretariat of the Pacific Community (SPC) contracted a team of five scientists with expertise in aquatic animal health, aquatic ecology and crustacean biology to undertake two risk analyses involving the proposed introduction of two crustaceans to SPC member countries for aquaculture

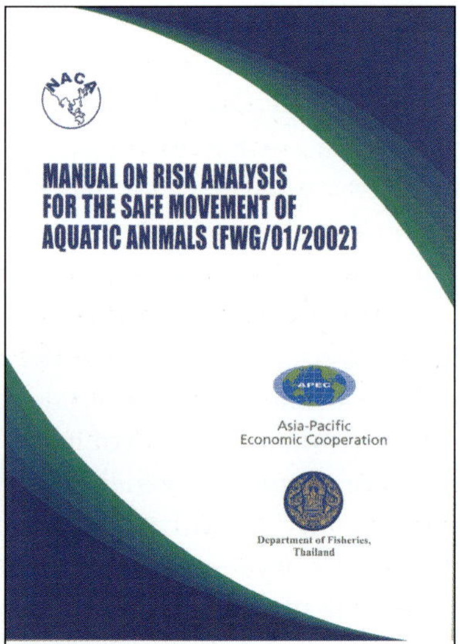

Import risk analysis procedures are elaborated

development. These included the proposed movement of postlarval giant river prawn (*Macrobrachium rosenbergii*) from Fiji to the Cook Islands, and of postlarval blue shrimp (*Litopenaeus stylirostris*) from Brunei Darussalam to Fiji (see Arthur *et al.*, 2004; Bondad-Reantaso *et al.*, 2004). The analyses have been completed and the full risk analysis reports are expected to be available in the near future from the SPC website (www.spc.org.nc).

- The Department of Fisheries, Government of Thailand, has recently completed a risk analysis for the importation of white shrimp (*Litopenaeus vannamei*) to Thailand. Unfortunately, the report is currently only available in the Thai language.
- In additional to a number of completed import risk analyses, the Government of Australia has several aquatic animal risk analyses in various stages of completion. These comprehensive analyses provide excellent examples of approaches to risk analysis and a wealth of information on hosts and pathogens for many species of concern to developing countries in the Asia-Pacific Region. Draft copies available from the AFFA website (www.affa.gov.au/content/publications.cfm) include:
  - Current import risk analysis: freshwater crayfish
  - Current import risk analysis: freshwater finfish
  - Current import risk analysis: non-viable bivalve molluscs
  - Current import risk analysis: prawns and prawn products

Health management initiatives

South East Asian Fisheries Development Center Aquaculture Department's (SEAFDEC-AQD) Regional Fish Disease Project

The goals of this project, which was initiated in 2000 and is funded under the Government of Japan's Trust Fund's Regional Fish Disease Control Project (see Nagasawa, 2004), are to promote disease-free aquaculture in Southeast Asia and healthy and wholesome trade of aquaculture products; to develop standardized diagnostic methods for important diseases of cultured organisms in Southeast Asia, and to establish a disease surveillance system. Phase I of the project, "Development of Fish Disease Inspection Methodologies for Artificially Bred Seeds", will complete in 2004, with Phase II of the project, entitled "Development of Fish Disease Surveillance System", expected to run from 2004 – 2008.

The project has the following components:

- research to develop standardized diagnostic methods for the region, disease control husbandry techniques, and monitoring methods for residual chemicals in aquaculture products;
- an international workshop for the regionalization of the standardized diagnostic methods, as well as disease control husbandry methods;
- hands-on training on diagnostic methods for important viral diseases in the region; and
- development of a surveillance system for disease problems in the region.

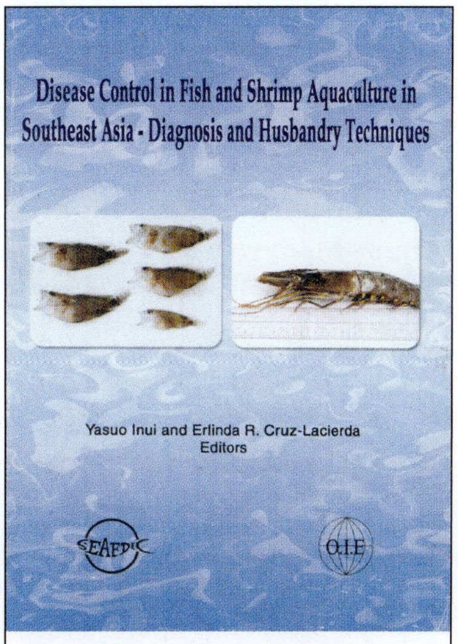

Disease control techniques are developed

Ongoing research includes studies on the establishment and standardization of diagnostic methods, the biology and pathogenesis of disease agents, disease prevention and control, and establishment of evaluation methods for residual pesticides in aquaculture products.

The project has organized two regional meetings:

- the "SEAFDEC-OIE Seminar-Workshop on Disease Control in Fish and Shrimp Aquaculture in Southeast Asia: Diagnosis and Husbandry

Techniques", held in Iloilo in December 2001 (see Inui and Cruz-Lacierda, 2002); and
- the "Meeting on Current Status of Transboundary Fish Diseases in Southeast Asia: Occurrence, Surveillance, Research and Training", held in Manila in July 2004 (see Lavilla-Pitogo and Nagasawa, 2004).

It also recently co-organized, with the Fisheries Research Agency of Japan (FRA), the Ministry of Agriculture, Forestry and Fisheries of Japan (MAFF) and the OIE, the "International Symposium on Koi herpes virus Disease, which was held in Yokohama in March of 2004.

One of the stated goals of the project is to coordinate its activities with the Food and Agriculture Organization of the United Nations (FAO) and the Network of Aquaculture Centres in Asia-Pacific (NACA), through presentation of meeting results at the invasive aquatic species meeting in Penang and the current workshop in Jakarta.

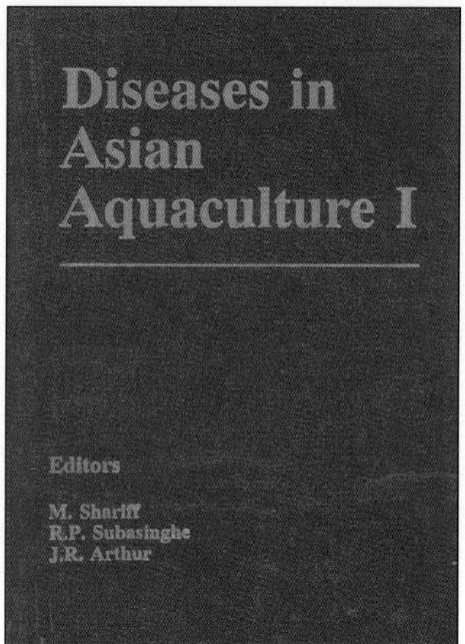

Regular conferences are held and proceedings published

The Fish Health Section, Asian Fisheries Society

The Fish Health Section (FHS), which was formed in 1989, organizes the triennial "Symposium on Diseases in Asian Aquaculture" series, with the next meeting, DAA VI, being planned for October 2005 in Sri Lanka.

It also publishes the Fish Health Section Newsletter (http://afs-fhs.seafdec.org.ph) as a means of keeping members current on aquatic animal health happening in the region and world-wide. The FHS also occasionally coordinates projects of interest to its members and publishes technical documents thorough its special reports series.

NACA/FAO activities

Much of the recent activities in aquatic animal health at the regional level are continuations or direct offshoots of FAO's and NACA's seminal and catalytic regional project TCP Project - "Assistance for the Responsible Movement of Live Aquatic Animals", which provided the countries of the region with detailed expert guidance for developing national and regional strategies for reducing the risks of disease due to transboundary movement of live aquatic animals. The TCP Project was an extensive consultative process, undertaken between 1998-2000, involving input from government-designated National Co-ordinators (NCs), NACA, FAO, OIE, and regional and international specialists. The primary output, the final Technical Guidelines, was unanimously endorsed at the Final Workshop on Asia Regional Health Management for the Responsible Trans-boundary Movement of Live Aquatic Animals, held in Beijing, PR China, 27–30 June 2000. The major outputs of the project were:

- The Asia Regional Technical Guidelines on Health Management for the Responsible Movement of Live Aquatic Animals and The Beijing Consensus and Implementation Strategy (FAO/NACA, 2000);
- the Manual of Procedures for the Implementation of the Asia Regional Technical Guidelines on Health Management for the Responsible Movement of Live Aquatic Animals. (FAO/NACA, 2001); and
- the Asia Diagnostic Guide to Aquatic Animal Diseases (FAO, 2001).

Most of the on-going supporting activities undertaken by NACA and/or FAO, with the assistance and participation of many other agencies and national governments, directly relate to one or more of the major components of the Technical Guidelines, i.e. disease diagnosis, surveillance and reporting; national and regional policy and planning; legislation, risk analysis, training and capacity building etc. Some examples include:

- The FAO/NACA/OIE Quarterly Aquatic Animal Disease Reports (Asia-Pacific Region)
- The Aquatic Animal Pathogen and Quarantine Information System (AAPQIS) (www.aapqis.org)
- The meetings of the Asia Regional Advisory Group (AG) on Aquatic Animal Health. This group of technical experts provides expertise and technical support to the Quarterly Aquatic Animal Disease Reporting System, to AAPQIS and to the Diagnostics Guide.
- Guidance on DNA-based molecular diagnostic techniques (see FAO, 2000)
- Guidance on disease surveillance and zoning (see FAO, 2004a)
- Guidance on emergency response to aquatic animal disease outbreaks (via the Regional Workshop on Preparedness and Response to Aquatic Animal Health Emergencies, Jakarta, September 2004 – this volume)
- Network on grouper diseases
- The Asia-Pacific Regional Programme on Mollusc Health Management
- Support to developing capacity and expertise in risk analysis (see above)
- Support for a series of fish parasite country checklists (Philippines, Bangladesh and Viet Nam have been completed (FAO 1997, 2002, 2004b); lists for Malaysia and Singapore are in progress)
- Various national TCP projects to support strategic planning, policy development, legislation, emergency response etc.
- Technical Guidelines for the Safe Transboundary Movement of Aquatic Animals, in support of FAO's Code of Conduct for Responsible Fisheries (CCFR)
- Initiatives to incorporate transboundary aquatic animal pathogens (TAAPs) into the mainstream of thought and activities related to aquatic IAS (see below).

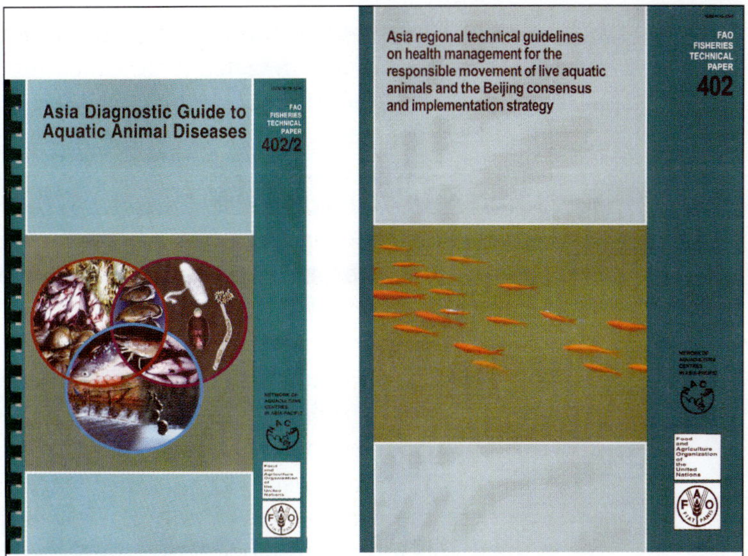

Health management guidelines and diagnostic manuals are prepared

TAAPs and aquatic IAS – a meeting of the minds

Until recently, scientists, environmentalists, policy-makers and others with concerns about free-living invasive aquatic species (fish, molluscs, crustaceans, plants etc.) and those working with exotic pathogens of aquatic animals (aquatic animal health specialists, epidemiologists etc.) had little contact and indeed, the two areas were treated as almost mutually exclusive. However, this situation is changing, as

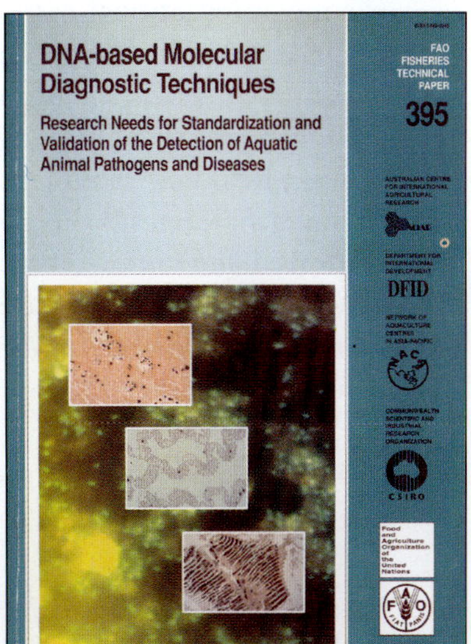

Research needs on diagnostics are evaluated

both groups have recently realized their many commonalties, and it is beginning to be accepted that TAAPs are, in fact, a large (albeit highly specialized) subgroup of invasive aquatic species. A recent meeting held in Malaysia has done much to bring the two groups closer together.

NACA/ASEAN/FAO/World Fish Center/United States Department of State Workshop on "Building Capacity to Combat Impacts of Aquatic Invasive Alien Species and Associated Trans-boundary Pathogens in ASEAN Countries"

This innovative workshop was held 12-16 July 2004 in Penang, Malaysia. The workshop, which was hosted by the Malaysian Department of Fisheries, brought together experts on TAAPs and those from the broader community of scientists, environmentalists and policy-makers dealing primarily with free living aquatic invasive alien species (aquatic IAS). The 75 participants included delegates from Association of South East Asian Nations (ASEAN) member countries, resource persons with experience in IAS and aquatic animal pathogens, and representatives of regional and international organizations, research institutes, universities and the private sector.

The workshop was convened specifically to better understand the relationship of aquatic IAS and pathogens and their impacts (both positive and negative), and to identify management and capacity building needs to reduce risks. The workshop built on the recommendations from a 2002 Bangkok workshop organized by the Global Invasive Species Program (GISP) and a 2003 workshop of countries sharing the Mekong watershed, particularly in promoting awareness, establishing coordination mechanisms and information exchange systems and identifying management strategies and risk mitigation measures for aquatic IAS.

While recognizing that positive social and economic benefits have come from the introduction of some alien aquatic species, the participants concluded that aquatic IAS and invasive aquatic animal pathogens (i.e. TAAPs) significantly impact aquaculture and have negative implications for aquatic biodiversity and the social and economic well being of people in the ASEAN region. The major recommendations of the workshop were:

- Management of aquatic IAS and associated pathogens is imperative and should be encouraged and implemented in all ASEAN countries.
- National strategies should be developed consistent with obligations under existing international treaties and instruments and in harmony with strategies for other IAS, including aquatic plants and ornamental fish. National strategies, coordinated through national focal points, should be based on impact assessment and management of alien species, where they are already established, and use of ecological and environmental risk analysis for proposed new introductions.
- National strategies should be implemented within a legitimate regional framework supported and endorsed by ASEAN. The recommendations in this Way Forward summary should be presented to the ASEAN Secretariat as a starting point for coordinated regional action, through the ASEAN Sectoral Working Group on Fisheries and other appropriate bodies.
- ASEAN member countries should have the necessary institutional and human resources to adopt a harmonized regional strategy. Bridging development gaps and capacity building across member countries is therefore necessary. Special attention should be given to capacity building among the Mekong basin countries of Cambodia, Lao PDR, Myanmar and Viet Nam.
- In-country IAS impact assessment and risk analysis training should be promoted and implemented to establish core expertise in these practices in all ASEAN countries. Experiences in risk analysis and impact assessment should be shared among ASEAN countries.

- Networking, information exchange and cooperation among concerned agencies, industry, trading partners and countries sharing common watersheds or waterways is recommended for cost-effective use of resources in support of ASEAN in achieving the goal of effective management of aquatic IAS and associated aquatic animal pathogens.
- Assistance should be sought from regional and international organizations to implement the workshop recommendations, including from the organizers and participants of this workshop and other regional and international organizations. Progress in implementing the workshop recommendations should be assessed in three years.

Future directions

Risk analysis, which has already been used informally or formally by several countries in the Asia-Pacific Region, will become a standard procedure for countries to assess proposals for the introduction or transfer of aquatic species. The lack of knowledge on the identities, geographic distributions and biology of many pathogens of major cultured species should lead to increased government and donor support to targeted studies on key species, for good risk analyses depend on the availability of good data. Likewise there are many knowledge gaps relating to the ecology of introduced aquatic species, such that prediction of their likely impacts in new ecosystems must be based on many uncertainties. International trade in aquatic animals should thus, by necessity, lead to increased support for studies on the biology and pathogens of the species to be traded.

Increasingly, the risk analysis process will become more integrated and standardized, encompassing analysis of ecological, genetic and pathogen risks within a single framework.

The use of specific pathogen free (SPF) species, so far only developed for marine shrimp, should be extended to other widely traded species (e.g. tilapias, giant river prawn, common and koi carps). The number of pathogens for which stocks can be certified as SPF should be increased, production procedures (including disease testing procedures) should become more standardized across the industry, and guarantees of freedom from specific pathogens more strongly written and demanded. A standardized regional certification procedure for SPF and/or high health (HH) production of broodstock and juveniles could provide developing countries with much needed assurances of disease status of imported animals and would assist in reducing risks due to pathogens to below national acceptable level of protection (ALOP). Thailand has already taken measures to implement, for a limited period of time, such a system for importations of broodstock of blue shrimp (*Litopenaeus vannamei*) at the national level.

Wider cooperation among trading partners in the Asia-Pacific will occur, insuring the accurate, comprehensive and timely information on country disease status is provided and that certification of production facilities is done to international standards. Smaller and/or developing countries in the region should increasingly pool limited resources with regards to expertise in areas like risk analysis and disease diagnostics. Initial steps in this direction have already been taken by SPC member countries and among countries in Southeast Asia.

Exporting countries that are not members of the OIE or that are OIE members but do not provide accurate or timely reporting of information on national disease status will increasingly be penalized via lost markets, as trading partners will determine that the importation of live aquatic animals produced by their hatcheries and farms entails an unacceptably high level of disease risk. This should lead to more timely and transparent sharing of information, and ultimately, to reduction of risks and pathogen transfer.

LITERATURE CITED

AFFA. 2001. *Guidelines for import risk analysis.* Draft September 2001. Canberra, Agriculture, Fisheries and Forestry–Australia, 119 pp. (www.affa.gov.au/content/publications.cfm).

Arthur, J.R., Bondad-Reantaso, M., Baldock, F.C., Rodgers C.J. & Edgerton, B.F. 2004. *Manual on risk analysis for the safe movement of aquatic animals (FWG/01/2002).* APEC/DoF/NACA/FAO, 59 pp. APEC Publ. No. APEC #203-FS-03.1.

Arthur, J.R., Hurwood, D., Bondad-Reantaso, M.G, Lovell, E.R. & Mather, P.B. 2004. Pathogen and Ecological Risk Analysis for the Introduction of Giant River Prawn, *Macrobrachium rosenbergii*, from Fiji to the Cook Islands. A consultancy report prepared for the Secretariat of the Pacific Community, Noumea Cedex, New Caledonia, under Contract Pro 7/54/8.

Arthur, J.R. & Reantaso, M.B. (eds.) 2004. *Capacity and awareness building on import risk analysis for aquatic animals (FWG/01/2002).* Report of the Joint APEC/FAO/NACA/OIE/DoF-Thailand/INP/CONPESCA/SAGARPA Workshops, Bangkok, Thailand 1-6 April 2002 and Mazatlan, Sinaloa, Mexico, 12-17 August 2002. Asia-Pacific Economic Cooperation, APEC Fisheries Working Group. 203 pp.

Arthur, J.R. and Subasinghe, R.P. 2002. Potential adverse socio-economic and biological impacts of aquatic animal pathogens due to hatchery based enhancement of inland open-water systems, and possibilities for their minimisation. In: J.R. Arthur, M.J. Phillips, R.P. Subasinghe, M.B. Reantaso, & I.H. MacRae, (eds.) *Primary aquatic animal health care in rural, small-scale, aquaculture development.* pp. 113-126. FAO Fisheries Technical Paper No. 406, Rome.

Bondad-Reantaso, M.G., Lovell, E.R., Arthur, J.R., Hurwood, D. & Mather, P.B. 2004. Pathogen and Ecological Risk Analysis for the Introduction of Blue Shrimp, *Litopenaeus stylirostris*, from Brunei Darussalam to Fiji. A consultancy report prepared for the Secretariat of the Pacific Community, Noumea Cedex, New Caledonia, under Contract Pro 7/54/8.

FAO. 1997. *Checklist of the parasites of fishes of the Philippines.* by J.R. Arthur & S.L. Lumanlan-Mayo. FAO Fisheries Technical Paper No. 369, 102 pp. Rome.

FAO. 2000. *DNA-based molecular diagnostic techniques: research needs for standardization and validation of the detection of aquatic animal pathogens and diseases.* P. Walker, & R. Subasinghe, (eds.) FAO Fisheries Technical Paper No. 395, 93 pp., Rome.

FAO. 2001. *Asia diagnostic guide to aquatic animal diseases.* by M.G. Bondad-Reantaso, S.E. McGladdery, I. East, & R.P. Subasinghe, (eds.) FAO Fisheries Technical Paper No. 402, Suppl. 2, 237 pp., Rome.

FAO. 2002. *Checklist of the parasites of fishes of Bangladesh.* by J.R. Arthur & A.T.A. Ahmed, FAO Fisheries Technical Paper No. 392/1, 77 pp., Rome.

FAO. 2004a. *Surveillance and zoning for aquatic animal diseases.* by R.P. Subasinghe, S.E. McGladdery & B.J. Hill, (eds.). FAO Fisheries Technical Paper No. 451, 73 pp. Rome.

FAO. 2004b. *Checklist of the parasites of fishes of Viet Nam.* by J.R. Arthur & B.Q. Te. FAO Fisheries Technical Paper No. 392/2, Rome. (In press).

FAO/NACA. 2000. *The Asia regional technical guidelines on health management for the responsible movement of live aquatic animals and the Beijing consensus and implementation strategy.* FAO Fisheries Technical Paper No. 402, 53 pp., Rome.

FAO/NACA. 2001. *Manual of procedures for the implementation of the Asia regional technical guidelines on health management for the responsible movement of live aquatic animals.* FAO Fisheries Technical Paper No. 402, Supplement 1, 106 pp., Rome.

Inui, Y. & Cruz-Lacierda, E.R. (eds.) 2002. *Disease control in fish and shrimp aquaculture in Southeast Asia – diagnosis and husbandry techniques.* Iloilo, Philippines, SEAFDEC Aquaculture Department, 215 pp.

Lavilla-Pitogo, C.R. & Nagasawa, K. (eds.) *Transboundary fish diseases in Southeast Asia: occurrence, surveillance, research and training.* Iloilo, Philippines, SEAFDEC Aquaculture Department,. 254 pp.

Murray, N. 2004. *Handbook on import risk analysis for animals and animal products.* Vol. 2. Quantitative risk assessment, Paris, OIE, 126 pp.

Murray, N., MacDiarmid, S.C., Wooldridge, M., Gummow, B., Morley, R.S., Weber, S.E., Giovannini, A. & Wilson, D. 2004. *Handbook on import risk analysis for animals and animal products*. Vol. 1. Introduction and qualitative risk analysis, Paris, OIE, 59 pp.

Nagasawa, K. 2004. Background and objectives of the Meeting on Current Status of Transboundary Fish Diseases in Southeast Asia: Occurrence, Surveillance, Research and Training. In C.R. Lavilla-Pitogo & K. Nagasawa, (eds.) *Transboundary fish diseases in Southeast Asia: occurrence, surveillance, research and training.* pp. 3-9. Southeast Asian Fisheries Development Center, Aquaculture Department, Iloilo, Philippines.

Institutional and regulatory frameworks for better preparedness for aquatic disease emergencies

Annick Van Houtte and Shalini Dogra
Legal Office
Food and Agriculture Organization of the United Nations
Viale delle Terme di Caracalla
00100 Rome, Italy
Annick.VanHoutte@fao.org

Van Houtte, A. & Dogra, S. 2005. Institutional and regulatory frameworks for better preparedness for aquatic disease emergencies. p. 133–145. In: Subasinghe, R.P.; Arthur, J.R. (eds.). Regional workshop on preparedness and response to aquatic animal health emergencies in Asia. Jakarta, Indonesia, 21–23 September 2004. *FAO Fisheries Proceedings*. No. 4. Rome, FAO. 2005. 178p.

ABSTRACT

This paper discusses the international and Asia regional context of emergency preparedness for serious aquatic animal disease outbreaks. Examples of national approaches to regulatory frameworks for emergency preparedness for aquatic animal disease outbreaks are drawn from several developed countries (Canada, Japan and Australia). A brief review of the current Indonesian situation is made and some recommendations for improving the ability of the country to deal with aquatic disease emergencies are made.

INTRODUCTION

No country can develop aquaculture practices that eradicate the chances of future diseases in its fish farming. Diseases in fish will inevitably occur, and thus fish-farming nations should understand that they cannot guarantee a permanently disease-free aquaculture and that they must therefore prepare themselves for disease outbreaks. When combating a disease in aquaculture, a state has two major objectives: (i) controlling the disease as soon as possible and (ii) minimizing its damages. Currently, various countries have, thorough their legislation, implemented strategies to achieve one or both of these goals. This paper will illustrate a number of approaches, each one providing certain benefits for better emergency response to disease in aquaculture.

Nowadays it would be erroneous to ignore the international context in which national regulation of fish health takes place. International (global, regional and subregional) issues have grown in importance in recent years because of the interdependence of states in the trade arena, namely because of the transboundary movement of aquatic animals (and plants) for aquaculture and the aquarium trade. This has also led to a growing recognition on the part of national governments of the need or the obligation to base their own principles and standards on those prepared under the auspices of international organizations and in harmony with those prepared in other countries. Efforts to find solutions to the problems caused by movements of live fish (in particular, the spread of fish disease) have also boosted interest in collaboration in the subregional, regional and global arena in the area of fish health. A number of regional and international organizations offer guidance or other forms of advice, and serve as fora for governments and other parties to discuss and resolve fish health related concerns. Their activities, although trade driven, play a role in facilitating prevention and control of fish disease occurrence and spread, thus including better preparedness for aquatic diseases emergencies.

Finally, this Regional Workshop takes place in the ambit of a TCP/INS/2905 project, the objectives of which are, *inter alia*, to enhance national regulatory frameworks and legislation, improve biosecurity measures and strengthen national disease surveillance and reporting to reduce the risk of movement of pathogens, both nationally and internationally, through the movement of live aquatic animals. It is therefore appropriate to say a few words about the legal and institutional framework in Indonesia, where the government has introduced aquatic animal quarantine procedures with a view to monitoring and controlling disease outbreaks, as well as to regulating the movement of aquatic animals both locally and internationally.

THE INTERNATIONAL CONTEXT

A few organizations serve as fora for governments and other interested parties to discuss and resolve fish health related concerns or which produce and disseminate guidelines or other forms of advice. Some of these have important implications for fish health related issues, in that they assist in formulating countries' laws and regulations on fish health management. Furthermore, international and regional approaches are essential in dealing with and identifying epidemiological responses to aquatic animal diseases.

World Trade Organization

The World Trade Organization (WTO) was created on 1 January 1995 following the latest and largest negotiation round, i.e. the Uruguay Round of Multilateral Trade Negotiations from 1986 to 1994. This round incorporated not only goods but also services and intellectual property. At the heart of the WTO are a series of trade agreements, ministerial decisions and declarations that provide the legal ground rules for international trade. Currently, there are about 60 such agreements, declarations and decisions in place. It is the Agreement on the Application of Sanitary and Phytosanitary Measures (SPS Agreement) that has the most important consequences for national fish health legislation.

The SPS Agreement sets out the rights and responsibilities of WTO members wishing to apply measures to protect human and animal life and health (sanitary measures) and plant life and health (phytosanitary measures). To minimize such measures' negative effects on trade, the SPS Agreement provides that they can be applied only to the extent necessary and must be based on an assessment of risk, taking into account scientific evidence, relevant processes and production methods, inspection, sampling and testing methods, specific diseases or pests, ecological and environmental conditions and, in the case of animal and plant life and health, relevant economic factors. Furthermore, national SPS measures must be applied in a nondiscriminatory manner, and they must be applied so that they do not constitute a disguised barrier to trade.

For animal and plant life and health, measures should be based on those standards adopted and recommended by the Office International des Épizooties (OIE, the World Organisation for Animal Health) and the International Plant Protection Convention (IPPC), respectively. Although the SPS Agreement acknowledges the limitations of means, it encourages the participation of Member States, in particular developing countries, in these international organizations, so that they can contribute to the formulation of sanitary and phytosanitary measures and have sufficient information to make decisions regarding the approval of international standards.

The main implication of the SPS Agreement for national legal frameworks is that as long as a Member State employs international standards in the formulation of its national measures, these are presumed to be consistent with the provisions of the SPS Agreement. However, member states are allowed to adopt measures that establish a higher level of protection than that provided by the relevant international standard if there is a scientific justification, based on risk assessment. Measures may not arbitrarily or unjustifiably discriminate between Member States where identical or similar conditions prevail, and importing Member States are obliged to accept the measures of other Member States as equivalent if the exporting country objectively demonstrates to the importing country that its measures achieve the importing country's appropriate level of protection (ALOP). The SPS Agreement also provides that Member States are to offer advance notice of any new or changed measures through national enquiry points, thus giving other Member States an opportunity to comment on them. Finally, Member States must take into account the special needs of developing countries, in particular the least developed countries, which are granted longer time frames for compliance with sanitary and phytosanitary measures.

In 2002, the World Bank and the WTO created the Standards and Trade Development Facility (STDF), a fund with the objective of enhancing the capacity of developing countries to participate in negotiations, to develop SPS standards and to implement those standards at the national level. The Food and Agricultural Organization of the United Nations (FAO), the World Health Organization (WHO) and the OIE, all with expertise in SPS issues, have joined the initiative. The STDF provides funds for technical assistance projects in developing countries that will draw on the expertise of these international organizations. Some of the projects have focused, for example, on strengthening the capacities of developing countries to participate in the development of plant and animal health measures, and by extension, helping them to meet those standards.

Office International des Épizooties

The Office International des Épizooties (OIE), or World Organisation for Animal Health, is an international organization created in 1924 and located in Paris, France. Its objectives are to guarantee the transparency of animal disease status in countries around the world and to collect, analyze and disseminate scientific veterinary information. OIE Member Countries, usually through their official veterinary services, commit to collecting information on animal diseases present in their territories, which the OIE then analyses and disseminates in order to facilitate prevention and control elsewhere. The OIE also provides expertise and technical support to Member Countries requesting assistance with animal disease control and eradication operations, including for diseases transmissible to humans (zoonoses). In addition, the OIE develops standards for international trade in animals and animal products.

Several commissions support the work of the OIE. Regional Commissions (Africa, Americas, Asia/Far East/Oceania, Europe and the Middle East) promote and organize activities at the regional level. Specialist Commissions study problems relating to epidemiology and the prevention and control of animal diseases and develop and revise OIE's international standards. The Specialist Commissions consist of members experienced in veterinary science and regulatory issues, elected by the International Committee and drawn from all regions. As such, the Fish Diseases Commission compiles information on diseases of fish, crustaceans and mollusks and their methods of control.

Historically, the international standards for animal health developed and adopted under the auspices of the OIE were not mandatory for its Member Countries.

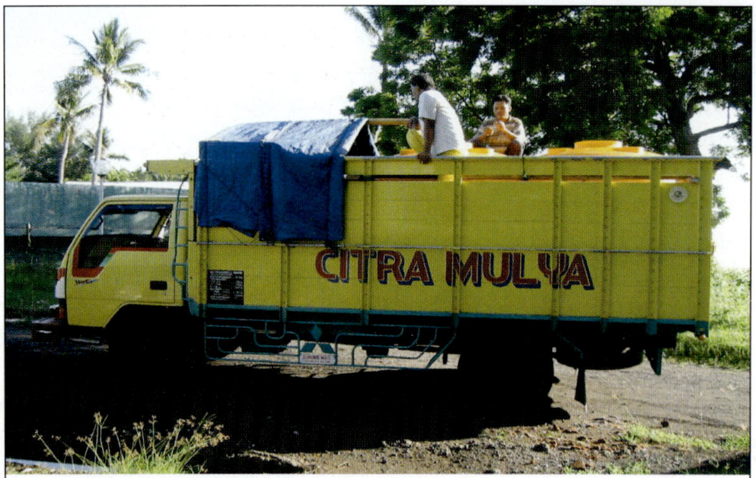

AGUS SUNARTO

Unregulated movement of aquatic species cause spread of diseases and pathogens

However, after the establishment of the WTO and the coming into force of the SPS Agreement, the OIE became the principal reference body for international standards concerning animal health and accordingly, standard-setting rose in importance as a primary task of the OIE alongside its traditional role of reporting disease information and disease control methods. Since all WTO members (i.e. most OIE Member Countries) must comply with the SPS Agreement, the implementation of OIE standards in national legislation has become essential. Different standards may be applied only where the importing country demonstrates scientifically to the exporting country that national animal health conditions require standards over and above those established by the OIE.

The OIE's animal health standards are developed and revised by the OIE Specialist Commissions and are the result of a consensus of experts from OIE Member Countries.

The international standards prepared by the OIE for aquatic animals are collected in the *Aquatic Animal Health Code* and the *Manual of Diagnostic Tests for Aquatic Animals* (OIE, 2003, 2004). They have been developed in acknowledgement of the fact that the epidemiology of aquatic diseases and the methods of disease control differ from those of land animals. The Aquatic Code gives detailed definitions of the minimum health guarantees required of trading partners in order to avoid the risk of spreading aquatic animal diseases, and includes sections on import risk analysis and import/export procedures. It also contains sections on health control and hygiene, and includes model international health certificates for trade in live and dead aquatic animals.

An important development has been the growing recognition within OIE of the importance of the interrelationship between animal health and food safety. The OIE has also begun to focus on the prevention of animal diseases from a food safety point of view, even where the diseases may not affect animals at all (but only humans). The OIE recently created the term "animal production food safety" to reflect this new field, which captures the importance of reducing risks to human health through effective measures imposed even before the slaughter of animals and the primary processing of their products. These developments have recently led towards greater collaboration between OIE and Codex and in particular, towards improving the current level of OIE input into Codex Alimentarius texts and to develop a method for the most effective utilization of Codex expertise in the work of OIE ad hoc groups. However, the likelihood for such developments to take place in the area of aquatic animal disease is very small, primarily because the aquatic animal diseases listed by the OIE are not diseases affecting human health.

International Organization for Standardization

The International Organization for Standardization (ISO), an international nongovernmental organization (NGO) that was created to "facilitate the international coordination and unification of industrial standards," is also active in areas related to fish health. Under development is ISO 22000, the Food Safety Management Standard, which will define the requirements for a food safety management system that covers the whole food chain from farm to fork. The extent to which this new development is likely to impact on fish health related matters is still to be seen.

Regional initiatives

Various initiatives have also been undertaken in Asia under the auspices of various organizations, including FAO, the Network of Aquaculture Centres in Asia-Pacific (NACA), OIE, and the Association of South East Asian Nations (ASEAN), as well as the South East Asian Fisheries Development Center (SEAFDEC) and the South East Asia Ministers of Education Organization (SEAMEO). Indonesia has been a strong participant in many international and regional activities aimed at preventing the transboundary spread of serious fish diseases. For instance, it participated in the FAO/NACA/OIE Regional Programme for the Development of National and Asia Regional Technical Guidelines on Health Certification and Quarantine for the Responsible Movement of Live Aquatic Animals and the ASEAN-organized Regional Seminar on the Harmonization of Quarantine Procedures for Live Fish, held 24-26 February 2003 in Penang, Malaysia, which led to the preparation of "Draft Guidelines for Harmonization of Quarantine Procedures of Live Fish among ASEAN Member Countries". There are also some on-going regional initiatives aimed at creating awareness and enhancing capacity building activities in the region. To illustrate this, there is the NACA/FAO/OIE Quarterly Aquatic Animal Disease (QAAD) Reporting System, which provides up-to-date information on important aquatic animal diseases in the Asia-Pacific Region. Such information is important as a "warning" and for purposes of risk assessment. Under the auspices of NACA, a Regional Advisory Group on aquatic animal health has been established. It meets annually and provides specialist advice, especially on emergency diseases of concern to governments (see www.enaca.org).

NATIONAL LEGISLATION AND PREPAREDNESS TO EMERGENCY SITUATIONS

A large number of countries have adopted legislation concerning fish health with the view to controlling disease outbreaks and limiting the damages thereof. We have identified three countries whose legal and institutional framework presents such characteristics and particularities as to enable them to prevent and control efficiently fish diseases and to be prepared for emergency situations.

Canada and the adoption of the precautionary approach

The best way to prepare for an emergency is to prevent one from ever occurring. In aquaculture, the way to prevent an emergency from occurring requires not letting a situation become an emergency. National authorities should take steps to try to predict accurately what diseases will most likely emerge in aquaculture. Hence, when the foreseen disease does hit, it won't be a real emergency; the country already knew it was coming and had prepared ahead of time. Rush decisions will be avoided. Thinking about a problem ahead of time lets the legislator think with a calmer mind and gives it time to consider all possible effects of a disease occurring in the fish farms. In other words, if a country adopts and carries out the precautionary principle or precautionary approach, it can maximize its reaction time to aquaculture disease and minimize the damages.

Canadian policies demonstrate proper execution of the precautionary approach. Explicitly evident in its *National Code on Introductions and Transfers of Aquatic Organisms*, the country systematically takes a precautionary approach towards aquaculture disease (see Anon., 2003). The legislator has not simply decided to sit down and wait. Instead, as explicitly stated on the Web site of Canada's Department of Fisheries and Oceans (DFO), its scientific research and international trade policies

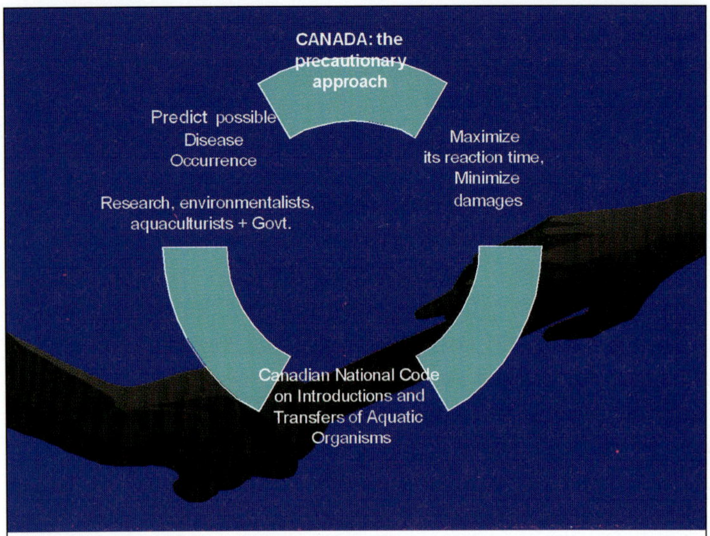

Canadian policies demonstrate proper execution of precautionary approach

are geared towards implementing efficient fish disease control procedures. The DFO proclaims it wants "Canada as the world leader in sustainable aquaculture". To achieve this goal, the fishery ministers of each province have mutually agreed to strive towards "technological advancements, capacity for innovation and a highly knowledgeable labour force" (see www.dfo-mpo.gc.ca/home-accueil_e.htm). Canada's DFO seems to realize that to prepare itself successfully ahead of time for fish diseases, it needs to have policies based on the best available technology and have scientific findings done by researchers who actually have knowledge in the field of aquaculture. There would be no point to foreseeing diseases if the predictions had no accuracy.

Obtaining different perspectives can help diffuse a stronger precautionary principle. Canada's DFO seeks to involve not only the government, but also environmentalists and aquaculturists in "maintaining the healthiest and most disease free environment for fish, either wild or cultured". By turning to different schools of thought, all of which have an interest in controlling fish disease, Canadian legislation avails itself to more sources of information. More information will likely form more accurate and well-thought out policies and assist the legislator in taking more factors into account. Given Canada's wide-ranging economic dependency on aquaculture, the DFO admits that it must take in as much information as possible when making decisions and passing regulations. If a national legislation considers as many factors as it possibly can before an actual disease occurs in its fisheries, the country will face less surprises and thus have less emergencies to overcome.

Japan: sharing power

National legislation can go beyond turning to nongovernmental sources for information. It can write laws that allocate some of the powers and responsibilities related to fish disease control to entities such as fishery associations or universities. Japan's legislative body exemplifies power-sharing. It displays how breaking down responsibility can benefit emergency response by minimizing the damages caused by a sudden disease outbreak.

Japan's national government shares powers relating to the management of fisheries, including aquaculture, as a mechanism to reach its aquaculturists. Aquaculture responsibilities are meted out to Japan's prefectural governments, which pass some of their authority on to fishery cooperatives. The 15 member fishery cooperatives consist of nine highly experienced fishers/aquaculturists, two local authority representatives and four scientists (see www.arc-corp.co.jp/JIFRS/English/CBFMinJapanFinal.htm).

A primary purpose behind fishery cooperatives is to have a governing body at the community level. Among their various duties that relate to fisheries, including aquaculture, the cooperatives exercise authority over aquaculture rights and issues relating to fish farming. Japan's national government takes advantage of the existence the local fishing/aquaculture community body and uses it as a tool for better emergency preparedness. Involving local, community-level entities in fish disease control is valuable because fish farmers have the closest and most consistent contact with the disease-stricken aquaculture. To control disease in aquaculture, a government ultimately will have to turn to the individuals who actually do the farming. To initially find out about the occurrence of disease in its aquaculture, a government most likely has to rely on its fish farmers for reports. To enforce its aquaculture regulations, a national government needs to make sure its community base, the fish farmers, carries them out. Just as a government needs its fish farmers in the daily enforcement of fish disease control, it needs them for emergency response situations.

Japan does not stop at involving its fishers/fishfarmers' communities. To combat fish farming diseases, Japan's national government has entrusted certain responsibilities to the Japan Fisheries Conservation Association (JFCA), the Japan Veterinary Medical Association and select graduate universities (see Inouye, 2003). The JFCA has the duty of "establishing uniform techniques for disease control". Under the umbrella of this duty, it has authority for technical extension, training and the inspection of imported live fish. In recent times, Japan's government has also started turning to the association to train fish disease technical workers. But for training specialists and technical workers, the government's Fishing Agency predominantly looks to the universities with veterinary or fishery faculties or to Japan's Veterinary Medical Association. In addition, Japan's national government relies on the scientific NGO, the Asian Fisheries Society, to distribute scientific journals and provide financial or technical assistance to fish disease researchers. By leaving the job of training specialists and assisting researchers to different nongovernmental entities, Japan's national government can expect a stronger emergency response system. By sharing responsibilities, the national authorities have fewer obligations and thus can concentrate more completely on the other aquaculture-related matters it needs to deal with. Also, entities such as the JFCA probably devote more time to studying and designing disease control tactics compared to what the national government would have available. As a result, it will likely come up with better thought out and coherently devised techniques. In Japan's system, each step in the process of aquaculture disease control separately grows strong under the relevant authority. For example, the veterinary faculties and the Japan Veterinary Medical Association are better equipped than a national legislative body to guide veterinary training. With each step going strong separately, ultimately the whole process becomes stronger. While Japan's legislation may not act under the precautionary principle, by sharing responsibility, it can at least address an emergency from different angles simultaneously and minimize the damages that come with diseases in fish farming.

Australia: specificity

Optimizing fish disease control doesn't stop at sharing responsibilities. Even after a legislator allocates some of the powers related to aquaculture management, it still has to tackle the duties it has left reserved for itself. To handle their fish disease control duties, some governments have decided to break them down as much as possible within their own legislation. By creating tailor-made laws for each type of fish disease, the legislator creates a model for how to deal with future diseases that are similar to the legislated one. While this method does not allow a government to necessarily foresee a fish disease, it does allow it to have a template to follow once a new disease emerges. When having to respond to an emergency fish disease, the government with a guiding template can react faster and be caught less off-guard.

INDONESIA

The National Strategy for Fish Health Management

Indonesia has developed its current policy with regard to fish health through its participation in the recent FAO/NACA/OIE Asia-Pacific Regional Programme for the Development of Asia Regional Technical Guidelines on Health Management for the Responsible Movement of Live Aquatic Animals (see FAO/NACA, 2000). The general objective of the National Strategy is to standardize Indonesia's fish health management programme in order to promote adequate disease control methods in aquaculture production systems, contribute to the development of sustainable aquaculture, and fulfil Indonesia's obligations as a member of the international community (Rukyani, Harjono and Sunarto, 2003).

The Government of Indonesia intends to develop and implement policies, legislation and practices that are both scientifically sound and generally accepted by regional trading partners and the broader international community. The draft National Strategy identifies ten programmes, or broad areas of concern, that need to be addressed:

1. Surveillance, Monitoring and Reporting of Fish Disease
2. Fish Quarantine
3. Regional and International Collaboration
4. Fish Disease Control (Contingency Planning)
5. Public Awareness
6. Research and Development
7. Rules and Regulations
8. Institutional Framework
9. Fish Resource and Environmental Management for Aquaculture
10. Funding Resource

For each of the ten components of the programme, the draft strategy outlines objectives and benefits, current status, key issues and an action plan; the latter is actually a brief listing of specific goals or objectives that are desired (see Arthur, 2003).

International context

Indonesia is a party to a number of international agreements and arrangements dealing with issues relevant to fish health and live fish movements and consequently, has obligations and rights under these agreements. Indonesia is a member of OIE, WTO, and the International Maritime Organization (IMO) and is a party to the Convention on International Trade in Endangered Species of Wild Fauna and Flora (CITES) and to the Convention on Biological Diversity (CBD). At the regional level, Indonesia is a member of NACA, SEAFDEC and SEAMEO, regional intergovernmental organizations concerned with preventing the international spread of fish disease.

Furthermore, Indonesia has participated in a number of regional initiatives developed respectively under the auspices of the FAO/NACA/OIE Regional Programme and ASEAN. The active participation of Indonesia on the international and regional scene witnesses its willingness to deal with the issues of fish health, live fish movement and preventing the spread of fish diseases.

Legislation related to fish health management

There are currently more than 50 laws and implementing regulations (mainly "decrees") dealing with fish health related issues (see Prayitno, 2003). Besides, draft subsidiary legislation exists, along with a number of codes and guidelines. The subsidiary legislation includes Government decrees, Presidential decrees, Ministerial decrees and Orders issued by the Directorate General for Aquaculture, as well as Center for Fish Quarantine Instruction Letters. Many of these regulations, however, are or may be obsolete, even though they are still technically in force, as they have never been formally repealed.

The Law No. 16 of 1992 concerning Animal, Fish and Plant Quarantine constitutes the framework law for the quarantine of animals, fish and plants for domestic and international movements. It sets the basic principles for the development and implementation of various quarantine actions with respect to the transit and import/export of live aquatic animals within and in and outside the country. This law has been implemented and is supplemented by the Government Decree No 15 of 2002 concerning fish quarantine. As its title suggests, it deals with fish quarantine and health certification. It goes much more into detail than the basic principles laid down in the Law of 1992. Composed of 12 Chapters, it consecutively deals with: General provisions; Quarantine requirements, Quarantine actions in case of entry, export, transit, mooring and landings in case of force majeurs etc.; Quarantine zones; Quarantine pests and diseases of fish and the carrier; Places of entry and exit/designation; Quarantine officers/competencies and installation; Quarantine Service tax; Development of quarantine awareness/community participation and Inter-country cooperation.

A quarantine action is defined as "the actions as the effort to prevent the introduction into, dissemination from one area to another within, or the exportation from, the territory of the Republic of Indonesia of quarantine pests and diseases of fish." Health certificates must accompany any introduction into the country of or the transport within the country from one area to another of a fish and/or other article capable of carrying quarantine pests and diseases of fish (called "a carrier"). They are issued in case of export of a carrier, if the importing country so requires.

Reference is made to risk analysis requirements (art.3) and factors that need to be taken into account for purposes of defining the distributional range of the pest or disease. These factors include namely whether the pest or fish disease outbreak occurred naturally; the impact of quarantine requirements and actions on trade and transport of people and articles, cost-benefit analysis and government capability to prevent the spread of pests and diseases.

Besides these two very basic instruments, there is a myriad of regulations pertaining to the scope of the quarantine activities, the operational aspects, the import and export of specific aquatic species (CITES related), the monitoring and control of the national and international spread of certain serious diseases (e.g. Koi herpes virus) and institutional matters. To illustrate the latter, Orders have been issued by the Directorate General for Aquaculture concerning the establishment of a national task force to overcome freshwater fish diseases.[1]

The current legal framework allows the Ministry of Marine Affairs and Fisheries (MMAF) to implement effectively a national policy for fish health management, including quarantine and certification procedures. The myriad of regulations expresses the concern of the ministry to deal with fish health related issues, whether operational or institutional, with a certain degree of specificity; however the approach taken is often piecemeal and ad hoc, as the problems arise.

Law enforcement (surveillance, control and fish inspection) is a major constraint to fish health management in Indonesia. The problem is often reported by officials. Lack of equipment and financial resources, lack of training in fish health matters by enforcement officers, insufficient coordination and cooperation between the MMAF and other national and regional authorities, absence of a surveillance and monitoring plan and lack of clarity in the roles and responsibilities of agencies and departments involved in surveillance and control activities have been reported as the major constraints to an effective control and enforcement scheme in Indonesia. There is no need to reiterate such findings, which are primarily policy issues, but some key legal issues need to be addressed in the basic legal framework on fish health management, namely the designation of relevant control/enforcement officers and the determination of their powers. Indeed, special attention should be given to enforcement provisions in the law.

---

[1] Directorate General of Aquaculture Decree No. 3750/DPBA/IK.220.DA/VIII/2002 Concerning the Formation of a National Team to Overcome Freshwater Fish Diseases; Decree of the Directorate General of Aquaculture No. 2101/2002 Concerning a National Task Force for Controlling Freshwater Fish Disease Problems (Carps, Gourami, and Others); Decree of the Directorate General of Aquaculture No. 2102/2002 Concerning the Establishment of a National Fish Health Commission.

Institutional framework: a myriad of institutions

A large number of national and provincial institutions are active in fish health management or have fish health related issues within their mandates. At the national level, within the MMAF, several primary units are mandated to deal with fish health:

- the Directorate for Fish Health and Environment under the Directorate General for Aquaculture;
- the Directorate of Fish Processing and Quality Control under the Directorate General for Capture Fisheries;
- the Center for Fish Quarantine under the Secretariat General;.
- the Agency for Marine and Fishery Research: Fish Disease Laboratory

A description of the respective mandates of these units can be found in the report of the International Consultant on Fish Health Management, Dr Arthur, under TCP/INS/2905 (see Arthur, 2003). Fish quarantine operational actions are conducted primarily by the Center for Fish Quarantine. The status of the latter is equivalent to the directorate. Suggestions were made to centralize the fish quarantine operational actions and related activities into one service, upgraded at the level of Directorate General, without distinction between capture fish and fishery products, aquaculture products or between import/export activities or movements within the country.

Some four expert commissions and committees have been established by the Directorate of Fish Health and Environment to address national fish health concerns; however, the purposes and tasks of these committees appear to be ill defined and overlapping.

Besides this central structure, there are a number (30) of Fish Quarantine Implementing Units (2 main fish quarantine stations, 7 regional fish quarantine stations, 10 fish quarantine stations Class I, 12 fish quarantine stations Class II and 1 Fish quarantine experimental unit). Some of these technical units are under both the Directorate General for Aquaculture and the Provincial Fisheries Services. In addition, there are some 380 checkpoints. These technical units are responsible for actual conduct of fish quarantine inspection and health certification. Quarantine checkpoints primarily check all shipments of live fish with a view to controlling the documentation, including the health certificates, accompanying the shipments. Discussions reported a need for development of expertise and capacity of the technical units to address fish health problems.

Other ministries play equally a role in international trade in live fish and products thereof. They are:

- the Ministry of Forestry, concerned with trade in endangered species and responsible for CITES-related matters;
- The Ministry of Health, concerned with fish food safety and fish as carriers of zoonotic diseases; and
- the Ministry of Trade, concerned with setting fees for trade in live fish and fishery products.

There are also some private developments, where ISO-approved companies are internationally recognized to issue health certificates.

Whether the implementation of the Autonomy Law has implications for the management of fish health is difficult to assess. However, uncertainty remains as to the nature and extent of the authority to be transferred from the central government to the various levels of local government. To ensure the success of the decentralization process, it is crucial that the relevant laws and regulations clearly spell out the nature and scope of the competence and powers to be transferred from the central government to provincial and district authorities. It is advisable that the MMAF prepares guidelines for the management of fish diseases and pests at the provincial level.

The primary weaknesses of the institutional structure lays in the lack of clear definition of the functions of the various authorities involved and the lack of communication

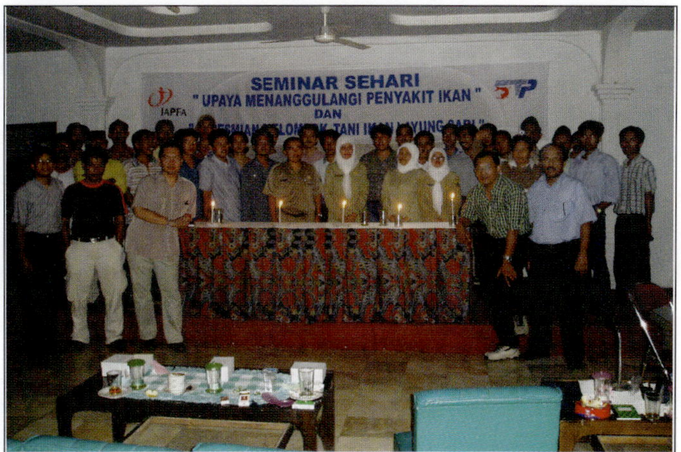

AGUS SUNARTO

Establishing farmer associations helped control of KHV outbreaks in Indonesia

between them. This seems to result in gaps and overlapping duties, from which interested parties (fish farmers, traders and others) benefit and suffer. Besides, several officers complained about the absence or lack of communication and networking between the various authorities involved. Lack of communication between the Directorate of Fish Health and Environment, the Center for Fish Quarantine and the Research Agency should be prevented if preparedness for emergencies has to be developed. Representatives of these institutions should meet on a regular basis to review progress made in dealing with important fish health related issues and generally speaking, once the National Strategy on Fish Health Management is adopted, to review its implementation. In other countries, universities (which provide scientific advice) and private-sector representatives have respective duties and opportunities to meet with government authorities with a view to addressing fish health related matters in order to increase the sustainability of aquaculture development and the industry's competitiveness in national and international markets and last but not least, prevent the occurrence of fish diseases and limit the damages caused by outbreaks. A forum should be identified where the private and public sectors could collaborate to use their findings in making decisions regarding regulations and industry practices, such as those relating to siting, feeding practices, introductions and transfers etc.

CONCLUSIONS

Guidelines and standards developed at the international level cannot be "imported" – they have to be tailored within specific national contexts. But regulatory problems can be shared among countries with similar circumstances, and so international and regional solutions devised and last but not least, trade can be improved. The last decade has witnessed a growing interest in the inter-relationship between food safety and other areas of agriculture, including fisheries, which were treated separately in earlier times, such as plant quarantine and animal quarantine. More recently, these topics happen to come under the heading "biosecurity," which is generally understood to mean protection from the environmental, economic and human health risks of potentially harmful organisms. At the national level, governments began to vest food safety, animal quarantine and plant quarantine authority in a single executive agency that carries out inspections "from farm to fork" and aims to protect animal, plant and human life and health. International developments have driven these changes. NACA further implemented, in collaboration with other international organizations, an APEC Fisheries Working-Group funded project (APEC FWG 01/2002) "Capacity and Awareness Building on Import Risk Analysis for Aquatic Animals." An important output is *the Manual on Risk Analysis for the Safe Movement of Aquatic Animals* (Arthur *et al.*, 2004).

Canada, Japan and Australia fall along the spectrum of emergency response. Canada seems the most ready. It structures its policies according to the precautionary principle. Together with an express aim of preventing diseases in aquaculture from occurring in the first place, it's Department of Fisheries and Oceans (DFO) reveals also elements of power-sharing and specificity. DFO involves environmentalists, aquaculturists and minority groups such as aborigines. With such a multifaceted approach, Canada strives to be the best equipped to deal with emergencies in fish farming because it maximizes its response time and minimizes disease-caused damages. While Canada tries to include all the possible actors related to aquaculture, including economists and environmentalists, Japan turns primarily to its fishers/aquaculturists. When Japanese fishery cooperatives make decisions about aquaculture, they rely on their members/fish farmers to compile information and report directly from the field. Japan, by sharing power, has prepared itself better for emergency situations because it will likely minimize damage. However Japan may not necessarily maximize its reaction time by sharing power. It can still be caught by surprise. Australia, on the other hand, through its very detailed and specified legislation, does save time because it creates guiding models for itself. Australia and Japan have focused efforts on what to do when a disease strikes fish farms. Canada, however tries to optimize its technology and research and policies ahead of time, before the disease occurs, so that it can be best equipped for when sickness does strike its fish farms.

Ultimately to succeed, emergency preparedness response legislation requires proper enforcement. Canada, Japan and Australia demonstrate what a country should do at the legislative level to prepare itself for diseases in aquaculture. But realistically, each one of these countries needs to have reliable enforcement techniques. For example, in the Canadian DFO, dedication to scientific advancement and research won't sufficiently guarantee the most up-to-date valid research; the scientists and researchers themselves need to display dedication and willingness to conduct research and undertake acute risk assessments. In Japan, looking to fishery association and fishery management organizations means trusting fish farmers to report occurrences of disease. While Canada, Japan and Australia may fall at different points along the spectrum of preparedness for emergencies in aquaculture, all three countries share one commonality: they must look to various actors for actual implementation. Scientists, enforcement officials and fish farmers need to be motivated to carry out relevant emergency preparedness response measures in aquaculture practices.

RECOMMENDATIONS FOR INDONESIA WITH REGARD TO FUTURE ACTIVITIES

Legislation may play a useful role to enhance responses to aquatic animal health emergencies. To this effect and with a view to promoting sound fish farming practices, combating fish disease occurrences and limiting their damage, the current laws and regulations of Indonesia should be carefully reviewed, reformulated and/or amended. Choices should be made: precautionary approach, power sharing, specificity or other? Such legislation should address a number of issues, like disease surveillance, control and eradication; contingency plans; new species introductions; domestic movement of live fish and their products; and fish inspection and quarantine. Besides, the challenge is also to design legislation that both enables and guides those (public and private sector) involved in fish health related activities. It should clearly redefine the duties of various authorities involved in matters of fish health at the national, provincial and district levels and promote effective coordination, power-sharing and communication between all those involved. The private sector should not be left behind. As providers of information and reports, fish farmers should be enabled to play a role in decision-making processes relating to the implementation of fish health management programmes.

The international agreements and regional guidelines set important parameters governing the adoption and implementation of fish health standards and measures.

LITERATURE CITED

Anon. 2003. *National code on introductions and transfers of aquatic organisms*. Department of Fisheries and Oceans Canada, September 2003, 53 pp. (www.dfo-mpo.gc.ca/aquaculture/ref/NCITAO_e.pdf)

Arthur, J.R. 2003. *Fish health management for Indonesia.* Report of international consultant on legislation. Project TCP/INS/2905(A). Health Management in Freshwater Aquaculture FAO, Rome. 55 pp.

Arthur, J.R., Bondad-Reantaso,M.G., Baldock, F.C., Rodgers, C.J. & Edgerton,B.F. 2004. *Manual on risk analysis for the safe movement of aquatic animals.* (FWG/01/2002). APEC/DOF/NACA/FAO, 59pp.

FAO/NACA. 2000 Asia regional technical guidelines on health management for the responsible movement of live aquatic animals and the Beijing consensus and implementation strategy. FAO Fisheries Technical Paper No. 402, 53 pp.

Inouye, K. 1996. An overview of health management of coldwater fish and shrimp in Japanese aquaculture. pp. 104-114. In: Subasinghe, R.P., Arthur, J.R. & Shariff, M. *Health management in Asian aquaculture*. FAO Fisheries Technical Paper No. 360.

OIE. 2003. *Manual of diagnostic tests for aquatic animals.* 4th Edn. Paris. (www.oie.int/eng/normes/fmanual/A_summry.htm)

OIE. 2004. *Aquatic animal health code*. 7th Edn. Paris. (www.oie.int/eng/normes/fcode/A_summry.htm)

Prayitno, S.B. 2003. *Legislation on fish health management: report of national consultant in legislation*. TCP/INS/2905(A). Health Management in Freshwater Aquaculture. FAO, Rome. 38 pp.

Rukyani, A., Hardjono & Sunarto, A. 2003. Status of quarantine procedures for live fish in Indonesia. Paper presented at the Regional Seminar on the Harmonization of Quarantine Procedures for Live Fish, 24-26 February 2003, Penang, Malaysia, 18 pp.

Capacity building for developing national and regional emergency prevention systems for transboundary aquatic animal diseases

C.V. Mohan and M.J. Phillips
Network of Aquaculture Centres in Asia-Pacific
Suraswadi Building, Department of Fisheries
Kasetsart University Campus
Ladyao, Jatujak, Bangkok 10900, Thailand
Mohan@enaca.org
Michael.phillips@enaca.org

Mohan, C.V. & Phillips, M.J. 2005. Capacity building for developing national and regional emergency prevention systems for transboundary aquatic animal diseases. p. 147–156. In: Subasinghe, R.P.; Arthur, J.R. (eds.). Regional workshop on preparedness and response to aquatic animal health emergencies in Asia. Jakarta, Indonesia, 21–23 September 2004. *FAO Fisheries Proceedings*. No. 4. Rome, FAO. 2005. 178p.

ABSTRACT

Transboundary movement of live aquatic animals is one of the principal reasons for increased disease emergencies in the Asia-Pacific Region. Disease emergencies may arise within a country in a number of ways: introductions of known exotic diseases, changes in the pattern of known endemic diseases or the appearance of unknown diseases. Contingency planning is critical to the effective management of such disease emergencies. A wide range of capacity and awareness building is required to effectively manage aquatic animal disease emergencies. This paper examines the capacity and awareness building needs of countries in the Asia-Pacific Region to deal with aquatic animal health emergencies and provides details of some of the key capacity and awareness building initiatives in the region. Further, the paper attempts to provide a general picture of responsibilities at the different stakeholder levels to implement effectively a contingency plan, and identifies the skills and capacity required to carry out the responsibilities.

INTRODUCTION

Threats to the sustainability of the aquaculture industry are numerous. Aquatic animal disease has been one of the most serious. Diseases caused by transboundary pathogens pose serious threats to aquaculture in many parts of the Asia-Pacific Region. Transboundary animal diseases are defined as epidemic diseases that are highly contagious or transmissible, with the potential for very rapid spread irrespective of national borders and which cause significant socio-economic and possibly public health consequences (Baldock, 2002).

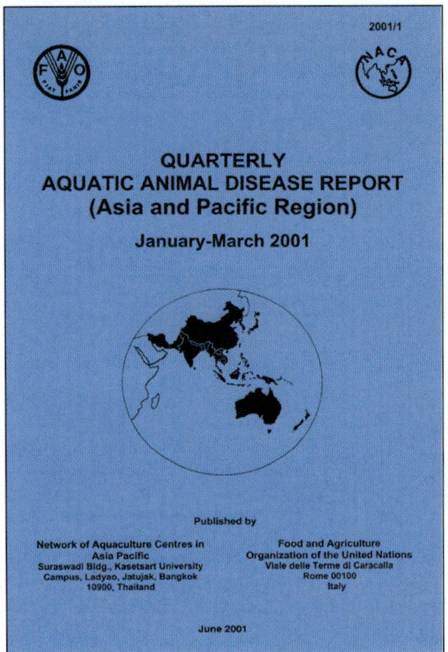

FAO/NACA quarterly disease report

Transboundary movement of live aquatic animals in the region is one of the principal reasons for increased occurrence and spread of several serious diseases (Subasinghe, Bondad-Reantaso and McGladdery, 2001; Bondad-Reantaso, 2004). Examples of diseases and pathogens introduced to new areas and hosts leading to serious consequences in the Asia-Pacific Region include epizootic ulcerative syndrome (EUS) in fresh- and brackishwater fishes, white spot syndrome virus (WSSV) and Taura syndrome virus (TSV) in cultured shrimp and viral encephalopathy and retinopathy (VER) in grouper. Common carp and koi mass mortalities in Indonesia since June 2002 and the confirmed outbreak of Koi herpes virus (KHV) in Japan (NACA/FAO, 2004) are further reminders of the dangers associated with the transboundary spread of pathogens. Important transboundary aquatic animal diseases positively reported based on the information recorded in 22 issues (1998 to 2003) of the Network of Aquaculture Centres in Asia-Pacific (NACA)/Food and Agriculture Organization of the United Nations (FAO)/World Organization for Animal Health (OIE) Quarterly Aquatic Animal Disease (Asia-Pacific Region) Reporting System (QAAD) is provided in Table 1. Careful examination of the history and spread of transboundary pathogens indicates how lack of effective surveillance systems and contingency plans can impact aquaculture and wild fisheries resources.

TABLE 1

Occurrence (+) of important finfish and crustacean transboundary diseases in the Asia-Pacific as reported in the NACA/FAO/OIE Regional Quarterly Aquatic Animal Disease (QAAD) Reporting System.

Disease[1]	EUS	VER	GID	KHV	WSD	TS
Country						
Australia	+	+				
Bangladesh	+				+	
Cambodia	+				+	
China PR					+	+
DPR Korea						
Hong Kong China		+	+			
India	+				+	
Indonesia	+	+	+	+	+	+
Iran					+	
Japan	+	+		+	+	
Lao PDR	+					
Malaysia	+	+			+	
Myanmar	+				+	
Nepal	+					
Pakistan	+					
Philippines	+	+			+	
Korea RO		+			+	
Singapore		+	+		+	
Sri Lanka	+				+	
Thailand	+	+			+	+
Viet Nam	+	+			+	+

[1] EUS=epizootic ulcerative syndrome, VER=viral encephalopathy and retinopathy, GID=Grouper iridoviral disease, KHV=koi herpes virus, WSD=whitespot disease, TS=Taura syndrome.

CAPACITY AND AWARENESS REQUIRED FOR CONTINGENCY PLANNING, EARLY WARNING AND EMERGENCY RESPONSE

A disease outbreak emergency exists when a population of aquatic animals is recognized as undergoing severe mortality events, or there is otherwise an emerging disease threat where urgent action is required. Infectious disease emergencies may arise within a country in a number of ways, for example: introductions of known exotic diseases, sudden changes in the pattern of existing endemic diseases or the appearance of previously unrecognized diseases. Contingency planning, early warning and early response are critical to the effective management of such disease emergencies. In simple terms, emergency response involves implementation of a well thought out and agreed technical response plan to identify and deal with an aquatic animal disease emergency event. Preparedness should happen during "peace time" (i.e. when there is no disease). When there is an emergency, the response should proceed according to the plans that have been developed.

Contingency planning is an agreed management plan and set of operational procedures that would be adopted in the event of an aquatic animal disease emergency. For mounting an effective emergency response, governments should have the capability to develop contingency plans and build the required operational capacity (e.g. human resources) to implement the plan effectively. Industry should be involved and ideally, also be encouraged to have "ownership" of the plans. Some of the important components of a contingency plan include: technical plans (e.g. manuals on disease strategy, general procedures), support plans (e.g. financial, resource) and operational plans (e.g. management manual, diagnostic resources, training resources), all with clearly designated responsibilities. Through a well-documented contingency action plan agreed upon by all major stakeholders, it should be possible to minimize the impact of an aquatic animal disease emergency.

The aim of early warning is to rapidly detect the introduction of an exotic pathogen or a sudden increase in the incidence of any disease. For establishing an effective early warning programme, a strong technical capability at the national level is fundamental in the areas of disease diagnostics, risk analysis, disease surveillance, zoning, epidemiological analysis, aquatic animal health information systems, national and international disease reporting, and information communication and sharing.

Emergency response is identified as all actions that would be targeted at rapid and effective eradication/containment/mitigation of an emergency disease outbreak. The responses may be of different types depending on the disease agent and the likely impact. Some responses (e.g. only monitoring) may not cause any disruption to the culture operation, while some may cause some disruption (e.g. movement control, treatment, increased surveillance). Drastic responses (e.g. destruction of stock, emergency harvest) will cause major disruption to farming practices. Operational capabilities at different levels (farm/village/province/national) are vital to mount an effective emergency response.

Australia has developed an effective emergency preparedness and response programme known as The Australian Aquatic Animal Diseases Veterinary Emergency Plan (see AQUAVETPLAN, 2002). It comprises a series of manuals outlining national emergency preparedness and response and control strategies. The manuals provide guidance based on sound analysis, linking policy, strategies, implementation, coordination and emergency management plans. The Control Centers Management manual outlines the organizational response during an aquatic animal disease emergency event, addressing legislative, management and resource issues. The Enterprise manual describes the emergency response options available for control and eradication of aquatic animal diseases. It also provides a framework for assessing which strategy to use, taking into account several factors (e.g. type of pathogen, management practices and effectiveness of treatment). The Destruction manual guides the decision to destroy the stock, and the choice and application of appropriate techniques based on several considerations (e.g. type of animal, disease and production system, their end use, possibility of the disease infecting human beings). The Disposal manual provides guidance for safe transport and disposal of carcasses, animal products and wastes. These manuals are aimed at government and industry personnel who may be involved in emergency disease preparedness and response. Closer examination of these manuals helps to understand the extent of technical capacity building, infrastructure and financial resources that are required to support an ideal national emergency preparedness and response programme.

STATUS OF CAPACITY FOR AQUATIC ANIMAL HEALTH MANAGEMENT IN THE ASIA-PACIFIC REGION

The guiding principles in the "*Asia Regional Technical Guidelines on Health Management and the Responsible Movement of Live Aquatic Animals*" (or the "Technical Guidelines") and their associated implementation plan, "*the Beijing Consensus and Implementation Strategy*" (BCIS) (FAO/NACA, 2000), was adopted as a regional strategy by 21 governments in the Asian Region in the year 2000. Within Asia, the Technical Guidelines provide the basic framework and guidance for national and regional efforts in reducing the risks of diseases due to transboundary movement of live aquatic animals. The main elements of the Technical Guidelines are: guiding principles, pathogens to be considered, disease diagnosis, health certification and quarantine measures, disease zoning, disease surveillance and reporting, contingency planning, import risk analysis, national strategies and policy frameworks, regional capacity building and an implementation strategy. The framework provided by the Technical Guidelines is a comprehensive one that includes all major requirements for managing aquatic animal disease emergencies associated with transboundary pathogens.

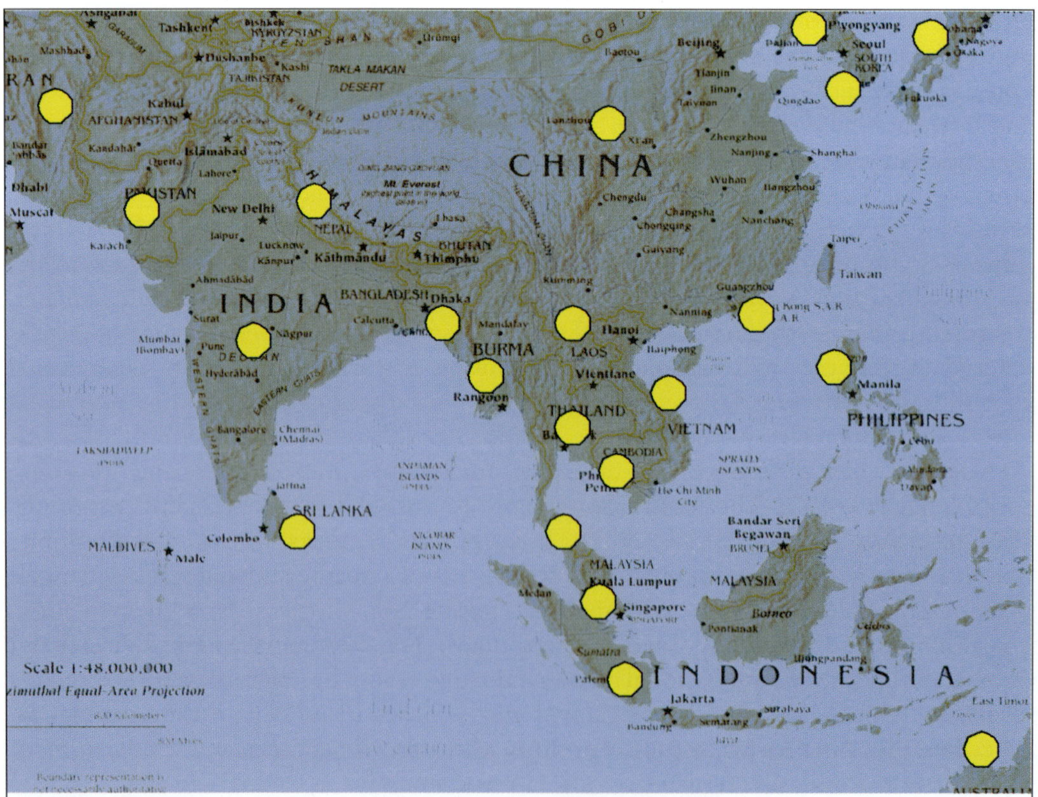

Twenty one Asian countries participate in the NACA/FAO regional aquatic animal health management programme

TABLE 2
Assessment of progress made in the Asia-Pacific Region towards implementation of the Technical Guidelines.

Elements in the Technical Guidelines	Progress Made (Number of Countries)		
	Good	Moderate	Low
Disease diagnosis	8	8	5
Health certification and quarantine measures	10	5	6
Disease zoning	3	3	15
Disease surveillance and reporting	6	9	6
Contingency planning	3	6	12
Import risk analysis	2	5	14
National strategies and policy frameworks	11	4	6

Countries in the region are at different stages of development of the national aquatic animal health strategies that contain the action plans of governments and that form the basis for the national-level implementation of the Technical Guidelines. Despite the considerable progress accomplished in the region, there are still areas that need to be seriously addressed. An assessment of the progress made in the Asia-Pacific in the implementation of the various elements contained in the Technical Guidelines shows the present status and highlights the regional capacity building needs (see Table 2).

This analysis suggests that contingency planning is one of the weak points where capacity building is required.

CAPACITY AND AWARENESS BUILDING NEEDS AT THE NATIONAL LEVEL

For some countries in the region, capacity-building activities should initially focus on developing and implementing simple and practical national aquatic animal health management strategies incorporating the key elements contained in the Technical Guidelines. For countries already having practical national strategies, it should be easier to target resources and build specialist capacity for early warning and early response to tackle aquatic animal disease emergencies. Early warning and early response programmes embrace all initiatives, mainly based on risk analysis, disease surveillance, reporting and epidemiological analysis. Mere establishment of emergency preparedness programmes and frameworks without appropriate skill and capacity development would be of little value. Capacity and awareness building is required at different levels to carry out the various responsibilities:

- contingency planning (e.g. developing disease strategy manuals, general procedure manuals, enterprise manuals, job descriptions, support plans and operational plans);
- early warning (e.g. risk analysis, disease surveillance, epidemiological analysis, aquatic animal health information systems, national disease reporting, international disease reporting) ; and
- early response (e.g. national and local disease control centers, information systems, laboratory procedures, field guides, trained field staff).

Table 3 attempts to provide a general picture of responsibilities at the different levels, and the skills and capacity required to carry out the responsibilities. A wide range of capacity and awareness building is required to effectively manage aquatic animal disease emergencies. It is clear from experience that for most countries in the region, it is going to be a very difficult challenge to develop an ideal emergency preparedness and response programme. The capacity is inadequate in many countries in Asia due to several factors, such as limited diagnostic capacities, lack of information, insufficient human resources and infrastructure, and lack of financial resources.

In such a scenario, there is a need to look to other options. Countries should target resources to develop simple and practical contingency plans to deal with high-risk diseases (e.g. Koi herpes virus disease, Taura syndrome) that are likely to be introduced. Management of an aquatic animal disease emergency will require a collaborative and team approach. Opportunities for optimizing the existing resources at the national level (e.g. promoting collaboration with livestock services, which are usually well experienced in managing terrestrial animal disease emergencies) should be seriously explored. At the regional level, countries with experience should be encouraged to share information with other countries and help bridge the development gap. Countries can also use regional reporting systems to be more aware of the new diseases that may pose risk.

Provision of adequate resources is crucial for the implementation of an emergency preparedness programme. Severe lack of resources at the level of policy development and at the operations level could significantly reduce the effectiveness of the response in the event of an aquatic animal disease emergency. Awareness building at the level of policy-makers is essential to improve their understanding of the seriousness of aquatic animal disease problems to secure adequate priority at the national level. Equally important is improving the understanding by both governments and industries of the benefits from investing in emergency response systems.

REGIONAL INITIATIVES TO SUPPORT EMERGENCY PREPAREDNESS

Several past and ongoing collaborative regional initiatives (e.g. training programmes, workshops, master classes) have supported capacity and awareness building on aquatic animal health. The following section briefly highlights some of the key capacity and awareness building initiatives in the region that assist countries in dealing with aquatic animal disease emergencies.

The NACA/FAO/OIE Quarterly Aquatic Animal Disease (QAAD) Reporting System, participated by 21 countries, is one such example. To date, 22 quarterly issues have been published and widely disseminated in the region. The NACA/FAO/OIE disease list includes all diseases listed by the OIE plus other diseases of concern to the region. The OIE *International Aquatic Animal Health Code* (2004) lists 35 diseases of finfish, molluscs and crustaceans based on three criteria (i.e. consequence, spread and diagnosis) and which should be reported to OIE by member governments. The NACA/FAO/OIE Quarterly Aquatic Animal Disease (Asia-Pacific Region) Reporting System lists 44 diseases, including a number which are non-OIE listed (e.g. Koi herpes virus disease, abalone viral mortality and grouper iridoviral disease). The information generated through the regional reporting system provides up-to-date information on important diseases in the Asia-Pacific Region, serves as an early warning system for emerging diseases (e.g. KHV, TS) and can be a valuable source of information to support risk analysis.

Recognizing the increasingly serious socio-economic impacts and the possible consequences for international trade arising from disease incursions due to the introduction and spread of transboundary pathogens through the irresponsible movement of live aquatic animals, an Asia Pacific Economic Cooperation (APEC) Fisheries Working Group (FWG)-funded project (APEC FWG 01/2002) "Capacity and Awareness Building on Import Risk Analysis (IRA) for Aquatic Animals" was successfully implemented by NACA during 2002–2004 in partnership with several regional and international organizations. The project provided valuable regional training and learning opportunities for APEC economies, NACA and FAO member governments and participating regional/international organizations. Capacity on aquatic animal health

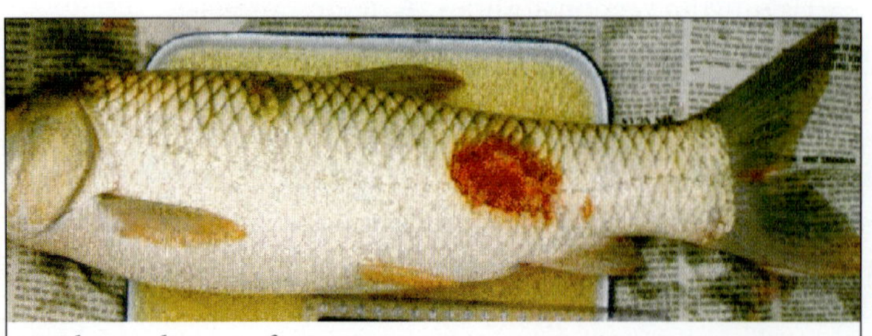
Red spot disease of grass carp may cause serious economic losses if not adequately controlled

CV MOHAN

management, particularly risk analysis, was enhanced, which could lead to improved aquatic animal health policies and practices in the region. Important outputs include two significant publications: (a) a technical report (Arthur and Bondad-Reantaso, 2004) and (b) a risk analysis manual (Arthur *et al.*, 2004) that provides a simplified overview of the risk analysis process to assist responsible individuals in formulating national policies and developing approaches to conduct risk analysis.

A regional Advisory Group (AG) on aquatic animal health established by the Governing Council of NACA in 2001 is functioning proactively to move forward the implementation of the Technical Guidelines. NACA provides institutional support, while FAO, OIE and the identified experts provide technical guidance. The AG meets annually, and through its meeting recommendations (NACA 2004) provides specialist advice, especially on emerging diseases of concern to governments in the region. The recommendations serve as an early warning to countries in the region with susceptible species.

With the aim to maximize the utilization of existing resources in the region, a Regional Aquatic Animal Health Resource Base is being identified under the ongoing NACA regional initiative. The resource base in aquatic animal health is being identified at three levels: regional resource experts (RRE), regional resource centres (RRC) and regional reference laboratories (RRL). RRE is the first level of resource, and the identified experts will provide specialist advice to the region in their fields of expertise, assist in developing diagnostic manuals and disease cards, and provide diagnostic assistance on disease emergencies in the region. The second level of resource, the RRC, will not be specific for a single disease but will have good experience in diagnosing and studying aquatic animal diseases and pathogens. RRL is the third level of resource that would be identified for diseases of regional concern not listed by the OIE but included in the QAAD list. A cohesive networking among RREs, RRCs and RRLs in the region will provide an effective, strong and broad network of diagnostic support that will assist to build capacity for implementation of the Technical Guidelines. The envisaged resource base within the Asia Region would provide national agencies with assistance in the diagnosis of key diseases on the regional disease list, provide more generalized support, assist in emergency response to new disease outbreaks and act as contact centers for advice and capacity building in close cooperation with institutions having a mutual interest in improving aquatic animal health.

Pathogens associated with aquatic animal disease emergencies do not respect borders and can spread very rapidly from country to country. Countries in the region are starting to cooperate more closely in their efforts to minimize the impact of aquatic animal diseases. The recent workshop hosted by the Government of Malaysia in July 2004 in Penang, Malaysia, entitled "Building Capacity to Combat Impacts of Aquatic Invasive Alien Species and Associated Trans-boundary Pathogens in ASEAN Countries" is an example of such cooperation. Unless this is done, the disease control efforts of individual countries will be continually frustrated. Part of this cooperation should be the rapid sharing of information on new disease occurrences and the spread of existing epidemic diseases to new areas, particularly near shared watersheds. Therefore, there is a need to continue the strong regional cooperation in aquatic animal health in the Asia-Pacific Region.

CONCLUSIONS

Aquaculture has suffered significant losses due to diseases, and increasing risks are foreseen in the future as aquaculture continues to expand. Enabling governmental policies and commitment among stakeholders will help in managing aquatic animal disease emergencies. Many countries in the region still face significant challenges in the practical implementation of health management strategies, especially in the areas of surveillance, reporting, zoning, contingency planning and risk analysis. This is mainly due to inadequate national capacity and awareness. Bridging development gaps and capacity building across member countries is necessary. As development and implementation of an effective emergency preparedness and response strategy is a long-term process, continuous efforts to motivate and support governments and private industry in initiating their health management programmes is required. Capacity and awareness building activities to suit the regional aquatic animal health management needs should be continuously undertaken to sustain the good momentum built in the region. In particular, further support to national and regional initiatives for capacity building is essential.

LITERATURE CITED

AQUAVETPLAN. 2002. *The Australian aquatic animal diseases veterinary emergency plan.* (www.affa.gov.au).

Arthur, J.R. & Bondad-Reantaso, M.G. (eds.) 2004. *Capacity and awareness building on import risk analysis (IRA) for aquatic animals.* Proceedings of the workshops, 1–6 April 2002, Bangkok, Thailand and 12–17 August 2002, Mazatlan, Mexico. APEC FWG 01/2002. NACA, Bangkok, 203 pp.

Arthur, J.R., Bondad-Reantaso, M.G., Baldock, F.C., Rodgers, C.J. & Edgerton, B.F. 2004. *Manual on risk analysis for the safe movement of aquatic animals* (FWG/01/2002). APEC/DoF/NACA/FAO, 59 pp.

Baldock, C. 2002. Health management issues in the rural livestock sector: useful lessons for consideration when formulating programmes on health management in rural, small-scale aquaculture for livelihood. In: J.R. Arthur, M.J. Phillips, R.P. Subasinghe, M.B. Reantaso &. I.H. MacRae, (eds.) *Primary aquatic animal health care in rural, small-scale, aquaculture development.* pp. 7-19. FAO Fisheries Technical Paper No. 406. Rome.

Bondad-Reantaso, M.G. 2004. Trans-boundary aquatic animal diseases/pathogens. In: J.R. Arthur & M.G. Bondad-Reantaso, (eds.) *Capacity and awareness building on import risk analysis for aquatic animals.* pp. 9-22. Proceedings of the workshops, 1–6 April 2002, Bangkok, Thailand and 12–17 August 2002, Mazatlan, Mexico. APEC FWG 01/2002, NACA, Bangkok.

FAO/NACA. 2000. *Asia regional technical guidelines on health management for the responsible movement of live aquatic animals and the Beijing consensus and implementation strategy.* FAO Fisheries Technical Paper No. 402, 53 pp., Rome.

NACA. 2004. Report of the second meeting of the Asia Regional Advisory Group on Aquatic Animal Health. NACA, Bangkok, 27 pp.

NACA/FAO. 2004. Quarterly Aquatic Animal Disease Report (Asia and Pacific Region). 2003/4, October to December 2003. NACA, Bangkok, 44 pp.

OIE. 2004. *International aquatic animal health code.* 6th edn. Office International des Épizooties, Paris, 165 pp. (www.oie.int/eng/normes/fcode/A_sum)

Subasinghe, R.P., Bondad-Reantaso, M.G. & McGladdery, S.E. 2001. Aquaculture development, health and wealth. In: R.P. Subasinghe, P. Bueno, M.J. Phillips, C. Hough, S.E. McGladdery & J.R. Arthur, (eds.) *Aquaculture in the third millennium. Technical proceedings of the Conference on Aquaculture in the Third Millennium.* pp. 167-191. Bangkok, Thailand, 20-25 February 2000. NACA, Bangkok and FAO, Rome.

TABLE 2

The responsibilities involved at different levels and the capacity building required for contingency planning, early warning and emergency response (the purpose of the table is mainly to show the enormity of capacity building that will be required at different levels to effectively prepare a contingency plan and run an early warning and emergency response system. The table however does not represent a complete job description and capacity requirements.)

Contingency Planning		
People	**Responsibilities**	**Capacity Required**
National committees/ responsible authorities (e.g. Ministry of Fisheries, Department of Fisheries, Department of Livestock, fisheries research centers, fisheries teaching institutions, extension departments, private sector)	• developing national aquatic animal health strategies • identifying diseases of national concern • commissioning risk analyses on high-priority disease threats • developing technical plans for emergency preparedness (disease strategy manuals, general procedure manuals, enterprise manuals, job descriptions) • developing support plans for emergency preparedness (e.g. financial, resource, legislation) • developing active disease surveillance & epidemiological analysis capabilities & emergency reporting systems • conducting training & awareness programmes	• qualified human resource with specialization in aquatic animal health (e.g. disease diagnostics, disease management, epidemiology, risk analysis, surveillance, zoning, disease treatments, biosecurity) • necessary laboratory infrastructure • access to information • financial resources
	• Ensuring operational capacity for early warning & emergency response (e.g. management manuals, diagnostic resources, capacity & awareness building)	• trained human resource for diagnostics (level II & III diagnostic capabilities), risk analyses, surveillance, epidemiology • adequate infrastructure • training resources • emergency field and laboratory services • adequate financial resources

Early Warning and Emergency Response				
People	**Responsibilities**	**Skills Required**	**Awareness Required to Support Skill Development**	**Capacity Required to Support Skill Development**
Pond/Farm Level (e.g. farmers, farmer associations, officers of the local disease control center)	• recognize a disease emergency • report to the concerned authority • initiate some early response • facilitate the implementation of response options suggested by the local/ national disease control centers	• ability to recognize an exotic disease • what constitutes a disease emergency? • skills to communicate the emergency to responsible authorities • skills to implement the suggested response options	• importance of disease emergencies & the need to report & initiate actions to contain such emergencies • socio-economic impacts of diseases, benefits of rapid containment	• Level I diagnostics (presumptive diagnosis based on history, clinical signs) • biosecurity principles • disinfection procedures • methods for safe destruction & disposal of affected animals
Village/District Level (e.g. extension staff, department officers, farmer leaders, research staff, officers of the local disease control center)	• recognize a disease emergency • report to the concerned higher authority • initiate some early response • implement the suggested response options	• knowledge of aquatic animal diseases • ability to recognize an exotic disease • what constitutes a disease emergency? • sampling & sample collection	• importance of disease emergencies & the need to report & initiate actions to contain such emergencies • socio-economic impacts of diseases, benefits of rapid containment	• Level I diagnostics (presumptive diagnosis based on history, clinical signs) • procedures for sampling & sample collection, preservation & transport • biosecurity • principles of monitoring & surveillance • disinfection methods • methods of safe destruction & disposal of affected animals

Early Warning and Emergency Response				
People	**Responsibilities**	**Skills Required**	**Awareness Required to Support Skill Development**	**Capacity Required to Support Skill Development**
State/Province Level (e.g. research personnel, officers of main line departments, officers of state & provincial & disease control centers)	• identify a disease emergency • identify risks with exotic pathogens • confirm a disease emergency • report to the national authority • ensure implementation of suggested response options	• disease diagnostics • risk analysis • surveillance • epidemiology	• importance of disease emergencies & the need to report & initiate actions to contain such emergencies • consequences of failure • importance of systematic surveillance, risk analysis, reporting	• advanced training on aquatic animal health at graduate/post graduate levels • level II and III diagnostics • principles of risk analysis • epidemiology • organizing general & targeted surveillance programmes
National Level (personnel from national research laboratories, main line departments, national disease control centers)	• confirm disease emergencies • organize & coordinate surveillance systems for early warning • organize & coordinate disease reporting mechanisms • conduct risk analysis • develop national contingency plans for dealing with aquatic animal disease emergencies • ensure effective implementation of contingency plans • organize disease zoning • organize training & awareness programmes	• disease diagnostics • risk analysis • surveillance • epidemiology • disease management • information management	• importance of surveillance, risk analysis, epidemiology, disease reporting, etc to management of aquatic animal disease emergencies	• Advanced training & specialization in aquatic animal health at degree/ postgraduate levels • level III diagnostics for listed diseases of concern to the country • designing & conducting risk analysis • designing & conducting surveillance programmes

National contingency plans for aquatic animal disease emergencies: the way forward for developing countries

Chris Baldock
AusVet Animal Health Services
PO Box 3180, South Brisbane Qld 4101
Australia
chris@ausvet.com.au

Baldock, C. 2005. National contingency plans for aquatic animal disease emergencies: the way forward for developing countries. p. 157–165. In: Subasinghe, R.P.; Arthur, J.R. (eds.). Regional workshop on preparedness and response to aquatic animal health emergencies in Asia. Jakarta, Indonesia, 21–23 September 2004. *FAO Fisheries Proceedings*. No. 4. Rome, FAO. 2005. 178p.

ABSTRACT

Infectious disease emergencies may arise within a country in a number of ways, for example: incursions of known exotic diseases, sudden changes in the behaviour of existing endemic diseases, or the appearance of previously unrecognized diseases. Contingency planning is critical to the effective management of such disease emergencies. A strong national approach is required to ensure that the necessary operational capability is in place so that early detection and effective responses are efficiently achieved. Recovery from an emergency disease response must be followed by measures to ensure that freedom from the particular disease is again maintained. This paper discusses each of these aspects.

INTRODUCTION

The epidemic spread and devastating impacts of white spot syndrome virus (WSSV) in cultured shrimp in Asia clearly demonstrated the vulnerability of aquaculture systems to wide-scale infectious disease emergencies. More recently, the widespread mass mortalities of koi and common carp in Indonesia have re-emphasized the impact that new diseases can have on local economies. Hopefully, the lessons learned from these experiences will result in better preparedness for, and improved responses to similar events when they occur in the future.

The role of contingency planning within a National Aquatic Animal Health Strategy is stressed in the "Asia Regional Technical Guidelines on Health Management for the Responsible Movement of Live Aquatic Animals and the Bejing Consensus and Implementation Strategy" (FAO/NACA, 2000) and preliminary guidance to developing countries on the development of contingency plans is provided in the "Manual of Procedures for the Implementation of the Asia Regional Technical Guidelines on Health Management for the Responsible Movement of Live Aquatic Animals" (FAO/NACA, 2001). This paper discusses the components of a national contingency plan in greater detail.

FIGURE 1
Framework for emergency disease preparedness

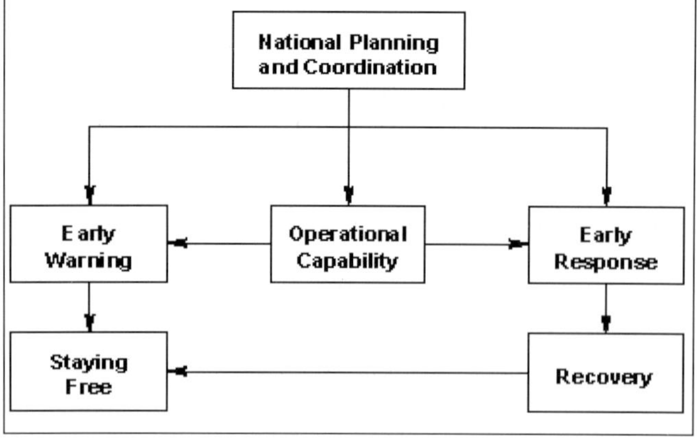

Infectious disease emergencies may arise within a country in a number of ways, for example: incursions of known exotic diseases, sudden changes in the behaviour of existing endemic diseases, or the appearance of previously unrecognized diseases. Early warning and early response are critical to the effective management of such disease emergencies. A strong national approach is required to ensure that the necessary operational capability is in place so that early detection and effective responses are efficiently achieved. Recovery from an emergency disease response is followed by measures to ensure that freedom from the particular disease is again maintained. Figure 1 shows the linkages among these different components. Each of these is explained in more detail in the following sections.

NATIONAL PLANNING AND COORDINATION

In order to have emergency preparedness planning recognized as an important core function of government services, and to have adequate funding and other resources allocated to these activities, the responsible authority should enlist the support of all interested parties. These will include the relevant minister and senior ministry officials, other government departments and agencies including national economic development planning authorities, farming and fishing communities and organizations, seafood marketing authorities, processors, traders and exporters.

Of these, the most important target groups are the government and the farming and fishing communities. In presenting a strong case for support for emergency preparedness planning, the identified disease risks should be described together with the potential socio-economic consequences of an incursion of the disease. Additionally, the benefits that will result from more rapid containment and eradication of the disease outbreak through preparedness should be forcefully presented. The case should preferably be supplemented by a formal socio-economic cost-benefit analysis.

Responsibility for aquatic animal disease emergencies

The Responsible Officer recognized by the Office International des Épizooties (OIE or World Organisation for Animal Health) for the particular country should have overall technical responsibility with regard to preparedness for and management of aquatic animal health emergencies. This may be the Chief Veterinary Officer (CVO) or equivalent, such as the Director of Fisheries of the country. The appropriate government minister would of course be ultimately responsible.

National emergency disease planning committee

A National Emergency Disease Planning Committee (NEDPC) should be appointed to facilitate and coordinate emergency planning. This committee should be directly accountable to the relevant minister such as the Minister of Fisheries and should be charged with the responsibility for developing and maintaining a high state of preparedness for animal disease emergencies. It should preferably be chaired by the Responsible Officer and should hold regular meetings to carry out the following functions:

- commissioning of risk analyses on high-priority disease threats and subsequent identification of those diseases whose occurrence would constitute a national emergency;

- appointment of drafting teams for the preparation, monitoring and approval of contingency plans and other documents;
- liaison with, and involvement of, relevant persons and organizations outside the government aquatic animal health services who also have a role in aquatic animal disease emergency preparedness planning. Where they exist, this would include industry groups, the national disaster management authority, departments of economic planning and finance, environment and wildlife;
- enhancement of the capabilities of emergency field and laboratory services, especially for specific high-priority disease emergencies;
- development of active disease surveillance and epidemiological analysis capabilities and of emergency reporting systems;
- staff training and fisherman/farmer awareness programmes;
- assessment of resource needs and planning for their provision during disease emergencies;
- drafting of legislation and development of financial plans;
- implementation of simulation exercises to test and modify disease emergency plans and preparedness; and
- overall monitoring of the national state of preparedness for disease emergencies.

The NEDPC should comprise the Responsible Officer as chairman, the National Emergency Disease Planning Officer (see below) as secretary, director of field services/ director of disease control (or equivalent), director of the national laboratory, head of the epidemiology unit, director of aquatic animal quarantine and directors of relevant state or provincial services.

In addition to these senior officials, representatives of other ministries that may have a substantial role in responding to aquatic animal disease emergencies, such as environment, wildlife services, economic planning and finance, should either be full members of the committee or should be co-opted as required. It is also highly desirable to have members drawn from the private sector, such as representatives of major fishing, farmer, processing and trading organizations.

National Emergency Disease Planning Officer

A National Emergency Disease Planning Officer (NEDPO) should be appointed. This officer should be a senior officer in the relevant department with training in epidemiology and wide field experience in the management of disease control programmes. If circumstances warrant it, a small unit of professionals should also be appointed to assist the NEDPO.

The planning officer would be both the adviser to, and the executive officer of the National Emergency Disease Planning Committee, and would be actively involved in all NEDPC programmes itemized above.

Aquatic animal disease emergencies as a component of the National Disaster Plan

Most countries have well-developed national disaster plans. These allow essential government and non-government services and resources to be rapidly mobilized in response to a disaster. Such plans may also allow these essential services to be given special powers to act in the emergency. The national disaster plan is usually aimed at specific natural disasters of an emergency nature such as major fires, floods, hurricanes, earthquakes and volcanic eruptions.

A strong case can be made for the official recognition of a disease emergency as a defined natural disaster situation that can be incorporated into the national disaster plan. An epidemic of an emergency aquatic animal disease, for example, has the same characteristics as other natural disasters: it is often a sudden and unexpected event, has the potential to cause major socio-economic consequences of national dimensions and even threaten food security, and requires a rapid national response.

EARLY WARNING

The aim of early warning is to rapidly detect the introduction of, or sudden increase in the incidence of any disease of aquatic animals that has the potential of developing to epidemic proportions and/or causing serious socio-economic consequences. It embraces all initiatives, mainly based on risk analysis and disease surveillance that lead to improved awareness and knowledge of the distribution and behaviour of disease outbreaks (and of infection) and which allow forecasting of the source and evolution of the disease outbreaks and the monitoring of the effectiveness of disease control campaigns.

Risk analysis

Risk analysis is something that we all do intuitively in our everyday life as well as in our professional work. Only recently has it developed into a more formal discipline and is increasingly used in many fields of endeavour. In aquatic animal health, it has perhaps been most widely applied in international trade to evaluate disease risks associated with imports. Import risk analyses are used in reaching decisions as to the most appropriate health certification and quarantine and other measures to be applied for imports into a particular country to produce an acceptable level of risk.

Risk analysis is a tool that can also be used to good advantage for animal disease emergency preparedness planning. International standards for import risk analysis are contained in the *Aquatic Animal Health Code* of the World Organisation for Animal Health (OIE, 2004) and a regional manual has recently been finalized (Arthur *et al.*, 2004).

Disease surveillance

Disease surveillance should be an integral and key component of all government aquatic animal health services. This is important for early warning of diseases, planning and monitoring of disease control programmes, provision of sound aquatic animal health advice to farmers, certification of exports, international reporting and verification of freedom from diseases. A comprehensive disease surveillance system provides a reliable picture of the health status of aquatic animal populations on an ongoing basis. It is particularly important for animal disease emergency preparedness.

Figure 2 provides a conceptual summary of the relationships among the broad components of a surveillance programme. This figure incorporates the OIE Code

FIGURE 2
Relationships among different components of a surveillance programme incorporating OIE Code concepts

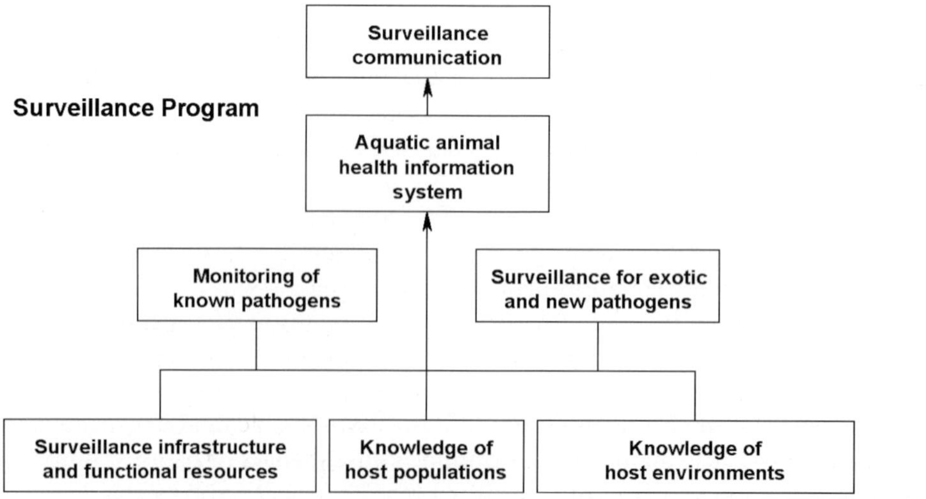

concepts of providing an effective surveillance infrastructure as well as including a description of host population and environmental characteristics.

EARLY RESPONSE

Early response is identified as all actions that would be targeted at rapid and effective containment of, and then possibly elimination of an emergency disease outbreak, thus preventing it from turning into a serious epidemic. There are three broad policy options for responding to emergency diseases; the option chosen for any particular disease will depend on many different factors. It may also be possible to use a combination of options in some instances. The options are:

- ***Eradication***. Initial eradication of disease with eventual total elimination of the pathogen from the country, including silent infections, if they occur. This is the highest level of response but may not always be possible, especially where the disease is well established prior to the initial detection (i.e. where early warning has essentially failed).
- ***Containment***.. Containment of the disease and pathogen to specified zones with control within infected zones and prevention of spread to uninfected areas of the country.
- ***Mitigation***. Reduction of the impacts of the pathogen by implementing control measures at the farm level which reduce the occurrence and severity of disease.

Contingency plans

Countries need to have in place well-documented contingency action plans for specific, high-priority emergency diseases, together with a series of generic plans for activities or programmes common to the various specific disease contingency plans (e.g. setting up national and local disease control centers). They also need to have resource and financial plans and proper legislative backing for all actions. These contingency plans need to be considered and agreed upon in advance by all major stakeholders, including the political and bureaucratic arms of government and the private sector, particularly farmer organizations. The contingency plans should be refined through simulation exercises and personnel should be trained in their individual roles and responsibilities. The components of a contingency plan are shown in Box 1.

The relationships among the different contingency plan components are shown in Figure 3.

BOX 1
Components of a contingency plan.

Summary document

Technical plans
- Disease strategy manuals (one for each high priority disease)
- General procedures manuals
- Enterprise manuals
- Job descriptions

Support plans
- Financial
- Resource
- Legislation
- Other agencies

Operational capability
- Management manuals
- Diagnostic resources
- Training resources
- Awareness and education
- Response exercises

Operational capability

Developing and maintaining an operational capability to effectively and efficiently deal with emergency disease events is a major and continuing challenge. It is simply not possible to be prepared for all possible contingencies, but countries should aim to have an immediate capability for small to moderate outbreaks. The emphasis should be on having key personnel who are well trained and stakeholders who are responsible and aware of the nature of emergency diseases. The capability of different components of the system should always be subject to testing and review.

Response management

Manuals should be prepared that provide a management structure and an information flow system for the handling of an emergency disease emergency at national and local levels. It should describe the operations of control centers, providing principles for the chain of command, functions of sections and role descriptions. Management manuals may be prepared for:

- organization and operation of the national disease control center;
- organization and operation of local disease control centers; and
- emergency disease reporting and information systems, including mapping.

Diagnostic resources

Once the particular disease has been recognized as an emergency, the capability to make both presumptive field diagnoses with subsequent confirmation in the laboratory must be available. For disease threats that are a high priority, this capability must be in place in advance of disease outbreaks. The initial diagnosis will need to be confirmed in a laboratory, possibly even an international reference laboratory. For large outbreaks, it may not be possible to confirm the field diagnosis on every occasion once control and eradication measures are underway.

Field resources

To respond effectively to an emergency disease, personnel with a range of skills and experience are required. These include persons with the ability to undertake thorough disease investigations, tracing of animals and products and supervise operations on infected premises.

Training

All staff should be thoroughly trained in their roles, duties and responsibilities in a disease emergency. Obviously more intensive training will need to be given to those who will be in key positions. It should also be borne in mind that any staff member, from the Responsible Officer downwards, may be absent or may need to be relieved during a disease emergency for one reason or another. Back-up staff should therefore be trained for each position. Training of aquatic animal health staff in early recognition of emergency diseases and collection and dispatch of diagnostic specimens is a key component of preparedness.

Awareness and education

This is one of the most critical, but sometimes neglected, aspects of preparedness planning for emergency diseases, and for fostering "ownership" and support for emergency disease control/eradication campaigns from farmers and other key stakeholders. It also engenders a "bottom up" approach to planning and implementation of disease control programmes, to complement the more traditional "top down" approach usually adopted by governments.

The communication strategies should aim to make stakeholders aware of the nature and potential consequences of important diseases and of the benefits to be derived from their prevention and eradication. Furthermore they should always have an element of rallying the community to the common cause of fighting a disease epidemic.

If at all possible, professional communicators and extension experts should be enlisted to help design and carry out awareness and publicity campaigns. Optimally, personal visits and discussions with farming and fishing communities, processors, traders etc are preferable, but media outlets such as newspapers, radio and television

FIGURE 3.
Relationships among different components of a National Aquatic Animal Disease Contingency Plan.

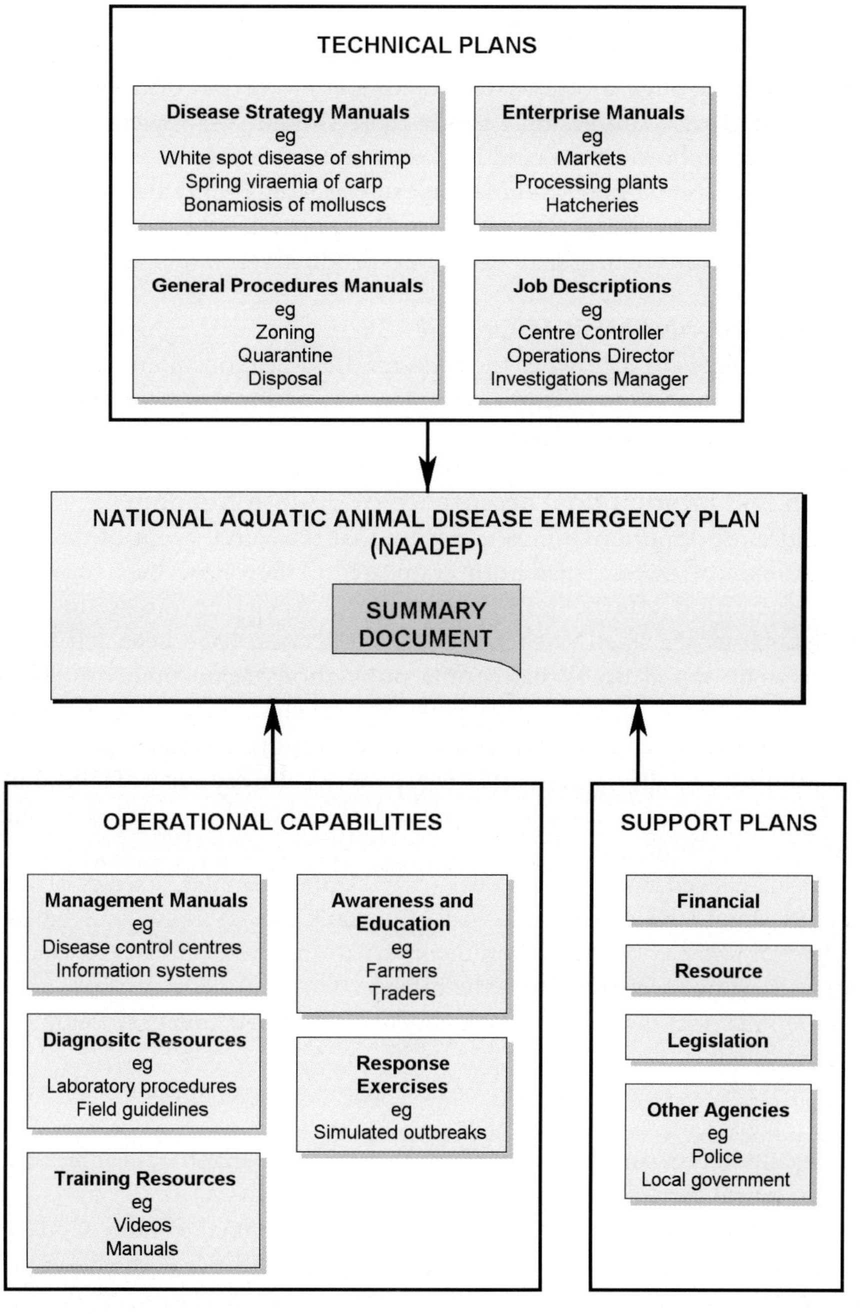

can reach a large target audience quickly. Radio programs have proven to be a very effective method for spreading the message. These should be broadcast at times of the day when most farmers could be expected to be listening to the radio - this may be early in the morning or at night.

Response exercises

Simulation exercises are extremely useful for testing and refining contingency plans in advance of any disease emergency. They are also a valuable means of building teams for emergency disease responses and for training individual staff.

Disease outbreak scenarios that are as realistic as possible should be devised for the exercises, using real data where possible (e.g. for farm locations, populations and trading routes). The scenario may cover one or more time phases during the outbreak with a possible range of outcomes. However, neither the scenario nor the exercise should be overly complicated or long. It is best to test just one system at a time (e.g. operation of a local disease control center). Simulation exercises may be carried out purely as a paper exercise or through mock activities – or a combination of both approaches. At the completion of each simulation exercise there should be a review to identify areas where plans need to be modified and further training is needed.

A full-scale disease outbreak simulation exercise should only be attempted after the individual components of the disease control response have been tested and proved. Earlier exercises of this nature may be counterproductive.

RECOVERY FROM AN EMERGENCY DISEASE

The process of recovery following the successful eradication of an emergency disease involves verification and international acceptance of national disease freedom as well as rehabilitation of farming communities.

Verification and international acceptance of disease freedom

The first and most important aim is to ensure that the causal agent of the disease (and not just the clinical disease) has been eradicated. There have been many occasions in which eradication efforts have been stopped when the disease seems to have disappeared. However small pockets of active infection have been left to smoulder. These have again flared up as susceptible populations again build up. This negates expensive control programmes.

It is therefore vital that as disease control measures diminish towards the end of the campaign, there be a shift of emphasis towards active disease surveillance to detect any residual infection. If vaccination has been used, this should be stopped so that there is no masking of infection.

When it is believed that infection has truly been eradicated, a series of verification programmes should be carried out. An important aim of these will be to provide objective proof to other countries and the international community as a whole that the country has regained freedom from the disease. This will provide the foundation for export trade in animals and animal products to be restored and/or developed.

This may involve:

- demonstration that the country has a capable aquatic animal health service and comprehensive disease surveillance programmes;
- statistically based surveys using laboratory tests for inapparent infection; and
- active clinical surveillance.

Reference should be made to the OIE Aquatic Animal Health Code for more specific guidelines on acceptable international disease freedom verification procedures for each disease.

Rehabilitation of farming communities

There will be a need to repopulate affected areas with disease-free animals, particularly if a "stamping out" campaign has been followed. The opportunity should be taken to introduce replacement animals that are not only free of the target disease but also of other important diseases. Consideration could also be given to upgrading genetic resources at the same time.

Special support mechanisms and programmes should be considered to allow affected farmers and farming communities to get back on their feet after a crippling disease outbreak. However, this could be regarded as a political rather than technical decision.

STAYING FREE

Lessons from the disease outbreaks and the campaigns to control and eradicate them should be learned so that the country will be in a better position to stay free of the disease and to respond more quickly and effectively to any further introductions.

A thorough review should be carried out while the events are still fresh in peoples' minds. This review should be led by the Responsible Officer and should include key representatives of both those involved in the disease control campaign (head office and local) and those affected by the disease outbreaks. Issues to be considered in the review include:

1. An epidemiological analysis of how the disease entered the country and the subsequent methods of spread with a view to strengthening quarantine and other preventive measures against the disease.
2. Based on the results of the above and on other experiences, a determination of how disease surveillance and other early warning procedures can be improved and on which geographical areas to concentrate efforts.
3. Revision of contingency plans for the disease.
4. Strengthening of public extension/education programmes.
5. Determination of whether legislative and other support frameworks need to be improved.
6. Further training programmes.

CONCLUSIONS

Having the capability to deal with emergency diseases involves a great deal of planning and training as well as having an appropriate level of resources mainly in the form of appropriately skilled personnel. Although a comprehensive capability in many countries will take a long time to achieve, foundations can be laid within the framework of whatever resources presently exist.

ACKNOWLEDGEMENTS

Material in this paper is consistent with the FAO Good Emergency Management Practices (GEMP) programme (www.fao.org/ag/AGA/AGAH/EMPRES/GEMP.htm), the OIE Aquatic Animal Health Code and the Australian emergency animal disease plans, AUSVETPLAN (www.aahc.com.au/ausvetplan/index.html) and AQUAVETPLAN (www.affa.gov.au/docs/animalplanthealth/aquatic/index.html).

LITERATURE CITED

Arthur, J.R., Bondad-Reantaso, M.G., Baldock, F.C. & Rodgers, C.J. 2004. Manual on pathogen risk analysis for the safe movement of aquatic animals (FWG/01/2001). APEC/DoF/NACA/FAO. 59 pp.

FAO/NACA. 2000. *The Asia regional technical guidelines on health management for the responsible movement of live aquatic animals and the Beijing consensus and implementation strategy.* FAO Fisheries Technical Paper No. 402, 53 pp., Rome.

FAO/NACA. 2001. *Manual of procedures for the implementation of the Asia regional technical guidelines on health management for the responsible movement of live aquatic animals.* FAO Fisheries Technical Paper No. 402, Supplement 1, 106 pp., Rome.

OIE. 2004. *Aquatic animal health code*, 7th Edn, Office International des Épizooties, Paris. (available at www.oie.int)

MSX disease emergency response: Canadian experience

Sharon E. McGladdery
Fisheries and Oceans Canada, Aquatic Animal Health Office
200 Kent Street, Ottawa, Ontario, K1A 0E6, Canada
mcgladderys@dfo-mpo.gc.ca
Mary F. Stephenson
Fisheries and Oceans Canada, Shellfish Health Unit
PO Box 5030, Moncton, New Brunswick, E1C 9B6, Canada
stephensonm@dfo-mpo.gc.ca

McGladdery, S.E. & Stephenson, M.F. 2005. MSX disease emergency response: Canadian experience. p. 167–178. In: Subasinghe, R.P.; Arthur, J.R. (eds.). Regional workshop on preparedness and response to aquatic animal health emergencies in Asia. Jakarta, Indonesia, 21–23 September 2004. *FAO Fisheries Proceedings*. No. 4. Rome, FAO. 2005. 178p.

ABSTRACT

Canada has had several disease emergencies emerge in its aquatic animals. The first came in the early 1900s before recognition of disease and the need for control activities was clearly understood for aquatic animals. This set the foundation for Canada's aquatic animal health learning curve that has increased exponentially over the last 20 years as aquaculture activities have intensified and diversified into new species and environments. The earliest Canadian aquatic animal disease case-history is presented, along with Canada's most recent experience in 2002 with the first-time detection of the oyster disease MSX, caused by the microscopic parasite *Haplosporidum nelsoni*, and a reportable disease listed by the World Organisation for Animal Health (OIE – Office International des Épizooties). Both are discussed in the context of theory and reality in dealing with aquatic animal disease emergencies that span multi-stakeholder interests and governmental jurisdictions.

INTRODUCTION

Canada has a long history of experience with aquatic animal disease management dating back to the 1915 emergence of Malpeque disease in oysters in Prince Edward Island (PEI). In the 1970s, Canada developed fish health protection regulations to provide health certification for the developing salmonid aquaculture industry. Parallel work was conducted with the International Council for the Exploration of the Sea (ICES) on wild fish diseases, on the management of outbreaks of infectious salmon anaemia (ISA) in the 1990s in New Brunswick and infectious haematopoietic necrosis (IHN) in Atlantic salmon in the Pacific, and on the study of aquaculture-wild disease interactions; up to Canada's most recent biosecurity challenge, returning once again to the oysters of Atlantic Canada, with the emergence of MSX disease caused by the protistan parasite *Haplosporidium nelsoni*.

The evolution of Canada's federal approach to aquatic animal biosecurity measures is based on these experiences and the increasing recognition of the need to be proactively prepared. The odds against successful disease eradication from open- or flow-through systems are low, but proactive response plans provide some assurance that the odds for a successful outcome are optimized.

CANADA'S INTRODUCTION TO AQUATIC ANIMAL HEALTH MANAGEMENT – MALPEQUE DISEASE

Canada's first experience of a significant aquatic animal disease pre-dates modern aquatic pathology, and aquaculture by almost 60 years. Mass mortalities of Eastern (American) oysters (*Crassostrea virginica*) occurred in Malpeque Bay, one of the major oyster-producing beds on Prince Edward Island (PEI) in 1915 (Needler and Logie, 1947). However, the mortalities were not recognized as being due to an infectious disease until it spread to neighbouring oyster beds on PEI via transplant activities in the 1930s. At this point, the disease became known as Malpeque Bay disease. Although the causative agent was not determined, the disease was reported to the Royal Society of Canada by Needler and Logie (1947) with the explanation: "*...this account is presented because of the rarity of recorded cases of mortalities in the sea attributable to contagious disease*". Ironically, the now internationally renowned "Malpeque oyster" derives its name from the same bay and from the survivors of the original Malpeque disease outbreak and 57 years later, mortalities in the sea caused by contagious disease are by no means rare.

Anecdotal evidence suggests that Malpeque disease may have been introduced via a massive transplantation of healthy oyster seed from New England in 1913–1914 (R.E. Drinnan, unpublished data). This was to help restore overfished oyster beds in Malpeque Bay. The first losses of over 99 percent of market-size oysters in Malpeque Bay occurred 12-18 months following the transplant. The fishery in the bay was closed and fishing effort moved to neighbouring oyster beds. Between 1935 and 1937, the oyster stocks in Malpeque Bay recovered to a level where they could be commercially fished again, and seed were transplanted into neighbouring bays. Malpeque disease re-emerged, virtually wiping out the remaining PEI oyster fishery, and indicating that an infectious agent was being carried by the apparently healthy oysters from Malpeque Bay. The first Canadian aquatic biosecurity control measure was put into place – a complete prohibition of any oyster transfers out of PEI (Needler and Logie, 1947).

By the mid-1950s, the PEI oyster beds had again recovered, and the first lesson in biosecurity risks was learned: human memory can rarely keep disease risk in perspective when high-risk stocks appear healthy. The jump of Malpeque disease from PEI to mainland Atlantic Canada in 1957 is attributed to unsanctioned transfers of oysters for processing in southwestern New Brunswick.

The response to this emergency was one that would attract strong debate today. Spread of the disease to neighbouring New Brunswick and Nova Scotia oyster beds was considered to be unpreventable because of southern Gulf of St. Lawrence hydrography and an inability to differentiate healthy carriers from uninfected oysters. Therefore, Malpeque disease-tolerant oysters from PEI were actively spread throughout the southern Gulf of St. Lawrence (Found and Logie, 1957; Drinnan, 1967). This was considered to be the most effective way of accelerating recovery of oyster stocks that were inevitably going to succumb to the disease.

This strategy worked, and the southern Gulf of St. Lawrence now produces ~7 000 tonnes of healthy, Malpeque disease-tolerant oyster populations, worth approximately CAD$ 10-15 million. Clinical signs of the disease are rare, and only naïve stocks from neighbouring Cape Breton waters (transplanted for experimental purposes) succumb to the disease, usually within 12-18 months (McGladdery and Stephenson, 1999, McGladdery and Bower, 1999).

Many organisms and aetiologies have been attributed to Malpeque disease (Li *et al.*, 1980), with current research indicating a possible cryptic viral or microcellular protistan aetiology (McGladdery and Bower, 1999); however, the causative agent has defied conclusive identification. Furthermore, the single generation inheritance of tolerance in offspring of the few survivors of initial exposure and the lack of a microscopically evident or culturable microbial agent have both complicated understanding of the disease. Recent transmission experiments, however, have demonstrated that the causative agent remains virulent for naïve oysters 40 years after the last clinical outbreaks (McGladdery and Stephenson, 1999). These transplant experiments, however, were abruptly halted in 2002 when MSX disease (caused by *Haplosporidium nelsoni*) was detected for the first time in oysters from inner Cape Breton waters.

In conclusion, Canada's introduction to aquatic animal health biosecurity is founded on an aetiological mystery.

EIGHTY-SEVEN YEARS LATER – MSX: AN EMERGENCY PREPAREDNESS CASE STUDY

The model contingency plan

In September 2002, a joint Fisheries and Oceans Canada (DFO) – Canadian Food Inspection Agency (CFIA) presentation was made at the Aquaculture Association of Canada's annual Aquaculture Canada^{OM} meeting, in Charlottetown, PEI.[1] A model contingency plan for a disease listed by the World Organisation for Animal Health (OIE - Office International des Épizooties OIE) that would pose a serious threat to a commercially significant species in Canada was presented. This was aimed at defining roles, responsibilities and resource requirements to address a disease emergency within the context of Canada's proposed National Aquatic Animal Health Partnership (NAAHP).

The model chosen was MSX disease of eastern oysters (*Crassostrea virginica*). This was considered to be a "worst case scenario" because detection of light infections is difficult using routine screening techniques (light microscope histology), mechanism(s) of transmission are unknown, and infections affect cultured and wild oyster populations. In addition, oyster production spans federal and provincial authorities, First Nations' traditional food fisheries, commercial fisheries, licensed aquaculture lease-holders, processing plants and brokerage operations, and roadside/retail marketer activities. In summary, control of MSX, if detected in open-water oysters, would be extremely "problematic" and involve a wide diversity of stakeholder interests.

Meanwhile back at the lab

Oyster samples from St. Patrick's Channel, Bras d'Or Lake (Figure 1), submitted to the DFO Shellfish Health Unit in Moncton due to reports of increasing levels of mortality over 2002, revealed plasmodia-like inclusions that had not been found previously in Canadian oysters. The high levels of infection (prevalence and intensity) along with intense haemocyte infiltration indicated that this was the likely cause of the mortalities being reported.

Histopathology samples were immediately sent to the Pacific Biological Station (PBS) in Nanaimo, British Columbia, and the Oxford Maryland Cooperative Laboratory. Histopathology and tissue samples preserved for molecular analyses were also sent to the OIE reference laboratory at the Virginia Institute of Marine Sciences (VIMS), Williamsburg, Virginia.

---

[1] McGladdery S.E., McVicar, A.H. & Warrell, W.S. Disease control models for the proposed National Aquatic Animal Health Program. Aquaculture CanadaOM 2002, October 21, 2002, Charlottetown, PEI.

FIGURE 1
Cape Breton, Nova Scotia and area where MSX was first detected

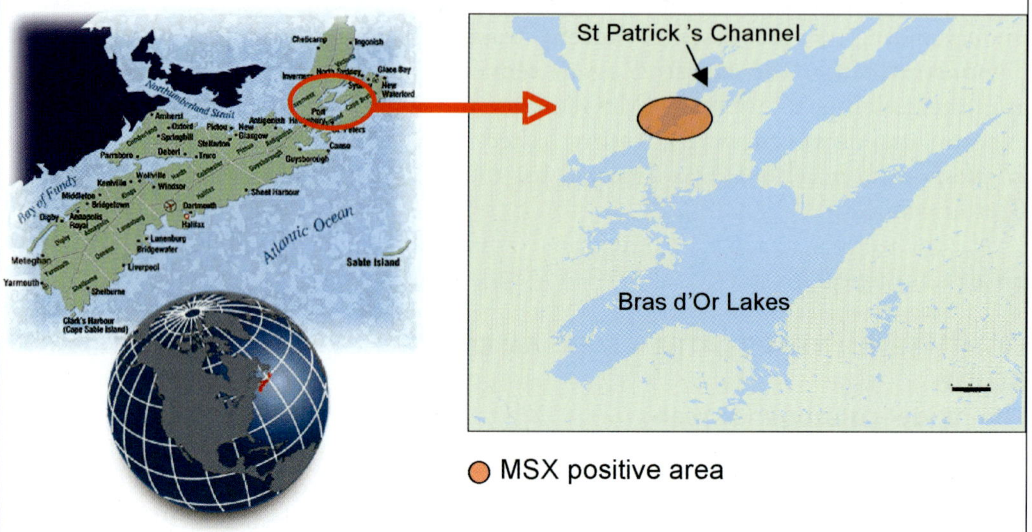

A working contingency plan

Initiation of the plan prior to diagnostic confirmation

The model contingency plan outlined at the Aquaculture Canada meeting was converted to a working contingency plan prior to official confirmation of the diagnosis. It contained actions required on "suspicion" of infection as well as those required on confirmation (or negation) of the diagnosis.

A critical first step was the appointment of a senior manager to compile the emergency response team (the MSX Task Group) and coordinate all activities. This person was selected on the basis of their knowledge of the industry and given the authority to make decisions and discuss options and recommendations directly with senior management (DFO regional and national management, as well as provincial aquaculture managers). The MSX Task Group consisted of key DFO and provincial personnel and was tasked with:

i) contacting the directly affected stakeholders; and
ii) preparing information for the public and for media communications.

This senior DFO coordinator was essential for permitting science expertise to concentrate on development of appropriate surveillance programmes and laboratory analyses protocols.

Conversion from suspect to confirmed diagnosis

As soon as MSX was confirmed by the OIE reference laboratory for molluscan diseases at VIMS, the Chief Veterinary Officer (CVO) for Canada was notified. The Office of the CVO immediately prepared an advisory note that was sent to OIE Headquarters in Paris. The report provided the known geographic extent of infection, mortality levels being reported, the contingency plan, and surveillance plans for delineating the exact geographic extent of the distribution of MSX in Canadian oysters. This advisory made Canada positive for MSX until the emergency surveillance could demonstrate which oyster stocks were not infected (Stephenson and McGladdery, 2002).

This model contingency plan doubled in size over the period of October 2002 to February 2003 from a six page document to the current plan, as results and tracking of stock movements evolved. Revisions are ongoing as results from positive, buffer and negative zones (established following the emergency targeted surveillance programme) continue to emerge.

Consultation and containment

A meeting was arranged close to the affected site with Cape Breton oyster growers, First Nations, and provincial and federal fisheries and seafood authorities. An overview of what was known about MSX was presented and the possible scenarios for introduction of the disease were discussed. This was considered to be an essential first step in getting to know the local faces involved and letting them know who the emergency response team were. It was also an important discussion for putting the outbreak into a socio-economic as well as epidemiological context. The history of who was working with whom, and moving which stock where, was an essential foundation for developing the surveillance programme required. It was also useful for identifying key stakeholder representatives to participate in the plethora of conference calls required to keep as many key people informed in as timely a manner as possible.

Based on an absence of evidence that MSX had been present historically (DFO surveillance of oyster mortalities since the 1930s), the hypothesis was of a recent introduction; however, surveillance data were needed to determine if this was linked to a point-source or to a wider-spread introduction. The appearance of MSX within the Bras d'Or Lakes system, which is more or less completely land-locked, suggested a link to human activities rather than climate change or oceanographic influences. Further, the known affected area is adjacent to a mining operation using cargo vessels carrying ballast from the eastern United States where MSX is endemic. Although the high mortalities and lack of historic evidence of infection were indicative of an exotic disease occurrence, this was considered insufficient alone to negate the possibility of a historic presence, especially of subclinical infections or unreported/unobserved oyster mortalities. An attempt to eradicate MSX from the affected sites was also discussed, but considered premature until the actual extent of infection was better known.

Pending collection of more data, it was important to contain spread from the known affected areas and areas that had direct oyster transfer links. Since the detection coincided with the peak period for harvest for the Christmas market, control of these activities was a priority. The commercial fishery was already closed for conservation purposes, so the only harvesting activity was by lease-holders and First Nations. Fisheries and Oceans and the Nova Scotia Department of Agriculture and Fisheries (NSDAF) agreed to withdraw harvest licenses and develop protocols that would permit oysters that were fit for market to be harvested safely. On finalization, these Harvest Protocols were posted on the DFO website to permit public access (www.dfo-mpo.gc.ca/science/aquaculture/msxdisease/msx_handle_e.htm). First Nations voluntarily stopped their food fishery for oysters.

Preparation of an emergency surveillance programme

Using the information on hand, surveillance was aimed at determining how far the disease could have spread outward from the known infection area. Surveillance priorities focused on current and recent oyster transfers within and out of Cape Breton waters. Transfer pathways into the southern Gulf of St. Lawrence and to PEI in the previous two years for live-holding, processing or depuration relay were also identified. Neighbouring provinces were alerted and included in surveillance collections.

As "controls" for possible transfer-activity related MSX spread, oyster samples from areas with no direct contact with Cape Breton oysters were included in the surveillance programme. Lastly, mussels (*Mytilus edulis*) close to oyster beds known to be positive for MSX were also included. This was due to concerns about the potential for non-oyster transfers with other Cape Breton aquaculture-related activities, notably those of mussels where leases are located in the same bays as oyster beds or aquaculture operations.

FIGURE 2
Histopathological detection of MSX in eastern oysters (*Crassostrea virginica*) from Cape Breton

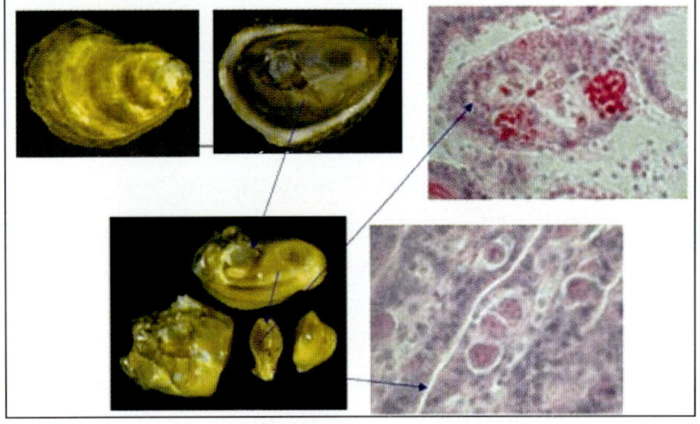

Emergency surveillance: sample collection and analysis

Sampling procedures and collection design were developed by the NSDAF in consultation with the DFO Shellfish Health Unit at the Gulf Fisheries Centre (GFC). Sites in Cape Breton farthest away from the known affected sites were sampled first. Two teams of personnel trained by the provincial veterinarian visited a maximum of two sites per day, using on-site wet gear, boats and harvesting equipment. All materials transferred between sites by the collection team, including vehicles, were disinfected between sites. New Brunswick and PEI provincial fisheries and aquaculture authorities assisted with collections from their provinces. These collections extended into winter months, despite the challenge of remote winter travel and sampling at sub-zero temperatures through ice. The samples were examined by shellfish pathologists at the DFO laboratory in Moncton and PBS Nanaimo. Sample receipt, processing, histopathological screening (Figure 2), data recording and polymerase chain reaction (PCR) subsample analyses were undertaken in accordance with detailed guidelines prepared in advance by the GFC Shellfish Health Unit. Equipment was standardized to ensure that effort and results between different inspectors and analysts were consistent. This included microscope objective magnifications, the number of runs through automatic staining machines for optimal counter-stain contrast and the reagents used for DNA extraction from tissue homogenates for PCR and for *in situ* hybridization analyses.

Due to winter temperatures being associated with lighter levels of infection in oysters in endemic waters along the eastern United States, confidence in negative results from routine microscopic examinations was low – especially those collected from beds close to known positive sites or with direct links to affected sites. Tissue samples from all oysters for the initial emergency surveillance were preserved for PCR using sterile technique to prevent cross-specimen contamination, prior to collection of tissues destined for both light and electron microscopy.

Histopathological examination procedures were developed to ensure coverage of the greatest geographic range as possible for heavy/conclusive infections. Thus, 30 oysters from each sample of 60 were examined at low and low-medium magnification – considered sufficient to detect heavy infections. Once all samples had been screened at this level, all negative samples were re-examined at high-dry magnification for light infections that could have been missed at the lower microscope magnifications. A third examination was made by another pathologist on any subclinical or inconclusive infections, for confirmation purposes. Some inconclusive samples were also sent to the OIE reference laboratory and Dr Susan Ford of the Haskin Shellfish Research Laboratory at Rutgers University, who was invited to meet with Cape Breton stakeholders by First Nations early in November 2002 to provide a first-hand account of dealing with MSX in the United States.

The remaining outstanding 30 oysters from samples that were negative after the low and high-power sweep were examined to confirm the absence of MSX from the tissue examples submitted. Lastly, subsamples of tissues preserved in 95 percent ethanol from negative oysters, along with all oysters showing inconclusive plasmodia-like tissue inclusions, were examined using PCR.

Throughout each analysis stage, a central logbook tracked sample possession and sample step. Positive infections indicated a positive sample, but further analysis for prevalence and intensity was deferred until all samples had been analysed.

FIGURE 3
Classic MSX and sub-clinical SSO oyster infections

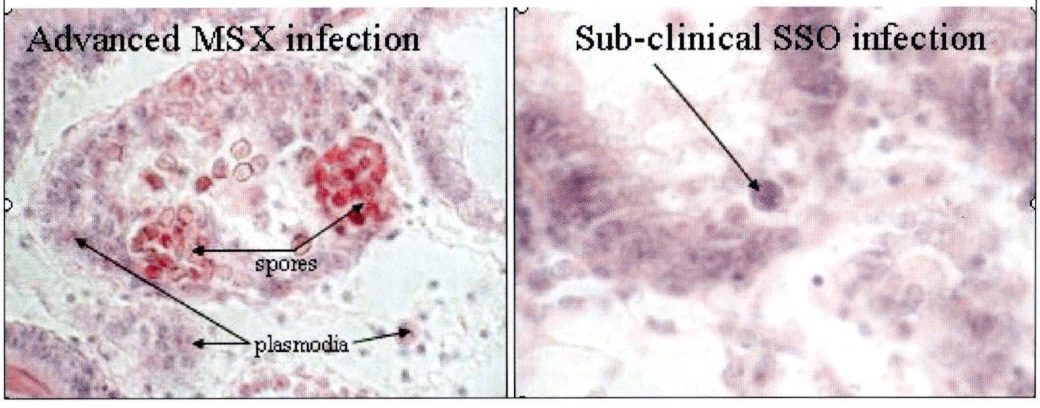

Communications and reporting of emergency surveillance results

Conference calls were held on a daily basis over the first few weeks while Harvest Protocols were finalized and surveillance collections were being made. Separate conference calls were needed for internal briefing of DFO (Ottawa and Area offices in Nova Scotia, New Brunswick and PEI); and for provincial and industry stakeholders. Up to five hours a day were spent ensuring everyone was briefed over October and November. The frequency of the calls was reduced over December and January to weekly and bi-weekly. Since March 2003, the calls have been limited to updates on results every few months or when new information is found.

The results from the initial emergency surveillance were completed in November 2002 and released according to a media communications plan. These showed two apparent levels of MSX infection. One was the classic MSX infection with plasmodial proliferation throughout the connective tissues and digestive tubules, some of which also showed spore development (Figure 3). These infections were found exclusively in oysters that had direct contact with the infected oysters in St. Patrick's Channel. A second type of infection, showing isolated plasmodia with no sign of proliferation or haemocyte infiltration response, was also detected. This was reported as "suspect MSX", but since MSX PCR analysis of these infections was all negative, it was emphasized that they required further investigation. Negative PCR results had also been obtained from lighter MSX infections, so the possibility of false negatives as well as false positives needed further analysis. The significance of the suspect infections was that they were outside Cape Breton, but in oysters that had transfer links (direct and indirect) with Cape Breton oysters.

Tests performed using the PCR primer for sea side organism (SSO) disease of oysters caused by *Haplosporidium costale*, a close relative of the MSX organism, confirmed the presence of the SSO parasite in oysters from PEI and the north shore of Cape Breton outside Bras d'Or Lakes. These infections were all light (1-3 plasmodia per tissue section) (Figure 3) and had no obvious links to the MSX outbreak in Cape Breton. PCR analysis of the first samples submitted from Cape Breton in late September used both MSX and SSO primers. Since SSO was listed by the OIE as one of a number of "other significant diseases" for molluscs in 2002, this was also reported to the OIE as a new finding for Canada. This was given the caveat that none of the infections were associated with clinical disease.

Additional samples were collected overwinter from wild and cultured oyster beds in Cape Breton, Nova Scotia, southwest Nova Scotia, the Bay of Fundy and the southern Gulf of St. Lawrence (New Brunswick, PEI and the Magdalen Islands, Québec). The results from all analyses, plus those conducted in early spring 2003, showed no change in the geographic distribution of MSX, but added more areas with subclinical SSO infections (Figure 4).

Control options and considerations

Given the apparently limited distribution of MSX, the feasibility of eradication was considered. A potential window of opportunity existed for oyster depopulation at affected sites in early May 2003, following the spring thaw and before temperatures and salinities rose to levels conducive to MSX proliferation (> 10 °C). However, eradication was judged unrealistic given that:

- all oysters (spat to adults) from affected areas would need to be removed,
- the intermediate host or reservoir of infection was unknown, and
- the method of introduction of MSX into Bras d'Or Lakes was unknown.

The high potential for failure via unharvested oysters, unknown reservoirs, and the inability to prevent subsequent re-introduction of the infection if eradication was successful, meant this would not be worth the effort. However, the decision not to pursue depopulation meant that Bras d'Or Lakes became an MSX-positive zone, encompassing both positive sites and those sites that had not tested positive.

Control options based on this MSX-positive zone designation had to be developed. Firstly, all Introduction and Transfers Committees (ITCs) were notified of the need to refuse transfer licenses for oyster movement out of Bras d'Or Lake waters. This reinforced the controls in place through the Harvest Protocols, since Bras d'Or Lakes are a naturally contained water body, nestled at the center of the Cape Breton Highlands with a narrow northern passage to surrounding Atlantic waters (Figure 1). This natural geographic containment is conducive to management of active transfer activities. Federal surveillance efforts would concentrate on a designated buffer zone surrounding Cape Breton, to ensure early detection of any emergence of MSX outside Bras d'Or Lakes.

With respect to control of oyster movements within Bras d'Or Lakes, "like to like" transfer is considered an acceptable risk for disease management, but required regional surveillance effort, with coordination between DFO Area Offices in Cape Breton and the Nova Scotia Department of Agriculture and Fisheries (NSDAF). DFO's Shellfish Health Unit has provided diagnostic guidance to the Unama'ki Institute of Natural Resources at Eskasoni and the NSDAF veterinary pathology laboratory at Truro to assist with oyster disease management within Bras d'Or Lakes. Consideration was given to mass transplantation of infected stock around Bras d'Or Lakes, for the same reasons applied to the question of management of Malpeque disease in the 1950s – i.e. to accelerate spread of the disease and depopulate remaining naïve stocks. However, with no concrete evidence of tolerance in surviving oysters in Cape Breton and over 40 years of research yielding mixed results from selective breeding for resistance to MSX in the United States (Sunila *et al.*, 1999, Ragone-Calvo *et al.*, 2003), the control option was considered to be premature.

FIGURE 4
2002-2003 distribution of MSX and SSO infections in Atlantic Canada

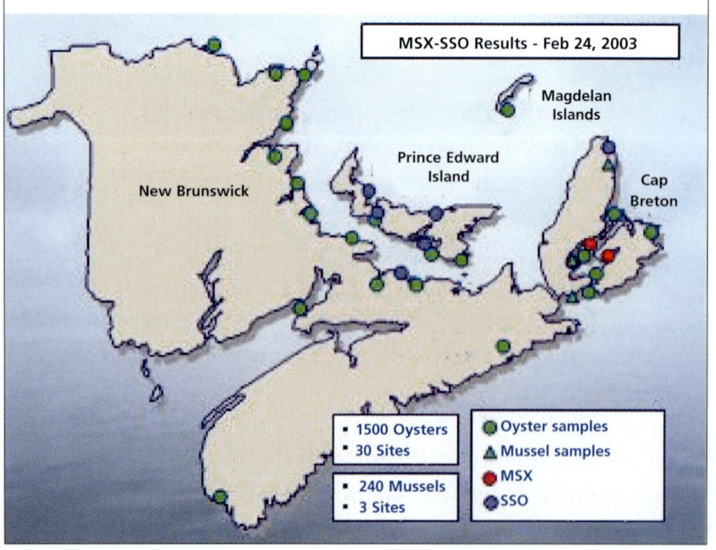

There also remained hope that the particularly severe winter of 2002/03 may have taken a natural toll on MSX, since 2003 proved to be the worst year in a decade for "winterkill". This flooded the diagnostic laboratory with samples for analysis in light of MSX concerns, with no MSX detected until its re-emergence in oysters from Bras d'Or Lakes in the early summer of 2003.

No restrictions of introduction and transfers of live oysters or shell were developed for oysters in areas determined to be positive for SSO. Surveillance efforts mapped subclinical infections at very low levels of prevalence (< 5 percent) and intensity (< 3 plasmodia/tissue section), along with their apparent diffuse distribution in oysters from around Atlantic Canada (including a single co-infection found in Cape Breton). These infections appear to pose no clear risk to apparently uninfected oysters in Atlantic Canada. The molluscan histopathology collection at GFC will be examined to determine whether or not SSO was present in Atlantic Canadian oysters prior to 2002, but unrecognized until the PCR analyses of 2002/03. A haplosporidian was reported from a single mussel from PEI in 2002, but this showed no molecular affinity to either MSX or SSO (Stephenson *et al.*, 2003).

One of the most challenging control debates centered on whether or not transfer restrictions should be applied to other species in the MSX-positive zone. This discussion is not new to Canada. Transfers of scallops from ISA-endemic areas and mussels from Malpeque endemic areas have been subject to similar debate. ISA screening of scallops used sensitive salmonid cell-lines. Malpeque disease risks from mussels used oyster "canary" sentinels. Neither proved positive for carriage of virulent infectious agents of the diseases of concern. However, mussel transfers were prohibited pending PCR analysis of mussels located near the most heavily MSX-positive oyster beds in late 2002, as well as in the summer of 2003. Neither these, nor samples examined from other locations in Cape Breton, showed any evidence of the presence of *H. nelsoni* or *H. costale.* Thus, no restrictions on movements of other molluscs out of the MSX-affected zone were made subject to normal conditions of transfer that include washing on site prior to transfer for processing, to reduce the risk of inadvertent transfer of fouling organisms (such as juvenile oysters) that might transmit these parasites.

Another control option that received detailed consideration was importation of resistant strains or species of oyster from the United States. However, physiological adaptation of a more southerly population to the growing conditions in Bras d'Or Lakes, along with concerns about introduction of other diseases, meant this option was considered premature.

Current status

The winter of 2002/03 was the hardest salt-water freeze-over experienced in Atlantic Canada for a decade. The spring thawing of the deep ice and snow cover reduced the salinities within the lakes to < 15 ppt until late into May-June in many bays. However, heavy infections were detected again in oysters from St. Patrick's Channel and other sites within Bras d'Or Lakes by June 2003. These infections have persisted into 2004.

No MSX has been detected in oysters sampled outside Bras d'Or Lakes waters. Thus, the remaining oyster-producing areas in Atlantic Canada are considered negative at the time of writing. Surveillance is being continued throughout Atlantic Canada, with emphasis on the buffer zone. All mortalities from these areas are examined for both MSX and SSO.

The controls put into place continue to restrict leaseholders to harvesting their oysters under stringent guidelines, although options have now been expanded to permit processing outside Cape Breton within a federally registered processing plant with effluent treatment controls. Signed agreement to these procedures is still required from both harvester and processing plant owner/manager. Marketing for direct human consumption is now permitted anywhere, including east of Québec City.

While the disease still exists, success in preventing spread is limited at best and vulnerable to ignorance or deliberate circumvention. Imposing restrictions on one sector of an industry with the significant economic impacts this incurs, while neighbours conduct business as usual, requires strong risk communication to avoid "mutiny" and non-compliance.

A post-mortem on the contingency plan: managing expectations

The technical aspects of the programme ran relatively smoothly, despite the emergence of SSO in the midst of the MSX-driven survey. The greatest problems arose (and continue to plague government) in managing expectations, especially those surrounding communications and the impacts that MSX controls have had on traditional oyster fishing and harvest practices.

Communications with the media, government departments and area offices, and senior management and with the laboratories involved centered on the two lead shellfish pathologists at the DFO Gulf Fisheries Centre (GFC). Despite strong coordination support from management, some stakeholders fell through the cracks. Initial focus was on Cape Breton and the principle affected lease-holders. On determining links to neighbouring provinces, they expressed concern that they had not been advised immediately. Likewise, the commercial harvesters were angry at not being included in the initial discussions, even though the fishery was closed. These would be considered to be oversights that need to be addressed in contingency plan revisions.

Another communication problem encountered was how to release results from the survey. Individual growers assisted greatly with the official collections and expected the Shellfish Health Unit to contact them individually as results were completed. Instead, it was decided to batch-release results, to permit DFO to prepare communications for senior managers, the media, the provinces and other stakeholders. This was seen as an unnecessarily stressful delay for the growers participating in the surveillance programme, and a lot of time was spent away from the microscope on the phone explaining the situation to individual growers, their family friends and neighbours! The historic accessibility of the shellfish pathologists, which served well in getting strong collaboration with initial harvest closures and surveillance protocols, was detrimental to the time needed for laboratory analysis. "Surge protection" for both communications as well as diagnostic work was considered to be a significant challenge that needs to be addressed for future emergency preparedness.

Batch results were released using a pre-agreed upon step-wise approach:

- Advise federal senior management.
- Advise internal DFO MSX working group – coordinator and area offices.
- Hold a DFO-Provincial conference call (provincial representatives advise senior provincial managers).
- Inform any stakeholders with positive or suspect results individually.
- Release results via conference call with key industry representatives.
- Release results to the media.

The hardest information to deal with was the inconclusive results in November. Ideally, these should not have been released, but pressure from government, industry and the media for follow-up to the October announcement of detection of MSX required as rapid a release of information as possible. The analyses undertaken were aimed specifically at detection of heavy (classic) infections and were given the strict caveat that no results were "truly" negative at this point. The detection of the cryptic plasmodial infections was unexpected. These could have been reported as "incomplete" rather than "suspect", but the fact that they demonstrated previously undetected plasmodia and indicated a potential broader distribution requiring precautionary measures (as applied on suspicion of MSX) meant they were reported as "inconclusive" and "very different from the MSX infections in Cape Breton". Expert opinion from the United States had confirmed that the plasmodia looked like MSX prior to the release of the results.

This conundrum was exacerbated by the fact that the PCR analyses were being field validated in the midst of the emergency surveillance. Inconclusive histology was reinforced by negative PCR. Experience from these analyses formed the basis for refinement of both the SSO and MSX primers recommended by the OIE.

As mentioned above, the shortage of experienced resources to cope with the "surge effect" generated by both laboratory and communication needs was a critical issue that needs to be addressed for any future disease emergencies. This is reflected in the three-phase surveillance approach that is being actively pursued by training more shellfish pathologists at local universities and the Unama'ki Institute of Natural Resources.

CONCLUSIONS

Canada's history of experience with Malpeque disease, as well as many other molluscan diseases on both coasts, served well in knowing the key stakeholders to involve. In addition, senior government management (federal and provincial) was quick to respond with support for the activities required. Likewise, the expertise from the United States, France and New Zealand all provided generous and invaluable support for technical discussions as well as review of risk assessments and control options.

The unknown issues that haunt molluscan health protection technically, epidemiologically and with respect to multi-user stakeholder interests also apply to new species (finfish, molluscs, crustaceans, echinoderms etc.) coming under increasing domestication and live transfer activities. It is hoped that some of the experience gained during this exercise is of use for the Koi herpes virus discussions in Indonesia.

ACKNOWLEDGEMENTS

Sincere thanks are due to many people who assisted during the course of the emergency response to MSX, including (but not limited to) Michelle Maillet, Anne Veniot, Susan Bower, Gary Meyer, Nancy Stokes, Eugene Burreson, Maurice Maillet, Gerard Blanchard, Brad Firth, Rene Lavoie, Dorothy Kieser, Gilles Olivier, Christiane Parcigneau, Dan Bedell, Pierre Gautreau, Janet Langille, Joan Reid, Allison MacIsaac, Charlie Dennis, Sheryl Denys, Roland Cusack, Andrew Bagnall, Lou Clancy, Darrell Harris, Crystal MacDonald, Florence Albert, Brian Muise and last, but not least, the grower whose diligent observations and open reporting helped detect this infection at an apparently early stage of its introduction into Canada and trigger as proactive emergency response as possible, Mr. James Crawford.

LITERATURE CITED

Drinnan, R.E. 1967. Rehabilitation of disease-depleted oyster populations in eastern Canada by large-scale transplants. International Council for the Exploration of the Sea C.M. 1967/E: 1-7.

Found, H.R. & Logie, R.R. 1957. Rehabilitation of disease-depleted oyster fisheries. Fish. Res. Board Can., Gen. Ser. Circ. No.29 (Biological Station of St. Andrews, N.B.), April 1959. 2 pp.

Li, M.F., Traxler, G.S., Clyburne, S. & Stewart, J.E. 1980. Malpeque disease, isolation and morphology of a *Labyrinthomyxa*-like organism from diseased oysters. International Council for the Exploration of the Sea C.M. 1980/F:15: 1-9.

McGladdery, S.E. &. Bower, S.M. 1999. Synopsis of infectious diseases and parasites of commercially exploited shellfish: Malpeque disease of oysters. (http://www-sci.pac.dfo-mpo.gc.ca/shelldis/pages/maldisoy_e.htm)

McGladdery, S.E. & Stephenson. M.F. 1999. Malpeque disease of American oysters (*Crassostrea virginica*) – transmission experiment results. Proceedings of the 9th International Conference of the European Association of Fish Pathologists, 19-14th September, Rhodes, Greece. P-008 (abstract).

Needler, A.W.H. & Logie, R.R. 1947. Serious mortalities in Prince Edward Island oysters caused by a contagious disease. *Trans. Roy. Soc. Can.* 41(2), Sect. 5: 73-89.

Stephenson, M.F. & McGladdery, S.E. 2002. Detection of a previously undescribed haplospordian-like infection of a blue mussel (*Mytilus edulis*) in Atlantic Canada. *J. Shellfish Res.* 21: 389 (abstract).

Stephenson, M.F., McGladdery, S.E., Maillet, M., Veniot, A.. & Meyer, G. 2003. First reported occurrence of MSX in Canada. *J. Shellfish Res.* 22: 355 (abstract).

PEDIATRIC DERMATOLOGY

Editors

Arun C Inamadar MD
Professor and Head
Department of Dermatology
Sri BM Patil Medical College and Hospital
BLDE University, Bijapur
Karnataka, India

S Sacchidanand MD
Registrar (Evaluation)
Rajiv Gandhi University of Health Sciences
Bengaluru, Karnataka, India
Formerly
Professor and Head
Department of Dermatology
Bangalore Medical College
Bengaluru, India

Assistant Editors

Aparna Palit MD
Associate Professor
Department of Dermatology
BLDEA's SBMP Medical College, Bijapur
Karnataka, India

S Ragunatha MD
Assistant Professor
Department of Dermatology
Sri BM Patil Medical College and Hospital
BLDE University, Bijapur
Karnataka, India

Jaypee Brothers

McGraw Hill Medical

© 2010, Jaypee Brothers Medical Publishers
First published in India in 2009 by

Jaypee Brothers Medical Publishers (P) Ltd.

Corporate Office
4838/24 Ansari Road, Daryaganj, **New Delhi** - 110002, India, +91-11-43574357

Registered Office
B-3 EMCA House, 23/23B Ansari Road, Daryaganj, **New Delhi** 110 002, India
Phones: +91-11-23272143, +91-11-23272703, +91-11-23282021,
+91-11-23245672, Rel: +91-11-32558559 Fax: +91-11-23276490, +91-11-23245683
e-mail: jaypee@jaypeebrothers.com, Website: www.jaypeebrothers.com

First published in USA by The McGraw-Hill Companies, 2 Penn Plaza, New York, NY 10121. Exclusively worldwide distributor except South Asia (India, Nepal, Sri Lanka, Bhutan, Pakistan, Bangladesh, Malaysia).

All rights reserved. No part of this publication may be reproduced, stored in a retrieval system, or transmitted, in any form or by any means, electronic, mechanical, photocopying, recording, or otherwise, without the prior permission of the publisher or in accordance with the provisions of the Copyright, Designs and Patents Act 1988 or under the terms of any licence permitting limited copying issued by the Copyright Licensing Agency, 90 Tottenham Court Road, London W1P 0LP.

ISBN-13: 978-0-07-166722-7
ISBN-10: 0-07-166722-9

Contributors

Anandan S
Professor and Head
Department of Dermatology
Sri Ramchandra Medical College
Chennai, Tamil Nadu, India

Anitha B
Senior Resident
Department of Dermatology
BLDEA's SBMP Medical College
Bijapur, Karnataka, India

Aparna Palit
Associate Professor
Department of Dermatology
BLDEA's SBMP Medical College
Bijapur, Karnataka, India

Arun C Inamadar
Professor and Head
Department of Dermatology
BLDEA's SBMP Medical College
Bijapur, Karnataka, India

Bindiya Fernandes
Department of Dermatology
Father Muller Medical College
Mangalore, Karnataka, India

Chitra S Nayak
Associate Professor
Department of Dermatology
BYL Nair Hospital and
TN Medical College
Mumbai, Maharashtra, India

Debabrata Bandyopadhyay
Professor and Head
Department of Dermatology
RG Kar Medical College
Kolkata, West Bengal, India

Deepankar De
Assistant Professor
Department of Dermatology
Venereology and Leprology
Postgraduate Institute of Medical
Education and Research
Chandigarh, India

Devinder Mohan Thappa
Professor and Head
Department of Dermatology
JIPMER
Pondicherry, India

Fiona Sequeira
Department of Dermatology
Father Muller Medical College
Mangalore, Karnataka, India

Hemanta Kumar Kar
Professor and Head
Department of Skin and STD
Dr Ram Manohar Lohia Hospital
New Delhi, India

Jayadev Betkerur
Professor and Head
Department of Skin and STD
JSS Medical College Hospital
Mysore, Karnataka, India

K Ravindra
Professor
Department of Dermatology
JJM Medical College
Devangere, Karnataka, India

KA Seetharam
Consultant Dermatologist
Hanuma Skin Center
Guntur, Andhra Pradesh, India

M Naeem Khan
Professor Emeritus
Plastic Surgery
Karachi, Pakistan

M Ramam
Professor
Department of Dermatology
AIIMS
New Delhi, India

Mangala HC
Department of Dermatology
Command Hospital
Bangalore, India

Manjunath Shenoy
Professor
Department of Skin and VD
KS Hegde Medical Academy
Mangalore, Karnataka, India

PVS Prasad
Professor and Head
Department of Dermatology, RMMC
Chidambaram, Tamil Nadu, India

Prabhakar Sangolli
Associate Professor
Department of Dermatology
Dr BR Ambedkar Medical College
Bangalore, Karnataka, India

Prafulla
Department of Dermatology
Father Muller Medical College
Mangalore, Karnataka, India

R Rajagopal
Professor and Head
Department of Dermatology
Command Hospital
Bangalore, Karnataka, India

Ragunatha S
Assistant Professor
Department of Dermatology
BLDEA's SBMP Medical College
Bijapur, Karnataka, India

Ramesh Bhat M
Professor
Department of Dermatology
Father Muller Medical College
Mangalore, Karnataka, India

Rashmi Mittal
Consultant Dermatologist
Kokilaben Hospital
Mumbai, Maharashtra, India

Rashmi Sarkar
Assistant Professor
Department of Dermatology and
Venereology
Maulana Azad Medical College
New Delhi, India

S Chidambara Murthy
Associate Professor
Department of Dermatology and Venereology, VIMS
Bellary, Karnataka, India

S Sacchidanand
Registrar (Evaluation)
Rajiv Gandhi University of Health Sciences
Bengaluru, Karnataka, India

Sandipan Dhar
Associate Professor
Paediatric Dermatology Division
Institute of Child Health and
Visiting Dermatologist
AMRI Hospitals
Kolkata, West Bengal, India

Sangeeta Amladi
Professor and Head
Department of Dermatology
TN Medical College and
BYL Nair Hospital
Mumbai, Maharashtra, India

Sanjeev Grover (Wg Cdr)
Professor
Department of Dermatology
Armed Forces Medical College
Pune, Maharashtra, India

Sanjeev Handa
Professor
Department of Dermatology, PGIMER
Chandigarh, India

Shankar Savant
Lecturer
Department of Dermatology
TN Medical College and
BYL Nair Hospital
Mumbai, Maharashtra, India

Shernaz Walton
Consultant Dermatologist/Clinical Director
Hull and East Yorkshire Hospitals NHS Trust
and Honorary Clinical Senior Lecturer
Hull York Medical School
Department of Dermatology
Princess Royal Hospital
Saltshouse Road
Hull, HU8 9HE
United Kingdom

Shirene Sequeira
Department of Dermatology
Father Muller Medical College
Mangalore, Karnataka, India

Sowmya Kaimal
Department of Dermatology
JIPMER
Pondicherry, India

Sudhansu Shukla
Department of Dermatology
Command Hospital
Bangalore, Karnataka, India

Sunil Dogra
Assistant Professor
Department of Dermatology
Venereology and Leprology
Postgraduate Institute of Medical Education and Research
Chandigarh, India

T Rajkamal
Department of Dermatology
Command Hospital
Bangalore, Karnataka, India

Thomas Oliphant
Specialist Registrar
Department of Dermatology
Princess Royal Hospital
Saltshouse Road, Hull HU8 9HE
United Kingdom

V Ramesh
Department of Dermatology
Safdarjung Hospital
New Delhi, India

VK Somani
Consultant Dermatologist
17- A, Journalist Colony
Jubilee Hills, Hyderabad, India

Veeranna S
Associate Professor
Department of Skin and STD
JSS Medical College and Hospital
Mysore, Karnataka, India

Vijay Kumar Garg
Professor and Head
Department of Dermatology and Venereology
Maulana Azad Medical College
New Delhi, India

Vijay Zawar
Consultant Dermatologist and Lecturer
Department of Dermatology
Nashik District Maratha Vidhya Prasarak Samaj
Medical College and Research Centre
Nashik, Maharashtra, India

Yasmeena Khan
Professor and Head
Department of Dermatology
Liaquat National Postgraduate Medical Centre
Karachi, Pakistan

Preface

Dermatology is an ever-expanding medical science. Subspecialties are growing at a rapid pace. Pediatric Dermatology is one such subspecialty which has grown on a global scale.

There has long been a need for a book on Pediatric Dermatology authored by dermatologists from around the world. This textbook is an attempt to present Pediatric Dermatology as viewed by the dermatologists with special interest in this subspecialty. We have attempted to incorporate a large number of clinical pictures and tables relevant to each chapter and condition.

Knowledge of Pediatric Dermatology will continue to grow rapidly, and it is essential to keep abreast of the current literature from the specialty journals.

We are honoured to have an opportunity to bring together experts in Pediatric Dermatology to write this book. We would like to thank each of the authors for their contributions. We are equally thankful to the contributors from United Kingdom and Pakistan.

We are especially appreciative of the contribution of our Assistant Editors Dr Aparna Palit and Dr S Ragunatha.

We thank the management of Jaypee Brothers Medical Publishers (P) Ltd, New Delhi for their neat and timely printing of this book.

We hope the readers will find this book useful in their practice. We wish, the postgraduate students would also find the book as an important tool for understanding and caring for the children with dermatological diseases.

Arun C Inamadar
S Sacchidanand

Contents

1

Structure and Functions of the Skin

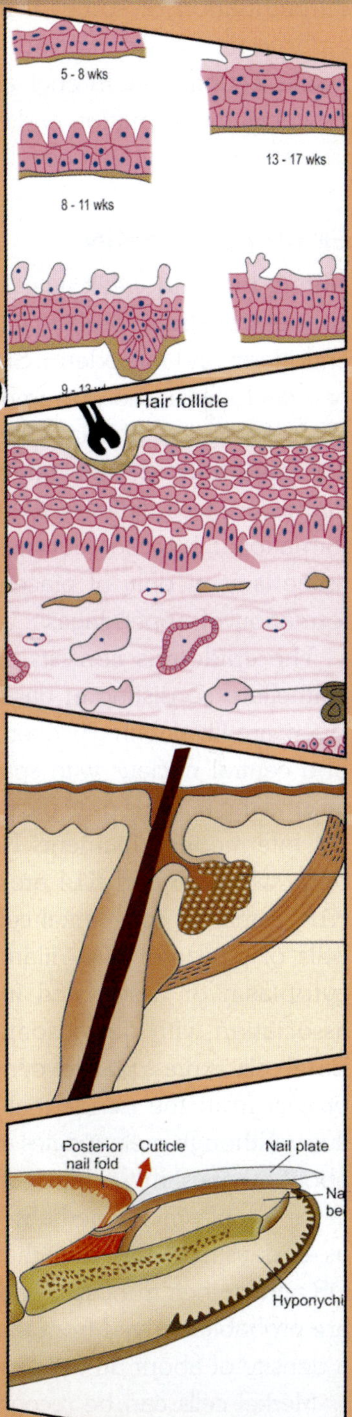

Chidambara Murthy S

EMBRYOGENESIS OF THE SKIN

Embryonic period corresponds to the age of conception until two months of estimated gestational age (EGA). Fetal period refers to the age between second month of EGA until birth. Initiation of histogenesis of all skin regions and differentiation of some of those tissues occur during embryonic period. Formation and differentiation of tissues is continuous through all the trimesters. This section describes the formation and development of skin during various phases of fetal development **(Table 1.1).**

EMBRYONIC SKIN

During the third week after fertilization, embryo undergoes gastrulation, resulting in the formation of ectoderm, endoderm and mesoderm. Shortly ectoderm divides into neuroectoderm and presumptive epidermis. At 30 days EGA, formation of skin is evident. By about six weeks the epidermis, dermo-epidermal junction (DEJ) and dermis are well delineated with nerve and blood vessel formation. Distinction between dermis and subcutaneous tissue is seen only at places. There is no evidence of formation of appendages.

The epidermis consists of simple, flat two-layered epithelium consisting of basal and periderm cells. Both layers are filled with glycogen. Both types of cells consist of a central nucleus with sparse cytoplasmic organelles around the nucleus or at the periphery of the cell. Keratin (K) intermediate filaments K19 and K8 are present in both, while K5 and K14 are expressed by basal layers. K18, a marker for Merkel cell, is also expressed by the cells of periderm. The filaments are dispersed in the cytoplasm or assembled in small, short bundles in association with desmosomes and hemidesmosomes. Basal cells express platelet-derived growth factor. Microvilli project from the peridermal surface into the amniotic fluid. Although melanocytes are found to be dendritic by about 50 days, there is lack of evidence of melanosomes in the cytoplasm. Langerhans' cells are recognized as early as 42 days EGA based on the presence of ATPase, HLA-DR and by their truncated or dendritic morphology. They are probably derived from the yolk sac or fetal liver with a density of about 50 cells/ mm^3.

Merkel cells can be recognized by 55-60 days using keratins K8, K18, K10 and K20. They are neuroendocrine cells distributed at a density of 130 cells/ mm^2. Merkel cells are derived from keratinocytes in situ.

The molecules and antigens characteristic of basal laminae (type IV collagen, laminin, heparan sulfate proteoglycan, nidogen/entactin) are expressed by 8 weeks. Skin-specific molecules are recognized during late first trimester. The antigens associated with the attachment structures are not recognized by light microscopy although keratinocytes have begun synthesizing them.

The dermis is highly cellular, but also contains extra cellular fibrous matrix proteins and type I, III, V and VI interstitial collagens. It consists of mesenchymal cells which are stellate and rich in glycogen. It also contains hyaluronic acid-rich proteoglycan matrix. Compact mesenchyme with a zone of sulfated proteoglycans, situated beneath the epidermis is rich in growth factors and receptors.

Elastic fibers are not detectable by light microscopy, although fibrillin and elastin can be recognized immunohistochemically and microfibrils by electron microscopy. Fine nerve fibers, arterioles; venules and capillaries are present within compact mesenchyme and deep dermis. The large nerve trunks and vessels are located in subcutaneous tissue.

Type IV collagen is present in basement membranes around the vessels, while type III and V collagen in vascular sheets. Autonomic nerves are not recognized.

Embryonic—Fetal Transition

The skin has a mucoid quality and is prone to errors in development at this stage. Transition from embryo to fetus also heralds the formation of appendages (discussed later). The hallmark of this stage is stratification of epidermis with an additional intermediate layer. Intermediate layer expresses K5 and K14 similar to basal layer. Additionally K1 and K10 are also present. Other markers of keratinocyte differentiation like pemphigus antigen, cornified cell envelope proteins; blood group antigens and cell surface glycoproteins are also expressed. This layer also contains glycogen. Genetic diseases involving mutation of keratins can be recognized by this period. At the same time cells of the periderm increase in size and develop microvilli-covered blebs.

Around 80 days EGA, melanocytes are present in maximal density (3000/mm^2). The number decreases towards birth. Melanosomes in these cells can be recognized by late first trimester. The knowledge about this helps in the prenatal diagnosis of tyrosinase-negative oculocutaneous albinism. By about 80 days, Langerhans'

TABLE 1.1: Major events and related diseases in the embryogenesis of skin

Major events	EGA	Vital proteins involved in the embryogenesis (diseases)
Epidermis		Bone Morphogenetic Proteins, Engrailed-1 (Aplasia cutis)
Epidermal specification:		
Presumptive epidermis	3 wks	
Periderm	6 wks	
Epidermal stratification:		
Intermediate layer	8 wks	p63 (AEC, EEC)
Epidermal keratinization:		
Follicular: Beginning	11-15 wks	
Completion	24 wks	
Interfollicular: Beginning	15 wks	K1, K10 (BCIE), K1, K9 (Vorner, Unna-Throst, Greither),
Completion	22-24 wks	Loricrin (NBCIE, Vohwinkle's), Transglutaminase-1(LI),
(Stratum granulosum and Stratum corneum)		Steroid sulfatase (X- linked ichthyosis), Fatty Aldehyde dehydrogenase (Sjögren-Larsson), Phytanoyl CoA Hydroxylase (Refsum disease), LEKTI (Netherton's)
Non keratinocytes:		
Melanocytes: in epidermis	8 wks	c-Kit (Peibaldism),PAX-3(Waardenburg's syndrome type 1)
Melanin	12-16 wks	
Transfer to keratinocytes	20 wks	
Langerhan's cells	6 wks	
Merckel cells	8-12 wks	
Cellular attachments:		
Desmosomes	8 wks	
Dermoepidermal junction		
Basement membrane	8 wks	K5, K14 (EB Simplex), Plectin (EB with MD), $\alpha6\beta4$
All basement membrane antigens	12 wks	(EB with PA), Laminin5 (Junctional EB), BPAG2 (GABEB), Collagen VII (Dystrophic EB)
Dermis		
Presumptive dermis	6-8 wks	Collagen 1 (Osteogenesis Imperfecta), Fibrillin (Marfan
Papillary and reticular dermis	12-15 wks	syndrome), elastin (Cutis laxa), MRP6 (Pseudoxanthoma
Elastic fibers	22-24 wks	elasticum)
Collagen bundles	12-16 wks	
Cutaneous vessels and nerves:		
Beginning	9 wks	TIE2 (venous malformations), Endoglein and Activin
Angiogenesis	20 weks-3 m postnatally	receptor-like kinase1 (Hereditary Hemorrhagic Telangiectasia)
Appendages		
Hair (Scalp): Beginning	9-12 wks	EDA (X-linked hypohidrotic ED), MSX1 (Witkop syndrome/
Visible hair	19-21 wks	tooth-nail syndrome)
Sebaceous gland maturation	13-16 wks	
Eccrine glands (palmoplantar):		
Beginning	8-9 wks	
Gland and dermal duct	16 wks	
Epidermal duct	22 wks	
Apocrine glands	24 wks	
Nail : Beginning	8-10 wks	Lmx-1B (Nail-Patella Syndrome), K6a/K16 (PC1), K6b/K17
Nail bed keratinization	11 wks	(PC2, Steatocystoma Multiplex)
Complete growth of nail plate	20 wks	
Hypodermis		
Fat lobules and fibrous septa	24wks	

Note: AEC- ankyloblepharon-ectodermal dysplasia-clefting, BPAG- bullous pemphigoid antigen, EB- epidermolysis bullosa, ED-ectodermal dysplasia, EDA- ectodysplasin A, EEC- ectrodactyly-ectodermaldysplasia-clefting, EGA- estimated gestational age, GABEB- generalized atrophic benign EB, K- keratin, MD- muscular dystrophy, NBCIE- non bullous congenital ichthyosiform erythroderma, PA- pyloric atresia, PC- pachyonychia congenita cells are highly dendritic, begin to express CD1a at the surface and develop Birbeck granules.

Merkel cells are located along the primary epidermal ridges of palmar skin and at a maximum density of 1400 cells/mm^2. They are found in association with developing hair follicles and sweat glands. They are also present in the dermis and are thought to originate from follicular or interfollicular epidermis. They may play a role in the organization of nerve fibers. Dense Core granules, characteristic marker for Merkel cells are absent.

DEJ has acquired adult features with well-developed hemidesmosomes, anchoring filaments and fibrils. Dermal and subcutaneous mesenchymal cells assume fibroblastic morphology and synthesize matrix molecules. Papillary and reticular dermis is demarcated based on increased cell density proximal to the epidermis, and larger collagen fibril diameter and fiber bundle size in reticular dermis. Adult vasculature is developed with one plexus at dermo-subcutaneous boundary and the other at the boundary between the papillary and reticular dermis interconnected by vertical plexuses. The nerve fibers are well formed. Collagen types III and V localize around vessels and nerves. Dilated channels of venous and lymphatic structures are seen in subcutaneous tissue.

Second Trimester

Important events that occur in second trimester include completion of the formation of lanugo hair, synthesis of the hair (17-19 weeks EGA), completion of nail (20-22 weeks EGA) and keratinization of interfollicular epidermis (22-24 weeks). Proliferation of basal cells results in addition of three intermediate cells which are flattened towards epidermal surface. At the end of this phase, interfollicular epidermis keratinizes. Cornified cell envelope and lamellar granules are found. Keratohyaline granules with profilaggrin and filaggrin are identified with formation of spinous layer. By 22-24 weeks EGA, cells similar to true stratum corneum and granular layers are identified.

Merkel cells at a density of 1700 Cells/ mm^2 and Langerhans' cells at 200 cells/ mm^2 are found in the epidermis. Melanosomes are transferred to keratinocytes in the fifth month of gestation. AF-1 and AF-2 associated with anchoring fibrils are recognized at this age. By 19-21 weeks hemidesmosomes, anchoring filaments and banded anchoring fibrils are well formed. In the dermis, interwoven, fibrous connective tissue, elastin and elastic fibers similar to elastin fibers of adult skin are recognized. Fibroblasts, mast cells, macrophages and smooth cells are also present.

In the hypodermis, by about 15-16 weeks, first stage of adipose tissue formation occurs. By 18 weeks, lipid droplets appear and at 20 weeks lobules of fat are formed. By the end of this stage, well-formed fetus with hair is present.

Third Trimester

The epidermis is fully keratinized. DEJ, dermis and adnexae are fully formed. Before 26 weeks, Langerhans' cells are localized only in the basal layer. From 27th week, they are also found in stratum spinosum. Large fat lobules are seen in hypodermis. Sweating response is limited but apocrine secretion begins. However, the structure and functions are not as matured as neonate. Babies may be born as preterm at this stage. The vasculature is less organized compared to the newborn.

UNIQUE FEATURES OF DEVELOPING SKIN

Periderm

Periderm is the outermost transient cellular layer shed into amniotic fluid at the end of the second trimester. It may take its origin from either the basal cells or the amnion or it itself may be the original ectoderm. It undergoes changes resulting in epidermis development **(Figure 1.1)**, but does not undergo keratinization. It is a layer that undergoes apoptosis.

Functions of periderm:

1. Exchange of substances between the fetus and the skin e.g. drugs.
2. It may add (secrete) materials into the amnion.
3. It may protect the developing epidermis.

Regionalization in Developing Skin

Regional differences as in adult skin are well documented. However, similar differences in the expression of diseases may indicate multiple biopsies for the prenatal diagnosis.

Keratinization

It occurs in different structures at different times of gestation. The timing appears to follow a rigidly specified program.

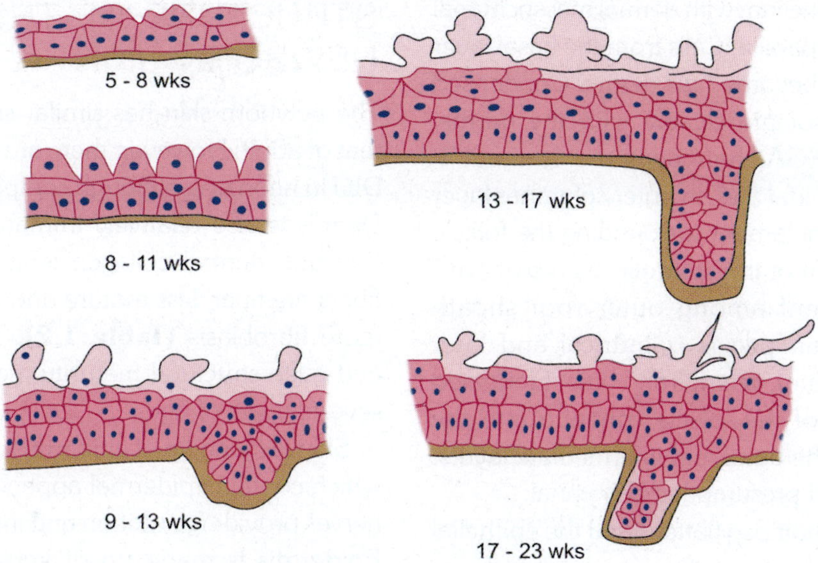

FIGURE 1.1: Development of epidermis

APPENDAGE FORMATION

By 10-11 weeks EGA, basal epidermal cells proliferate to form buds at specifically patterned sites. These buds grow into the dermis as hair germs and sweat ducts or fold to result in nail fold. This occurs in response to epithelial-mesenchymal interactions. Apart from this the nerves, vessels and adhesion molecules also play a role. The dermis is responsible for initiation and assembly, while epidermis determines the type of appendage.

Nail Formation

By 70 days, the boundaries of the nail folds are established by proximal, lateral and distal folds. By 90 days, the dorsal ridge is formed. The nail fold invaginates deeply into the dermis resulting in dorsal and ventral layers. The ventral fold becomes the nail matrix. Nail is the earliest structure to keratinize in utero. By 15 weeks, a fragile nail consisting of cells form nail bed and by about 19 weeks, cells from both nail bed as well as matrix form nail.

Eccrine Gland Formation

By around 10-12 weeks EGA, sweat glands are initiated on the palms and soles. Primary epidermal ridges organize from the basal layer. Mounds of mesenchyme form volar pads. These are transient and disappear by the end of first trimester. Sweat glands develop on the body late in the second trimester.

Pilosebaceous Apparatus

Formation of hair follicle begins on the head and face around 70-80 days EGA and proceeds cephalo-caudally. There are different stages of formation of hair follicle (**Figure 1.2**). The induction, development, maintenance and regression in adults are dependent upon an

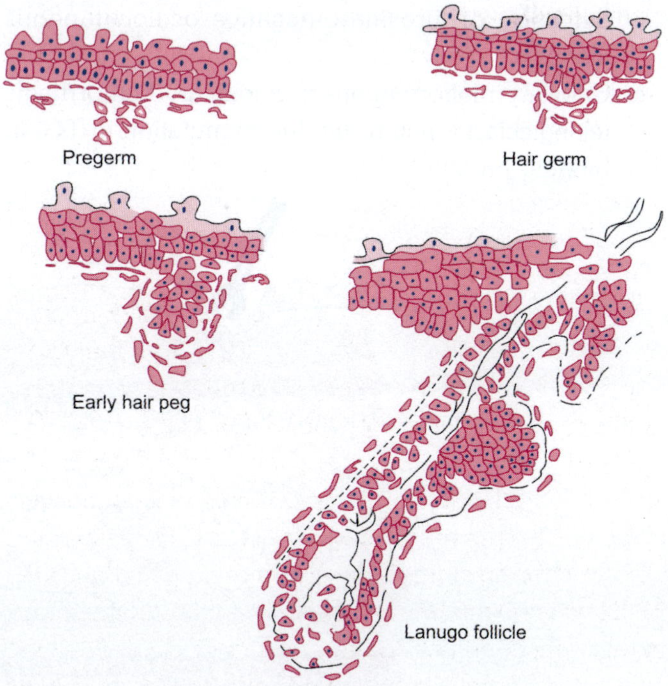

FIGURE 1.2: Stages of hair formation

association of follicle epithelium with dermal mesenchymal cells which form dermal papilla. Cells from the basal layer bud into the dermis to become hair germs. Condensed mesenchymal cells associate closely with the germs. Around 13-14weeks EGA, hair pegs are formed. It consists of an inner cuboidal and an outer columnar layer associated with the basal lamina surrounding the follicle and continuous with that of the interfollicular epidermis. Merkel cells are present among outer root sheath keratinocytes. Each hair peg is cylindrical and later develops into infundibulum, isthmus and bulb. Elongated core cells in the neck of the follicle continue into the epidermis, in between the basal and intermediate layers. This is the hair tract and presumptive hair canal.

The distal end of the hair peg flattens and the epithelial cells along this basal border elongate to form matrix. Inner root sheath and hair cone are formed. Melanocytes aggregate in the matrix and produce melanin ahead of other sites. Between 15 and 17 weeks, bulbous hair peg and bulges for arrector pili muscle, sebaceous gland and apocrine glands are formed.

Applied Importance

a. Disorders of keratinization can be identified by using chorionic villus biopsy, amniocentesis and fetal skin biopsy at various stages of development.
b. Density of melanocytes can be useful in early detection of tyrosinase-negative oculocutaneous albinism.
c. Capillary malformations in hereditary hemorrhagic telangiectasia may result due to mutation in TGF-β binding protein.

STRUCTURE OF THE NEWBORN SKIN

The newborn skin has similar structural composition as that of adult. However, there are a few salient differences. DEJ in neonates, although complete, is flat without ridges. Dermis is also relatively immature compared to adults. Reticular dermal collagen is in smaller bundles, elastic fibers are finer, less mature and it is cellular consisting of more fibroblasts **(Table 1.2).** Functional, biochemical and even structural maturity may not be achieved until several years of age.

Skin is made up of epidermis and dermis (**Figure 1.3**) which contain epidermal appendages, blood vessels and nerves providing nutrition and integration to these tissues. Epidermis is made up of keratinocytes, Merkel cells, melanocytes and Langerhans' cells. DEJ is a complex structure which supports epidermis and transports molecules bi-directionally. Dermis consists of mast cells, blood vessels, lymphatics and appendages.

EPIDERMIS

Keratinocytes form more than 90% of the cells. Epidermis comprises of basal, spinous, granular and horny layers. Melanocytes, Merkel cells and Langerhans' cells are present among them.

Basal Layer

It is known as stratum basale or germinativum. The basal keratinocyte is a columnar cell, which rests on basement membrane (hemidesmosome). It has desmosomal junctions, gap junctions, adherens junctions with other

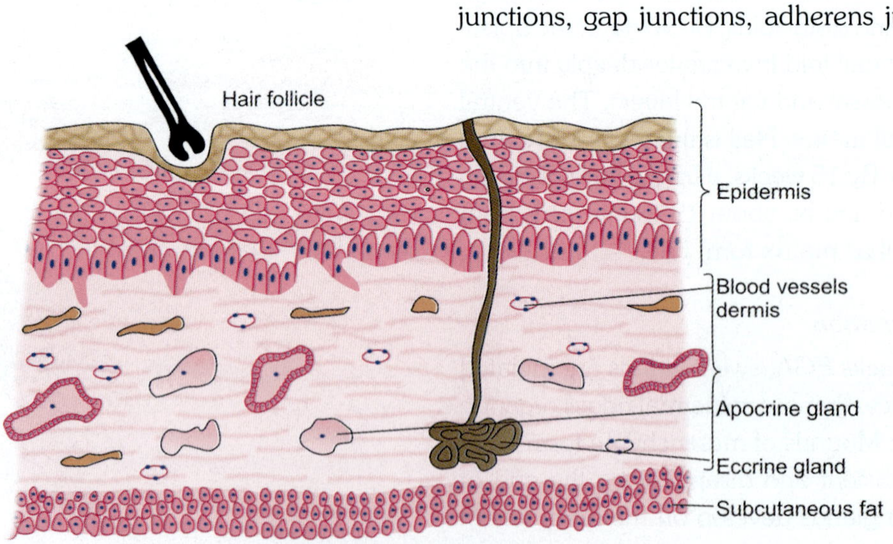

FIGURE 1.3: Structure of the skin

TABLE 1.2: Structural and functional difference between adult, term and preterm infant skin

Structure/function	Adult	Term infant	Preterm infant	Significance
Epidermal thickness	50 µm	50 µm	27 µm	↑TEWL, Percutaneous toxicity
Barrier maturity	Mature	Mature	Attains maturity in 2-3 wks, in VLBW maturity is slow, 8 wks	↑TEWL, Percutaneous toxicity and infection
Surface area to weight ratio	Normal	Five times more than adults	Seven times more than adults	↑Percutaneous toxicity
TEWL	Normal	Two-third of total insensible water loss	10-15 times greater than term infants	Fluid loss as much as 30% of body weight in 24 hrs, heat loss, ↑calorie loss (580 calories/ ml)
Antimicrobial defense	Normal	Normal	impaired expression of antimicrobial cationic peptides and antibacterial acid mantle	↑Percutaneous infections
Melanosomes	Normal	Fewer	One-third of term infant	↑risk of photosensitivity
Collagen	Normal	↓collagen	↓↓collagen	↑skin fragility and blistering
Elastin and elastic fiber	Normal	↓in papillary dermis with finer fibers	↓↓ in papillary dermis with finer fibers	↑skin fragility and blister formation (e.g. syphilis)
Brown fat	Absent	Present	Present	Non shivering thermogenesis
Hair	Normal	Synchronized growth phase	Synchronized growth phase, persistent lanugo hairs	Neonatal alopecia, estimation of gestational age
Sweat response				
Thermal stress	Normal	Greater thermal stimulus is required	Same as that of term infant	↑insensible water loss in infants on phototherapy/ under radiant warmer
Emotional	Normal	Well developed	Not well developed	
Thermoregulatory response (neural/ endocrine)	Normal	Present	Present but less pronounced	↑Susceptibility to cold and heat stress

Note: TEWL- transepidermal water loss, VLBW- very low birth weight, ↑- increased, ↓- decreased

basal keratinocytes and spinous keratinocytes, and desmosomal junctions with Merkel cells. It also borders Langerhans' cells and melanocytes. Keratins K5 and K14 are hallmarks, although K15 can be present in small amounts. This acts as a renewing source for life-time of an individual.

Spinous Layer

Stratum spinosum consists of 3 to 4 layers of more flattened cells containing large bundles of keratin filaments. In addition to the keratin filaments of basal layer, newly synthesized K1 and K10 are present. Desmosomes are prominent and shrinkage of tissue during processing gives spine-like appearance. Lamellar granules are 300-500 micrometers in diameter, membrane-bound organelles formed in the Golgi bodies. These contain carbohydrate complexed with proteins, lipids and hydrolytic enzymes. These help in barrier function.

Granular Layer

In stratum granulosum the cells are arranged in two to three layers and contain keratohyalin granules. Lamellar granules are released which fuse and aggregate with the plasma membrane in between granular and horny layers.

Filaggrin forms in this layer and may have a role in aggregating keratin filaments. Transitional layer in between granular and horny layer comprising of cells with heavily convoluted nucleus may be present. Apoptosis is initiated in this layer.

Horny Layer

This is the outermost layer of cells comprising of dead cells. It varies form 15 layers on general skin up to hundreds of layers on palms and soles. The thickness is similar in children and adults. Within plasma membrane, a highly cross-linked structure 'the cornified cell envelope', formed by epidermal transglutaminase, loricrin, keratins, pancornulin and other proteins is present. Epidermal ceramides are cross-linked across the cell membrane to the envelope which may stabilize the extracellular lipid layer.

NONKERATINOCYTES

Melanocytes

In the epidermis, Melanocytes are located in the basal layer. Each melanocyte is linked with 36 basal and spinous cells forming epidermal melanin unit (EMU). Melanocyte is a round to oval cell with refractile brown granules in the cytoplasm. Melanosomes are complex organelles and the site of melanin production. They contain tyrosinase and lysosomal enzymes. They are divided into four stages based on the pigmentation.

Langerhans' Cells

Langerhans' cells are regularly distributed suprabasally at a density of 460-1000 cells/mm^2. They have a convoluted nucleus and the Birbeck granules. Surface markers include class I and II HLA-antigens, S-100 protein and others.

Merkel Cells

Merkel Cells these are located individually in basal layer or in larger groups as touch receptors in association with myelinated nerves in epidermis, hairs and mucosae. They contain dense core granules and simple keratins. K20 is relatively specific for these cells.

APPENDAGES

Hair

Hair follicle is divided into four segments, infundibulum, isthmus, stem and bulb **(Figure 1.4)**. The pilosebaceous duct in the infundibulum is lined by a stratified keratinzed epithelium. The bulge is the site of expansion of outer root sheath cells and is at the insertion of the arrector pili muscle. This is the site of stem cell population of the follicle. The bulb contains the germinal cells of the follicle, melanocytes, langerhans' cells and Merkel cells. Dermal papilla is located in the concavity of the bulb. The inner root sheath ends at the junction between the isthmus and the infundibulum. The cells of the innermost sheath synthesize trichohyalin but the outer root sheath cells do not keratinize. Fully formed hair consists of inner and outer cuticular layers, cortex and medulla. Hair provides protection, sensory perception and adds to the cosmetic appearance.

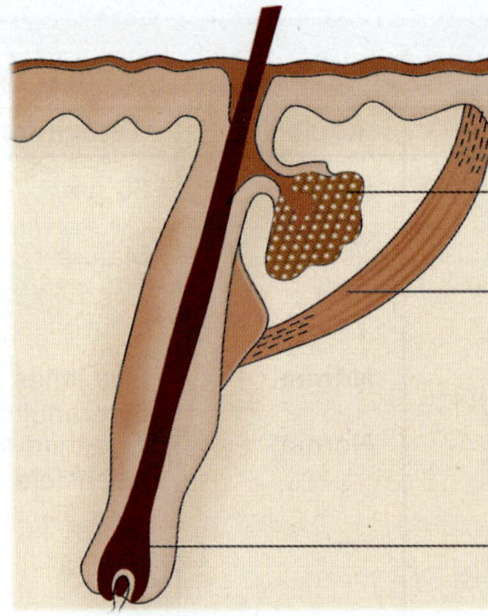

FIGURE 1.4: Structure of the hair

Nail

Nail consists of nail matrix, nail bed, nail plate, lateral and posterior folds, lunula, cuticle and hyponychium **(Figure 1.5)**. Nail matrix differs from epidermis and hair

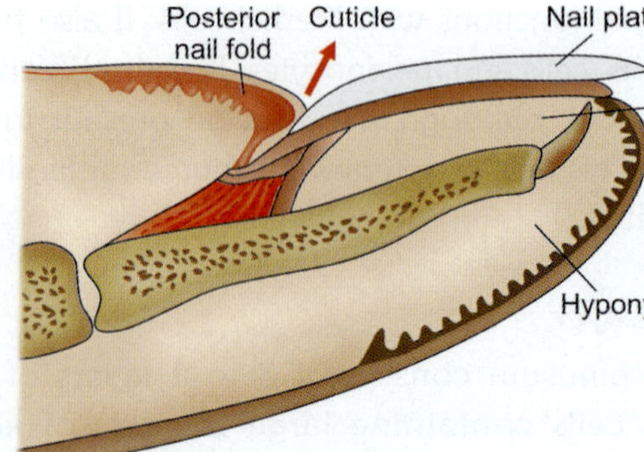

FIGURE 1.5: Structure of the nail

in producing cells that retain nuclei. Melanocytes are present in the lower two to four layers of matrix. It protects the underlying structures from physical trauma as well as infections. Nails can be used for scratching.

Eccrine Glands

They are distributed all over the body. The highest density is on the palms, soles and the forehead. The secretory coil is in the reticular dermis or subcutaneous tissue. The secretory portion consists of pyramidal, clear, dark and myoepithelial cells. Clear cells secrete water and electrolytes. The eccrine duct has two layers in the dermis. The intraepidermal portion of the duct lining is keratinized at the outermost sweat pore. The outer cells have prominent microvilli and mitochondria for reabsorption. The innermost cells form a "cuticular border" with microvilli, microfilaments and intermediate filaments. Clinically, sweating starts on 1st day after life.

Apocrine Glands

These are large, coiled tubular glands situated deep in the dermis. They occur over face, scalp, axilla and anogenital regions. Modified glands are present in eyelids (Moll's gland), ear canal and areola. It consists of secretory and myoepithelial cells. The duct contains three layers of cells.

Sebaceous Glands

They are associated with hair follicle. The density is highest over face, scalp and upper chest. Modified glands may be present in eyelids, lips, buccal mucosa, glans and prepuce. They secrete sebum which is oily.

Dermo-epidermal Junction (Figure 1.6)

This consists of dermal ridges and papillae. Electron microscopy shows lamina lucida, lamina densa, anchoring filaments, anchoring fibrils, the reticular lamina and subepidermal region of the papillary dermis. Hemidesmosomes span the cytoplasm of keratinocyte and portions of lamina lucida. It includes the bullous pemphigoid antigens.

Dermis

Dermis consists of papillary and reticular zones. Reticular lamina (compact zone) in superficial papillary dermis consists of fine dense collagen. In contrast, reticular dermis has elastic fibers, thicker collagen bundles and a higher density of vessels than papillary dermis. They contain fibroblasts and dermal dendrocytes. Fibroblasts are the source of the extra-cellular structural molecules of the dermis.

FUNCTIONS OF THE NEWBORN SKIN

MECHANICAL FUNCTIONS

Skin protects against the trauma due to blunt objects. Dermis plays a major role, although stratum corneum and subcutaneous tissue also play a part.

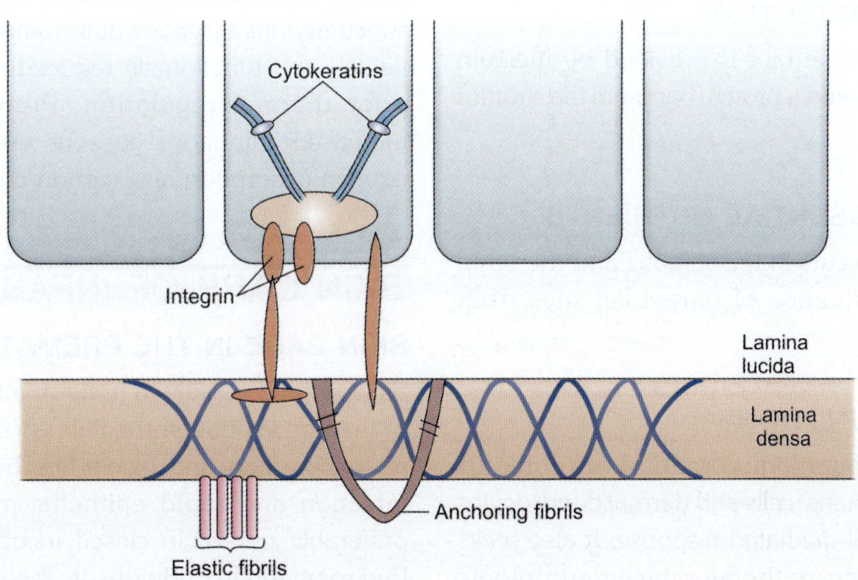

FIGURE 1.6: Dermo-epidermal junction

PHYSICAL FUNCTIONS

Stratum corneum acts as an effective physical barrier to prevent entry of toxic substances into the skin. Although the thickness and layers of stratum corneum in neonates is comparable to that of adult, it is functionally immature. Hence care should be taken during topical applications of soaps, aniline dyes, hexachlorophene, phenol and other toxic substances. Further, infants have three times more surface area per unit weight compared to adults, resulting in toxicity of topical applications.

CHEMICAL FUNCTIONS

An intact stratum corneum prevents invasion by microorganisms. Sebaceous lipids are known to have antibacterial properties. Anti Microbial Peptides (AMPs) such as defensins and cathelicidins present in the epidermis can destroy gram-positive and gram-negative organisms.

MAINTENANCE OF HOMEOSTASIS

Skin plays an important role in thermoregulation by heat loss or conservation. Heat can be lost through radiation, convection, conduction and evaporation. Dermal vasculature plays an important role. In high environmental temperatures, eccrine sweating plays a role. In neonates, since the barrier function is immature, the rate of heat loss by evaporation may exceed the baby's heat production.

ULTRAVIOLET PROTECTION

Protection from ultraviolet rays is provided by melanin barrier in the epidermis and a protein barrier in the stratum corneum.

SYNTHESIS OF ESSENTIAL NUTRIENTS

Vitamin D synthesis occurs in the spinous and the basal layers, under the influence of ultraviolet rays from sunlight.

IMMUNOLOGIC FUNCTIONS

Skin acts as an immunologic organ, as it contains macrophages, Langerhans' cells and dermal dendrocytes participating in the cell-mediated response. It also seeks to check the invading pathogens by immunologic mechanism.

SKIN OF THE PREMATURE INFANT

A premature infant is the one who is born before 37 weeks of gestation. It also refers to infants with less than 2.5 kg of weight. Extreme prematurity refers to babies with less than 1.25 kgs of body weight. The skin of the premature infant is that of the third trimester fetus. The skin is immature in both structural and physiologic properties. The skin of a newborn infant of 26 weeks' gestation is pink and relatively transparent; the underlying blood vessels are readily seen with moist surface. The epidermis although structurally complete, is relatively thin with only 5-6 layers of cells in stratum corneum and is poorly keratinized. Glycogen is still retained and barrier is poorly developed. Also, as the surface area per unit weight is seven times that of an adult, absorption and toxicity of topically applied medications can occur. Lack of enzymatic activities to detoxify substances, also adds to this. Nonspecific factors such as increased permeability of the skin and decreased gastric acid content of the stomach also may reduce neonatal immunity. Transepidermal water loss is also increased in preterm skin. It is inversely proportional to gestational age. There are only a few mature Melanosomes in the melanocytes. The development of DEJ is complete but flat. The papillary dermis is edematous and the bundles of collagen fibrils are smaller and more widely spaced. The dermis is about three-quarters of the thickness of adult dermis. Fine collagen fibers and small-sized collagen fiber bundles give the dermis a highly cellular and delicate appearance. Elastic fibers are tiny, sparse and immature. Lack of subcutaneous fat, poor autonomic control of cutaneous vessels and functionally reduced sweating contribute to poor thermal regulation. Premature infants have increased cutaneous gaseous exchange i.e. increased oxygen absorption and carbon dioxide evaporation.

SKIN CARE OF INFANTS

SKIN CARE IN THE PREMATURE INFANT

Skin matures rapidly in preterm infants after birth. Goals of therapy include immediate access to the infants, heat retention, fluid and electrolyte balance, prevention of infection and rapid epithelial maturation. They are preferably nursed in closed incubator and kept warm. Environmental conditions in these units are potentially harmful, resulting in scarring. Cosmetically or functionally significant lesions may be caused by different procedures including skin stripping due to adhesive tape. Neonatal staff must be aware of this potential long-term complication.

Preventive Measures

Disinfection: Catheter-related septicemia is most commonly caused by coagulase-negative Staphylococci. To prevent this, hand washing by staff and parents must be advocated. Two consecutive10 second wipes with chlorhexidine, alcohol or povidone-iodine or a longer duration of cleaning for about 30 seconds is more effective than a single 10 second wipe.

The Incubator: Regular change of infants' posture reduces the risk of skin erosions and bedsores. Fingers and toes must be kept visible. Catheters or needles should be secured with a transparent tape to detect extravasation. Scarring alopecia can occur after extracorporeal membrane oxygenation or hypoxaemia-hypoperfusion. Non-blanchable erythema and disruption of epidermis are early indicators of pressure sore and demands postural change.

Transcutaneous oxygen monitors: These should not be left in place for more than one hour without surveillance. Non-blanchable erythema and hyper pigmented skin craters following prolonged contact can occur. Karaya electrodes seem to be less traumatic. Placement of electrodes on the limbs may facilitate frequent auscultation.

Minimal use of tape and adhesive: Tapes and adhesives should be used on small areas of skin and removed gently with warm water soaked gauze and diluted soap but not alcohol, which may irritate. A pectin-based skin barrier may be used, when frequent application and removal of adhesives is needed.

Emollients: Emollients are safe and effective in neonatal peeling and scaling dermatitis. They decrease fragility, improve wound care and help to protect infants. Vegetable oil (e.g. olive oil), lanolin and petrolatum – based ointments reduce scaling and fissure, and enhance cutaneous hydration.

Transparent cover: Use of a transparent covering over the isolette on small premature infants may help to decrease insensible water losses.

Reduction of water loss: Water loss can be reduced by humidification of the surrounding air, use of plastic bubble blankets, heat shields or topical application of paraffin.

NEONATAL SKIN CARE

After birth, neonatal skin is exposed to air, temperature changes, friction, microbes etc. Maintaining skin integrity and preventing exposure to toxic substances in childhood assures healthy skin for several years ahead.

At birth, microbial colonization of skin is nil. Within a few days, aerobic flora colonizes over the groins, axillae and scalp. Coagulase-negative Staphylococci (Staphylococcus epidermidis) is the commonest followed by *S. aureus*. The latter is usually due to contamination by the mother or nursing staff.

SKIN CARE AT BIRTH

Removal of Vernix Caseosa

At birth, newborn skin is coated with vernix caseosa, blood, meconium and cellular debris. Premature infants tend to have less vernix than term babies and the post mature little or none. There is considerable inter-individual variation. It is unclear whether vernix gives mechanical or microbial protection. It is wiped off with a clean towel after birth.

Washing and Bathing

A bath cleans the infant completely. It should not last for more than five minutes. Infants may be bathed immediately after birth. The water should be sterilized by boiling, but the temperature of the bath -water should not exceed 37° C. A solid or liquid soap or a syndet may be used to clean the baby. Bubbles bath used can irritate or dry the skin. Soap should be thoroughly rinsed, and the baby patted dry especially in folds.

Napkin Changes

Napkin should be changed frequently, at least at each nursing and feeding time. Baby should be washed in lukewarm water and dried thoroughly. Partial occlusive agent like mineral oil application can act as a physiological barrier. Skin should be thoroughly air-dried each time the diaper is changed. Powder may be applied in the skin folds after drying. Soaps should preferably be avoided or they should be mild. Nappies should be home laundered with mild detergents. Nappy pads with cotton padding are more suited.

Scalp

Shampoos may be rarely used. On first signs of seborreic dermatitis, application of mineral or animal oil limits the spread.

Nails

They should be trimmed short and kept clean.

The Ears

Cotton swabs soaked in boiling water may be used without injury to the canals.

Umbilicus

After birth, the umbilical cord dries out and falls within 5-10 days. Certain products containing eosin or other stains are applied. They act as drying agents rather than as antiseptics.

SKIN CARE OF THE TERM BABY AND INFANT

A large number of over-the-counter cosmetics for children are available in the market. In addition to the prescribed medical treatment, infants' skin is at risk by these cosmetics.

Role of Cosmetic Products

Several types of products are used like detergents in the form of soaps or shampoos, antiseptics, emollients etc.

Detergents: Detergent is a substance capable of cleaning the skin by removing impurities like dust, greasy substances and micro-organisms. These act by reducing surface tension between water and air, creating a foaming effect. Foaming power is directly proportional to skin damage. Its usage should be followed by a thorough rinsing.

Soaps are alkalis with delipidating effect on the skin. In hard water, soaps tend to precipitate.

Syndets: These are composed of tensioactive cleansing agents with detergent quality, produce little foam and minimal irritation. They should be used with moisture as an additive.

Bubble Bath Products: Prolonged bath may irritate the genital mucosa.

Shampoos: These contain anionic tensioactive agents which ensure adequate cleansing. The pH should be equivalent to that of tears and have low ocular irritation index. Medicated shampoos containing selenium sulphide, zinc pyrithione and ketoconazole may be used for seborreic dermatitis.

Antiseptics: Risk of toxicity due to absorption is high with these topical medications, due to increased surface area, immature barrier and other factors. Biguanides and amidines are better for use in infants. Dilution, application time and rinsing conditions need to be determined since the action is time-dependent.

Emollients: Emollients can be applied on normal as well as pathologic skin and reduces imperceptible water loss.

Protective creams: Protective creams are used to reduce the risk of irritation, particularly napkin rash. These contain a fatty phase, an aqueous phase, a surfactant, zinc oxide, scents and preservatives. They can paradoxically increase occlusion and cause napkin dermatitis. Early sensitization can occur with certain preservatives.

Powders: These are used to prevent maceration over the skin folds in infants. Excessive use may cause miliaria

Role of Massage

Touch helps in growth and development of the child. Massage with oil is better than without. The oil should be smooth, of optimum viscosity, frictionless and non-occlusive. Mineral oil is one of the best ingredients. Gentle massage can be practiced from 10th day till 10th year of life. Massage given by the mother helps in developing bondage between the mother and the baby. Complete head to toe massage can be given daily.

BIBLIOGRAPHY

1. Akiyama M, Smith LT, Yoneda K, et. al. Expression of transglutaminase 1 (TG1) and cornified cell envelope (CCE) proteins during human epidermal development. J Invest Dermatol 1997;108:598.
2. Borradori L, Sonnenberg A. Structure and function of hemidesmosomes:more than simple adhesion complexes. J Invest Dermatol 1999; 112:411-8.
3. Burgeson RE. Type VII collagen, anchoring fibrils and epidermolysis bullosa. J Invest Dermatol 1993; 101:252-5.
4. Caputo R, Monti M. Children's skin and cleansing agents. Wien Med Wochenschr (Suppl) 1990; 108:24-5.

5. Dhar S. Newborn skin care revisited. Indian J Dermatol 2007; 52:1-4.
6. Drijkoningen M, Dewolf–Peeters C, Van DerSteen K, et. al. Epidermal Langerhans' cells and dermal dendritic cells in human fetal and neonatal skin:an immunohistochemical study. Pediatr Dermatol 1987; 4:11-17.
7. Elias PM. Epidermal lipids, barrier function and desquamation. J Invest Dermatol 1992; 98:270.
8. Fairley JA, Rasmussen JE. Comparison of stratum corneum thickness in children and adults. J Am Acad Dermatol 1983; 8:652.
9. Fine JD, Smith LT, Holbrook KA, Katz SI. The appearance of four basement membrane zone antigens in developing human fetal skin. J Invest Dermatol 1984; 83:66-9.
10. Foster CA, Holbrook KA. Ontogeny of Langerhans' cells in human embryonic and fetal skin:cell densities and phenotypic expression relative to epidermal growth. Am J Anat 1989; 84:157- 64.
11. Harpin VA, Rutter N. Barrier properties of the newborn infants' skin. J Pediatr 1983; 102:419-25.
12. Holbrook KA, Dale BA, Smith LT, et. al. Markers of adult skin expressed in the skin of the first trimester fetus. Curr Prob Dermatol 1987; 16:94-108.
13. Holbrook KA, Underwood RA, Vogel AM, et. al. The appearance, density and distribution of melanocytes in human embryonic and fetal skin revealed by the anti-melanoma monoclonal antibody, HMB-45. Anat Embryol 1989; 180:443-55.
14. Kim D-G, Holbrook KA. The appearance, density and distribution of Merkel cells in human embryonic and fetal skin:their relation to sweat gland and hair follicle development. J Invest Dermatol 1995; 104:411-6.
15. Lane AT. Development and care of the premature infants' skin. Pediatr Dermatol 1987; 4:1-5.
16. Malathi I, Millar MR, Leeming JP, et. al. Skin disinfection in preterm infants. Arch Dis Child 1993; 69:312-6.
17. Malloy MB, Perez-Woods RC. Neonatal skin care:prevention of skin breakdown. Pediatr Nurs 1991; 17:41-8.
18. Messenger A. The control of hair growth:an overview. J Invest Dermatol 1993; 101:4-9S.
19. Moll I, Kuhn C, Moll R. Cytokeratin 20 is a general marker of cutaneous Merkel cells while certain neuronal proteins are absent. J Invest Dermatol 1995; 104:910-5.
20. Paus R, Cotsarelis O.The biology of hair follicles. N Engl J Med 1999 ; 341:491-7.
21. Salomon D, Saurat J-H, Meda P. Cell-to-cell communication within intact skin. J Clin Invest 1988; 82:248.
22. Smith LT, Holbrook KA. Embryogenesis of the dermis. Pediatr Dermatol 1986; 3:271-80.
23. Zaias N. Embryology of the human nail. Arch Dermatol 1996; 87:37-53.

2

Neonatal Dermatology

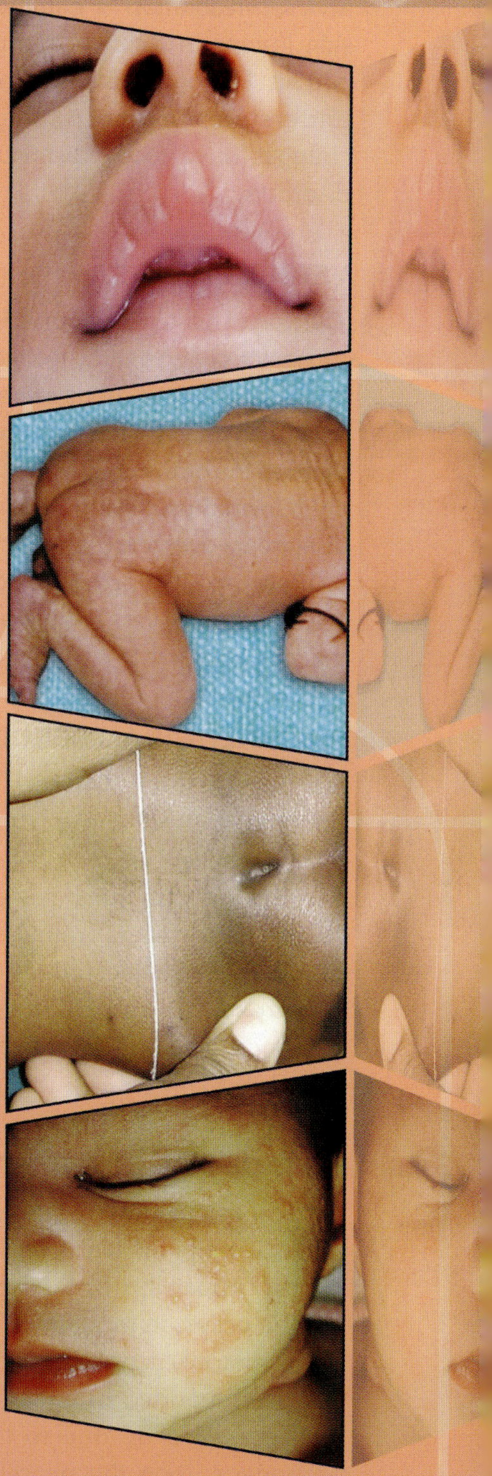

Ramesh Bhat M, Fiona Sequeira
Shirene Sequeira, Prafulla, Bindiya Fernandez

TRANSIENT NEONATAL DERMATOSES

Transient neonatal dermatoses are benign conditions seen in neonates, which reflect immaturity and transition from the intra uterine life. Most of these are normal and self-resolution is common. However, presence of skin lesions in a newborn may create concern among parents. Pathogenesis of some of these conditions is poorly understood. Some of these transient cutaneous changes have to be distinguished from more serious disorders.

VERNIX CASEOSA

The skin of full-term neonates is covered by a white, greasy substance giving a slimy feeling, known as vernix caseosa. It consists of sebaceous secretion, shed epithelium and lanugo hair and this coating on fetal skin facilitates passage through the birth canal. Vernix caseosa may provide some antibacterial protection and should be left 'as it is' till it disappears over few days after birth. Pre- and post mature babies usually lack this coating. Yellowish brown discoloration of vernix may indicate hemolytic disease of the newborn.

PHYSIOLOGICAL DESQUAMATION

Scaling of the skin may be physiological in the neonatal period and is pronounced in post-mature (40-42 weeks) babies. However, term babies may also develop this within first few days of life. The peeling of superficial skin starts around ankles, palms and soles and may be more widespread to involve the lower trunk **(Figures 2.1A and B)**. In cases with excessive desquamation, it may be mistaken as congenital ichthyosiform disorders.

SEBACEOUS GLAND HYPERPLASIA

Sebaceous gland hyperplasia (SGH) is characterized by multiple, pinpoint, white / yellowish papules on the nose, cheeks, upper lips and forehead of neonates **(Figure 2.2)**. It occurs in more than 50% of term newborns and less commonly in preterm infants. An incidence of 21.4% has been reported in an Indian study. Its occurrence is considered to be due to the influence of maternal androgens upon the pilosebaceous unit of the baby. Lesions usually resolve spontaneously in a few months.

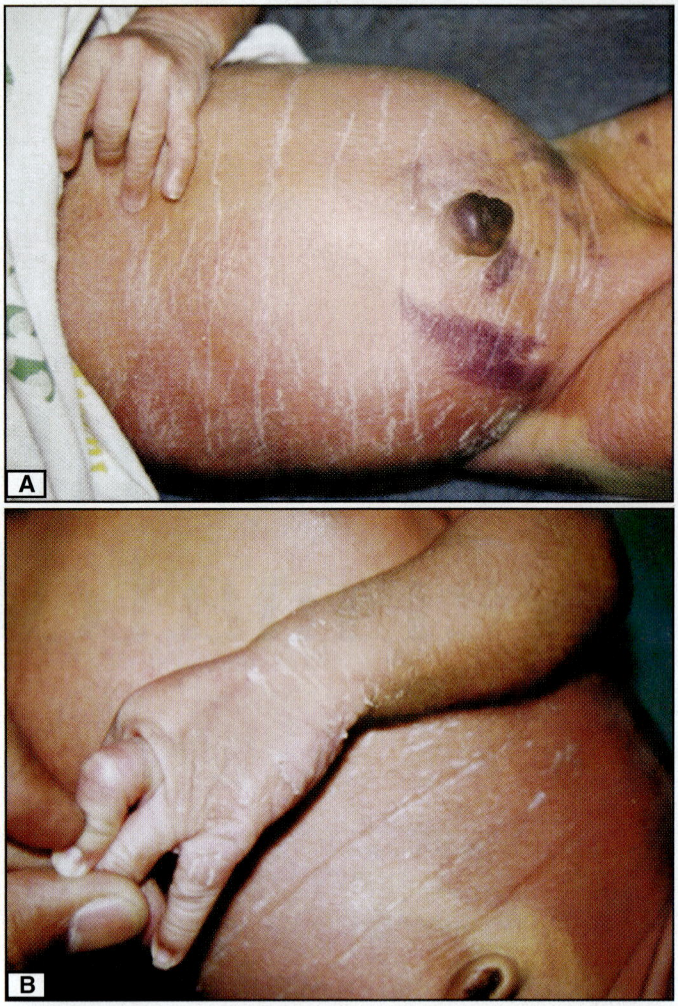

FIGURES 2.1A AND B: Physiological desquamation

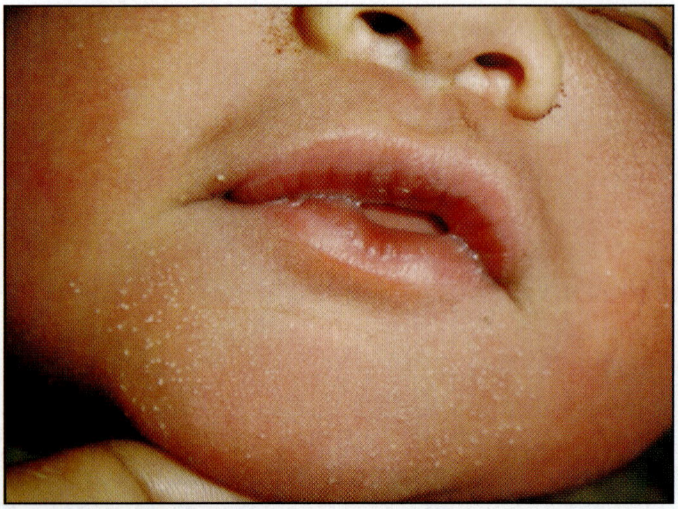

FIGURE 2.2: Sebaceous gland hyperplasia

MILIA

Milia are small epidermal cysts found on the facial skin and scalp of newborns. These consist of few, 1-2 mm, yellowish-white papules distributed commonly on forehead, peri-ocular area and cheeks. In one Indian study, the incidence of milia has been reported as 23.8%. These generally resolve spontaneously by the first month of life. Persistent milia beyond this age or numerous lesions may be associated with underlying disorders like Orofacial-digital syndrome, Marie-Unna hypotrichosis and Bazex-Dupré-Christol syndrome.

ERYTHEMA TOXICUM NEONATORUM (ERYTHEMA NEONATORUM ALLERGICUM, DYSPEPTIC ERYTHEMA, TOXIC ERYTHEMA OF NEWBORN)

Erythema toxicum neonatorum (ETN) is a benign, transient, self-limiting, asymptomatic condition seen in full-term neonates. It affects 30-70% of newborns without gender or racial predilection. In one Indian study, the incidence of ETN was found to be 21%.

The exact etiology of ETN is unknown. Some authors attempted to correlate the occurrence of ETN with peripheral blood eosinophilia and others proposed it to be a minor form of graft *vs.* host disease. In a more recent study it has been found that there is over-expression of human antibacterial peptides LL-37 and b defensin-1 in skin biopsies from ETN lesions; it was considered that it is an inflammatory response representing activated antimicrobial defense system soon after birth. Rarity of ETN in premature infants may be because of the incomplete maturation of this defense system.

ETN occurs anytime from birth to two weeks of age, maximum incidence being during the first 4 days of life. The eruption is evanescent (persists 2-3 days) and characterized by asymptomatic papules, vesicles and occasionally pustules present on an erythematous background (**Figures 2.3A and B**). In 70% cases, the lesions have a 'flea-bitten appearance' presenting as erythematous patches topped with yellowish-white papules, distributed on forehead, face, trunk and extremities. In the remaining 30% cases, pustular eruptions, surrounded by erythema are seen predominantly on the trunk. Palms and soles are usually spared.

Diagnosis is clinical and laboratory investigations are not required. Differential diagnosis includes transient neonatal pustular melanosis, candidiasis, bacterial infections, herpes simplex virus (HSV) infections and miliaria. In case of diagnostic confusion, microscopic examination of the smear (Gram stain) prepared from pustular lesions may be performed, which reveals numerous eosinophils.

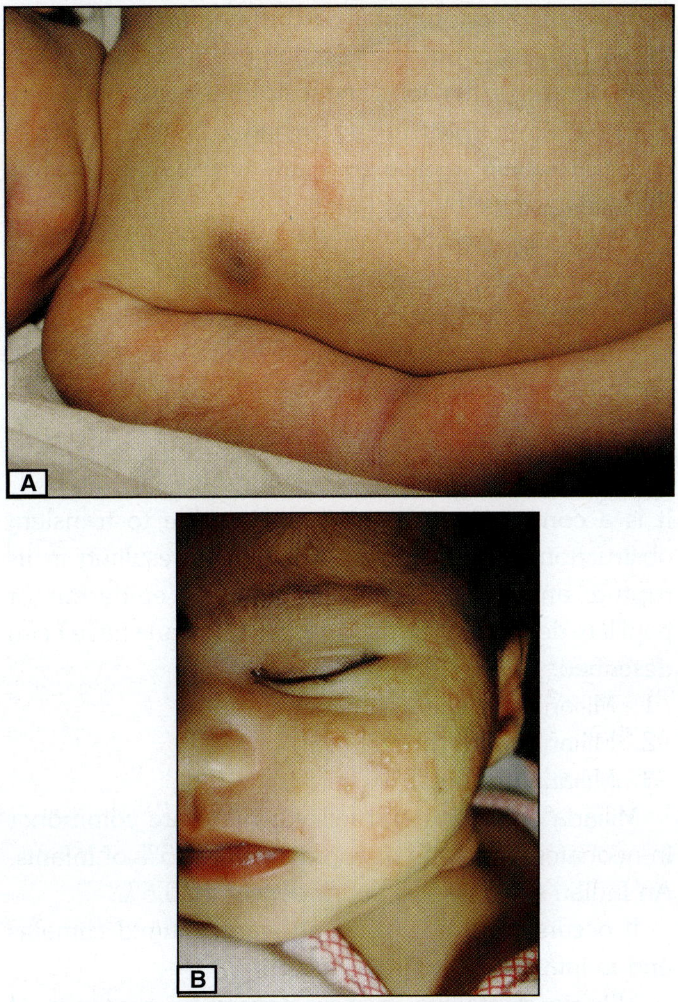

FIGURES 2.3A AND B: Erythema toxicum neonatorum

As it is a self-limiting condition, treatment is not required.

TRANSIENT NEONATAL PUSTULAR MELANOSIS (NEONATAL PUSTULAR MELANOSIS, PUSTULAR MELANOSIS)

It is a benign condition seen in term infants characterized by pustules or vesicles on normal-appearing skin present at birth, which may resolve with hyperpigmentation.

Etiology of this condition is also unknown. It is commoner among black infants (4.4%), compared to white infants (0.2%) , which may be due to accelerated stimulation of melanocytes in black races.

The lesions are always present at birth. Clinically it is characterised by flaccid vesicles/ pustules (1-3 mm) on normal skin distributed over chin, chest, back and buttocks. The lesions may be clustered around nipples or at pressure points. Unlike erythema toxicum neonatorum, palms, soles and scalp may also be involved. The vesiculo-pustules rupture leaving collaret of fine scales or crusts which resolve over few weeks with residual freckle-like hyperpigmentation.

Microscopic examination of the contents of the pustule shows presence of neutrophils. Differential diagnosis includes ETN, which may co-exist at times, bacterial, viral or candidal infections and miliaria. No therapy is required for this self-limiting condition.

MILIARIA

It is a common condition occurring due to transient obstructions of the eccrine sweat ducts resulting in its rupture and leakage of sweat in to the epidermis or papillary dermis. Three clinical types of miliaria have been described:

1. Miliaria crystallina (sudamina)
2. Miliaria rubra (prickly heat)
3. Miliaria profunda

Miliaria crystallina and miliaria rubra are commoner in neonates, occurring in approximately 15% of infants. An Indian study quotes an incidence of 20.6%.

It occurs more commonly in warm, humid climates and in infants treated in incubators.

Miliaria crystallina is characterized by presence of asymptomatic, superficial, non-inflammatory pin-point to pin-head-sized, clear vesicles which appear like dewdrops on the skin **(Figure 2.4)**. Here, the level of blockage of the eccrine duct is at the level of the stratum corneum.

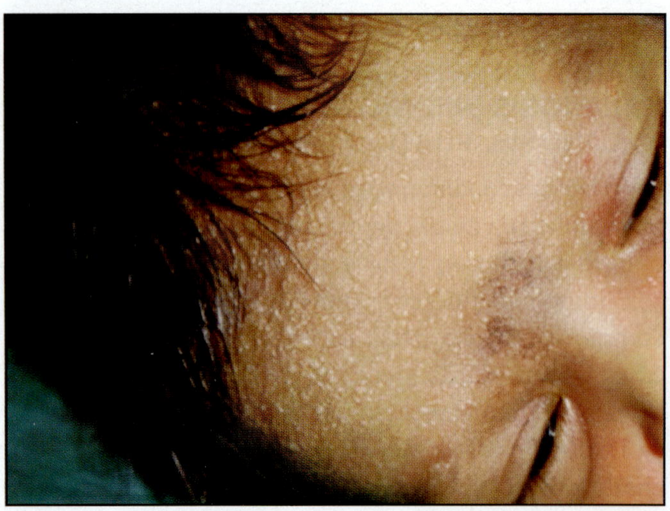

FIGURE 2.4: Miliaria crystallina

In miliaria rubra, the level of obstruction is lower in the epidermis. It is characterized by erythematous, non-follicular papules (1-3 mm), vesicles and rarely pustules (miliaria pustulosa). Miliaria crystallina appears at the end of the first week of life, whereas miliaria rubra is usually seen beyond this period (11th-15th day). Commonly affected sites are forehead, scalp, intertriginous areas, neck and trunk. The lesions subside with fine desquamation.

The differential diagnosis includes erythema toxicum neonatorum, varicella, HSV infection, pityrosporum folliculitis and transient neonatal pustular melanosis.

Warm, humid environment should be avoided in children with miliaria. Cool bathing and air-conditioning are helpful in severe cases. No specific therapy is required.

NEONATAL ERYTHEMA

Generalized erythema is a common finding in most of the newborns and persists for few hours after birth. It is indicative of cutaneous vasodilatation with resultant hyperemia as the infant gets adjusted to the external environment.

ACROCYANOSIS

Bilateral acral cyanosis is observed in many neonates, which may be intermittent and variable in intensity. It gradually subsides by few weeks of life and is of no pathological significance. It is more pronounced in winter months and hypothermic neonates.

The cyanotic appearance may be due to dilatation of the dermal vasculature in the acral parts, resulting in hemostasis and formation of desaturated hemoglobin. The cyanosis resulting from congenital heart disease is more intense and generalized, involving tongue, lips and other body parts.

HARLEQUIN COLOR CHANGE

Harlequin color change (HCC) is a transient erythema involving the dependent part of the body of a lying infant, with simultaneous paleness of the upper half, with a sharp demarcation at the mid-line. HCC may be attributed to poorly-developed neural control on cutaneous vasculature.

Premature and low-birth-weight infants are more prone (15%) to develop HCC. It usually develops on 3rd to 4th day of life. The erythema shifts on turning the baby to opposite side, which may take 30 seconds to 20 minutes. Head and genitalia are not usually involved and mucosal surfaces are spared. It is a benign condition and subsides by third week of life.

CUTIS MARMORATA

Cutis marmorata (CM) is a transient, bluish, reticulate/ mottled pattern of cutaneous discoloration found in premature as well as full-term infants **(Figure 2.5)**. This phenomenon is thought to be due to exaggerated cutaneous vasomotor response to environmental temperature changes, the core temperature remaining unaltered. The condition is commoner in winter months. Warming of the infant helps in normalizing the condition.

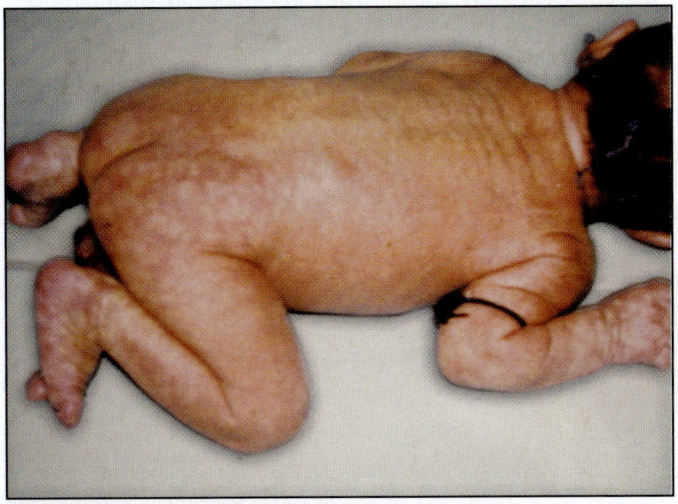

FIGURE 2.5: Cutis marmorata

Though CM is a benign condition, severe or persistent involvement should raise the suspicion of certain conditions like Down syndrome, congenital hypothyroidism and Cornelia de Lange syndrome. Cutis marmorata telangiectatica congenita (CMTC) is another clinical entity where the infant shows CM at birth, which is not reversible with warming. Telangiectasia, phlebectasia, atrophy and ulceration may develop subsequently and CMTC may be associated with many other congenital deformities. Infants with neonatal lupus may present with mottled appearance of skin due to associated livedo reticularis.

SUCTION BLISTER

These are the blisters developed due to self-sucking of the skin by the infant. These are seen on the body parts accessible to the infants' mouth such as hands and feet. The lesions may be present at birth, representing onset of such sucking during intra-uterine life. Clinically it is characterized by presence of bulla, erosion or calluses on normal looking skin **(Figure 2.6)**. It may be mistaken for lesions of epidermolysis bullosa, which may also present with bullae on distal extremities. The lesions resolve without sequelae. If the blister ruptures, a topical antibiotic may be used to prevent secondary infection.

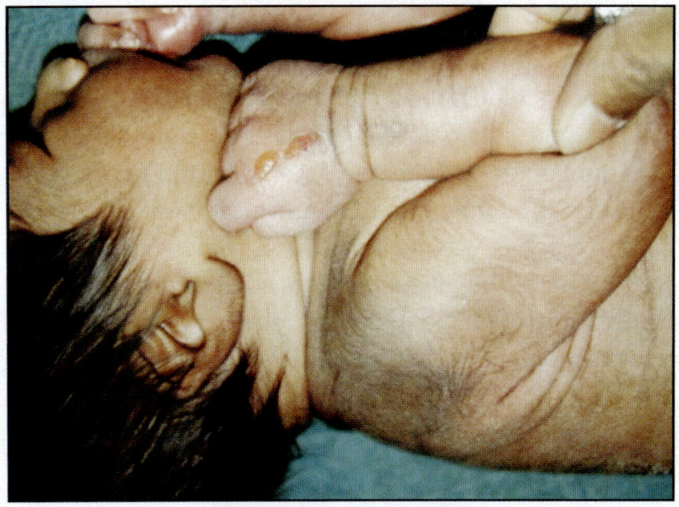

FIGURE 2.6: Suction blister

SUCKING PADS / CALLUSES

These are localized or diffuse thickening of the lip present in neonates at or soon after birth. When present at birth **(Figure 2.7)**, probably these result from vigorous sucking in the intrauterine life. Following birth, these are related to breast feeding. These are more prominent in black neonates. There is spontaneous resolution after few weeks.

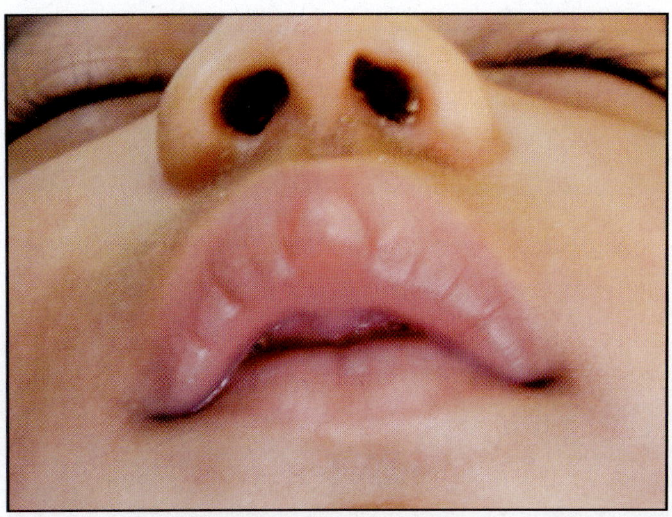

FIGURE 2.7: Sucking pads

EPSTEIN'S PEARLS

These are equivalent to milia occurring in the oral cavity along the median palatal raphe, especially at the junction of hard and soft palate. Lesions are usually multiple. These are epidermal inclusion cysts occurring in 60-85% of newborn infants. In an Indian study the incidence of Epstein's pearls was recorded 61%. When such lesions are present at the alveolar margins, these are termed as **Bohn's nodules**. No therapy is required as most lesions resolve spontaneously within the first few weeks of life.

MINIATURE PUBERTY

Miniature puberty is a conglomeration of clinical features found during the neonatal period, simulating pubertal secondary sexual characters, due to effect of maternal and placental androgens during fetal life.

The clinical features include enlargement of breast tissues, prominent linea nigra (a vertical, hyperpigmented line extending from lower end of umbilicus to mons pubis) and pigmentation of genitalia (dark pigmentation of scrotum/labia majora). The pigmentary changes are more prominent is dark-skinned infants. In female infants there is clitoral enlargement and transient vaginal bleeding (3rd-4th day of life) may be seen. There may be thick milk-like secretion (witches milk) from the breast, which subsides with normalization of the breast tissue (end of first month) **(Figures 2.8A to C)**.

Presence of features of miniature puberty does not warrant any therapeutic intervention. Rarely, stagnant milk in enlarged breast tissue may result in mastitis, which has to be treated promptly.

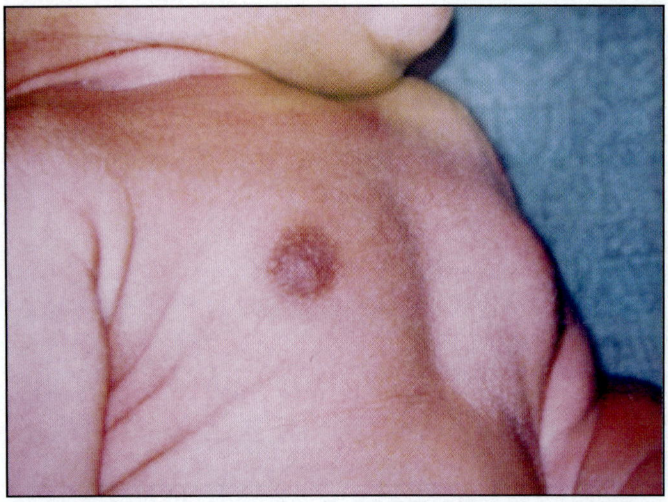

FIGURE 2.8A: Enlargement of breasts (miniature puberty)

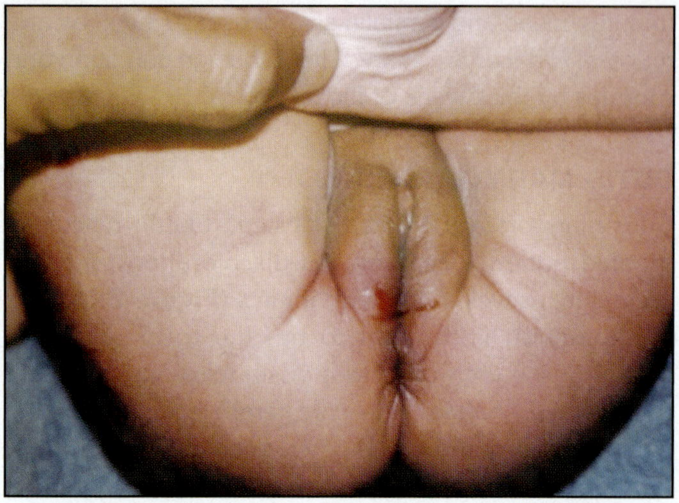

FIGURE 2.8B: Vaginal bleeding (miniature puberty)

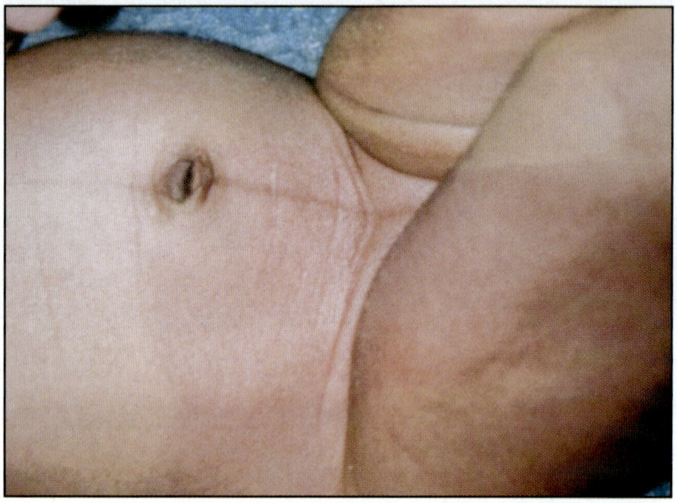

FIGURE 2.8C: Linea nigra (miniature puberty)

ACNE NEONATORUM

Acne is not rare in the neonatal period and is characterized by presence of papules, pustules and comedones mainly on the face **(Figure 2.9)**. It is commonly mild and transient. In an Indian study the incidence is reported to be 5.4%. It is considered to be due to stimulation of sebaceous glands by maternal and neonatal androgenic hormones. There are case reports of correlation between neonatal acne and familial hyperandrogenism. Transient neonatal cephalic pustulosis is a condition which resembles pustular acne neonatorum, is a superficial pustular infection caused by *Malassezia* species.

Acne neonatorum is a self-limiting condition. However, topical anti-acne preparations may be used sparingly to hasten the clearance of the lesions.

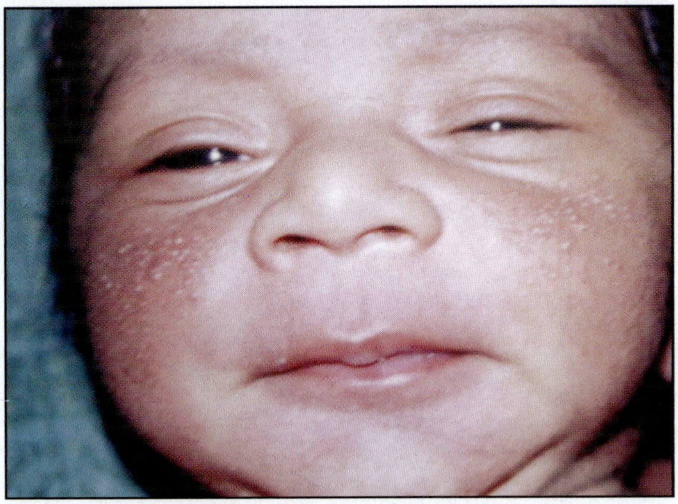

FIGURE 2.9: Acne neonatorum

DEVELOPMENTAL ABNORMALITIES

Some defects during embryogenesis results in developmental abnormalities recognized during neonatal period. These may be major or minor congenital anomalies or sometimes a developmental variant. Some common developmental anomalies, present at birth or during infancy have been described below.

CYSTS

Thyroglossal Duct Cysts

Thyroglossal duct cysts are the most common cause of midline anterior neck swelling in children, which may be found anywhere along the length of this duct. There may be familial occurrence. It has to be differentiated from dermoid and bronchogenic cysts. Treatment is by surgical excision.

Bronchogenic Cysts

Bronchogenic cysts are congenital anomalies occurring in the chest or mediastinum and rarely on the skin. Usually it presents as a subcutaneous swelling near to suprasternal notch. It may discharge mucous through a fistula. Treatment is by surgical excision.

Dermoid Cysts

Dermoid cysts are unusual, congenital subcutaneous growths that occur along the embryonic fusion lines. These often present during childhood with outer orbit being the most commonly affected site. There may be an intracranial extension. Histopathologically these are encapsulated and the wall contains keratinized, stratified squamous epithelium. The lumen may contain lipid material and hair. With complete excision, recurrence is rare.

BRANCHIAL CLEFTS AND SINUSES

Branchial cleft abnormalities may present as cystic masses, which may be infected, draining sinuses or fistulae. Defects in the second cleft are the most common. Anomalies of first branchial cleft present as pre-auricular cysts and sinuses. Accessory tragus, congenital midline cervical clefts with or without associated defects may also occur. Complete surgical excision is the treatment of choice with preceding course of antibiotic in presence of infection.

APLASIA CUTIS CONGENITA AND SCALP DEFECTS

Aplasia cutis congenita is a rare congenital disorder affecting the scalp. The scalp skin, bone and underlying dura may be absent; however, the majority of the cases are limited to the dermis and epidermis. The rare larger defects are prone to complications like hemorrhage and infection. Conservative treatment is preferred, however, sometimes grafting may be required to cover larger defects.

AMNIOTIC BAND SYNDROME

Amniotic band syndrome refers to the infrequent occurrence of congenital deformities presumably due to entanglement of fetal parts in strands of ruptured amniotic sac. A wide spectrum of clinical deformities is encountered and range from simple ring constrictions to major craniofacial and visceral defects. Constriction band of a distal extremity in a circumferential manner may cause lymphedema or even amputation of the distal part. Surgical correction is the only available treatment option.

BENIGN NEOPLASM

Gliomas, hemangiomas, smooth muscle hamartomas and melanocytic nevi may also be present during birth. Nasal gliomas are rare tumors present as bluish or red swellings at the nasal root. Smooth muscle hamartomas present as hyperpigmented plaque with hypertrichosis. Hemangiomas are common tumors occurring in neonates and more commonly present in premature infants.

MISCELLANEOUS

Encephalocele is the herniation of brain tissue through the skull and present as soft swellings.

Congenital lip pits are of three types and these are:

a. Commissural lip pits, the commonest variant, bilateral
b. Midline cysts of upper lip, a very rare entity.
c. Lip pit located on the paramedian lower lip, solitary/ bilateral

The first and the third variants may be familial. All these pits end in a short, blind tract and may secrete mucoid material. Congenital lip pits may be associated with cleft palate and lips, pre-auricular sinuses or communication to parotid duct. 'Van der Woude's syndrome' is an autosomal dominant condition presenting with congenital lip pits, cleft lip and palate with variable expressivity and high penetrance. Surgical excision is the only treatment option.

CUTANEOUS SIGNS OF SPINAL DYSRAPHISM

Spinal dysraphism (SD) is easy to diagnose when the manifestation is overt. However, frequently this congenital deformity of the spine is occult and becomes difficult to detect. There are certain cutaneous markers which may be indicative of an occult SD. It is important to detect these signs so as to halt the progressive neurological impairment of the affected child. Following are the cutaneous signs of spinal dysraphism:

Skin dimples: Usually occur above the gluteal fold, on midline; the possibility of underlying SD is more if the dimple is wider / deeper. Other cutaneous markers of SD may co-exist **(Figure 2.10)**.

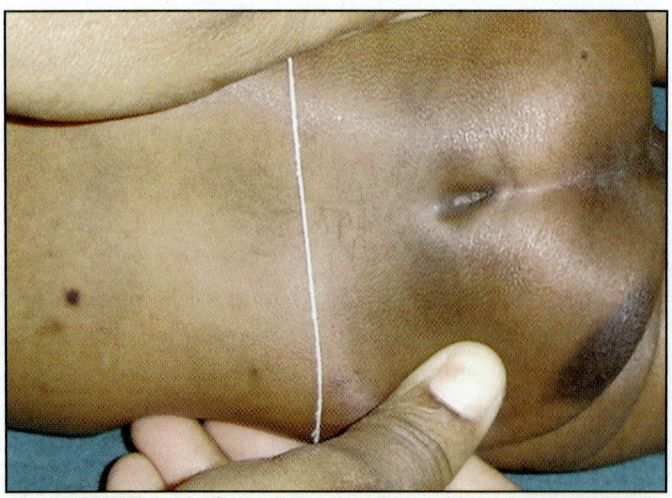

FIGURE 2.10: Sacral dimple with multiple congenital melanocytic nevi

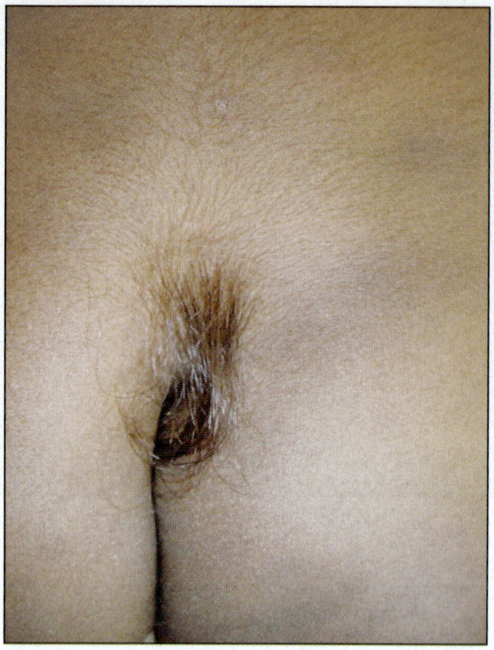

FIGURE 2.11: Tuft of hair (sign of occult spinal dysraphism)

Tuft of hair: This is the commonest cutaneous sign of occult SD. It may present as long, coarse, terminal hairs (faun-tail) or a patch of lanugo/vellus hairs **(Figure 2.11)**.

Aplasia cutis: A scar-like defect in the lumbo-sacral area may represent aplasia cutis and may be a marker of SD.

Sacral hemangioma: Capillary malformations in the lumbosacral area may be associated with SD.

Human tail: Vestigial tails in the lumbo-sacral or sacro-coccygeal areas may be indicative of underlying SD.

Other lower-back, midline lesions which may indicate the presence of SD are congenital lipoma, sinus tracts, dermoid cysts, melanocytic nevi, localized telangiectasia, sacro-coccygeal teratoma, etc. Among all these lesions skin dimples, tufts of hair, human tail, lipoma, dermoid cysts / sinus and aplasia cutis are the skin markers indicating high risk of SD.

CUTANEOUS MANIFESTATIONS OF CONGENITAL INFECTIONS

Intrauterine infection of the fetus by microbial agents results in congenital infections. The effects of congenital infection may be quite distinct and more severe than the effects of the same acquired during childhood. Congenital infections are usually caused by viruses and affect the fetus at any time during pregnancy till the time of delivery.

ETIOLOGY

a. Viruses: Cytomegalovirus (CMV), herpes simplex virus (HSV), parvovirus B-19, enteroviruses, hepatitis B virus, varicella zoster virus (VZV), human immunodeficiency virus (HIV) and rubella.
b. Bacteria: *Treponema pallidum*, *Mycobacterium tuberculosis*, *Salmonella typhi*, *Campylobacter*, *Borrelia burgdorferi*
c. Fungi: *Candida albicans*
d. Protozoa: *Toxoplasma gondii*, *Plasmodium* and *Trypanosoma cruzi*

The acronym 'TORCH' is in use to denote congenital infections namely toxoplasmosis, rubella, cytomegalovirus and herpes simplex virus infection. Clinical manifestations of common congenital infections are described below.

CANDIDIASIS

Candidiasis in infancy may be congenital or acquired in the neonatal period. These are caused mostly by *C.albicans* but other species may also be involved.

Congenital candidiasis is acquired *in utero* and may lead to grave consequences like premature birth or intrauterine death. Here the clinical manifestations are present at birth / first day of life as diffuse, erythematous papules and pustular eruptions. Palms, soles, and nails may also be involved but diaper area and oral cavity is usually spared. In premature infants there may be a diffuse, scaly involvement or a scalded appearance. Systemic involvement is rare in this form of the disease.

Neonatal candidiasis is acquired during passage through an infected birth canal or during postnatal period. It manifests after initial few days or weeks after birth. Here the lesions are localized involving the oral mucosa, diaper area or other intertriginous areas. Skin lesions are present as erythematous patches with satellite pustules and peripheral scaling.

TORCH INFECTIONS

Toxoplasmosis

Toxoplasmosis is caused by intracellular protozoa *Toxoplasma gondii*. Congenital infection is possible from acute infection in the mother due to transmission of the organism during gestational period. Incidence of infection is directly and severity inversely proportional to the gestational age of the fetus. Severe clinical manifestations are seen only in 10% of the infected offsprings. Chief clinical findings in patients with congenital toxoplasmosis include chorioretinitis, central nervous system abnormalities (microcephaly, hydrocephalus, encephalomyelitis, seizures and mental retardation), icterus with hepatosplenomegaly, anemia and thrombocytopenia.

Cutaneous features are non-specific like maculopapular rash, petechiae and ecchymoses, vascular lesions simulating 'blueberry muffin' and calcifications, involving any body part. Skin lesions are usually present at birth but may appear within few weeks and gradually subside by another few weeks.

Rubella

Congenital rubella syndrome is a symptom complex comprised of intra-uterine growth retardation (IUGR), microcephaly and microphthalmia, visceral and skin involvements in varying combinations. The infection may be subclinical without manifestations at birth. Severity of the infection is more if acquired in first trimester. Children with congenital rubella have a reduced life-span.

Cutaneous manifestations at birth and early neonatal period (20-50%) are secondary to hematological involvement. There is extramedullary hematopoiesis giving rise to dark blue / red macules which are gradually enlarged to form papules simulating 'blueberry muffin.' Associated thrombocytopenia may attribute a hemorrhagic component to the lesions giving rise to a 'cranberry muffin' appearance. The lesions may persist for several weeks and gradually fade thereafter.

Older infants may develop maculopapular rash, cutis marmorata, hyperpigmentation and recurrent urticaria. Affected infants may be infective till six months of age. Treatment of congenital rubella is mostly supportive.

Cytomegalovirus Infection

Congenital CMV infection is one of the most common TORCH infections. Clinical manifestations are present at birth only in 5-10% of the infected cases. The most common clinical manifestations include IUGR, microcephaly, hepatosplenomegaly, chorioretinitis, deafness and thrombocytopenia. Cutaneous features include showers of petechiae, purpura and 'blueberry muffin' lesions. Mental retardation may develop later.

CMV infection may be acquired much more commonly during passage through birth canal, through breast-feeding or through blood transfusion

Herpes Simplex Virus Infection

Intrauterine infection of the fetus, i.e. congenital HSV infection is rare (4-5%). When occurs, it may either be transplacental, from a viremic mother or an ascending infection from a mother with active herpes genitalis. Premature birth is common. Clinical manifestations are evident within first 48 hours as widespread vesiculo-bullous lesions, erosions and scars. Scalp may show areas of absence of skin, simulating aplasia cutis congenita.

Other features include microcephaly or hydrocephalus, microphthalmia and chorioretinitis.

Most infections are acquired during birth (neonatal infection). The chances of acquiring infection is more (50%) if mother has primary genital herpes, compared to recurrent disease (5%). Three clinical patterns are known to occur:

- Localized mucocutaneous infection
- Disseminated infection
- CNS infection ± mucocutaneous infections

Cutaneous lesions include vesicles on erythematous base, which may be few, localized or multiple and generalized, but lack the classical grouping seen in herpetic infection. Distribution of lesions is determined by fetal presentation during birth; initial vesicles appearing on face and scalp in cephalic presentation and on buttocks in breech presentation. Lesions subside by crusting. Oral lesions are present as ulcers.

The infant is usually ill with fever, irritability/lethargy, hypotonia and poor feeding. The cutaneous lesions may recur till 5 years of age and multiple recurrences (>3/year) is associated with increased risk of CNS involvement.

Prognosis of neonatal HSV infection is better than congenital infection, more so if the disease is localized. Treatment includes intravenous acyclovir (15 mg/kg/day, 8 hourly).

VARICELLA ZOSTER VIRUS INFECTION

Varicella zoster infection during pregnancy may affect the fetus / neonate in different ways as follows:

- Fetal varicella syndrome
- Neonatal varicella
- Infantile H. Zoster.

Fetal varicella syndrome (congenital varicella syndrome/varicella embryopathy) is a rare entity occurring due to transmission of the infection during early gestational period. Maternal varicella has a higher risk of such transmission than herpes zoster. The syndrome represents severe multi-system anomalies involving CNS, eye, musculoskeletal, gastrointestinal and genitourinary systems and skin. Microcephaly, seizure, psychomotor retardation, microphthalmia, chorioretinitis, hypoplastic limbs are the prominent clinical features. Cutaneous lesion includes dermatomal cicatricial areas, which may be associated with ipsilateral limb hypoplasia.

Maternal varicella in late gestational period may give rise to perinatal infection within 10 days of birth, known as *neonatal varicella* **(Figure 2.12)**. The disease may also be transmitted while the mother is still in incubation period and develop the skin rash during or immediately after delivery. The neonatal disease is severe with disseminated skin rash (with hemorrhagic and coalescent vesicles), encephalitis, hepatitis and pneumonia. Mortality is very high. Infants of mothers who develop varicella within 5 days before to 2 days after delivery are administered varicella zoster immunoglobulin (VZIG), 125 units. Lesional contact with the baby has to be avoided.

Infants developing varicella beyond 10 days of birth is considered to be acquired due to postnatal exposure.

Human Immunodeficiency Virus Infection

If the mother has HIV infection, the fetus has 25% chance of being infected by the virus. The fetus is more likely to be infected if the mother has a low CD4+T cell count or AIDS. Other risk factors include vaginal delivery and preterm birth.

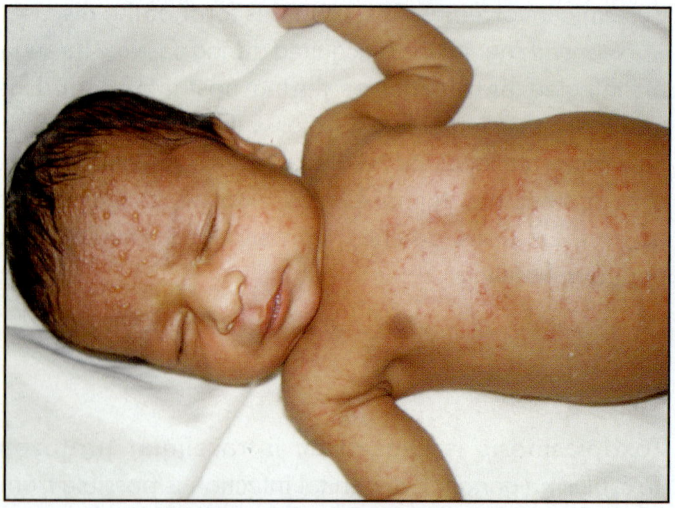

FIGURE 2.12: Neonatal varicella

The clinical features depend upon the effects of the virus on an immature and naïve immune system. Infants with vertically acquired HIV infection are usually clinically normal during the neonatal period. 'Congenital HIV syndrome' manifesting as microcephaly, flattened nasal bridge, short nose, and patulous lips has been described. Cutaneous manifestations during neonatal period include recurrent abscesses, and oro-pharyngeal candidiasis. Details of management of neonatal HIV infection have been discussed in respective chapter.

CONGENITAL SYPHILIS

Congenital syphilis is a rare infection now-a-days. The detailed clinical feature of this disorder has been described in respective chapter. The muco-cutaneous manifestations of early congenital syphilis are briefed below.

Maculo-papular lesions are commonly seen in early congenital syphilis, which may be coppery-red in color, with or without scales and distributed symmetrically, predominantly on the palms, soles and diaper areas. Lesions may be generalized also. Bullous lesions are encountered rarely which may be present at birth. Condyloma lata are raised, flat moist lesions present at the ano-genital region, angles of the mouth, around the nostrils, fingers and toes. Healing of skin lesions leads to characteristic radiating scars of rhagades observed around the mouth or anus.

Syphilitic rhinitis produces a serous nasal discharge with or without blood tinge (snuffles), which may be present at birth and is highly infectious. Subsequently this may produce perforation of the nasal septum with flattening of the nasal bridge, resulting in saddle nose. Mucous patches and moist erosions may be present in the buccal and genital mucosa. Lesions of pharynx and larynx leads to a characteristic hoarse cry and cough.

Patchy hair loss at sides of the back of the scalp is seen. Alopecia affecting eyebrows in infants may suggest syphilis. Rarely infant may present with an abundance of coarse hair, which may stop short of the hair margin, the so called 'syphilitic wig'.

Papules at the base of the nail may involve the nail bed causing 'syphilitic onychia'.

BIBLIOGRAPHY

1. Benjamin LT, Trowers AB, Schachner LA. Giant aplasia cutis congenita. Pediatr Dermatol 2004;21(2):150-3.
2. Dash K, Grover S, Radhakrishnan S, Vani M. Clinico epidemiologic study of cutaneous manifestations in the neonate. Ind J Dermatol Venereol Leprol 2000; 66: 26-28.
3. Demmler GJ. Congenital cytomegalovirus infection treatment. Pediatr Infect Dis J 2003; 22(11):1005-6.
4. Jones J, Lopez A, Wilson M, Congenital toxoplasmosis. Am Fam Phys 2003.
5. Kimberlin DW. Herpes simplex virus infections in neonates and early childhood. Semin Pediatr Infect Dis 2005; 16(4): 271-81.
6. Mianda SB, Delmaestro D, Bertoli R, Marinho T, Lucas E. Focal dermal hypoplasia with exuberant fat herniations and skeletal derformities. Pediatr Dermatol 2005; 22(5): 420-3.
7. Peirno SP, Waldhausen JH, Congenital cervical cysts, sinuses and fistulae. Otolaryngol Clin North Am. 2007; 40(1):161-76.
8. Riyaz N, Riyaz A, Chandran R, Rakesh S.V, Focal dermal hypoplasia (Goltz syndrome). Ind J Dermatol Venereol Leprol 2005;71:279-81
9. Sachdeva M, Kaur S, Nagpal M, Dewan SP. Cutaneous lesions in new born. Ind J Dermatol, Venereol, Leprol 2002; 68:334-7.
10. Sudheer MS, Silveira MP. Congenital syphilis. Indian Pediatrics 2002;39:972-3.
11. Thomas J. Neonatal dermatoses: An overview–Indian J Dermatol Venereol Leprol 1999;65:99-103.

3

Geno-dermatoses

- Principles of genetics
- Prenatal diagnosis of hereditary disorders of skin
- Inherited vesicullo-bullous disorders
- Ectodermal dysplasia
- Hereditary disorders of keratinization
- Hereditary disorders of pigmentation
- Hereditary disorders of the immune system
- Hereditary disorders of photosensitivity
- Hereditary disorders of metabolism
- Multiple tumor syndromes
- Hereditary disorders of connective tissue
- Premature aging syndromes
- Chromosomal disorders
- Skin gene therapy

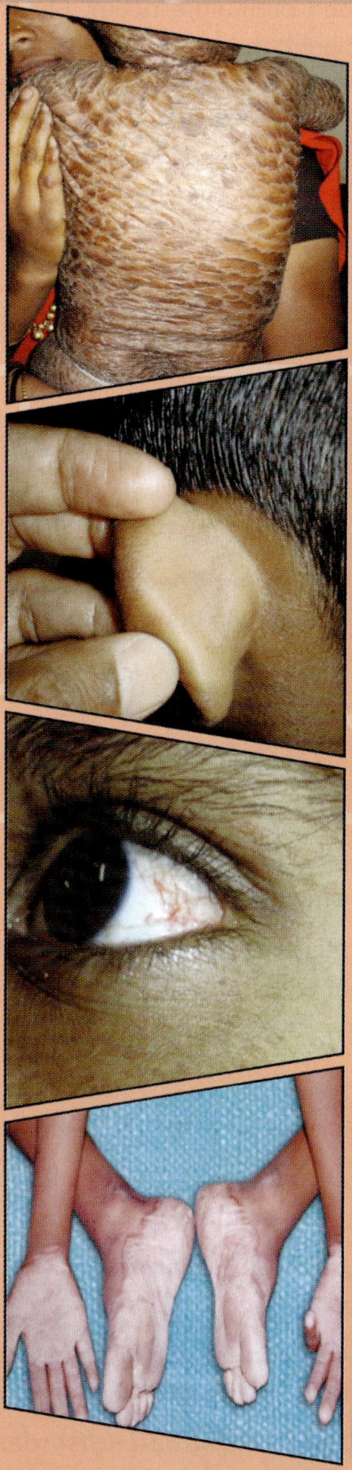

Aparna Palit, Arun C Inamadar
Ragunatha S

INTRODUCTION

A significant portion of pediatric dermatological disorders are of genetic origin. Majority of these disorders are multi-systemic and persists throughout the life. Some of these disorders are associated with risks of early malignancy and premature death. Other cause disfigurement and parents bring these children to the dermatologist for their unusual appearance. Management of these disorders involves the patient as well as the family. Services to be rendered to such a family include determining the inheritance pattern of the particular disease, genetic counseling to prevent further such occurrence and motivating the parents for prenatal diagnosis in case of future pregnancy. The following section includes basic principles of genetic transmission of diseases and the terms related to it.

PRINCIPLES OF GENETICS

Following are some of the terminologies used for understanding of principles of genetic transmission.

Genotype: The characters of an individual transmitted through the genes

***Phenotype*:** Physical expression of the genetic characters in an individual.

Autosomal characters are borne by autosomes (22 pairs of chromosomes) and sex-linked characters are carried by sex chromosomes (X/Y). Genes are located at particular chromosome loci as alleles, which determine genetic characters of an individual.

Heterozygosity: Two different alleles at a particular locus of a chromosome pair

Homozygosity: Identical alleles at chromosome loci.

***Hemizygous*:** Males with expression of X-linked characters (unpaired allele) are termed as hemizygous.

Dominant character: A character, whose phenotypic expression is possible in heterozygous state.

Recessive character: A character, which manifests only in homozygous state.

Congenital character: A character, which is present at or before birth.

Familial character/disorder: It is defined as occurrence of a character in a family clearly in excess of its expected occurrence in the same population.

MAJOR PATTERNS OF GENETIC TRANSMISSION

- Autosomal dominant (AD),
- Autosomal recessive (AR),
- X-linked dominant (X-L-D),
- X-linked recessive (X-L-R).
- Holandric transmission: It indicates sex-linked transmission through Y chromosome.

Mitochondrial Inheritance

Transmission of some disorders is related to mitochondrial DNA (mt DNA). These show a maternal inheritance which simulate X-linked inheritance pattern. All the sons and daughters of an affected woman are affected but father-to-offspring transmission does not occur. Increased maternal age is an important factor in mitochondrial inheritance of characters. Palmoplantar keratoderma with sensori-neural deafness (mutation of MTTS1) follows this type of inheritance pattern.

Sporadic Disorder

Some disorder with known genetic transmission may arise in a family as a *de novo* spontaneous mutation. Family history of the genetic disease may be negative in such cases. Increased paternal age has been noticed in some sporadic AD disorders. Rarely, single case of a recessive disorder may occur in a family.

Penetrance and Expressivity

These are the properties of a genotype, which determines phenotypic expression. Penetrance and expressivity of a character may be variable. Some characters have high or low penetrance and some are non-penetrant. Similarly, expressivity may be high or low.

Heterogeneity

Different genotypic or phenotypic expression is commonly observed in many of the genodermatoses, designated as heterogeneity. This may be of different types;

Clinical heterogeneity: Distinct phenotypes produced by different mutations in the same gene results in clinical heterogeneity. Mutations at the XPD gene producing xeroderma pigmentosum (XP), XP in association with Cockayne syndrome and trichothiodystrophy is the classical example of this type.

Genetic heterogeneity: Similar disease phenotype occurs due to mutation of different underlying genes. Tuberous sclerosis, resulting from mutations of 2 genes, TSC1 and TSC2 is an example of genetic heterogeneity.

Locus heterogeneity/Non-allelic heterogeneity: Mutations of genes at different chromosomal loci can cause the same phenotype; mutation of either keratin-5 or keratin-14 gene in epidermolysis bullosa simplex is an example of this type.

Allelic heterogeneity: Mutations at the different alleles of one locus determines the clinical severity in a disease spectrum, e.g. milder Weber-Cockayne and more severe Dowling-Meara types of epidermolysis bullosa simplex.

Contiguous Gene Syndromes

Large genomic deletions involving several neighboring genes may give rise to combinations of different disorders. Deletions of varying sizes within chromosome X-p22.3 results in varying combinations of X-linked-ichthyosis, Kallman's syndrome, chondrodysplasia punctata, ocular albinism, mental retardation and short stature.

Cutaneous Mosaicism

Cutaneous mosaicism is an interesting phenomenon manifesting in some patients with genodermatoses. It is caused by post-zygotic, somatic mutation involving only a percentage of the cells and is easily recognizable in the skin. Occurrence of mosaicism in a disorder is suspected when a patient's clinical features are milder than the usual. Functional mosaicism is observed in all females with regard to their X chromosomes, one of which is inactivated in early embryonic life, known as lyonization. Cutaneous mosaicism may adopt several clinical patterns as follows:

a. Blaschkoid, e.g. incontinentia pigmenti, McCune-Albright syndrome
b. Checker-board pattern, e.g. speckled lentiginous nevus, Becker nevus
c. Phylloid pattern, e.g. phylloid hypomelanosis
d. Large patches without mid-line separation, e.g. acquired melanocytic nevi,
e. Lateralization pattern, e.g. CHILD nevus.

Chromosomal disorders: This result from aberrations, like deletion, translocation, alteration in number and instability involving autosomes or sex-chromosomes. Some of these possess cutaneous manifestations.

GENETIC COUNSELING

Communication and education addressing concerns relating to the development and/or transmission of a hereditary disorder is known as genetic counseling. It is provided to the couples with family history or earlier history of child-birth with genodermatoses.

A specialist with adequate knowledge in the field can undertake genetic counseling.

The discussion should be in simple, comprehensible language, with due regard to the cultural and religious beliefs and sympathy to the affected family.

Consequences of consanguineous marriages are to be explained to the families and should be discouraged.

PRENATAL DIAGNOSIS OF HEREDITARY SKIN DISORDERS

Intrauterine diagnostic techniques have made the definitive prenatal diagnosis of several genetic skin disorders easier. These include chorionic villus biopsy, amniocentesis, fetoscopy and fetal ultrasonography (USG). Fetoscopy or USG guided fetal skin biopsy sample can be studied by light, electron or immunofluorescent microscopy in some rare disorders like epidermolysis bullosa. Other techniques include collection of fetal blood through transabdominal route (USG-guided cordocentesis) and maternal serum screening. Recent advances in the prenatal diagnosis of diseases include DNA-based mutation analysis, antenatal PCR analysis, fluorescent *in situ* hybridization (FISH) technique and pre-implantation genetic diagnosis (PGD). However, these recent techniques are expensive and not widely available.

The couple seeking genetic counseling should choose from the options offered for prenatal diagnosis and take the ultimate decision. Informed written consent should be obtained before any procedure is performed.

CLASSIFICATION OF GENODERMATOSES

Genodermatoses encompasses a wide variety of disorders, some of which will be discussed in the following section;

1. **Inherited mechano-bullous disorders**
   Epidermolysis bullosa of different groups.

2. **Ectodermal dysplasias and disorders of ectodermal appendages**
   Anhidrotic ectodermal dysplasia
   Hidrotic ectodermal dysplasia
   EEC syndrome
   Rapp-Hodgkin syndrome
   Dyskeratosis congenita
   Incontinentia pigmenti
   Oral-Facial-Digital syndrome
   Johanson-Blizzard syndrome
   Schöpf-Schulz-Passarge syndrome
3. **Disorders of keratinization**
   Ichthyosis and ichthyosiform syndromes
   Palmoplantar keratoderma
   Erythrokeratoderma
3. **Hereditary disorders of pigmentation**
   Piebaldism
   Waardenburg syndrome
   Oculocutaneous albinism
   Hermansky Pudlak syndrome
   LEOPARD syndrome
   Carney complex
4. **Hereditary disorders of immune system**
   Ataxia telangiectasia
   Chronic mucocutaneous candidiasis
   Chédiak Higashi syndrome
   Complement deficiency disorders
   Chronic granulomatous disease of childhood
   DiGeorge syndrome
   Hyper IgE syndrome
   Immunoglobulin deficiency
   Severe combined immunodeficiency
   Wiskott-Aldrich syndrome
5. **Hereditary disorders of photosensitivity**
   Porphyrias
   Inherited DNA repair disorders and chromosome instability syndromes
6. **Hereditary disorders of metabolism**
   Phenylketonuria
   Homocystinuria
   Tyrosinemia II
   Alkaptonuria
   Hartnup disease
7. **Familial multiple tumor syndromes**
   Neurofibromatosis I & II
   Tuberous sclerosis complex
   Gardner syndrome
   Cowden syndrome
8. **Hereditary disorders of connective tissue**
   Pseudoxanthoma elasticum
   Cutis laxa
   Marfan syndrome
   Buschke-Ollendorff syndrome
   Ehlers-Danlos syndrome
   Osteogenesis imperfecta
9. **Premature ageing syndromes**
10. **Chromosomal disorders.**

INHERITED VESICULO-BULLOUS DISORDERS

INTRODUCTION

Inherited vesiculo-bullous disorders comprise mechanobullous group of diseases, e.g. epidermolysis bullosa (EB), which are precipitated by minor trauma and present at birth or soon thereafter. Köebner (1886) first described a milder form of this disorder. There are three major clinico-pathologic variants of this disorder; EB simplex, junctional EB and dystrophic EB. Each of these variants includes different sub-types, some of which are relatively rare. The milder variant of the disorder, e.g. EB simplex is self-limiting whereas the severe variants may be fatal. Whatever may be the severity, this group of disorders is associated with immense morbidity in terms of altered appearance and inability to perform daily activities. In the following section, major types of epidermolysis bullosa will be discussed.

CLASSIFICATION

Each major variant of EB results from specific cleavage at the basement membrane zone. Individual groups have been subdivided depending upon inheritance pattern, focal or generalized distribution of skin lesions and common or rare occurrence of the disorders.

Commoner and major groups of EBs have been presented in **Table 3.1**.

EPIDERMOLYSIS BULLOSA SIMPLEX (EBS)

The inheritance pattern in EBS is mostly autosomal dominant except in a few families, where autosomal recessive transmission has been recorded. There is dissolution of the infra-nuclear portion of basal keratinocytes forming intra epidermal vesicle **(Figures 3.1A and B)**. Some variants, Weber-Cockayne, Köebner, Dowling-

TABLE 3.1: Classification of epidermolysis bullosa

1.	**Epidermolysis bullosa simplex** (AD /AR) **Commoner variants:** Localized: EBS-Weber-Cockayne Generalized: EBS- Dowling-Meara (Herpetiformis) EBS-Koebner (AD, rarely AR) **Less common variants:** EBS with muscular dystrophy (letalis), (AR) EBS-superficialis EBS with mottled pigmentation (X-L-R) EBS-Mendes da Costa EBS-Ogna
2.	**Junctional epidermolysis bullosa** (AR) **Commoner variants:** Herlitz (Gravis) Non-Herlitz (Mitis) **Less common variants:** JEB with pyloric atresia Inverse Progressive Cicatricial Localized
3.	**Dystrophic epidermolysis bullosa (AD / AR)** **AD** **Commoner variants:** Dystrophic DEB **Less common variants:** Pretibial EB-pruriginosa Bart's disease Transient bullous dermolysis of newborn **AR** **Commoner variants:** Hallopeau-Siemens (severe, generalized, mutilating) Mild, non-mutilating Less common variants: Inverse

Meara and EBS with mottled pigmentation are caused by mutation of the genes encoding basal cell keratins 5 and 14. In EBS-Dowling-Meara, the mutation may occur *de novo* resulting in sporadic cases, which thereafter is transmitted as an AD trait. EBS with muscular dystrophy and Ogna variant are caused by mutation of the plectin gene.

Clinical Features

EBS-Weber-Cockayne: This is one of the commoner, localized variant of the disease. Skin lesions start appearing any time between birth and puberty. Painful, tense bullae are present mainly over palms and soles. Palmoplantar hyperhidrosis and very rarely mucosal bullae are present.

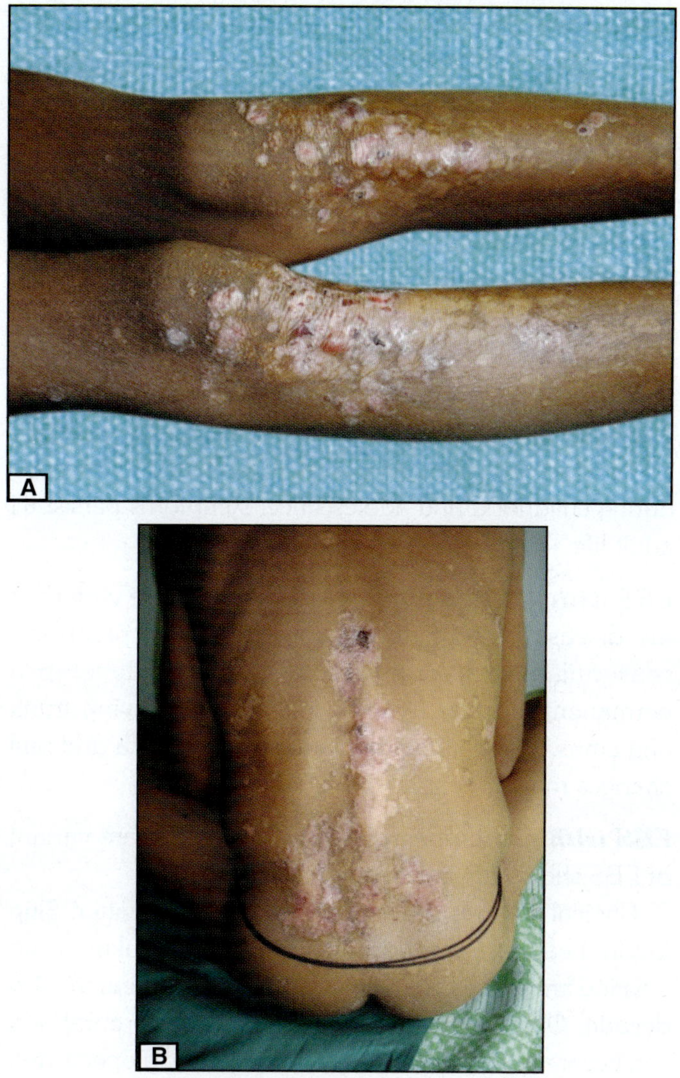

FIGURES 3.1A AND B: Epidermolysis bullosa simplex

Skin lesions are precipitated by trivial trauma during daily work or walking and exacerbated in warm weather. Nail, hair and teeth remain uninvolved. Lesions heal without scarring. The condition is self-healing and improves with age. However, it causes great morbidity in childhood in terms of restricted mobility and daily activities.

EBS-Köebner: This variant of the disease resembles Weber-Cockayne type except the earlier onset of clinical features and involvement of other body parts. In infancy, occiput, back and legs are commonly involved, thereafter predominant involvement of palms and soles are seen. Intraoral bullae are commoner and more severe in these patients. Summer months and friction from clothing are important precipitating factors. Improvement is seen around adolescence and adult life.

EBS-Dowling-Meara (Herpetiformis): This is the most severe form of EBS resembling junctional and dystrophic variants. Skin lesions are present at birth involving the whole body. After initial months, bullae tend to appear in groups on trunk and limbs assuming a herpetiform appearance. Skin lesions heal without scarring but post-inflammatory hyperpigmentation may be a sequelae. Major mucosal involvement occur involving oral cavity and larynx giving rise to hoarse cry during early childhood. Palmoplantar keratoderma, nail dystrophy and periodic nail shedding are common. Friction from clothing is an important precipitating factor but seasonal variation is not observed. Though there is a tendency to improve during childhood and adolescence, symptoms persist till adult life.

EBS with mottled pigmentation: It is a rare variant of the disease present during childhood with recurrent, seasonal, non-scarring bullae. Patients develop a permanent macular hyperpigmentation involving trunk and limbs. Punctate palmoplantar keratoderma and nail changes may appear later in life.

EBS with muscular dystrophy: This very rare variant of EBS shows AR transmission.

Clinical features start at birth or soon thereafter. Skin lesions heal with scarring and milia. Muscle weakness and wasting may start any time between first year to 4th decade. Other associated features may be cerebral and cerebellar atrophy, urethral stricture, scarring alopecia and nail dystrophy.

EBS-Ogna: Traumatic, seasonal, bullae formation occurs on hands and feet. A generalized, non-episodic, skin fragility is present, manifesting as bruising, hemorrhagic bullae and erosions. Nail dystrophy and onychogryphosis of great toe nail is common.

EBS-superficialis: In this rare type of EBS, the cleavage occurs in the subcorneal layer. Hence the bullae are transient, leaving behind erosions and crusts.

JUNCTIONAL EPIDERMOLYSIS BULLOSA (JEB)

This group of epidermolysis bullosa is the rarest of the three main types. AR transmission is observed in all variants of the disease.

The plane of cleavage is at the lamina lucida of basement membrane zone. Hemidesmosomes are sparse and small with indistinct or attenuated sub-basal dense plate. There is mutation of any of the 3 genes (LAMA3, LAMB3 and LAMC2) encoding for anchoring filament protein laminin 5. The mutations are less disruptive in non-Herlitz type of disease. Some cases of non-Herlitz disease result from mutation of the genes encoding collagen 17 of hemidesmosome (COL17A1 or 180 kDa bullous pemphigoid antigen genes). In JEB-pyloric atresia, there is mutation of the gene for $\alpha 6 \beta 4$ integrin, another hemidesmosomal protein.

Clinical features

JEB-Herlitz: Skin lesions are present at birth as generalized tense bullae and widespread mucosal involvement. Occasionally the degree of blistering may be minimal at birth, later progressing to full-blown disease. Characteristic features include bullae on buttocks and pinna. Lesions heal without scarring and milia. Hoarseness of voice occurs due to laryngeal involvement. Paronychia, nail dystrophy and total loss of nails are seen. There is associated anemia, nutritional deficiency and failure to thrive leading to death by 6 months of age. If patients survive beyond this age, a distinctive, persistent, perioral and occipital erosions with granulation tissue is seen. Other features at this stage are non-scarring alopecia and dental pitting. Death may result from septicemia or sudden blockage of larynx or trachea due to presence of bullae.

JEB-non-Herlitz: This is a milder form of JEB where survival till adulthood is possible. Extensive, generalized bullae formation is seen during infancy. Formation of perioral granulation tissue is less prominent than JEB-Herlitz. Post-inflammatory hyperpigmentation, scarring, atrophy, alopecia, nail dystrophy and dental enamel hypoplasia are common. Though less severe, all mucosae may get involved resulting in oral erosion, hoarse voice, esophageal stricture and urethral meatal stenosis. Conjunctival scarring and corneal erosion may lead to blindness. Squamous cell carcinoma may arise on scarred skin.

JEB-pyloric atresia: This is a rare variant of JEB. Widespread skin lesions and pyloric atresia are present at birth. The pyloric atresia requires surgical correction but recurs subsequently. Musosal involvement in the genito-urinary tract may lead to stricture and hydronephrosis in later life. Pregnancy with a fetus suffering from this disorder is usually complicated with polyhydramnios.

DYSTROPHIC EPIDERMOLYSIS BULLOSA (DEB)

This variant of EBS is characterized by marked scarring, milia formation and deformities. These follow AD or AR modes of transmission. The plane of cleavage is in the sublamina densa of basement membrane zone. There is mutation of the gene (COL7A1) encoding type VII collagen, the predominant component of anchoring fibrils. These are morphologically altered, reduced in number or absent. In transient bullous dermolysis of newborn, type VII collagen is retained in the cytoplasm of basal and suprabasal keratinocytes. In Bart's syndrome, ultrastructural findings are poorly formed anchoring fibrils and cleavage below the lamina densa. Genetic linkage studies in the original family with Bart's syndrome, mapped the gene for the disease to chromosome 3p at or near the site of the gene encoding type VII collagen. Clinical features of DEB are as follows.

DEB with AD Inheritance

Dominant dystrophic epidermolysis bullosa (DDEB): This is the commonest type of dystrophic EB. Earlier subdivisions 'Cockayne-Touraine' and 'Pasini' types are considered obsolete currently. Clinical features are highly variable even within a single family. Vesicles and bullae are either present at birth or appear by 5 years of age. The classical sites of involvement are bony prominences on extremities. Healing occurs with atrophic scarring and milia formation. Dystrophic nails and total anonychia are common. Albopapuloid lesions are commonly seen on lower back as well-circumscribed areas of hypopigmented, atrophic, wrinkled skin studded with ivory-white papules.

Mucosal involvement may occur and in about one fourth of the cases, result in sequelae like microstomia, dysphagia, constipation etc. Unlike other generalized forms of EB, tracheobronchial and ocular involvement, anemia and growth retardation are unusual in this type. Disease severity decreases through adult age but disfiguring skin lesions result in significant psychological morbidity.

Pretibial DDEB: It is a rare condition presenting with recurrent blistering of the pretibial region, healing with scarring and milia formation. Onset may be early or delayed to second or third decade of life. Associated nail dystrophy is usual. Both autosomal dominant and recessive transmission may occur.

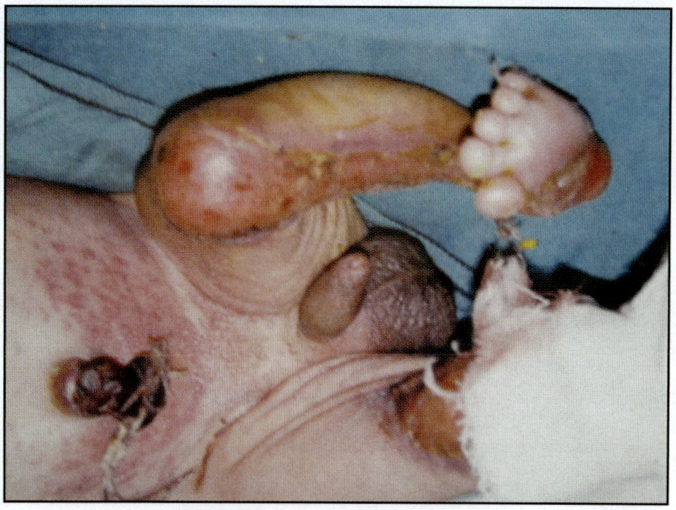

FIGURE 3.2: Bart's syndrome

Congenital, localized absence of skin (Bart's syndrome): This is present at birth as a denuded area, usually over the pretibial area **(Figure 3.2)**. Similar clinical feature may be associated with other forms of EB like all the three variants of EBS, JEB-Herlitz, RDEB-Hallopeau-Siemens and very rarely non-Hallopeau-Siemens RDEB. Recently, ultrastructural study of skin from different members of the original family with Bart's syndrome has proved it to be a subtype of DDEB. Nail dystrophy is usually associated. Scarring and milia formation at the site of lesion and persistence of skin lesion till adult life has been recorded.

Epidermolysis bullosa pruriginosa: This disorder is clinically distinct by presence of intensely itchy, lichenified nodules and plaques with occasional bullae formation on trauma-prone areas. Lesions may be linear with excoriations and milia formation. Nail dystrophy may be associated. Both autosomal dominant and recessive transmission may occur.

Transient bullous dermolysis of the newborn: This is a rare variant of DEB, present with extensive vesiculo-bullous lesions at birth. During infancy, there is marked improvement in the blistering tendency.

DEB with AR Inheritance

Recessive dystrophic epidermolysis bullosa (RDEB)—Hallopeau-Siemens type:
It is a rare, severely scarring form of the disease. Generalized vesicles and bullae are present at birth and aggravated by friction **(Figures 3.3A and B)**. There is severe cutaneous and mucosal scarring and loss of nails

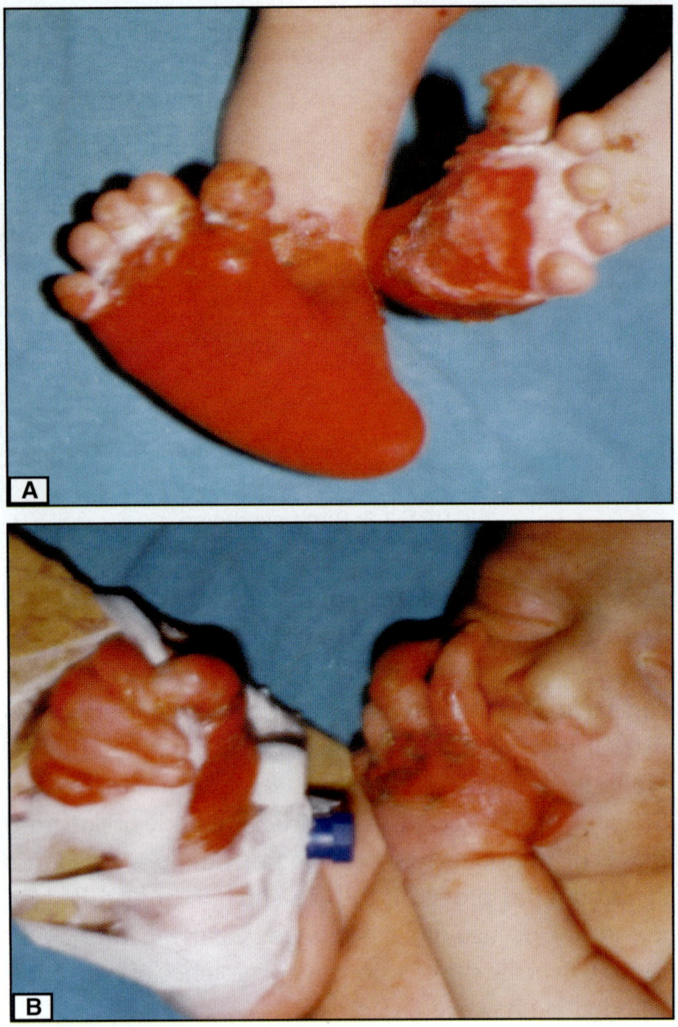

FIGURES 3.3A AND B: Autosomal recessive DEB

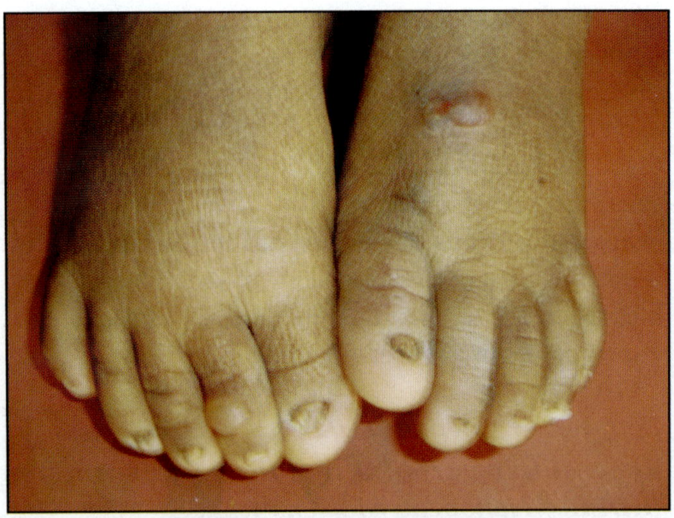

FIGURE 3.4: Nail changes in DEB

(Figures 3.4 and 3.5). Scarring leads to progressive flexion contracture and fusion of the digits (pseudosyndactyly) resembling hands and feet encased in mitten.

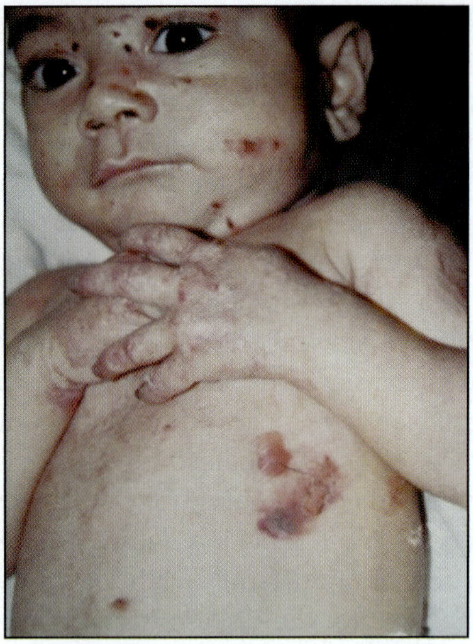

FIGURE 3.5: Hemorrhagic blisters scarring and milia in DEB

Other joints may also develop flexion contracture leading to immobilization. Irreversible alopecia and deformity of pinnae are present. There is a high incidence of squamous cell carcinoma and melanoma occurring at an early age. Mucosal involvement is common predominantly involving the gastrointestinal tract and eye. Even gentle brushing precipitates oral erosions and bullae formation followed by scarring. This gives rise to microstomia, inability to maintain oral hygiene and dental caries **(Figure 3.6)**. There are frequent occurrence of ankyloglossia, dysphagia, esophageal dysmotility, web or stricture formation and constipation. Corneal erosion and ectropion may occur.

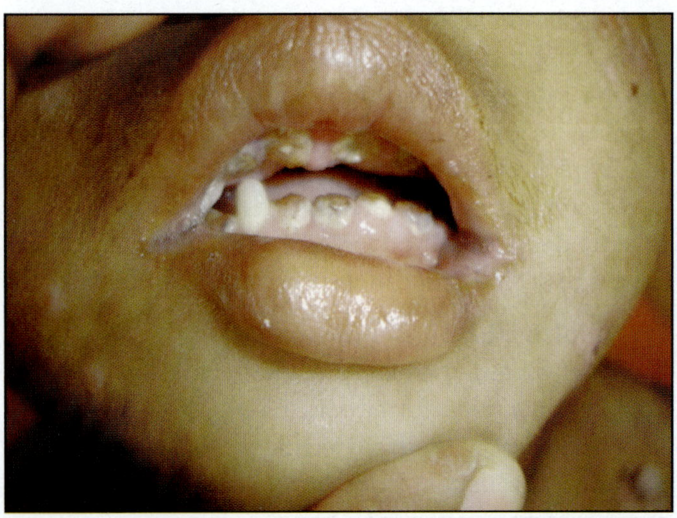

FIGURE 3.6: Dental anomalies in DEB

RDEB is associated with very high morbidity in terms of complete immobility by adolescence. Anemia results from the combined effects of inadequate diet, frequent gastrointestinal bleeding, chronic illness and associated malignancy. Death is frequent by puberty.

Mild, non-mutilating RDEB: Here clinical features are similar to Hallopieu-Siemens type, but with less severity and a milder course. Skin lesions improve by adolescence and flexion contractures are seen in fingers rather than mutilation.

RDEB-inverse form: The predominant sites of involvement in this type are acral parts as well as intertriginous areas like axillae and groins. Bullae and erosions are common in these areas. Scarring of hands and feet with flexion deformities, loss of nails and oral and esophageal mucosal involvements are common.

COMPLICATIONS OF EPIDERMOLYSIS BULLOSA

Infection of denuded areas and risk of septicemia is a continuous threat for children suffering from EB. Scarring skin lesions, deformity of acral parts, loss of nails and joint contracture impair daily activities and result in severe psychological impact in older children and adolescents. Mucosal involvement hampers regular food intake resulting in anemia and malnutrition. Malignancies may complicate the course of some variants of the disease. Death may occur in infancy or early childhood.

DIFFERENTIAL DIAGNOSIS OF EPIDERMOLYSIS BULLOSA

Simpler treatable conditions should be excluded at birth and in early neonatal period. These include suction blister, bullous impetigo, staphylococcal scalded skin syndrome, disseminated neonatal herpes, candidiasis and congenital syphilis. Rare disorders which may simulate EB are incontinentia pigmenti, epidermolytic hyperkeatosis, immunobullous disorders like neonatal pemphigus and bullous pemphigoid and porphyrias.

In preschool children, in addition to some of the above disorders, bullous scabies, bullous erythema multiforme, Stevens-Johnson syndrome, chronic bullous disease of childhood, acrodermatitis enteropathica and bullous mastocytosis should be ruled out. In older children and adolescents, rare disorders like epidermolysis bullosa acquisita and porphyrias are to be excluded.

When a clinical diagnosis of EB has been made, it may be difficult to determine the type, as overlapping features may be present. EBS-Dowling-Meara may resemble JEB or RDEB and definitive diagnosis can be made by ultrastructural study.

INVESTIGATIONS OF EPIDERMOLYSIS BULLOSA

Skin biopsy is the main investigation done for EB. Light microscopic examination helps in differentiation from some other bullous disorders. To determine the plane of cleavage and type of EB, ultrastructural and immunohistochemical studies are required.

Preferably, a fresh intact vesicle should be biopsied within 24 hours of eruption. Otherwise, edge of an older lesion can be sampled. In absence of suitable skin lesion for biopsy, in severe variants of the disease, bulla formation can be induced by gentle rubbing of the uninvolved area with a pencil eraser. Perilesional skin should be biopsied for immunohistochemical study.

Ultrastructural study by electron microscopy remains the gold-standard for diagnosis. In absence of this facility, antigen mapping at the level of split (e.g. bullous pemphigoid antigen-1, laminin, collagen VII) by immunohistochemical study is helpful. These techniques exclude immunobullous disorders confirmatively. Gene mutational analysis can be undertaken at specific research centers.

MANAGEMENT OF EPIDERMOLYSIS BULLOSA

Treatment of all forms of epidermolysis bullosa is mainly symptomatic with an aim to prevent occurrence of new lesions and deformity. In localized variants of EBS, hands and feet are to be kept cool and dry, especially during summer. Associated hyperhidrosis can be managed with topical antiperspirants like aluminium chloride hexahydrate (20%). School-going children should use well-fitted, soft, leather shoes with cotton socks. Change-over to a different design of shoe is required at regular intervals to avoid continuous pressure at one site.

In neonates with skin lesions at birth, handling by attendees should be minimal and a soft pad can be used for this purpose. Puncturing the intact bullae reduces discomfort and the blister roof should be retained as biological dressing to hasten healing. Denuded areas should be treated with a mixture of white soft and liquid paraffin. Adhesive tapes should never be used over the skin of these patients; instead, dressings can be retained with roller bandage. Depending on availability and affordability, non-occlusive, hydrocolloid fiber dressing or autologous epidermal skin grafts can be chosen for wound management. Potassium permanganate soaks and antibiotic ointments are helpful for infected lesions. In older infants, hands and feet can be covered with mitten and socks to prevent self-inflicted injury.

In infants with mucosal involvement, care should be taken while breastfeeding to prevent trauma. Lips are to be smeared with vaseline and nipple lubricated. Use of nasogastric tube is better avoided and pacifiers, if used, should be devoid of ring which may cause occlusion around mouth. In older children and adolescents with gross esophageal involvement, adequate nutritional support is required.

School going children and adolescents suffering from EB, as well as their family members require psychological support and repeated counseling to attain a positive attitude towards this highly morbid condition. In families with history of EB, genetic counseling should be provided to the couples planning pregnancy. DNA-based prenatal diagnosis of JEB and DEB is possible by chorionic villous sampling and amniocentesis.

Control of existing infection and pain and prevention of infection of denuded areas should be undertaken enthusiastically. Patients with Hallopeau-Siemens RDEB should be screened at frequent intervals for evidence of malignancy. There is no specific therapy to treat these conditions. Phenytoin and isotretinoin have been used without substantial evidence of being effective. In future, gene therapy may bring hope to treat this group of debilitating diseases.

ECTODERMAL DYSPLASIA

Structural and functional anomalies involving one or more ectodermal structures like hair, teeth, nail and sweat glands give rise to a rare, heterogeneous group of disorders, designated as ectodermal dysplasia (ED). The defects are present at birth, and are non-progressive.

In the classification system of ED (Pinheiro and Freire-Maia, 1994) there is numerical designation of the involved structures, which are combined to represent organ involvements in a given disorder (e.g. 1-2, 1-3, 1-4, 2-3, 1-2-4, 2-3-4, 1-2-3-4 etc, when 1 represents hair, 2, teeth, 3, nail and 4, sweat gland). Alternatively, these disorders can be named according to the affected structures, like, tricho-odontic, tricho-onychial, tricho-dyshidrotic etc.

X-LINKED HYPOHIDROTIC/ANHIDROTIC ECTODERMAL DYSPLASIA (CHRIST-SIEMENS-TOURAINE SYNDROME)

Commonest disorder among this group is hypohidrotic ectodermal dysplasia (HED). Males are the main sufferers (>90%) and female carriers present with incomplete features of the disease. All the ectodermal derivatives are involved.

Genetics

The principal inheritance pattern is X-L-R. The involved gene ED-1 (X-q12-13.1) encodes a protein ectodysplasin A (a member of the tumor necrosis factor family). It plays an important role in the genesis of ectodermal structures. Though rare, HED may follow AD or AR inheritance patterns. The autosomal gene is located on chromosome 2q11-q1 (ED-3). Autosomal recessive HED results from mutation of 'crinkled' gene. This form of HED is characterized by complete clinical manifestations in both male and female patients. Mosaic forms can also occur. Patients with AR disease are clinically indistinguishable from the classical X-L-R disease. Sweating abnormality is milder in patients with AD inheritance pattern.

Clinical Features

Male children develop classical clinical features of the disease. Presentation is in early childhood with prolonged and episodic high pyrexia (as high as 108°F) and heat intolerance, especially following exertion, hot food or drinks or febrile convulsion. These result from lack of sweating. Hair and skin are involved at or soon after birth. The skin is thin, smooth, dry and finely wrinkled, especially in periorbital area, giving a prematurely aged look. Dermatitis may be present. Scalp hair may be sparse or absent at birth. In older children hair is thin, light colored and sparse with almost total absence of eyebrows and eyelashes. Parallel dark bands across the full width of the hair-shaft (bar-code appearance) may be present.

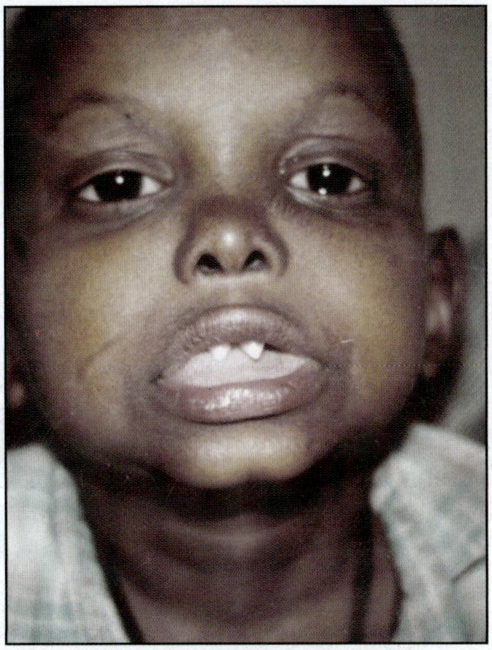

FIGURE 3.7: Sparse hair and conical teeth in anhidrotic ectodermal dysplasia

The facies is characteristic with frontal bossing, depressed nasal bridge, prominent malar bones, sunken cheeks and pointed chin. This mid-facial hypoplasia gives rise to a 'dish-face' appearance in profile. Full, everted lower lips, pseudo-rhagades, conspicuous nostrils and prominent, low-lying ears are frequent. Older children look identical to each other because of similar facies.

Both temporary and permanent teeth are affected, There is partial or total anodontia and the existing teeth are deformed and conical **(Figure 3.7)**. Maxillary hypoplasia results in low-arched, flat palate. Nails are brittle, thin and ridged and dermatoglyphic patterns are distorted.

Mucosal involvement gives rise to dry mouth, atrophic rhinitis, sinusitis, dysphagia, hoarse voice and bronchitis. Ocular manifestations include corneal opacity, cataract, subluxation of lens and absence of lacrimal puncta, which is characteristic. Other features include conductive deafness, hypoplasia or aplasia of breasts, atopic dermatitis, asthma and susceptibility to recurrent infections. Intelligence is usually normal. Life expectancy is normal or just below average.

Clinical features are incomplete in carrier females. They present with missing or conical teeth, sparse hair, abnormal dermatoglyphics or focal hypohidrosis following Blaschko's lines.

Diagnosis

Prolonged undiagnosed fever with characteristic facies in a male neonate is the pointer to the diagnosis. Mother or other female family members should be examined for some features of the disease which may be present in 2/3rd cases. Demonstration of hypohidrosis is possible by some standard techniques like sweat pore counts (by silicone rubber plastic imprints), starch-iodine test and quantitative pilocarpine iontophoresis. 'Valerio Ventruto technique' is an easy method of sweat pore counting from the palmer skin of the fingertips of the patient by using X-ray film, which is compared to a control. These tests help in quantitative assessment of disease severity.

Histopathology of hypothenar palmer skin biopsy shows partial development or sparse/total absence of sweat glands in the dermis. Sebaceous glands and hair follicles are also decreased in other body areas. Suspected carriers may need sweat testing or skin biopsy for diagnosis.

Differential Diagnosis

Occasionally, the affected babies simulate collodion baby at birth. Other ectodermal dysplasias have similarities with HED but can be distinguished by typical features.

Management

These patients should be managed at cool, ambient temperature. Light clothing, repeated cold water sprays, air-conditioned housing and avoidance of hot food and undue exertion prevent repeated episodes of hyperpyrexia. Affected children may participate in sports and other physical activities with the help of special cooling devices. Maintainance of oral hygiene prevents caries and early loss of teeth. Hair and dental prosthesis should be provided so that the child's self-esteem and social communication abilities are restored. In addition to above measures affected children may need psychological support.

Involved families need genetic counseling. Fetal skin biopsy after 24 weeks of gestation, allow appreciating the sweat gland structure which may be shriveled or absent. The involved gene can be located by DNA-probing techniques on chorionic villus biopsy specimen.

HIDROTIC ECTODERMAL DYSPLASIA (CLOUSTON'S SYNDROME)

The triad of clinical features in hidrotic ectodermal dysplasia (HED) includes palmoplantar keratoderma, generalized hypotrichosis and nail dystrophy.

Genetics

The transmission is autosomal dominant. The affected gene ED2 is in the pericentromeric region of chromosome 13q11-q12.1, which encodes for connexin-30. The later is a member of the gap junction family and mediates diffusion of ions and metabolites between adjacent cells. Homozygous state of HED may be lethal.

Clinical Features

Short, discolored, dystrophic nails dominate the clinical picture. This is associated with painful, bulbous fingertips. Other changes include thin and brittle nail with slow growth and persistent infective paronychia. Hair is normal at birth but gradual change occurs thereafter; it becomes pale, sparse, brittle and total alopecia may occur by puberty.

Eyebrow and eyelashes are thin and sparse and other body hairs are absent in adults.

Palmoplantar keratoderma is diffuse with deep fissures and variable transgradiens. There are localized skin-thickening over pressure points and also beneath the nails. Oral leukoplakia may be present. Sweat glands are not affected.

Teeth may be normal or involved with caries early. Bony changes include thickening of the skull bones and tufting of the terminal phalanges of the fingers and toes. Structural anomalies include syndactyly and polydactyly. Physical and mental retardation may be associated. Life expectancy is usually normal.

Diagnosis

A relatively normal facies, normal sweating and teeth and associated palmoplantar keratoderma differentiates this condition from HED.

Management

Keratolytic agents and emollients are helpful for palmoplantar keratoderma. In severe cases, systemic retinoids can be administered but require long-term treatment.

ECTRODACTYLY-ECTODERMAL DYSPLASIA-CLEFT LIP/PALATE (EEC SYNDROME)

Both ectodermal and mesodermal derivatives are involved in this very rare syndrome. Three clinical types, EEC-1, EEC-2 (OMIM 602077) and EEC-3 (OMIM 604292) have been described.

Genetics

EEC follows AD inheritance pattern. The gene locations are 7q11.2-q21.3 (EEC-1), chromosome 19 (EEC-2) and 3q27 (EEC-3).The mutated gene in EEC-1 is p63, which is essential for maintaining the progenitor cells for genesis of limbs and cranio-facial regions in fetal life.

Clinical Features

Split hand and feet (lobster claw deformity) and cleft palate and lip are present in 70-100% cases and are the distinctive feature. Tetramelic deformity of limbs is commonest (75%) and 3rd and 4th digits are most commonly involved. Nails are hypoplastic and dystrophic.

The affected children have typical facies with hypoplastic maxillae, short philtrum and broad nasal tip. Recurrent keratitis with epiphora results from naso-lacrimal duct obstruction. This may result in blindness in the long run. Hair is involved in all which appear dry, sparse, hypopigmented and wiry. Other features include choanal atresia, oligodontia, anodontia, peg-shaped teeth, dry, scaly skin, scalp dermatitis and mild hypohidrosis.

Other abnormalities which may be associated in varying combinations include conductive deafness, glandular hypospadius, urethral reflux and hydronephrosis, hypothalamic-pituitary dysfunction, mental retardation and hamartoma of the tongue.

Diagnosis

Major diagnostic criteria:

- Ectodermal dysplasia,
- Ectrodactyly,
- Cleft lip/palate,
- Lacrimal duct anomalies

Minor diagnostic criteria:

- Renal anomalies,
- Deafness,
- Mental retardation
- Choanal atresia.

Absence or hypoplasia of metacarpals and metatarsals are seen in radiography of hands and feet.

Management

Deformities are recognizable by prenatal USG. Early repair of cleft lip/palate should be undertaken. Multidisciplinary approach is needed for management of other anomalies.

RAPP-HODGKIN SYNDROME/HAY-WELLS SYNDROME (AEC SYNDROME)

There is significant clinical overlap between Rapp-Hodgkin syndrome and Hay-Wells syndrome. Though earlier considered different, now these two entities are recognized as same. There is AD inheritance pattern with variable expressivity. Heterozygous, missense mutation occurs in the SAM domain of p63.

Erythroderma is present at birth in 90% cases. Skin erosions may be present which run a chronic course. Older children develop marked hypohidrosis and heat intolerance. Sparse, light-colored hair with a 'steel-wool' texture is seen and there may be other hair shaft anomalies like pili torti/canaliculi. A distinctive facies results from prominent forehead, maxillary hyperplasia, narrow nose and small mouth. Fusion of the eyelids is a distinctive feature in this disorder.

Nail dystrophy, cleft lip/palate and hypodontia or conical teeth may be associated.

Additional anomalies include hypospadius, supernumerary nipples, syndactyly, auricular deformities, lacrimal duct atresia, microphthalmia and ventricular septal defect.

Management should focus on surgical correction of the eyelids and management of hyperhidrosis.

DYSKERATOSIS CONGENITA (ZINSSER-COLE-ENGMAN SYNDROME)

It is a rare disorder characterized by reticulate skin pigmentation, nail dystrophy, leukokeratosis and hematological abnormalities. The principal inheritance pattern is X-linked (MIM 22430), but AD (MIM 127550) and AR (MIM 22430) modes of transmission have been reported. There is missense mutation of DKC1 gene (Xq28), encoding a protein dyskeratin. Chromosomal instability and T-cell instability is found in this disorder resulting in predisposition to malignancy.

Cutaneous features are most consistently present and appear by first year of life. There is grayish brown, reticulated pigmentation, atrophy and telangiectasia involving neck, upper chest and proximal arms. Nail involvement is present in 98% cases, usually by first year of life in the form of thinning, longitudinal grooves, pterygium formation or total atrophy. Loss of dermatoglyphics is characteristic. Palmoplantar keratoderma and hyperhidrosis, bullae precipitated by minor trauma, alopecia and premature graying of hair are other features.

Leukokeratosis may involve any mucosae including that of gastrointestinal and genitourinary tracts. Ocular features include continuous epiphora resulting from lacrimal duct atresia, blepharitis and conjunctivitis. Hematological abnormality includes pancytopenia, which manifests by 10 years of age but may appear later.

Hemorrhagic tendency and infections due to bone marrow failure results in early mortality. Patients are prone to develop malignancy by third decade of life, especially squamous cell carcinoma on leukokeratotic areas and Hodgkin's lymphoma.

Close monitoring of these patients is required for bone marrow failure and development of malignancy. Excessive sun exposure should be curtailed to reduce the risk of malignancy. Repeated blood transfusions, granulocyte colony stimulating factors and bone marrow transplantation are of help to prolong life span.

INCONTINENTIA PIGMENTI (BLOCH-SULZBERGER DISEASE)

Incontinentia pigmenti (IP) is a rare X-L-D disorder, usually lethal in males. Cutaneous involvement is multiphasic, and multisystem involvement is present.

GENETICS

There is mutation (deletion) of NEMO gene, located in Xq28, which is required for activation of transcription factor NF-κB, necessary for immunological, inflammatory and apoptotic pathways.

CLINICAL FEATURES

Cutaneous manifestations appear in following stages which may be overlapping.

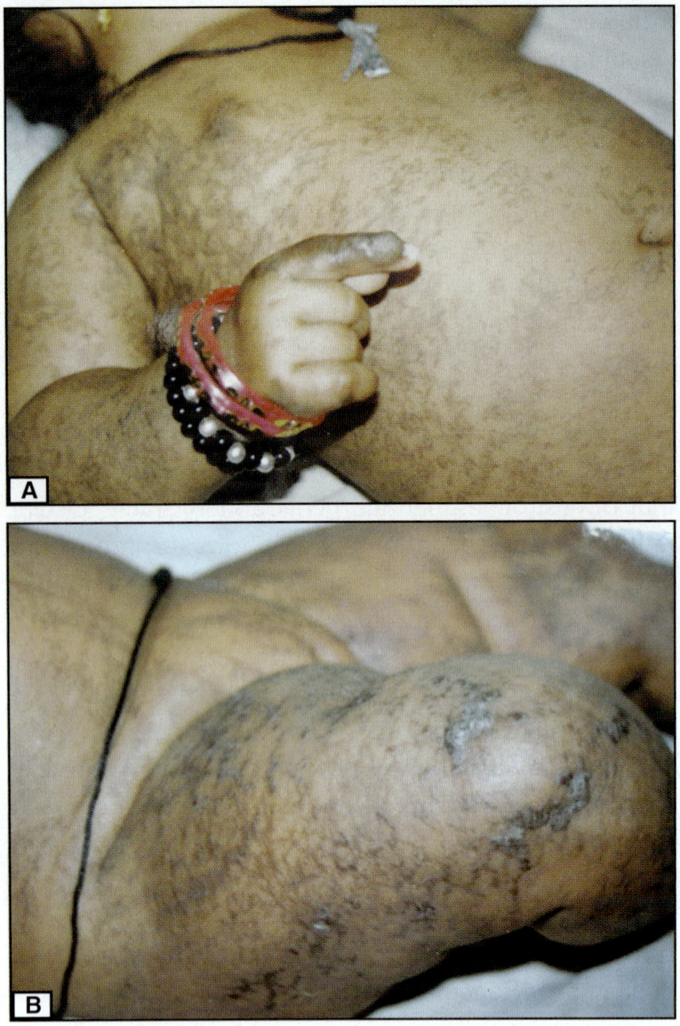

FIGURES 3.8A AND B: Hyperkeratosis and whorls of hyperpigmentation in incontinentia pigmenti

- Stage 1: Vesicle and pustule on erythematous base, present on any body parts except face.
- Stage 2: Papule, verrucous lesions and hyperkeratosis, in streaks/whorled pattern, involving mainly lower limbs.
- Stage 3: Localized hyperpigmentation in whorls/streaks on trunks and extremities.
- Stage 4: Hypopigmented, hairless streaks with atrophy and scarring, present on lower limbs.

Cutaneous manifestations may start in intrauterine life and skin lesions of first or second stage may be present at birth. However, vesicular lesions may continue to appear till adult life and warty lesions may persist till adolescence. The hyperpigmented skin lesions of third stage appear in childhood and disappear by the end of second decade. This is the most consistently present skin lesions in these patients **(Figures 3.8A and B)**. Stage 4 develops in minority of patients in adult life. Mothers of affected or yet asymptomatic patients may show lesions of stage 4. Focal anhidrosis is a hallmark feature of this disorder. Ridging and pitting of nails and cicatricial alopecia may be present.

Other systemic involvements include ocular (mainly retinal vascular involvement), neurological (seizure, spastic paralysis, psychomotor retardation), dental (anodontia, conical teeth, delayed eruption) and skeletal abnormalities. Congenital heart diseases may be associated. Breast hypoplasia is commoner in this group of individuals.

INVESTIGATIONS

The initial vesicular lesions are associated with intense tissue and peripheral blood eosinophilia. Histopathological features of skin lesions are characteristic of each stage of disease. In first stage, there is spongiosis, intraepidermal blister formation, eosinophilia and dyskeratotic cells. Second stage is characterized by hyperkeratosis, dyskeratosis and occasional eosinophils. Marked pigment incontinence is the main feature of third stage. Fourth stage is characterized by fibrosis and absence of pigment.

Hypohidrotic skin lesions in patients and their mothers can be identified by starch-iodine test.

DIAGNOSIS

Diagnosis is mainly clinical. Diagnostic criteria for IP are listed below.

Major criteria:
- Typical neonatal skin lesions with erythema, vesicles and eosinophilia
- Streaks of hyperpigmentation along Blaschko's lines, fading by adolescence.
- Linear, atrophic, hairless lesions.

Minor criteria:
- Alopecia/wooly hair
- Dental anomalies
- Ocular anomalies

Presence of at least one of the major criteria is essential for clinical diagnosis of IP. This is further supported by histopathological features.

DIFFERENTIAL DIAGNOSIS

The vesiculo-pustular eruptions present at birth or soon thereafter are to be differentiated from neonatal herpes simplex, candidiasis, impetigo, erythema toxicum neonatorum and infantile pustular melanosis. The linear hyperkeratotic lesions resemble verrucous epidermal nevus. In hyperpigmented stage, nevoid and whorled hypermelanosis has to be ruled out by proper history about evolution of skin lesions. The initial vesicular lesions are associated with intense tissue and peripheral blood eosinophilia.The hypopigmented streaks of fourth stage are to be differentiated from hypomelanosis of Ito.

MANAGEMENT

The skin lesions should be treated symptomatically by prevention of infection and regular use of emollients. Regular ophthalmologic and neurological screening is mandatory in childhood for early diagnosis of any involvement.

Oral-Facial-Digital Syndrome (OFD)

Four distinct variants of this disorder exist; OFD-I (Papillon-Léage-Psaume syndrome)

OFD-II (Mohr syndrome)

OFD-III

OFD-IV

OFD I has X-L-D inheritance whereas the other three types follow AR transmission pattern. These conditions are of rare occurrence and can be distinguished by characteristic features.

Johanson-Blizzard Syndrome

The inheritance pattern is AR. Congenital membranous aplasia cutis of the scalp present as small stellate defects on the frontal area. Others are absence of permanent teeth buds, hypoplastic alae nasi, sparse hair and deafness. Dwarfism, mental retardation, hypotonia and genital abnormalities may be associated. Endocrinological abnormalities include hypothyroidism, pancreatic insufficiency and diabetes.

Schöpf-Schulz-Passarge Syndrome

AR inheritance is usual in this form of ectodermal dysplasia but rarely, AD transmission may also occur. Cysts at the eyelid margins, palmoplantar keratoderma and hypotrichosis are the distinguishing clinical features. Hypodontia, brittle and furrowed nails and benign and malignant tumors of palm and soles are frequent.

HEREDITARY DISORDERS OF KERATINIZATION

ICHTHYOSIS

Introduction

The term 'ichthyosis' has been derived from the Greek word 'ichthys' meaning fish-scale. This descriptive term refers to the similar appearance of the skin seen in this group of disorders resulting from abnormal keratinization. Ichthyosis consists of heterogenous disorders, including severe congenital forms, different ichthyosiform syndromes and acquired form, induced by drugs and disease states. A classification of ichthyosis has been presented in **Table 3.2**. Clinical expression of these disorders is greatly variable ranging from mild ichthyosis vulgaris to severe, lethal harlequin ichthyosis. There are certain clinical pointers to diagnose individual conditions; however, confirmative diagnosis is possible only by ultrastructural study.

Ichthyosis Vulgaris

Ichthyosis vulgaris is a common variant of the disease. It is commoner in atopic individuals. The transmission is autosomal dominant with variable penetrance. However, cases without family history are commonly seen. Some authors believe it to be a polygenic disorder, sharing common genetic predisposition as atopic dermatitis

Pathogenesis: The skin of patients with ichthyosis vulgaris is deficient in histidine which is a basic molecule necessary for synthesis of profilaggrin and filaggrin. Profilaggrin is not available for keratin synthesis, impairing the formation of keratohyalin granules and keratin filament. Stratum corneum ceramide level may be decreased in these patients.

Clinical features: Ichthyosis vulgaris manifests during first few months of life and clinical features are mild. There is light-gray colored scale involving extensor extremities and trunk **(Figure 3.9)**. The flexures, such as the axillae, groins and antecubital and popliteal fossae are spared. The condition is asymptomatic and family history may be positive. Though reduced in severity, it persists till adult life. In cases with associated atopy, keratosis pilaris, hyperlinearity of palms and soles and pruritus may be present.

Histopathology: Histopathology reveals compact orthohyperkeratosis and granular layer is almost absent.

TABLE 3.2: Classification of congenital ichthyosis

Ichthyosis	
Autosomal dominant	
Generalized	Ichthyosis vulgaris
Localized	Bullous Ichthyosiform erythroderma
Autosomal recessive	Ichthyosis bullosa of Siemens
	Ichthyosis hystrix
	Lamellar ichthyosis
	Non-bullous Ichthyosiform erythroderma
X-linked	Harlequin ichthyosis
	Multiple sulphatase deficiency
	X-linked recessive ichthyosis
Ichthyosiform syndromes	Sjögren-Larsson syndrome
	Refsum's disease
	Conradi-Hünermann-Happle syndrome
	Chanarin-Dorfman syndrome
	KID syndrome
	CHILD syndrome
	Netherton's syndrome
	IBIDS syndrome

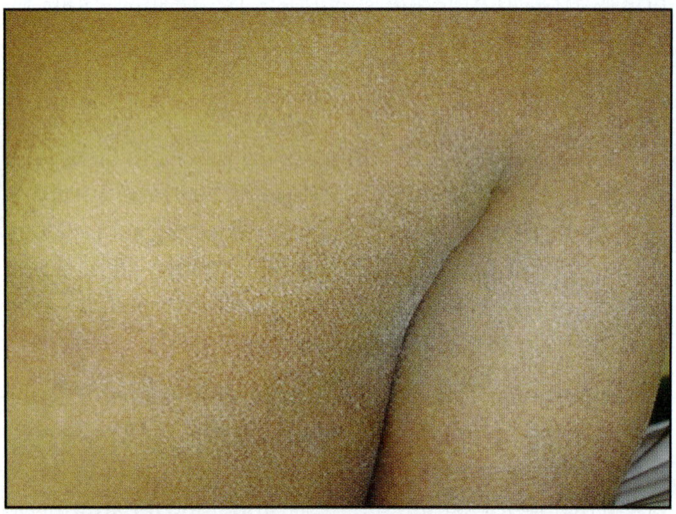

FIGURE 3.9: Branny scale of ichthyosis vulgaris

Occasional follicular hyperkeratosis is observed. Other features include small and reduced eccrine sweat and sebaceous glands and mononuclear infiltrate in the upper dermis. Electron microscopy shows fragmented keratohyaline granules.

X-linked Recessive Ichthyosis (XLRI)

XLRI is the second common variant of ichthyosis with X-linked recessive transmission. It is unique among congenital ichthyosis by presence of extracutaneous manifestations.

Pathogenesis: Two molecular pathways are involved in the pathogenesis in XLRI. The prime factor is the lack of steroid sulfatase (isomer of aryl sulfatase C, a membrane bound microsomal enzyme) in affected patients. This enzyme is normally present in the leukocytes, keratinocytes and fibroblasts and is responsible for epidermal hydrolysis of cholesterol sulfate to cholesterol. In deficiency of steroid sulfatase, there is accumulation of cholesterol sulfate in the epidermis. This results in barrier instability by non-lamellar phase separation in the stratum corneum interstices. The high level of cholesterol sulfate also delays the corneodesmosome degradation which results in corneocyte retention. High Ca++ in the stratum corneum of patients with XLRI may be another contributory factor, which enhances corneocyte retention.

The gene encoding steroid sulfatase is located at Xp22.3 which is particularly susceptible to deletions. Complete deletion of the steroid sulfatase gene is seen in most cases (>90%), and it is one of the genetic disorders with highest chromosomal deletions. Contiguous gene syndromes may occasionally result when deletions extend to the neighboring genes. Examples of these include XLRI in association with Kallmann syndrome, ocular albinism type 1, X-linked recessive chondrodysplasia punctata, short stature, and mental retardation. Point mutations may also occur in steroid sulfatase gene, leading to amino acid substitutions in the polypeptide chain.

Clinical features: The baby may be born with collodion membrane or clinical features start within few weeks of birth. The scales are typically large, polygonal, dark in color and firmly attached, especially over extremities, neck and pre-auricular area of the face. Over the sides of the trunk and back of the neck, the scales give a dirty appearance. Flexural involvement may be seen in some cases. Palms and soles are not involved. Clinical features persist till adult life.

Main extracutaneous manifestations of XLRI are corneal opacities (25-50 %) and cryptorchidism (10-20 %). Rarely, mental deficiency or hypogonadism may be present. Numerous corneal opacities (dots or commas), without hindering the vision are present in adult patients and carrier females. These are demonstrable by slit-lamp examination. There is an increased risk of testicular cancer in these patients which may involve even normally descended testis. Female patients and carriers may develop obstetric complications like prolonged labour due to inadequate cervical dilatation resulting from deficient placental steroid sulfatase.

Histopathology: Histopathological features are non-specific with normal or prominent granular layer. Sebaceous glands are present. Electron microscopic findings include numerous keratohyaline granules which may be smaller or normal.

Multiple Sulfatase Deficiency

It is a very rare disorder of childhood, where neurological manifestations are the predominant clinical feature. There is deficiency of all the seven types of sulfatases, however, the relatively milder cutaneous manifestations indicate partial deficiency of steroid sulfatase. The transmission is AR.

Neurological manifestations simulate late infantile metachromatic leukodystrophy. Clinical features start during second year as psychomotor retardation, limb hypotonia and unsteady gait which are progressive. In late stage the child is bed-bound and blindness supervenes. Ichthyosis starts during third year, resembles XLRI, but is less severe.

Lamellar Ichthyosis (LI)

Lamellar ichthyosis is a severe form of disorder transmitted as autosomal recessive trait. Rarely, a clinically indistinguishable form with AD inheritance has been reported.

Pathogenesis: Patients with LI have deranged process of cornification and desquamation resulting from mutations in TGM1 gene located on chromosome 14q11. This leads to abnormal keratinocyte transglutaminase1 (TGase 1) enzyme, which catalyze calcium dependent amide cross linking between amino acid residues on precursor proteins forming the impermeable layers of epidermal cell envelope. Moreover, this enzyme helps in formation of lipid envelope by linkage of epidermis-specific omega hydroxyceramides to the plasma membrane. Hence, in absence of the enzyme, synthesis of protein and lipid envelope of keratinocytes is disturbed.

Clinical features: LI presents at birth and is one of the causes of collodion baby. The ichthyosis is generalized with involvement of face, flexures, palms and soles. The scales are large, quadrilateral, dark- brown in color, free and raised at the edges and adherent at the centre. Deep fissures are present in between the scales. The overall appearance is that of a tree bark **(Figures 3.10A to C)**. There is intense tautness of skin, resulting in ectropion, eclabium **(Figure 3.11)**, hypoplasia of nose and pinna and flexion contracture of limb joints and digits. Occlusion of sweat ducts lead to loss of sweating and heat intolerance. Scarring alopecia may be present, especially over scalp margins. Nail changes include ridging, thickening and nail dystrophy. Ectropion may lead to conjunctivitis and keratitis.

'Bathing-suit ichthyosis' is a distinct type of autosomal recessive congenital ichthyosis, seen among South African black children. Skin lesions are present at birth and may present as collodion baby. There is diffuse scaling of scalp, trunk and proximal parts of the upper limbs sparing face and distal extremities. The number of reported cases of this rare disorder is less than fifteen.

Histopathology: Histopathological study reveals marked orthohyperkeratosis, mild acanthosis and regular papillomatosis. Electron microscopic findings include elongated cholesterol clefts and lipid droplets in the stratum corneum. Minimized or absent cornified cell envelope has been reported.

Harlequin Ichthyosis (HI)

HI is a very rare, severe form of congenital ichthyosis with autosomal recessive inheritance. Sporadic cases may also occur. It is associated with high perinatal mortality and the survivors experience high morbidity due to subsequent development of severe erythroderma and other deformities.

Pathogenesis: In patients with HI, there is abnormal localization of epidermal lipids and lamellar granule

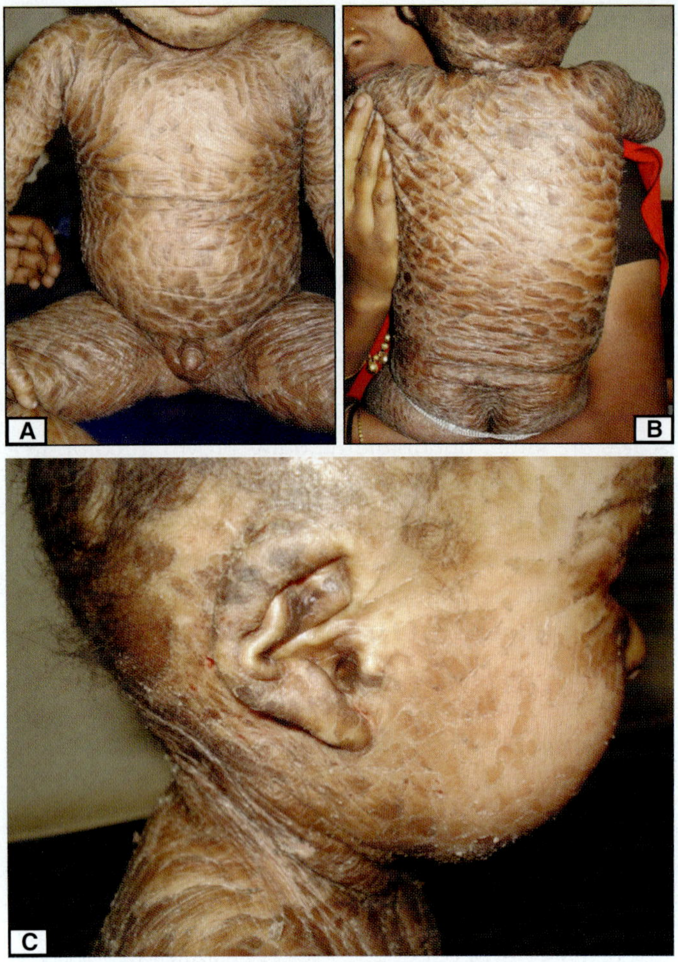

FIGURES 3.10A TO C: Lamellar ichthyosis

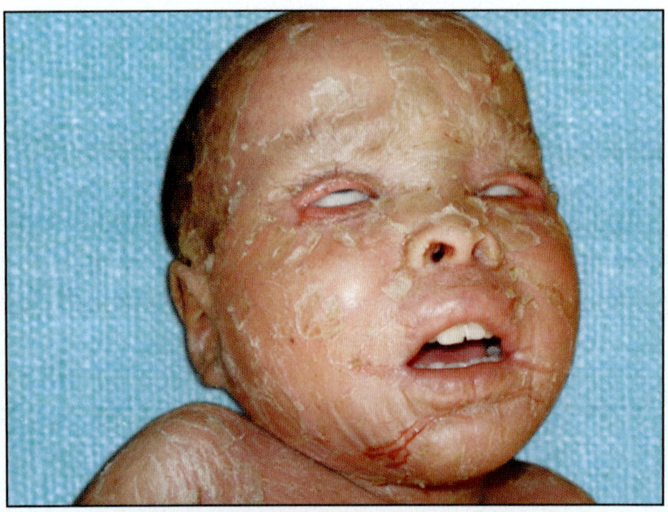

FIGURE 3.11: Ectropion and eclabium

formation is defective. There is mutation in the ABCA12 gene encoding an adenosine triphosphate-binding cassette (ABC) transporter. ABCA12 is associated with lipid transport in lamellar granules and loss of this function leads to a defective lipid barrier in the stratum corneum. Posttranslational block in conversion of profilaggrin to filaggrin leads to deficiency of the later. Genetic heterogeneity is observed in HI. Depending upon the pattern of keratin expression, there are three types. Type I (normal keratin, profilaggrin staining +), type II (hyperproliferation of suprabasal keratin, K6/K16), type III (hyperproliferation of suprabasal keratin, K6/K16 and negative profilaggrin staining).

Clinical features: Preterm delivery and stillbirth are common in this disorder. The affected newborn is encased in "armor"-like thick, yellow plate-like scales with deep red fissuring. The skin is stretched tightly over face resulting in a grotesque appearance. The facial features include ectropion, loss of eyelashes and eyebrows, eclabium and flattening of the ears and nose. Presence of constriction bands leads to swelling of the limbs and flexion of the digits which may become hypoplastic and rudimentary. Live born infants develop multiple systemic complications. These include respiratory insufficiency due to constriction of chest wall, esophageal stenosis leading to hypoglycemia and dehydration and temperature regulation. Death within first few days of life is usual resulting from these complications.

Histopathology: Light microscopic findings are non-specific.

Epidermolytic Hyperkeratosis (EHK)

EHK (bullous ichthyosiform erythroderma), is a rare autosomal dominant disorder of keratinization associated with blister formation. Autosomal recessive and sporadic forms may also occur.

Pathogenesis: In suprabasal keratinocytes committed to terminal differentiation, the intermediate filaments are composed of keratin 1/keratin 10 heterodimers. In EHK there are mutations in epidermal keratin 1/keratin 10 genes resulting in abnormal keratin-intermediate filament cytoskeleton. This results in abnormal clumping of suprabasal keratinocytes and impaired tonofilament network in the differentiating epidermal cells.

Clinical features: Skin lesions are present at birth as generalized flaccid bullae and extensive areas of denudation. This is provoked by friction resulting from passage through the birth canal. With time, tendency to extensive vesiculation decreases and hyperkeratotic skin lesions supervene. In older children and adolescents, there are dirty brown, spiny skin ridges, especially distributed over joints, flexures, back, scalp, periumbilical and peri-areolar regions. However, episodes of focal vesiculation are common, precipitated by friction, trauma or infection. In severe cases with generalized hyperkeratosis, skin has a cobblestone appearance which may be shed in large plates revealing underlying erosion. Erythroderma with peeling and scaling may be present. In the neonatal period, sepsis and fluid-electrolyte imbalance are the potential causes of mortality.

Palmoplantar keratoderma may be present and depending on the presence or absence of this feature, six phenotypes of EHK have been identified (PS-1,2,3 and NPS-1,2,3). Palmoplantar keratoderma is diffuse with sharply demarcated, erythematous border. The keratoderma may be severe with fissuring and digital contractures (PS-2), or rarely cerebriform (PS-3). NPS types have normal palms and soles except NPS-3, where hyperlinearity is the feature. Limited spiny lesions in the nevoid form simulating ichthyosis hystrix may be present over flexures and extremities. Severe scalp involvement resulting in encasement of hair shafts with scale is a common feature. Nails may be dystrophic. Mucosae and teeth are normal.

Histopathology: Epidermal changes include marked hyperkeratosis and acanthosis. Multiple perinuclear vacuoles and large clumps of keratohyaline granules are present in the granular and upper spinous layer cells. Bullae results from suprabasal splits. These combined histopathological features are known as 'epidermolytic hyperkeratosis'. Mild perivascular lymphocytic infiltrate is present in the upper dermis. Electron microscopy reveals perinuclear clumping of tonofilaments and variable desmosomal disruption with cleft formation.

Ichthyosis Bullosa of Siemens

Ichthyosis bullosa of Siemens (IBS) is a superficial variant of epidermolytic hyperkeratosis characterized by lack of erythema and palmoplantar involvement. The epidermolysis in IBS correlates with sites of expression of K2e gene and several mutations involving this gene have been reported. The transmission is AD.

Symptoms start during neonatal period and may persist till adult life. Flexures, shin and lower abdomen are commonly involved areas. Initial lesions are bullae which rupture shortly with annular peeling of the involved skin with collaret-like border (mauserung or moulting). Subsequently, circumscribed areas with grayish, rippled scales develop. Rarely, hypertrichosis and palmoplantar blistering with hyperhidrosis may be associated. Histopathological changes are similar to classic EHS, but more superficial, confined to granular and upper spinous layers with normal suprabasal and basal cells. Areas of blistering show intracorneal split surrounded by orthohyperkeratosis. Electron microscopy reveals bundles and clumps of tonofilaments in the granular layer.

Ichyhyosis Hystrix

Ichyhyosis hystrix (IH) resembles EHK due to presence of spiny scales. However, here the lesions are localized and there is no skin fragility or bullae formation. There is no evidence of epidermolysis in histopathology. Skin lesions may be present at birth or appear during childhood and include muddy, spiny hyperkeratosis on extensor extremities and trunk with or without mild erythema. Lesions may follow Blaschko's lines. Diffuse, mutilating palmoplantar keratoderma may be present.

Vacuolated and bi-nucleate cells in the upper epidermis are a characteristic feature. Ultrastructural findings are perinuclear tonofilament shells forming cytoplasmic compartments in granular and upper spinous cell layers, surrounded by a ribosome-rich region.

Nonbullous Ichthyosiform Erythroderma

Nonbullous ichthyosiform erythroderma (NBIE) is a rare type of ichthyosis with AR transmission, present at birth. AD inheritance pattern has been reported in some families.

Pathogenesis: There is extensive genetic heterogeneity in this disorder. Some patients with NBIE have transglutaminase-1 deficiency (mutation in TGM-1), resulting in abnormal cornified cell envelope and impaired skin-barrier.

Clinical features: Presentation at birth is mostly as a collodion baby. In infancy and thereafter, there is a persistent erythroderma with thin, white, small, semi adherent scales. However, degree of erythema and scaling is highly variable, even among affected family members. Scarring alopecia, nail dystrophy and hypohidrosis and heat intolerance may be present.

Histopathology: Light microscopic findings are non-specific. Ultrastructural findings reveal lipid droplets in the stratum corneum resulting from retained, abnormal lamellar bodies in the corneocytes. Intercellular lipid lamellae are highly disorganized.

Collodion Body

This term is used for a transient appearance of neonates, born with some congenital ichthyosis. The newborn is encased in a shiny, taut membrane, which sheds thereafter and gradually clinical features of a definitive ichthyosis becomes apparent. NBIE is the commonest condition (60-80%) resulting in collodion baby, followed by lamellar ichthyosis. Some ichthyosiform syndromes like, Sjögren-Larsson syndrome, Conradi-Hünermann syndrome, trichothiodystrophy may also present with collodion membrane at birth.

These neonates are usually born preterm. A parchment-thin, yellowish, plastic-like membrane covers the whole body, tethering at the body orifices **(Figure 3.12)**. The appearance is typical with ectropion, eclabium, flat pinna, absence of skin creases and sausage-shaped digits. Limb movements are restricted. Following birth the membrane dries up with fissures around the flexures and completely shed in few weeks. Thereafter the clinical features of specific ichthyosis become evident. In 10-20% patients, the condition is transient and the child subsequently develops normal skin. This condition is termed as 'self-healing collodion baby' or 'lamellar ichthyosis of newborn.'

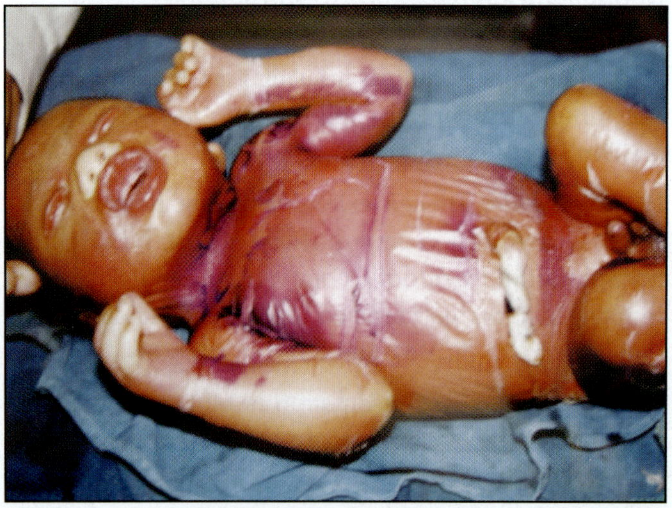

FIGURE 3.12: Collodion baby

Complications: Complications are common with all types of ichthyosis. Recurrent bacterial infections are common in these patients which may lead to fatal sepsis in some cases. Erythroderma due to LI and NBIE and Harlequin ichthyosis may lead to hypothermia, fluid, electrolyte imbalance and metabolic disturbances. Severely erythrodermic children are prone to develop protein energy malnutrition and stunted growth. Ocular complications in the form of exposure dermatitis and dystrichiasis are common in presence of poorly managed ectropion. Dysmorphic appearance results in severe psychological impact to children suffering from ichthyosis.

Differential diagnosis: Mild ichthyosis vulgaris may be mistaken as the xerosis of atopic children, especially when these conditions are co-existing. Individual types of ichthyosis can be differentiated from each other by detailed history, meticulous clinical examination and electron microscopic features of skin biopsy specimen. In all cases, other systemic involvements must be looked for to rule out ichthyosiform syndromes.

Investigations: Though minor differences may exist, light microscopic examination of skin biopsy specimen is non-specific and usually non-contributory. Electron microscopic features are distinct and this is mandatory to categorize the type of ichthyosis. In patients with XLRI, testing steroid sulfatase activity provides confirmative diagnosis; however the testing is cumbersome and not available in all the centers. An alternative screening test for these patients is serum electrophoresis, where the electromobility of beta-lipoprotein is enhanced due to accumulation of cholesterol sulfate to this fraction. Pregnant women with risk of carrying a fetus with XLRI and multiple sulfatase deficiency can be screened by estimation of maternal serum and urinary estriol, which are low in such cases.

Prenatal diagnosis is advisable in all severe forms of congenital ichthyosis. Ultrastructural study of amniotic fluid cells or fetal skin during second trimester helps in determining characteristic findings. DNA-based studies from chorionic villus or amniotic fluid cells help to localize the mutation as early as 10-12 weeks.

Management: The cornerstone of management of any type of ichthyosis is hydration and lubrication of skin and prevention of recurrent infection. The defective keratinization can be normalized with help of retinoids. Long-term therapy is required; hence an effective but least toxic therapeutic regimen should be opted for.

Patients should be bathed daily with repeated application of bland emollients like white petrolatum or liquid paraffin. Use of soaps containing antibacterial agents may help in preventing colonization by microorganisms. In patients with EHK, avoidance of mechanical trauma is important, which may precipitate fresh bulla formation.

Soft, non-occlusive clothes and shoes are preferable for these children. Existing erosions should be covered with paraffin soaked protective dressing. Protein-rich diet and oral fluid supplementation should be provided for neonates and children with erythroderma. Physical activities should be restricted in summer months to prevent heat intolerance in children with secondary hypohidrosis.

Ointments containing keratolytic agents like salicylic acid, lactic acid and urea are effective in reducing the scale. However, these should not be used over extensive areas in infants and small children because of risk of toxicity due to percutaneous absorption. Topical tretinoin, tazarotene and vitamin D3 derivatives can be used for exposed body parts. Systemic retinoids are very effective in this group of disorders except in EHK, where it may enhance skin fragility **(Figures 3.13A and B)**. Treatment with etretinate or acitretin is usually started at a lower dose with gradual building up of a minimum effective dosage. Patients should be monitored carefully for side-effects related to use of systemic retinoids for prolonged period.

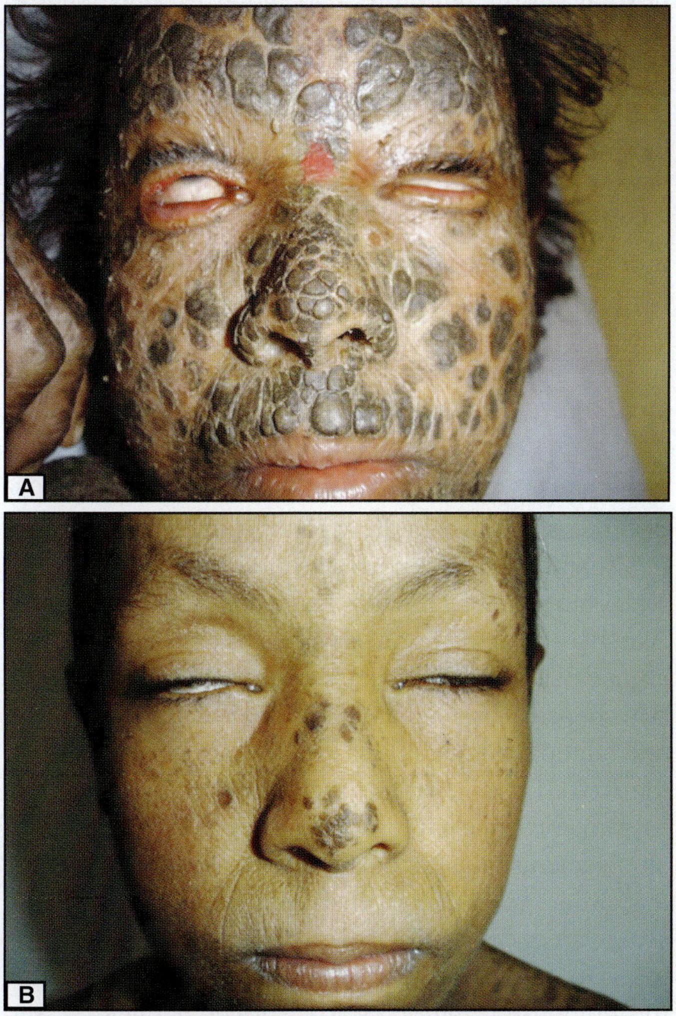

FIGURES 3.13A AND B: Lamellar ichthyosis before and after treatment with systemic retinoids

Patients with Harlequin ichthyosis, extensive EHK and collodion babies are to be managed in dermatology intensive care units with barrier nursing. Warm, humidified environment is maintained. Cleansing with lukewarm water, application of bland emollients, nasogastric feeding and maintenance of fluid and electrolytes are the key factors to be monitored. Patients should be monitored for development of sepsis and antibiotics are to be used when necessary. Use of ophthalmic lubricants, regular cleansing of nasal and oral cavity and release of constricting bands are necessary to prevent complications.

The disfigurement resulting from ichthyosis, especially in severe forms, causes severe psychological impairment. Counseling of the parents and school teachers is mandatory to ensure an improved social interaction for these children. Members of the affected family should be encouraged to undergo prenatal diagnosis.

ICHTHYOSIFORM SYNDROMES

Sjögren-Larsson Syndrome

Sjögren-Larsson syndrome (SLS) is an autosomal recessive disorder characterized by the clinical triad of congenital ichthyosis, neurological impairment and mental retardation. Mutation of the ALDH3A2 gene located on chromosome 17p11.2 results this condition. This gene encodes fatty aldehyde dehydrogenase (FALDH), which catalyzes oxidation of medium and long chain fatty aldehyde to fatty acids. Abnormal lipid accumulation in skin and brain, results in cutaneous and neurological symptoms.

The ichthyosis is present at birth which may rarely present as collodion baby. Scales are variable, ranging from fine white to large, plate-like **(Figure 3.14)**. Associated pruritus is a distinct feature in this type of ichthyosis. Neurological manifestations appear by 2–3 years of age as progressive, spastic, di- or tetraplegia accompanied by speech deficits and mental retardation. A pathognomonic feature in SLS is perifoveal glistening white dots in the retina.

Diagnosis is possible by measurement of fatty aldehyde dehydrogenase in cultured fibroblasts from skin biopsies. PCR assay helps in identifying the mutations. Prenatal diagnosis is also possible by using these techniques.

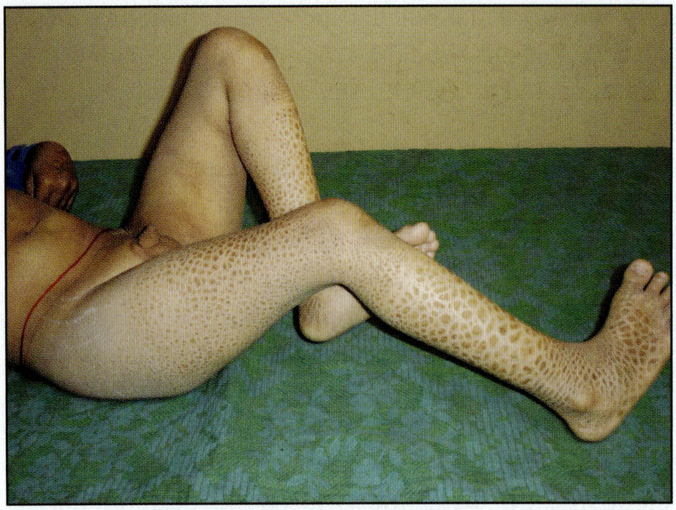

FIGURE 3.14: Sjögren-Larsson syndrome

Patients with SLS need multispecialty approach involving dermatologist, neurologist, ophthalmologist and physiotherapist. Enthusiastic physiotherapy improves the mobility of affected patients and thus reduces morbidity. Gene therapy is a potential future treatment option for these patients. Delivery of human FALDH into keratinocytes of SLS patients using recombinant adeno-associated virus-2 vectors results in augmentation of FALDH activity.

Chanarin-Dorfman Syndrome

It is a rare, autosomal recessive, neutral lipid storage disease with ichthyosis. There is accumulation of triglycerides in all tissues. Generalized ichthyosis is present at birth. Other clinical features are sensorineural deafness, cataract, myopathy, hepatosplenomegaly and growth retardation. The diagnostic feature is numerous lipid-vacuoles in the circulating granulocytes and monocytes demonstrable in freshly prepared peripheral blood smear. Special staining of fresh, frozen skin biopsy specimen shows cytoplasmic lipid droplets in various cells of dermis and epidermis. There is mutation of CGI-58 gene on chromosome 3p21.

Prognosis of the disorder depends on extent of hepatic involvement. Systemic retinoid therapy is helpful in ichthyosis.

Refsum Disease

It is an AR, neurocutaneous disorder, clinically characterized by cerebellar ataxia, peripheral polyneuropathy, atypical retinitis pigmentosa and ichthyosis. Neurological and visual impairments start insidiously during childhood. The ichthyosis is adult-onset, mild, with small, white scales, simulating ichthyosis vulgaris. Other organ involvements may also occur. The disease runs a progressive course with periods of exacerbation and remission.

There is deficiency of peroxisomal enzyme phytanoyl CoA hydroxylase; hence the affected patients are unable to degrade phytanic acid, derived from dietary chlorophyll. This metabolic defect leads to accumulation of excessive phytanic acid in tissues and body fluids. Two genes, PHYH (PAHX) located on chromosome10p, and PEX7, have been identified to be responsible for Refsum disease.

Histopathological examination of skin reveals lipid containing vacuoles in basal keratinocytes. Liquid gas chromatography of plasma reveals very high levels of phytanic acid. Severely diminished phytanic acid oxidase activity is demonstrable in cultured fibroblasts. Heterozygous carriers also show low enzyme activity, but normal serum phytanic acid level. Protein level in cerebrospinal fluid is elevated in affected individuals.

Prenatal diagnosis is possible by assessing phytanic acid oxidation in cell-culture done from chorionic villus biopsy or amniocentesis.

Restriction of dietary phytanic acid (<5mg/day) is advised which prevents acute exacerbations of the disease and arrest organ involvements, especially damage of peripheral nerves. This may be combined with plasma exchange during acute episodes.

Conradi-Hünermann-Happle Syndrome

This is a rare X-linked-dominant, multisystem disorder, affecting skin, bone and eye. The other name for this disorder is X-L-D chondrodysplasia punctata.

Usually the child is born with erythroderma. Often the scales are arranged in swirls and whorls along the lines of Blaschko. Scaling improves within the first few months of life and persists as mild ichthyosis on the extremities. Other skin changes observed are follicular atrophoderma, hyper and hypopigmentation and localized scarring alopecia of the scalp. Other characteristic feature of the disorder is asymmetrical skeletal and ocular involvement. Skeletal involvements may not be apparent at birth but manifests thereafter. Limb-length discrepancies, severe kypho-scoliosis, congenital dislocation of hip and facial dysplasia are seen. Radiologically, there is punctate calcification of the epiphyseal region of long bones. Unilateral and sectorial cataracts are typical ophthalmic signs.

CHILD Syndrome

It is an acronym for congenital *h*emidysplasia, *i*chthyosiform nevus and *l*imb *d*efects. It is usually present at birth. The inheritance is probably X-linked dominant with exclusively female phenotype and lethality in male embryos. The characteristic feature is the strictly unilateral inflammatory nevus with overlying yellowish, waxy scales. In some cases it may follow Blaschko's lines.

The ichthyosis is limited to one half of the body and there is ipsilateral hypoplasia or aplasia of the bony structures and the viscera. Epiphysial stippling is the characteristic radiological feature seen in early infancy. The majority of the reported cases are females, suggesting an X-linked dominant gene, lethal in hemizygous males.

KID Syndrome

It is a very rare syndrome comprising of the clinical triad of *k*eratitis, *i*chthyosis and *d*eafness. Majority of the cases are sporadic, but both AD and AR mode of inheritance have been reported. This disorder is considered as a type of ectodermal dysplasia by some authors. Mutation in the connexin gene may be involved in the pathogenesis of this condition.

At or soon after birth, there may be a transient erythroderma. Later, well-defined, fixed, hyperkeratotic plaques develop on erythematous base, especially on elbow, knee, palms and soles and sometimes on face. There may be a generalized, rippled hyperkeratosis with palmoplantar keratoderma. Diffuse, scarring alopecia is almost always present. Leukonychia and nail dystrophy may be seen. There is high incidence of squamous cell carcinoma in these patients.

Extracutaneous manifestations include congenital, bilateral, sensorineural deafness and progressive photophobia resulting from keratitis. Ocular involvement progresses to result in corneal vascularization and blindness.

Netherton Syndrome

Netherton syndrome is a rare AR disorder characterized by ichthyosis, hair shaft disorder and atopy. The patients may present with congenital or neonatal erythroderma. Later, some patients develop erythematous, polycyclic skin lesions with double-edged scaling, which may resemble skin lesions of atopic dermatitis. These skin lesions are classically known as ichthyosis linearis circumflexa. The classical hair abnormality seen in these patients is trichorrhexis invaginata (bamboo hair), which may appear later in childhood.

Less commonly, trichorrhexis nodosa or helical hairs may be present. Asthma, elevated serum IgE level, recurrent sino-pulmonary infections and bacterial and viral skin infections may be associated. Malnutrition and growth retardation are common in these children. The patients are prone to develop multiple skin cancers and vulval carcinoma.

There is impaired permeability barrier due to altered lamellar body membrane. Mutation in SPINK5 (chromosome 5q 32) is involved in the pathogenesis of Netherton syndrome as well as atopy. Though scanning electron microscopy gives a clearer picture, light microscopic examination of scalp or eyebrow hair can be done for easy diagnosis of trichorrhexis nodosa. Hydration and repeated use of moisturizers are helpful to restore barrier function of skin. Low dose systemic retinoids or phototherapy is helpful in some cases.

IBIDS Syndrome

Some cases of IBIDS syndrome are associated with lamellar ichthyosis, and in such cases the term IBIDS syndrome is used; the first letter 'I' stands for ichthyosis. IBIDS syndrome has been further subdivided; some cases associated with photosensitivity and a defect in UV-induced DNA repair is grouped into the PIBIDS syndrome, the letter 'P' denoting photosensitivity.

Acquired Ichthyosis

Common causes of acquired ichthyosis in children are malnutrition, leprosy, in endemic countries like India and malignancy like Hodgkin's lymphoma. Clinically the scaling simulates ichthyosis vulgaris.

ERYTHROKERATODERMA

Erythrokeratoderma is a rare group of disorder characterized by stationary or transient and migratory, erythematous, hyperkeratotic plaques. There are few syndromes included in this disorder. These are transmitted mostly as AD trait. Skin lesions may be precipitated by factors like emotional stress and change in temperature. Hair and nails are normal. There are several rare variants of the disease, like erythrokeratoderma with ataxia, progressive, partially symmetric, erythrokeratoderma with deafness, erythrokeratoderma annularis migrans and ichthyosiform erythroderma with changing pattern of annular erythema.

Erythrokeratoderma Variabilis (Mendes da Costa Syndrome)

Skin lesions of erythrokeratoderma variabilis (EKV) are usually present at birth or early infancy, though occurrence may be delayed till early adult life. AD inheritance is classical, but families with AR transmission have also been reported. There is a defect in gap junction connexin proteins Cx31 and Cx30.3 expressed in the granular layer of epidermis, resulting from mutations in GJB3 and GJB4 genes respectively. There remain some cases without demonstrable connexin mutations, suggesting genetic heterogeneity.

Clinical features are highly variable in a family, even in an individual. Two morphological types of skin lesions may occur. Transient, asymmetrical, bizarre, erythematous patches may be present at birth and change the site and configuration in hours to days. Localized or generalized, well defined, fixed, brownish, hyperkeratotic plaques appear later and distributed mainly on extensor surfaces **(Figures 3.15A and B)**. Skin lesions may be pruritic. EKV tends to improve during puberty and there may be exacerbation during pregnancy.

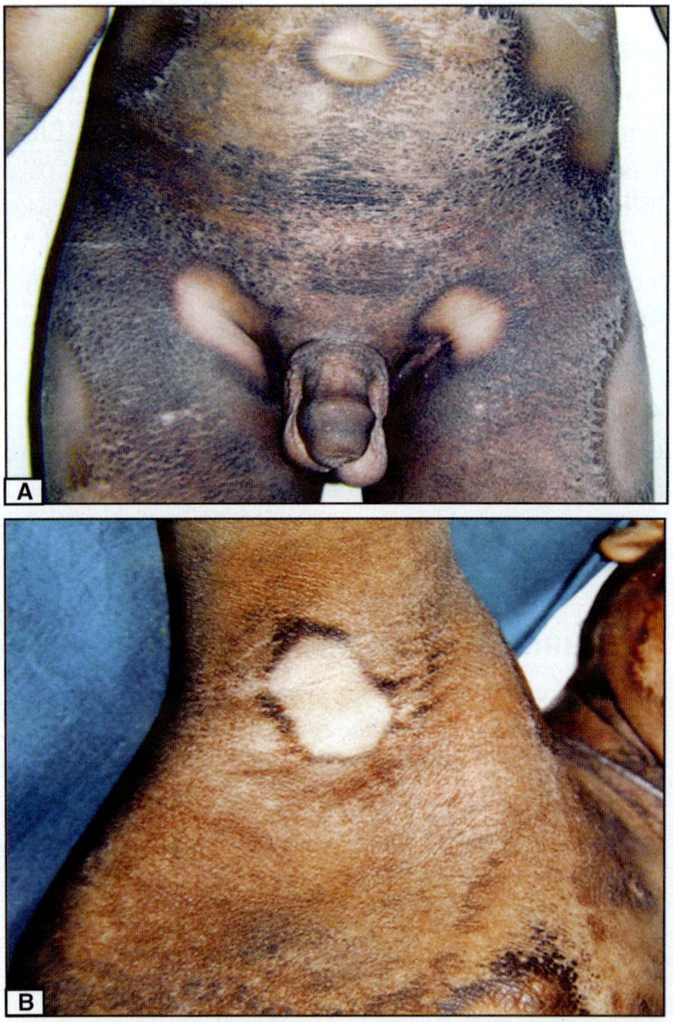

FIGURES 3.15A AND B: Erythrokeratoderma variabilis

Symmetric Progressive Erythrokeratoderma of Darier-Gottron (Gottron's syndrome)

Clinical features appear within first year of life as symmetrical, erythematous, hyperkeratotic plaques on face, extremities and buttocks. These are usually asymptomatic or may be associated with mild itching. The lesions are persistent and gradually progress to involve proximal parts of limbs. Rarely, these may involute at puberty.

Whether progressive symmetric erythrokeratoderma exists as a distinct entity is controversial. Some cases resemble a variant of Vohwinkel syndrome and loricin mutations have been found in them. Other cases have features overlapping with EKV.

Erythrokeratoderma En Cocardes of Degos (Dego's syndrome)

Skin lesions are in the form of large, round, erythematous, concentric plaques resembling targets. The lesions are present at birth and resolute and recur at intervals.

Topical treatment consists of emollients, retinoids and mild keratolytic agents. Topical tazarotene has been used effectively to treat EKV. Systemic retinoids may bring a total clearance of skin lesions as long as the treatment is continued.

PALMOPLANTAR KERATODERMA

Palmoplantar keratoderma (PPK) is a heterogenous group of disorder characterized by hyperkeratosis of the palms and soles. Majority of the disorders in this group are hereditary, some are part of other dermatoses and few are acquired. The pathogenesis in hereditary cases involves various components of the epidermal cells, namely, keratins, cornified envelope components, e.g., loricrin and transglutaminase, desmosome, connexin and cathepsin C, involved in transmembrane signal transduction. A classification of PPK and the salient features have been given in **Table 3.3**.

TABLE 3.3: Classification and salient features of PPK						
Type	**Inheritance pattern**	**Mutation**	**Age of onset**	**Trans gradiens**	**Erythema -tous edge**	**Other features**
Diffuse						
Non-transgradient						
1. Vörner's	AD	K9	Infancy	-	+	HP- epidermolysis
2. Thost-Unna	AD	K1 / K2	Infancy / childhood	-	+	Hyperhidrosis,nail thickening
Transgradient						
1. Camisa Syndrome	AD	Loricrin	Childhood	+	-	Honeycomb pattern, pseudo-ainham of digits, ichthyosis
2. Vohwinkel's syndrome	AD	Connexin 26	Childhood	+	-	Honeycomb pattern, starfish hyperkeratosis, pseudo-ainham
3. Greither's Syndrome	AD	1p, in some cases4q23	Gradual at 8-10 yrs	+	+ / -	Hyperhidrosis + / - very rare, scleroatrophy, severe nail changes, risk of SCC,
4. Huriez Syndrome	AD -	SLURP-1	Childhood	+	-	Hyperhidrosis, maceration, Malodor, digital constriction, nail changes
5. Mal de Meleda	AR	Early	Childhood	+	+	Rare, flexion contracture of digits, periorificial hyperkeratosis, alopecia
6. Olmsted's Syndrome	Sporadic / ?AR		Infancy	+	+	Periodontosis with loss of teeth, recurrent pyogenic infections
7. Papillon-Lefevre syndrome	AR	Cathepsin G	Childhood	+	+	
Focal						
1. Focal PPK with oral leukokeratosis	AD	Keratin 16	-	-	-	Nail changes
2. Striate PPK	AD	18q12.1,	Puberty	-	-	Cardiac disease, wooly hair desmoglein- 1gene, 6p21
3. Punctate PPK	AD		10-45 yrs			Carcinoma colon

Diffuse Palmoplantar Keratoderma

Diffuse PPK may be associated with transgradiens or without this feature. The two major non-transgredient diffuse PPK are Vörner's keratoderma (epidermolytic PPK) and Thost-Unna keratoderma (non-epidermolytic PPK). Both the conditions follow AD pattern of inheritance. The child is normal at birth but palmoplantar involvement is evident by the age of 1 year. There may be history of similar affection in several family members. Vörner's keratoderma is the commonest type of diffuse

PPK. History of blistering or fissuring of palms and soles may be present. Uniform, thick, yellowish hyperkeratosis involving entire palms and soles with sharp erythematous cut-off borders is present in both the conditions. Hyperhidrosis is common in Thost-Unna variant resulting in frequent dermatophyte infections, pitted keratolysis and associated malodor.

Histopathologically, Vörner's keratoderma shows evidence of epidermolysis in suprabasal cells. Electron microscopic examination reveals aggregated tonofilaments. The histopathological features in Thost-Unna keratoderma are non-specific hyperkeratosis and acanthosis.

Diffuse transgradient keratodermas **(Figures 3.16)** are characterized by encroachment of the hyperkeratotic border beyond palms and soles on the dorsal aspects and flexor aspect of wrist. Involvement of elbows, knees and tendo-Achilles may also be seen. Different syndromes in this group have been described below.

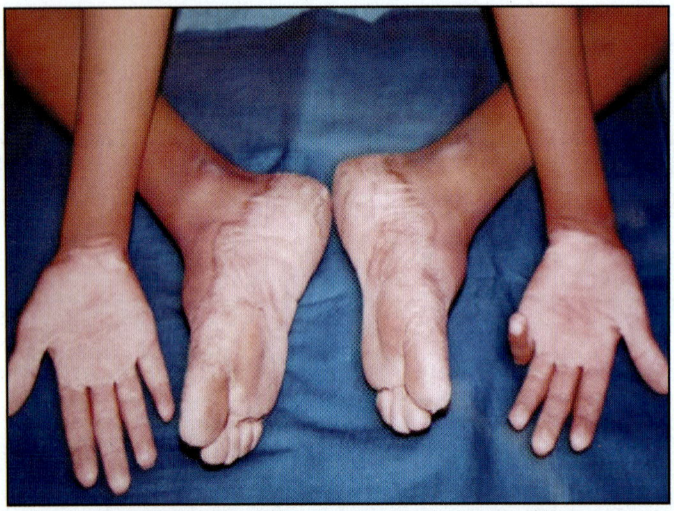

FIGURE 3.16: Diffuse PPK with transgradiens

Greither's Syndrome

Onset of this AD disorder is during infancy. It is progressive thereafter with florid manifestation in late childhood and may improve in adulthood. Histopathology is non-specific with orthohyperkeratosis. An early onset, more severe form with pseudo-ainham formation and auto amputation of digits may occur, known as Sybert's keratoderma.

Vohwinkel's Syndrome (Cicatrizing keratoderma with hearing impairment)

Cutaneous changes of this autosomal dominant disorder include honeycomb-like palmoplantar keratoderma, pseudo-ainham of digits leading to autoamputation and stellate keratoses of the knuckles and other extensor surfaces. The lesions on extensor surfaces are relatively warty with spiky projections showing characteristic 'starfish' appearance. Sensorineural deafness may be associated. It is present since birth, non-progressive and may not be detectable in early life.

Camisa's Syndrome (Loricrin keratoderma/variant Vohwinkel's syndrome)

This PPK is associated with mild ichthyosis which may present as collodion baby at birth. Other features like honeycomb keratoderma, star-shaped hyperkeratosis and pseudo-ainham of digits are similar to the classic disease. Light microscopy reveals thick stratum corneum with retained nuclei. Presence of loricrin in these nuclei is evident by immunno-electron microscopy.

Mal de Meleda (Keratoderma palmoplantaris transgrediens)

This rare autosomal recessive PPK has been named after the Croatian island Meleda from where the first patients were described. There is mutation in the ARS gene, which encodes SLURP-1 (secreted Ly-6/uPAR related protein 1), involved in transmembrane signal transduction. It starts in early childhood as erythema of palms and soles followed by appearance of patchy, wax-like, yellow hyperkeratosis, extending on to extensor surface including malleoli and tendo-Achilles. Hyperhidrosis, malodorous maceration and fungal superinfections are common. Sclerodactyly of the fingers, digital constrictions and nail changes are seen.

Keratoderma with Scleroatrophy (Huriez syndrome)

This is a very rare syndrome, characterized by keratoderma, scleroatrophy of the fingers and a high frequency of squamous cell carcinoma in the affected skin. The condition may be present at birth. The keratoderma is diffuse and dense and dermatoglyphics may be absent. Palms are more severely affected than soles. The skin over distal extremities is atrophic, parchment-like. Nails show hypercurvature, longitudinal ridging, koilonychia and onychorrhexis.

Olmsted Syndrome

This is a very rare, severe form of transgredient PPK. The cases are sporadic or follow autosomal recessive transmission. There is defect in expression of K1 and K10 in the involved epidermis along with persistence of acidic keratins K5 and K 14. Onset is during first year of life. Bilateral mutilating keratoderma and periorificial hyperkeratotic plaques are the hallmark of this disorder.There is well defined, erythematous, diffuse hyperkeratosis of the palms and soles associated with fissuring and flexion deformities of the digits, which may lead to constriction and spontaneous amputation. Other features include generalized alopecia and linear hyperkeratotic papules over the flexor aspects of limbs. Nail and teeth abnormalities, joint laxity and corneal dystrophy have been reported. The condition is slowly progressive and malignant change of involved areas may occur. Occurrence of this rare disorder has been recorded in India.

Papillon Lefevre/Haim-Munk Syndrome

This syndrome includes PPK with progressive periodontosis, transmitted as autosomal recessive trait. This may result from homozygous mutation of the gene encoding lysosomal protease cathepsin C. The disease usually manifests during second or third year of life as transgradient, hyperkeratosis of the palms and soles associated with intense erythema. Soles are more severely affected, with hyperhidrosis and malodor. Hyperkeratotic plaques may be present on Achilles tendon, knees and elbows. Progressive periodontosis and gingivitis result in loss of deciduous as well as permanent teeth by puberty and the patients are edentulous by the age of 15 years. Recurrent pyogenic infections of skin and internal organs are common. Evidence of disturbed immune function is present in these patients in the form of impaired neutrophil phagocytosis. Calcification of the falx cerebri, though inconsistently present, is a characteristic finding.

Haim-Munk syndrome is a variant of this disorder, observed only in some families in the state of Kerala, India. In addition to the above features, these patients have arachnodactyly and atrophic nail changes.

FOCAL PALMOPLANTAR KERATODERMA

Focal PPK are more evident on areas of mechanical trauma, i.e. on soles. Most of this disorders show AD inheritance pattern. While evaluating patients with focal PPK, it should be remembered that any diffuse PPK may present with focal lesions initially.

Watchers Keratoderma (PPK varians)

This variant includes different subtypes with considerable variability. Different patterns of lesions like areate, nummular, linear or striate may occur and coexist. Manifestations start when the child starts walking. Severity depends on exogenous factors like mechanical trauma. This condition is also termed as 'hereditary painful callosities'.

Striate Keratoderma

This appears late during adolescence, as linear keratotic streaks along sides of fingers and palms. Sole lesions may be well-circumscribed and nummular. There may be associated anomalies like sensorineural deafness, mental retardation, spastic paraplegia, pili torti and abnormal teeth.

Punctate Keratoderma

This variant is rare in children and clinically characterized by numerous, discrete, hard, slightly elevated keratotic papules (2-5 mm) on the palms and soles. Lesions on soles may be painful. Some papules may fall out leaving a circular depressed crater, where the lesion reappears. The condition may coexist with other forms of focal keratodermas.

Marginal papular keratoderma (Acrokeratoelastoidosis of Costa)

This condition is characterized by development of small, round, firm, umbilicated papules along the lateral margins of the hands and feet. It usually appears during early childhood and progresses slowly. Histopathology reveals dermal elastorrhexis.

Focal Keratoderma with Oral Leukokeratosis

It is an autosomal dominant condition associated with leukokeratosis of tongue and buccal mucosa. Mild nail changes in the form of splinter hemorrhage and wide onychocorneal band are present. A mutation involving K16 gene has been identified and it is considered as a milder variant of pachyonychia congenita.

PPK in Association with Other Disorders

Diffuse and focal PPK may be part of several other disorders like, epidermolysis bullosa, bullous ichthyosiform erythroderma, hypohidrotic ectodermal dysplasia, Weary-Kindler syndrome, pachyonychia congenita, type II tyrosinemia (Richner-Hanhart syndrome), etc. Though rare in childhood, some commoner diseases like psoriasis, pityriasis rubra pilaris, hyperkeratotic dermatitis, confluent viral warts, (immunocompromised children), Norwegian scabies may present with PPK. Warty arsenic toxicity in older children may be an important cause of PPK in many parts of India.

Complications

In the pediatric age group, any type of PPK may delay the initiation of walking, because of associated discomfort and pain. Painful fissures and callosities may alter the gait of the child. Contracture of fingers may develop because of prolonged lack of use of hands. The odd look and inability to perform daily activities cause great psychological morbidity in school-going children.

Diagnosis

Diagnosis is guided by clinical pattern and mode of inheritance. Light microscopic examination of skin biopsy specimen is usually non-contributory except in Vörner's syndrome, where evidence of suprabasal epidermolysis is present. Ultrastructural and immunohistochemical studies help in diagnosis of some cases with typical findings. In Vörner's syndrome, immunostaining reveals increased expression of cornified envelope proteins like transglutaminase 1, loricrin, involucrin and also filaggrin. In Camisa's syndrome, immunoelectron microscopy reveals abnormal loricrin distribution with sparse labeling of the cornified envelope and strongly labeled intranuclear granules in granular and cornified layers. Genetic mapping is confirmatory in the syndromes with known site of mutation.

Management

Treatment is not required for mild, asymptomatic cases. Most of the parents are familiar with the features as several family members are affected. Severely affected, mutilating cases should primarily be managed with mild keratolytic agents (salicylic acid, lactic acid, urea) and repeated application of emollients. Topical retinoids are helpful in improving focal lesions in some cases. Paring of hyperkeratotic area and sealing of painful plantar fissures help the child resume walking. Oral retinoids, like acitretin and isotretinoin are helpful in severe cases and in preventing ainham formation and autoamputation. However, intermittent therapy is recommended to avoid side effects. All affected children need psychological support to cope up with the stress associated with this group of disorders.

Peeling Skin Syndrome

This is a rare disorder, characterized by continual shedding of the entire stratum corneum in sheets. Two variants of the disorder are recognized, non-inflammatory (type A) and inflammatory (type B). The inflammatory variant shows clinical overlap with Comel-Netherton syndrome. Disease confined only to palms and soles (acral peeling skin syndrome) has been reported. Occasionally, bullous lesions may be seen in these patients. The pathognomonic histopathological feature is cleavage within or below the stratum corneum. This disorder may be associated with hair shaft and nail anomalies, hypogonadism, growth retardation and aminoaciduria.

HEREDITARY DISORDERS OF PIGMENTATION

Hereditary pigmentary disorders include hypo or hyperpigmentation which may be localized or generalized. Systemic involvement is present in almost all of these disorders. In the following section, important disorders in each category will be discussed.

DISORDERS WITH HYPOPIGMENTATION

Piebaldism

It is a rare disorder with AD inheritance pattern. There is mutation of c-kit proto-oncogene on chromosome 4q12 which is pivotal for melanocyte survival. Skin lesions are present at birth as polygonal, depigmented patches on trunk and extremities. White forelock (poliosis) and leukotrichia of mid-portion of eyebrows is common. These lesions are usually static but may increase in size or repigment. Though inconsistently present, a distinctive feature of piebaldism is presence of hyperpigmented macules on the borders of depigmented patches as well as on normal skin. Histopathologially, depigmented skin lesions show reduced number or absence of melanocytes. Waardenburg syndrome show similar cutaneous features but associated with systemic involvement.

Waardenburg Syndrome

Waardenburg syndrome (WS) is a rare AD disorder with variable expressivity. Four clinical types, WS-1,2,3 and 4 have been recognized. There is deranged neural crest differentiation affecting melanocytes in skin and eye, Organ of Corti and stria vascularis in inner ear and facial bones and cartilages. There are mutations in the genes controlling neural crest differentiation, e.g. *Pax3* (WS-1 and 3) and gene encoding MITF transcription factor (WS-2). Mutations in several genes regulating development of neural crest are involved in the genesis of WS-4.

Clinical features are present in the neonatal period. Cutaneous features include white forelock and piebald macules. Dysmorphic facial features include broad root of the nose, dystopia canthorum and synophrys. Unilateral or bilateral sensorineural deafness is present in 10-40% cases and this may be the presenting feature where cutaneous features are subtle. Ocular manifestations include heterochromia irides (20%) and segmental fundal hypopigmentation.

Patients with WS-2 will have relatively normal look because of absence of dystopia canthorum. However, deafness is commoner in this type. WS-3 is also known as Klein syndrome and has associated musculoskeletal anomalies involving shoulder girdle. WS-4 (Shah-WS), is associated with megacolon, resulting from agangliosis of distal bowel and vaginal agenesis.

Diagnosis is evident from typical facies, cutaneous features and deafness. Premature graying of scalp, eyebrow and eyelash hairs may occur in early adult life. Hearing aids should be provided early to improve the auditory handicap.

Oculocutaneous Albinism

Oculocutaneous albinism (OCA) is an inborn error of metabolism involving the enzyme tyrosinase in the melanogenic pathway. The mode of transmission is AR. Hypopigmentation of skin, hair and eyes is characteristic of this disorder. There are various types of the disease with varying severity. Earlier classification system was based on tyrosinase activity (negative/positive). The salient features of different types of OCA have been presented in **Table 3.4**.

OCA can occur in all ethnic population and among both white and dark individuals. The commonest type observed is OCA2, particularly among non-Caucasians. The most severe form of the disease is OCA1A, with absolute absence of enzyme activity throughout life. Brown albinism is milder than OCA1 and OCA2.

Histopathological and ultrastructural studies reveal normal structure and count of melanocytes. However, there is failure of maturation of melanosomes and significant reduction of melanin content. In rufous albinism, melanocytes contain eumelanosomes and pheomelanosomes at various stages of maturation. Estimation of tyrosinase activity in hairbulbs of affected individuals is diagnostic.

The patients with OCA1A are at significant risk for development of UV light-induced cutaneous malignancies **(Figure 3.17)**. Such risks are lower in other variants. There is no definitive treatment for this group of disorders. Stringent photoprotection and protective eyewear is mandatory for management of these patients.

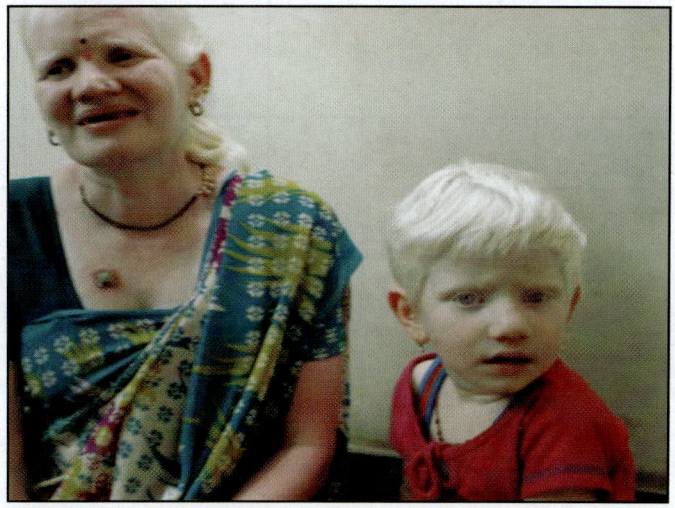

FIGURE 3.17: Tyrosinase negative oculocutaneous albinism (mother & child); mother having a squamous cell carcinoma on chest

Hermansky-Pudlak Syndrome

It is a multisystem, AR disorder, characterized by tyrosinase positive OCA, bleeding diathesis and accumulation of ceroid-like substance in the reticuloendothelial system. There is mutation in the HPS1 gene which encodes a protein involved in trafficking of proteins to lysosome and melanosome.

The cutaneous manifestations are greatly variable; some patients are severely affected as in OCA1, others show a pale tan and straw-colored hair. Photoexposed areas may show freckles and lentigines. Ocular findings include iris translucency, spotty or absent retinal pigmentation, photophobia, nystagmus and decreased visual acuity. Platelet aggregation defect results from absence of platelet-dense granules, resulting in a life-long bleeding diathesis. This may range from bruising, epistaxis and menorrhagia

TABLE 3.4: Salient features of different OCA

Type	Chromosome locus and mutation	Tyrosinase activity and pigment	Presentation at birth	Ocular feature	Skin	Hair
OCA1	11q14-21, gene encoding tyrosinase					
OCA1A		Tyrosinase-negative, Complete lack of pigment	Complete absence of Pigment.	Gray-blue irides, red reflex, foveal hypoplasia, Photophobia	White	White
OCA1B	Same as OCA1, milder mutation	Residual enzyme activity	Skin, hair white at birth	Less severe than OCA1A	Yellowish later	Yellowish red later.
OCA1TS		↓ enzyme activity at 35-37°C.			Normal pigmentation on cooler parts, head and limbs; rest body parts depigmented.	
Platinum OCA			Same as OCA1	Metallic tinge develop later		Metallic tinge develop later
OCA1 MP			Same as OCA1	Pigment develops later	Depigmented	
OCA2	15q11-12, P gene (pinkeyed-dilution) mutation	Tyrosinase positive	Some pigment at birth	Less severe than OCA1A	Pigment ↓ with age, multiple lentigines on photoexposed parts	Yellow to light brown
Brown albinism	P gene mutation			Blue-green to brown irides, ↓ retinal pigment, nystagmus	Cream to light tan, multiple lentigines on photoexposed parts	Beige to light brown
Rufous albinism	TYRP1 mutation			Mild. Reddish brown to brown eye, fundal pigment, nystagmus, photophobia, ↓ visual acuity	Reddish brown skin pigmented nevi & freckles	Mahogony red/deep red

in adult females to life-threatening hemorrhage. Other organ involvements include interstitial pulmonary disease, granulomatous colitis, cardiomyopathy and renal failure. Recurrent pyogenic infections and lupus erythematosus may be associated.

Hair-bulb tyrosinase activity is present. Bleeding time is prolonged but platelet count and all other coagulation parameters are normal. Histopathological examination of skin reveals incomplete and immature melanosomes and occasional macromelanosomes. However, the melanosome number remains normal. Biopsy from the involved viscera shows ceroid-like deposits in histiocytes.

Photoprotection, management of episodes of bleeding and avoidance of factors which may potentiate such hemorrhage are the mainstay of care for these patients. Premature death is caused by pulmonary infections and should be treated aggressively.

Other disorders with diffuse hypopigmentation, Chédiak Higashi syndrome and Griscelli syndrome will be discussed in other section.

DISORDERS WITH HYPERPIGMENTATION

Leopard Syndrome

This is a AD disorder with high penetrance, also known as 'multiple lentigines syndrome.' LEOPARD is acronym for *L*entigines, *E*CG abnormalities, *O*cular hypertelorism, *P*ulmonary stenosis, *A*bnormalities of genitalia, *R*etardation of growth and *D*eafness.

Lentigines are present at birth and increase to numerous in number by puberty. Common sites of distribution are face, neck and upper trunk. Multiple Café au lait spots are present. Cardiac anomalies include conduction defects, pulmonary or subaortic stenosis. Genital abnormalities include gonadal hypoplasia, cryptorchidism and hypospadias. Affected children have short stature, delayed puberty and a typical facies with hypertelorism and prognathism. Sensorineural deafness is profound and may appear late.

Skin biopsy from lentigines show increased melanocytes and giant Melanosomes. ECG abnormalities are the hallmark of this disorder. Care should be taken for deafness and cardiac anomalies.

Carney Complex

The disorders under this condition are NAME syndrome (Nevi, Atrial myxoma, Myxoid neurofibroma, Ephelids) and LAMB syndrome (Lentigines, Atrial myxoma, Mucocutaneous myxoma and Blue nevi). Currently these are considered to be the same entity and termed as Carney complex. Additional features include endocrine overactivity and hyperplasia or neoplasia of various endocrine glands.

HEREDITARY DISORDERS OF IMMUNE SYSTEM

Many of the congenital immunodeficiency disorders present with mucocutaneous manifestations. Recognizing the underlying immunodeficient state is important in these cases to take prophylactic and preventive care. In the following section, congenital immunodeficiency disorders of dermatological importance will be discussed.

ATAXIA TELANGIECTASIA

Ataxia telangiectasia (AT) is an AR disorder characterized by progressive ataxia, oculo-muco-cutaneous telangiectasia, selective immunodeficiency and chromosomal instability. There are several mutations involving the 'ataxia-telangiectasia mutated' (ATM) gene which encodes a protein acting as early sensor of DNA damage. Translocations of T cell receptor genes on chromosome 14q11, 7q14 and 7q35 make these patients prone to develop lymphoreticular malignancies.

The presenting feature is cerebellar ataxia, which manifests as the child learns walking. Dysarthric speech, myoclonic jerks, choreoathetosis may be observed in older children. The telangiectasias appear on bulbar conjunctiva by 3 to 6 years of age **(Figure 3.18A)**. Subsequently, mucocutaneous telangiectasias start appearing mainly on ear **(Figure 3.18B)**, eyelids, malar

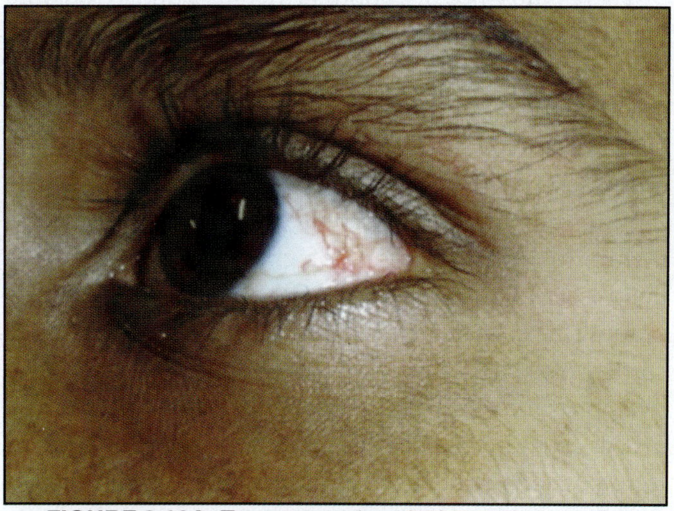

FIGURE 3.18A: Tortuous conjunctival vessels in ataxia telangiectasia

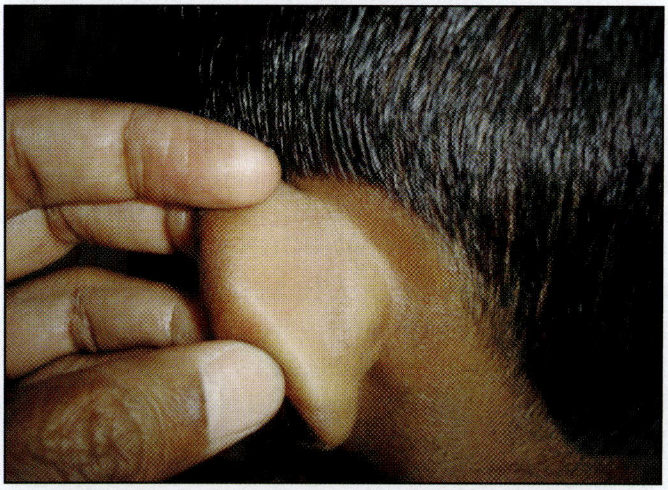

FIGURE 3.18B: Telangiectatic blood vessels (ataxia telangiectasia)

areas, neck, popliteal and cubital fossae and palate. Accentuation of these lesions may occur following sun-exposure. In 90% of the affected children, loss of subcutaneous fat, atrophic and sclerotic skin and premature graying of hair gives rise to a senile look. By the initial years of second decade, the patients are wheel-chair bound with a mask-like facies.

Recurrent sino-pulmonary infections occur in more than 80% cases and are the leading cause of death. Psychomotor retardation and endocrine abnormalities are seen. If the patients survive till teen age, there are increased risks of leukemia (70%), lymphoma (200%) and carcinomas (40%). Unaffected family members and heterozygous carriers are at increased risk of developing malignancy, especially breast cancer.

There is deficiency of IgA (70%) and variable abnormalities of IgE, IgM and IgG.

There is absence or abnormal thymus gland in majority of the patients and increased T-suppressor and decreased T-helper cells.

Cytogenetic study reveals spontaneously occurring chromosomal anomalies like fragmentation, breaks and gaps, observed in cultured fibroblasts and lymphocytes 2-18 times more frequently, suggestive of chromosomal instability. Development of chromosome break in fibroblasts following sun exposure and ionizing radiation are indicator of defective repair process. Heterozygous carriers also show such anomalies.

Approximately 10% of phytohemagglutinin-stimulated T cells in these patients demonstrate the above stated translocations, which are predictors of lymphoreticular malignancies seen in these patients.

There is no specific therapy for AT. Avoidance of sun exposure and use of sunscreen is recommended. Early institution of physiotherapy helps in preventing contracture of extremities. Patients have short life span up to late childhood or early teenage. Commonest causes of death are respiratory tract infections and malignancy.

CHRONIC MUCOCUTANEOUS CANDIDIASIS

Chronic mucocutaneous candidiasis (CMC) is characterized by recurrent and progressive infection of skin, hair and nail most commonly caused by *Candida albicans*. Deficiency of T cell in these patients prevent effective handling of infection by *Candida sp.*This disorder show AR inheritance pattern in familial cases, others are sporadic.

Cutaneous features are variable. There may be recurrent, therapy-resistant orogenital candidiasis and dystrophic nails to severe, generalized, granulomatous lesions. Intertriginous, periorificial and scalp lesions are common. Acute paronychia is common and in long-term, nails are brittle, dysrtrophic and scarring alopecia are present. Mucosal infection is commonest in the oral cavity, but any other mucosa may get involved. Cutaneous dermatophytic and pyogenic infections are common but there is no tendency to develop systemic candidiasis.There is several subgroups of the disorder as described below.

1. Familial CMC: Oral candidiasis is evident by 2 years of age, skin and nail infections are less common.
2. Chronic localized candidiasis (candidal granuloma): This type manifests by 5 years of age as localized, thick, adherent crust on face and scalp. There is associated oral candidiasis.
3. Autoimmune polyendocrinopathy-candidiasis-ectodermal dysplasia (APECED): Candidal infections start by 5 years and consist mostly of granulomatous lesions on face and scalp. Endocrinological manifestations start around teenage; most commonly hypoparathyroidism (88%), followed by hypoadrenocorticism (60%). Several other endocrinopathies and autoimmune disorders may be associated. Patients may also demonstrate autoantibodies like rheumatoid factor, antithyroglobulin, antimelanocyte, and antimicrosomal antibodies.
4. CMC with keratitis: Patients develop photophobia due to keratitis by 2 years and oral and vaginal candidiasis by 5 years of age. The mode of inheritance may be AD in some families.
5. Late-onset CMC: Candidal infections start late by 10 years or early teenage. Clinical features are milder.
6. CMC associated with other immunological disorder: CMC may be associated with severe combined immunodeficiency, DiGeorge syndrome and hyper IgE syndrome.
7. CMC associated with other non-immunological disorder: KID syndrome, multiple carboxylase deficiency, acrodermatitis enteropathica and EEC syndrome may be associated with CMC.

Candida is demonstrable by scraping and culture from the skin and mucosal lesions.

There is impaired candida-specific cell mediated immunity in the affected individuals. Abnormalities noted against candida antigens are lack of response in skin tests, reduced lymphocyte blastogenic transformation response, and abnormal lymphokine production. In addition, presence of serum inhibition factors that alter the response to candida, impaired chemotaxis, phagocytosis and intracellular killing, depressed IgA and complement function have been noted. However, about one quarter of patients with CMC do not have any demonstrable immunological defect.

Repeated systemic antifungal therapy with fluconazole or itraconazole is necessary. Patients should be evaluated for endocrine dysfunction.

CHÉDIAC HIGASHI SYNDROME

Chédiak Higashi syndrome (CHS) is a rare AR disorder characterized by pigmentary dilution, photophobia and severe recurrent infections. There is mutation of lysosomal trafficking regulator gene LYST resulting in defective secretory processes of lysosome and melanosomes. There are giant granules in leukocytes, melanocytes, hair, renal tubular epithelium, neurons of CNS and many other tissues which are incapable of discharging their enzyme content into phagocytic vacuoles. The immunological defect in CHS includes impaired chemotaxis of leukocytes and reduced function of suppressor T cells and NK cells.

The patients present with light colored skin, hair and iris. The hairs may have a silvery sheen. Loss of pigmentation of iris result in increased red reflex and photophobia. Neurological involvement include abnormal gait, paresthesia, peripheral and cranial neuropathy, nystagmus. Recurrent infections of skin and respiratory tract are frequent, caused by common pyogenic organisms.

An accelerated, lymphoma-like phase of the disease can occur in 85% of patients with lympho-histiocytic infiltration of viscera, resulting in organomegaly, lymphadenopathy, pancytopenia, jaundice and varied neurological symptoms. Associated immunodeficiency and Epstein-Barr virus infection may contribute to the occurrence of this phase.

Management of CHS is mainly supportive, by prompt treatment of infections. In the accelerated phase combination therapy with vincristine, cyclosporin A and prednisolone is required. Bone marrow transplantation improves the immunodeficiency but features of pigment dilution persist. Mean life span of affected children is 6 years. CHS has to be differentiated from other two silvery hair syndromes, Griscelli and Elejalde syndrome.

COMPLEMENT DEFICIENCY DISORDERS

Complement deficiency disorders are rare. Most are inherited as AR trait. This group of disorders present with features of autoimmune disorders or recurrent infections. Deficiency of the early components of classical pathway, i.e., C1, C4 and C2 present with SLE-like symptoms in childhood. Patients with deficiency of alternate and terminal pathway components develop recurrent infections with meningococci and other pyogenic organisms. Many children with complement deficiency may remain normal.

C2 Deficiency

C2 deficiency is the commonest of this group of disorders encountered in clinical practice. Two types are known; type 1, resulting from gene translation and type 2, resulting from defective secretion. SLE-like clinical picture is more common (60%) in homozygous female children. Clinical features of other disorders which may be associated are juvenile rheumatoid arthritis (heterozygous girls), dermatomyositis, Henoch-Schönlein purpura, Hodgkin's disease, inflammatory bowel disease, etc.

The classical cutaneous feature of C2 deficiency is a photosensitive, papulosquamous rash, simulating SCLE or DLE or malar erythema. Arthritis is associated in 80% cases. Fever, leucopenia and oral ulcers are present in 50% cases. Less frequently, any other systemic involvement similar to SLE may be present in these cases. Patients are susceptible to recurrent pulmonary infections by pneumococcus and other capsulated bacteria.

Anti-Ro antibody is present in 75% patients and it is the commonest laboratory finding. Antinuclear and anti-DNA antibodies are present in low titer or absent. The cutaneous lesions are difficult to control. Photoprotection, use of sunscreens, topical and systemic steroids and chloroquin as and when necessary are the mainstay of management.

Important dermatological manifestations of other complement deficiency include Leiner's disease (seborrheic dermatitis and diarrhea) in patients with C3 deficiency and C5 dysfunction. Cephalothoracic lipodystrophy may be present in C3 deficient patients. Patients with deficiency of membrane attack complex (C5-C9) develop recurrent infections by pneumococci since childhood and by gonococci and meningococci, starting around puberty. Patients with C7 deficiency may have features of CREST syndrome.

Reduced or deficient CH50 is a marker for complement deficiency disorders. Individual deficiency of complements can be assessed by radioimmunodiffusion assay. Early use of antibiotics is essential for patients with infections. Fresh plasma transfusion may replenish the deficient complements but carry the risk of immune complex deposition by activation of C3 and C5.

'Leiner's disease phenotype' is a condition characterized by infantile-onset severe seborrheic dermatitis, diarrhea, failure to thrive and recurrent Gram-negative bacterial and candidal infections. The condition is familial with probable AD inheritance pattern. There is defective yeast opsonization due to C5 dysfunction. However, this phenotype may be observed in other immunodeficiency disorders like severe combined immunodeficiency, hypogammaglobulinemia and hyper IgE syndrome.

CHRONIC GRANULOMATOUS DISEASE OF CHILDHOOD

Chronic granulomatous disease (CGD) encompasses a group of disorders characterized by abnormal phagocytosis of leukocytes resulting in recurrent, severe infections.

These disorders are rare, mostly affecting males (90%). Genetic transmission is X-linked in majority of the cases, rest follow AR pattern. There is impaired function of the enzyme NADPH oxidase, resulting in defective respiratory burst and inability of the leucocytes to generate oxidative metabolites to kill intracellular organisms.

Cutaneous manifestations may be present at birth as periocular and perioral abscesses. These are recurrent and gradually extensive lesions with regional lymphadenopathy develops. The main causative organism is *S. aureus*. Others are Gram negative bacteria like *Pseudomonas, Klebsiella, E.coli* and fungi like *Aspergillus, Candida* and *Cryptococcus*. Nodular and necrotic granulomatous lesions develop at the areas of infection. Other features include seborrheic dermatitis, aphthous-like oral ulcers and occasionally, skin lesions simulating SLE or DLE.

Other organ involvement occurs, commonest being lymph nodes. Suppurative lymphadenitis and abscess involving cervical lymph nodes is frequent, but any other group of lymph nodes may be involved. Bronchopneumonia is very frequent and hepatic abscess, osteomyelitis, recurrent diarrhea may occur. Granulomatous lesions may develop in parenchyma of liver and spleen and mucosa of gastro-intestinal and genitourinary tracts. Intestinal obstruction and malabsorption are the sequelae. These patients are at increased risk of developing non-infectious, inflammatory disorders like inflammatory bowel disease and auto-immune disorders. Severity and complications are more in X-linked forms of CGD.

Screening for CGD is done by nitroblue tetrazolium (NBT) reduction test. Leucocytes from normal individuals are able to reduce NBT during phagocytosis converting it blue from the original yellow color. In patients with CGD this test remains negative, as only 5-10% of the leucocytes retain this property of reducing NBT during phagocytosis. Other more specific tests include ferri-cytochrome C reduction assay and chemiluminescence/fluorescent assays. Tests for leucocyte chemotaxis and phagocytosis remain normal. Early diagnosis and treatment of any infection is crucial for management of these patients. Interferon-α brings clinical improvement in these patients by enhancing oxidant-independent antimicrobial pathway. Leucocyte transfusion may be helpful in overcoming an infectious crisis. Visceral obstruction caused by granulomas may be relieved by short course of systemic steroid. Bone marrow transplantation is helpful.

DIGEORGE SYNDROME

This syndrome is characterized by congenital agenesis of thymus and consequent T cell defect. There is deletion of chromosome 22 (22q11), which may be present in some other disorders. The T cell dysfunction may be milder in some patients (partial DiGeorge syndrome), who may attain adequate antibody response.

Facial dysmorphism result from defective development of third and fourth pharyngeal pouches, characterized by short philtrum, cleft palate, low-set, malformed ears and hypertelorism is present in affected patients. Cutaneous features are non-specific; recurrent mucocutaneous candidiasis and viral infections since neonatal period, and persistent, non-infectious granulomas are usual. Other systemic abnormalities include congenital heart disease (septal defects, anomalous aortic arch and blood vessels), aplastic parathyroid glands giving rise to hypoparathyroidism and neonatal tetany.

Transplantation of thymus gland and HLA identical bone marrow transplantation are treatment options for affected patients.

HYPERIMMUNOGLOBULIN E SYNDROME

Hyper IgE syndrome (HIE) is characterized by severe dermatitis, recurrent cutaneous and sino-pulmonary infections and very high serum level of IgE. The condition is AD with variable expressivity. The affected gene is located in chromosome 4q.

Episodes of infections start within first few months of life. Large abscesses occur in any body part, which may be non-tender (cold abscess), with minimal or no fever at all. Recurrent furuncle, cellulitis, lymphangitis are common, mainly caused by *S. aureus*. Chronic mucocutaneous candidiasis is very frequent. Extremely pruritic and lichenified eczema is present since infancy, which improves by late childhood. Pulmonary involvement includes empyema, bronchiectasis and pneumatoceles with related complications. Typically, patients with HIE have a coarse facies; broad nose with fleshy tip, prominent forehead, enophthalmos and ill-proportioned cheeks and jaw associated with huge facial abscesses. Other features include scoliosis, hyperextensible joints, dental anomalies and susceptibility to repeated fractures due to osteopenia.

Very high level of IgE (>2000 IU/ml in adults, lower in children) is characteristic in these patients. Other immunological parameters are usually normal, though abnormalities of chemotaxis and cell mediated immunity are observed intermittently. Altered response in skin testing by candida and tetanus antigen is seen.

Because of extensive dermatitis, HIE is often misdiagnosed as atopic dermatitis or Wiskott-Aldrich syndrome. Abscesses need prompt drainage and antibiotic therapy. Administration of gammaglobulin decreases IgE level and the severity of dermatitis. Recombinant interferon-α improves leucocyte chemotaxis and prevents recurrent infections.

Job syndrome is considered as a variant of HIE, which is commoner in females. In addition to the usual features this patients will have fair skin, red hair and joint hyperextensibility.

IMMUNOGLOBULIN DEFICIENCY

Selective IgA deficiency is the commonest disorder in this group though clinical features are evident in 10-15% cases. Respiratory tract infections and gastroenteritis caused by *Giardia* are common. Cutaneous manifestations include SLE-like skin lesions, chronic mucocutaneous candidiasis, vitiligo and severe dermatitis.

Selective IgM deficiency is extremely rare. Recurrent bacterial infections, extensive large warts and severe eczema are the clinical features.

X-linked hypogammaglobulinemia with hyper IgM is characterized by recurrent infections, autoimmune disorders like hemolytic anemia and thyroiditis and lympho-reticular system involvement, like hepato-splenomegaly and lymphadenopathy. Mucocutaneous lesions include pyoderma, extensive warts and oral ulcers. There is reduced level of IgA, IgG and IgE and neutropenia. IgM level is increased.

Pan-hypogammaglobulinemia is a rare disorder. Two variants have been reported, infantile-onset X-linked hypogammaglobulinemia and adult-onset common variable immunodeficiency (CVI). Recurrent, multiple pyoderma, eczema and non-infectious granuloma are the usual cutaneous features. Few patients may develop dermatomyositis-like clinical features. There is increased susceptibility to hepatitis B, echovirus enteritis and meningoencephalitis and recurrent respiratory tract infection.

SEVERE COMBINED IMMUNODEFICIENCY (SCID)

SCID is a rare, heterogenous disorder of immunodeficiency. Both AR and X-L-R modes of transmission have been observed. Clinical manifestations start by 6 months of age. Majority of the affected patients (75%) are boys. There is profound deficiency of T lymphocytes and low absolute lymphocyte count. There are different subsets of the disease depending upon presence or absence of B lymphocytes and NK cells.

Presenting features are mucocutaneous candidiasis, recurrent pyogenic infections, viral gastroenteritis and pneumonia. Maculopapular rash, seborrheic dermatitis like picture and cutaneous features like all stages of graft *vs.* host disease may be present. Patients may present with exfoliative dermatitis.

SCID has to be differentiated from other causes of severe immunodeficiency like HIV infection. However, these patients do not demonstrate the virus, anti-HIV antibody and altered CD4: CD8 ratio. Untreated patients of SCID usually die by 1 year of age. Administration of live vaccines and non-irradiated blood products should be prohibited in these patients. Patients should be kept in isolated environment. HLA-identical bone marrow transplant brings remission in 90% patients by reconstitution of T cells.

WISKOTT- ALDRICH SYNDROME

Wiskott-Aldrich syndrome (WAS) is a rare immunodeficiency disorder characterized by recurrent pyogenic infections, platelet dysfunction and deficiency and severe dermatitis. Transmission is X-L-R and males are affected mostly.

Platelet dysfunction is the most consistent finding in these patients manifesting since birth as petechiae and multiple ecchymosis. There may be episodes of epistaxis, hematemesis, melena and hematuria. The dermatitis appears within next few months and clinically indistinguishable from atopic dermatitis. Erythroderma is very common in these patients. Recurrent bacterial infections of skin, otitis media, sinusitis and pneumonia also start during this time. Patients are at risk of developing meningitis and septicemia. Older children are susceptible to develop viral infections also.

Lymphadenopathy, hepatosplenomegaly and arthritis are other manifestations. Lympho-reticular malignancy, particularly non-Hodgkin's lymphoma is common in these patients appearing by second decade. Average life expectancy is 15 years and patients die due to hemorrhage, infections or malignancy.

Persistent thrombocytopenia is a feature, platelet count ranging from 1000 – 80,000/ mm^3. In addition, platelets are small with defective structure and aggregation. Though total serum immunoglobulin level is normal, IgM level is low. Delayed hypersensitivity reactions to skin test antigens are absent. Coomb's positive hemolytic anemia, leucopenia and impaired leucocyte chemotaxis have been reported. The immunodeficiency results from primary T cell abnormality leading to defective cell mediated and humoral immunity.

Appropriate antibiotic and intravenous gammaglobulins are helpful in controlling infections. Platelet transfusions are required before surgical procedures. Bone marrow transplantation is the treatment of choice.

HEREDITARY DISORDERS WITH PHOTOSENSITIVITY

The two major groups of hereditary disorders with photosensitivity are porphyrias and inherited DNA-repair disorders. There are some other genetic disorders which may also present with photosensitivity since early childhood. These include pigmentary disorders like albinism and metabolic disorders like phenylketonuria and Hartnup disease. Clinical manifestations of hereditary disorders usually start during infancy or early childhood. All these conditions are to be differentiated from other acquired and late-onset disorders with photosensitivity in childhood. Thorough clinical and laboratory evaluation is needed for appropriate diagnosis of these patients.

PORPHYRIAS

Porphyrias are a group of disorders arising from specific enzyme deficiency in different steps in the pathway of heme biosynthesis. Absence of a particular enzyme results in accumulation of the precursor metabolite giving rise to specific type of porphyria. The usual cutaneous findings in these disorders are intense photosensitivity, vesiculation and scarring.

The porphyrins are potent photosensitizers by virtue of their property to become activated by visible spectrum of light (400-410nm or above) and emit fluorescence. During this process, there is production of free radicals and singlet oxygen which cause cell death and damage to tissue. The immediate effects are erythema, edema, purpura and skin pain. Delayed effects are skin fragility giving rise to vesiculation followed by scarring.

Classification

The initial classification of porphyrias, proposed by Günther (1911) was based on the clinical features and the type of porphyrin present in blood, urine and feces. Recent classification is based on the organ source of the accumulated porphyrin. **Table 3.5** presents the classification of porphyrias. Porphyrias with predominant

TABLE 3.5: Classification of porphyrias and their inheritance pattern

Type	Inheritance pattern
Erythropoietic porphyrias	
Congenital erythropoietic porphyria (CEP)	AR
Erythropoietic protoporphyria (EPP)	AD
Congenital erythropoietic coproporphyria (ECP)	
Hepatic porphyrias	
Acute intermittent porphyria (AIP)	AD
Variegate porphyria (VP)	AD
Hereditary coproporphyria (HCP)	AD
Porphyria cutanea tarda (PCT)	AD
ALA-dehydrogenase porphyria (ALADP)	AR
Hepatic / Erythropoietic porphyrias	
Hepatoerythropoietic porphyria (HEP)	AD
Harderoporphyria	

TABLE 3.6: Accumulation of precursor porphyrins in various tissues and their excretion in major types of porphyrias

Porphyria	RBCs	Plasma	Urine	Feces
CEP	Uroporphyrin ++, Coproporphyrin, Protoporphyrin	Uroporphyrin ++, Coproporphyrin	Uroporphyrin ++, Coproporphyrin	Uroporphyrin +, Coproporphyrin++
EPP	Protoporphyrin++	Protoporphyrin++ (free form)	—	Protoporphyrin+ / ±
PCT	—	Uroporphyrin +	Uroporphyrin ++, Coproporphyrin	Coproporphyrin +, Isocoproporphyrin ++, Protoporphyrin ±
VP	—	—	Uroporphyrin +, Porphobilinogen ++, In acute attack, Coproporphyrin + Δ-amino levulinic acid	Protoporphyrin++, Coproporphyrin +
HEP	Protoporphyrin++	Uroporphyrin +, Coproporphyrin +	Uroporphyrin ++, Coproporphyrin +, Isocoproporphyrin +	Coproporphyrin +, Isocoproporphyrin ++
HCP	—	Coproporphyrin ± / + (acute attack)	Coproporphyrin ++, Porphobilinogen ++, Δ-aminolevulinic acid + (acute attack)	Coproporphyrin ++
AIP	—	Porphobilinogen ++, Δ-aminolevulinic acid ++	In acute attack, Porphobilinogen ++, Δ-aminolevulinic acid ++	—

dermatological manifestations have been discussed in the following section. **Table 3.6** presents the various precursors accumulated in tissues in different types of porphyrias and the routes through which these are eliminated.

Congenital Erythropoietic Porphyria

Congenital erythropoietic porphyria (CEP, Günther's disease) was the first recognized 'inborn error of metabolism," and the first described porphyria (Schultz, 1874). It is an AR disorder resulting from the mutation of UROS gene located on 10q25.2-26.3, encoding the enzyme uroporphyrinogen III synthase. The disorder is phenotypically heterogeneous resulting from different mutations at this site. Severe clinical manifestations are present in homozygous individuals. Heterozygous individuals have partial deficiency of the enzyme. Some genotypes develop milder disease even in homozygous state.

Pathogenesis: There is deficiency of the enzyme uroporphyrinogen III synthase resulting in accumulation of porphyrins in bone marrow which is distributed to skin resulting in photosensitivity and chronic photodamage. Avid binding of porphyrins to calcium phosphate of dentine gives rise to fluorescent teeth. The porphyrins may have a toxic effect on bone marrow itself and may contribute to hemolytic anemia, which in turn lead to hyperactivity of bone marrow. Effect of accumulated porphyrin as well as compensatory expansion of marrow space may contribute to frequent fracture of bones.

Clinical features: The clinical features start in early infancy or childhood or may be present at birth. Red staining of the diapers is the earliest feature resulting from urinary excretion of porphyrins. Rarely, the disorder starts manifesting in late childhood or adult life.

Cutaneous manifestations of CEP are most severe of all porphyrias. There is intense photosensitivity and the affected children may scream when exposed to sunlight. There is painful vesiculation, scarring and mottled pigmentation of all exposed parts. Vesicles are filled with reddish fluid containing porphyrins. Long term changes include hypertrichosis of the exposed body parts, mutilation of ear lobules, eyelids, nose and hands.

Cicatricial alopecia of scalp and nail changes like pigmentation and onycholysis are seen. The hallmark finding of CEP is erythrodontia, reddish to dirty brown, fluorescent teeth.

There is severe ocular involvement in the form of photophobia and features of ocular photo damage like keratoconjunctivitis, corneal ulceration and scarring, ectropion and cataract. Other systemic involvements include intermittent hemolytic anemia, splenomegaly and severe thrombocytopenia. Bony involvements include osteoporosis, frequent fractures, including compression fracture of vertebrae, acro-osteolysis and soft tissue calcification.

Erythropoietic Protoporphyria

Erythropoietic protoporphyria (EPP) is a milder type of disease showing AD inheritance with variable penetrance. There is mutation of FECH gene located on chromosome 18q21.3, encoding the enzyme ferrochelatase.

Pathogenesis: There is deficiency of the enzyme ferrochelatase resulting in accumulation of excess of free protoporphyrin in RBCs and plasma and excretion of these in bile and feces. Since protoporphyrin is water-insoluble, it is not excreted in urine.

Clinical features: EPP is one of the commonest types of porphyria seen in children. Clinical features start during childhood as intense photosensitivity and the child usually cries inconsolably when exposed to sunlight. Older children complain itching, burning and stinging sensation following sun-exposure. Clinical examination reveals urticarial lesions, vesicles and occasional purpura. Symptoms are aggravated in summer months and spring. In the long run, skin on exposed body parts show evidence of photo-damage. These include shallow, linear and elliptical scars on prominent parts of the face, like forehead, tip of nose **(Figure 3.19A)**, cheeks and chin. The skin on dorsa of the hands shows pebbling and there may be perioral linear furrows **(Figure 3.19B)**. Photo-onycholysis may be present. There is spontaneous improvement of the symptoms during second decade of life.

Systemic involvements include anemia, cholelithiasis and hepatitis. Hepatic involvement is usually mild but there may be hepatic cirrhosis resulting in fulminant hepatic failure, and death. Gallstones, composed of protoporphyrins are common at an early age.

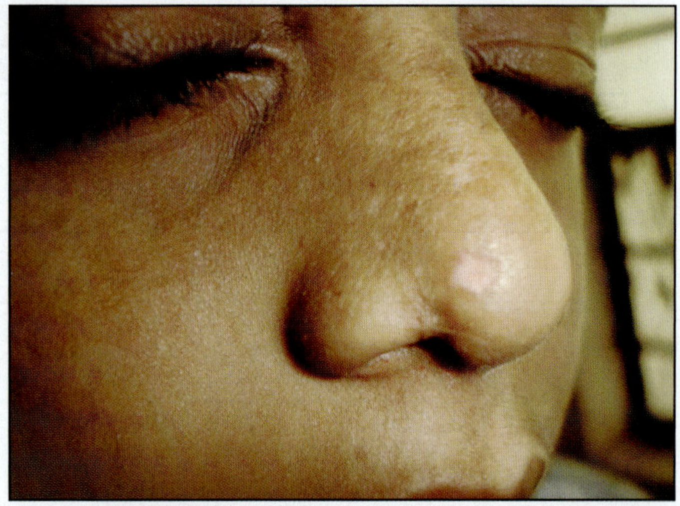

FIGURE 3.19A: Shallow elliptical scar on nose (erythropoietic protoporphyria)

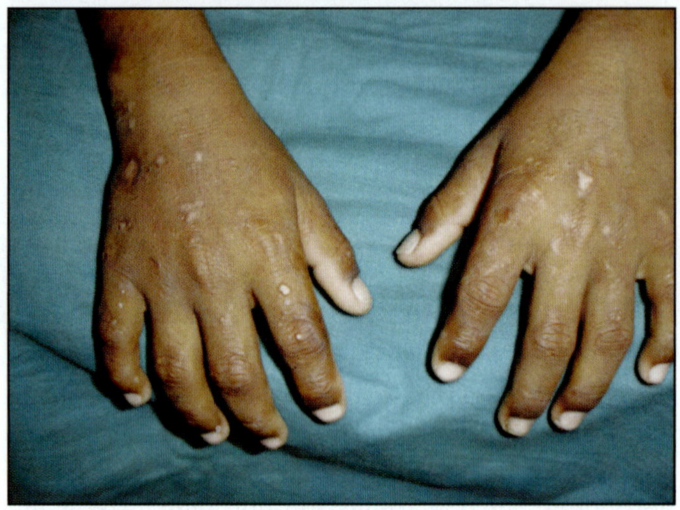

FIGURE 3.19B: Scarring on dorsa of hands (erythropoietic protoporphyria)

Regular monitoring of liver function tests is necessary for these patients.

Erythropoietic Coproporphyria

Erythropoietic coproporphyria is the rarest and only countable cases have been reported to date. The onset is in childhood and clinically it resembles EPP. Increased erythrocyte coproporphyrin and protoporphyrin are seen in these cases. Enzyme inflicted or the genetic defects are not clear.

Porphyria Cutanea Tarda

Porphyria cutanea tarda (PCT) is the commonest type of porphyria. There are two variants of this disorder, sporadic (type I) and familial (types II and III). The familial types show AD inheritance. The affected gene is located at 1p34. The sporadic form is genetically heterogenous and manifests under conditions of hepatic damage by exogenous factors like drugs, alcohol, viral infections or being influenced by endogenous factors like estrogen and iron overload.

Pathogenesis: There is partial deficiency of hepatic uroporphyrinogen decarboxylase in type I PCT. Both hepatic and erythrocyte enzyme activity is decreased in type II and only hepatic enzyme is decreased in type III. There is accumulation of uroporphyrins and coproporphyrins in liver and plasma and increased excretion in urine, and feces.

Clinical features: The sporadic form of the disease manifests in middle age. The familial variant can manifest at any age including in childhood. There is photosensitivity which gets worse during summer months. Vesiculo-bullous lesions along with crusting are seen on photo-exposed parts which heal very slowly. Photo-onycholysis is a feature. Skin fragility is evidenced by erosions resulting from minor trauma. After certain duration, skin becomes atrophic, with mottled pigmentation and scars studded with milia. Facial hypertrichosis is a common finding, especially in females. Pseudosclerodermatous plaques are seen both on exposed and covered body parts but unusual in children.

Degenerative eye changes like pterygium and pinguecula are common. Complications of iron overload are the usual sequelae. These include hepatic siderosis and hepatocellular carcinoma. Incidence of diabetes and lymphoma are increased in these patients.

There may be spontaneous remission with age.

Hepatoerythropoietic Porphyria

It is an extremely rare disorder with a combination of clinical features of CEP and biochemical pictures of PCT. Dark colored urine and extreme photosensitivity is present since birth and there is severe cutaneous photo-damage. Urine and feces contain high levels of uroporphyrin and coproporphyrin. Serum iron level is normal.

Acute Intermittent Porphyria

Acute intermittent porphyria (AIP) is a rare disorder with AD inheritance pattern.

There is deficient activity of porphobilinogen deaminase. Clinical manifestations start during puberty and mainly neuro-visceral; the classical triad includes acute, colicky abdominal pain, neuro-psychiatric symptoms and dark urine. Predominantly motor neuropathy is a feature. Cutaneous features are absent in AIP as the accumulated precursors (Aminolevulinic acid and porphobilinogen) do not possess photosensitizing property.

Variegate Porphyria

Variegate porphyria (VP) is rare with AD inheritance pattern, seen mainly among South African population. There is mutation of the gene PPOX, located on 1q22, encoding the enzyme protoporphyrinogen oxidase. Deficient activity of this enzyme leads to accumulation of protoporphyrin and coproporphyrin in plasma and feces.

VP is rare in pediatric age group. Clinical features start during puberty and are admixtures of AIP and PCT. Acute neuro-visceral symptoms simulating AIP are common in women. Cutaneous manifestations simulating PCT are commoner in men.

Chester Porphyria

This porphyria is named so because of its initial description from a family in Chester, England. It is an acute variant simulating AIP and without photosensitivity. There is deficiency of both porphobilinogen deaminase and protoporphyrinogen oxidase and porphyrin excretion patterns may simulate either AIP or VP or a combination of both.

Hereditary Coproporphyria

Hereditary coproporphyria (HCP) is a rare AD porphyria with combined features of AIP and PCT. Some authors consider it as a variant of VP, but HCP has a world-wide distribution. There is decrease in activity of the enzyme coproporphyrinogen oxidase. The patients present during childhood with photosensitivity, blistering, hypertrichosis and hemolytic anemia. Acute episodes of neuro-visceral symptoms may occur but are less recurrent than AIP.

Investigations in Porphyrias

There are increased precursor porphyrins in the system like blood (erythrocytes/plasma), liver, bone marrow or skin and increased excretion of these in urine and feces. These are demonstrable by Wood's lamp or other lights of specific wave length because of their property of fluorescence.

In CEP, there is accumulation of uroporphyrin I and coproporphyrin I, which are excreted in urine and feces, demonstrable as reddish pink fluorescence under Wood's lamp examination. Peripheral blood RBCs and normoblasts in bone marrow show red fluorescence under fluorescent microscope. The plasma protoporphyrin in EPP is free unlike some other conditions where zinc-bound protoporphyrin is present. Examination of blood smears with a lamp emitting 400nm wavelength light shows transient coral red fluorescence. Demonstration of fecal protoporphyrin is inconsistent and urine does not show any fluorescence in EPP. In PCT, urine shows coral red fluorescence under Wood's lamp examination. Sensitivity of the test can be enhanced by acidification of urine or by adding talc, which adsorbs porphyrins. Increased fecal level of porphyrins is diagnostic of VP but not usually demonstrable before puberty. The plasma fluorescence is demonstrable at light wavelength of 626 nm, specific for VP.

Fluorescence of teeth is demonstrable by Wood's lamp in CEP, PCT and some other types which simulate clinical features of these.

Histopathological examination of skin reveals sub-epidermal bullae and mild dermal infiltrate. There is deposition of PAS positive amorphous material in upper dermis and perivascular area. Immunofluorescence reveals deposition of IgG.

Liver function tests are usually abnormal in EPP and gallstones composed of protoporphyrins are common.

Differential Diagnosis of Porphyria

Porphyrias are to be differentiated from other causes of childhood photosensitivity and disorders with skin fragility. These include inherited DNA repair disorders, metabolic disorders like phenylketonuria and Hartnup disease and epidermolysis bullosa. Moreover, differentiation from other types of porphyrias is important. Milder variants of porphyrias may be mistaken with acquired photodermatoses.

Severely photosensitive child with features of mutilation and pink staining of diapers is quite characteristic of CEP. In mildly affected older children with CEP, EPP may be a differential diagnosis, but demonstration of elevated porphyrins in both urine and RBC rules out the later. Late onset CEP may be mistaken as PCT.

EPP can be clinically differentiated from CEP by absence of vesicles, pigmentary changes, hypertrichosis and mutilation The skin lesions of EPP may be mistaken as polymorphous light eruption, solar urticaria and actinic prurigo. Some conditions like iron deficiency anemia, lead-poisoning and some other forms of porphyrias may show increased level of plasma protoporphyrin, but unlike EPP, these are zinc-bound protoporphyrin.

Epidermolysis bullosa constitute important differential diagnosis for PCT due to presence of skin fragility, vesiculation, scarring and milia formation. However, photosensitivity and hypertrichosis are not present in the former.

In presence of sclerodermoid skin changes present in some porphyrias, localized or generalized morphea and other causes of pseudoscleroderma are to be ruled out

Management of Porphyrias

Management of porphyrias is mostly symptomatic. Absolute photoprotection by physical means (protective clothes, hat, and sunglass) is necessary for these patients. Modification of daily activities (attending night school) adds to the protective measures for the affected children.

Topical sunscreens are not of much help as these patients are sensitive to visible spectrum of sunlight. Opaque physical sunscreens (titanium oxide) may be helpful in some cases of EPP.

Systemic photo protective agents like oral beta carotene in the dosage of 50-200 mg/day gives variable response approximately after 4-12 weeks. Cysteine, in the dosage of 500 mg twice daily offers protection against photosensitivity. In patients with EPP, phototherapy (PUVA, UVB, NB-UVB) provides protection against photosensitivity by hardening and hyperpigmentation of skin.

In presence of severe hemolytic anemia as in CEP, splenectomy is advised. Associated liver disease in EPP can be treated with cholestyramine which reduces hepatic protoporphyrin level and improves photosensitivity. Some other means like blood transfusion, oral iron and bile acids may reduce hepatic protoporphyrin level.

Avoidance of hepatotoxic drugs and preventive measures for viral hepatitis are important measures to manage patients with PCT. Measures which have been used to reduce iron load and excess porphyrins in PCT include phlebotomy, desferioxamine, low-dose chloroquine (3 mg/Kg) or hydroxychloroquine and plasmapheresis.

Bone marrow and liver transplantations provide temporary improvement in CEP and PCT, but there are reports of relapse. Cord blood stem cell transplantation or gene therapies for the affected enzyme are the newer and promising therapeutic modalities for patients with porphyria.

INHERITED DNA-REPAIR DISORDERS AND CHROMOSOME INSTABILITY SYNDROMES

High level of spontaneously occurring chromosomal abnormalities are seen in this group of disorders which is distinct for each entity. Some disorders of dermatological importance has been discussed in the following section. Early-onset photosensitivity and malignancy are the hallmark of these disorders.

Bloom Syndrome (Congenital Telangiectatic Erythema and Stunted Growth)

Bloom syndrome (BS) is a rare disorder characterized by clinical triad of photosensitivity, growth retardation and early malignancies. High rate of sister chromatid exchange (SCE) is a distinct cytogenetic feature. BS is prevalent among Ashkenazi Jews, but has also been reported among many other races, including Indians.

Genetics: There is AR inheritance pattern. The affected gene 'BLM' is located on chromosome 15q 26.1. Clinical manifestation occurs only in homozygous state and heterozygous individuals are asymptomatic carriers. History of parental consanguinity is common. A mosaic form of BS exists (low-SCE), who are born exclusively of unrelated parents.

Pathogenesis: Excessive chromosomal instability and breakage are seen in these patients which predispose them to malignancy. BLM, a member of RecQL gene, is a DNA helicase involved in replication and repair of DNA. Mutated BLM abolish the usual suppressive effect on homologous recombination of chromosomes. In addition, UV resistance power of cells is impaired. This results in photosensitivity. Uncontrolled cell proliferation and premature cell death makes the affected individual prone to malignancy and results in stunted growth.

Clinical features: Photosensitive rash is the earliest feature, developing in infancy or early childhood.

Marked erythema, telangiectasia, vesiculation and crusting are present on sun-exposed skin. Multiple café-au-lait macules may be present mainly over the trunk. Conjunctival telangiectasia may rarely be present.

Severe growth retardation is the hallmark of BS. It starts in the intrauterine life leading to IUGR and low birth weight. After birth, though growth occurs proportionately, the child's stature remains below average these children are markedly smaller than siblings. There is striking resemblance to each other because of a characteristic facies, constituted of dolichocephaly, long, narrow, keel shaped face, sharp nose and low-set ears. IQ is below normal. Patients usually have a shrill voice.

There are recurrent episodes of fatal diarrhea, respiratory tract and ear infections resulting from underlying immunodeficiency. These cause significant morbidity and mortality. Type 2 diabetes mellitus may occur at a young age. Gonadal dysfunction is common in male children. Minor structural anomalies include clinodactyly, syndactyly, congenital heart disease and annular pancreas.

One or several organs develop malignant tumors (risk increased 150 - 300-fold) in BS patients. Leukemia and lymphoma are the commonest among these. Visceral malignancies, involving gastrointestinal tract, lungs, breast, uterus and cervix may be seen at an early age. Average life-span is up to second or third decade.

Diagnosis: Clinical diagnosis of BS is easy in presence of photosensitivity, stunted growth, recurrent episodes of infection and early onset malignancies. Histopathological examination of skin reveals non-specific features like thinned-out epidermis, hydropic degeneration of basal cells and pigmentary incontinence. Absence of immune deposits at the dermo-epidermal junction in direct immunofluorescence study of skin differentiates this condition from SLE.

Cytogenetic study is diagnostic. There is frequent spontaneous chromosomal breakage and 5 to 10-fold increased SCE (50-100/metaphase as compared to < 10 in normal individuals). In some patients with BS, SCE rate is normal. Approximately 1% quadriradial configuration in mutagen induced cultured lymphocytes is characteristic of this disorder. Cytogenetic study of carriers is normal.

Differential diagnosis: Other causes of childhood photosensitivity like Rothmund-Thomson syndrome, Cockayne syndrome, xeroderma pigmentosum, ataxia telangiectasia, erythropoietic protoporphyria and Hartnup disease are to be ruled out.

Management: Photoprotective measures like opaque sunscreen, full-sleeve clothing and wide-brim hat are mandatory for these children. Infections should be treated promptly. Periodic screening should be undertaken for evidence of malignancy.

Xeroderma Pigmentosum

Xeroderma pigmentosum (XP) is characterized by photosensitivity, freckling on skin and eye and early neoplasia. Incidence of XP is highest in Japan. The disorder is heterogenous with seven subtypes (complementation groups A-G) and a variant, XP-V. Commonest subtype worldwide is XP-C. XP-A is seen most frequently among Japanese population. B, E and G subgroups are extremely rare. Occurrence of XP-D and XP-F are intermediate.

Genetics: The inheritance pattern of XP is AR. A form with AD inheritance pattern exists.

Affected children are born of obligate heterozygote carriers without any clinical manifestation. Genetic heterogeneity exists in XP as evidenced by various subgroups. The gene locations of XP are;

- XPA (9q22.3),
- XPB (2q21),
- XPC (3p25),
- XPD (19q13.2-13.3),
- XPE (11p12-p11),
- XPF (16p13.3-13.13),
- XPG (13q33).

Pathogenesis: In normal individuals nucleotide - excision-repair (NER) pathway is engaged in removal and replacement of damaged DNA. This pathway is defective in patients with XP. Hence the cells exposed to UVB are not subjected to the regular repair process. This results in photosensitivity and carcinogenesis in patients with XP.

Clinical features: Skin, eyes and nervous system bear the main impact of the disorder. Growth retardation and short stature are common. Patients are normal at birth; by the age of 6 months to 3 years they develop persistent facial erythema, acute sun-burn, widespread, progressive and permanent freckling on exposed body parts and xerosis. Conjunctiva, lips and covered body parts are gradually involved. The freckles are dark brown and pinpoint to 1 cm in size. In addition, there are numerous atrophic hypopigmented macules and multiple telangiectasia on skin and mucosa giving a mottled appearance of skin **(Figure 3.20)**.

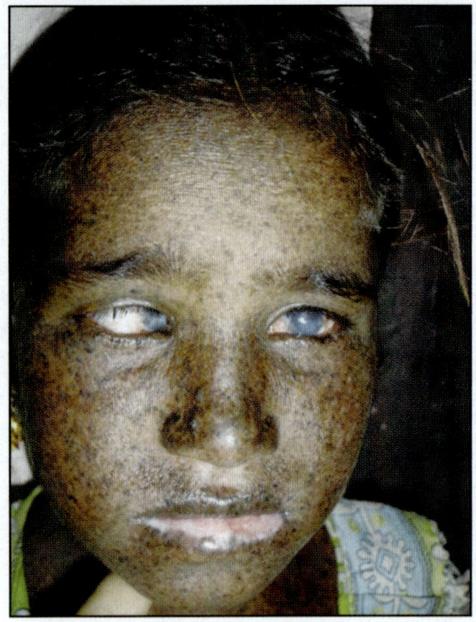

FIGURE 3.20: Xeroderma pigmentosum

Premalignant (e.g. keratoacanthoma, actinic keratoses) and malignant tumors are common in these patients. Multiple, pigmented basal cell carcinoma appear by 3rd or 4th year of life. Squamous cell carcinoma and malignant melanoma are also common and concurrent occurrence of different tumors is seen. Anterior tongue may be involved with leukoplakia and SCC.

Ocular involvement is present since infancy (80%) as photophobia, conjunctival xerosis and recurrent conjunctivitis. Changes like scarred eyelids, loss of eyelashes, symblepharon and ectropion develop gradually as evidence of photo-damage. Freckles in bulbar conjunctiva, vascular pterygium, corneal opacities, ocular keratoacanthoma and epithelioma of the eyelids may also occur.

In 20% patients with XP, neurological manifestations start during infancy. Mental retardation, areflexia/ hyporeflexia, spasticity, ataxia and sensorineural deafness occur in varying combinations. Immune-deficiency may be present in some cases

Malignant visceral tumors occur more frequently (10 to 20-fold increased risk) in patients with XP. Medulloblastoma and astrocytoma of the brain, bronchogenic, gastric, pancreatic, uterine, testicular and breast carcinomas are commonly encountered. Recurrent infections, neurological complications and metastatic malignancy increase the morbidity and mortality. Majority of the severely affected patients die within second decade.

Clinical features are variable. Cutaneous manifestations are severe in XP-A, XP-C, XP-D and XP-G. Neurological manifestations are common among XP-A and XP-D, occasionally present among XP-C and XP-G. Neurological manifestations are early onset (<7 years) in XP-A, whereas it manifests late (>7 years) in XP-D. Milder clinical features are seen in XP-E, XP-F and the dominant variant of the disorder.

XP-CS complex is the association of XP with Cockayne's syndrome. XP-B, XP-D and XP-G may have such association. Affected patients are photosensitive but freckling, pre malignant skin lesions and skin cancers are absent. Systemic lupus erythematosus may occur in association with XP.

Diagnosis: Early onset photosensitivity, photophobia and freckling are characteristic of XP. In advanced cases histopathological features include flattening of the epidermis with distinctive irregular proliferation of rete pegs, heavily laden with pigments. Basophilic degeneration of dermal collagen, solar elastosis and increased vascularity are other features.

The confirmatory diagnostic method in XP is unscheduled DNA synthesis (UDS) assay following UV-irradiation. It is done on skin fibroblasts, lymphocytes or epidermal cells in culture to demonstrate DNA repair defects. Cells from XP patients show low UDS values compared to controls and low recovery of RNA synthesis (RRS).

Demonstration of DNA repair defects in amniotic fluid cells help in prenatal diagnosis. Other methods include DNA analysis of trophoblast cells, polymerase chain reaction and alkaline comet assay. Successful prenatal carrier detection for XP-A has been possible by DNA-based study of chorionic villus cells.

Differential diagnosis: XP can be differentiated clinically from other causes of childhood photosensitivity by presence of freckling. Early onset multiple BCC may also be seen in basal cell nevus syndrome.

Management: Absolute photoprotection should be adopted since early age using physical sunscreens, wide-brim hats and full-sleeve garments. School goers need alteration of daily schedules in the form of admission to night school and evening play-time. Early detection of premalignant and malignant lesions is possible by regular medical supervision. Any of the following measures; topical 5-fluorouracil, cryotherapy, dermabrasion, excision and skin grafting or intralesional interferon alpha, can be used to manage recurrent episodes of such lesions.

Day time ophthalmic care includes use of sunglasses with side-shields. Already damaged eye requires artificial tears, soft contact lenses and corneal transplant, in case of corneal opacity.

Oral isotretinoin (1mg/Kg /day) reduce the incidence of cutaneous malignancies in these patients. A newer therapeutic modality is topical liposomal lotion of microbial enzyme T4 endonuclease V. This helps the affected cells to bypass developing DNA repair defect s and thus helpful in reducing the incidence of actinic keratoses and BCC.

De Sanctis-Cacchione Syndrome

It is a subtype of XP, where the classic cutaneous and ocular features of XP is associated with microcephaly, dwarfism, severe mental retardation, deafness, hypogonadism, shortening of tendo-Achilles, and neurological abnormalities like choreoathetosis and cerebellar ataxia. It is usually seen in sufferers of XP-A. Severe neurological impairment results from loss of neurons in cerebral cortex and cerebellum leading to inability to speak, termed as xerodermic idiocy. CT scan reveals cerebro-cortical atrophy, ventricular dilatation and small brain-stem in these patients.

XP-variant

In some cases (20%) of XP, the defect lies in the alternative pathway (post-replication/daughter-strand repair) instead of NER. These patients are considered as XP variant. This result in defective DNA synthesis in UV-irradiated cells, which are low molecular weight, and there is delay in the production of intact high molecular weight DNA strands. Clinically these patients are indistinguishable from XP-C. Cutaneous and ocular manifestations are present but there is no neurological deficit.

Pigmented Xerodermoid

Some patients with clinical features of XP manifest late in the third or fourth decade of life. NER pathway is normal in functioning but there is almost total depression of DNA synthesis after UV radiation.

Cockayne Syndrome

Cockayne syndrome (CS) is a very rare disorder characterized by photosensitivity, psychomotor retardation, senile look and progressive ocular and neurological abnormality. It is categorized into two complementation groups; CS-A (type-I) and CS-B (type-II). Eighty percent of the reported cases are CS-B. This is the more severe form starting in intrauterine life. CS-A, the classical form starts after birth.

Genetics: CS follows AR inheritance pattern. The mutated genes are ERCC8 (CS-A), located on chromosome 5, and ERCC6 (CS-B), located at 10q11-q21. These belong to 'excision-repair-cross-complementation' group.

Pathogenesis: The defect in CS is in the transcription-coupled repair (TCR) pathway, a variant of NER pathway. Intact TCR pathway is essential for removal of damaged portions of transcribed DNA. This defect results in profound photosensitivity and neurodegeneration.

Clinical features: Clinical manifestations start after 6 months of age as photosensitivity, psychomotor retardation and failure to thrive.

Photosensitivity is evident as persistent erythema of the butterfly area of the face which may exacerbate on inadvertent sun-exposure. This improves with age. In Cs-A, photosensitivity is milder and appear during late childhood or adolescence. Patients look cachectic and senile due to generalized loss of subcutaneous fat and premature graying of hair. Loss of orbital fat gives rise to enophthalmos **(Figure 3.21A)**. Physical features include stunted growth, long limbs and disproportionately large hands and feet. Large, protruding ears gives rise to a 'mickey mouse' like appearance **(Figure 3.21B)**. Dental caries may be seen more frequently.

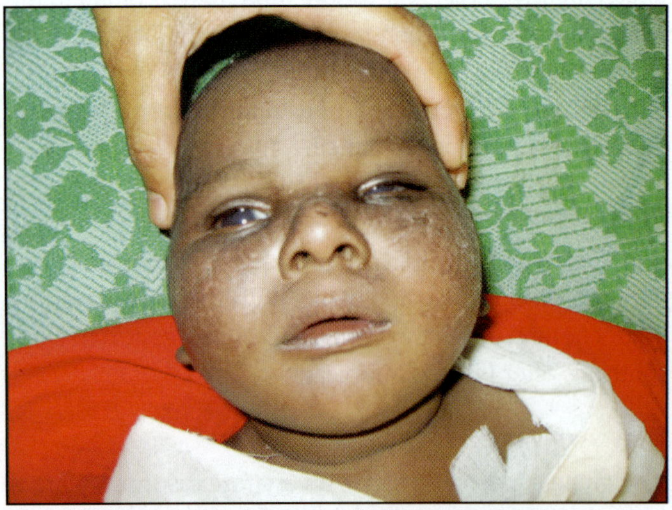

FIGURE 3.21A: Photosensitivity, microcephaly and enophthalmos (Cockayne syndrome)

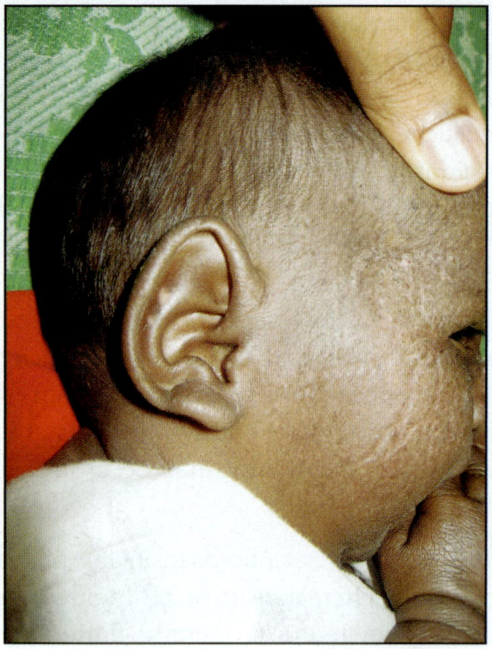

FIGURE 3.21B: Large pointed ear (Cockayne syndrome)

"Salt and pepper" appearance of the retina on fundoscopy is the hallmark feature of CS, present in 60-100% cases. Other findings include optic disc pallor, optic atrophy and cataract. The latter may be present at birth or develop by 3 years of age and cortical, nuclear or posterior subcapsular types may be present.

Normal pressure hydrocephalus, hyperreflexia, cerebellar ataxia, intention tremors, incontinence and sensorineural deafness are the usual neurological manifestations. There may be severe mental retardation. Other systemic involvements include nephropathy, hypertension, hepatomegaly and endocrine disturbances like adrenal failure, hyperinsulinemia and growth hormone deficiency.

Ocular and neurological features are progressive. Poor prognostic factors include presence of cataracts at birth, microphthalmia and iris hypoplasia. Severely affected patients survive till second decade.

Diagnosis: The characteristic description of a patient with CS is 'a cachectic dwarf with mickey mouse facies and severe mental retardation'. CT or MRI scan of the brain reveals calcifications in the basal ganglia, lateral ventricles or frontal lobes, which is considered as characteristic for CS. Other radiological features include demyelination of peripheral nerves and central nervous system. Meningeal and skull bone thickening may be present.

RRS until 24 hours after UV radiation is deficient and this is diagnostic of CS. The UDS assay following UV-irradiation of skin fibroblasts in culture is negative. Prenatal diagnosis is possible by RRS test from amniotic fluid cells or chorionic villus biopsy sample.

Differential diagnosis: Photosensitivity in CS is not as pronounced as BS and XP and improves with time. Freckles are absent. Unlike Rothmund Thomson syndrome, covered body parts are not involved. Malignant tumors are not seen in this disorder. CS may be mistaken as progeria because of the senile look.

Management: Photoprotection and symptomatic treatment of ocular and neurological manifestations are important in patients with CS.

Rothmund-Thomson Syndrome (Poikiloderma congenitale)

Rothmund-Thomson syndrome (RTS) is a rare disorder characterized by photosensitivity, poikiloderma, cataract, growth retardation and predisposition to malignancy. It has been reported among all ethnic groups including Indians.

Genetics: Inheritance pattern of RTS is AR. In 50% cases, there is mutation in a DNA-helicase gene *Rec*QL4 located on chromosome 8q.24.3. There is variable expression of the clinical features suggestive of genetic heterogeneity.

Pathogenesis: *Rec*QL4 is a member of the DNA-helicase family which maintains the integrity of DNA-repair pathways following UV-exposure. When this is mutated in RTS, DNA repair capacity following UV-exposure is impaired resulting in photosensitivity and carcinogenicity.

Clinical features: Cutaneous manifestations start by 3-6 months of age and definitely present by second year. Photosensitivity is the earliest feature. There is persistent erythema, edema and vesiculation of face, 'V' of neck and distal extremities. Subsequently there is dull-brown pigmentation along with speckled hypopigmentation, telangiectasia and atrophy, known as poikiloderma **(Figure 3.22A)**. Covered body parts like thighs and buttocks are also involved. The facies is typically bird-like, with prominent forehead, depressed nasal bridge, beaked nose and pointed chin. Subsequently, the skin over extremities become markedly atrophic with telangiectasia **(Figure 3.22B)** and some patients develop verrucous hyperkeratotic lesions on these sites.

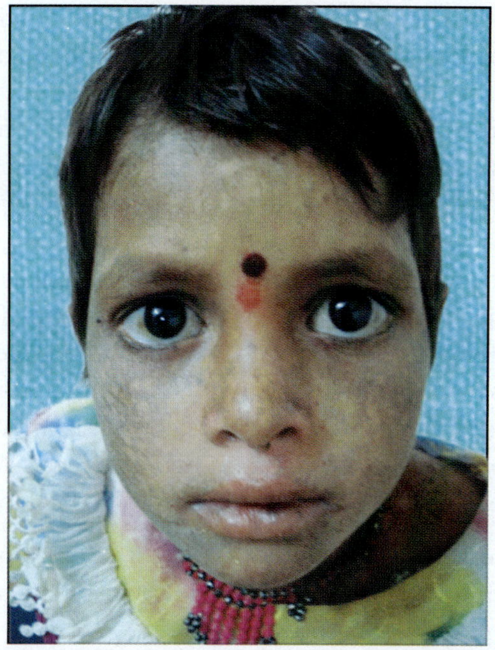

FIGURE 3.22A: Photosensitivity with poikilodermatous change (Rothmund-Thomson syndrome)

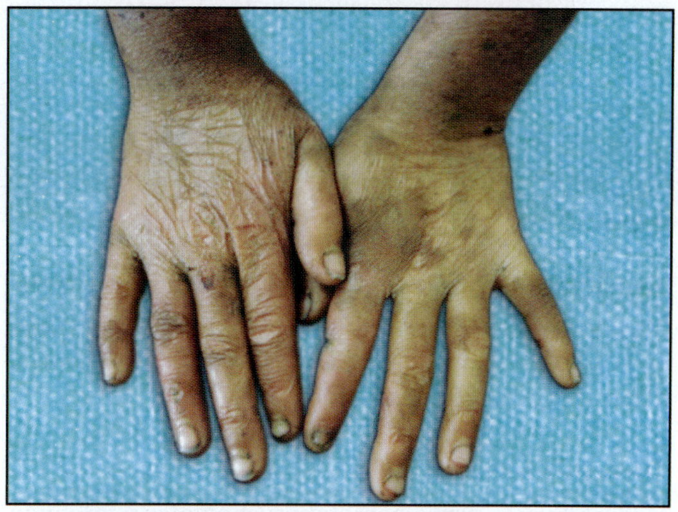

FIGURE 3.22B: Atrophic parchment-like skin on dorsa of hands (Rothmund-Thomson syndrome)

Anterior subcapsular cataracts are present bilaterally in >70 % patients. It is developed very rapidly and may be present during first year or usually detected by 3-7 years of age. Other ocular findings include photophobia, keratoconus, bilateral glaucoma, retinal coloboma, chorioretinal atrophy and blue sclera. Hair is thin and sparse or absent all over the body. Mild nail and dental changes are present. These are dystrophic, brittle nails (30%) and small, conical teeth with predisposition to caries (40%).

Bone age is lower than the chronological age of the patients and there is a proportionate dwarfism. There are multiple bony anomalies involving extremities like thumb hypoplasia, radial ray defect, absent radii, brachydactyly, syndactyly and clinodactyly. Mild to severe hypogonadism is present in both sexes but adult females may have successful pregnancy. Intelligence is normal. Various cutaneous and systemic malignancies develop in these patients. These include Bowen's disease, BCC, osteosarcoma, myelodysplastic syndromes, acute myeloid leukemia, Hodgkin's disease and malignant fibrous histiocytoma. Other disorders and anomalies which may be present in association with RTS are hyperparathyroidism, Addison's disease, osteogenesis imperfecta, osteoporosis, annular pancreas and duodenal stenosis. Life expectancy is normal in absence of malignancies.

Diagnosis: Poikiloderma, cataract and growth retardation form the characteristic clinical triad of RTS. Karyotyping is usually normal.

Differential diagnosis: Poikiloderma involving even covered body parts along with early onset photosensitivity are the differentiating points from other poikilodermatous disorders like dyskeratosis congenita and Werner syndrome.

Management: The child should be protected from sunlight since childhood. Suspicious skin lesions should be removed by keratolytics, topical 5-Fluorouracil or dermabrasion. Poikiloderma and telangiectasia may be improved with vascular pulsed dye laser. Cataract should be treated early. Regular follow-up is mandatory for early detection of malignancies.

Trichothiodystrophy

Mild ichthyosis, brittle hair and psychomotor retardation are the main clinical features of trichothiodystrophy. These may be present at birth in variable combination. Photosensitivity is present in 50% cases. Ocular involvements are frequent and include multiple punctate opacities in lens and rarely retinal degeneration.

There is AR inheritance pattern. The mutated genes are similar to that of XP-B and XP-D, of which the later is more commonly affected. There may be clinical overlap with XP and patients with photosensitivity demonstrate excision repair defects. A yet uncloned gene TTD-A may also be involved in the pathogenesis.

A sulfur-deficient hair protein gives rise to brittleness of hair. Alternate dark and light bands in hair shaft are evident by polarized microscopy, described as 'tiger-tail' appearance. DNA test in fibroblast culture is diagnostic. Fetal eyebrow biopsy or hair analysis helps in prenatal diagnosis.

HEREDITARY DISORDERS OF METABOLISM

Hereditary metabolic disorders include following groups;

- Disorders of amino acid metabolism
- Organic acidurias
- Transport defects, e.g. Hartnup disease
- Lysosomal storage disease
- Mucopolysaccharidosis
- Hyperlipoproteinemia

Disorders with predominant cutaneous involvement have been discussed in the following section.

DISORDERS OF AMINO ACID METABOLISM

Phenylketonuria

Phenylketonuria (PKU) is the first well-defined inborn error of amino acid metabolism. There are different subtypes of the disorder. The classical type will be described here. The transmission is AR. There is mutation of the gene encoding phenylalanine hydroxylase, located at 12q24.1.

Pathogenesis: Deficient phenylalanine hydroxylase results in inability to convert phenylalanine to tyrosine. There is increased plasma phenylalanine and increased urinary excretion of phenylpyruvic acid and phenylacetic acid. Pigment dilution results from inhibitory effect of phenylalanine hydroxylase on tyrosinase.

Clinical features: The affected infants are normal at birth and clinical features start manifesting within 4 months to 2 years of age. Psychomotor retardation and vomiting are the earliest features. There is severe and progressive mental retardation. There are behavioral abnormalities like irritability, hyperactivity and self destructive attempts.

Cutaneous manifestations include a dermatitis, which appears in 20%-50% affected children within first year of life and may resemble that of atopic individuals. The skin color is pale in 90% children with blond hair and blue eyes. There is moderate photosensitivity. Sclerodermoid change of extremities sparing the distal parts is characteristic of this disorder. A mousy odor emanates from patients' body due to excretion of phenylacetic acid in sweat and urine.

Microcephaly, stunted linear growth, recurrent pyogenic infections and cataract are other features in these patients. Neurological manifestations include seizure, hypertonia, increased tendon reflexes and abnormal gait. In mothers with uncontrolled PKU, phenylalanine crosses the placental barrier and results in microcephaly, congenital mental and growth retardation and infantile epilepsy.

Investigations: Serum phenylalanine level starts rising by 3rd/4th postnatal days. In established cases it is 10-50 times higher than normal ($\geq$ 20 mg /dl). Plasma tyrosine level is normal or raised. Urinary phenyl pyruvic acid is elevated, demonstrable by ferric chloride test (a green discoloration on addition of 10% ferric chloride). However this test may be negative in initial weeks of life and is not recommended as a diagnostic test for neonates. Guthrie test is a semi-quantitative microbiological assay to estimate phenylalanine level in capillary blood and this test is utilized for neonatal screening of phenylketonuria in several countries.

Histopathological examination of skin reveals normal melanocytes but reduced number of mature melanosomes. CT scan of brain may reveal intracranial calcification.

Management: Early diagnosis of PKU is of immense importance as early institution of dietary therapy can halt the progression of this debilitating disorder. A synthetic, low-phenylalanine diet (250-550 mg/day) throughout life is the mainstay of management in these patients. There should be fine balance as high phenylalanine causes neurological abnormality and very low dietary concentration of this amino acid causes growth retardation.

Cutaneous manifestations are reversible with such diet. Early institution of dietary restriction can prevent mental retardation and a low to normal IQ can be expected. The patients on such diet do not develop behavioral abnormalities. Regular monitoring of serum phenylalanine level (by Guthrie test; twice weekly in neonates, weekly in infants, biweekly in toddlers and monthly thereafter) throughout life is required in patients with such diet.

Supportive care is needed in presence of mental retardation and behavioral abnormalities.

Homocystinuria

It is an autosomal recessive disorder resulting from deficiency of the enzyme cystathione-β-synthase. There is increased urinary excretion of homocystine and methionine. Clinical features are evident in childhood and the major organs affected are central nervous system, blood vessels and bones. Seizure and psychomotor retardation are common. Bony involvements include stiff joints, osteoporosis and bony deformities like genu valgum and scoliosis. There are high risks of early thromboembolism, atherosclerosis, renovascular hypertension and cerebrovascular accident. The hallmark clinical feature is downward dislocation of the lens due to disruption of zonular fibers connecting lens and ciliary body.

Cutaneous manifestations include a pale complexion, blond, coarse, brittle hair, a distinctive malar flush, livedo reticularis of lower limbs and tissue paper scars.

Detection of urinary homocystine by cyanide-nitroprusside test helps in diagnosis.

Some patients are responsive to pyridoxine (250-500 mg/day) and early institution of this therapy reduces the risk of thromboembolism and brings change to hair color and texture. Methionine restricted diet, started in childhood may halt mental retardation and reduces the incidence of lens dislocation and seizure.

Tyrosinemia II (Richner Hanhart Syndrome)

This is a very rare AR disorder resulting from deficiency of cytoplasmic tyrosine aminotransferase (TAT), a rate-limiting enzyme in tyrosine catabolism. The mutated gene is located in chromosome 22q-24q. There is increased serum level of tyrosine. Urinary excretion of tyrosine and its metabolites are increased.

The systems affected are eye, skin and central nervous system. Painful, herpetiform/dendritic corneal ulcers develop within first few months of life and leads to intense photophobia and subsequent corneal scarring. Cutaneous features develop thereafter as focal, painful fissuring and hyperkeratosis of palms and soles making the child unable to walk and perform daily activities. Movement disorders and tendency of self-mutilation are present.

Increased serum tyrosine level in absence of elevated phenylalanine is diagnostic of the condition. Maintenance of daily protein intake to 2-3 g/Kg/day along with dietary restriction of tyrosine and phenylalanine are helpful.

Alkaptonuria (Ochronosis)

Alkaptonuria is a rare AR disorder resulting from deficiency of the enzyme homogentisic acid oxidase involved in the metabolism of phenylalanine and tyrosine. The mutated gene (AKU) is located in chromosome 3q21-q23. The term ochronosis refers to the deposition of a brownish-black, melanin-like pigment derived from oxidized homogentisic acid in connective tissues.

Pathogenesis: The enzyme homogentisic acid oxidase, located in liver and kidney, cleaves homogentisic acid into maloylacetoacetic acid, the end product in this metabolic pathway. In deficiency of the enzyme, there is excess of homogentisic acid which is oxidized and polymerized by the enzyme homogentisic acid polyphenol oxidase resulting in formation of a pigment. This pigment binds irreversibly to collagen and elastic fibers and accumulated in macrophages. Deposition of the pigment in ear cartilage and ocular structures gives the characteristic color. In joint cartilages, it facilitates deposition of calcium pyrophosphate dehydrate which initiates osteoarthritis.

Clinical features: The clinical picture of alkaptonuria varies with age. Within first few days of life, there is a brownish discoloration of the diapers due to urinary excretion of homogentisic acid. The other findings in childhood are black cerumen, brownish/greenish blue pigmentation of axillary skin and pigmentation of sweat gland pores.

Other clinical features of alkaptonuria like ochronotic discoloration of different body parts, arthropathy, renal calculi and cardiac involvement start manifesting from third decade onwards. The disease is slowly progressive. Morbidity due to disability is very high in this disorder but life expectancy is normal.

Investigations: The urine is normal or grayish while voiding, but immediately turns dark on exposure to air or alkalinization. Liquid-gas chromatography of urine detects urinary homocystine. Histopathological examination of pigmented skin demonstrates deposition of the dark pigment which is difficult to differentiate from melanin.

Differential diagnosis: Staining of diapers is observed in other conditions like porphyria, hemoglobinuria, myoglobinuria and hematuria. Hemochromatosis and Addison's disease may give rise to dark pigmentation of skin but the distribution is distinct of each disorder.

Treatment: Oral administration of ascorbic acid, an antioxidant, may prevent future damage of connective tissues. Avoidance of high protein diet to restrict the intake of phenylalanine and tyrosine may be helpful. However, a balanced, normal diet during childhood is recommended to attain normal growth. 2 (-2-nitro-4-trifluoromethyl-benzoyl)-1,3-cyclohexanedione (NTBC), an inhibitor of *p*-hydroxyphenylpyruvate dioxygenase which mediates the formation of homogentisic acid from p-hydroxyphenylpyruvic acid has been recognized as a treatment modality for alkaptonuria.

Hartnup Disease

Hartnup disease is a rare autosomal recessive disorder characterized by pellagrous skin lesions and cerebellar ataxia. The mutant gene is located on 5p15.

Pathogenesis: There is a transport defect of neutral amino acids across the brush bordered epithelium of small intestine and renal tubular epithelium. Failure of intestinal absorption of tryptophan results in deficiency of nicotinic acid giving rise to the clinical features simulating pellagra. Bacterial action on unabsorbed tryptophan results in formation of indole compounds which are excreted in urine. The defect in the renal tubule results in amino-aciduria.

Clinical features: A pellagrous dermatitis involving malar area of face, neck and forearms, starts by 3 years of age or earlier **(Figure 3.23A)**. Following sun exposure, the lesions are acute onset with well demarcated erythema, vesiculation and oozing. In chronic cases, the lesions are dry and scaly with pigmentary changes **(Figure 3.23B)**.

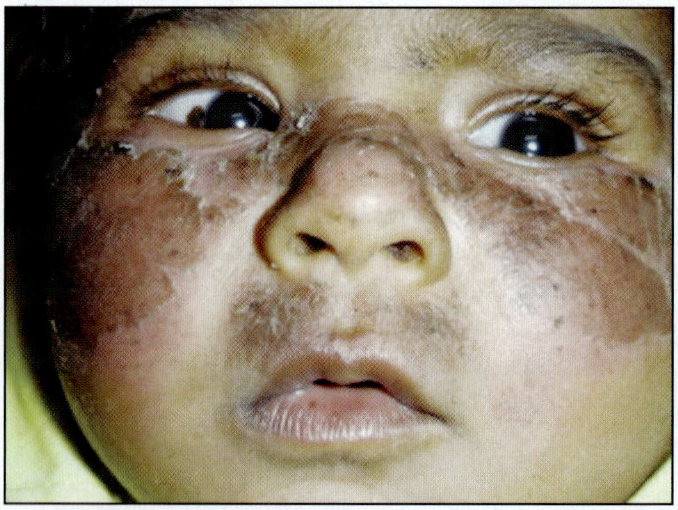

FIGURE 3.23A: Acute photosensitivity in Hartnup disease during infancy

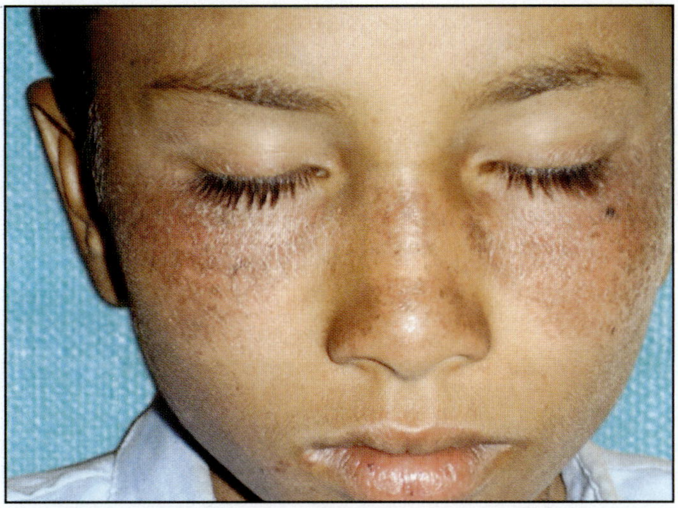

FIGURE 3.23B: Milder photosensitivity in an older boy with Hartnup disease

Neurological manifestations follow the dermatitis and include mild mental retardation, emotional lability, intermittent cerebellar ataxia, nystagmus and tremor involving extremities and tongue. Clinical features show exacerbation during spring and early summer. Other manifestations include glossitis, hypoproteinemic edema and diarrhea. Clinical manifestations tend to become milder as the child grows older.

Investigations: Urine chromatography reveals neutral aminoaciduria, comprising mostly of threonine, tyrosine, histidine, proline, cystine and lysine which is diagnostic.

Differential diagnosis: Other causes of childhood photosensitivity are to be ruled out in patients with Hartnup disease. Pellagra resulting from nutritional deficiency can be differentiated by absence of neurological symptoms.

Treatment: Treatment includes supplementation of oral nicotinic acid (200-400 mg/day), which helps to resolve the skin lesions rapidly and the neurological symptoms are improved to some extent.

MULTIPLE TUMOR SYNDROMES

NEUROFIBROMATOSIS

Neurofibromatosis (NF) is characterized by benign growths of the peripheral nerve sheaths, and *Café au lait* macules (CALM) in combination with various other cutaneous and systemic abnormalities. There are eight clinical variants of which Type I (von-Reckling Hausen's disease) and type II (bilateral vestibular schwannoma) are commonly encountered. Segmental form of the disease (type V) is known to occur.

Neurofibromatosis I (von-Recklinghausen's Disease)

NF1 is a multi-system disorder with AD inheritance pattern. Incomplete or monosymptomatic forms may occur. The re is mutation of a tumor-suppressor gene, NF1 (17q11.2), which encodes a protein neurofibromin involved in inactivation of *ras* proto-oncogene.

Expression of the disease is variable in a family and all generations are affected. Transmission of the disease from maternal side has more severe manifestations. Homozygous state is not encountered with as it may be lethal. Sporadic cases may occur.

Mucocutaneous features: *Mollusca fibrosa* are cutaneous neurofibromas with all-over distribution. These are soft, violaceous, sessile/pedunculated papules and nodules of varying size with button-hole appearance of the larger lesions. Deeper lesions have a firm consistency. There is rapid increase in the number of lesions during puberty suggesting hormonal influence and in females of this age group the lesions may be aggregated over the areola of the breast. Sudden pain and enlargement of individual neurofibroma may indicate hemorrhage or malignant transformation.

Plexiform neurofibromas are large, diffuse, elongated lesions with a bag-of-worms feeling **(Figure 3.24A)**. These are common along the branches of trigeminal and cervical nerves. The lesions may be hyperpigmented (giant CALM) with or without overlying hypertrichosis.

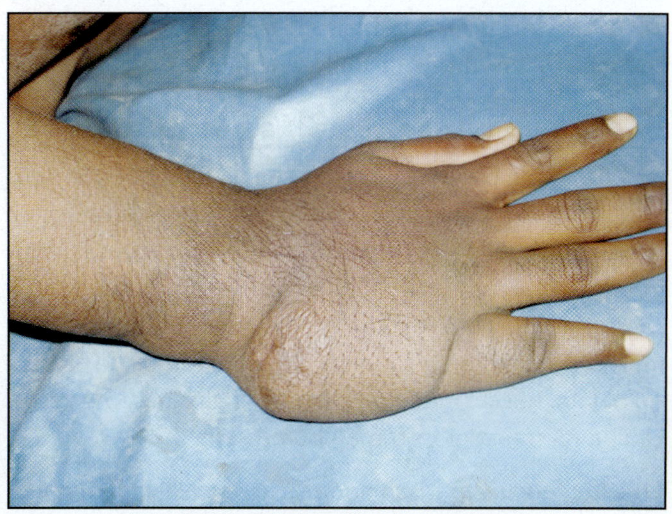

FIGURE 3.24A: Plexiform neurofibroma

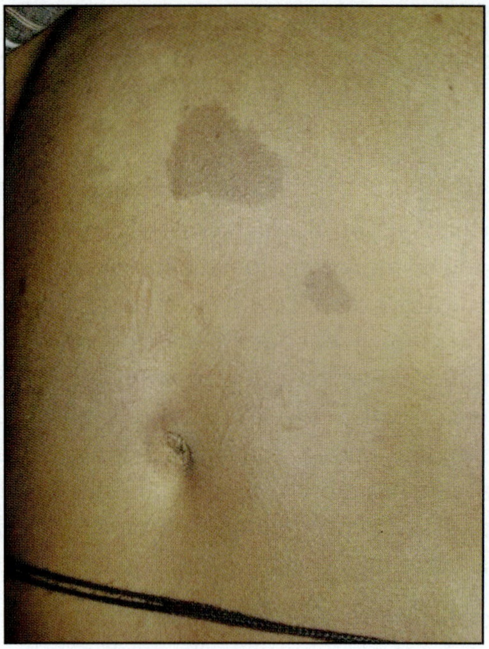

FIGURE 3.24B: Café au lait spots

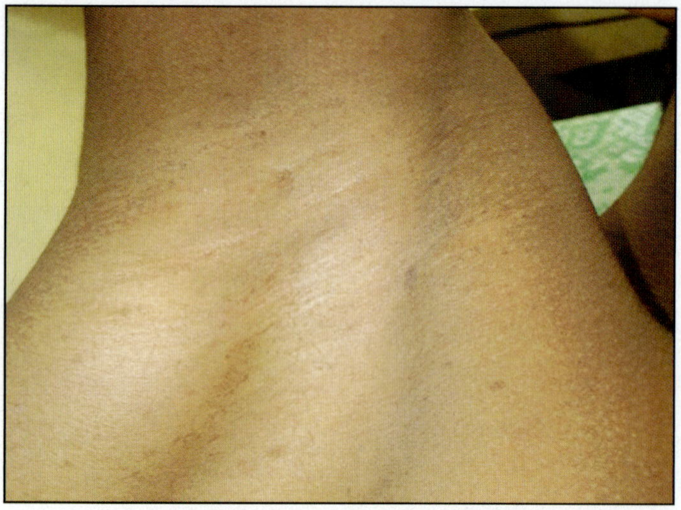

FIGURE 3.24C: Axillary freckling

'Elephantiasis neurofibromatosa', is a disfiguring pendulous mass with wrinkled surface, usually over a limb. This occurs due to diffuse involvement of nerve trunks with overgrowth of the adjacent subcutaneous tissue.

Neurofibroma arising from dorsal root ganglia may grow through the spinal foramina causing spinal cord compression.

Café-au-lait macules are well-circumscribed, light-brown lesions of varying size (0.5-50 cm) present in 90% cases of NF1 **(Figure 3.24B)**. These may be present at birth as the earliest sign of the disease. The lesions increase in size and number as the child grows. Few CALMs may occur in normal individuals. Presence of six or more lesions (0.5cm/more in children and 1.5 cm/more in adults) is suggestive of NF.

Freckles appear later than the CALM and are present in 70% of the patients. Crowe's sign is a pathognomonic feature of NF1, which is intertriginous localization of freckles in axillae **(Figure 3.24C)**, groins and infra-mammary area.

Pruritus may be a feature of NF1, resulting from diffuse mast cell infiltration of the skin. Papillomas may be present on palate, buccal mucosa, tongue and lips in some cases. Unilateral macroglossia may be present.

Ocular features: *Lisch nodules* are small, well-defined, dome shaped, pigmented hamartomas of the iris. The lesions are asymptomatic, better appreciated in slit lamp examination and increase with age. It is present in 30% of children below 6 years of age and 90% of adults.

Skeletal features: Bony abnormalities of NF1 include kyphoscoliosis, asymptomatic pseudoarthrosis of long bones (1%) and dysplasia of the sphenoid wing resulting in weak orbital wall. The later feature is distinct and though harmless, may result in pulsating exophthalmos. Short stature, macrocephaly and hypertelorism may be present in some patients. Kyphoscoliosis may give rise to cardio-respiratory disorders in later life.

CNS features: Speech impairment and learning difficulties are common in affected children.

Epilepsy may be an associated feature. However, convulsion may also result from intracranial tumors like optic nerve glioma, astrocytoma and schwannoma.

Endocrine manifestations: Acromegaly, Addison's disease, hyperparathyroidism and pheochromocytoma may be present in patients with NF1. There may be precocious puberty and gynecomastia in male children. There are various other systemic features in association with NF1. These include reno-vascular hypertension in children, cardiovascular anomalies, pulmonary hypertension, recurrent gastro-intestinal bleeding and constipation resulting from dysfunction of colonic musculature. Several malignancies may occur; these include leukemias, Wilm's tumor, rhabdomyosarcoma, retinoblastoma and malignant melanoma. Poor prognostic indicators are early onset, rapid progression of the disease before puberty and extensive systemic involvement.

TABLE 3.7: Diagnostic criteria for NF1 (National Institute of Health Consensus Development Conference, 1988)

	Presence of two /more of the following criteria are needed for diagnosis:
1.	Six / more CALMs, > 5 mm in greatest diameter at prepubertal age and >15 mm in greatest diameter in adults.
2.	Two / more neurofibroma of any type or one plexiform neurofibroma.
3.	Axillary or inguinal freckling.
4.	Optic glioma.
5.	Two / more Lisch nodules.
6.	A distinctive osseous lesion, e.g. sphenoid dysplasia/ thinning of cortex of long bones with / without pseudoarthrosis.
7.	First-degree relative (parent, sibling, offspring) with NF1 by the above criteria

Diagnosis: The diagnostic criteria of NF1 have been presented in **Table 3.7**. Patient and relatives should be examined in detail as diagnosis is mainly clinical. Histopathological examination of neurofibromas shows arborizing Schwann cells in collagenous stroma. Screening of the eye for Lisch nodules should be done by silt lamp examination and patients as well as asymptomatic relatives should be tested. Depending upon the clinical features, X-Ray, CT scan or MRI are advised. Prenatal diagnosis is possible with an accuracy of >95%.

Differential diagnosis: CALMs may be present in some other conditions like tuberous sclerosis, Bloom syndrome, Cowden's disease, Fanconi anemia, McCune-Albright syndrome, Watson syndrome, Silver-Russell syndrome as well as in10-20% of normal individuals. Plexiform neurofibroma may simulate congenital melanocytic nevus during childhood.

Treatment: Individual neurofibroma may be excised when these attain large size, become painful or disfiguring, or rapidly progressive. Ablation through CO2 laser can be done. Surgical debulking of plexiform lesions can be performed. Drugs like pirfenidone (antifibrotic agent), interferon α-2b, methotrexate and vinblastine are under trial for treating plexiform lesions.

Segmental NF-1: Post-zygotic mutation of NF-1 gene gives rise to segmental disease representing somatic mosaicism. Cutaneous neurofibroma, CALM and intertriginous freckling localized to one body area is the presenting manifestation. Isolated plexiform neurofibroma or tibial pseudoarthrosis may be the only feature of segmental NF-1. Full manifestation of the disease may be present in subsequent generation.

Neurofibromatosis II (Bilateral acoustic schwannoma)

NF-2 is a disorder manifested by 3rd decade of life. It follows AD inheritance pattern and normally the affected gene (22q11.21) encodes a protein schwannomin (neurofibromin-2/merlin). There are bilateral vestibular schwannomas and other meningeal and glial tumors involving the CNS. Patients present with vertigo, tinnitus and impaired hearing. Few neurofibromas and CALM may be present. The later lesions are larger, pale and five or less in number. Posterior subcapsular cataract may be present since childhood. Though the intracranial tumors are benign, these are associated with early mortality.

TUBEROUS SCLEROSIS COMPLEX (BOURNEVILLE'S DISEASE, EPILOIA)

Tuberous Sclerosis Complex (TSC) is a hamartomatosis. Multi system involvement is there and affected patients develop lesions in the skin, eye, central nervous system, heart, lungs, kidneys and bones.

Genetics

There is AD inheritance pattern. The expressivity of TSC is highly variable even among the members of the same family. There is a wide variety of mutations in TSC1 (9q34) and TSC2 (16p13) genes which encode two proteins hamartin and tuberin respectively. Tuberin bears similarity to neurofibromin of NF1 which possesses tumor suppressor property. In lack of tuberin activity, there is activation of Rap1 (a GTPase-activating protein involved in cell proliferation and cell cycle regulation), which leads to unregulated cell growth and formation of hamartomas. In addition to the hereditary form, sporadic cases may result from TSC2 mutation. Mosaic form of the disorder can occur. TSC2 is located in close proximity to the gene for polycystic kidney disease, PKD1.

Clinical Features

Cutaneous features:

1. *Cutaneous angiofibromas (adenoma sebaceum)* are 1-10 mm, reddish pink, dome-shaped papules present symmetrically over nasolabial folds, cheeks, chin and sometimes on eyelids, forehead, ears and scalp **(Figure 3.25A)**. These usually appear at 3-4

years of age and become florid during puberty. Lesions may be subtle, confined only to nasolabial furrows or rarely, large cauliflower-like. Mosaic form of TSC may present with unilateral angiofibromas.

2. *Ash-leaf spots* are lanceolate, hypopigmented lesions (1-3 cm), present in patients with TSC (90%) **(Figure 3.25B)**. In most of the cases these lesions are the first manifestation of TSC, present at birth or appear during infancy. Lesions vary in number from few to > 75. In fair-skinned individuals, ash-leaf spots are better visualized with Wood's lamp.
3. *Fibrotic plaque/nodules* may be present at birth. Common sites of occurrence are forehead, cheek and scalp. The lesions are skin-colored, firm and may be large.
4. *Shagreen patches (peau chagrine lesions, truncal plaques)* are relatively uncommon lesions (14-20%) appearing concurrent with angiofibromas. The lesions are skin-colored, soft, irregular plaques with multiple follicular prominences simulating orange-peel **(Figure 3.25C)**. The lesions are solitary or multiple and variable in size, reaching up to several inches surrounded by smaller satellite lesions. Lumbo-sacral region is the commonest site of occurrence, followed by back and breast.

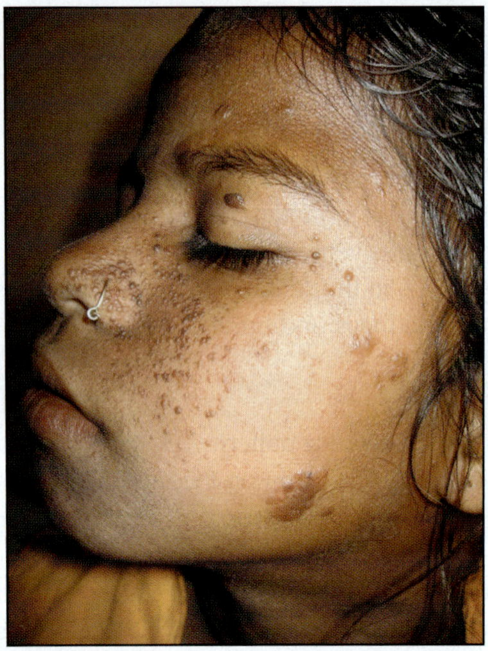

FIGURE 3.25A: Cutaneous angiofibromas and fibrotic plaque (Tuberous sclerosis)

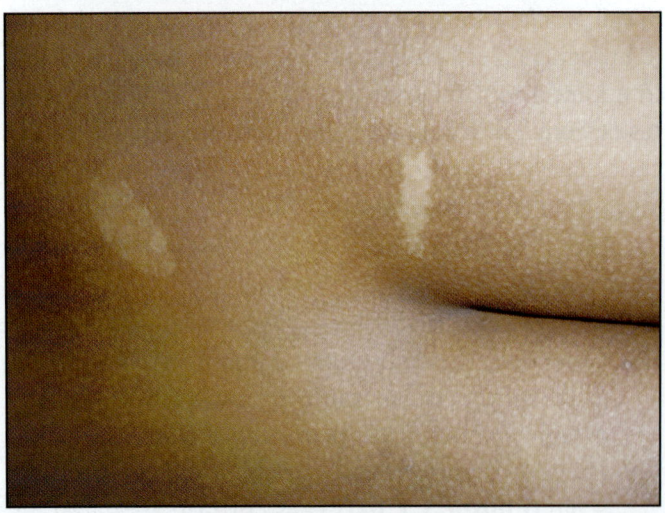

FIGURE 3.25D: Ash leaf spots

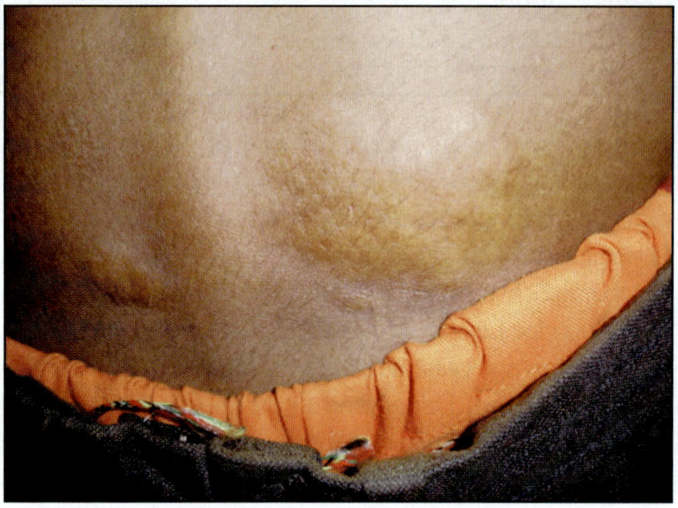

FIGURE 3.25C: Shagreen patch

5. *Koenen's tumors* are periungual/subungual fibromas appearing around puberty, occurring in up to 50% patients. These are smooth, skin-colored, firm projections (5-10 mm), arising from nail-bed and projecting through nail-folds.
6. Poliosis of scalp hair/eyelash, CALM, diffuse bronzing of skin, gingival fibromas, mucosal neuroma and small dental pits are present occasionally.

Ocular features:

1. *Retinal hamartomas* are flat, gray/yellow streaks along blood vessels or elevated, multi-nodular lesions resembling mulberry. These are seen in 50-76% of patients and are usually asymptomatic. Rarely, these may result in scotomas or amaurosis.
2. Other ocular lesions include pedunculated tumor of palpebral conjunctiva, glial hamartomas at the optic disc (giant drusen), retinal angiomas and colobomas at different levels. White spots on iris or retina may occur, which are analogous to ash-leaf spots in skin

CNS features: Cerebral cortex (gyri/floor and walls of ventricles) is involved with sclerotic areas and subependymal nodules (tubers) which may undergo calcification. Symptoms include obstructive hydrocephalus, seizure, mental retardation, behavior disorders and psychosis.

Cardiac lesions: Approximately 50% patients with TSC develop rhabdomyoma of cardiac muscle during infancy or at puberty in female patients. The lesions may lead to arrhythmias and sudden infant death or may remain asymptomatic and regress spontaneously.

Renal lesions: Overall, renal involvement is seen in 15% patients with TSC. Commonest renal lesions are angiomyolipoma. These are asymptomatic unless >4 cm in size. Bilateral, multiple renal cysts occur next in the order of frequency and may result due to simultaneous affection of TSC2 and PKD-1 on chromosome 16. Other renal lesions include malignant angiomyolipoma, renal cell carcinoma and oncocytoma.

Pulmonary lesions: These are rare and manifests during second decade, especially in females. Recurrent spontaneous pneumothorax is common and chylothorax may result from pulmonary lymphangioleiomyoma.

Colonic polyposis, cysts in solid viscera, pituitary-adrenal dysfunction and bony abnormalities may be observed. Life expectancy of severely affected children is low. Common causes of death are seizure, intracranial tumors or cardiac failure.

Diagnosis: **Table 3.8** presents the diagnostic criteria for TSC (revised by National Institutes of Health Consensus Conference).

There is little diagnostic problem when the complete syndrome is present. In infants and children, seizure, psychomotor delay and behavioral abnormalities are the commonest presenting features and screening for TSC is essential in childhood convulsions/mental retardations provided common causes are ruled out. Cutaneous markers of the disease present at birth are ash-leaf spots and forehead plaque. Screening tests for TSC in young children include Wood's lamp examination for ash-leaf spots (white-skinned patients), ophthalmoscopic examination, CT/MRI scanning of the brain and neonatal 2-D echocardiography. Cardiac lesions can be diagnosed *in utero* by fetal echocardiography.

In older patients, organ-specific characteristic findings are revealed by imaging techniques. Skull X-Ray may reveal calcification in 50% cases. Calcifications at the floor of the lateral ventricles are seen as curvi-linear opacities. Calcified peri-ventricular shadows in CT/MRI of the brain are one of the characteristic findings in TSC. Cortical tubers (brain stones), hypo-attenuated parenchymal mass and dilatation of the lateral ventricles are other features. Renal lesions are detected by abdominal ultrasonography/CT. Cystic lesions of the phalanges and cortical thickening of metatarsals/carpals may be present in X-Ray of the hands and feet.

TABLE 3.8: Diagnostic criteria for TSC

Major features:
Facial angiofibromas / forehead plaque, Non-traumatic, ungual / peri-ungual fibroma, Hypomelanotic macules (>3), Shagreen patch, Multiple, nodular, retinal hamartomas, Cortical tuber, Sub-ependymal nodule, Sub-ependymal giant cell astrocytoma, Cardiac rhabdomyoma, single / multiple, Lymphangiomyomatosis, Renal angiomyolipoma.
Minor features:
Multiple randomly distributed dental enamel pits, Hamartomatous rectal polyps, Bone cysts, Cerebral white matter migration lines, Gingival fibromas, Non-renal hamartomas, Retinal achromic patch, "Confetti" skin lesions, Multiple renal cysts.
Definite diagnosis: 2 major features / 1 major + 2 minor features. **Probable diagnosis:** 1 major feature + 1 minor feature. **Possible diagnosis:** Either 1 major feature or 2 / more minor features.

Differential diagnosis: Normal neonates may sometimes have few ash-leaf spots and does not indicate presence of the disease. Angiofibroma at puberty may be mistaken as acne, trichoepithelioma, verrucae, and milia. Reddish hue of these lesions and histopathological features of capillary dilatation and dermal fibrosis are characteristic. Intracranial calcifications may be the feature of other conditions like Sturge-Weber syndrome, congenital toxoplasmosis and cytomegalovirus infection, hyalinosis cutis et mucosae and basal cell nevus syndrome.

Management: Obstructive hydrocephalus and brain neoplasms need neurosurgical intervention and such procedures improve life-expectancy of these patients. Pulsed dye vascular laser and carbon dioxide laser are helpful for removing angiofibromas.

GARDNER SYNDROME

Gardner syndrome is characterized by multiple epidermoid cysts, pre-malignant intestinal polyps, osteoma and fibrous tumors of skin and other organs.

Genetics: There is AD inheritance, with high penetrance and variable expressivity. The mutated gene APC (Adenomatous Polyposis Coli) is located on 5q21q22. It is a proto-oncogene from *ras* family, which normally inhibits signal transduction functions of cells and the mutation leads to uncontrolled growth.

Clinical features: Clinical features start appearing in infancy and childhood. Numerous epidermoid cysts are present, mostly on face, scalp and extremities, and few on trunk.

Osteomas are small, asymptomatic lesions, usual on skull bones like, maxilla, mandible and sphenoid and rarely long bones are involved. By puberty, 50% patients have multiple osteomas. Asymptomatic intestinal polyps start appearing by second decade, which may undergo malignant change in later life.

Other cutaneous and visceral lesions include desmoid tumors, fibromas, lipomas and leiomyomas. Congenital hypertrophy of the retinal pigmented epithelium is frequently present at birth and may be helpful in screening of the patients. Carcinoma may occur in the viscera in later life.

COWDEN SYNDROME (MULTIPLE HAMARTOMA SYNDROME)

Multiple hamartomas of ectodermal, endodermal and mesodermal origin are the characteristic feature of this rare syndrome. There is AD inheritance with variable expression. Mutation of tumor suppressor gene PTEN (10q22-23), results in abnormal cell proliferation and predisposition to malignancy.

Clinical features appear usually in second or third decade of life. Muco-cutaneous lesions are universal. Skin-colored, small, lichenoid papules (trichilemmomas) are present around eyes, mouth and chin giving a cobblestone appearance. Similar is the finding in mucosa, where multiple, 1-3 mm, papillomatous lesions are present

Acrokeratosis verruciformis-like lesions are present on hands and wrists and umbilicated, punctate keratoses are present on palms and soles. Thyroid and breast neoplasms are frequent in these patients.

Craniofacial anomalies like craniomegaly, high-arched palate and adenoid facies gives a typical look to the patients. Skeletal anomalies include kyphoscoliosis, pectus excavatum and defective digits. Visceral neoplasms include polyposis of the gastro-intestinal tract, ovarian cysts, uterine leiomyomas, etc. Skin lesions are treated with topical 5-fluoro uracil, systemic retinoids and laser therapy. Female patients are to be screened for lesions in breast.

HEREDITARY DISORDERS OF CONNECTIVE TISSUE

This group of multi-system disorders involves collagen and elastin tissue present in different structures like skin, eye and blood vessels. The inheritance pattern is autosomal dominant or recessive. In some of these disorders clinical manifestations are evident during adult life. Cutaneous features may be subtle whereas serious systemic manifestations may result from visceral involvement. Following disorders will be discussed in this section:

1. Pseudoxanthoma elasticum
2. Cutis laxa
3. Marfan syndrome
4. Buschke-Ollendorff syndrome
5. Ehlers-Danlos syndrome
6. Osteogenesis imperfecta

PSEUDOXANTHOMA ELASTICUM (GRÖNBLAD-STRANDBERG SYNDROME)

Pseudoxanthoma elasticum (PXE) is a disorder involving elastic tissues of skin, eye and cardiovascular system. The clinical features are subtle or yet to develop during childhood and gradually manifest through adolescence and adult life.

There has been controversy regarding inheritance pattern of PXE. Recent molecular studies indicate the principal mode of inheritance is AR and there is no definite evidence of AD transmission.

Pathogenesis

There is mutation of the ABCC6 gene (16p13.1), which encodes a transmembrane ATP-binding cassette (ABC) transporter. Exact role of ABCC6 in maintaining integrity of elastic tissue is unknown. However, such mutation may lead to accumulation of metabolic products resulting in progressive degeneration and calcification of elastic fibers.

Clinical Features

The full-fledged disorder consists of distinctive skin lesions, retinal changes and vascular disorder.

Skin lesions are typically small (1-3 mm), yellowish papules, often coalesced to form reticulate/confluent plaque, distributed on the sides of the neck, axillae, groins and periumbilical area. In childhood these asymptomatic lesions are usually overlooked and the involved areas gradually attain a cobblestone (Moroccan leather/plucked chicken skin) appearance and in the elderly, there are redundant skin folds. Similar changes may also occur in the lips, buccal mucosa and visceral mucous membrane.

The characteristic ophthalmologic change includes angioid streaks which are grayish brown, ill-defined, linear bands in the retina, present bilaterally, without causing visual impairment. This results from visualization of the choroids through torn Bruch's membrane. This is a finding in adulthood (87%), but has been reported in children. Other ocular changes include, drusen, leopard spotting and pigmented dots on a string of pearls pattern.

Degeneration and calcification of the internal elastic lamina of visceral blood vessels may result in serious consequences like renovascular hypertension, coronary artery disease and gastrointestinal hemorrhage during adolescence. Late vascular complications include myocardial infarction, intermittent claudication and cerebrovascular accident.

There is increased incidence of first trimester fetal loss due to improper placental development. Mothers may develop cardiovascular complications during pregnancy.

Diagnosis

When cutaneous features are full blown, clinical diagnosis and histopathological confirmation are easy. Histopathological features from involved skin include irregular swelling and clumping of the degenerated elastic fibers in the mid and lower dermis (appears slightly basophilic on H&E stain and black with van Giesson/von Kossa stain). Areas of calcium deposition may be seen. Collagen in the surrounding area may be reduced. Similar changes involving elastic fibers are also present in blood vessels and other organs.

In absence of classical cutaneous manifestations use of diagnostic criteria for PXE is prudent **(Table 3.9)**. X-Ray and ultrasonography may reveal calcification in soft tissue and viscera.

TABLE 3.9: Diagnostic criteria for PXE

Major criteria
1. Yellow cobblestone-like lesions on flexures 2. Characteristic histopathological changes in lesional skin (Van Gieson and von Kossa stain) 3. Angioid streaks in retina
Minor criteria
1. Characteristic histopathological changes in lesional skin 2. Family history of PXE (first-degree relatives)

Management

There is no specific treatment for PXE. Preventive measures like avoidance of smoking, and counseling for cardiovascular risk factors may be started early in life.

CUTIS LAXA (GENERALIZED ELASTOLYSIS)

Cutis laxa is characterized by lax, pendulous skin, with loss of dermal elastic tissue demonstrable histopathologically. It may be hereditary or acquired or may occur as part of some other genetic disorders. Hereditary form of the disease may show AD or AR (more severe disease) inheritance pattern.

Pathogenesis

The AD cases result from mutations in the gene encoding elastin. Mutation of fibulin 5/ DANCE, a microfibrillary protein critical for synthesis and stabilization of elastic tissue has been found to be responsible for AR cutis laxa.

Clinical Features

The AD form of the disease is insidious onset, manifesting in adult life, without systemic involvement and a normal life expectancy. The recessive form of the disease presents during infancy as intrauterine growth retardation, delayed closure of fontanels and laxity of ligaments.

Cutaneous manifestations start within first 2 months of life and there is a prematurely aged look by the end of second year. There is characteristic downward slant of palpebral fissures with ectropion, broad, flat nose, sagging cheeks and large ears, described as 'bloodhound facies' **(Figure 3.26)**. Skin in general is loose, hanging in

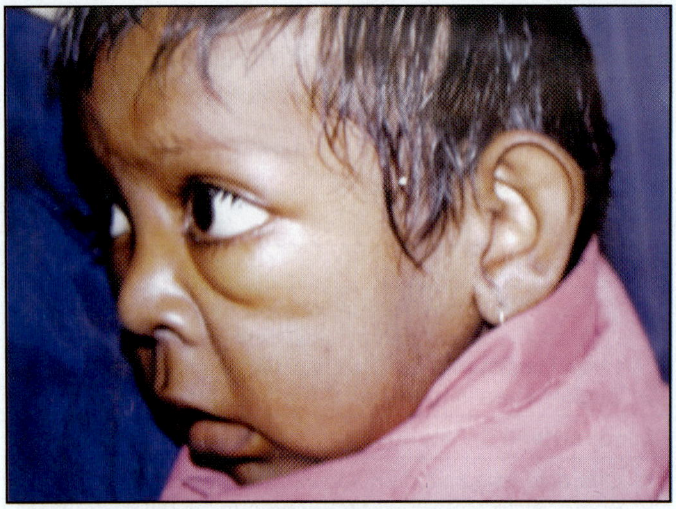

FIGURE 3.26: Lax, pendulous skin (bloodhound facies) in cutis laxa

pendulous folds on face, neck, abdomen, thigh and knee and recoils only slowly following stretching. Skin laxity facilitates the formation of multiple hernias.

Systemic involvements in AR cutis laxa include pulmonary emphysema, resulting in cor pulmonale, aortic aneurysm, gastrointestinal and genitourinary diverticula, osteoporosis and dental caries. Uterine and rectal prolapse and hiatal hernia are other complications Male children usually have gonadal maldevelopment and are impotent with infantile genitalia during adulthood. Life span is shortened due to pulmonary complications and the average life span is up to 4th decade.

Diagnosis

Diagnosis of cutis laxa is mostly clinical by presence of loose skin with a slow recoiling property. Histopathological examination of skin biopsy reveals sparse, short, fragmented and clumped elastic fibers with granular degeneration in the upper dermis. Electron microscopic findings include separation of the elastin microfibrills from the matrix, aggregation, fragmentation and clumping of the fibers, and a “wood-grain” pattern.

Management

Management of cutis laxa is mostly symptomatic. Plastic surgical repair may be helpful in improving the physical appearance of the patient. Appropriate investigations and timely intervention for the systemic involvements is mandatory.

Acquired Cutis Laxa

Acquired form of cutis laxa may occur at any age and is associated with a myriad of disorders. Skin laxity may be confined to a localized area or widespread. The disorders which may give rise to cutis laxa are urticaria and angioedema, systemic lupus erythematosus, severe rheumatoid arthritis, sarcoidosis, syphilis, multiple myeloma and Klippel-Trenaunay syndrome. Children may develop cutis laxa following exposure to drugs like penicillin, d-penicillamine and isoniazid.

Cutis laxa may be a part of de Barsey syndrome, SCARF syndrome, Costello syndrome and Lens-Majewski hyperostotic dwarfism.

MARFAN SYNDROME

This is an autosomal dominant disorder of elastic tissue affecting skeletal, ocular and cardiovascular system.

Pathogenesis

There is mutation in the fibrillin-1 (FBN1) gene (15q21.1), which is involved in the synthesis of components of elastin-associated microfibrills. This results in increased susceptibility of elastic fibers to protease degradation and altered elastin homeostasis.

Clinical Features

The clinical features are predominantly skeletal, highly variable and may not be evident until adolescence. The stature is tall with disproportionate extremities which is more prominent distally. There are long, sinuous digits (arachnodactyly), long hallux, dolichocephaly, high-arched palate and large paranasal sinuses. Kyphoscoliosis, pectus excavatum and flat feet are common. Laxity of joint capsules gives rise to unstable, hypermobile joints. Dislocation of hip may be the presenting feature of Marfan syndrome during neonatal period.

Ocular abnormality includes ectopia lentis (upward dislocation), present in 50-70% cases, tremulousness and heterochromia of iris, myopia and retinal detachment. Ocular manifestations result from affection of the zonular fibers of the lens.

Aortic dilatation may start appearing during childhood. In adult life, aneurismal dilatation of the ascending aorta is the commonest cardiovascular involvement. Both mitral and aortic valvular incompetence is common. Mitral valve prolapse may occur in around 80% cases.

Cutaneous lesions are not very common. The various changes that have been observed are elastosis perforans serpiginosa, striae atrophicans, skin hyperextensibility and papyraceous scars.

Prognosis is determined by the extent of cardiac involvement and death may occur in childhood.

Diagnosis

Early diagnosis of Marfan syndrome is crucial in view of the serious cardiac sequelae, especially occurring in children while participating in sports. In presence of full clinical manifestations, diagnosis of Marfan syndrome is easy. Incomplete forms may pose diagnostic difficulty. There are few simple clinical screening tests, helpful in detecting the hypermobility of joints:

- *Thumb sign (Steinberg sign):* positive if the tip of the fully opposed thumb extends past the ulnar border of the clenched fist.
- *Wrist sign:* positive if thumb and little fingers overlap when encircled around the opposite wrist **(Figure 3.27)**.
- *Body segment ratio*: a low upper segment (vertex to pubis) to lower segment (pubis to sole) ratio at puberty.
- *Increased arm span*: fingertip to fingertip length exceeding individual's height.

Whenever suspected clinically, echocardiography and slit lamp examination of the eye should be performed for confirmation of diagnosis. Other family members should be screened for presence of suggestive clinical features.

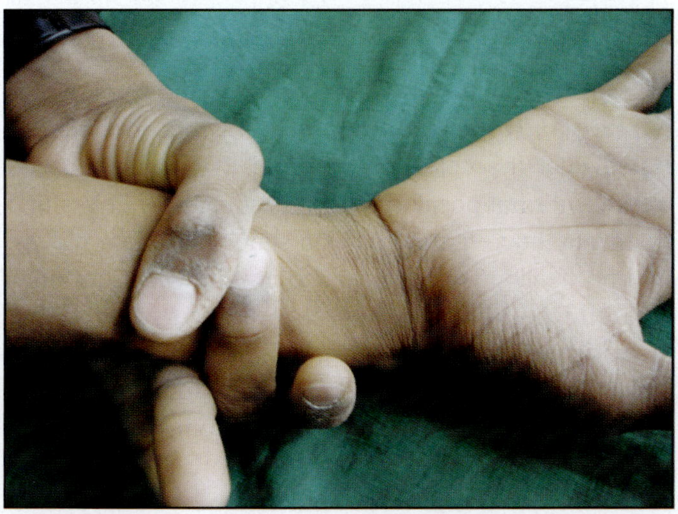

FIGURE 3.27: Positive wrist sign in Marfan syndrome

Management

Measures should be adopted since childhood to prevent occurrence of cardiac morbidity and related mortality. These include avoidance of undue physical exertion, isometric exercise, etc. Prosthetic replacement of the aortic root and defective heart valves, once the child's growth is complete increases the life expectancy. Regular ophthalmologic check-up is required for symptomatic lens dislocation. Surgical procedures may be undertaken in cases with profound spinal and other skeletal deformities.

BUSCHKE-OLLENDORFF SYNDROME (DERMATOFIBROSIS LENTICULARIS DISSEMINATA)

This syndrome consists of connective tissue nevus of the skin and osteopoikilosis. There is increased elastin production as evidenced by raised elastin mRNA levels in cultured fibroblasts. The inheritance is AD with variable expressivity.

Clinical Features

The commoner skin lesion is juvenile elastoma. These are asymmetric, yellowish nodules/plaques which are usually symptomless but may rarely present with mild pain or pruritus. The other type of skin lesion includes monomorphic, asymptomatic, small lichenoid papules, distributed on buttocks, proximal trunk and extremities. These may simulate skin lesions of PXE and are designated as dermatofibrosis lenticularis disseminata. The skin lesions start appearing during childhood and are present by puberty. Some lesions may disappear subsequently while new skin lesions appear.

Bony involvement is evident radiologically as multiple, circumscribed, small (1-10 mm) round to oval opacities, particularly conspicuous in phalanges, carpal and tarsal bones, epiphysis and metaphysis of long bones and flat bones of pelvis and scapula. These lesions grow over the years and are present by puberty.

Incomplete clinical picture is observed among family members who may have either skin lesions or osteopoikilosis.

Diagnosis

Histopathology of the skin lesions show thick, interlacing elastic tissue fibers in the reticular dermis lying among normal collagen demonstrable by elastic tissue stain.

TABLE 3.10: Salient features of different types of EDS

Type	Inheritance	Genetic defect	Cutaneous changes	Joint hypermobility	Others
Classical	AD	Mutations in COL5A1, COL5A2, COL1A1	Hyperextensibility, Bruising	++, subluxation of large joints	Blue sclera, genu recurvatum, kyphoscoliosis
Hypermobility	AD	Unknown	Variable hyperextensibility	+, dislocation, joint pain	Resistamce to topical / intradermal local anesthetic
Vascular	AD	Mutations in COL3A1,	Thin, translucent skin with easy bruising. Elastosis perforans serpiginosa.	Minimal, limited to digits	Spontaneous rupture of large vessels, colon and gravid uterus. Pneumothorax
Kyphoscoliosis	AR	Mutations in PLOD gene	Soft, velvety & hyperextensible. Marfanoid habitus	+	Scoliosis, microcornea, glaucoma, keratoconus
Arthrochalasia	AD	Mutations in COL1A1 (type A) COL1A2 (type B)	Soft & hyperextensible ± abnormal scarring	++ Multiple dislocations of both large & small joints. Bilateral hip dislocation	Chubby face due to lack of facial tissue and depressed nasal bridge.
Dermatosparaxis	AR	Mutation in type I collagen N-peptidase	Severe fragility, sagging, Wound healing, normal Skin redundancy	–	Umbilical hernia, blue sclera

Electron microscopy reveals clumping of elastin and swollen endoplasmic reticulum in the fibroblasts. Bone lesions are foci of tightly meshed trabeculae.

Several other anomalies may be associated. These include muscle fibrosis and contractures, skeletal anomalies like short stature, otosclerosis, spinal stenosis, supernumerary vertebra and ribs.

Management

As it is an asymptomatic condition, treatment is not necessary.

EHLERS-DANLOS SYNDROME (CUTIS HYPERPLASTICA)

Ehlers-Danlos Syndrome (EDS) is an inherited disorder of collagen characterized by hyperextensible, fragile skin and hypermobility of joints.

Classification

There are six clinical types of EDS. The salient features of these types have been presented in **Table 3.10**. There are other rarer and less well-known variants of the disease which are not further elaborated here.

Clinical Features

Skin hyperextensibility, fragility and joint hypermobility are the universal findings in all clinical types of EDS **(Table 3.10)**. However, the clinical expression is highly variable from almost unrecognizable to severe debilitating disease.

In general, the skin is thin, velvety and hyperelastic but not lax **(Figure 3.28A)**. The hyperextensibility is tested over the volar forearm and the skin is recoiled back to normal position following stretching. Palms and soles may have redundant skin simulating loose gloves. Wound healing is poor resulting in thin, wide, atrophic, cigarette paper-like (papyraceous) scars over bony prominences. Minor trauma causes gaping, "fish mouth" wounds and there are chances of wound-dehiscence post operatively. Approximately 50% (as compared to 10% in normal individuals) of patients with EDS are able to touch the tip of the nose with tongue (Gorlin's sign) **(Figure 3.28B)**.

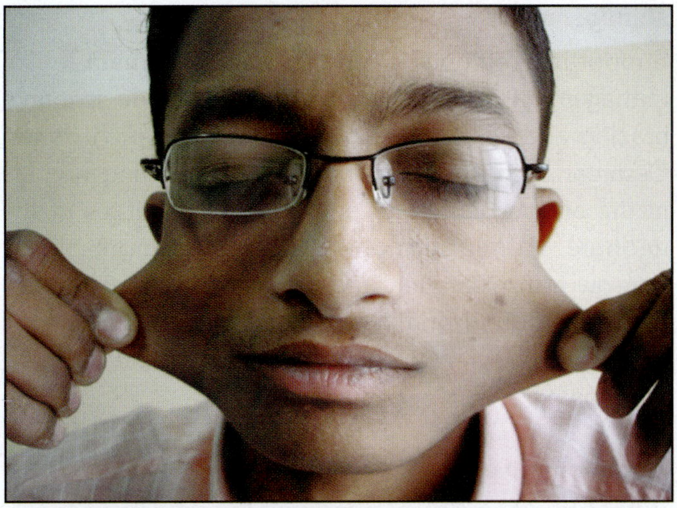

FIGURE 3.28A: Hyperextensible skin in Ehlers-Danlos syndrome

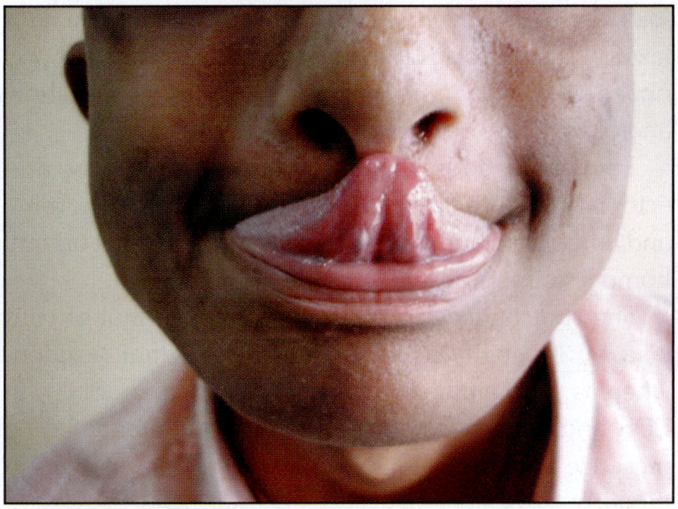

FIGURE 3.28B: Gorlin's sign in Ehlers-Danlos syndrome

Patients in classical type of EDS may have a typical facies with widely spaced eyes, broad nose and epicanthic folds. The sclerae may be blue. Molluscoid pseudotumors are bluish-grey, spongy swellings, arising from subcutaneous collection of connective tissue.

Marked joint mobility, subluxation of large joints and pain are characteristic of hypermobility type of EDS **(Figure 3.28C)**. In ecchymotic type, easy bruisability is common.

The skin is not hyperextensible in vascular type of EDS and joint involvement is minimal. Premature birth and low birth weight, resulting from rupture of placental membrane are common. Two clinical phenotypes 'acrogeric' and 'ecchymotic'may occur. A prematurely aged look with hollowed eyes, peaked nose and thin lips with fragile skin is the feature of the former.

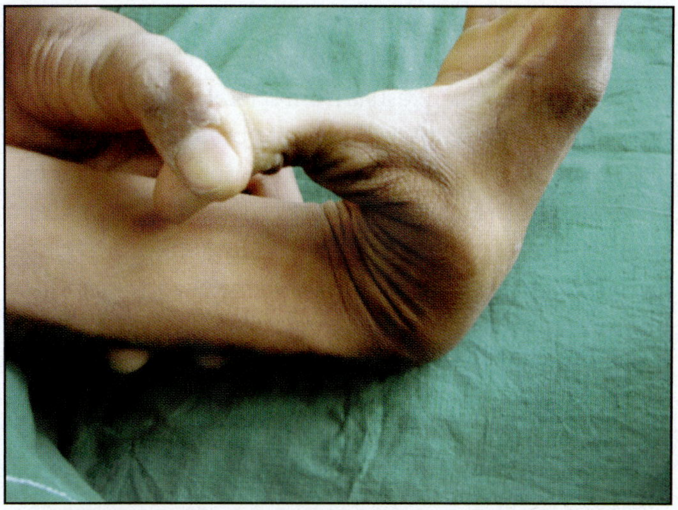

FIGURE 3.28C: Hypermobile joint in Ehlers-Danlos syndrome

Diagnosis

Diagnosis of EDS is mostly clinical. Subtype categorization requires electron microscopic study of dermal collagen, cultured fibroblast analysis and mutation analysis. Chorionic villus biopsy may help in prenatal diagnosis.

Management

There is no specific treatment for EDS. Preventive measures include avoidance of trauma, physical contact sports and careful, planned surgical procedures if required. Bleeding episodes should be treated conservatively. Oral ascorbic acid may help in kyphoscoliosis type of EDS, by regulating collagen biosynthesis.

OSTEOGENESIS IMPERFECTA

Osteogenesis imperfecta (OI) is a heterogenous group of disorder involving type I collagen. The principal organs of involvement are the skeletal system, eye, teeth and heart. Joint hypermobility and cutaneous changes may be present.

Pathogenesis

There is mutation involving type I collagen genes (COL1A1 or COL1A2) in about 90% cases. The mutations are variable and differ in families.

Clinical Features

Clinical features of OI are variable. Multiple fractures start during intrauterine life and may lead to bony deformities.

Skin is thin, translucent and fragile. Mild joint hypermobility is present. China blue sclera (90%) is distinctive of this disorder which results from scleral thinning, making the choroid pigment visible. Easily breakable, yellow to gray colored teeth, susceptible to caries (dentinogenesis imperfecta) is present in some cases. Deafness results from otosclerosis, starting during second to third decade of life. Cardiovascular system involvement includes mitral and aortic valve dilatation, regurgitation, prolapse and arterial fragility. Depending upon clinical severity OI can be categorized into 4 major subtypes, I (A & B), II, III & IV. All the types of OI are AD, but type III may rarely follow AR inheritance pattern.

Type IA (Classic form): This is the commonest clinical type (>50%). Affected patients present during childhood with multiple fractures, deafness, persistent blue/grey sclera and easy bruising. Bony deformities are uncommon and patients attain almost normal height at adulthood. Mitral valve prolapse or aortic incompetence may be present.

Type II (Lethal perinatal form): This is the rarest clinical type of OI. Multiple fractures occur in intrauterine life and the infant is either still born or survives only few days after birth. There is low birth weight and severe attenuation of limbs (micromelia). Radiological screening of an affected neonate reveals features like beaded ribs, crumpling of femur and calcification of skull.

Type III (Progressively deforming): Early fracture is a feature of this type which occurs during intrauterine life or during birth. With age, the child develops crippling deformities like scoliosis and bowing of the long bones of the extremities. Blue sclera is present at younger age, which becomes normal by adult life. Abnormal scar formation, resembling that of EDS may be present. There is high mortality associated with this clinical type.

Type IV (Mild form): This is a milder condition with AD inheritance. Dental involvement is frequent and blue sclera is absent.

Diagnosis

Diagnosis is mostly clinical. Bone fragility since early childhood, short stature and limbs with crippling deformities are characteristic. Blue sclera, though characteristic, is not pathognomonic of OI and may occasionally be seen in EDS, Marfan syndrome and iron deficiency anemia.

Management

Supportive orthopedic measures are the mainstay of management of these patients. These include splinting, bracing and surgical straightening of deformed bones. Cesarean section is recommended for expecting mothers in the affected family to prevent bone fractures of the neonate. Administration of growth hormone, bone marrow transplantation and bisphosphonates (alendronate and pamidronate) are some of the therapeutic measures to increase longitudinal growth and reducing bone pain.

Differential Diagnosis

Yellowish, pebble-like skin on flexural areas is characteristic of PXE. In older age group, localized, redundant skin folds are seen, which has to be differentiated from cutis laxa, where the skin laxity is generalized and childhood onset. Some patients with α-thalassemia may show angioid streaks.

Thin, long body habitus, bony abnormalities and ectopia lentis are the features of both Marfan syndrome and homocysteinuria. However, increased level of urinary homocysteine is observed in the later.

The stretchable skin in EDS differs from that of cutis laxa by its ability to spring back to normal position, whereas it remains lax in the later. Joint hypermobility in EDS and Marfan syndrome are to be differentiated by presence of ectopia lentis and abnormal body habitus in the later.

Easy bruisability in ecchymotic EDS is often mistaken as a primary coagulation disorder or child abuse. Similarly, multiple bony fractures in OI may be considered as child abuse.

PREMATURE AGEING SYNDROMES

There are varied causes for a prematurely aged look in children. It encompasses conditions which gives rise to generalized lipoatrophy or lax and hyperextensible skin resulting in older appearance than the expected look for that age. There are four categories in this group of disorders:

- True premature ageing,
- Conditions with skin atrophy/lipoatrophy
- Conditions with skin laxity
- Conditions with aged appearance of the individual

TRUE PREMATURE AGEING

Hutchinson-Gilford Syndrome (Syn: Progeria)

Hutchinson-Gilford syndrome (HGS) is a rare condition characterized by premature ageing, short stature and very short life span with death at teenage. The incidence is estimated to be 1: 8,000,000.

HGS results from AD transmission or sporadic mutation. There is mutation of lamin A, responsible for configuration of nuclear lamina; hence the nuclear structure is distorted. Abnormal metabolism of hyaluronic acid (probably an anti-ageing factor) may be responsible for the occurrence of clinical features.

Clinical features: The disorder is slightly commoner in males (M: F = 1.5:1). Low birth weight is common as growth rate of affected children is half the normal. The patients present during the first two years of life, skin changes starting within initial 6 months. Skin is atrophic, hyperpigmented and shiny in some areas like lower trunk and thigh, giving rise to sclerodermoid appearance but wrinkled and dull at other sites. Mid-facial dusky discoloration is an early feature. Sweating is diminished. Prominent veins are seen on scalp and thigh with sparse to absent scalp hair, eyebrows and eyelashes.

Craniofacial changes include macrocephaly (large cranium relative to the face), fronto-parietal bossing, thin, beaked nose with grooved nasal tip, prominent eyes, protruded ears with small or absent lobule, micrognathia and crowded teeth. Voice is high pitched and creaky.

Other features include narrow chest, protuberant abdomen, prominent, stiff limb joints with mild flexion at knees (horse riding stance), resulting in wide-based gait. Bony changes are shortened clavicle and terminal phalanges. Osteoporosis and fractures are frequent. Premature death occurs due to coronary artery disease or cerebrovascular accidents, resulting from athero-sclerosis.

Diagnosis: Urinary hyaluronic acid is increased consistently and in combination with clinical features, is extremely helpful in diagnosis of HGS. X-Ray demonstrates resorption of terminal phalanges and distal clavicle.

Histopathological features of skin include epidermal atrophy and network of thick and irregular elastin fibers in reticular dermis with hyaline fibrosis.

Cockayne syndrome, Werner syndrome and Hallerman Streiff syndrome should be differentiated from HGS.

Management: Multidisciplinary approach involving cardiologist, orthopedician, rheumatologist and dentist is required for these patients.

Werner Syndrome

Werner syndrome (WS) is the classical example of accelerated ageing characterized by sclerodermoid skin changes, short stature and hypogonadism. The inheritance is AR. The affected gene (WRN, a member of DNA helicase enzyme family) is located at 8p12. There are increased incidence of chromosome breakage and mutations. Skin fibroblasts show reduced growth potential and life span demonstrable *in vitro*.

Clinical features: The incidence is 1–20/1,000,000 with equal sex ratio. Clinical features start at puberty and patients present at third to fourth decade of life. There are sclerodermoid changes over acro-facial areas with atrophy, mottled pigmentation, telangiectasia, soft tissue calcification and leg ulceration. Craniofacial features include bird-like facies, beaked and pinched nose, inelastic ears and taut circumoral skin. Widespread loss of subcutaneous fat, progressive, premature hair loss and canitis are observed.

Musculoskeletal features include short stature due to growth arrest at puberty, thin spindle-like extremities due to muscular wasting and osteoarthritis with osteoporosis. Juvenile posterior sub capsular cataract and high pitched hoarse voice are other features. Patients tend to develop diabetes and hypogonadism with reduced fertility. Premature death occurs by fourth to sixth decade due to malignancy, myocardial infarction or cerebrovascular accident.

Rothmund Thomson syndrome (RTS), progeria and scleroderma should be considered as differential diagnosis. RTS has earlier age of onset compared to WS. Acrometageria and mandibular dysplasia are other conditions confused with WS.

Investigations: Estimation of blood sugar level, urinary hyaluronic acid assay and X Ray of the extremities help to support clinical diagnosis.

Management: Symptomatic treatment by specific specialists is required. Human insulin like growth factor 1 resulted in increase in bone mineral density but did not ameliorate other symptoms of WS.

Cockayne Syndrome

Subcutaneous fat loss on the face with resultant sunken eyes gives aged appearance.

Rothmund Thomson Syndrome

RTS is a disorder with early childhood poikiloderma, short stature, juvenile cataract and skeletal anomalies giving prematurely aged appearance.

CONDITIONS WITH SKIN ATROPHY/ LIPOATROPHY

Wiedman-Rautenstrauch Syndrome (Syn: Neonatal progeroid syndrome)

Wiedman-Rautenstrauch syndrome (WRS) is a premature ageing syndrome characterized by intrauterine growth retardation, short stature, typical facies, and lipoatrophy with paradoxical caudal fat accumulation. The inheritance is AR. Skin manifestation consists of progeroid appearance at birth, psuedohydrocephaloid appearance, sparse hair, prominent scalp veins, wide anterior fontanelle and malar hypoplasia. Natal teeth are almost always present. Generalized lipoatrophy is seen. Lifespan of the affected patients is uncertain.

DeBarsy Syndrome

The syndrome shows AR inheritance pattern and consists of progeroid appearance, growth and mental retardation, cutis laxa, corneal clouding, cataract and athetoid movements. Prominent forehead, nasal bridge, and thin lips are characteristic.

Acrometageria

Clinical manifestations are limited to the skin and skeleton. Atrophy of hands and feet, atrophic nose tip are seen in acrogeria. Cutaneous findings in metageria are seen in limbs as well as other structures. Generalized limb lipoatrophy with early onset diabetes and premature atherosclerosis is noted. Lifespan is dependant on the severity of these metabolic conditions.

Mandibulo acral dysplasias, Lenz – Majewski syndrome, Mulvihil – Smith syndrome, Lenaert syndrome are the other conditions where premature ageing is part of other symptom constellation.

CONDITIONS WITH SKIN LAXITY

Conditions associated with lax skin may also give the individual an aged appearance. Following are some of the important clinical conditions in this category of diseases.

Cutis Laxa

Inherited or acquired loose skin which tends to hang in folds is characteristic of cutis laxa giving the child an aged look.

Wrinkly Skin Syndrome

This is a rare AR disorder characterized by wrinkled skin on the hands, feet and abdomen. Microcephaly and relatively expressionless, asymmetric face is characteristic. Prominent venous pattern on the chest, hands and feet is the striking cutaneous finding.

Cutis laxa like skin features are seen in Costello syndrome and EDS-like skin changes are seen in Hernandez syndrome.

CONDITIONS WITH AGED APPEARANCE OF THE INDIVIDUAL

Marfanoid ageing syndrome with Marfanoid habitus and premature ageing is reported. Premature ageing is also seen in Lee syndrome and Berlin syndrome.

CHROMOSOMAL DISORDERS

Chromosomal abnormalities are common (1 in 150-250 neonates) and may involve autosome or sex chromosome. These aberrations result in spontaneous abortion in majority of the cases causing repeated fetal wastage.

There are two broad categories:

- Abnormalities of chromosome number, e.g. aneuploidy/polyploidy.
- Abnormalities of chromosome structure, e.g. deletion, duplication, translocation or ring formation.

Chromosomal disorders are characterized by multiorgan congenital anomalies, mental retardation, microcephaly, facial dysmorphism, maldevelopment of gonads and related infertility.

Study of chromosomal anomalies is known as karyotyping. Peripheral blood lymphocytes are most commonly used for this purpose. Skin, bone marrow, chorionic villi or amniotic cells are other choice. Lymphocytes are grown in phytohemagglutin containing media. Colchicine is added to the culture to arrest the growth of the cells at metaphase and fixed and stained by G (giemsa) banding technique. The resultant preparation is called 'metaphase spread' as it allows visualization of chromosomes in metaphase when these are easily visible because of maximum condensation.

AUTOSOMAL DISORDERS

Trisomy is the commonest numerical chromosomal anomaly occurring during first stage of maternal meiosis. Incidence of trisomy increases proportionately with increased maternal age (35 years/older).

Down's Syndrome (Mongolism)

Down's syndrome is the first recognized chromosomal anomaly (1866) and also the commonest autosomal disorder occurring at a frequency of 1 in 700 lives.

Etiology: There are three recognizable mechanisms of development of Down's syndrome;

- *Trisomy of chromosome 21*: non-disjunction of maternal cell during meiosis gives rise to an extra chromosome and this is the commonest cause (95%) of Down's syndrome. Its occurrence is related to increased maternal age.
- *Translocation*: translocation between chromosomes 13, 14 and 15 or chromosomes 21 and 22 (Robertsonian translocation) results in a rare (3%), familial variant of Down's syndrome. It is inherited from either of the clinically normal parents and the chromosome number of the affected children remains 46.
- *Post-zygotic mosaicism*: Some cases of Down's syndrome (2%) result from post-zygotic mosaicism. These patients have a mixed population of cells, normal and trisomic.

Clinically, the first two variants are indistinguishable. The third type has less florid manifestations.

Clinical features: Facial features are present since birth or gradually become evident during childhood. These are as follows:

- Microcephaly with flat face,
- Slanting palpebral fissures, and epicanthic folds,
- Thick, fissured lips,
- Short nose with flat nasal bridge and small ears,
- Scrotal tongue.

The skin is soft and velvety with cutis marmorata present at birth and infancy. Mild to moderate xerosis and childhood atopic dermatitis may be present. Hair is fine, sparse and hypopigmented. Extensive, treatment-resistant, alopecia areata may occur in these children. Dermatoglyphics are grossly abnormal and include simian palmar crease, single flexion crease in little finger and ulnar loops.

Other anomalies include congenital heart defects, duodenal atresia, cataract, Brushfield's spots in iris, hypothyroidism and epilepsy. Skeletal abnormalities include short stature, short, cone-shaped fingers, clinodactyly and unstable atlanto-axial joint. Severe mental retardation is present (except in cases with post-zygotic mosaicism) and the affected children develop simple language skills. Life expectancy is short in the presence of serious malformations.

Characteristic clinical features in a child of elderly mother are diagnostic. Karyotyping helps in confirmation of the diagnosis. Prenatal diagnosis is possible by karyotyping of the tissue samples of chorionic villus and ultrasonographic measurement of fetal nuchal-pad thickness.

SEX-CHROMOSOMAL DISORDER

Turner Syndrome (Gonadal Dysgenesis)

The phenotype of Turner syndrome is female. This chromosomal disorder leads to spontaneous, first trimester abortion in 95% cases. The frequency of live-birth is 1 in 2500 to 3000 female children.

Etiology: The underlying defect is missing or structural anomaly of one of the X-chromosomes. The resultant genotype is 45X0. When there is partial deletion of the involved X chromosome the genotype may be 46XX with milder Turner phenotype. Various mosaic forms can occur.

Clinical features: Growth retardation starts in intrauterine life and continued through post-natal period. Short stature, webbed neck (pterygium colli), broad, shield-shaped chest with wide-spaced nipples, cubitus valgus, kyphoscoliosis and high-arched palate constitute the clinical features which are fully manifested in adults. Coarctation of aorta and other cardio-vascular defects are present. Absence of secondary sexual characters and primary amenorrhea are evident at puberty. Patients are infertile.

In neonatal period, cutaneous features include a redundant skin-fold around neck and lymphedema of hands and feet. Cutaneous laxity over neck and back, low posterior hair-line, hypoplastic nails and keloidal tendency are seen. There are an increased number of melanocytic nevi which may turn to malignant melanoma.

Other minor anomalies include short fourth and/or fifth metacarpals and metatarsals, and minor ocular defects like squint or ptosis. Intelligence is usually normal.

Patients present at puberty for primary amenorrhea. Physical features may be subtle at this stage. Hormonal assay reveals increased pituitary gonadotrophins, reduced estrogen level and high urinary FSH. Buccal smear is chromatin negative. Prenatal diagnosis is possible by karyotyping of the amniotic fluid cells.

Normal height can be achieved by treatment with human growth hormone. Estrogen replacement therapy improves secondary sexual characters.

Klinefelter's Syndrome

Patients with Klinefelter's syndrome have male phenotype. The incidence is 1 in 600 live male births.

Etiology: There is duplication of 'X' chromosome and genotype of the affected patient is 44XXY, with a chromosome number 47. Male gonadogenesis is improper with fibrous seminiferous tubules interfering with the development of secondary sexual characters.

Clinical features: Clinical features are evident at puberty. The patients are tall and obese with gynecomastia. Genitalia are normal male type but testicles are small and fibrotic. Secondary sexual characters do not develop. Psychiatric anomalies may be present without mental retardation.

Incontinentia pigmenti, which is usually lethal in males, has been reported in association with Klinefelter's syndrome. This may be because of existence of an extra X chromosome in affected individuals. There is an increased risk of leg ulceration.

Diagnosis may be suspected from characteristic clinical features. Buccal smear is chromatin positive. Definitive diagnosis is possible by karyotyping. Testosterone replacement therapy helps in development of secondary sexual characters.

SKIN GENE THERAPY

The insertion or introduction of a desired gene into the skin in order to express the gene product is called skin gene therapy. There are two forms of genetic modification of cells, germ line gene therapy and somatic gene therapy. The former modifies germ line cells which will once and for all remove the chances of the genetic defect in the progeny of that person. The latter refers to modification of different cells which is possible in all accessible somatic cells (Blood, skin, muscle, and endothelial cells, etc.). Since skin is an easily accessible organ, skin diseases are the obvious choice for gene therapy. With increasing knowledge of genetic basis of skin disorders, it is possible to treat these disorders by expressing normal gene or, by blocking the expression or by deleting abnormal mutated gene from the cells. Therefore, the skin gene therapy is an ultimate treatment modality for genodermatoses. However, gene therapy can also be used for polygenic disorders like psoriasis.

GOALS OF SKIN GENE THERAPY

1. Delivery of the desired gene to a high percentage of target cells
2. Persistent expression of the desired gene for a suitable period of time

TARGET CELLS FOR SKIN GENE THERAPY

1. *Epidermal keratinocytes:* The first goal of skin gene therapy can easily be accomplished by introducing the desired gene into epidermal keratinocytes because these cells are easily obtained and expanded in culture, and the inserted gene can be modulated and monitored in the graft. Keratinocytes are also potent growth factor secreting cells. However, the second goal cannot be accomplished as keratinocytes are continually proliferating and differentiating cells.
2. *Epidermal stem cells:* To achieve persistent expression of inserted gene, the epidermal stem cells should be targeted because these cells have unlimited capacity for self-renewal and the inserted gene not only persist indefinitely in the epidermis but also transferred to all progeny cells of stem cell. However, the identification, enrichment and targeting of these cells are difficult.
3. *Fibroblasts:* These cells are targeted when there is increased requirement of growth factors (wound healing) or collagen (Collagen V[22] in dystrophic epidermolysis bullosa).

APPROACHES TO SKIN GENE THERAPY

1. *In-Vivo approach:* In this approach the desired gene is directly inserted into the skin. It is simple and direct. However, the gene is inserted into a limited number of cells and the expression of gene is transient. The stem cells are difficult to target by this approach.
2. *Ex-Vivo approach:* In this approach the target cells are cultured from a skin biopsy specimen and the desired gene is inserted into them while they are propagated in tissue culture. Epidermal stem cells can also be targeted by this approach. However, it is more complicated and time-consuming.

TECHNIQUES TO INSERT THE GENE INTO THE CELLS

Various techniques **(Table 3.11)** have been used to insert desired gene (DNA) in the in-vivo and ex-vivo approaches. For efficient insertion of DNA, the vector should possess some ideal characteristics **(Table 3.12)**.

TABLE 3.11: Techniques to insert the gene into the cells

A. Physical methods (In-vivo approach)
a. Microinjection of DNA coated microscopic gold particles by electroporation (Biolistic method)
b. Direct injection of naked DNA
B. Chemical transfection methods (Ex-vivo approach)
a. Liposome mediated DNA transfer
b. Endocytosis of DNA trapped in fine precipitate of calcium phosphate
c. Receptor mediated endocytosis of DNA conjugated with galactose
C. Biological methods or Replication deficient viral vectors (Both in-vivo and ex-vivo approach)
a. Retrovirus (Integrates DNA directly into cellular chromosome of dividing cells)
b. Adenovirus (Enters non dividing cells but do not integrate the DNA into cellular chromosome)
c. Adeno-associated virus (Enters non dividing cells and also integrates into cellular chromosome)

TABLE 3.12: Characteristics of ideal vector

• Should protect the DNA
• Should deliver DNA easily through cell membrane into the nucleus
• Should be non-toxic and non-immunogenic
• Should persist in host nucleus
• Should be possible to produce in large quantities

CANDIDATE DISEASES FOR SKIN GENE THERAPY

The diseases that are amiable to skin gene therapy include both skin and systemic diseases. Among skin diseases both genetic and non genetic diseases are potential candidates for the skin gene therapy **(Table 3.13)**. The genodermatoses with recessive inheritance, and in which the defective gene is identified and cloned have the better chance of successful gene therapy. In recessive disease the insertion of single normal gene (allele) is enough to carry out the function of defective gene. However, in dominant disease the defective gene (allele) is dominant over the normal allele. Therefore, only deletion or blocking the expression of defective allele can restore the function of the gene. The skin gene therapy to be successful in non genetic dermatoses, it is crucial to delineate the role played by cytokines, growth factors or other molecules in the pathogenesis of disease. Once determined, the genes for molecules which inhibit the pathogenesis can be inserted to control the disease (e.g. psoriasis). In case of cutaneous malignancies like melanoma, the host immune system against the cancerous cells can be stimulated by inserting the immunotherapy genes (e.g.interleukin-2).

TABLE 3.13: Candidate diseases for skin gene therapy

Skin diseases
Genetic diseases
1. Epidermolysis bullosa
2. Lamellar ichthyosis
3. Xeroderma pigmentosum
Non genetic diseases
1. Psoriasis
2. Melanoma
3. Wound healing
Systemic diseases
1. Severe combined immunodeficiency (Adenosine deaminase deficiency)
2. Disorders of coagulation (Hemophilia)
3. Diabetes mellitus (Insulin)
4. Growth hormone deficiency

LIMITATIONS OF SKIN GENE THERAPY

1. Persistent expression of desired gene in high percentage of cells has been difficult in animal models.
2. Risk of development of unwanted immune response against normal protein.
3. Difficulty in identifying and targeting stem cells.

BIBLIOGRAPHY

1. Ablin DS. Osteogenesis imperfecta: a review. Can Assoc Radiol J 1998; 49:110-1
2. Abuelo D. Chromosome disorders. In: Alper JC, editor. Genetic disorders of the skin. St.Louis: Mosby Year Book 1991;44-63.
3. Ahluwalia J, Pattari S, Trehan A, Marwaha RK, Garewal G. Accelerated phase at initial presentation: An uncommon occurrence in Chediak-Higashi syndrome. Pediatr Hematol Oncol 2003;20:563-7.
4. Ahmed I. Childhood porphyrias.Mayo Clin Proc 2002;77: 825-36.
5. Alapetite C, Benoit A, Moustacchi E, Sarasin A. The comet assay as a repair test for prenatal diagnosis of xeroderma pigmentosum and trichothiodystrophy. J Invest Dermatol 1997;108:154-9.
6. Al-Khenaizan S. Hyperpigmentation in Chediak-Higashi syndrome. J Am Acad Dermatol 2003; 49: S244-S246.
7. Alter BP, Gardner FH, Hall RE. Treatment of dyskeratosis congenita with granulocyte colony-stimulating factor and erythropoietin. Br J Haematol 1997;97: 309-11.
8. Arita K, Akiyama M, Tsuji Y, Onozuka T, Shimizu H. Erythrokeratoderma variabilis without connexin 31 or connexin 30.3 gene mutation: immunohistological, ultrastructural and genetic studies. Acta Derm Venereol 2003;83:266-70.
9. Au KS, Rodriguez JA, Finch JL, Volcik KA, Roach ES, Delgado MR, *et al.* Germline mutational analysis of the TSC-2 gene in 90 tuberous sclerosis patients. Am J Hum Genet 1998;62:286-94.
10. Baraitser M, Hodgson SV. The Johanson-Blizzard syndrome. J Med Genet 1982;19:302-3.
11. Batta K, Rugg EL, Wilson NJ, *et al.* A keratin 14 "knockout" mutation in recessive epidermolysis bullosa simplex. Br J Dermatol 2000;143:621-7.
12. Berlin AL, Paller AS, Chan LS. Incontinentia pigmenti: a review and update on the molecular basis of Pathophysiology. J Am Acad Dermatol 2002;47: 169-87.
13. Bloom D. Congenital telangiectatic erythema resembling lupus erythematosus in dwarfs. Am J Dis Child 1954;88: 754-8.
14. Boeshans KM, Mneser TC, Ahvazi B. A three-dimensional model of the human transglutaminase 1: insights into the understanding of lamellar ichthyosis. J Mol Model. 2007;13:233-66.
15. Bohr VA. Werner syndrome and its protein: clinical, cellular and molecular advances. Mech Ageing Dev 2003;124:1073-82.
16. Brilliant MH. The mouse p (pink-eyed dilution)and human P genes, oculocutaneous albinism type 2 (OCA2) and melanosomal pH. Pigment Cell Res 2001;14:86-93.
17. Broughton BC, Berneburg M, Fawcette H, *et al.* Two individuals with features of both xeroderma pigmentosum and trichothiodystrophy highlight the complexity of the clinical outcomes of mutations in the XPD gene. Hum Mol Genet 2002;10: 2539- 47.
18. Bruce AJ, Ahmed I. Childhood-onset porphyria cutanea tarda: Successful therapy with low-dose hydroxychloroquine (Plaquenil). J Am Acad Dermatol 1998;38: 810-4.
19. Buckley RH, The hyper-IgE syndrome. Clin Rev Allergy Immunol 2001;20: 139-54.
20. Buckley RH. Molecular defects in human severe combined immunodeficiency and approaches to immune reconstitution. Annu Rev Immunol 2004;22: 625-55.
21. Burrows NP. The molecular genetics of the Ehlers-Danlos syndrome. Clin Exp Dermatol 1999;24:99-106.
22. Byers PH. Osteogenesis imperfecta: perspectives and opportunities. Curr Opin Pediatr 2000;12:603-9.
23. Camacho F, Ferrando J, Pichardo AR, Sotillo I, Jorquera E. Rapp-Hodgkin syndrome with pili canaliculi. Pediatr Dermatol 1993;10:54-57.
24. Celli J, Duijf P, Hamel BC, Bamshad M, Kramer B, Smits AP, *et al.* Heterozygous germline mutations in the p53 homolog p63 are the cause of EEC syndrome. Cell 1999;143-53.
25. Chamlin SL, McCalmont TH, Cunningham BB, et al.Cutaneous manifestations of hyper-IgE syndrome in infants and children. J Pediatr 2002;141:572-5.
26. Chao SC, Chung CH, Yang CC, Yang MH, Lee JY. Mutation analysis of X- linked hypohidrotic ectodermal dysplasia in a Taiwanese family. J Formos Med Assoc 2003;102:412-7.
27. Cleaver JE, Volpe JP, Charles WC, Thomas GH. Prenatal diagnosis of xeroderma pigmentosum and Cockayne syndrome. Prenat Diagn 1995;14:921- 8.
28. Collod Beroud G, Bolleau C. Marfan syndrome in the third millennium. Eur J Hum Genet 2002;10:673-81.
29. Common JE, O'Toole EA, Leigh IM, Thomas A, Griffiths WA, Venning V, et al. Clinical and genetic heterogeneity of erythrokeratoderma variabilis. J Invest Dermatol 2005;125: 920-7.
30. Crawford TO. Ataxia telangiectasia. Semin Pediatr Neurol 1998;5:287-94.
31. Cserhalmi-Friedman PB, Garzon MC, Guzman E, et al. Maternal germ-line mosaicism in dominant dystrophic epidermolysis bullosa. J Invest Dermatol 2001;177:1327-8.
32. Dale BA, Kam E. Harlequin ichthyosis. Variability in expression and hypothesis for disease mechanism. Arch Dermatol 1993;129:1471-7.
33. Davies DR, Armstrong JG, Thakkar N, Horner K, Guy SP, Clancy T, *et al.* Severe Gardner syndrome in families with mutations restricted to a specific region of the APC gene. AM J Hum Genet 1995;57:1151-8.
34. de Paula Rodrigues GH, das Eiras Tamega I, Duque G, Spinola Dias Neto V. Severe bone changes in a case of Hutchinson – Gillford syndrome. Ann Genet 2002;45:151-5.
35. Denyer J. Management of severe blistering disorders. Semin Neonatal 2000; 5: 321-4.
36. Di Cristofano A, Pesce B, Cordon-Cardo C, Pandolfi PP. PTEN is essential for embryonic development and tumor suppression. Nature Genet 1998;19:348-55.
37. Di Giovanna JJ. Retinoid chemoprevention in patients at high risk of skin cancer. Med Pediatr Oncol 2001;36:564-7.
38. Dollfus H, Porto F, Caussade P, Speeg-Schatz C, Sahel J, Grosshano E, *et al.* Ocular manifestations in the inherited DNA repair disorders. Surv Ophthalmol 2003;48:107-22.
39. Dollfus H, Porto F, Caussade P, Speeg-Schatz C, Sahel J, Grosshans E, *et al.* Ocular manifestations in the inherited DNA repair disorders. Surv Ophthalmol 2003;48:107-22.
40. Downs AMR, Kennedy CTC. Scleroatrophic syndrome of Huriez in an infant. Pediatr Dermatol 1998;15:207-9.
41. Dupuis-Girod S, Medioni J, Haddad E, et al. Autoimmunity in Wiskott-Aldrich Syndrome: Risk factors, clinical features and outcome in a single-center cohort of 55 patients. Pediatrics 2003;111:E622-7.

42. Eady RAJ, McGrath JA. Prenatal diagnosis of genetic skin disease. In: Burns T, Breathnach S, Cox N, Griffiths C, editors. Rook's Text Book of Dermatology. Oxford: Blackwell Science; 2004;7(1):13.1-13.13.
43. Elder GH. Hepatic porphyrias in children. J Inherit Metab Dis 1997;20:237-46.
44. Elias PM, Crumrine D, Rassner U, Hachem JP, Menon GK, Man W, et al. Basis for abnormal desquamation and permeability barrier dysfunction in RXLI. J Invest Dermatol 2004;122:314-9.
45. Ellis NA, German J. Molecular genetics of Bloom's syndrome. Hum Mol Genet 1996;5:1457-63.
46. Falabella MF, Valencia IC, Eaglstein WH, Schachner LA. Tissue-engineered skin (Apligraft) in the healing of patients with epidermolysis bullosa wounds. Arch Dermatol 2000;136:1225-30.
47. Fernandez B, Ruas E, Machado A, Figueiredo A. Ectrodactyly-ectodermal dysplasia-clefting syndrome (EEC): report of a case with perioral papillomatosis. Pediatr Dermatol 2002; 19:330-2.
48. Fine JD, Fady RAJ, Bauer EA, *et al.* Revised classification system for inherited epidermolysis bullosa: report of the second international consensus meeting on diagnosis and classification of epidermolysis bullosa. J Am Acad Dermatol 2000;42:1051-66.
49. Foran SE, Abel G. Guide to porphyrias. A historical and clinical perspective. Am J Clin Pathol 2003;119: S86-S93.
50. Gennery AR, Cant AJ, Jeggo PA. Immunodeficiency associated with DNA repair defects. Clin Exp Immunol 2000;121:1-7.
51. Gennery AR, Cant AJ. Diagnosis of severe combined immunodeficiency. J Clin Pathol 2001;54:191-5.
52. German J. Bloom Syndrome: A Mendelian prototype of somatic mutational disease. Medicine 1993;72:393-406.
53. German J. Bloom's syndrome. Dermatol Clin 1995;13:7-18.
54. Geronemus RG. Treatment of the cutaneous vascular component of the Rothmund- Thomson syndrome. Pediatr Dermatol 1996;13:175.
55. Ghosh D. Mutations in X-linked ichthyosis disrupt the active site structure of estrone/DHEA sulfatase. Biochim Biophys Acta 2004;1739:1-4.
56. Goldsmith LA, Epstein EH Jr. Genetics in relation to the skin. In: Freedberg IM, Eisen AZ, Wolff K, Austen KF, Goldsmith LA, Katz SI, editors. Fitzpatrick's Dermatology in General Medicine. New York: McGraw-Hill; 2003;6(1):47-58.
57. Gomber S, Dewan P, Dua T.Homocystinuria: A rare cause of megaloblastic anemia.Indian Pediatr 2004;41:941-3.
58. Gordon N. Sjogren-Larsson syndrome. Dev Med Child Neurol 2007;49:152-4.
59. Goto M. Werner's syndrome: from clinics to genetics. Clin Exp Rheumatol 2000;18:760-6.
60. Guenther LC. Inherited disorders of complement. J Am Acad Dermatol 1983;9: 815-39.
61. Guerriero C, Albanesi C, Girolomoni G, DeSimone C, Capizzi R, Amerio P, et al. Huriez syndrome: case report with a detailed analysis of skin dendritic cells. Br J Dermatol 2000;143;1091-6.
62. Hampel H, Peltomaki P. Hereditary colorectal cancer: risk assessment and management. Clin Genet 2000;58:89-97.
63. Harper JI, Trembath RC. Genetics and genodermatoses. In: Burns T, Breathnach S, Cox N, Griffiths C, editors. Rook's Text Book of Dermatology, 7th edn, Vol-1. Oxford: Blackwell Science; 2004; 12.1-12.85.
64. Haug S, Braun-Falco M. Restoration of fatty aldehyde dehydrogenase deficiency in Sjögren-Larsson syndrome. Gene Ther 2006;13:1021-6.
65. Hazan C, Orlow SJ, Schaffer JV. X-linked recessive ichthyosis. Dermatology Online Journal 2005;11:12.
66. Headon DJ, Emnal SA, Ferguson BM, Tucker AS, Justice MJ, Sharpe PT, et al. Gene defect in ectodermal dysplasia implicates a death domain adaptor in development. Nature 2001; 414: 913-6.
67. Hengge UR. Progress and prospects of skin gene therapy: A ten year history. Clin Dermatol 2005; 23: 107-14.
68. Herod J, Denyar J, Goldman A, Howard R. Epidermolysis bullosa in children: Pathophysiology, anaesthesia and pain management. Paediatr Anaesth 2002; 12:388-97.
69. High WA, Miller MD. Localized epidermolytic hyperkeratosis of the female genitalia: a case report and review of an under appreciated disorder of women. Med Gen Med 2005;7:33.
70. Hoffman B, Stage H, Ruzicka T, et al. Effect of topical tazarotene in the treatment of congenital ichthoses. Br J Dermatol 1999; 141: 642-46.
71. Hom HM, Tidman MJ. The clinical spectrum of epidermolysis bullosa simplex. Br J Dermatol 2000;142:468-72.
72. Hu X, Plomp AS, van Soest S, Wijnholds J, de Jong PT, Bergen AA. Pseudoxanthoma elasticum. A clinical, histopathological and molecular update. Surv Ophthalmol 2003; 48:424-38.
73. Huang JL, Zaider E, Roth P,Garcia O,Pollack S, Poh-Fitzpatrick MB. Congenital erythropoietic porphyria: clinical, biochemical and enzymatic profile of a severely affected infant. J Am Acad Dermatol 1996;34:924-7.
74. Huizing M, Gahi WA. Disorders of vesicles of lysosomal lineage. The Hermansky-Pudlak syndrome. Curr Mol Med 2002;2:451-67.
75. Huizing M, Hess R, Dorward H, Claassen DA, Helip-Wooley A, Kleta R, et al. Cellular, molecular and clinical characterization of patients with Hermansky-Pudlak syndrome type 5. Traffic 2004;5:711-22
76. Hyman MH, Whittemore VH. National Institutes of Health Consensus Conferences: Tuberous Sclerosis Complex. Arch Neurol 2000;57:662-5.
77. Inamadar AC, Palit A, Athanikar SB, Sampagavi VV, Deshmukh NS. Rothmund thomson syndrome, report of 3 cases. Ind Jl Dermatol Venereol Leprol 2003;69:56-8.
78. Inamadar AC, Palit A, Athanikar SB, Sampagavi VV, Deshmukh NS. What syndrome is this? Olmsted syndrome. Pediatr Dermatol 2004;21:603-5.
79. Inamadar AC, Palit A. Bloom syndrome in an Indian child. Pediatr Dermatol 2005;22:147-50. Erratum in: Pediatr Dermatol. 2005:285.
80. Inamadar AC, Palit A. Cutaneous signs in heritable disorders of the connective tissue. Ind Jl Dermatol Venereol Leprol 2004;70:253-5.
81. Inamadar AC, Palit A. Peeling skin syndrome with aminoaciduria. Pediatr Dermatol 2005;22:314-6.
82. Inamadar AC, Palit A. Photosensitivity in children: an approach to diagnosis and management. Ind J Dermatol Venereol Leprol 2005;71:71-9.

83. Irvine AD, McLean WHI. The molecular genetics of the genodermatoses: progress to date and future directions. Br J Dermatol 2003;148:1-13.
84. Irvine AD, Paller AS. Inherited disorders of keratinization. Curr Probl Dermatol 2002; 71-116.
85. Irvine AD, Rugg EL, Lane EB, et al. Molecular confirmation of the unique phenotype of epidermolysis bullosa simplex with mottled pigmentation. Br J Dermatol 2001;144:40-5.
86. Itin PH, Burgdorf WHC, Happle R, Paller A, König A, Pierini A, *et al.* Genodermatoses. In: Schachner LA, Hansen RC, editors. Pediatric Dermatology. Edinburgh: Mosby; 2003;3: 263-384.
87. Jablonska S, Blaszczyk M. Scleroderma-like disorders. Semin Cutan Med Surg 1998;17:65-76.
88. Jansen GA, Waterham HR, Wanders RJ. Molecular basis of Refsum disease: sequence variations in phytanoyl-CoA hydroxylase (PHYH) and the PTS2 receptor (PEX7). Hum Mutat 2004;23:209-18.
89. Judge MR, McLean WHI, Munro CS. Disorders of keratinization. In: Burns T, Breathnach S, Cox N, Griffiths C, editors. Rook's textbook of dermatology. Oxford, Blackwell Science 2004;7:34.1-34.111.
90. Kalfa VC, Roberts RL, Stiefem ER. The syndrome of chronic mucocutaneous candidiasis with selective antibody deficiency. Ann Allergy Asthma Immunol 2003;90:259-64.
91. Kavanagh GM, Jardine PE, Peachey RD, Murray JC, De Berker D. The scleroatrophic syndrome of Huriez. Br J Dermatol 1997;137:114-8.
92. Keane FM, Mellerio JE, Ellison J, et al. Treatment of anaemia in dystrophic epidermolysis bullosa with intravenous iron (III) hydroxide-sucrose complex. Br J Dermatol 2000;143 (Suppl:57):51-2.
93. Khumalo NP, Joss DV, Huson SM, Burge S. Pigmentary anomalies in ataxia Telangiectasia. A clue to diagnosis and an example of twin spotting. Br J Dermatol 2001;144:369-71.
94. King RA, Willaert RK, Schmidt RM, Pietsch J, Savage S, Brott MJ, et al. MC1R mutations modify the classic phenotypeof oculocutaneous albinism type2 (OCA2). Am J Hum Genet 2003;73:638-45.
95. Kirkpatrick CH. Chronic mucocutaneous candidiasis. Pediatr Infect Dis J 2001; 20:197-206.
96. Kirschner LS, Carney JA, Pack SD, Taymans SE, Giatzakis C, Cho YS, *et al.* Mutations of the gene encoding the protein kinase A type -I-alpha regulatory subunit in patients with the Carney complex. Nature Genet 2000;26;89-92.
97. Kitao S, Shimamoto A, Goto M, Miller RW, Smithson WA, Lindor NM, *et al.* Mutations in *Rec*QL4 cause a subset of cases of Rothmund-Thomson syndrome. Nat Genet 1999; 22:82-4.
98. Knight SW, Heiss SS, Vulliamy TJ,Greschner S, Stavrides G, Pai GS, et al. X-linked dyskeratosis congenita is predominantly caused by missense mutations in the DKC1 gene. Am J Hum Genet 1999;65:50-8.
99. Ladda RL. Principles of genetics. In: Alper JC, editor. Genetic disorders of the skin..Louis: Mosby Year Book;1991.p.1-34.
100. Lamartine J, Munhoz Essenfelder G, Kibar Z, Lanneluc I, Callouet E, Laoudj D, et al. Mutations in GJB6 cause hidrotic ectodermal dysplasia. Nat Genet 2000;26;142-4.
101. Lambert WC, Kuo HR, Lambert MW. Xeroderma pigmentosum. Dermatol Clin 1995;13:169-209.
102. Lambert WC, Lambert MW. Diseases associated with DNA and chromosomal instability. In: Alper JC, editor. Genetic disorders of the skin. St.Louis: Mosby Year book 1991;320-58.
103. Landau M, Krafchik BR. The diagnostic value of *café-au-lait* macules. J Am Acad Dermatol 1999;40:877-90.
104. Landolt MA, Nuoffer JM, Steinmann B, Superti-Furga A. Quality of life and psychologic adjustment in childrenand adolescents with early treated phenylketonuria can be normal. J Pediatr 2002;140:516-21.
105. Larralde M, Markan PA, Peruffo L, Calb I, Magarinos G. Yellowish papules on flexural areas of a child. Pediatr Dermatol 2002;19:557-9.
106. Lilic D. New perspectives on the immunology of chronic mucocutaneous Candidiasis. Curr Opin Infect Dis 2002; 15:143-7.
107. Lindor NM, Furuichi Y, Kitao S, Shimamoto A, Arndt C, Jalal S. Rothmund-Thomson syndrome due to *Rec*QL4 helicase mutations: report and clinical and molecular comparisons with Bloom syndrome and Werner syndrome. Am J Med Genet 2000;90:223-8.
108. Listernick R, Charrow J. Neurofibromatosis-1 in childhood. In: James WD, Cockerell CJ, Hwang ST, Maloney ME, Paller AS, editors. Advances in Dermatology. Philadelphia: Mosby 2004;20:75-115.
109. Liu W, Prayson RA. Dura mater involvement in ochronosis (alkaptonuria). Arch Pathol Lab Med 2001;125:961-3.
110. Loeys B,Van Maldergem L,Mortier G,Coucke P, Gerniers S, Naeyaert JM, et al. Homozygosity for a missense mutation in fibulin -5(FBLN5) results in a severe form of cutis laxa. Hum Mol Genet 2002;11:2113-8.
111. Luo G, Santoro IM, McDaniel LD, Nishijima I, Mills M, Youssoufian H, *et al.* Cancer predisposition caused by elevated mitotic recombination in Bloom-mice. Nat Genet 2000;26:424-9.
112. Math A, Frank J, Handisurya A, Poblete-Gutierrez P, Slupetzky K, Fodinger D, et al. Identification of a de novo keratin 1 mutation in epidermolytic hyperkeratosis with palmoplantar involvement. Eur J Dermatol 2006;16:507-10.
113. Maynard TM, Haskell GT, Lieberman JA, LaMantia AS. 22q11 DS: genomic mechanisms and gene function in DiGeorge/ velocardiofacial syndrome. Int J Dev Neurosci 2002;20:407-19.
114. McGrath JA, Duijf PN, Doetsch V, Irvine AD, deWall R, Vanmolkot KR, et al. Hay-Wells syndrome is caused by heterozygous missense mutations in the SAM domain of p63. Hum Mol Genet 2001;10:221-9.
115. Mellerio JE, Pulkkinen L, McMillan JR, et al. Pyloric-atresia-junctional epidermolysis bullosa syndrome: mutation in the β4 gene (TGβ4) in two unrelated patients with mild disease. Br J Dermatol 1998;139:862-71.
116. Monk BE, Pieris S, Soni V. Schöpf-Schulz-Passarge syndrome. Br J Dermatol 1992;127:33-5.
117. Mueller RF, Young ID, editors. Chromosomes and cell division. In: Emery's elements of medical genetics,11th edn. Edinburgh: Churchill- Livingstone 2001;29-53.
118. Mueller RF, Young ID. Genetic Counseling. In: Mueller RF, Young ID, editors. Emery's elements of medical genetics. Edinburgh: Churchill-Livingstone 2001;11:241-8.
119. Mueller RF, Young ID. Prenatal diagnosis of genetic disease. In: Mueller RF, Young ID, editors. Emery's elements of medical

genetics. Edinburgh: Churchill- Livingstone 2001;11:303-11.
120. Muller CR, Fregin A, Srsen S, et al. Alleleic heterogeneity of alkaptonuria in Central Europe. Eur J Hum Genet 1999; 7:645-51.
121. Muller FB, Huber M, Kinaciyan T, Hausser I, Schaffrath C, Krieg T, et al. A human keratin 10 knockout causes recessive epidermolytic hyperkeratosis. Hum Mol Genet. 2006; 15:1133-41.
122. Munoz F, Lestringant G, Sybert V, Frydman M, Alswaini A, Frossard PM, et al. Definitive evidence for an autosomal recessive form of hypohidrotic ectodermal dysplasia clinically indistinguishable from the more common X-linked disorder. Am J Hum Genet 1997;61:94-100.
123. Nakano A, Chao SC, Pulkkinen L, et al. Laminin 5 mutations in junctional epidermolysis bullosa: molecular basis of Herlitz *vs.*non-Herlitz phenotypes. Hum Genet 2002;110:41-51.
124. Nanda A, Kanwar AJ, Kapoor MM, Thappa DM, Radotra BD, Vaishnavi C, *et al.* Rothmund-Thomson syndrome in two siblings. Pediatr Dermatol 1989;6:305-8.
125. Nellist M, van Slegtenhorst MA, Goedbloed M, van den Ouweland AM, Halley DJ, van der Sluijs P, *et al.* Characterization of the cytosolic tuberin-hamartin complex. Tuberin is a cytosolic chaperon of hamartin. J Biol Chem 1999;274: 35647-52.
126. Notarangelo L, Casanova JL, Fischer A, Puck J, Rosen F, Seger R, et al. Primary immunodeficiency diseases: an update. J Allergy Clin Immunol 2004;114:677-87.
127. Nuytinck L, Freund M, Lagae L, Pierard GE, Hermanns-Le T, De Paepe A. Classical Ehlers-Danlos syndrome caused by a mutation in type I collagen. Am J Hum Genet 2000;66:1398-1402.
128. Omerod AD, White MI, McKay E, Johnston AW. Incontinentia pigmenti in a boy with Klinefelter's syndrome. J Med Genet 1987;24:439-41.
129. Paller AS, Manzini AJ. Hereditary disorders of the dermis. In: Paller AS, Manzini AJ,editors. Hurwitz Clinical Pediatric Dermatology, 3rd edn. Philadelphia: Elsevier Saunders; 2006;129-44.
130. Pavithran K, Nair RP, Dharmaratnam AD. Symmetrical progressive erythrokeratoderma. Indian J Dermatol Venereol Leprol 1983;49:36-8.
131. Pianigiani E, De Aloe G, Andreasi A, Rubegni P, Fimiani M. Rothmund-Thomson syndrome (Thomson type) and myelodysplasia. Pediatr Dermatol 2001;18:422-5.
132. Pignault V, Bondurand N, Lemort N, et al. A heterozygous endothelin 3 mutation in Waardenburg-Hirschsprung disease: is there a dosage effect of EDN3/EDNRB gene mutations on neurocristopathy phenotypes? J Med Genet 2001;38:205-9.
133. Pinheiro M, Freire-Maia N. Ectodermal dysplasias. A clinical classification and a causal review. Am J Med Genet 1994; 53:153-62.
134. Rantamaki T, Kaitila I, Syvanen AC, Lukka M, Peltonen L. Recurrence of Marfan Syndrome as a result of parental germ-line mosaicism for an FBN1 mutation. Am J Hum Genet 1999; 64:993-1001.
135. Reddy BSN, Kochar AM, Anitha M, Bamezai R. Bloom's syndrome-a first report from India. Int J Dermatol 2000; 39:760-73.
136. Refsum H, Fredriksen A, Meyer K, Ueland PM, Kase BF. Birth prevalence of Homocystinuria. J Pediatr 2004;144:830-2.
137. Ringpfeil F, Pulkkinen L, Uitto J. Molecular genetics of pseudoxanthoma elasticum. Exp Dermatol 2001;10:221-8.
138. Rizzo WB. Sjögren-Larsson syndrome: Molecular genetics and biochemical pathogenesis of fatty aldehyde dehydrogenase deficiency. Mol Genet Metab 2007;90:1-9.
139. Ruggieri M, Huson SM. The clinical and diagnostic implications of mosaicism in the neurofibromatoses. Neurology 2001;56:1433-43.
140. Sampson J, Maheshwar M, Aspinwall R, Thompson P, Cheadle JP, Ravine D, *et al.* Renal cystic disease in tuberous sclerosis: role of polycystic kidney disease 1 gene. Am J Hum Genet 1997;61:843-51.
141. Schalkwijk J, Zweers MC, Steijlen PM, Dean WB, Taylor G, van Vlijmen IM, *et al.* A recessive form of the Ehlers-Danlos syndrome caused by tenascin-X deficiency. N Eng J Med 2001;345:1167-75.
142. Schnur RE, Grace K, Herzberg A. Buschke-Ollendorff syndrome, otosclerosis and congenital spinal stenosis. Pediatr Dermatol 1994;11:31-4.
143. Segal BH, Leto TL, Gallin JL, et al. Genetic, biochemical, and clinical features of the chronic granulomatous disease. Medicine 2000;79:170.
144. Shaw PH, Mancini AJ, McConnell JP, Brown D, Kletzel M. Treatment of congenital erythropoietic porphyria in children by allogeneic stem cell transplantation: A case report and review of the literature. Bone Marrow Transplant 2001; 27:101-5.
145. Siegel DH, Howard R. Molecular advances in genetic skin diseases. Curr Opin Pediatr 2002;14:419-25.
146. Smahi A, Hyden-Granskog C, Peterlin B, et al. The gene for the familial form of incontinentia pigmenti (IP2) maps to the distal part of Xq28. Hum Mol Genet 1994;3:273-8.
147. Sonea MJ, Moroz BE, Reece ER. Leiner's disease associated with diminished third component of complement. Pediatr Dermatol 1987;4: 105-7.
148. Spacey SD, Gatti RA, Bebb G. The molecular basis and clinical management of ataxia telangiectasia. Can J Neurol Sci 2000; 27:184-91.
149. Spacey SD, Gatti RA, Bebb G. The molecular basis and clinical management of ataxia-telangiectasia. Can J Neurol Sci 2001; 27:184-91.
150. Spritz RA. Piebaldism, Waardenburg syndrome and related disorders of melanocyte development. Semin Cutan Med Surg 1997; 16:15-23.
151. Starink TM, Van der Veen JPW, Arwert F, deWall LP, deLange GG, Gille JJ, *et al.* The Cowden syndrome: a clinical and genetic study in 21 patients. Clin Genet 1986;29:222-33.
152. Sullivan KE. DiGeorge syndrome/chromosome 22q11.2 deletion syndrome. Curr Allergy Asthma Rep 2001;1:438-44.
153. Sybert VP. Ectodermal dysplasias. In: Freedberg IM, Eisen AZ, Wolff K, Austen KF,Goldsmith LA, Katz SI, editors. Fitzpatrick's Dermatology in General Medicine. New York: Mc Graw-Hill; 2003: 6(1):515-22.
154. Taback SP, Collu R, Deal CL, Guyda HJ, Salisburg S, Dean HJ, *et al.* Does growth hormone supplementation affect adult height in Turner's syndrome? Lancet 1996;348:25-27.

155. Taylor AMR. Chromosome instability syndromes. Best Pract Res Clin Haematol 2001;14:631-44.
156. Thomas AC, Cullup T, Norgett EE, Hill T, Barton S, Dale BA, et al. ABCA12 is the major harlequin ichthyosis gene. J Invest Dermatol 2006;126:2408-13.
157. Thrasher AJ, Kinnon C. The Wiskott-Aldrich syndrome. Clin Exp Immunol 2000;120:2-9.
158. Thunell S, Harper P, Brun A. Porphyrins, porphyrin metabolism and porphyrias. IV.Pathophysiology of erythropoietic protoporphyria- diagnosis, care and monitoring of the patient. Scand J Clin Lab Invest 2000;60:581-604.
159. Toyofuku K, Wada I, Spritz RA, Hearing VJ. The molecular basis of oculocutaneous albinism type 1 (OCA1): sorting failure and degradation of mutant tyrosinases results in a lack of pigmentation. Biochem J 2001;355 (Pt 2): 259-69.
160. Vennos EM, Collins M, James WD. Rothmund- Thomson syndrome: review of the world literature. J Am Acad Dermatol 1992;27:750-62.
161. Ventruto V. A simplified method for observing and recording dermatoglyphic patterns, including counting sweat pores. Clin Genet 1986; 30: 525-7.
162. Vogel JC, Walker PS, Hengge UR. Gene therapy for skin diseases. Advances in Dermatology 1996;11:383-98.
163. Ward DM, Shiflett SL, Kaplan J. Chediak-Higashi syndrome: A clinical and molecular view of a rare lysosomal storage disorder. Curr Mol Med 2002;2: 469-77.
164. Wienecke R, Konig A, Declue JE. Identification of tuberin, the tuberous sclerosis-2 product. Tuberin possesses specific RAP1 GAP activity. J Biol Chem 1995;270;16409-14.
165. Wolkenstein P, Frèche B, Zeller J, Revuz J. Usefulness of screening investigations in neurofibromatosis type 1. A study of 152 patients. Arch Dermatol 1996;132:1333-6.
166. Yap S. Classical homocystinuria: Vascular risk and its prevention. J Inherit Metab Dis 2003;26:259-65.
167. Yarosh D, Klein J, O'Connor A, Hawk J, Rafal E, Wolf P. Effect of topically applied T4 endonuclease V in liposomes on skin cancer in xeroderma pigmentosum: a randomized study. Lancet 2001;357:926-9.
168. Yoo S, Simzar S, Han K, Takahashi S, Cotliar R. Erythrokeratoderma variabilis successfully treated with topical tazarotene. Pediatr Dermatol 2006;23:382-5.
169. Zeitlin L, Rauch F, Plotkin H, Glorieux FH. The effects of intravenous pamidronate on the bone tissue of children and adolescents with osteogenesis imperfecta types I, III and IV. Pediatrics 2003; 111: 1030-6.
170. Zibolen M, Srsnova K, Srsen S. Increased urolithiasis in patients with alkaptonuria in childhood. Clin Genet 2000;58:79-80.

4

Eczemas

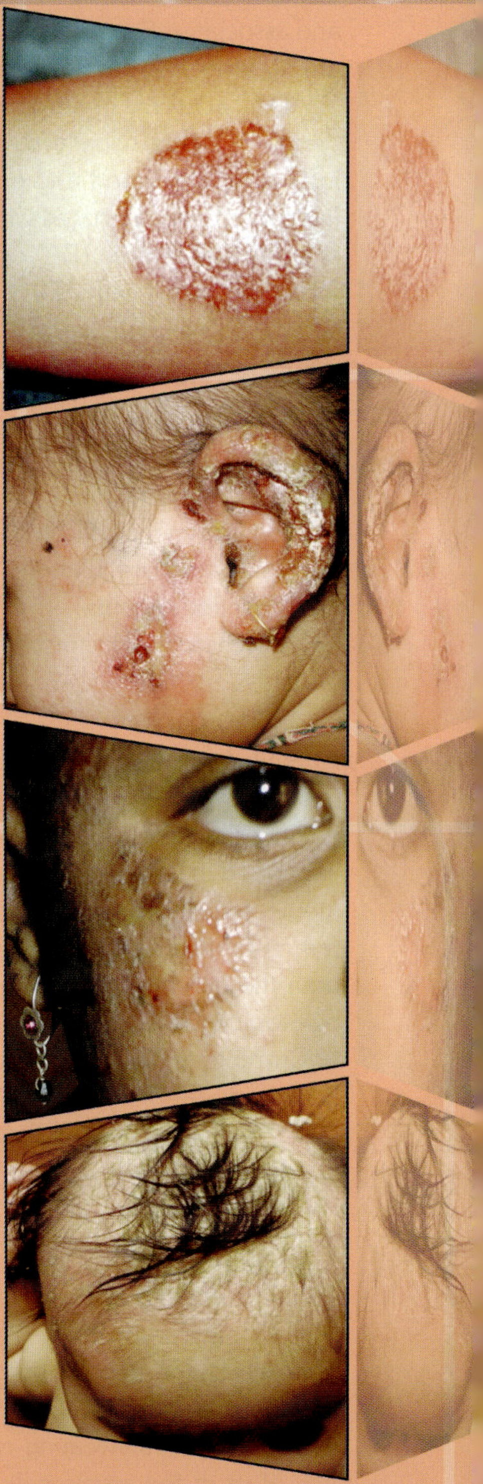

Atopic Dermatitis
Sandipan Dhar

Eczemas other than Atopic Dermatitis
Sanjeev Handa

ATOPIC DERMATITIS (SYN: ATOPIC ECZEMA, BESNIER'S PRURIGO)

INTRODUCTION

The term 'atopy' was coined by Coca and Cooke. The disease was named as 'atopic dermatitis' by Sulzberger and associates. Besnier in 1892 described the association of hay fever and asthma with atopic dermatitis (AD)

AD is a chronic or chronically relapsing inflammatory dermatosis that usually manifests for the first time in infancy or childhood and gradually improves with age. It is commonly associated with either allergic rhinitis (AR) or bronchial asthma (BA) or both, which may precede, follow or coexist with AD.

ETIOPATHOGENESIS

Various etiological factors implicated in the pathogenesis of AD are:

1. Hereditary factors
2. Environmental factors
3. Immunodysregulation
4. Infectious agents
5. Psychological factors

Hereditary Factors

A family history of 'atopy' can be obtained in approximately 43-73% of the cases with AD. Studies have shown a concordance of 85% for AD in monozygotic twins as compared to 20% in dizygotic twins. When the mother is atopic, the offsprings are more likely to get the disease rather than when the father is affected. However, when both the parents are atopic, the chances of the child to be atopic increase several folds.

Currently it has been documented that the control of IgE production lies on chromosome 11q13 marker D11S97. The genes implicated are divided into class I and II as follows.

Environmental Factors

Atopic dermatitis is supposed to be more common in urban than rural set up. This is probably because of industrialization and changed lifestyle. In general AD is known to aggravate during winter. However, heat and exercise induced sweating can increase the pruritus of AD. Most of the atopic individuals usually sweat much more as compared to their non-atopic counterparts. Cholinergic hyper responsiveness may, thus be responsible for influencing the course of AD.

Immunodysregulation

Th2 cells play a significant role in the immunopathogenesis of AD. Raised IgE levels and an increased number of eosinophils are found in the blood of AD patients. In addition, blood of patients with AD is rich in allergen specific T-cells, which produce IL-4, IL-5 and IL-13. These cytokines not only promote antibody response but also inhibit the production of Th1 cytokines IFN-γ, IL-2 and TNF-α by the T-cells. Increased expression of cAMP phosphodiesterase (PDE) in immune cells leading to increased production of PDE2 and IL-10 by monocytes and eventual interference with the production of IFN-γ is seen in AD.

Infectious Agents

The increased incidence of carriage state of *Staphylococcus aureus* has been a subject of interest in patients with AD. Several studies, including one by the author have also demonstrated increased carriage state of *S. aureus* in both involved and uninvolved skin in patients with AD. Exacerbation of AD is reported to be induced when the density of *S. aureus* is greater than 10^6 CFU/cm^2 (colony forming unit). It is advisable to try treatment with oral anti-staphylococcal antibiotic in any child with moderate to severe atopic dermatitis.

Psychological Factors

AD has a tremendous psychological effect on various aspects of life of an affected individual. In children, it has been found that a hyper-responsive hypothalamic-pituitary-axis (HPA) blunts the body's capability to produce cortisol during the period of stress. The resultant inability to suppress inflammatory response leads to aggravation of the eczema. It is quite well known that children suffering from AD usually have a swinging mood with frequent fluctuations. Many a times such mood fluctuations correlate well with the severity of AD. Menarche often precipitates AD for the first-time.

PREVALENCE AND INCEDENCE OF AD

Recently there have been concerns over the increase in the global incidence of AD. Around 10-20% of children in developed countries suffer from AD. In a study in India of duration over 7.5 years (January 1987 to June 1994) by the author, an incidence of AD among total dermatology outpatient attendees in a tertiary care hospital was recorded to be 0.42%. Cases of AD comprised 28.46% of the total number of cases of pediatric skin disease. In India though the prevalence of full blown AD is low, minor forms of AD, e.g., pityriasis alba, juvenile plantar dermatitis, infra/retroauricular fissuring occur quite frequently.

DIAGNOSTIC FEATURES

Hanifin and Rajka proposed a systematic approach towards the standardization of the diagnosis of AD by incorporating 3 major/basic and 23 minor features **(Figures 4.1 to 4.6)**. They suggested that a diagnosis of AD can be established if 3 of the major and 3 of the minor criteria are present. These are highlighted in **Tables 4.1 and 4.2**.

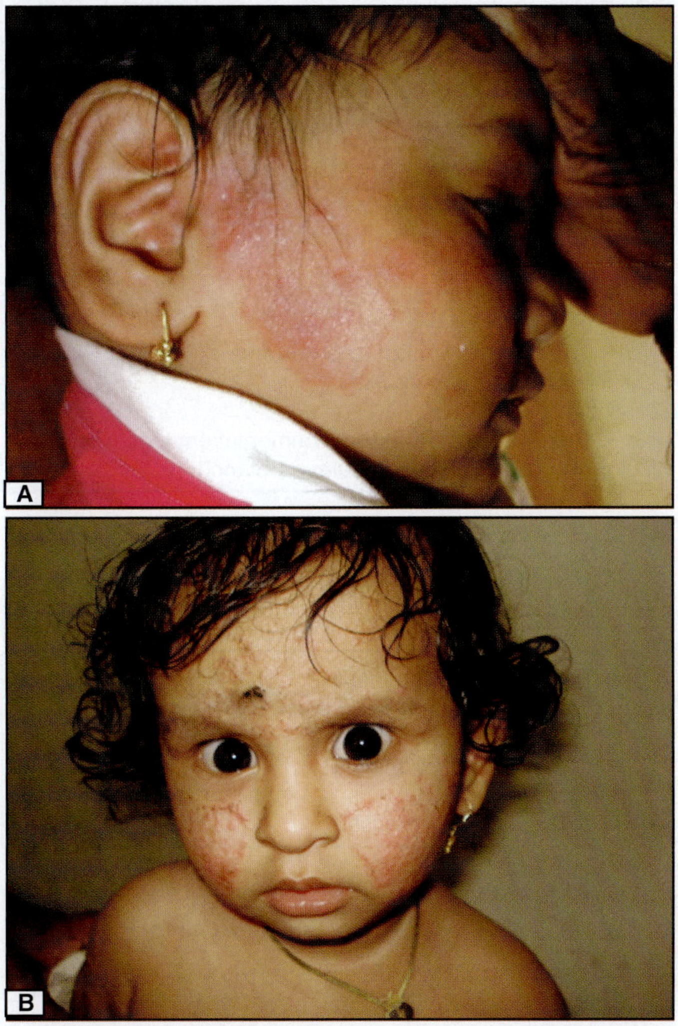

FIGURES 4.1A AND B: Facial involvement in infantile AD

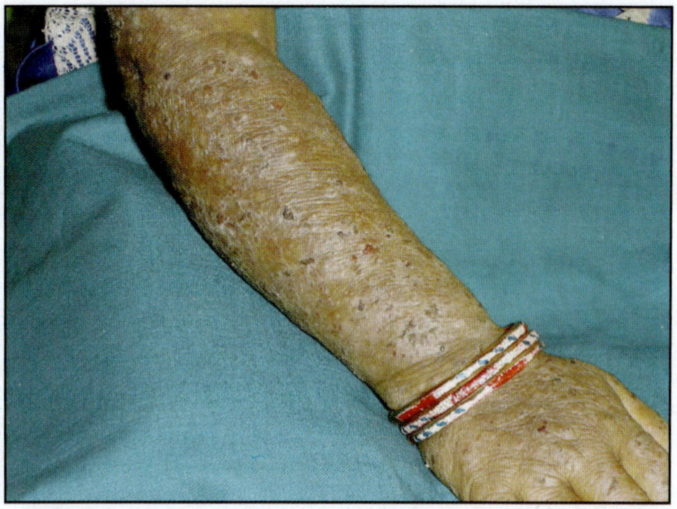

FIGURE 4.2: Crusted papules and lichenification involving extensor extremity

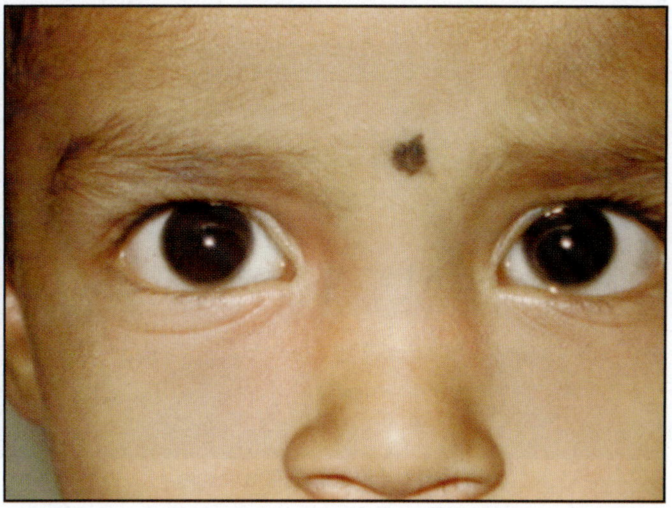

FIGURE 4.3: Dennie-Morgan fold

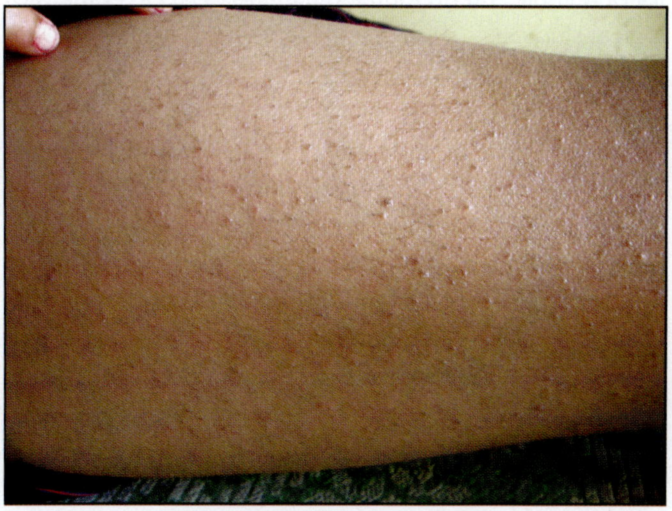

FIGURE 4.4: Keratosis pilaris

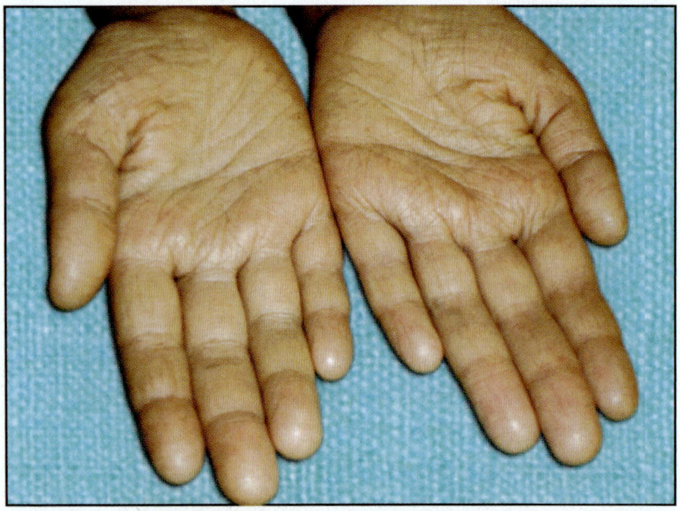

FIGURE 4.5: Hyperlinearity of palms

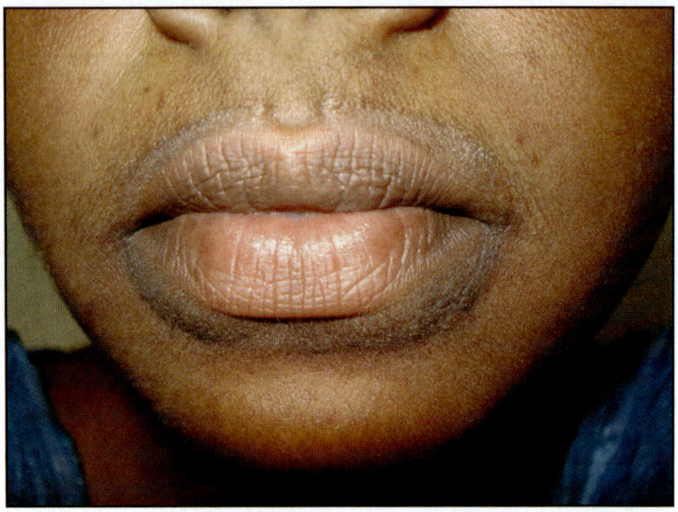

FIGURE 4.6: Lipstick cheilitis

The recently formulated UK working party's diagnostic criteria **(Table 4.3)** are aimed at developing a minimum list of reliable criteria for the diagnosis of AD in epidemiological studies.

The Key Steps to Diagnose AD

History: Personal and family history of atopic manifestations are important for the diagnosis of AD. The risk of developing AD is proportional to the number of family members affected. The history of associated asthma (mean age at onset 4-5 years) and allergic rhinitis (mean age at onset 9-10 years) is important in later part of childhood. The onset of AD is usually below 2 years of age. The lesions are invariably very itchy and may impair night's sleep. Precipitation of itching by sweating and worsening of eczema by emotion and anxiety are classical features of AD.

TABLE 4.1: Major/ Basic features for the diagnosis of atopic dermatitis

1. Pruritus
2. Typical morphology and distribution: flexural lichenification or linearity in adults, facial and extensor involvement in infants and children.
3. Chronic or chronically relapsing dermatitis.
4. Personal or family history of atopy (asthma, allergic rhinitis, atopic dermatitis)

TABLE 4.2: Minor/less characteristic features for the diagnosis of atopic dermatitis

1. Xerosis
2. Ichthyosis/palmar hyperlinarity/keratosis pilaris
3. Immediate (type 1) skin test reactivity.
4. Elevated serum IgE
5. Early age at onset
6. Tendency towards cutaneous infections (esp. *Staphylococcus aureus* and *Herpes simplx*)/impired cell mediated immunity
7. Tendency towards nonspecific hand or foot dermatitis
8. Nipple eczema
9. Cheilitis
10. Recurrent conjunctivitis
11. Dennie-Morgan infraorbital folds
12. Keratoconus
13. Anterior subcapsular cataracts
14. Orbital darkening
15. Facial pallor/facial erythema
16. Pityriasis alba
17. Anterior neck folds
18. Itch when sweating
19. Intolerance to wool or lipid solvents
20. Perifollicular accentuation
21. Food intolerance
22. Course influenced by environmental/emotional factors
23. White dermographism/delayed blanch

TABLE 4.3: UK working party's diagnostic criteria of AD

1. History of flexural dermatitis
2. Onset under the age of 2 years
3. Presence of an itchy rash
4. Personal history of asthma
5. History of a dry skin
6. Visible flexural dermatitis

Clinical presentations: The diagnosis of a classical full blown case of AD is not difficult. However, the manifestations of AD may not always be classical and presentation may be with only a few minor features. This is particularly so among Indian children. Only a high degree of suspicion and awareness about it can pick up these minor forms of AD known as 'atopic diathesis.' In day-to-day practice, the diagnosis of AD is made on the basis of eczematous lesions, usually multiple and pruritic, with associated personal history of 'atopy'. The skin of these infants and children is almost always dry and they usually experience pruritus all over the body. The children are usually a little hyperactive and restless but intelligent.

The clinical manifestations of AD among Indian children are less severe compared to the western counterparts. This could be because of the following facts:

- The practice of prolonged breastfeeding,
- Different climate,
- Different food habits in mothers and babies,
- Clothing
- Under-developed industrialization,
- Different lifestyle
- Genetic factor.

Laboratory investigations: Total serum IgE is elevated in >80% of patients with AD. A positive correlation with the extent and severity of the disease as well as respiratory atopic disease has been found. However, IgE may be raised in a host of other conditions apart from 'atopy'. It does not predict the course and long term prognosis of the disease. Moreover in 20-40% of the patients having pure AD, IgE values may be normal. The author had investigated this aspect of AD in India.

Specific IgE antibodies against environmental antigens can be detected in most patients with AD. Children with associated respiratory atopy have up to 100% positive RASTs for airborne allergens, and 80% positive for foods. In children with pure AD, specific IgE can only be found in about 20% of the cases.

DIFFERENTIAL DIAGNOSIS

In an individual patient one must consider a number of other conditions which may simulate AD. In infants, seborrheic dermatitis is the most common differential diagnosis. At times it may be difficult to differentiate between these two entities because of some overlapping features. Pruritus, age at onset and a family history of atopy cannot reliably differentiate between these two conditions. Lesions over forearms and shins, specific serum IgE to egg white and milk favors a diagnosis of AD. In infantile seborrheic dermatitis, the lesions are found in axillae and/or in napkin area.

Scabies in babies often undergoes eczematization, particularly over the face, quite closely simulating AD. A history of acute-onset pruritus among the family contacts, presence of burrows, inflamed papules and nodules over the genital and axillary areas support a diagnosis of scabies with eczematization.

There are a number of genetic and metabolic disorders where an eruption resembling AD (with or without other atopic disorders) may be seen or these are associated with a raised IgE level. Many such conditions are primary immunodeficiency disorders **(Table 4.4)**.

TABLE 4.4: AD like conditions with immunocompromised state

1.	Agammaglobulinaemia
2.	Anhidrotic ectodermal dysplasia
3.	Ataxia-telangiectasia
4.	Coeliac disease
5.	Cystic fibrosis (heterozygote)
6.	Histidine depletion (experimental)
7.	Hurler's syndrome
8.	Hyper IgE syndrome
9.	Hypereosinophilic syndrome
10.	Jung's disease
11.	Nephrotic syndrome
12.	Netherton's syndrome
13.	Phenylketonuria
14.	Wiskott-Aldrich syndrome

COMPLICATIONS

Complications may be encountered in all patients with AD **(Figures 4.7 and 4.8)**. However, these are more common in patients with extensive eczema. Various complications encountered are:

1. Extensive staphylococcal pyoderma.
2. Kaposi's varicelliform eruptions from disseminated herpes infection
3. Extensive molluscum contagiosum lesions.
4. Extensive verruca vulgaris or common warts.
5. Disseminated dermatophytic infections.
6. Disseminated candidal infections.
7. Various psychological complications.

NATURAL HISTORY AND PROGNOSIS

Studies on the natural history of atopic dermatitis have produced variable results. In one study, 90% of the children were found to undergo spontaneous resolution by 10 years of age. However, other studies have shown that in only 60% of the affected children the disease cleared by 16 years of age. Overall, when started in

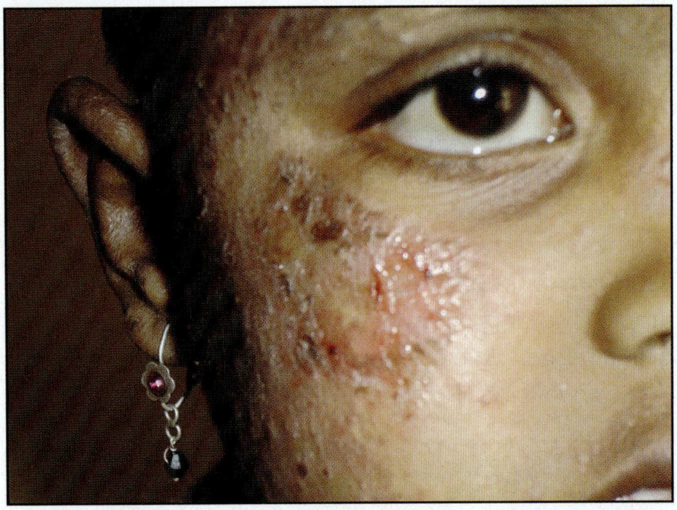

FIGURE 4.7: Atopic dermatitis with secondary bacterial infection

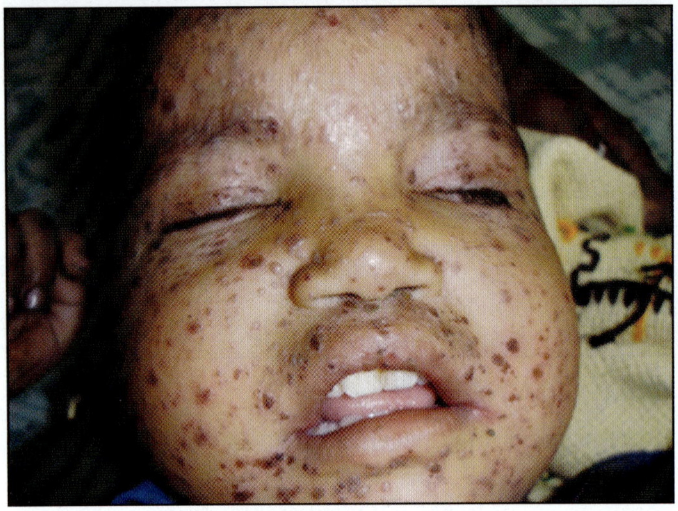

FIGURE 4.8: Eczema herpeticum

infancy, the disease follows a stepwise reduction in the severity over next 10-12 years and by 12-15 years it heals completely. However, true clearance rate may actually be far from these figures. Many children or individuals probably relapse at some stage in adulthood either in the form of irritant hand eczema or pompholyx or dyshidrotic eczema of the hands. Factors which may indicate a poor prognosis include severe childhood disease, early onset and concomitant family history of asthma/hay fever.

MANAGEMENT OF ATOPIC DERMATITIS

Successful management of AD requires a systematic, multi-pronged approach that incorporates skin hydration, topical glucocorticoid therapy and identification and elimination of flare factors such as irritants, allergens, infectious agents and emotional stress. The treatment schedule is categorized into two broad groups:

(i) General measures
(ii) Specific measures

General Measures

As atopic dermatitis often shows flare-ups, measures should be taken to identify the trigger factors for itch; this improves sleep and family interactions and reduces absenteeism from school.

Most children have a dry skin. In tropical countries where sweating is excessive, overuse of soap predisposes the skin to irritation. Soap should be less alkaline (pH 5.5) and not to be used very frequently. However twice a day regular use is beneficial as far as the skin cleaning is concerned.

Avoiding contact of woolen and synthetic garments with the skin is another important aspect. These cause irritation when in contact with dry skin precipitating the itch-scratch cycle. Parents should be advised to put cotton lining or undergarments beneath such dresses.

It is seen that house dust mite antigen promotes a flaring up reaction. The most common house dust mite is *Dermatophagoides pteronyssinus*. Animal danders can also aggravate AD. In patients with AD, allergic to dust-mite, prolonged avoidance of dust has been found to result in improvement of skin lesions. Avoidance measures include use of dust mite proof encasings on pillows, mattresses, and box springs, washing the beddings in hot water weekly, removal of bedroom carpets and decrease indoor humidity levels with air conditioning. The family must be discouraged to keep furry pets.

If there is definite history of aggravation of eczema after intake of some kind of foods, e.g. egg or fish, it should be omitted from the diet. However, in infants and children with a strong family history of 'atopy', it is advisable to avoid cow's milk, wheat, soy, peanuts and egg up to at least 2 years of age. Patients should be advised about the risk of *Herpes simplex* infection in a child with atopic dermatitis and told to avoid contact of active cold sores with the child's skin.

Specific Measures

This includes institution of appropriate therapy according to the severity of the disease, in addition to the general measures. Conventionally there are three lines of management depending upon the severity of illness and extent of involvement of skin by the disease process.

First line of therapy: It is intended for patients with milder disease and includes application of emollients, topical corticosteroids, with or without antibiotics and oral antihistamines.

Emollients: Emollients, e.g. petrolatum jelly are occlusive agents which make the skin soft and pliable by increasing the hydration of stratum corneum. These are used in the management of AD. After a short bath (approximately 5 minutes) in tepid water, the skin is patted with a soft towel in such a way that a thin film of water remains on the skin. Immediately an emollient is applied over the wet skin. The idea is to trap the water in the skin to maintain hydration. Two to three such applications of emollient a day will keep the skin soft and supple. Bath oils are used in the west. In India, however, body massage with coconut oil before bath can be advocated as an effective alternative to costly bath oils.

Bath: It is true that soaps and detergents used during bathing remove the lipid and oil from skin surface and exert a drying effect exacerbating eczema. But regular bathing is advantageous as it allows removal of dirt and debris from the skin and thereby reduces the chance of infection. Bathing also helps to keep a thin film of emollient over the skin surface when a moisturizing soap is used.

The water for bathing should be lukewarm. Addition of antiseptics to bath water may reduce the commensal bacteria on skin-surface, thus increasing chances of infection by pathogenic organisms. Use of coaltar or ketoconazole containing shampoo is useful in reducing excessive scaling over the scalp in atopic children.

Cleansing products: Soaps are the commonly used cleansing agents. The alkalinity induced by soaps can alter the pH of skin surface. In hard water, soap may form a precipitate of calcium and magnesium salts. This will get deposited on the hair and skin. 'Syndets' (synthetic detergents) can be produced at desired pH. It requires preservation for stability. Unless emollient is a constituent, like soaps, these can also cause dryness.

Compress: Compresses are wet dressings used effectively in the management of acute eczema. There are different types; such as saline compresses, medicated compresses wherein potassium permanganate, silver nitrate or hydrogen peroxide can be used as additive. 'Wet wraps' may be useful in extensive oozing lesions.

Topical corticosteroids: Topical corticosteroids still remain the first line of treatment for treating majority of the cases of AD. However, AD is a chronic disease frequented by relapses; hence topical corticosteroids need to be prescribed from time to time to control the eczema.

Priority should be given to the desired potency of the steroid. The decision is based on the patient's age and the type, severity, extent, location and the duration of eczema. **Table 4.5** gives a guideline of this and **Table 4.6** highlights some commonly used topical corticosteroids in AD. Fluticasone and mometasone, though potent, have less potential for causing local skin atrophy and adrenal suppression from systemic absorption. Fluticasone is approved by US FDA for use in infants above 3 months of age.

1. Whether to choose ointment, cream, gel or lotion?
Vehicles are an important consideration while opting for topical corticosteroid therapy. Ointments have an oily base, hence gives an occlusive effect (like emollients) after application. Hence the penetration of the drug is better and potency increases. Thick lichenified areas are best sites for using ointments. Creams have watery base, best applied on non lichenified mild eczematous areas. Lotions and gels are best for intertriginous and hairy areas. Lotions are also used over oozy areas. Gels can give rise to stinging sensation and better avoided in small children.

2. How much to apply?
Finger tip unit (FTU): A fingertip unit is the amount of ointment expressed from a tube with a nozzle of 5 mm diameter, applied from the distal skin crease to the tip of the palmar aspect of the index finger. One FTU weighs 0.49 g and covers 312 cm^2 in adult males. In adult females, it weighs 0.43 g and covers 257 cm^2. A guideline given in **Table 4.7** shows the required FTUs in different body parts at various ages. Usually twice daily application is sufficient.

Topical calcineurin inhibitors: Long-term use of topical steroid is associated with local atrophy and telangiectasia. In addition, there may be percutaneous absorption resulting in systemic side effects. Hence, for long-term maintenance therapy of AD, topical calcineurin inhibitors like tacrolimus and pimecrolimus are in use. Of the two, tacrolimus is more effective as well as cheaper.

Tacrolimus: The long-term efficacy of tacrolimus (0.03%) ointment has been studied in large, multicentric trials in

TABLE 4.5: Considerations for chosing a topical corticosteroid (TCs) product

Potency (Class)	Type of dermatoses	Extent of dermatoses	Duration of TCs usage	Location of dermatoses	Usage in infants & children	State of the epidermis
Super-potent (I)	Dermatoses resistant to intermediate or high potency TCs	Avoid extensive application (>50g weekly)	For short term use only; 2-3 weeks at a time	Do not use on face, axilla, submammary area of groin	Avoid use in infants & children <12 yrs	Best for thick lichenified/ hypertrophic skin
High (II & III)	Severe	Avoid extensive application (>50g weekly)	For short term use if extensive application to atrophy prone areas	Do not use over face, axilla, submammary area or groin	Avoid use in infants & children <12 yrs.	Best for thick lichenified or hypertrophic skin; avoid on thin skin.
Intermediate (IV & V) moderately potent	Mild to Moderate	Best for short term treatment of extensive AD	Avoid extended use (>1-2 weeks) in infants and children	Best on trunk and extremities	Avoid extended use (>1-2 wks) in infants & children	Safer for short term use on thin skin. Less effective on thicker skin
Low (VI & VII) potent	Mild	Preferred for treatment of large areas	Best if long term treatment is required	Best choice for face, axilla, groin, and other moist occluded areas	Infants & children	Best for thin skin not effective on thick skin

TABLE 4.6: Some commonly used corticosteroid preparations according to their potency

Superpotent	**Moderately Potent**
Clobetsol propionate 0.05% ointment	Mometasone furoate cream 0.1%
Betamethasone dipropionate 0.05%	Fluticaone propionate ointment/ cream (0.05%) Prednicarbate cream 0.25% Betamethasone valerate (0.05%)
Highly potent	**Mildly potent**
Mometasone ointment 0.1%	Clobetasone butyrate 0.05%
Betamethasone diproprionate cream 0.5%	Aclometasone diproplonate 0.05%
Beclomethasone	Hydrocortisone acetate 0.1%
Dipropionate 0.025%	
Prednicarbate 0.25% ointment	

TABLE 4.7: Estimation of the necessary amount of topical corticosteroid for children

Anatomic area	FTU required to cover			
	3-6 month	1-2 year	3-5 months	6-10 years
Face & neck	1	1.5	1.5	2
Arm & hand	1	1.5	2	2.5
Leg & foot	1.5	2	3	4.5
Anterior trunk	1	2	3	3.5
Posterior-trunk & buttocks	1.5	3	3.5	5

children with moderate to severe AD. Tacrolimus ointment (0.03%) was applied to all affected areas twice daily for up to 12 months in children with AD. It was found to be significantly more effective than placebo. The adverse effects of topical tacrolimus may be local or systemic. These include burning and erythema at the application-site, pruritus and stinging, allergic reaction at a distant site, herpes simplex infection at the site of application as well as non-application site, folliculitis, flu-like syndrome, headache etc. However, these are usually mild and transient and majority disappear on continuation of treatment.

Pimecrolimus (SD2 ASM 981): Topical pimecrolimus is applied as 1.0% cream twice daily over the eczematous lesions. It reduces pruritus and controls flare and inflammation. It has been evaluated in randomized double blind vehicle controlled clinical trials in infants, children and adults with mild to severe AD.

Adverse effects are usually mild and transient, e.g., burning, pruritus at the local site, herpes simplex or herpes zoster virus infections.

Systemic Therapy

Majority of the cases of AD can be controlled with topical therapy, oral antihistamines and oral anti-staphylococcal antibiotics. This is particularly so for Indian patients with AD, in whom severe grades of the disease is uncommon. Systemic therapy may be required to treat AD under following circumstances:

1. Non-response to topical therapy
2. Widespread eczema/erythroderma due to AD
3. Frequent relapses
4. Patients requiring frequent courses of systemic steroids.
5. Significant compromise in quality of life (QOL), e.g., sleep disturbance, school-absenteeism, etc.

Various systemic therapies include immuno-suppressants, immune response modifiers, anti-inflammatory agents etc. **Table 4.8** enumerates the systemic therapeutic modalities.

TABLE 4.8: Systemic modalities for AD

Immunosuppressants
i. Oral corticosteroids
ii. Cyclosporine
iii. Azathioprine
iv. Methotrexate
v. Mycophenolate mofetil
Immune response modifiers
vi. Gamma interferon
vii. Leucotriene inhibitors
viii. Inti IgE antibodies (Omazulimab)
ix. High dose intravenons immuoglobulin (hdIvIG)
Miscellaneous agents
x. Oral antihistamines
xi. Evening primrose oil
xii. Antibiotics antifungals, antivirals
xiii. Traditional Chinese herbal medicine

Antihistamines: These have an important role in the management of atopic dermatitis. The conventional class 1 (First generation) H1-antihistamines are the mainstay of treatment because of their additional sedative effect. Agents like promethazine, trimeperazine or hydroxyzine, given 1 hour prior to bedtime can be useful when there is severe nocturnal itching. However, in infants, these may sometimes result in paradoxical excitation. These are best used for short duration, as tachyphylaxis occurs with prolonged use. Cetirizine can be used long-term (6 to18 months) to reduce the severity of itching with a secondary effect of improvement or subsidence of the dermatitis. The author prefers to use cetirizine in infants (>6 months old) and children in this way. Most studies conclude that non-sedating 2nd generation antihistamines are of little value for the pruritus of atopic dermatitis.

Systemic corticosteroids: Systemic corticosteroids control the inflammation and eczema very rapidly and severity of the disease is reduced quickly and effectively. However, liberal use of systemic steroids is limited by relapses on withdrawal, long-term serious adverse effects and steroid dependence. Systemic steroids are used to tide over the crisis of acute flares of AD. It is usually given at a dose of 1mg/Kg body weight/day and tapered off by 2-3 weeks. If there is a tendency of rebound flare, it is better to add a steroid-sparing agent like azathioprine, which helps to curtail the dose of steroid and keep the disease under control.

Cyclosporine (CyA): CyA has been extensively studied for the treatment of severe AD in children and is currently considered as the first line therapy for treating severe and extensive AD in the western countries. The drug is started at a dose of 3-5 mg/Kg body weight/day in 2 divided doses. The response is observed by 2-3 weeks of initiation of treatment. The dose can be subsequently tapered off to 1mg/kg every alternate week to stop it completely by 3-6 months. Although there are reports of long-term remission of AD with CyA, relapses within few weeks of stoppage of treatment occurs in majority of the patients. The author has a personal experience of treating 25-children with moderate to severe AD with cyclosporine. The median duration to control the disease was 2.5 weeks. Relapses occurred in 18 of 25-children after 3-6 weeks of stoppage of the drug. Hypertrichosis was observed in 5 of the 14 girls after a variable period of 2-4 months of CyA use.

Immunomodulators: Methotrexate has been used in children at a dose of 2.5 mg (or 5 mg in larger adolescents) daily for 4 days sequentially in a week for a period of 1-2 months. It needs a weekly complete blood count and monthly liver function test monitoring.

Azathioprine has been found to work quite effectively in children with severe recalcitrant dermatitis given over a period of 3-4 months.

Interferon gamma at a dose of 50 ug/m^2 daily or on alternate days has shown promising results in some pediatric patients with AD.

Desensitization: Desensilization with the allergens is not a very useful and practicable modality. This plays a very limited role in the management of AD even when an allergic factor has been firmly established clinically.

Complementary treatments: *Probiotics* significantly reduce the risk of development of AD during the first 4 years of life in infants whose mothers received *Lactobacillus rhamnosus(Lactobacillus GG)* during pregnancy and lactation. Addition of *Lactobacillus* GG and *Lactobacillus reuteri* to children up to 13 years of age improved the patients' evaluation of their dermatitis.

Montelukast, a leucotriene antagonist has by and large been found ineffective.

Chinese herbal medicine was found to significantly reduce eczema, inflammation, erythema and pruritus in patients with AD. The beneficial response is however, short-lived even on continuation of treatment. The possibility of toxicities on long term use of the drug is a matter of concern. Hepatitis has been reported following the ingestion of Chinese herbs and could be either because of the chemicals or contaminants in the herbs. There is recent report of corticosteroid contamination in Chinese herbal treatment. A very recent controlled trial failed to find any benefit of Chinese herbal therapy in recalcitrant AD.

Counseling and Psychotherapy

Stress aggravates AD: On the other hand, a severly affected child is also a source of stress to the entire family. A patient hearing, a bit of empathetic attitude and encouragement can ease the children and their parents by listening to family problems, problems of working mother of a AD child or a father's anxiety and disappointment about handling such children. A doctor can relive their tension a lot by spending a little more time with the patients/parents. 'Hypnotherapy' and 'massage therapy' basically work by bringing about psychological wellbeing of the children.

ECZEMAS OTHER THAN ATOPIC DERMATITIS

The term eczema means "boil out". It refers to the morphology of erythema, scaling and crusting. The term dermatitis is often used synonymously, though it is a wider and all inclusive term for inflammation of the skin that appears as erythema, erythema and scaling or erythema, scaling and crusting.

CLASSIFICATION

The easiest and practical classification to date is that of two broad groups, exogenous and endogenous eczemas depending upon whether the causative factors are external or internal. It has to be clearly understood that several exogenous factors have a role in precipitating or aggravating the endogenous eczemas as will be clearer in the subsequent text.

Exogenous eczemas - Diaper dermatitis
Contact dermatitis
Phytodermatoses

Endogenous eczemas - Seborrheic dermatitis
Autosensitization dermatitis
Perioral dermatitis
Asteatotic eczema
Nummular eczema
Pityriasis alba
Pompholyx
Lichen simplex chronicus,
Prurigo
Juvenile plantar dermatosis

Eczematous eruptions represent a significant proportion of the dermatologic disease burden in the neonates and children. Their exact incidence is unknown. In an Indian study 24% patients aged up to 17 years had eczema. We shall discuss each entity in the later part of this chapter.

DIAPER DERMATITIS (Syns: Napkin Dermatitis, Nappy Rash)

Dermatitis localized to the diaper area is known as diaper dermatitis. It is a common condition that occurs in otherwise healthy infants. It is not only seen in infants using diapers but also incontinent adult patients using diapers. In a series of 1089 napkin wearing children the prevalence of napkin dermatitis was found to be 50%. It causes discomfort to infants, anxiety to parents and caregivers and contributes to the load on the health care system. A large variety of napkins, both disposable and non-disposable, are available and used. Earlier thought to be due to the irritant effect of ammonia released by the urea splitting bacteria, it is now known to be more complex in etiology. Moist environment inside the diaper is the basic factor which leads to maceration of the skin, increased bacterial growth and increased local pH. In this alkaline environment the fecal lipases and proteases have a marked irritant effect. Candida albicans often invades secondarily.

CLINICAL FEATURES

Diaper dermatitis is characterized by glazed red erythematous skin of the convexities of the buttocks, medial aspect of thighs, scrotum and the labia majora where the contact with the diaper is the greatest. The deep folds of the groins and over the thighs are spared. When it begins to resolve it leaves wrinkled skin. The condition may also start with just a mild perianal erythema following diarrhea. Two variants are described. The edges of the napkin may lead to erythematous marks on the thighs and abdomen known as tide mark dermatitis or the more severe form of papuloerosive dermatitis known as Jacquet's dermatitis.

DIAGNOSIS AND DIFFERENTIAL DIAGNOSIS

It is based upon the morphology and the location of the rash. *Allergic contact dermatitis* is considered as a possible diagnosis if the rash worsens with treatment. Contact allergy may arise due to parabens, neomycin, lanolin, detergents used to wash cloth napkins or to rubber components used in the elastic waistband and around proximal thighs. *Atopic dermatitis* generally is associated with eczema at other sites, family history of atopy, severe pruritus and a chronic course. *Napkin psoriasis* is rare and typically presents as chronic, sharply marginated, slightly scaly, erythematous plaques, involving both the deep folds and the convex surface of the buttocks and thighs. Classic lesions elsewhere and nail involvement may help in the diagnosis. *Seborrheic dermatitis* presents as scaly erythematous plaques involving the inguinal folds. The lesions are sharply demarcated with greasy, yellowish scales. Involvement of other sites like the scalp, forehead, posterior auricular folds and umbilicus may aid in the diagnosis. *Candidal napkin dermatitis* presents with intensely red, scaly plaques with satellite papules and pustules. There is often a history of antibiotic use. *Perianal streptococcal disease* is caused by group A beta hemolytic streptococcus and presents as well defined bright red erythema in the perianal area. There is associated pruritus and pain due to perirectal fissuring. It may coexist with a more recently described entity streptococcal intertrigo characterized by macerated foul smelling erythema of the inguinal, axillary, popliteal and neck folds. *Acrodermatitis enteropathica* is a rare disease caused by inherited or acquired zinc deficiency. It occurs at the time of weaning in breast fed infants and is characterized by periorificial and acral rash which also involves the napkin area. It is an eczematous rash which becomes psoriasiform in chronic cases. *Biotin responsive multiple carboxylase deficiency* is another rare disorder with an acrodermatitis enteropathica like picture and other features like alopecia, seizures and ataxia. *Letterer–Siwe disease* should be suspected in intractable cases with a rash like seborrheic dermatitis. Infiltrated papules with hemorrhagic crusting are classical. *Congenital syphilis* may present with perianal moist eroded condyloma lata lesions. There may be other signs and symptoms to suggest congenital syphilis.

MANAGEMENT

The management of diaper dermatitis can be divided into general measures and specific treatment.

General measures include proper cleaning of the perianal area with tap water after passing faeces, keeping the diaper area dry, avoidance of occlusive pants, use of a protective emollient ointment (white soft paraffin) or barrier creams (containing zinc oxide, titanium dioxide or dimethicone) once irritation develops, frequent change of diapers, use of absorbent napkins and avoiding antiseptics while washing cloth napkins. There is however not enough evidence to support or refute the use and type of disposable napkins for the prevention of napkin dermatitis in infants. Advances in diaper technology have however contributed significantly to the reduction of diaper dermatitis. From the 80's till date, basic cellulose diapers have been replaced by the absorbent gelling materials (AGM) and now by microbreatheable diapers.

Specific treatment includes the use of topical antifungal steroid combinations containing imidazole and 1% hydrocortisone for 1-2 weeks. If the rash is complicated by bacterial infection topical antimicrobial agents like benzalkonium chloride or triclosan may be used. Systemic antifungal therapy (nystatin suspension) is rarely indicated in recalcitrant cases. Tar preparations are no longer used and talcum powders are also best avoided.

CONTACT DERMATITIS

Allergic contact dermatitis (ACD) was thought to be uncommon in children till some years ago due to the lack of knowledge about contact factors operative in children. ACD increases with age, and a prevalence of between 13.3% and 24.5% has been reported. It is generally accepted that ACD is rare in the first years of life, and with increasing age (by the age of 10 years) reaches the incidence seen in adults. Evaluation of eczemas in children nowadays routinely involves considering allergens as possible causative agents. This is because sensitization to contact allergens has been seen to begin in children as young as 6 months of age. It is likely that allergen exposure in children has changed with time. The reported incidence of ACD among children, in particular nickel and rubber allergy, appears to be increasing, which may relate to changing fashions and hobbies. The variation in the patch test results in children is a reflection of the temporal, geographic, age and sex difference in the populations studied. Patch testing infants may be difficult and false-positive reactions may occur.

CLINICAL FEATURES

Contact allergy should be considered in all children with dermatitis, particularly with eyelid or hand dermatitis. The clinical features of allergic contact dermatitis are similar as in adults. The site of involvement rather than the morphology may give the clue to it being allergic in origin. Involvement of the site of skin contact, skin piercing in nickel allergy **(Figure 4.9)**; airborne pattern in compositae dermatitis; streaky lesions in plant dermatitis and generalized involvement in systemic contact dermatitis due to ingestion of the allergen may be seen. Some experts believe that the pattern of presenting dermatitis in children should not determine referral for patch testing and any child with a persistent eczema should be referred for patch testing.

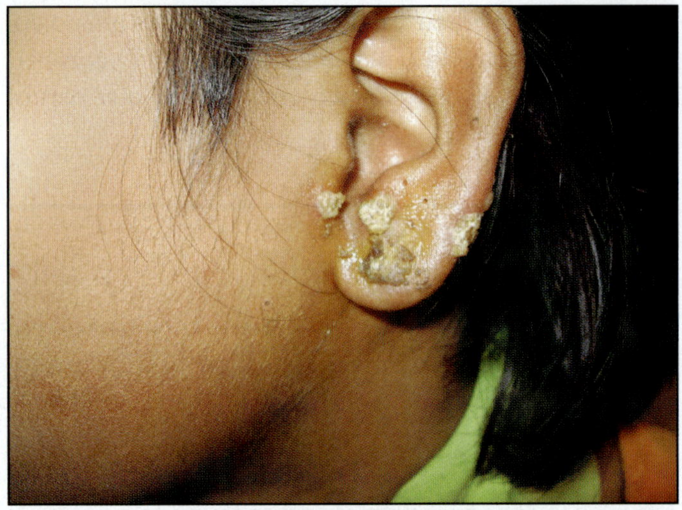

FIGURE 4.9: Allergic contact dermatitis to artificial jewellary

PATCH TESTING

Patch testing is needed to identify the responsible allergens and should be performed in children. It is the only objective method of screening for contact allergy. Patch test results from different countries have revealed certain similarities in the allergens responsible for allergic contact dermatitis in children, namely nickel, cobalt, chromate, mercurial compounds (thimerosal/thiomersal) rubber chemicals, fragrance chemicals and neomycin. Several less common, but emerging, allergens have also been reported recently including para-phenylenediamine in henna tattoos, cocamidopropyl betaine in 'no tears' shampoos and cleansers, and disperse dyes in clothing materials. A panel of 12 allergens has been recommended as a standard series in children recently by the German Contact Dermatitis research Group. Since sensitization rates to different allergens show variations over time, periodic evaluations of patch test results in children is necessary in order to update the test trays. Finn chambers or TRUE test system may be used. Doubtful reactions may be checked by performing the repeated open application test (ROAT).

MANAGEMENT

Once the relevance of an allergen is established, the patient is advised to avoid coming in contact with the allergen. Since children are already exposed at an early age to well-known allergens, therefore, strategies of avoidance have to gain or regain importance and should start as early as possible. The active eczema is managed with antihistamines and topical steroids like mometasone or fluticasone. Systemic steroids are rarely required for intractable cases not managed with topical steroids.

AUTOSENSITIZATION DERMATITIS

The development of acute widespread dermatitis at a site distant to the local inflammatory focus is known as autosensitization or autoeczematization. It is not a well accepted term.

CLINICAL FEATURES

It occurs suddenly as a widespread, symmetrical, papular or papulovesicular erythematous rash which is pruritic. The lesions may coalesce and form oozy crusted eczematous plaques. They tend to persist till the original inflammatory focus is treated. Over the palms the lesions may simulate pompholyx. In the clinical context it is seen in association with stasis/chronic eczema of the legs and also as generalized exfoliative dermatitis subsequent to a local dermatitis. Excited skin syndrome may be considered an example of this condition in relation to contact eczema. Increased circulating activated T cells have been reported along with an elevated T helper to T suppressor ratio. This is probably due to the cytokines produced at the site of local inflammation.

MANAGEMENT

It involves treatment of the local inflammatory inciting stimulus. Oral antibiotics for infection, antihistaminics and systemic steroids help to clear the rash.

SEBORRHEIC DERMATITIS

Seborrheic dermatitis (SD) is common in early childhood. The overall age- and sex-adjusted prevalence of seborrheic dermatitis has been seen to be 10.0% in boys and 9.5% in girls. It is highest in the first 3 months of life, decreasing rapidly by the age of 1 year. Cradle cap occurs in up to 41.7% of the children examined and is usually categorized as minimal to mild. SD is a distinct inflammatory eruption that involves the scalp and intertriginous areas. The disease is most common in the first 4-6 weeks of life, but may occur up to 6-9 months. Both sexes are equally involved. Unlike atopic dermatitis it is associated with very little pruritus. There is a significant overlap between SD, psoriasis and atopic dermatitis (AD). Patients diagnosed to have typical SD have gone on to develop typical AD. However, it is unlikely that infants with SD will go on to develop SD as adults. Pityrosporum ovale has been implicated in the etiology of SD. There are also reports of impaired activity of the enzyme delta-6-desaturase, leading to an abnormality of essential fatty acids. In children with active dermatitis levels of EFA 18:1w9 are increased, levels of 18:2w6 decreased, whereas 20:4w6 levels remained normal. The rare EFA 20:2w6 levels are also increased in significant amounts.

CLINICAL FEATURES

The scalp is generally the first site to be involved in the form of a cradle cap, which is greasy yellow scaling on the vertex **(Figure 4.10)**. Hair loss is not a feature. Such

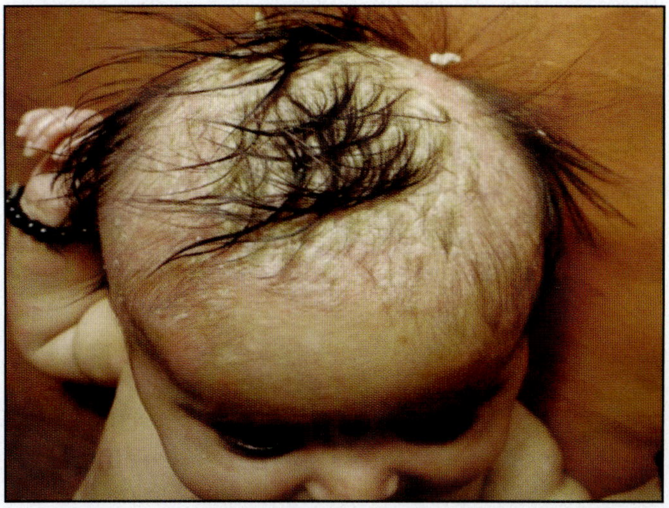

FIGURE 4.10: Cradle cap

scaling may appear in infancy in babies with a clear scalp at birth. The retroauricular creases are commonly affected. Lesions also occur on the face, primarily the central forehead, glabella, eyebrows, malar eminences, nasolabial folds and external ears with erythema and a yellow greasy scale. Lesions may also be seen in the axillae, inguinal and intergluteal folds. In the napkin area SD presents as sharply marginated erythematous plaques with a tendency to coalesce, resulting in large red infiltrated patches. Lesions may also occur over the trunk, the presternal and interscapular areas.

DIAGNOSIS AND DIFFERENTIAL DIAGNOSIS

The diagnosis is essentially clinical. Histology is not diagnostic and consists of subacute dermatitis. The presence of neutrophils is more suggestive of SD. The differential diagnosis includes several disorders like AD, Psoriasis, Contact dermatitis and Langerhans cell histiocytosis (LCH). *Atopic dermatitis* generally is associated with eczema at other sites, family history of atopy, pruritus and a chronic course. *Napkin psoriasis* is rare and typically presents as chronic, sharply marginated, slightly scaly, erythematous plaques, involving both the deep folds and the convex surface of the buttocks and thighs. Classic lesions elsewhere and nail involvement may help in the diagnosis. *Allergic contact dermatitis* occurs only in a small number of exposed and sensitized individuals. It is considered as a possible diagnosis if the rash does not improve or worsens with treatment. In *LCH* the individual lesions are erythematous purpuric macules and papules. Scaling is common and the scalp is often involved with hemorrhagic crusts and scales. Anemia, hepatosplenomegaly, lymphadenopathy and diarrhea, are the other features

MANAGEMENT

Mild topical steroids like hydrocortisone 1% along with emollients are the mainstay of treatment. Topical antibacterial and antifungal agents separately or combined with steroids may be indicated in some cases. The topical calcineurin inhibitors (TCIs) pimecrolimus and tacrolimus are approved for atopic dermatitis but have been used successfully for SD also. Owing to the possible role of Pityrosporum ovale in the etiopathogenesis of SD ketoconazole, ciclopirox olamine and bifonazole 1% shampoo are recommended as effective and safe treatment for lesions of scalp seborrheic dermatitis in infants and young children. For cradle cap baby oil should be massaged on to the scalp prior to bathing. In refractory cases, emulsifying ointment should be used to soften the scales and then rinsed out after several hours.

PERIORAL DERMATITIS

Perioral dermatitis is a papulosquamous eruption occurring symmetrically around the mouth. The condition is seen in both adults as well as children. It appears at all ages in childhood and adolescence. A granulomatous variant has also been described. The exact etiology of perioral dermatitis is unknown. The role of Demodex folliculorum in perioral dermatitis is not satisfactorily explained. The increased density of D. folliculorum in perioral dermatitis is most likely a secondary phenomenon, associated with topical steroid therapy. Use of strong topical steroids is thought to predispose to the development of perioral dermatitis. In cases not induced by steroids a specific etiology can often not be found. It has also been proposed to be a variant of rosacea. But it lacks the flushing and telangiectasia associated with rosacea.

CLINICAL FEATURES

The condition is characterized by small erythematous papules on a background of erythema leaving a clear uninvolved zone between the vermilion border and the affected skin. In more severe forms small vesicopustules may become evident. The granulomatous form is characterized by discrete small dome shaped skin colored papular lesions. It lacks pruritus though a burning sensation may be present. Lesions may also occur around the perinasal and periocular areas. There are remissions and relapses in the course of the disease. The lesions may heal with pinpoint scarring.

DIAGNOSIS AND DIFFERENTIAL DIAGNOSIS

Histopathology: it is indistinguishable from rosacea and reveals a mixed lymphohistiocytic inflammatory infiltrate around hair follicles. In the granulomatous form of the disease non-caseating granulomas may be seen. The differential diagnosis includes contact dermatitis, rosacea, lip lick dermatitis and demodex folliculitis. The granulomatous form may be confused with sarcoidosis and lupus miliaris disseminata faciei.

MANAGEMENT

Topical treatment alone is ineffective. A patient using topical steroids needs to be weaned off the steroids gradually by replacing them with mild preparations or bland emollient creams. Patients have to be cautioned about a possible flare up of their disease on stopping strong topical steroids. Other suspected contactants like fluoride containing toothpaste and cosmetics should be avoided. Oral tetracycline 250 mg twice per day is very effective but should not be given to children less than 9 years of age. Oral erythromycin is preferred for children along with topical metronidazole. Topical erythromycin, clindamycin and azelaic acid are also efficacious. Recently the TCIs tacrolimus and pimecrolimus have been tried and found effective.

ASTEATOTIC ECZEMA (Syn. Eczema craquele, Pruritus hiemalis, Xerotic eczema)

Dry, scaly and itchy eczema seen in winters in the elderly is classically known as asteatotic eczema. It may also be seen in children with a xerotic skin. It occurs due to factors like a decrease in skin lipids, excessive use of soap with a tendency to chapping, malnutrition, zinc deficiency and low humidity combined with overheated rooms. Drugs like cimetidine and even topical corticosteroids have been implicated. There is a defect in the epidermal barrier with increased transepidermal water loss and a decreased ability to repair the barrier. Xerosis precedes asteatotic eczema.

CLINICAL FEATURES

In eczema craquele (EC) the skin is dry, flaky and very itchy. The pruritus is more marked over the shins and arms. The skin over the pretibial region bilaterally develops fine cracks within the eczematous patch. Widespread EC, topical corticosteroid resistance, and deep red and inflammatory fissures have been significantly correlated with neoplasia. Generalized eczema craquele is associated with several malignancies like lymphoma, gastric adenocarcinoma, spheroidal cell carcinoma of the breast and angioimmunoblastic lymphadenopathy.

DIAGNOSIS

Histopathology reveals features of a mild or subacute eczema.

MANAGEMENT

Treatment consists of avoidance of excessive use of soap and hot dry rooms with a low ambient humidity and lubrication of the skin after bathing with lukewarm water with oils or creams. Antihistaminics along with bland emollient creams like white soft paraffin are helpful in controlling the pruritus. Ammonium lactate lotion (12%) has also been used. Products containing urea, lactic acid and alpha hydroxy acids are best avoided because they cause a stinging sensation and their toxic effects with prolonged use are unknown. Rarely hydrocortisone 1% or other mild steroid creams may be required when the skin is inflamed.

NUMMULAR ECZEMA (Syn. Discoid eczema)

Nummular eczema (NE) is characterized by coin shaped well defined eczematous lesions. It is mostly seen in the first two years of life. The exact etiology is unknown. Bacterial hypersensitivity, nutritional deficiencies, dryness of the skin, contact allergy and irritants are some of the etiological possibilities. It has been considered a variant of atopic eczema but its relationship to atopy is not clear and serum IgE levels may be normal. The incidence of atopy is not higher in patients of nummular eczema. Substance P (SP) and calcitonin gene-related peptide (CGRP) but not vasoactive intestinal polypeptide (VIP) fibres were more frequent in lesional than in nonlesional papillary dermis of both AD and NE. Since mast cells are also increased in number in lesions of NE they are able to maintain neurogenic inflammation through activation by SP and CGRP. The increased SP/CGRP nerves in the epidermis of NE lesions may stimulate keratinocytes to release cytokines which affect various cell types enhancing the inflammation.

CLINICAL FEATURES

Nummular eczema presents as well defined coin shaped lesions of variable size ranging from 1-5 cm. The lesions are mostly localized to the extremities and trunk. In the

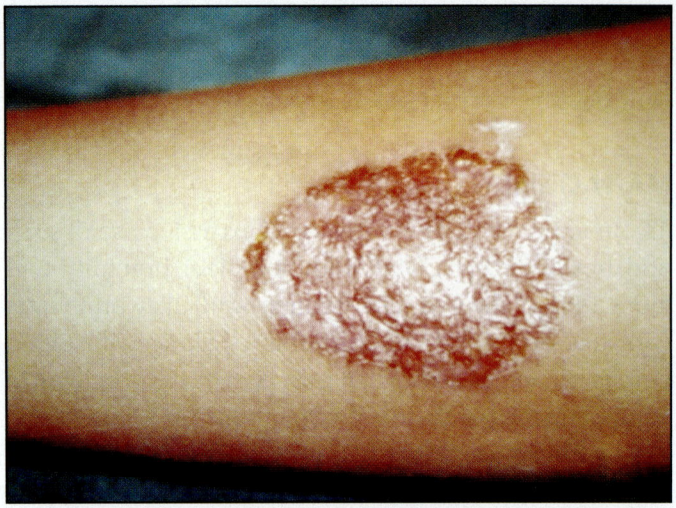

FIGURE 4.11A: Nummular eczema (acute, oozy lesion)

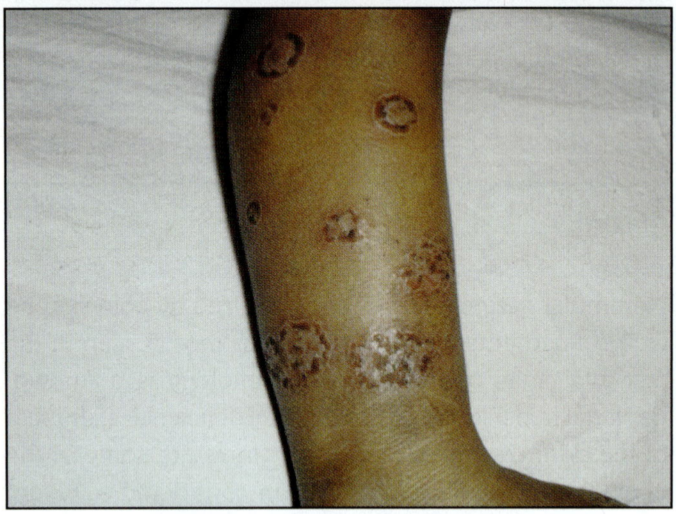

FIGURE 4.11B: Dry discoid eczema

acute phase the lesions are edematous, bright red, oozy with crusting at places **(Figures 4.11A and B)**. They are formed by a coalescence of minute papules and vesicles and are intensely itchy. They heal with scaling and no pigmentary change. Dry skin tends to exacerbate the disease. The condition tends to persist over several months and has remissions and relapses.

DIFFERENTIAL DIAGNOSIS

Nummular eczema has to be differentiated from tinea corporis in the chronic and impetigo in the acute stage. Psoriasis, lichen simplex chronicus and contact dermatitis may at times also have discoid lesions.

MANAGEMENT

General measures like avoiding extremes of temperature, avoidance of excessive use of soap and woolen clothing which irritates the skin, use of lukewarm water for bathing and rubbing of bath oil on the wet skin help. Oozing lesions may benefit with potassium permanganate compresses. Once the disease remits liberal use of emollients helps prevent a relapse. *Specific treatment* includes the use of antihistamines and steroid creams like mometasone or fluticasone for acute lesions. Ointments are better suited for dry chronic lesions. A course of systemic antibiotics is often very helpful and for numerous lesions a short course of systemic steroids may also be required.

INFECTIOUS ECZEMATOID DERMATITIS

Infectious eczematoid dermatitis (IED) is possibly an example of autosensitization. The nosological status of this term is unclear. Though the mechanism by which the microorganisms cause the dermatitis is not known, rapid response to antimicrobial drugs is ample proof of their etiologic role. A bacterial antigen may be producing a cytotoxic reaction or toxins produced by the bacteria may be functioning as superantigens and causing a widespread T cell mediated immune response. Poor hygiene, sweating and maceration all act as aggravating factors.

CLINICAL FEATURES

Certain criteria are used to establish the diagnosis of IED-firstly the condition arises from a primary lesion that is exudative, for example an ulcer, sinus, abscess, discharging ear or an infected wound and secondly the area involved is in direct contiguity with the primary lesion **(Figure 4.12)**. The dermatitis may be acute, streaky lesions along the path of the discharge. In acute IED the lesions are vesicopustular and exudative and also accompanied by pruritus. In the subsiding form the lesions are relatively dry, scaly and fissured.

DIFFERENTIAL DIAGNOSIS

IED has to be differentiated from impetigo and infected eczemas, like infected AD. Increased levels of C reactive protein may offer a useful clue. Infective dermatitis is a distinct entity that has been described in Jamaican children with HTLV 1 infection and in children from Peru. Onset is in early childhood. It is characterized by a severe eczematous rash involving the scalp, ear, retroauricular

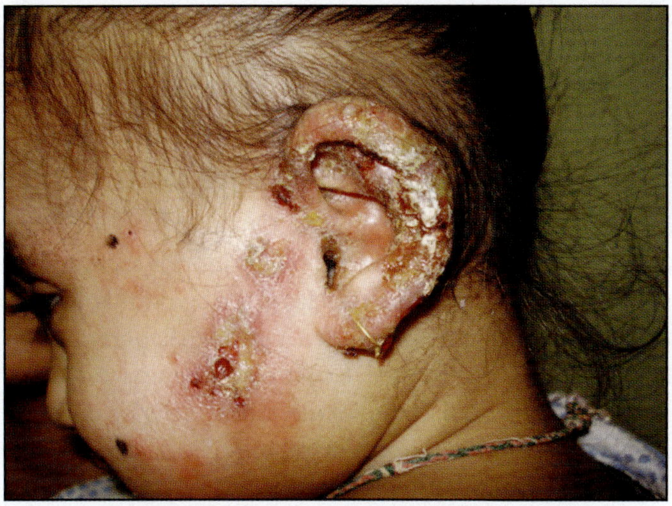

FIGURE 4.12: Infectious eczematoid dermatitis

areas, eyelid margins, axillae, groin and the neck. A watery nasal discharge may also be present. The children respond well to antibiotics, but recurrence is the rule.

TREATMENT

The local focus of infection has to be treated with appropriate oral antibiotics after sensitivity testing. Antihistaminics and a short course of systemic steroids given along with is beneficial. Topical steroid antibiotic combinations are indicated only for mild cases. Potassium permanganate bath as an antiseptic and emollients are encouraged as general measures.

PITYRIASIS ALBA (Syn. Pityriasis sicca faciei, Pityriasis simplex faciei)

Pityriasis alba (PA) is characterized by hypopigmented round to oval scaly patches occurring most commonly over the face in children around the age of 3 years and adolescents. The point prevalence has been seen to be 8.4%. Its etiology and pathogenesis are still poorly understood. Recent studies have found direct correlations between the incidence of PA and atopy, amount of sun exposure and the lack of sunscreen use. It is considered a minor criterion of atopic dermatitis.

CLINICAL FEATURES

A few hypopigmented round to oval scaly patches occur most commonly over the face in children and adolescents

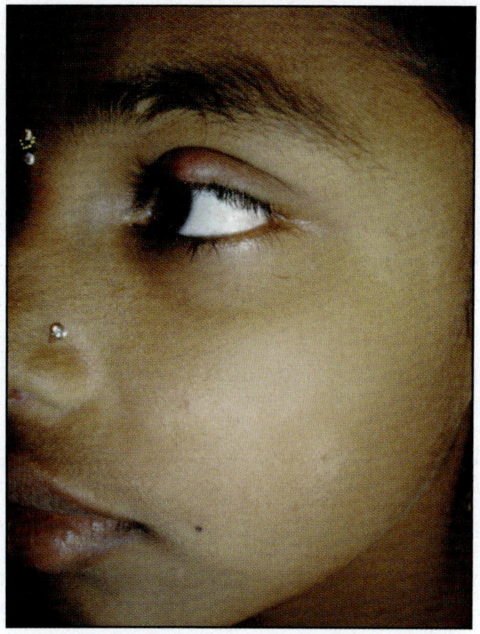

FIGURE 4.13: Pityriasis alba

(Figure 4.13). The margins of the lesions are not very well defined and they may also occur over the arms, neck or trunk in extensive disease. The patches of PA may be slightly erythematous at times and usually vary in size from one to few centimeters in diameter. The lesions have fine loosely adherent scale and are asymptomatic. The condition is self limiting with an excellent prognosis. Extensive pityriasis alba is probably identical with progressive macular hypomelanosis (PMH). Extensive pityriasis alba is histologically and clinically different from classical pityriasis alba, which is basically an eczematous disorder. PMH is characterized histologically by diminished pigment in the epidermis and a normal-looking dermis. Electron microscopy shows a shift from large melanosomes in normal-looking skin to small aggregated, membrane-bound melanosomes in hypopigmented skin. Propionibacterium acnes bacteria living in hair follicles are the cause of PMH as a result of production of a hypothetical depigmenting factor.

DIAGNOSIS AND DIFFERENTIAL DIAGNOSIS

Histopathology shows non-specific changes like hyperkeratosis, parakeratosis, acanthosis, exocytosis and reduced melanin in the basal layer. Mild perivascular inflammatory cell infiltrates are seen in the dermis. The thickened stratum corneum reduces the penetration of UV light which probably accounts for the hypopigmentation.

Vitiligo (depigmented lesions), tinea corporis and leprosy (hypopigmented anesthetic macules) figure in the differential diagnosis of PA.

MANAGEMENT

The lesions tend to clear spontaneously over some months. Emollients and bland oils at the time of bathing should be encouraged. Mild topical steroids are useful. Cases with extensive lesions may require oral PUVA. Tacrolimus has also been tried recently with good results.

POMPHOLYX (Syn. Dyshidrotic eczema, Dyshidrosis)

Pompholyx is an eczema characterized by discrete vesicles on the palms and soles, and along the sides of the fingers and toes. When the palms are involved it is known as cheiropompholyx, when feet podopompholyx and when both, cheiropodopompholyx. The name dyshidrosis is not preferred and is in fact is a misnomer because there is no involvement of the eccrine sweat ducts. The exact etiology of pompholyx is unknown. The gene for a rare autosomal dominant form of pompholyx maps to chromosome 18q22.1-18q22.3. Pompholyx is thought to be related to emotional stress, atopic diathesis (a personal or family history of atopy is present in 40-50% of the patients) and as a manifestation of nickel allergy (oral administration of nickel can induce pompholyx like lesions). Other allergens implicated in the pathogenesis of pompholyx are primula, PPD, benzoisothiazolones, dichromates, perfumes, balsam, dyes and rubber. Drugs like aspirin and contraceptives and an active focus of dermatophyte or Candida infection are some other etiological factors considered by some authors.

CLINICAL FEATURES

Classically it presents as a sudden eruption of bilaterally symmetrical tense vesicles by the sides of the fingers and toes. The palms and soles may also be involved. The lesions are described as 'sago grain like'. The occurrence of the lesions may be accompanied by pruritus or a pricking sensation. Smaller lesions may coalesce to form large multiloculated bullae. It may occur at any age but is rare below 10 years of age. The vesicles may get infected leading to the development of pustules. The lesions do not rupture being deep seated and dry up instead over time when the skin peels off. Usually an attack subsides with in 2-3 weeks but the course is variable. It is difficult to predict the frequency and severity of the attacks.

DIAGNOSIS AND DIFFERENTIAL DIAGNOSIS

Diagnosis is essentially clinical. On histopathology the changes are not specific and evolving lesions show foci of spongiosis and spongiotic vesicles in the epidermis, edema of the papillary dermis and a superficial perivascular lymphocytic infiltrate. Eosinophils may be seen occasionally. The differential diagnosis includes diseases localized to the hands and feet like infantile acropustulosis, palmoplantar pustulosis and hand foot and mouth disease. *Infantile acropustulosis* occurs during the first few months of life and is characteristically a pustular eruption. Histologically eosinophils and neutrophils are observed. *Palmoplantar pustulosis* similarly has pustular lesions. *Hand, foot and mouth disease* has oval vesicles along the palmar creases, lilac border to the lesions and involvement of the mouth to help to differentiate.

MANAGEMENT

General measure include avoiding the precipitating cause, local hygiene, compresses with potassium permanganate (1:10 000 dilution) and treatment of an infective focus if any.

Specific treatment includes the use of antihistamines, potent topical steroids and a course of antibiotics if indicated. Severe case may require a course of systemic steroids for 7-10 days. Patients having a contraindication to the use of steroids or unwilling to use steroids may be benefited by the use of dapsone. Tacrolimus and pimecrolimus have also been tried and found useful by some authors. Several other therapies which have been used in adult patients include methotrexate, mycophenolate mofetil, azathioprine, intradermal botlinum toxin, UVA1 therapy, tap water iontophoresis and eternacept.

LICHEN SIMPLEX CHRONICUS (Syn. Neurodermatitis)

Lichen simplex chronicus (LSC) is a reactive change to the stimulus of repeated skin scratching. It manifests as an asymmetrical localized area of lichenified skin. LSC is considered as a localized form of AD or the end stage of several other itchy dermatoses. However, it is seen even in patients who do not have an atopic diathesis. The etiology of LSC is unknown. Repeated rubbing or scratching as a result of intense pruritus precipitated by a minor irritant or an existing itchy skin condition like AD or CD results in LSC. The areas involved are mostly accessible to a patient's hand-like the back of neck, shins or the ankles. It is believed that the itch threshold is lower in patients of LSC and their itching is more intense during periods of stress. Common triggers for the development of the disease include psychological distress, and local environmental problems such as heat, sweating, and excess dryness. The incidence in dermatology practice is said to be around 3%.

CLINICAL FEATURES

LSC is uncommon in children. The peak incidence is between 30-50 years of age. Women are more frequently affected than men. Well circumscribed lichenified plaques are pathognomonic of LSC. These plaques due to the lichenification have a thickened, erythematous, hyperpigmented skin with accentuation of skin markings **(Figure 4.14)**. Slight scaling and excoriation marks are the other clinical features. The sites of involvement are the nape of the neck, dorsum of the feet, ankles and the wrists. Scrotum and vulva are the other areas to be routinely involved. Lichen simplex chronicus may also develop as a superimposed condition in the presence of other anogenital diseases such as candidiasis, psoriasis, lichen sclerosus, tinea cruris, and neoplasia. The pruritus is irresistible and paroxysmal and not relieved until a sensation of burning or pain is induced by violent scratching. The course is chronic with partial remissions. Polysomnographic findings of patients with LSC have revealed that the sleep pattern is disturbed in these patients by arousals and awakenings related to scratching bouts during sleep.

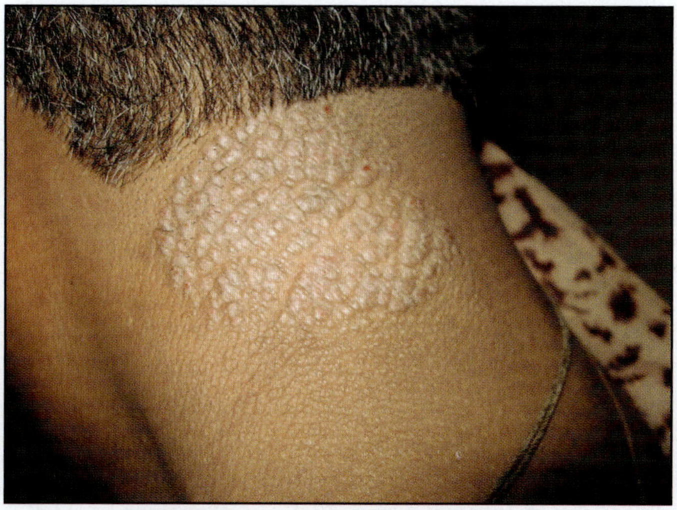

FIGURE 4.14: Lichen simplex chronicus

DIAGNOSIS AND DIFFERENTIAL DIAGNOSIS

Histopathologic findings are those of a chronic eczema in the form of hyperkeratosis, lengthening of rete ridges and vertically arranged collagen bundles in a thickened papillary dermis. A sparse perivascular lymphohistiocytic infiltrate may be present in the superficial dermis. Proliferation of Schwann cells may be seen in a significant number of cases.

Other itchy dermatoses like atopic, contact and stasis dermatitis may develop secondary lichenification. Hypertrophic lichen planus, psoriasis, and lichenified dermatophytosis may be the other differential diagnosis.

MANAGEMENT

Successful therapy requires attention not only to trigger factors, but also to repair of the damaged barrier layer, reduction in inflammation, and break-up of the itch-scratch cycle. Avoidance of precipitating factors and management of stress are important in the management. High potency topical steroids like clobetasol in an ointment base are preferred along with older generation sedating antihistamines. Tacrolimus and pimecrolimus are other alternatives to steroids. Topical or systemic antibiotics may be used as the case may be when infection is suspected. Tricyclic antidepressants may be used with benefit where stress is a known factor. The help of a child psychologist must be sought in the presence of a psychopathology. Topical aspirin/dichloromethane and botulinum toxin type A are other newer therapies.

PRURIGO

The term prurigo lacks a definite nosologic status. It is a reactive skin change to repeated scratching manifesting as papular or nodular lesions. It is seen mostly in patients with an atopic diathesis. Other trigger factors are insect bites, photosensitivity, stress and Hodgkin's lymphoma. Depending upon the trigger or etiologic factors it has been classified into –

1. Prurigo simplex (Syn. Chronic prurigo, Subacute prurigo, Chronic pruritic dermatoses of unknown cause, Papular dermatitis, Itchy red bump disease, Rosen's papular eruption). It is a disease more of the middle aged. Both the sexes are equally involved. The characteristic lesion is the prurigo papule which is a dome shaped papular lesion topped by a vesicle. The intact vesicle is hardly seen due to the severe pruritus and crusted papules are the norm. The papules are in various stages of evolution and polymorphic lesions are seen. The extremities and trunk are symmetrically affected. The lesions appear in crops. Topical corticosteroids and antihistamines form the mainstay of treatment. PUVA or UVB may be required for recalcitrant disease.
2. Atopic prurigo (Syn. Besnier's prurigo) (beyond the scope of this chapter)
3. Actinic prurigo (beyond the scope of this chapter)
4. Prurigo nodularis. It is characterized by chronic intensely pruritic nodules 0.5 -2 cm in diameter, localized to the extensor aspect of the lower extremities in both children and adults. The surface is keratotic and crusting or scaling may be a feature. The lesions are usually pigmented, but hypopigmentation may be seen in some of the lesions. The lesions heal with pigmentary change and scarring. The surrounding skin generally remains normal except in atopics when it may become lichenified. The exact etiology is unclear. It may be seen in response to insect bites, mycobacteria, hepatitis C, atopic diathesis, local trauma, or pruritus due to underlying systemic disorders like Hodgkin's disease, anemia, chronic renal failure, leukemia, polycythemia rubra vera, carcinoid syndrome, obstructive biliary disease, parasitic infections, diabetes mellitus, etc. An increased number of Merkel cells and dermal nerves have been seen in the lesions. Increased numbers of CGRP and substance P immunoreactive nerves have been detected. Histopathology shows marked hyperkeratosis, and acanthosis, mixed inflammatory cell infiltrate composed of lymphocytes, histiocytes, mast cells and eosinophils. Increased nerve growth factor in the lesions is responsible for the neurohyperplasia. The differential diagnosis is limited to hypertrophic lichen planus which may have lesions of classic lichen planus elsewhere. The goal of treatment remains control of pruritus and proper emolliation of the skin. Sedating oral antihistamines combined with potent topical steroids, sometimes under occlusion, remain as the treatment of choice. Topical capsaicin and tacrolimus have also been tried. Few lesions may be managed with intralesional steroids or cryotherapy. Oral cyclosporine and thalidomide have been shown to improve both appearance of the skin and pruritus. Systemic regimens involving the use of psoralen + UVA (PUVA), erythromycin, arotinoid acid, chloroquine, dapsone, minocycline, naltrexone and azathioprine are used for the treatment of this condition. Complete and/or remarkable regression of prurigo nodularis has been reported with roxithromycin and tranilast in combination within 4 to 6 months of use. Habit reversal training can be tried for the itch-scratch cycle associated with prurigo nodularis.
5. Sutton's summer prurigo (beyond the scope of this chapter).
6. Prurigo pigmentosa (beyond the scope of this chapter).

JUVENILE PLANTAR DERMATOSIS (Syn. Forefoot eczema, Atopic winter feet)

Juvenile plantar dermatosis (JPD) is an eczematous condition involving the undersurface of the anterior part of the feet in children. It is seen at different ages and the peak incidence is between 4-7 years of age. It is seen more commonly in boys; is seasonal and there is an exacerbation of the disease during winter in almost 50% cases. A personal or family history of atopy is seen in up to 50% of patients. Several factors are considered to play a role in the etiopathogenesis. Use of sports shoes with rubber sole is incriminated as the most likely cause resulting in occlusion and maceration. The other factors are abnormalities of the sweat glands, use of tight nylon socks, repeated friction and alternating maceration and dehydration of the feet.

CLINICAL FEATURES

The disease generally involves children less than 15 years of age as a glazed red symmetrical erythema of the undersurface of both the forefeet. Hyperkeratosis in the form of scaling and fissuring occurs. The fissures may be deep and walking may be painful. Children should be discouraged from picking off the scales to prevent the occurrence of small wounds and secondary infection. The weight bearing areas of the sole are involved along with the plantar surface of the toes. This is also the area which bears the brunt of the physical forces. Rarely their may be extension up to the heels. The interdigital areas and the arch of the foot are invariably spared. The course is prolonged and is characterized by remissions and relapses. Acanthosis nigricans (AN) has been seen to be associated more frequently in patients with juvenile plantar dermatosis.

DIAGNOSIS AND DIFFERENTIAL DIAGNOSIS

The histopathologic findings are nonspecific. Epidermal changes consist of acanthosis, alternating parakeratosis and orthokeratosis. There is no spongiosis. The dermis shows mononuclear cell infiltrate around the capillaries and sweat ducts. The sweat ducts show changes in the form of uncoiling or breakage in the epidermis. The differential diagnosis includes contact dermatitis, plantar psoriasis and involvement of the feet in atopic dermatitis. *Contact dermatitis* to footwear is an oozy condition in the acute phase, besides being intensely pruritic. Also contact dermatitis may involve the lateral aspect and dorsa of the feet. *Plantar psoriasis* is characterized by scaly plaques with fissuring and involvement of the arch of the foot. Lesions elsewhere, on the knees and elbows may be seen. *Atopic dermatitis* involves the dorsum of the feet and toes with very itchy papulovesicular lesions. Involvement of other sites like the cubital and popliteal fossae may aid in the diagnosis. Tinea pedis is mostly unilateral and involvement of the nails is common. Superficial scaling and a positive mycological examination help confirm the diagnosis.

MANAGEMENT

The treatment can be divided into preventive measures like avoidance of occlusive footwear and the use of cotton socks. Specific therapy includes the use of moderate steroid creams to control the inflammation and emollient creams after removal of the shoes. Tacrolimus has also been tried. Use of emollients after soaking the feet in tap water gives better results.

PHYTODERMATOSES (Syn. Dermatitis venenata)

A large number of plants are potential causes of dermatitis including flowers, grasses, vegetables, fruits and weeds.

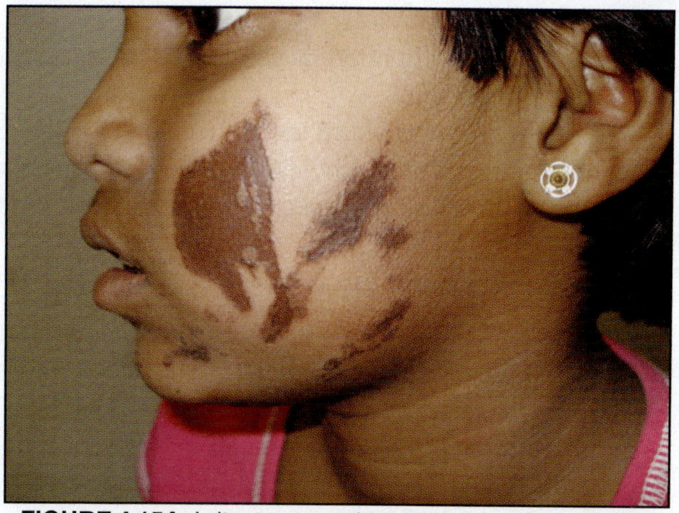

FIGURE 4.15A: Irritant contact dermatitis due to mango juice

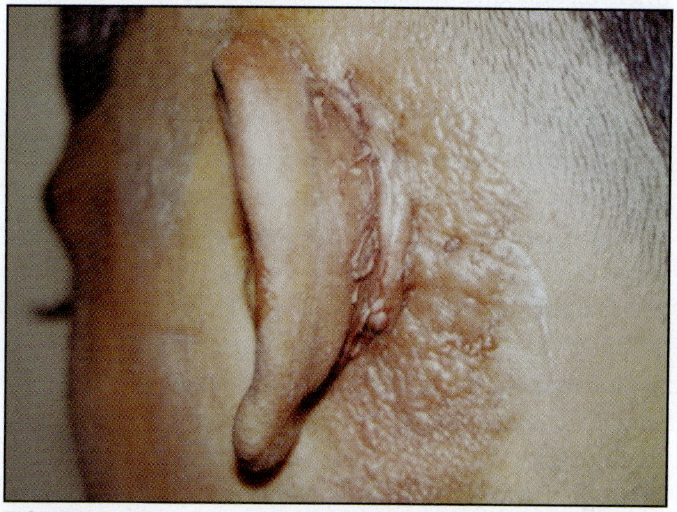

FIGURE 4.15B: Irritant contact dermatitis due to povidone-iodine

The plants may cause two types of reactions irritant and allergic.

IRRITANT REACTIONS

Irritant reactions **(Figures 4.15A and B)** are due to the thorns, spines or hair on the plants producing a mechanical irritant contact dermatitis or due to chemical irritation. Cactus hair (glochids) upon penetration into the skin can give rise to pruritus. Secondary infection may occur following this exposure, for example infection by sporotrichosis or mycobacteria following penetrating injuries. Plants can also induce chemical irritation of the skin due to –

- Calcium oxalate crystals (ejected from the cells into the skin or mucosa by Dieffenbachia picta (dumb cane or leopard lily))
- Thiocyanates (Mustard, Horseradish)

- Capsaicinoids (Chillies)
- Phorbol esters (Euphorbiaceae family produces a highly irritant latex).

Hair on the plants of Urtica species (stinging nettle) inject histamine and acetylcholine into the skin causing tingling and numbness at the site.

HYPERSENSITIVITY REACTIONS

Hypersensitivity reactions manifest as urticaria and angioedema, i.e. Immediate type 1 hypersensitivity due to naturally derived proteins in plants (peanuts, kiwi fruit, banana and rubber latex protein), and airborne pollens (mulberry and grasses). Investigations include skin application food test (SAFT), patch testing to grass family, prick testing and a RAST test. Management includes avoidance of the offending antigen and antihistaminics.

ALLERGIC CONTACT DERMATITIS

Allergic contact dermatitis can be caused by several plants of family anacardiaceae, leguminosae, gramineae, compositae, pinaceae, araliaceae, ginkgoaceae and styraceae. It is less common in children. The lesions are pruritic, streaky and vesiculobullous. They develop within 1-3 days after exposure and evolve gradually. Lesions are localized to the area of contact to begin with but may spread. They heal with minimal pigmentary change. The diagnosis of ACD requires careful history and patch testing. Treatment is with potent topical steroids, antihistamines or systemic steroids if the rash is extensive. Physical methods of plant destruction, weed killers, barrier creams and preparations meant to prevent percutaneous penetration (polymine, salts of a linoleic acid dimmer and quaternium-18 bentonite lotion) are of limited value. Hyposensitization may be hazardous.

PHYTOPHOTODERMATITIS

Phytophotodermatitis is the phototoxic reaction produced by furocoumarins (psoralens; naturally occurring fungicides) in many plants when they come in contact with the skin that is then exposed to UVA light. It is common in children and the uncovered or sunexposed areas are only involved. A burning erythema, followed by edema and painful linear vesiculation occurs some hours after the exposure. The lesions heal with hyperpigmentation which may take several months to resolve. Children are at risk while playing in the gardens and parks. The lesions are localized only to the area of contact and have a sharp cut off. Diagnosis of phytophotodermatitis is not difficult and differential diagnosis includes the battered baby syndrome which also may have similar streaky linear lesions. The plants which produce such a phototoxic reaction belong to the following families –

- Umbelliferae (Parsley, celery, parsnip, giant Russian hogweed)
- Rutaceae (Bergamot, Dictamnus, Rue, anise scented berry Pelea anisata)
- Moraceae
- Compositae

Phytophotodermatitis is totally preventable. The treatment consists of relief of pain by analgesics, aspiration of large bullae, potassium permanganate compresses and the application of aqueous ceams or soothing calamine lotion. Topical steroids help to reduce inflammation and may help to resolve the pigmentary changes faster. For extensive involvement systemic steroids may be indicated for a few days. Superadded infection may be treated with a course of antibiotics.

BIBLIOGRAPHY

1. Aschoff R, Wozel G. Topical tacrolimus for the treatment of lichen simplex chronicus. J Dermatolog Treat 2007;18:115-7.
2. Baer EL, Davies MW, Easterbrook KJ. Disposable nappies for preventing napkin dermatitis in infants. Cochrane Database Syst Rev 2006;3:CD004262.
3. Beattie PE, Green C, Lowe G, Lewis-Jones MS. Which children should we patch test? Clin Exp Dermatol 2007;32:6-11.
4. Brar Kamal Jeet, Shenoi SD, Balachandran C, Mehta VR. Clinical profile of forefoot eczema: a study of 42 cases. Indian J Dermatol Venereol Leprol 2005;71:179-81.
5. Bruckner AL, Weston WL, Morelli JG. Does sensitization to contact allergens begin in infancy? Pediatrics 2000;105(1):e3.
6. Chang TT, Stevens SR. Atopic dermatitis: The role of recombinant interferon-α therapy. Am J Clin Dermatol 2002; 3: 175-83.
7. Chen JJ, Liang YH, Zhou FS, Yang S, Wang J, Wang PG, Du WH, Xu SJ, Huang W, Zhang XJ. The gene for a rare autosomal dominant form of pompholyx maps to chromosome 18q22.1-18q22.3. J Invest Dermatol 2006;126:300-4.
8. Clayton TH, Wilkinson SM, Rawcliffe C, Pollock B, Clark SM. Allergic contact dermatitis in children: should pattern of dermatitis determine referral? A retrospective study of 500 children tested between 1995 and 2004 in one U.K. centre. Br J Dermatol 2006;154:114-7.
9. Cox H, William OCM, Harper J. Genetics of Atopic dermatitis. In: Harper J, Oranje A, Prose N.(eds). Text book of Pediatric Dermatology. Blackwell Science, Oxford, 2003; 169-77.
10. Del Rosso JQ. The use of topical azelaic acid for common skin disorders other than inflammatory rosacea. Cutis 2006;77:22-24.

11. Dhar S, Kanwar AJ, Epidemiology and clinical pattern of atopic dermatitis in north Indian paediatric population. Pediatr Dermatol 1998; 15: 347-51.
12. Dhar S, Kanwar AJ, Kaur S, et al. Role of bacterial flora in the pathogenesis and management of atopic dermatitis. Ind J Med Res 1992; 95: 234-8.
13. Dhar S, Kanwar AJ. Grading of severity of atopic dermatitis in north Indian children. Ind J Dermatol 1995; 40: 67-72.
14. Dhar S, Malakar R, Chattopadhyay S, Dhar S, Banerjee R, Ghosh A. Correlation between the severity of atopic dermatitis with peripheral eosinophil count and serum IgE. Indian J Dermatol Venereol Leprol 2005; 71: 246-9.
15. Diepgen TL, Fartasch M. Recent epidemiological and genetic studies in atopic dermatitis. Acta Dermatol Venereol (Suppl). 1992;176:13-8.
16. Diepgen TL. Long-term treatment with cetirizine of infants with atopic dermatitis: A multi-country, double-blind, randomized placebo-controlled trial(the ETAC trial) over 18 months. Pediatr Allergy Immunol 2002;13:278-86.
17. Dogra S, Kumar B. Epidemiology of skin diseases in school children: a study from northern India. Pediatr Dermatol 2003;20:470-3.
18. Dolenc-Voljc M, Pohar M, Lunder T. Density of Demodex folliculorum in perioral dermatitis. Acta Derm Venereol 2005;85:211-5.
19. Edmonds EV, Riaz SN, Francis N, Bunker CB. Nodular prurigo responding to topical tacrolimus. Br J Dermatol 2004;150:1216-7.
20. Eichenfield LF, Hanifin JM, Beck LA,et al.Atopic Dermatitis and asthma :parallels in the evolution of treatment. Pediatrics 2003;111:608-16.
21. Engler R J, Kenner J, Leung D Y.Smallpox vaccination : Risk considerations for patients with atopic dermatitis.J Allergy Clin Immunol 2002; 110:357-65.
22. Erasala GN, Merlay I, Romain C. Evolution of disposable diapers and reduction of diaper dermatitis. Arch Pediatr 2007;14:495-500.
23. Fleicher J. Treatment of atopic dermatitis: role of tacrolimus ointment as a topical noncorticosteroidal therapy. J Allergy Clin Immunology 1999; 104: S126-30.
24. Foley P, Zuo Y, Plunkett A, Merlin K, Marks R. The frequency of common skin conditions in preschool-aged children in Australia: seborrheic dermatitis and pityriasis capitis (cradle cap). Arch Dermatol 2003;139:318-22.
25. Gambichler T, Hyun J, Sommer A, Stücker M, Altmeyer P, Kreuter A. A randomised controlled trial on photo (chemo) therapy of subacute prurigo. Clin Exp Dermatol 2006;31:348-53.
26. Gibbs NF. Juvenile plantar dermatosis. Can sweat cause foot rash and peeling? Postgrad Med 2004;115:73-5.
27. Gonzalez-Otero F. Cyclosporin in children with severe atopic dermatitis. J Am Acad Dermatol 1997; 36: 1029-30.
28. Goodyear HM, Harper JL. 'Wet wrap' dressings for eczema: an effective treatment but not to be misused.Br J Dermatol 2002;146:59.
29. Goon AT, Goh CL. Patch testing of Singapore children and adolescents: our experience over 18 years. Pediatr Dermatol 2006;23:117-20.
30. Grover JK,Vats V,Gopalakrishna R, Ramam M. Thalidomide: a re-look. Natl Med J India 2000;13:132-41.
31. Gupta AK, Skinner AR. Management of diaper dermatitis. Int J Dermatol 2004;43:830-4.
32. Hafeez ZH. Perioral dermatitis: an update. Int J Dermatol 2003;42:514-7.
33. Hanifin J, Gupta A K. Rajagopalan R. Intermittent dosing of fluticasone propionate cream for reducing the risk of relapse in atopic dermatitis patients. Br J Dermatol 2002;147:528-37.
34. Hanifin JM, Chan SC, Cheng JB, et al. Type 4 phosphodiesterase inhibitors have clinical and in vitro anti-inflammatory effects in atopic dermatitis. J Invest Dermatol 1996; 107: 51-6.
35. Harper JI, Ahmed I, Barclay G, et al. Cyclosporin for severe childhood atopic dermatitis: short course versus continuous therapy. Br J Dermatol 2000; 142: 52-8.
36. Hill D J , Heine RG, Hosking C, S et al. IgE with food sensitization in infants with eczema attending a dermatology department. J Pediatr 2007; 151:331-3.
37. Horiuchi Y, Bae S, Katayama I. Uncontrollable prurigo nodularis effectively treated by roxithromycin and tranilast. J Drugs Dermatol 2006;5:363-5.
38. Humphrey S, Bergman JN, Au S. Practical management strategies for diaper dermatitis. Skin Therapy Lett 2006;11:1-6.
39. Inamadar AC, Palit A. The genus Malassezia and human disease. Indian J Dermatol Venereol Leprol 2003;69:265-70.
40. Järvikallio A, Harvima IT, Naukkarinen A. Mast cells, nerves and neuropeptides in atopic dermatitis and nummular eczema. Arch Dermatol Res 2003;295:2-7.
41. Johansson O, Liang Y, Emtestam L. Increased nerve growth factor- and tyrosine kinase A-like immunoreactivities in prurigo nodularis skin — an exploration of the cause of neurohyperplasia. Arch Dermatol Res 2002;293:614-9.
42. Kalliomaki , Salminen S, Poussa T,et al. Probiotics and prevention of atopic disease: 4-year follow-up of randomized placebo-controlled trial. Lancet 2003;361:1869-71.
43. Kanwar AJ, Dhar S. Severity of atopic dermatitis in north India. Br J Dermatol 1994; 131: 733-4.
44. Koca R, Altin R, Konuk N, Altinyazar HC, Kart L. Sleep disturbance in patients with lichen simplex chronicus and its relationship to nocturnal scratching: A case control study. South Med J 2006;99:482-5.
45. Krupa Shankar DS, Shrestha S. Relevance of patch testing in patients with nummular dermatitis. Indian J Dermatol Venereol Leprol 2005;71:406-8.
46. Kütting B, Brehler R, Traupe H. Allergic contact dermatitis in children: strategies of prevention and risk management. Eur J Dermatol 2004;14:80-5.
47. Lan CC, Lin CL, Wu CS, Chai CY, Chen WT, Chen GS. Treatment of idiopathic prurigo nodularis in Taiwanese patients with low-dose thalidomide. J Dermatol 2007;34:237-42.
48. Lee MR, Shumack S. Prurigo nodularis: a review. Australas J Dermatol 2005;46:211-8.
49. Leung D Y .Atopic dermatitis and the immune system.The role of superantigens and bacteria. J Am Acad Dermatol 2001;45:s13-6.
50. Leung D Y, Bieber T. Atopic Dermatitis. Lancet 2003; 361:151-60.
51. Lin RL, Janniger CK. Pityriasis alba. Cutis 2005;76(1): 21-4.
52. Lofgren SM, Warshaw EM. Dyshidrosis: epidemiology, clinical characteristics, and therapy. Dermatitis. 2006;17:165-81.

53. Lovell CR. Phytophotodermatoses. In:Harper J, Oranje A, Prose N, eds. Textbook of Pediatric Dermatology. Massachusetts: Blackwell Publishing, 2006:357-66.
54. Luger T, Van Leent EJM, Grabber M, et al. SDZ ASM 981: an emerging safe and effective treatment for atopic dermatitis. Br J Dermatol 2001: 144; 788-94.
55. Malakar S, Dhar S. Menarche precipitating the onset of atopic dermatitis. Pediatr Dermatol 1998; 15: 242-4.
56. McAlvany JP, Sherertz EF. Contact dermatitis in infants, children and adolescents. Adv Dermatol 1994;9:205-23.
57. Militello G, Jacob SE, Crawford GH. Allergic contact dermatitis in children. Curr Opin Pediatr 2006;18:385-90.
58. Misago N, Nakafusa J, Narisawa Y. Childhood granulomatous periorificial dermatitis: lupus miliaris disseminatus faciei in children? J Eur Acad Dermatol Venereol 2005;19:470-3.
59. Murphy LA, Atherton D. A retrospective evaluation in severe childhood atopic eczema, using thiopurine methyltransferase levels to exclude patients at high risk of myelosuppression. Br J Dermatol 2002; 147: 308-15.
60. Nguyen V, Eichenfield LF. Periorificial dermatitis in children and adolescents. J Am Acad Dermatol 2006;55:781-5.
61. Ong P Y , Ohtake T, Brandt C,et al.Endogenous antimicrobial peptides and skin infections in atopic dermatitis. N Eng J Med 2002 ;347 :1151-60.
62. Ong Py, Hamid QA, Travers JB, et al. Decreased IL-15 may contribute to elevated IgE and acute inflammation in atopic dermatitis. J Immunol 2002; 168: 505-10.
63. Prasad HR, Srivastava P, Verma KK. Diapers and skin care: merits and demerits. Indian J Pediatr 2004;71:907-8.
64. Relyveld GN, Menke HE, Westerhof W. Progressive macular hypomelanosis: an overview. Am J Clin Dermatol 2007;8:13-9.
65. Rigopoulos D, Gregoriou S, Charissi C, Kontochristopoulos G, Kalogeromitros D, Georgala S. Tacrolimus ointment 0.1% in pityriasis alba: an open-label, randomized, placebo-controlled study. Br J Dermatol 2006;155:152-5.
66. Rodríguez-Martín M, Sáez-Rodríguez M, Carnerero-Rodríguez A, Rodríguez-García F, Cabrera de Paz R, Sidro-Sarto M, Guimerá F, Sánchez R, García-Bustínduy M, Noda-Cabrera A. Treatment of perioral dermatitis with topical pimecrolimus. J Am Acad Dermatol 2007 Mar;56:529-30.
67. Rudzki E, Samochocki Z, Releandel P, et al. Frequency and significance of major and minor clinical features of Hanifin and Rajka among patients with atopic dermatitis. Dermatology 1994; 189: 41-6.
68. Sanjana VD, Fernandez RJ. Lichen simplex chronicus - A Psychocutaneous disorder? Indian J Dermatol Venereol Leprol 1995;61:336-8.
69. Sayal SK, Bal AS, Gupta CM, Pattern of skin diseases in pediatric age group and adolescents. Indian J Dermatol Venereol Leprol 1998;64:117-9.
70. Scheinfeld N. Diaper dermatitis: a review and brief survey of eruptions of the diaper area. Am J Clin Dermatol 2005;6:273-81.
71. Schnopp C, Remling R, Mohrenschlager M, Weigl L, Ring J, Abeck D. Topical tacrolimus (FK506) and mometasone furoate in treatment of dyshidrotic palmar eczema: a randomized, observer-blinded trial. J Am Acad Dermatol 2002;46:73-77.
72. Schurmeyer-Horst F, Luger TA, Bohm M. Long-term efficacy of occlusive therapy with topical pimecrolimus in severe dyshidrosiform hand and foot eczema. Dermatology 2007; 214:99-100.
73. Seidenari S, Giusti F, Pepe P, Mantovani L. Contact sensitization in 1094 children undergoing patch testing over a 7-year period. Pediatr Dermatol 2005;22:1-5.
74. Shipley DR, Kennedy CT. Juvenile plantar dermatosis responding to topical tacrolimus ointment. Clin Exp Dermatol 2006;31:453-4.
75. Sidbury R and Hanifin JM. Systemic therapy of atopic dermatitis. Clin Exp Dermatol 2002; 25: 559-66.
76. Sparsa A, Boulinguez S, Liozon E, Roux C, Peyrot I, Doffoel-Hantz V, Labrousse F, Vidal E, Bordessoule D, Bonnetblanc JM, Bédane C. Predictive clinical features of eczema craquelé associated with internal malignancy. Dermatology 2007;215:28-35.
77. Valia RG. Etiopathogenesis of seborrheic dermatitis. Indian J Dermatol Venereol Leprol 2006;72:253-55.
78. Vinod S, Singh G, Dash K, Grover S. Clinico epidemiological study of pityriasis alba. Indian J Dermatol Venereol Leprol 2002;68:338-40.
79. Vocks E, Busch R, Frohlich R, et al. Influence of weather and climate on subjective symptom intensity in atopic eczema. Int J Biometerol 2001; 45: 27-33.
80. Wallengren J. Prurigo: diagnosis and management. Am J Clin Dermatol 2004;5:85-95.
81. Wananukul S, Chindamporn A, Yumyourn P, Payungporn S, Samathi C, Poovorawan Y. Malassezia furfur in infantile seborrheic dermatitis. Asian Pac J Allergy Immunol 2005;23: 101-5.
82. Warner M, Camisa C. Topical corticosteroids. In: Wolverton SE (ed.). Comprehensive Dermatologic Therapy. WB Saunders company 2001; 548-77.
83. Wellington K, Jarvis B. Spotlight on topical pimecrolimus in atopic dermatitis Am J Clin Dermatol 2002: 3; 435-8.
84. Williams H, Robertson C, Stewart A, et al. Worldwide variations in the prevalence of symptoms of atopic eczema in international study of asthma and allergies in childhood. J Allergy Clin Immunol 1999; 103: 125-38.
85. Williams HC, Durney PDJ, Hay RJ, et al. The UK working party's diagnostic criteria for atopic dermatitis: derivation of a minimum set of discriminators for atopic dermatitis. Br J Dermatol 1994; 138: 383-96.
86. Williams HC. Epidemiology of atopic dermatitis: recent advances and future predictions. Curr Probl Dermatol 1999; 28: 9-17.
87. Wollina U. The role of topical calcineurin inhibitors for skin diseases other than atopic dermatitis. Am J Clin Dermatol 2007;8:157-73.
88. Worm M, Aberer W, Agathos M, Becker D, Brasch J, Fuchs T, Hillen U, Höger P, Mahler V, Schnuch A, Szliska C; German Contact Dermatitis Research Group (DKG). Patch testing in children—recommendations of the German Contact Dermatitis Research Group (DKG). J Dtsch Dermatol Ges 2007;5:107-9.
89. Yosipovitch G, Sugeng MW, Chan YH, Goon A, Ngim S, Goh CL. The effect of topically applied aspirin on localized circumscribed neurodermatitis. J Am Acad Dermatol 2001;45:910-3.
90. Zaki I, Emerson R, Allen BR. Treatment of severe atopic dermatitis in childhood with cyclosporin. Br J Dermatol 1996; 135: 21-4.
91. Zalaudek I, Di Stefani A, Ferrara G, Argenziano G. Childhood granulomatous periorificial dermatitis: a controversial disease. J Dtsch Dermatol Ges 2005;3:252-55.

5

Bacterial Infections

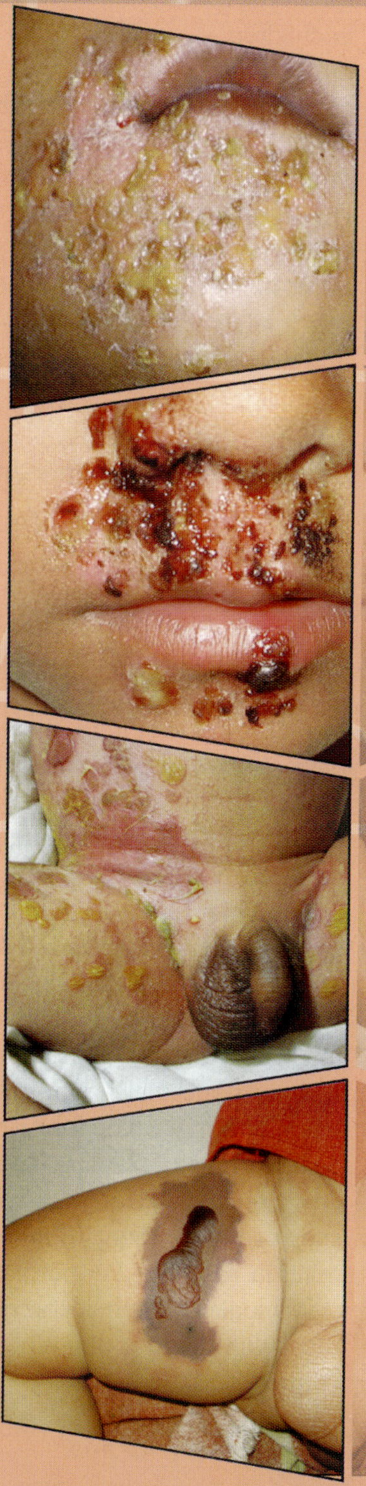

Arun C Inamadar

Bacterial infections of skin are common in pediatric age group. The two gram – positive cocci (*S.aureus* and group A beta-hemolytic *Streptococci*) account for majority of the primary pyodermas. Toxin mediated severe life-threatening conditions like staphylococcal scalded skin syndrome (SSSS) and meningococcemia are also frequent in children.

IMPETIGO

Impetigo is the most common bacterial skin infection of children. It is a contagious, superficial skin infection produced by *Streptococcus pyogenes, Staphylococcus aureus*, or a combination of both. It usually follows minor skin injuries such as an insect bite. Warm, moist climates and poor hygiene predisposes to this infection.

TYPES

Clinically two different presentations are seen:
- Bullous impetigo
- Non-bullous impetigo.

Bullous Impetigo

Bullous impetigo (BI) is caused by an epidermolytic toxin produced by phage group II staphylococci at the site of infection, causing intra epidermal cleavage by targeting desmoglien 1, a cell – cell adhesion molecule. It presents as flaccid, thin-walled bullae. The center of the bullae collapses but peripheral area may retain fluid as inner tube rim. Varnish like crusts may appear at the center, which when removed, reveal eroded base and collarets of moist scale **(Figures 5.1A and B)**. The lesions have little or no surrounding erythema, usually seen in streptococcal impetigo. It typically occurs on the face, but may affect diaper area also. Impetigo circinata is a clinical type or stage of BI characterized by circinate, crusted lesions which develop following the rupture of large fragile bullae **(Figure 5.2)**. This is more commonly seen in warm environment. Axilla, groin and hands are the predilected sites of involvement. *S.aureus* can colonize lesions of miliaria resulting Periporitis staphylogenes. Periporitis staphylogenes staphylococcal sweat gland abscess, found mostly on the face of young children in summer season **(Figure 5.3)**.

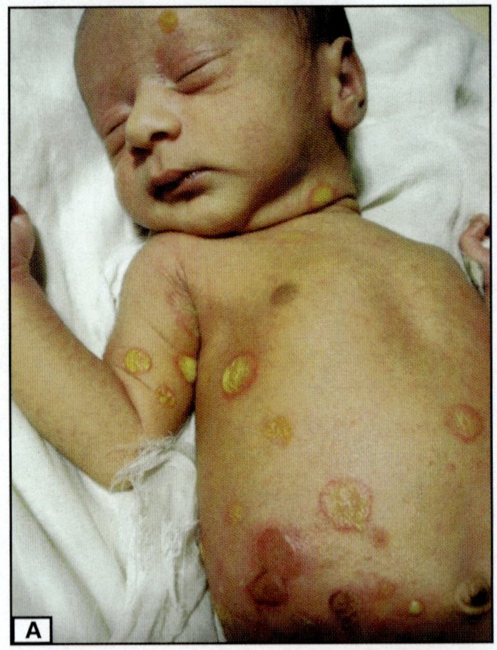

A

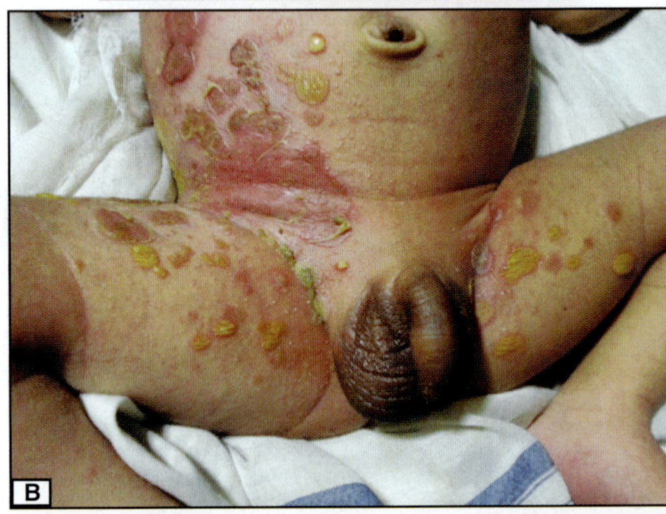

B

FIGURES 5.1A AND B: Bullous impetigo

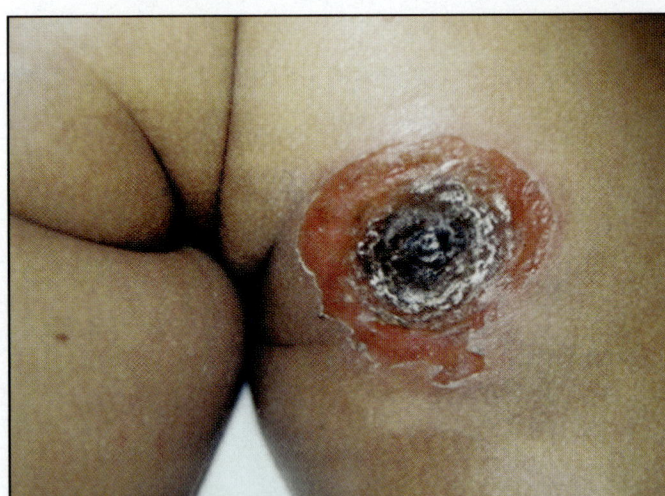

FIGURE 5.2: Circinate impetigo

Non-bullous Impetigo

Non-bullous impetigo (NBI) is more common (> 70%). NBI was once thought to be primarily a group A beta

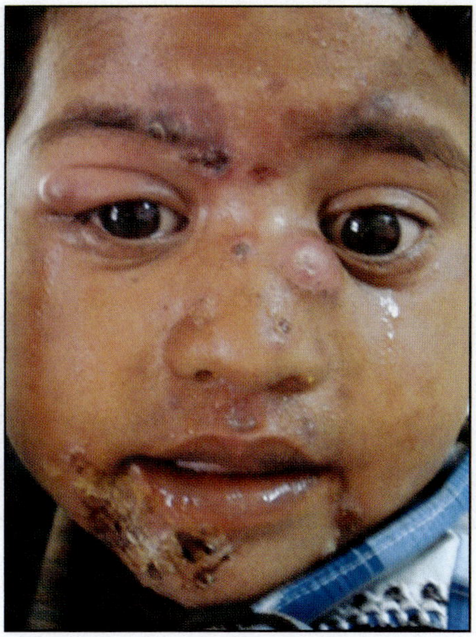

FIGURE 5.3: Periporitis staphylogenes

hemolytic streptococcal (GABHS) disease, but now appears to be caused by *S.aureus* also. Surrounding erythema, satellite lesions, fever and regional lymphadenopathy are characteristic of streptococcal infection. It originates as small vesicle or pustule that ruptures to expose a red, moist base **(Figure 5.4)**. The dried cloudy yellow fluid forms a honey-colored crust, the hallmark of NBI **(Figure 5.5)**. Satellite lesions appear beyond the periphery. Individual lesions may extend peripherally with central clear area, resulting in annular or gyrate morphology. Preceding minor skin trauma is must, as intact skin is resistant to the entry of *Streptococci*. The sites most commonly affected are skin around nose and mouth. The palms and soles are not affected.

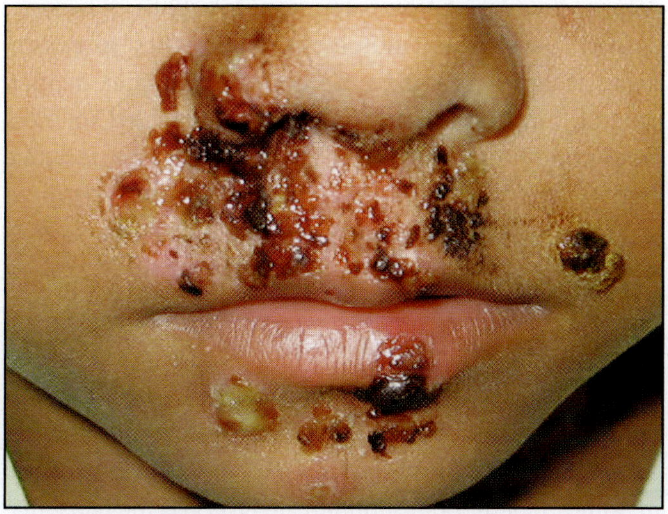

FIGURE 5.4: Impetigo contagiosa

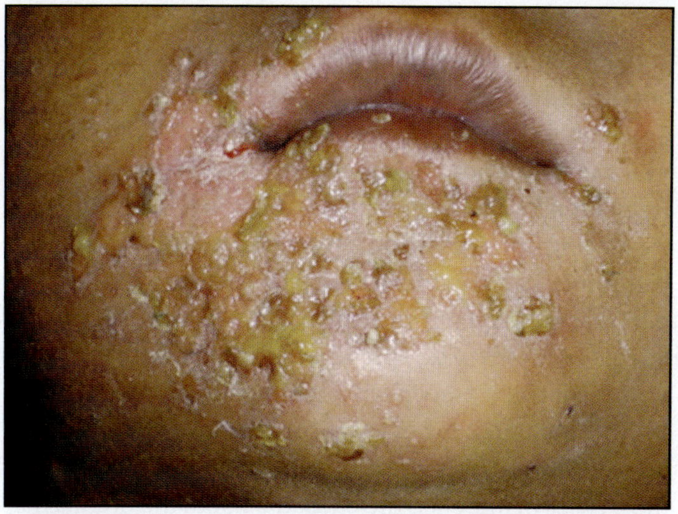

FIGURE 5.5: Honey-colored crust in impetigo contagiosa

Systemic symptoms are infrequent. Complications like sepsis, osteomyelitis, septic arthritis, lymphadenopathy and pneumonia are seen with both NBI and BI in infants. Acute glomerulonephritis (PSGN) and scarlet fever may follow streptococcal infection. The incidence of PSGN increases in the presence of nephritogenic strains of GABHS (10-15%). PSGN is common in children aged 6 to 10 years. Infants younger than 18 months are rarely affected. Rheumatic fever does not occur following streptococcal skin infection. Changing bacteriology of skin infections, more often by staphylococci rather than streptococci, has greatly reduced the concern about PSGN.

DIAGNOSIS

Diagnosis of BI and NBI is based on history and typical clinical presentation. Gram stained smears are adequate in proving the diagnosis. Culture is rarely required, unless methicillin resistance (MRSA) is suspected and also to evaluate carrier status. Evidence of previous streptococcal infection can be assessed by anti-Dnase B titers and anti-hyluronidase titers. ASLO (anti-streptolysion O) titer is low or absent, hence not of much significance in evaluating PSGN.

The disease may resolve spontaneously or become chronic. If untreated it may spread and last for weeks to months. Systemic complications are rare.

TREATMENT

Treatment of impetigo consists of: local therapy, topical antibiotics, oral antibiotics, prevention of recurrent attacks, care of carriage status and management of MRSA.

Crusts should be removed to facilitate better penetration of topical antibiotics by wet cloth compress. For limited localized infections, mupirocin 2% ointment or cream is used three times daily for 7 to 10 days. Local treatment does not treat lesions that evolve in other areas. Retapamulin 1% ointment has been approved for the treatment of impetigo. Retapamulin is the new pleuromutilin class of antibacterial and acts as a potent inhibitor of bacterial protein synthesis. Oral therapy is indicated, when wide spread infections (satellite lesions) are present with associated lymphadenopathy and fever. Erythromycin is a better choice in areas with a low prevalence of erythromycin resistant *S.aureus*. Because most cases of impetigo are caused by both the organisms, a 5–10 day course of penicillinase–resistant semisynthetic penicillin like cloxacillin, dicloxacillin, amoxicillin plus clavulinic acid is indicated. Cephalosporins (Cephalexin 20-40 mg/kg/day divided three times daily) can also be used.

In severe and recalcitrant cases MRSA infection must be considered. MRSA isolates are susceptible to clindamycin and co-trimoxazole. Children with recurrent impetigo should be evaluated for carriage of staphylococci. As nose is a common site of carriage, mupirocin application to the nasal vestibule twice daily for 5 days is significantly effective in managing such cases. This course is repeated monthly for a minimum of three months.

ECTHYMA

Ecthyma is a deep or ulcerative type of primary pyoderma, covered by adherent crusts. These are commonly seen over lower extremities and gluteal region. Ecthyma is initiated by GABHS. Thick crusts (oyster-shell like) and underlying pain full ulcer, healing with scar are characteristic clinical features for diagnosis **(Figure 5.6)**. Treatment consists of warm compresses and a 7-10 day course of dicloxacillin or cephalosporins.

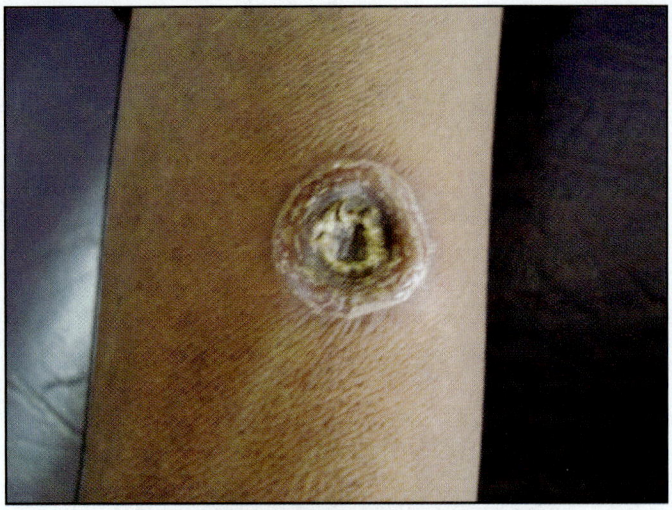

FIGURE 5.6: Ecthyma

ECTHYMA GANGRENOSUM

Ecthyma gangrenosum is seen in children with *Pseudomonas aeruginosa* bacteremia. It is characterized by haemorrhagic papules that progress to bullae, ulceration with eschar formation. Appearance of such lesions in infants should prompt a thorough investigation for occult immunodeficiency. Diagnosis is confirmed by gram stain and blood culture. Treatment is with aminoglycosides or antipseudomonal penicillins.

FOLLICULITIS

Folliculitis is an inflammation of the hair follicle. Bacterial folliculitis includes follicular impetigo and sycosis barbae. Superficial folliculitis, otherwise termed as 'Bockhart's impetigo' is common in children. It is usually seen on the buttocks and thighs. Lesions are painless yellow-white pustules with hair shaft protruding from the center. The condition usually responds to cleansing with antibacterial soap and topical antibiotics. Extensive and resistant cases need to be treated with systemic anti-staphylococcal antibiotics, like cloxacillin, dicloxacillin and clindamycin.

FURUNCLES AND CARBUNCLES

A furuncle evolves from superficial folliculitis. It is deep, painful, perifollicular abscess with tendency to central necrosis and suppuration. Carbuncles are larger, deeper, painful, interconnected aggregates of infected follicles. Both conditions are rare in children. Therapy includes antistaphylococcal antibiotics and minor surgical procedure like incision and drainage.

CELLULITIS

Cellulitis is an acute infection of dermis and subcutaneous tissue. It is clinically characterized by fever, erythema, edema and pain. It is caused by GABHS and staphylococci in adults. *Haemophilus influenzae* type B is the causative agent in children.

BUCCAL CELLULITIS (BLUE CELLULITIS)

H.influenzae type B (Hib) is commonly implicated in buccal cellulitis often seen in children below 2 years. It characteristically presents as dusky red to blue discoloration of the involved skin, hence the name blue cellulitis/ 'bruised cheek syndrome'. Meningitis is the dreaded complication associated with buccal cellulitis. Blood culture is diagnostic. Therapy must be prompt. Cefotaxime and ceftriaxone are effective as these have good CSF penetrance. Rifampicin prophylaxis should be considered for the entire family of an index case, especially when the family includes a child younger than 4 years.

PERIORBITAL AND ORBITAL CELLULITIS

Periorbital cellulitis is more common in children. It is also termed as pre septal cellulitis. It presents with erythema and edema of the eyelid, conjunctivitis, chemosis, normal vision, and preservation of ocular motility. *H. influenzae* is the common causative agent in children. With the advent of Hib immunization, Hib is being replaced by streptococcal species (GABHS and *S. pneumoniae*) and *S.aureus.* When the infection traverses the orbital septum it results in **orbital cellulitis.** It presents as proptosis, orbital pain, restricted movements of the eyes and chemosis. Complications like cavernous vein thrombosis are observed. Intravenous antibiotics are indicated for the treatment. Cefuroxime is effective as it has better CSF penetrance, thereby reducing the likelihood of meningitis. Surgical intervention is indicated when there is radiological evidence (CT scan) of intracranial involvement, a sub periosteal or orbital abscess, decreasing vision and worsening ocular movement or no response to IV antibiotics in 24 to 48 hours period.

PERIANAL CELLULITIS

It is caused by GABHS, commonly seen in children. There is moist, edematous, pink skin around the anus along with itch and pain. Topical mupirocin and semi-synthetic penicillin bring relief to the condition.

ERYSIPELAS

It is an acute inflammatory form of cellulitis that differs from the other forms by presence of lymphatic involvement evident as erythematous streaks. It has a sharp upper margin as compared to cellulitis **(Figure 5.7)**.

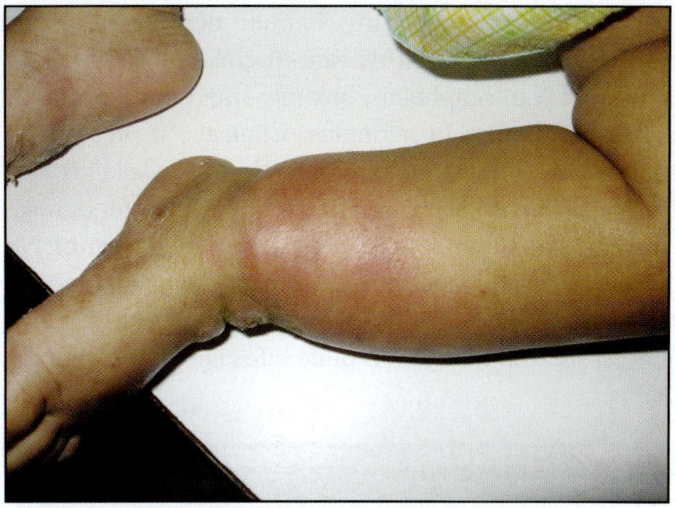

FIGURE 5.7: Erysipelas

Children often do not develop erysipelas. Rarely *H.influenzae* may cause it.

BLISTERING DISTAL DACTYLITIS

It is a condition characterized by a large fluid-filled lesion, later with purulent material, occurring on the fingertip. It is usually caused by GABHS and is more common in children. It responds to antibiotics (erythromycin / penicillin) and incision drainage.

NECROTIZING FASCIITIS

Necrotizing fasciitis (NF) is a rapidly progressive infection of the subcutaneous tissue resulting in destruction of subcutaneous fat and fascia **(Figure 5.8)**. It is associated with severe systemic toxicity like hypotension, renal

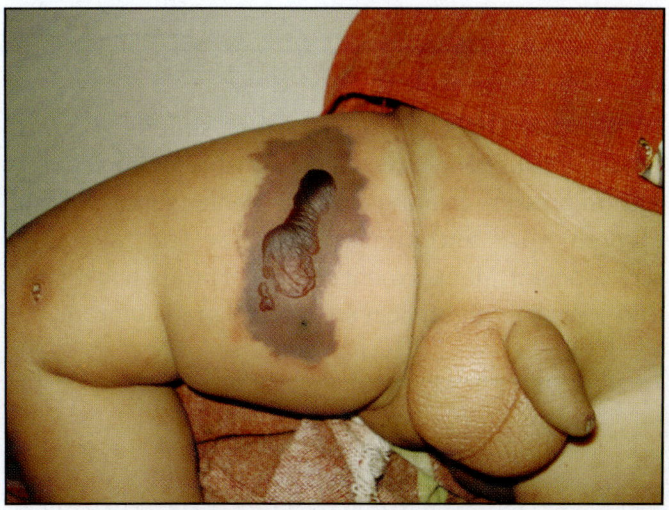

FIGURE 5.8: Necrotizing fasciitis

impairment, coagulopathy, hepatic derangement and respiratory distress. NF is rare in children. It has been observed with omphalitis, balanitis, mammitis, and fetal scalp monitoring in neonates. Clinically it presents as painful swelling with exquisite tenderness. Cellulitis with return of fever; tachycardia and severe skin tenderness are the signs that should prompt the diagnosis of NF. Overlying skin is anesthetic, which is very characteristic. Immediate surgical debridement of necrotic tissue is necessary. Clindamycin is quite effective in treating NF.

ERYTHRASMA

Erythrasma is a superficial bacterial infection caused by *C.minutissimum*. It is non inflammatory, uniformly brown, scaly, half-moon shaped plaque without advancing border. Incidence is less common in children. Common locations include groin, axillae and interdigital spaces. It shows characteristic coral red fluorescence under Wood's lamp examination. It responds well to oral erythromycin, topical miconazole, clotrimazole and topical clindamycin.

TRICHOMYCOSIS AXILLARIS

It is a superficial bacterial infection of axillary and pubic hair caused by *C. tenuis*. It appears as adherent white to yellow nodules consisting of bacterial elements embedded in an amorphous matrix. It is seen only in post pubertal children. Shaving of the part and topical application of erythromycin/ clindamycin is curative.

PITTED KERATOLYSIS

It is caused by *Corynebacterium sedentarius* and *Dermatiphilus conglensis*. Clinically it presents as shallow pits on pressure bearing areas of plantar surface of feet. Hyperhidrosis and immersion of the feet favours its development. Management consists of promoting dryness and topical erythromycin solution or oral erythromycin.

STAPHYLOCOCCAL SCALDED SKIN SYNDROME (SSSS)

SSSS is a bacterial disease caused by staphylococcal epidermolytic toxin (ET). Other names of the disease are Ritter's disease and pemphigus neonatorum. It is more common in children younger than 2 years. The reasons for such age preference are thought to be lack of immunity to the toxins and renal immaturity in children leading to poor clearance of the toxins.

Pathogenesis is related to epidermolytic toxins elaborated by *S. aureus*. Recent studies have indicated that the three isoforms of ETs, i.e., ETA, ETB, and ETD are glutamate-specific serine proteases that specifically and efficiently cleave a single peptide bond in the extracellular region of human and mouse desmoglein 1 (Dsg1), a desmosomal intercellular adhesion molecule found in the superficial epidermis. Its rarity in adult is explained by the fact that 75% normal people older than 10 years will have ET antibodies. Outbreaks of SSSS have been reported in neonatal intensive care units due to handling of babies by infected or asymptomatic carriers of staphylococci.

Clinically SSSS (**Figures 5.9A and B)** begins with localized infection of the conjunctiva, throat, nares, perineum or umbilicus. A scarlatiniform eruption appears followed by a tissue paper like wrinkling of the epidermis. The eruption is more marked over flexures. The characteristic facial appearance consists of separation of perioral crusts leaving behind radial fissures around the mouth. The Nikolsky's sign is positive. Generalized denudation of skin leads to complications like fluid loss,

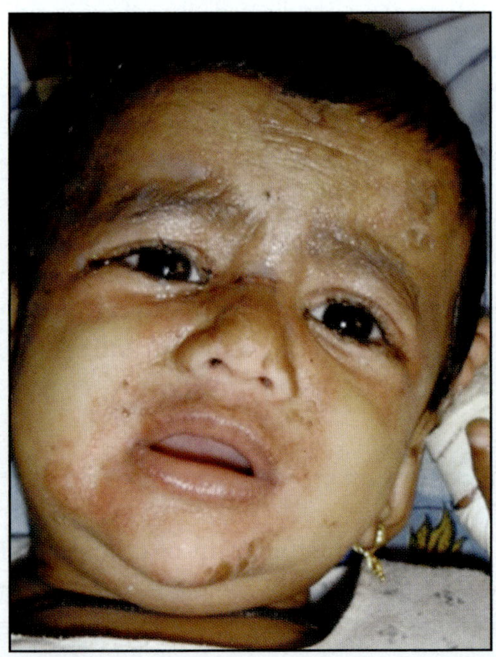

FIGURE 5.9A: SSSS (early stage with erythema)

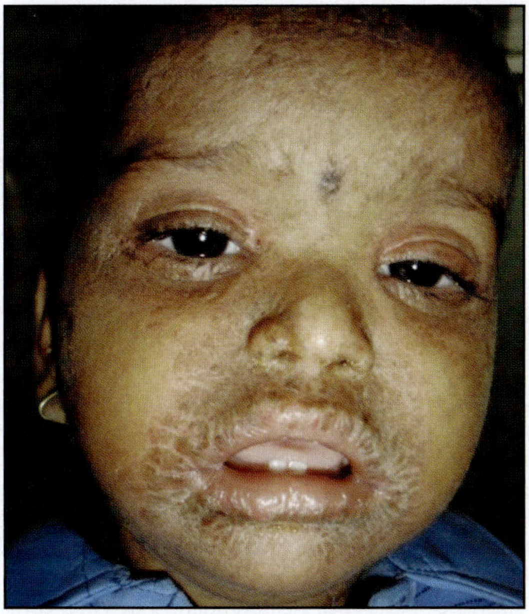

FIGURE 5.9B: SSSS (following initiation of treatment)

dehydration and decreased thermoregulation. Fever, malaise, irritability and poor feeding develop subsequently. Risk of secondary infection and sepsis also increases. With appropriate management, skin heals within 7-10 days. Re-epithelialization is rapid because of the high level split in the epidermis.

Diagnosis of SSSS is based on clinical features. Clinically main differential diagnosis is toxic epidermal necrolysis (TEN). TEN is more common in adults and is always secondary to drug, with high mortality rate. Mucosal involvement is more prominent. Histopathologically, TEN shows dermo-epidermal separation rather than the granular split seen in SSSS.

Diagnosis is confirmed by isolation of *S.aureus*. Culture specimen should be taken from the eye, nose, throat, or pyogenic foci on the skin. Exfoliated skin and intact blisters will not yield any organism as these are caused by hematogenous spread of ETs. Biopsy shows splitting of the epidermis in the stratum granulosum.

Hospitalization and intravenous antibiotic therapy are must for extensive cases. Attention to fluid and electrolyte balance, infection control measures and pain management should be given. A penicillinase-resistant penicillin (Nafcillin 100-200 mg/kg daily), first or second generation cephalosporins or clindamycin are all good initial choices. Children infected with MRSA need treatment with vancomycin. For milder form and diseases in older children, ambulatory treatment is advised.

MENINGOCOCCEMIA

Meningococcemia is an acute septicemia caused by the Gram negative bacteria *N.meningitidis*. It progresses faster than any other infectious disease due to shock and disseminated intravascular coagulation (DIC).

It is very common in children under 5 years of age. More than 50% of the cases among infants younger than 1 year are caused by serogroup B. Incidentally, there is no vaccine available for this serogroup. Endotoxin released by *N.meningitidis* invades small blood vessels and causes damage by releasing cytokines. There is associated severe hypotension, low cardiac output, organ anoxia and DIC.

Clinically, up to 75% of children develop a skin eruption, a petechial rash and ecchymosis specific for meningococcal disease. The petechiae are small, stellate with a raised border and slightly depressed vesicular or pustular center. Trunk and lower extremity are common sites of involvement. In severe cases, these may progress to bullae, necrosis with sloughing and eschar formation. Consumptive coagulopathy in the form of purpura fulminans **(Figure 5.10)** may be the end-stage with poor prognosis.

The differential diagnosis includes: Henoch-Schonlein purpura, rickettsial diseases and other bacterial septicemias or meningitides. The diagnosis is confirmed by blood and CSF culture. Gram stained smears from petichial lesions show diplococci. Lesional biopsy shows dermal vessel thrombi and evidence of vasculitis.

Treatment consists of administration of penicillin G, chloramphenicol (penicillin allergic patients), and

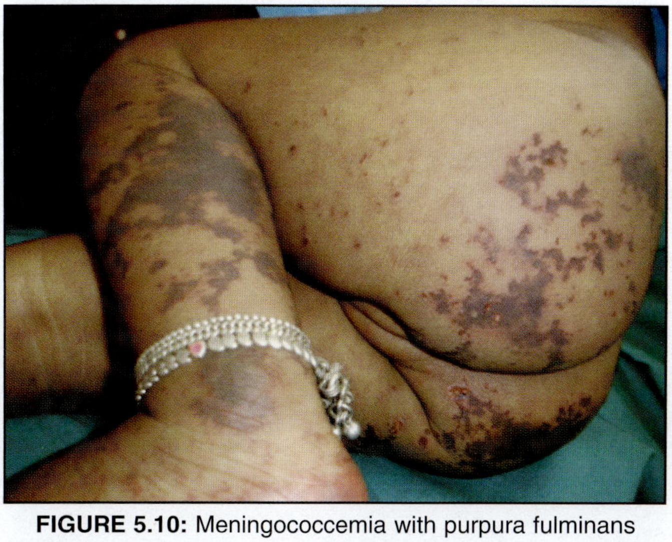

FIGURE 5.10: Meningococcemia with purpura fulminans

cephalosporins (ceftriaxone, cefotaxime and cefuroxime). In presence of DIC, fresh plasma transfusion is needed. Debridement of necrotic skin and subcutaneous tissue is a necessity if poor tissue perfusion is the complication.

Antimicrobial prophylaxis should be given within 24 hours after identification of an index case. Rifampicin is the ideal drug in neonates, children, as well as in adults. The dosage for infants of age <1 month is, 5 mg/ kg every 12 hours for 2 days; for infants older than 1 month, the dose is 10 mg / kg every 12 hours for 2 days. Adult dosage is 600 mg every 12 hour for 2 days.

BIBLIOGRAPHY

1. Bernard P. Management of common bacterial infections of the skin. Curr Opin Infect Dis 2008;21:122-8.
2. Durupt F, Mayor L, Bes M, Reverdy ME, Vandenesch F, Thomas L, et al. Prevalence of Staphylococcus aureus toxins and nasal carriage in furuncles and impetigo. Br J Dermatol 2007;157:1161-7.
3. Gabillot-Carré M, Roujeau JC. Acute bacterial skin infections and cellulitis.Curr Opin Infect Dis 2000;20:118-23.
4. HanakawaY, Selwood T, Woo D, Lin C, Schechter NM, Stanley JR. Calcium-dependent conformation of desmoglein 1 is required for its cleavage by exfoliative toxin. Journal of Investigative Dermatology 2003; 121:383-9.
5. Jacobs MR. Retapamulin: a semisynthetic pleuromutilin compound for topical treatment of skin infections in adults and children. Future Microbiol 2007;2:591-600.
6. Koning S, van der Wouden JC, Chosidow O, Twynholm M, Singh KP, Scangarella N. Efficacy and safety of retapamulin ointment as treatment of impetigo: randomized double-blind multicentre placebo-controlled trial. Br J Dermatol 2008;158:1077-82.
7. Ladhani S, Garbash M. Staphylococcal skin infections in children: rational drug therapy recommendations. Paediatr Drugs 2005;7:77-102.
8. Nishifuji K, Sugai M, Amagai M. Staphylococcal exfoliative toxins: "molecular scissors" of bacteria that attack the cutaneous defense barrier in mammals. J Dermatol Sci 2008; 49:21-31.
9. Orange AP, Chosidow O, Sacchidanand S, Todd G, Singh K, Scangarella N, et al. Topical retapamulin ointment, 1%, versus sodium fusidate ointment, 2%, for impetigo: a randomized, observer-blinded, noninferiority study. Dermatology 2007;215:331-40.
10. Pandit AM, Siddaramappa B, Choudhary SV, Manjunath-swamy BS. Ecthyma gangrenosum in a new born child. Indian J Dermatol Venereol Leprol 2003;69:52-3.
11. Parish LC, Parish JL. Retapamulin: a new topical antibiotic for the treatment of uncomplicated skin infections. Drugs Today (Barc) 2008;44:91-102.
12. Raghavan M, Linden PK. Newer treatment options for skin and soft tissue infections. Drugs 2004;64:1621-42.
13. Vayalumkal JV, Jadavji T. Children hospitalized with skin and soft tissue infections: a guide to antibacterial selection and treatment. Paediatr Drugs 2006;8:99-111.
14. Yang LP, Keam SJ. Retapamulin: a review of its use in the management of impetigo and other uncomplicated superficial skin infections. Drugs 2008;68:855-73.

6

Viral Infections and Exanthems

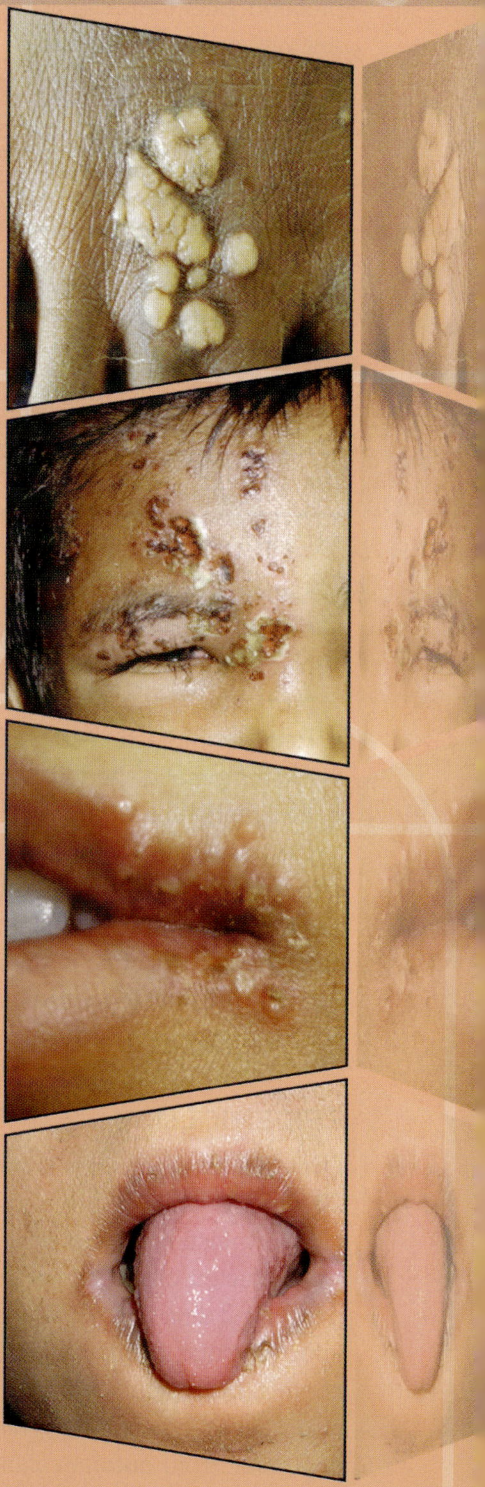

Viral Infections

K A Seetharam

Viral Exanthems

Vijay Zawar

HERPES VIRUSES

Herpes viruses are DNA viruses, mostly infect animal species and universally distributed. There are eight types of herpes viruses **(Table 6.1)**, known to infect humans. This group of viruses characteristically produces primary infection, after that establishes latent infection in host and reactivates at a later stage.

TABLE 6.1: Types of herpes viruses

Alpha viruses
Herpes simplex virus Type 1 and 2
Varicella zoster virus (HHV 3)
Beta viruses
Cytomegalo virus (HHV 5)
Gama viruses
Epstein- Barr virus (HHV 4)
Human herpes virus-6
Human herpes virus-7
Human herpes virus- 8

HERPES SIMPLEX VIRUS (HSV)

- Hepes simplex viruses, Type 1 and 2 produce varied clinical manifestations.
- Neonatal HSV infection has high morbidity and mortality.
- Recurrent infections are less severe than primary.
- Asymptomatic shedding occurs intermittently.
- Early initiation of antiviral therapy is useful.

Herpes simplex virus has two types. Type 1 is usually responsible for nongenital infections and Type 2 causes genital infections. Herpes simplex viruses have the unique property of replicating in the nervous tissue and remains latent, mostly the trigeminal ganglia for HSV-1 and sacral nerve ganglia in HSV-2.

EPIDEMIOLOGY

Primary HSV-1 infection is generally a childhood disease, 20-35% of children are infected by the age of 5 years. HSV-1 infections, most often result from direct contact with infected oral secretions of lesions. The incubation period is 2 days to 2 weeks. HSV-2 causes mostly genital infections and commonly acquired with intimate sexual contact, but a significant number of genital infections are also caused by HSV-1. While genital HSV-1 infections can result from autoinoculation of virus from facio-oral lesions, sexual abuse should always be considered in prepubertal children with genital HSV-2 infections. Neonatal HSV infection occurs in 1 per 3000 deliveries and is mostly caused by HSV- 2, during birth through an infected maternal genital tract. Ascending *in utero* infection can result in congenital HSV infection.

CLINICAL FEATURES

Herpes simplex viruses produce an array of clinical manifestations in children **(Table 6.2)**. True primary infections in a person without prior exposure are usually quiet severe. They are associated with regional lymphadenitis. They run a clinical course of 1-3 weeks. Recurrent infections are less severe and heal quickly.

TABLE 6.2: Clinical presentations caused by HSV

Primary herpetic gingivostomatitis
Primary herpetic lesions on skin
Primary neonatal HSV infection
Herpes genitalis
Herpetic eye infection
Herpetic whitlow
Herpetic gladiatorum
Recurrent herpes infections
Erythema multiforme minor

Gingivostomatitis

This is most often seen in infants and young children. The children are febrile, irritable, refuse to eat and drink. Erythematous, painful, tense, superficial ulcerations, covered with exudates are seen **(Figure 6.1)**. There may be perioral cutaneous lesions. Tender submandibular lymphadenopathy is common. It lasts from 7 to 14 days. As oral intake is poor hospitalization may be required.

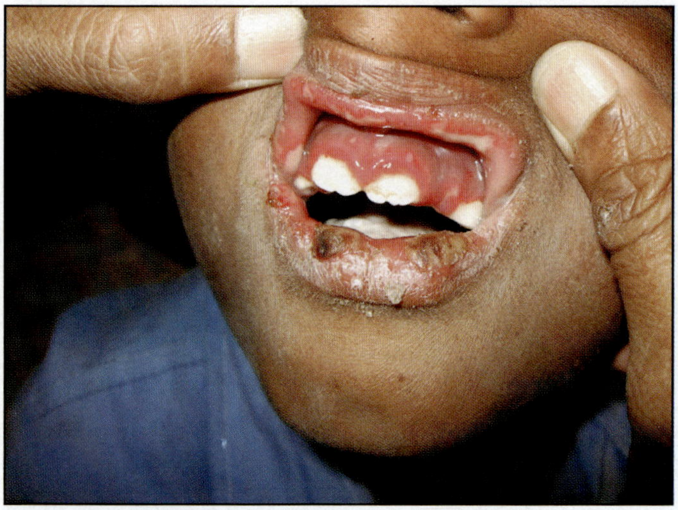

FIGURE 6.1: Herpetic gingivostomatitis

Herpes Simplex Lesions on Skin

Primary HSV lesions on skin (fever blisters, cold sores) are characterized by grouped vesicles or erosions on an erythematous base. They often coalesce and produce large ulcers with a scalloped edge. The lesions are most common on face and extremities.

Neonatal Herpetic Infection

Neonatal HSV infection is seen 1 in 3000 live births. It tends to manifest within first 4 weeks of life, mostly in first week. 75-80% infections are caused by HSV-2 and the rest by HSV-1. Three patterns, SEM (Skin, Eye, and Mouth disease), CNS disease and disseminated infection are described. Multiple vesicles, grouped and disseminated, erosions and ulcers, especially at places of trauma occur. Lesions can turn into pustular, bullous and necrotic. Children with SEM disease should be carefully evaluated and followed for CNS or disseminated infections as they may be delayed. Neonates with CNS infection develop focal encephalitis and meningoencephalitis, associated with fever, seizures and coma. CSF shows lymphocytic pleocytosis. Disseminated infections involve multiple organs, liver, lung, brain, and adrenals causing jaundice, respiratory insufficiency, and neurologic deterioration and disseminated intravascular coagulation. It is often severe with high morbidity and 50% mortality and there is significant chance of permanent sequelae among its survivors. Perinatal HSV infection is a part of TORCHES (toxoplasmosis, other agents—varicellazoster virus, parvovirus B19, rubella, cytomegalovirus, herpes simplex, enteroviruses, Epstein-Barr virus, syphilis) syndrome.

Herpetic Eye Infection

HSV-1 is a leading cause of keratoconjunctivitis with associated corneal opacity and visual loss. It is associated with pain, edema of eyelids, burning, blurred vision, conjunctivitis and uveitis. Dendrite ulcers of cornea are a classic finding. Acute retinal necrosis is rare, but serious and commonly occurs with HSV-2.

Inoculation HSV Infection

Direct inoculation of virus into abrasion or into normal skin can cause indurated papules, vesicles and large bullae. Herpetic whitlow, typically involves fingertips, most common in thumb suckers and dental surgeons with inoculation from oral lesions. Herpes gladiatorum occurs in wrestlers as multiple crops of vesicles, pustules or plaques, erythema of face, scalp and upper trunk, simulating pyogenic infections.

Eczema Herpeticum

Eczema herpeticum refers to a widespread cutaneous infection with HSV, in a patient with pre-existing disease. The pre-existing disease could be any, but mainly atopic dermatitis, Darier's disease, burns, contact dermatitis, ichthyoses and other inflammatory dermatoses. Kaposi's varicelliform eruption refers to eczema herpeticum (HSV infection), eczema vaccinatum (caused by vaccinia) and also infections by other viruses like Coxasackie A16.

The majority of eczema herpeticum cases are primary infections, multiple widespread vesicles erupt in crops, rapidly become pustular. They may be confined to abnormal skin, but may be disseminated **(Figure 6.2)**. Face is edematous and is associated with severe constitutional symptoms like fever, malaise, pain and irritability. The fever subsides in 4-5 days and pustules become crusted and heal with scarring. Rarely do they progress to potential fatal infection.

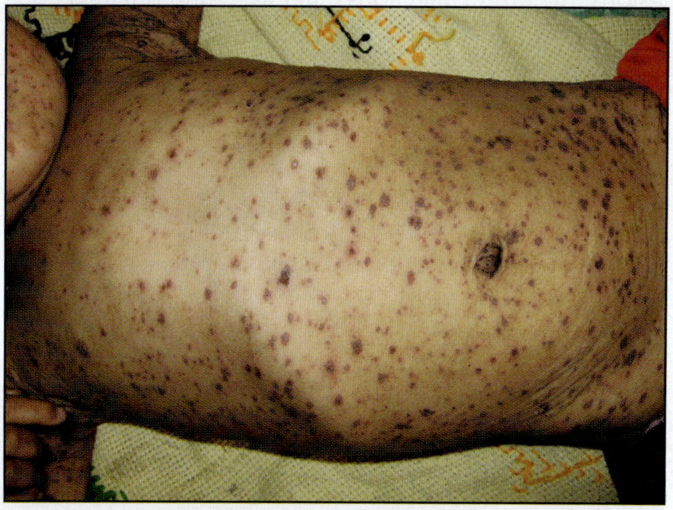

FIGURE 6.2: Eczema herpeticum

Herpes Genitalis

Herpes genitalis is usually caused by HSV-2, occasionally by HSV-1, occurs after the onset of sexual activity. Grouped vesicles, painful shallow ulcers occur on genitalia and perineal areas. Herpes genitalis occurring in children should be investigated for sexual abuse.

Recurrent Infections

After primary infection, the virus remains latent in sensory ganglia. Reactivation is triggered by emotional stress,

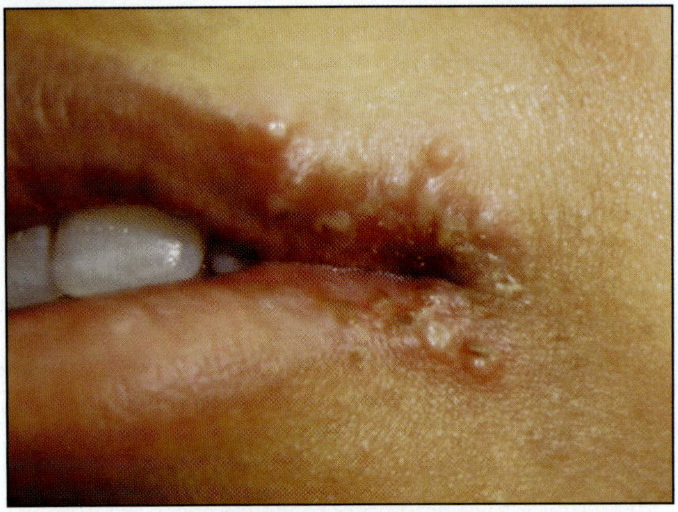

FIGURE 6.3: Herpes labialis

trauma, sunburn, menses, fever and infections. They are less severe than primary and heals rapidly. Recurrences are more common with HSV-2 infections (90%) compared with HSV-1(50%). Reactivation occurs at any site of primary infection. Patients often report itching or burning in the affected area prior to the appearance of lesions. Recurrent infections differ from primary infections in the smaller size of vesicles and the absence of constitutional symptoms and heal rapidly without scarring **(Figure 6.3)**.

Erythema Multiforme

Recurrent erythema multiforme minor can occur with recurrent herpes infections, usually 1-2 weeks after HSV infection **(Figure 6.4)**.

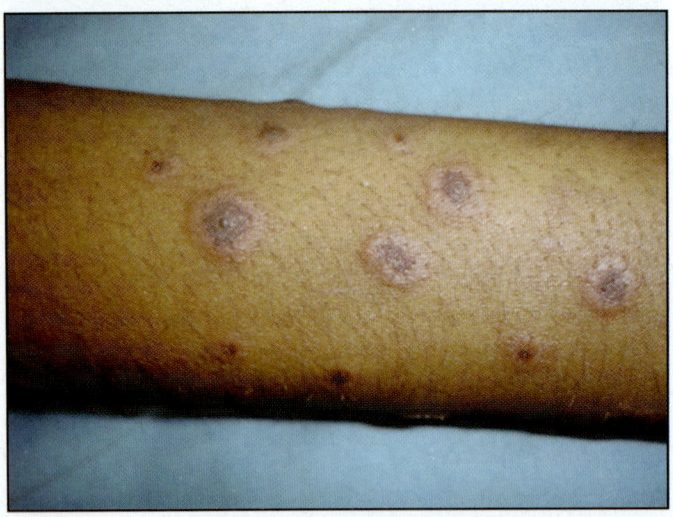

FIGURE 6.4: Erythema multiforme

Asymptomatic Shedding

In individuals with HSV, virus may be present at the site of infection, even in the absence of clinically evident lesions. This is known as asymptomatic shedding. The viral titre is lower than during clinically active disease. Transmission can occur with asymptomatic shedding.

LABORATORY INVESTIGATIONS

Cytologic smear from the base of vesicle stained with Giemsa or Wright's stain show multinucleated keratinocytes, molding of nuclear borders and nuclear inclusions (Tzanck smear). The virus can be easily and rapidly grown in culture from the vesicular fluid in 24-48 hours. Skin biopsy reveals intraepidermal bulla, ballooning degeneration of cells and large multinucleated giant cells with intranuclear inclusions. Neutralizing antibodies will rise after the first week of primary infection. If facilities available, immunofluorescent and immunoperoxidase techniques demonstrate and differentiate Type 1 and Type 2 on tissue specimens. Polymerase chain reaction (PCR) test is rapid and sensitive with HSV infections and more frequently used for CNS infection.

TREATMENT

In many instances, supportive therapy, and antibiotics to prevent secondary bacterial infection may be sufficient. Cool compresses with tap water or Burrow's solution for 10 minutes 3 times daily are helpful. However, specific antiviral treatment is desired for severe outbreaks, recurrent infections and neonatal HSV infections.

There are three systemic antiviral agents, useful for HSV infections: acyclovir, valacyclovir and famcyclovir. Valacyclovir is valyl ester of acyclovir and its bio-availability is 3-5 times greater than acyclovir. Famcyclovir is the deoxy analogue of pencyclovir and is well observed and has a long intracellular life. All these types are generally safe and highly effective because of their specific antiviral activity. They are converted into active form by the viral enzyme thymidine kinase and inhibit viral DNA synthesis with little impact on host cell. Valacyclovir and famcyclovir have the advantage of BID dose compared to acyclovir. However famcyclovir and valacyclovir have not been approved by FDA for children.

Acyclovir, 20 mg/kg, divided into 5 times daily given for 7 days has shortened the duration of lesions, decreased morbidity and duration of the viral shedding. Acyclovir is more effective, if started at the time of prodrome in recurrent infections or with in 24-48 hours of the appearance of lesions. Acyclovir is highly safe and free of side effects except in rare cases of rapid IV administration of the drug, where transient renal dysfunction may occur.

Topical acyclovir applied 5 times daily shows modest effect on primary and recurrent infections as well. In many clinical trails, topical acyclovir alone was found ineffective. Topical 1% penciclovir, topical 1.8% tetracaine and 10%, docosanol are useful in relieving the itching, pain and discomfort. Ethyl ether, chloroform, alcohol, idoxiuridine, silver sulphadiazine have been shown to be ineffective. Foscarnet is the only antiviral, useful and approved for the acyclovir resistant HSV infections in AIDS patients as it does not require HSV thymidine kinase. Herpetic eye infection should be treated with trifluridine, poloxuridine or adenosine arabinoside.

Women with active genital HSV had to be delivered by 'C-section', preferably within 4-6 hours of membrane rupture. In severe recurrent infections suppressive therapy for longer period for one year or more is helpful.

PROGNOSIS

The mucocutaneous infections in children regress excellently. Untreated Neonatal CNS infections result in residual deformity and death. SEM often results in good outcome.

VARICELLA-ZOSTER VIRUS (HHV-3) INFECTIONS

- Varicella-zoster virus (VZV) produces varicella as primary infection and herpes zoster on reactivation.
- In varicella, lesions of different stages are present at the same time.
- Varicella vaccine is highly efficacious.
- Herpes zoster is unilateral and localized in immunocompetent, bilateral and disseminated in immunosuppressed.
- Post herpetic neuralgia is rare in children.

Varicella-zoster virus is a double-stranded DNA virus. It causes chicken pox as a primary infection and herpes zoster (shingles) on reactivation.

CHICKENPOX (VARICELLA)

EPIDEMIOLOGY

Chickenpox is benign, but highly contagious infection, caused by varicella-zoster virus. Ninety percent of cases occur in children less than ten years of age. 96% of children will have varicella within one month of exposure to the index case. The incubation period is 10 to 23 days (average 14-16 days). It is common in late winter and early spring. It spreads mainly by person to person contact and respiratory droplets. The disease is infectious from 2 days before the onset of rash to 5-6 days after onset or until all lesions crust. Crusts are non-infectious. The disease in adults is more severe and morbidity is high compared to children. After the infection immunity is usually lifelong. HIV infected patients have more severe wide spread atypical varicella with disseminated pox-like lesions.

PATHOGENESIS

Varicella caused by varicella-zoster virus (HHV-3) and produce infection within keratinocytes with epidermal cell death.

CLINICAL FEATURES

Varicella is basically a vesicular exanthem with low grade fever and mild systemic symptoms. It begins abruptly as discrete erythematous macules, papules over thorax, scalp, and mucous membranes. Lesions progress rapidly into vesicles, surrounded by erythema. This appearance is named 'dew drops on a rose petal'. Vesicles enlarge become umbilicated, turns into pustules and crusts in 2-4 days **(Figure 6.5)**.

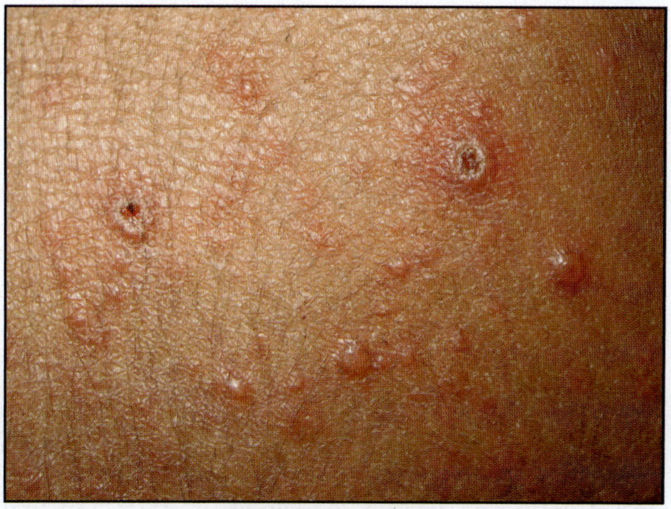

FIGURE 6.5: Varicella

Crusts fall in 1-3 weeks without scarring. Lesions of different stages are seen in the same area at same time. Generally children have less severe form of the disease, compared to adolescents and adults, who have more severity and morbidity with more complications, commonly varicella pneumonia. Pruritus is common, sometimes severe. Secondary bacterial infection of skin lesions may occur. Sometimes the vesicles enlarge into large bullae, become hemorrhagic and rupture, mimicking impetigo. This is termed as varicella bullosa, develops due to superinfection with toxin producing *S. aureus* which causes epidermolysis. Oral lesions occur over hard palate, uvula and tonsillar pillars as vesicles, which rapidly develop into sharp ulcers with surrounding halo. Recurrence of varicella in immunocompetent children is very rare, though there are some recent reports, where 14 normal children with 2 episodes of varicella have been reported. In immunocompromised children with lymphoma, leukemia and HIV-infection, severe life-threatening forms may occur. Lesions may last longer, sometimes even for few months. Congenital varicella syndrome can occur with fetal infections *in utero* (first and second trimester) and results in varicella embryopathy with limb atrophy, scarring, cataract formation, microcephaly and cortical atrophy.

LABORATORY INVESTIGATIONS

Investigations are rarely necessary in uncomplicated varicella. Tzanck smear from the base of vesicle reveals multinucleated giant cells and inclusion bodies. Viral cultures, immunofluoprescence and serologic methods may be helpful in differentiation. Skin biopsy shows ballooning degeneration, multinucleate giant cells and nuclear inclusions.

TREATMENT

In normal children supportive care is sufficient. Antihistamines are helpful in relieving pruritus and antibiotics to prevent secondary infection. Soothing lotions like calamine relieve discomfort. Oral and perineal lesions are treated by saline rinses and compresses.

Oral acyclovir is not recommended routinely for uncomplicated varicella in healthy children. Acyclovir, 20 mg/kg/day in 4-5 divided doses for 5 days is given for children more than 2 years of age with chronic cutaneous and pulmonary disease. Acyclovir, if started in first 24 hours of onset, for 5 to 7 days has shortened the duration of disease, decreases itching and heals rapidly. Valacyclovir and famcyclovir have not been evaluated in primary varicella infection. In immunocompromised, intravenous acyclovir is recommended (5-10 mg/kg/8 hourly) for 7 to 10 days.

VARICELLA ZOSTER IMMUNOGLOBULIN (VZIG)

VZIG may be indicated in highly susceptible and high risk individuals with leukemia, lymphoma and children receiving chemotherapy. If it is given within 72 hours of exposure, it may not prevent the disease, but modify the disease course to less severe form. New born, whose mothers developed varicella 5 days before delivery or within 2 days after delivery should be given VZIG.

VARICELLA VACCINE

Varicella vaccine, a live attenuated vaccine is approved for use in varicella since 1995 and is highly effective. Single dose is advised for healthy children from 12 months to 12 years. In children more than 13 years of age and in adults, 2 doses are recommended at the interval of 4-8 weeks. Seroconversion is 97%. The possibility of vaccine induced varicella or herpes zoster is low. Adverse reactions include fever, injection-site reactions and rash.

PROGNOSIS

Recovery is excellent in healthy children. Immunosuppressed children have high rate of complications. Virus persists in latent form and causes herpes zoster on reactivation. School children can return to school, once all the existing lesions are crusted and there are no more new lesions.

HERPES ZOSTER (SHINGLES)

Zoster means girdle. It is named so because of the characteristic rash that forms like a belt around thorax in many patients. It is a self-limiting localized disease that causes discomfort for several days but heals without complications in most cases.

EPIDEMIOLOGY

Herpes zoster is due to reactivation of latent infection, caused by varicella-zoster virus. Patients had previous varicella infection or vaccine. There are no racial, sexual or seasonal preferences for zoster. It may occur at all ages, mostly after 40 years of age and the incidence in children is low. Varicella vaccine induced herpes zoster has been reported in both normal and immunocompromised individuals, but it is very rare.

CLINICAL FEATURES

Zoster lesions are often preceded by pain, paresthesias, tenderness or itching. Depending on the location, the severity of pain may be confused with pleurisy, cardiac disease, cholecystitis, appendicitis and renal colic. But in children, these prodromal symptoms are rare. About 3 to 5 days after the prodrome, the eruption appears over the affected segment. The eruption is commonly unilateral, involving 1-3 dermatomes. Erythematous macules, papules and plaques appear first, soon evolve into grouped vesicles, and rarely to blisters with in 24-48 hours **(Figures 6.6A and B)**. The vesicles become pustules, crust and fall with in 1-2 weeks. In more than 50%, zoster involves thoracic nerves. In children thoracic nerves and ophthalmic branch of trigeminal nerve are frequently involved. Lesions on tip of nose indicate involvement of nasociliary branch of ophthalmic division of trigeminal nerve, suggesting possibility of scleritis and kerto conjunctivitis (Hutchinson's sign). Involvement of maxillary division of trigeminal produces vesicles on uvula and tonsillar fossa, while mandibular division involvement produce vesicles on anterior part of tongue, floor of mouth, and buccal mucosa. Motor paralysis is more common than thought previously. Zoster involving the facial nerve at the geniculate ganglion produces vesicles on pinna, severe ear ache and ipsilateral facial plasy. This triad is known as the Ramsay-Hunt syndrome.

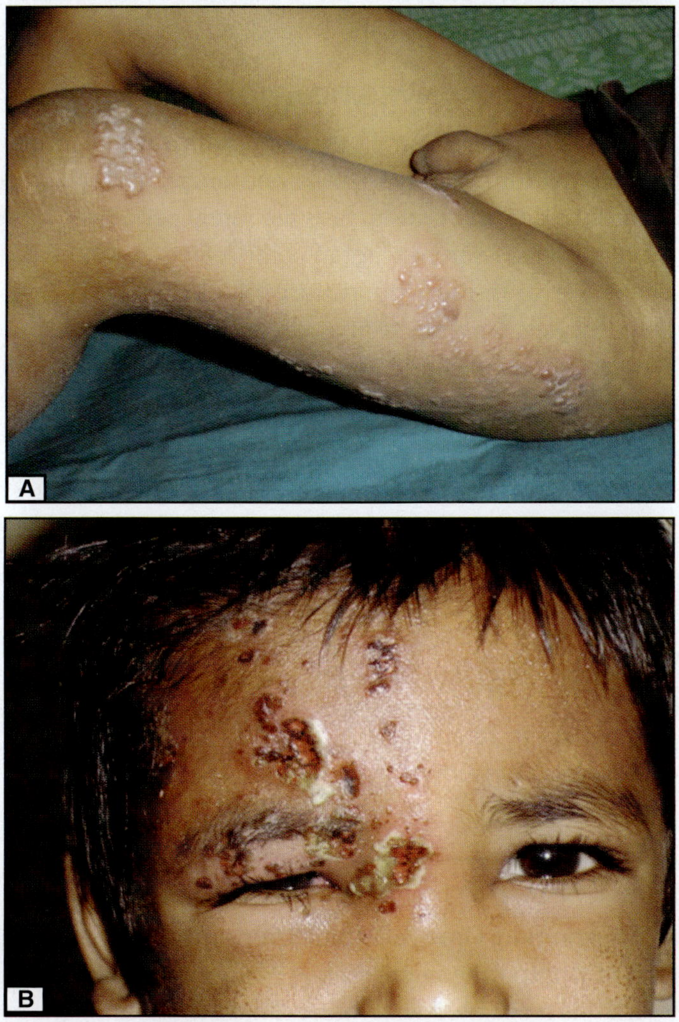

FIGURES 6.6A AND B: Herpes zoster

Discrete, scattered lesions of zoster can occur (15-20) in normal individuals. If more than 20-25 zoster vesicles occur, scattered all over body, it is called disseminated zoster and is seen in immuncompromised. Internal organ involvement may occur in those individuals. Zoster involves normally 1-3 dermatomes, unilaterally. But in immunocompromised (children with lymphoma, leukemia and HIV infection) multiple dermatomes are involved. They may be contiguous or noncontiguous, unilateral or bilateral. This is known as *zoster multiplex*. In these individuals, lesions may be hemorrhagic, bullous, and necrotic and heal slowly with scarring. Lesions may be disseminated all over body. Sometimes lesions may be persistent as hyperkeratotic papules. Occasionally varicella zoster virus on reactivation produces only pain and tenderness in the affected dermatome without clinical lesions. This is termed as *Zoster sine herpete*. Post herpetic neuralgia, which is more common in more than 50 years of age, is very rare in children.

Usually herpes zoster does not recur, in normal individuals except in rare occasions (5%). Recurrent zoster in the same dermatome or different dermatomes is seen in immunocompromised.

LABORATORY INVESTIGATIONS

In most cases, no laboratory tests are needed to confirm the diagnosis. Tzanck smear from the base of fluid shows similar findings as in HSV infections. Skin biopsy also cannot differentiate between HSV and VZV. Direct fluorescent antibody testing, using the swab from the base of vesicle is very useful, highly sensitive and can differentiate between HSV and VZV. Virus can be cultured from vesicle fluid.

TREATMENT

In most cases therapy is supportive. Analgesics and antibiotics are sufficient in most cases. Salicylates are to be avoided in children for the risk of Reye's syndrome. Systemic steroids are thought to decrease post herpetic neuralgia in patients older than 50 years, but PHN is very rare in children. Topical acyclovir, 4-5 times daily, applied for 10 days promotes healing of localized zoster, but ineffective in reducing pain and preventing post herpetic neuralgia. Oral acyclovir, 15 to 20 mg/kg/day in 4-5 divided doses, if started within 24-48 hours, reduces pain, shortens the duration of lesions, promotes healing and prevents post herpetic neuralgia. Valacyclovir and famcyclovir are more bioavailable products, but not approved for treatment in children. In immunosuppressed or in severe disseminated zoster intravenous acyclovir therapy is recommended. Acyclovir resistant varicella zoster virus infections are reported in AIDS patients and foscarnet is helpful in those cases (40 mg/kg/ every 8 hours for 10 days).

Ocular involvement has to be evaluated by ophthalmologist. Varicella zoster virus keratitis should be distinguished from HSV keratitis as the treatment is entirely different. VZV keratitis is treated with topical corticosteroids, whereas HSV keratitis is treated with antivirals.

PROGNOSIS

In normal individuals herpes zoster spontaneously improves without scarring. In immunosuppressed, healing takes longer time and causes scarring and the lesions may be persistent as keratotic papules.

EXANTHEM SUBITUM

Synonyms: Roseola infantum, sixth disease

- Caused mostly by human herpes virus-6.
- Fever subsides, rash appears.
- Only symptomatic treatment is required.

Exanthem subitum is mostly caused by Human herpes virus (HHV)-6, especially by B type and occasionally by Human herpes virus-7. HHV 6 and 7 establish latency after primary infection like other herpes viruses, mainly in salivary glands and peripheral blood lymphocytes.

EPIDEMIOLOGY

Most cases of exanthem subitum are seen between 6 months and 3 years of age. It can occur at any time of year, but more common in spring. Transmission is airborne, mostly through salivary and respiratory secretions. The incubation period is 9-10 days.

CLINICAL FEATURES

High fever (101°-106° F) starts abruptly and lasts for 3 to 5 days. The child is otherwise well with few symptoms. As the temperature falls, rash appears. The initial rash includes discrete pink, rosy macules, morbilliform eruption, not itchy, mostly starts on neck and trunk, gradually spreads to face, arms and legs. After 1-2 days, the rash fades away without scarring or pigmentation. Periorbital edema and hematuria are seen occasionally. Erythematous papules may occur on mucosae of soft palate in 65% of patients (Nagayamai's spots). Occipital and cervical lymph nodes are enlarged. Febrile seizures may occur and encephalitis is rare.

LABORATORY INVESTIGATIONS

Clinical picture is usually specific with lack of other symptoms during febrile phase and eruption begins as fever subsides. Laboratory tests are rarely performed and usually unnecessary, except in complicated cases. HHV-6 can be identified by culture of peripheral blood lymphocytes. Serological titres and PCR are available but they are time consuming and expensive.

TREATMENT

Only symptomatic measures are required. Antipyretics, tepid sponge baths are necessary to control the high fever. In complicated CNS disease, gancyclovir and foscarnet are helpful.

PROGNOSIS

It is benign in infants. By the age of 4 years, almost all individuals are seropositive.

EPSTEIN-BARR VIRUS (HHV-4)

- Epstein-Barr virus (EBV) infections are asymptomatic and nonspecific in children.
- EBV is associated with many clinical manifestations in adults.

- Fever, sore throat, fleeting rash and lymphadenopathy are characteristic of infectious mononucleosis.

Epstein-Barr virus, a member of herpes virus family, selectively infects B lymphocytes and certain squamous epithelial cells. The virus persists in latent state in infected B cells but not in epithelial cells. Many clinical conditions are reported in association with Epstein-Barr virus **(Table 6.3)**. EBV infection is universal. The type of infection acquired, depends on the age at the time of primary infection. EBV infections are usually asymptomatic or nonspecific in infants and young children, but in adults results in infectious mononucleosis.

TABLE 6.3: Clinical conditions associated with Epstein-Barr virus

Infectious mononucleosis
Burkitt's lymphoma
Nasopharyngeal carcinoma
Hairy leukoplakia
Non-Hodgkin's lymphoma
Smooth muscle tumors
Angioimmunoblastic lymphadenopathy
special to infants and young children
Giannotti-Crosti syndrome
Kawasaki disease
Granuloma annulare like lesions
EBV associated lymphomas (in immunosuppressed)

INFECTIOUS MONONUCLEOSIS SYNONYM: GLANDULAR FEVER

Infectious mononucleosis is caused by Epstein-Barr virus in 90% of cases. 5-10% is caused by cytomegalo virus, *Toxoplasma gondii*, adeno virus and rubella virus.

EPIDEMIOLOGY

Infectious mononucleosis is transmitted via close contact through oral secretions (kissing disease) and by blood transfusion. Early childhood infection is less frequent. Primary infection is more common in early adult life. The incubation period is 10-60 days. Virus replicates in cells of pharynx and seropositive individuals shed virus in saliva. Asymptomatic carrier stage is common.

CLINICAL FEATURES

Fever, sore throat and lymphadenopathy are the characteristic triad of infectious mononucleosis. Multiple petechiae at the junction of hard and soft palate is a characteristic sign, seen in 3-13% of patients and usually appear on second or third day of fever. Pink, fleeting morbilliform maculopapular rash is seen in 5-15% of cases and lasts for 1-5 days. Nausea, malaise, headache, abdominal pain, jaundice are observed. Periorbital edema is seen in 30% of cases. In severe cases hepatomegaly, splenomegaly and occasionally splenic rupture can occur. 90 to 100% of patients treated with ampicillin or amoxycillin, develop an extensive maculopapular eruption, 1-2 days after initiating therapy. Acrocyanosis, cold urticaria, erythema nodosum and erythema multiforme are described. Extreme fatigue may persist for three months.

LABORATORY INVESTIGATIONS

Lymphocytosis with 10% atypical lymphocytes is seen in first and second weeks of infection. Neutropenia, thrombocytopenia, elevated transaminases and increased alkaline phosphatase are observed. Occasionally leukemoid reaction (30,000–50,000 cells/mm^3) is reported. Positive monospot test (Heterophile antibody test, Paul-Bunnel test) is confirmatory and highly sensitive, but seen in third week of illness. But in children less than 4 years of age, false negative reactions are more common. Viral capsid antigen (VCA)–IgG antibody is found in high titres. IgM anti-VCA antibody is useful in identifying acute infection. PCR or culture of saliva or peripheral blood mononuclear cells yields positive results.

DIFFERENTIAL DIAGNOSIS

Rash may be confused with other exanthems, but the characteristic triad differentiates it. In older children, EBV infection must be differentiated from streptococcal pharyngitis. In some, periorbital edema may be confused with dermatomyositis.

TREATMENT AND PROGNOSIS

Treatment is generally supportive. Acyclovir inhibits EBV replication and reduces viral shedding. It is not indicated because clinical manifestations are not due to replication of virus, but are secondary to immune response to virus. Corticosteroids are not indicated in uncomplicated but given in serious cases, 2-3 mg/kg/day for 3 days. Ampicillin, penicillin and tetracyclines are avoided. Avoid strenuous activity, contact sports, where abdominal injury may cause splenic rupture. If there are no complications, recovery is excellent.

Other cutaneous manifestations of EBV infections like hairy leukoplakia, Gianotti-Crosti syndrome are discussed in appropriate sections.

CYTOMEGALOVIRUS INFECTIONS (HHV-5)

- Cytomegalo virus (CMV) is DNA virus of herpes family.
- 5-10% congenital CMV infections are symptomatic.
- Viral isolation is the gold standard to diagnose CMV infection.

Cytomegalo virus (CMV) is the DNA virus of herpes family. CMV infections occur world wide and are usually unapparent. Primary infection is followed by life-long carriage of virus with intermittent shedding in almost all secretions—saliva, milk, urine, semen and vaginal secretions.

EPIDEMIOLOGY

CMV infection of new born is common. It can occur congenitally *in utero*, perinatally through birth and postnatally through breast milk. Children may acquire CMV from oral secretions or urine of other infected infants. In adults sexual transmission is important. Blood transfusion is also a source of CMV infection.

CLINICAL FEATURES

The clinical manifestations are different in congenital and acquired CMV infections.

Congenital CMV Infection

Mothers infected with CMV will deliver infants with CMV infection in approximately 40% of cases. Only 5-10% of affected infants are symptomatic. The classical findings are petechiae, purpura, hepatosplenomegaly, intrauterine growth retardation, hyperbilirubinemia, thrombocytopenia, chorioretinitis, deafness, microcephaly and finally mental retardation. Extramedullary hemopoiesis presents as purple or red papules and nodules (blueberry muffin spots). Vesicles are rare. The hair, nails, and teeth are normal.

Acquired CMV Infections

Cutaneous manifestations are rare in children with acquired CMV. Infectious mononucleosis like rash with lymphadenopathy and fever has been reported. CMV has been suggested as a precipitating factor in scleredema and Gianotti-Crosti syndrome. In immunosuppressed individuals, cutaneous ulcers, and generalized morbilliform, urticarial and petechial eruptions, indurated pigmented nodules and plaques are described. Hepatitis, pneumonia, choreoretinitis, GI ulcerations and Gullian–Barre syndrome can occur.

LABORATORY INVESTIGATIONS

Viral isolation is the best method to diagnose CMV infection. A fresh urine specimen is excellent as systemic CMV infection is always associated with viruria. When virus is cultured, serologic confirmation is required to demonstrate acute infection, because of persistent viral shedding in carrier state. CMV- specific IgM and a four-fold rise in complement fixation titers can confirm the acute infection.

TREATMENT

In most cases, CMV does not require specific therapy. In severe infections, Gancyclovir and foscarnet are effective. Acyclovir is not effective as CMV lacks thymidine kinase. Cidofovir has been tried and found effective, but not recommended in children.

PROGNOSIS

Most of congenital CMV infections are asymptomatic. Five percent of those will develop sequelae especially sensory deafness. Congenital CMV infections can not be cured, but suppressed. With acquired infections in healthy children recovery is good. In immunosuppressed, morbidity and mortality is high.

POX VIRUSES

Pox viruses are complex DNA viruses that replicate in the cytoplasm of epidermal cells. They are the largest viruses, slightly smaller than bacteria. Man is infected by three kinds of pox viruses: Orthopox viruses (variola, vaccinia), Parapox viruses (ORF, MIlker's nodule) and intermediate viruses (molluscum contagiosum, tenapox).

MOLLUSCUM CONTAGIOSUM

- Molluscum contagiosum(MC) is caused by DNA virus of pox family.

- Skin colored umbilicated and translucent papules.
- MC can be widespread, multiple and giant in immunosuppressed.
- Lesions are self-limited: treatment should be individualized.

Molluscum contagiosum (MC) is the common cutaneous viral infection in children. It is caused by DNA Poxvirus, largely affecting human beings. Four subtypes have been identified and Type 1 is the commonest, affecting children.

EPIDEMIOLOGY

The disease is worldwide and it can occur at any age. It is common in young children and sexually active adults. The peak incidence is in children less than 5 years of age, with a prevalence of 25%. The MC infection is spread by skin to skin contact, by fomites and autoinoculation. Outbreaks at swimming pools are known, especially with heated pools, as it is presumed warm water enhances the spread. The incubation period is 2 to 8 weeks, may be maximum for 6 months. It is infectious as long as lesions are present. MC is a common opportunistic infection in AIDS and often a marker for advanced disease.

PATHOGENESIS

MC virus is a brick shaped particle 200-300 nm, replicates in cytoplasm of infected epidermal cells of all layers. The cells turn over and epidermal transit time is increased. The basal cell layer remains intact. Cells at the upper layers, especially malphigian layer undergo distortion and ultimately destroyed, forming large hyaline bodies, containing cytoplasmic masses of virus material (molluscum bodies).

CLINICAL FEATURES

MC lesions are discrete, dome-shaped, pearly white, waxy papules with central umbilication **(Figure 6.7)**. They appear vesicular because of translucent nature. The size may vary from 1 to 5 mm, the giant one being as large as 10-15 mm. Lesions can occur anywhere on body, but mostly on face, axillae, sides of trunk and genitalia in children. Palms and soles are rarely involved. Mucosal lesions may occur. Lesions in the genital area in adolescents and adults are usually sexually transmitted but in children, it may not be the cause. However, sexual abuse is considered, if other supporting evidence is present. Lesions usually resolute spontaneously by forming erythema, pus and crusting. Individual lesions last several weeks or months. Eczematous dermatitis occur around the molluscum in 10% of cases (molluscum dermatitis) and it disappears spontaneously, when molluscum regress. Multiple and widespread lesions are reported in atopic individuals and in immunosuppressed. In AIDS, lesions may be numerous, giant and confluent. MC, confined to hair follicles, molluscum folliculitis has been reported in HIV infection. Lesions on eyelids may produce conjunctivitis and /or keratitis.

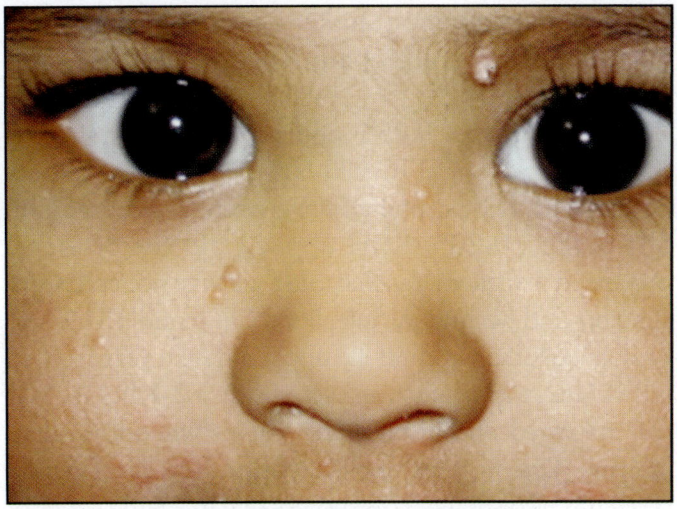

FIGURE 6.7: Molluscum contagiosum

LABORATORY INVESTIGATIONS

MC is diagnosed mostly on clinical grounds. Smears, made from the cheesy material expressed from the lesion is crushed between two slides and stained with Giemsa or Wright's stain show homogeneous pear-shaped molluscum bodies. Skin biopsy reveals epidermal hyperplasia and many epidermal cells contain large, intracytoplasmic inclusion bodies (Henderson-Paterson bodies). The dermis is normal except in rare instances, where molluscum body ruptures and produces pronounced inflammatory infiltrate.

TREATMENT

Molluscum, even if untreated, it nearly always resolves spontaneously; but may take few weeks to years. This fact should be given due consideration, especially in young children. Simple scratching of the lesion by mother may produce inflammation and the lesion may resolve. Varieties of topical preparations are reported with success.

Topical tretinoin 0.05% applied twice daily showed some success. Topical TCA 25-50%, iodine 10%, benzoyl peroxide and liquid phenol have been found useful. In one study 10-20% KOH applied bid for 30 days, produced excellent results. Side effects noticed were stinging and secondary infection. Cantharidin 0.9% in flexible collodion is carefully applied by the physician to individual lesions and washed off after 2-4 hours. It is well tolerated and resolves the lesions without residual scarring. One to three applications of 40% silver nitrate paste has also shown 97% success rate in a large series of patients. Topical imiquimod 5%, applied daily for 4 weeks or 3 times weekly for 14-16 weeks has reported 50-78% success. Occasional irritation is produced and may precipitate new lesions. Topical cidofovir 3% has been found effective in immunodeficient individuals in 3-6 weeks. Burning, erosion and post inflammatory hyperpigmentation are noted sometimes. Oral cidofovir has not been approved for use in children.

Currettage with a dermal curette or needling of the lesion is the best. Anesthesia is often not necessary. EMLA, applied for 1-2 hours before treatment is good. The dose of EMLA cream should be limited in neonates and infants because of the risk of methemoglobinemia. Lignocaine cream may be helpful in anxious children. CRYO therapy has been used as first line treatment by some. A brief freeze of lesion with a surrounding thin rim is adequate. If the lesions are giant, rapidly progressive, and in periocular areas, general anesthesia may be necessary. As the new lesions continue to appear for some weeks, lesions should be removed every 2-4 weeks until cleared completely. Common bathing, sharing towels and use of swimming pools are to be avoided. Photodynamic therapy was used recently in HIV+ individuals with substantial reduction of lesions. Electron beam and pulsed dye laser were used for recalcitrant lesions in immunocompromised. Oral cimetidine, 40 mg/kg/day in divided doses has been found effective, but cautioned because of many systemic drug interactions.

PROGNOSIS

Most mollusci are self-limited in 6 months to 1 year. Some persist for years.

ORF

Synonyms: Sheep pox, Ecthyma contagiosum

- Caused by parapox virus
- Seen in sheep handlers and veterinary surgeons
- One to several lesions develop on hands and feet
- Generally resolve without therapy in 4-6 weeks

ORF is caused by a parapox virus. The disease is widespread in sheep and goats.

EPIDEMIOLOGY

Human infections are common in sheep handlers, veterinary surgeons and farmer's wives, who bottle-feed lambs. They are caused mainly by direct contact. Fomites and feeding troughs also play a role. The incubation period is 5 to 6 days.

CLINICAL FEATURES

Initially a small, firm tender red papule appears and slowly enlarges to form hemorrhagic pustule or bullae. Central umbilication may occur and often crusts. They may be single or few in number with the size varying from 2 cm to 5 cm. Fingers and hands are commonly affected. Regional lymphadenitis is not uncommon. A fully developed lesion may show a grayish white ring around central crusting, further surrounded by erythema. Pyogenic granulomas like lesions are reported in children, especially with atopic dermatitis. Erythema multiforme occasionally appears, 1- 2 weeks after the onset of ORF.

DIAGNOSIS

Clinical lesions with appropriate history may make the diagnosis easy. Histology reveals inter- and intracellular edema of epidermis, vacuolization and ballooning degeneration. Dermis shows dense cellular infiltrate, mainly of histocytes, macrophages, lymphocytes, and plasma cells.

TREATMENT

Spontaneous recovery occurs in 6–8 weeks. Secondary infection is treated and spontaneous recovery is awaited. Excision of the lesion may enhance healing. 40% idoxuridine has been claimed effective.

MILKER'S NODULE

Synonyms: Pseudocowpox, paravaccinia.

EPIDEMIOLOGY

Milker's nodule is caused by parapox virus with same morphology as of ORF virus. The calves are affected with ring sores and ulcers in the mouth. Milkers and veterinarians, who examine the mouth of calves, are infected accidentally. Human to human spread does not occur. Incubation period is 1-2 weeks.

CLINICAL FEATURES

Flat red tender papules appear initially. As they enlarge they crust in the center with secondary erythema. Lymphangitis may occur. Lesions regress without scarring in 4–6 weeks. They are common on hands, but may be seen on face. Usually solitary but multiple lesions can occur. The nodules are very vascular and are confused with pyogenic granuloma. Differentiation from ORF is difficult and history is more helpful.

TREATMENT

Secondary infection is controlled and spontaneous recovery is awaited.

HUMAN PAPILLOMA VIRUSES

- DNA viruses belonging to Papovaviridae family.
- More than 200 types are known and 100 have been sequenced.
- Mostly cause different verrucous lesions.
- Spontaneous regression is seen in 1-2 years.
- Recurrences are common and multiple treatments are needed.
- Malignant transformation is seen with certain HPV subtypes .

INTRODUCTION

More than 200 types are known and 100 have been sequenced. These viruses cause species specific cutaneous and mucous membrane infections **(Table 6.4)**. Certain HPV types are oncogenic, particularly HPV 16 and 18.

EPIDEMIOLOGY

Human papilloma viruses are transmitted mainly by direct skin to skin contact. Autoinoculation can occur, mainly in intertriginous areas, causing kissing warts. Indirect transmission by fomites, clothing, contaminated articles and swimming pool surfaces can occur. Condylomata acuminata and laryngeal papilloma can be acquired during birth from the infective lesions of maternal birth canal. Immunocompromised like renal transplant patients and individuals with AIDS have widespread infections. Incubation period is 1-12 months, average 2-3 months.

TABLE 6.4: Clinical Infections of HPV subtypes

Infection	HPV Types
Common warts (Verruca vulgaris)	1,2,4,7
Plantar, palmar warts	1,4
Flat warts	3,10,28
Anogenital warts (Condylomata acuminata)	6,11,16,18
Epidermodysplasia verruciformis	3, 5, 8, common. (many other types)
Heck's disease (Focal epithelial hyperplasia)	13,37
Laryngeal papilloma	6,11
Verrucous carcinoma	16,18

PATHOGENESIS

HPV enters the basal keratinocytes through the broken skin. The virus replicates in the nucleus and migrates upwards through epidermis. It is difficult to grow *in vitro*. Polymerase chain reaction, DNA probe techniques and molecular nucleic acid hybridization have separated many HPV subtypes.

CLINICAL FEATURES

Common Warts (Verruca vulgaris)

Common warts are mainly caused by HPV 1, 2, 4, and 7. They are dome-shaped papules, nodules with finger-like projections, giving cauliflower like appearance **(Figure 6.8)**. They are usually skin colored and sessile. They can be solitary or in groups, sometimes form plaques. They present commonly on hands, around nails, but may occur anywhere on body, including lips and mouth. Atopic individuals have more prevalence and more numerous lesions.

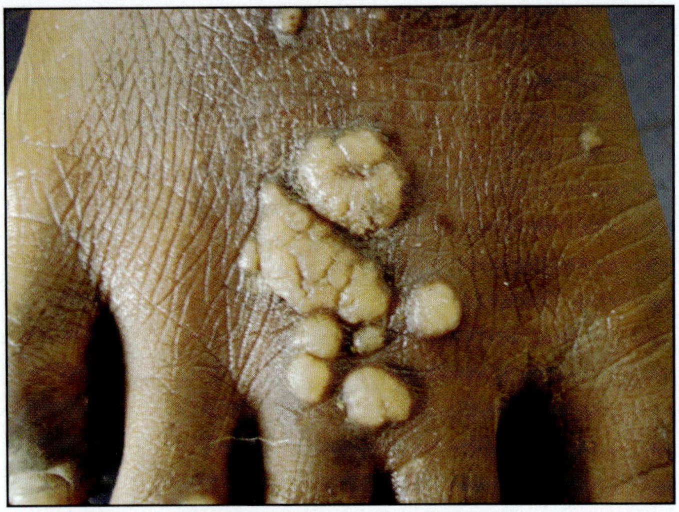

FIGURE 6.8: Verruca vulgaris

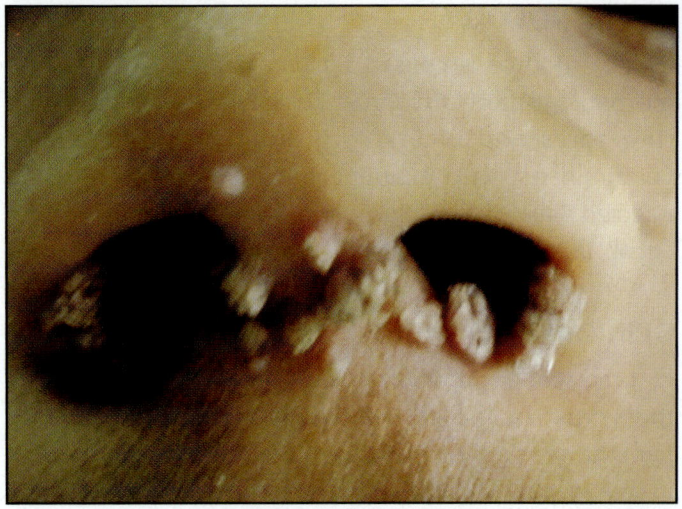

FIGURE 6.9: Filiform warts

Flat Warts (Verruca plana)

Plane warts are mostly associated with HPV 3, 10 and 28. They are most common on face. They are small, multiple, broad based, smooth and flat topped.

Plantar Warts

Plantar warts are mainly associated with HPV 1 and 4. They occur on weight bearing areas and are extremely painful. They are hyperkeratotic and can be extensive, forming mosaic warts. They interrupt natural skin lines; as opposed to calluses. The return of skin lines is a sign of complete resolution of wart. They may simulate calluses, but, removal of the superficial layers of stratum corneum reveals bleeding points in warts, which represent extravasated RBC and thrombosed capillaries and helps to differentiate from other lesions on the soles. Corns and calluses are more painful with direct pressure, where as warts are more painful with lateral pressure. HPV 60, a less common form is associated with plantar warts with cystic component.

Filiform Warts

Filiform warts are slender, soft, thin finger like growths, mainly seen on face and neck **(Figure 6.9)**. Digitate warts occur in small groups usually on scalp.

Anogenital Warts (Condylomata acuminata)

They are caused by HPV 6, 11, 16 and 18. The incubation period is 3–8 months, but it may occur as long as 1-2 years after exposure. They are asymptomatic papules, less verrucous and vary in color from pink to brown. They can be solitary, multiple and confluent. In males, they are seen on shaft of penis, urethral meatus, scrotum and perineal areas. In females, they present on labia, vagina, cervix and perianal areas. In children less than three years of age, they occur mainly because of vertical transmission from the infected secretions of maternal birth canal. In children more than three years of age, vertical transmission is unlikely and sexual abuse could be the cause.

LABORATORY INVESTIGATIONS

Generally laboratory tests are not needed to confirm the diagnosis of verrucae. Skin biopsy may show hyperkeratosis, focal vertical parakeratosis, papillomatosis, koilocytosis (vacuolated epidermal cells) and benign acanthosis. Koilocytes with eosinophilic inclusions is a typical finding of papilloma virus infection.Polymerase chain reaction, DNA probes and advanced southern blot molecular biology techniques can be used for typing of HPV.

DIFFERENTIAL DIAGNOSIS

Common warts are sometimes confused with molluscum contagiosum, umbilication in molluscum helps to differentiate. Plantar warts have to be differentiated from calluses (see plantar warts section). Anogenital warts are to be differentiated from candylomata lata(syphilis). C.lata are more pink and moist, VDRL and TPHA tests are positive.

TREATMENT

Nongenital warts frequently resolve spontaneously in 1–2 years without causing any residual change. Controlled trials in children suggest that about 30% respond to topical placebo within three months and more than 50-60% undergo remission without therapy within two years. These facts should be considered and it seems appropriate, especially in young children to reassure and observe or to use least traumatic forms in treating these lesions. Hypnosis has been said to be effective, but it is difficult to evaluate its effectiveness with the high rate of spontaneous remission. It is important to remember that warts are benign cutaneous growths and therapy should also be benign.

Topical Therapy

Topical modalities are non traumatic, lengthy and not successful always. Topical tretinoin 0.025% and 0.05% may be helpful in flat warts. Salicylic acid preparations (5-20%) in plaster forms or liquids along with lactic acid in collodion base are useful in common warts and plantar warts. Repeated paring after salicylic acid application may hasten the resolution. The regression depends on the size of warts. Usually it takes 6 to 8 weeks or longer to resolute. Good compliance from the patient is required for better results.

Topical trichloroacetic acid 50%, once or twice weekly is also useful. A necrotic crust that forms should be removed and the remaining lesion should be retreated. This method is painless, but relatively slow.

Cantharidin, extracted from blister beetle (*Cantharis vesicatoria*), alone or in combination with salicylic acid has been found effective in common warts and in plantar warts. Wart should be painted with cantharidin, covered with occlusive tape after drying. Tape is left on for 24 hours or until the area hurts. A blister will form crusts and falls of in 7 to 14 days. If any residual part is there, it should be retreated. It is effective and does not cause pain and more useful in children.

Podophyllin resin, imiquimod and cidofovir have been tried, but they are most successful in genital warts. Localised heat therapy (50°C) for 30-60 sec, for 1-4 treatments led to 80% success rate. 20% formalin (3% formaldehyde), 10% glutaraldehyde in aqueous ethanol solution have been tried with moderate results. Appropriate therapy should be considered depending upon number, size, location, convenience and cost.

Ablative Therapies

Electrodessication, curettage, liquid nitrogen (-195°C), CO_2 laser, pulsed dye laser are useful. Electrodessication of few lesions may make others to resolve, especially in flat warts. Liquid nitrogen can be applied for multiple lesions rapidly without anesthesia and with less scarring and less fear of pigmentary charges. It has been said best in plantar and periungual warts. It is extremely painful and sometimes may destroy nail matrix permanently. Enucleation by dissection is excellent in palms and periurgual areas, if one or few lesions are present. CO2 laser, pulsed dye laser have shown 70-90% clearance rate, especially in recalcitrant warts. Alexandrite, 755 nm has been tried recently with success.

Systemic Treatments

High dose of oral cimetidine 30-40 mg/kg/day in 3-4 divided doses for six weeks are effective in children; but not so useful in adults. Side effects include diarrhea and headache. Ranitidine has shown variable results. Combination of levamisole and cimetidine is more effective. Interferons α–2b, intralesionally and systemically, has been tried, one million units 3 times/ week for three weeks, has been found effective, in both nongenital and anogenital warts. High incidence of adverse systemic side effects limits its use. A clinical trail of etretinate 1 mg/kg/day in 20 children led to complete regression of extensive warts in 80% with 2 years follow-up.

Genital warts are best treated with 25% podophyllin resin in compound tincture benzoin, protecting the surrounding skin with petrolatum. It is best used under supervision with weekly applications. The medicine should be washed after 4-6 hours. Self application should be avoided because of high irritation and ulceration. Podophilox 0.5%, a purifed form of podophyllin twice daily for 3 days weekly for 4 weeks is convenient to use for self application and yields good results.

Imiquimod 5%, 2-3 times per week for 16 weeks has been successful. Over night application is more effective. Irritation and erythema are expected. It has no systemic side effects. It has been approved for children more than 12 years of age. It is best effective in C. acuminata and found successful in common warts. Cidofovir 3%, liquid nitrogen, surgical excision, laser also are helpful in treating genital warts.

Contact immunotherapy with diphenyl cyclopropenone (DCP), Squaric acid dibutylester(SADBE) have cure rates of 50-80% in recalcitrant warts in children.

HPV Vaccine

A quadrivalent (6, 11, 16, 18) recombinant vaccine is available to prevent cervical cancers and genital warts. It is given for females between 9 to 26 years. Vaccine is given as 3 doses at 0, 2 and 6 months. It is administered before first sexual activity; it will reduce the risk of cervical cancer and genital warts considerably.

PROGNOSIS

Most warts regress. Some persist for years. Recurrences are common and multiple treatments are needed.

EPIDERMODYSPLASIA VERRUCIFORMIS

- Mostly caused by HPV 3,5, 8.
- Autosomal recessive.
- Cell mediated immunity is impaired.
- Mostly the lesions are flat warts and tinea versicolor like.
- Malignant change occurs in about 10% cases.

Epidermodysplasia verruciforms(EDV) is rare inherited disorder, generalized and persistent.

EPIDEMIOLOGY

EDV is mostly associated with HPV 3,5,8 subtypes, though many other types 9,10,12,14,15,17,19-25,28,38,47,49 are also reported. Many EDV patients are infected with multiple HPV types. Most cases are autosomal recessive, but autosomal dominant and X-linked dominant forms are also reported. High incidence of consanguinity is present in the affected families.

CLINICAL FEATURES

The cutaneous lesions are mainly flat warts, reddish brown scaly macules resembling tinea versicolor or pityriasis rosea **(Figure 6.10)**. The lesions mainly occur on the sun exposed area, but may be generalized all over body. Oral mucosa is spared. The lesions start during childhood and puberty but may appear at any age. EDV lesions are remarkably persistent and may remain unchanged for decades. Impairment of cell immunity is found. But patients are not susceptible to other viral and bacterial infections. Malignant change occurs in about 10% cases, but metastasis is uncommon. The risk of

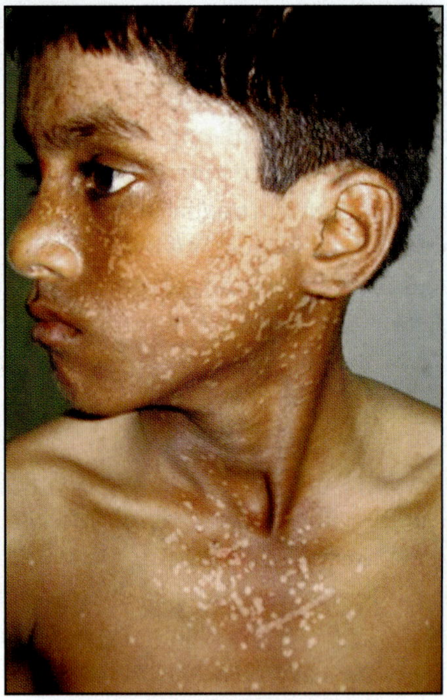

FIGURE 6.10: Epidermodysplasia verruciformis

neoplasia is more with HPV 5 and 8. The combination of HPV infection, relative immunosuppression and sunlight are potent carcinogenic combination.

DIAGNOSIS

Skin biopsy shows swollen keratinocytes with vacuolation which contain basophilic granules. Dysplastic changes may be found. EDV has to be differentiated from acrokeratosis verruciformis. In acrokeratosis, flat warty papules occur on the back of hands and feet, and on knees and elbows. The palms are diffusely thickened and show punctiform breaks. There is no vacuolation in keratinocytes.

TREATMENT

There is no effective treatment. Cidofovir has been found effective. Etretinate 1 mg/kg/day is helpful in some cases, but the lesions recur. Liquid nitrogen destruction of the lesions on sun exposed areas decreases the risk of malignancy. Sun protection measures are essential to prevent neoplasia.

HECK'S DISEASE

Heck's disease is otherwise known as focal epithelial hyperplasia. Heck's disease is mostly caused by HPV 32 and HPV 13. It is commonly seen in children and young adults and familial predisposition is observed. Painless, diffuse, soft, flattened, multiple sessile papules, usually white in color, occur in oral mucosa and cannot be scrapped off. The underlying mucosa may be swollen, producing cobblestone appearance. The lesions are not precancerous and self-limiting.

VIRAL EXANTHEMS

INTRODUCTION

The term 'exanthem' means a skin eruption occurring as a symptom of acute infectious disease, commonly due to viral infections (sometimes due to cocci as in scarlet fever) *Exanthema=breaking out* (Greek) *anthos=blossom* of flower.

This term viral exanthem implies that it is a chain of clinical observations on the skin that follow a typical pattern occurring more or less specific to the given viral illness.

Viral exanthema is a frequent finding in dermatology outpatients. Its accurate diagnosis is important not only for the patients but also for their contacts, parents and the schools because some diseases are highly contagious and may have significant impact on the health of the affected individual. Diagnosis of certain viral exanthema in pregnancy viz. erythema infectiosum and rubella may have adverse outcome on fetus, suggesting careful work up and follow up. Systemic features in viral exanthem are equally important because of their bearing on patient's complete treatment and prognosis. Generally, most viral exanthemas are diagnosed on clinical grounds. Therefore, in addition to appropriate history and careful clinical examination, a perfect knowledge of various clinical presentations and diagnostic criteria is essential for accurate diagnosis. In certain situations, however, it might be difficult to label the rash due to atypical or incomplete presentations, thus requiring further clinical observations, appropriate investigations and follow up.

This chapter is an attempt to describe several common, uncommon and comparatively newer viral exanthemas.

TRADITIONAL EXANTHEMS

Since a long time in the history of medical literature, several typical exanthems are commonly described during infancy and childhood. Following table depicts six classical traditional exanthems and their common medical terminologies **(Table 6.5)**.

TABLE 6.5: Classical Viral exanthems

Traditional label	Common clinical label
First disease	Measles
Second disease	Scarlet fever
Third disease	Rubella
Fourth disease	*Duke's disease
Fifth disease	Erythema infectiosum
Sixth disease	Roseola infantum

*It must be noted that Fourth Disease i.e. Duke's disease, is non-existent entity now because the original descriptions for this disease were actually overlapping with the other classical exanthems.

ERYTHEMA INFECTIOSUM (EI)
SYNONYMS: FIFTH DISEASE

Salient features:

- Slapped cheek appearance followed by reticular truncal rash triggered by sunlight, temperature, physical or mental stress caused by Parvovirus B19.
- Disease loses infectivity with the appearance of rash.
- Aplastic anemia in patients with hematological disorders and immunodeficiency
- Pregnant women are at risk for fetal loss.

Historical Aspects

Anderson et al in 1983 identified human parvovirus B19 as the causative agent of EI.

Etiology

EI is caused by human parvovirus B19 belonging to family *parvoviridae*, genus *erythroviridae*. Parvovirus is a single-stranded DNA unenveloped virus.

Epidemiology

School-going children are the most affected, mainly between 4 and 10 years. The distribution is worldwide. The outbreaks in schools occur in late winter and early spring. The disease spreads via droplet infection by saliva, sputum or nasal discharge. The incubation period is 4-15 days.

Pathogenesis

The disease is transmitted commonly via aerosol (and less commonly by blood products). The virus multiplies in respiratory epithelium, which is followed by viremia. Thus, the infection is likely to be transmitted before the rash erupts. Cutaneous and rheumatological findings develop only after production of enough antibodies against parvovirus B19. Hence, the skin manifestations are thought to be due to multisystem immune complex deposition. Other hypothesis is that these could be due to triggering of inflammatory reaction to parvovirus antigens on skin. Hematological manifestations are explained due to specific affinity of the organism towards erythroid progenitor cells.

Clinical Features

A prodrome of low grade fever, malaise, myalgia, pharyngitis, nausea, diarrhea or arthralgia may be present in few patients before the onset of the characteristic rash described as, "*slapped cheek appearance*". The latter consists of a macular or occasionally plaque of bright erythema involving the cheeks. Sparing of periorbital areas and the nasal bridge is said to be characteristic. The patient is infectious up to one week before the rash appears. The onset of rash renders the child non-infective in normal patients. However, in those with aplastic crisis, the infectious phase may last longer up to few weeks. The rash on cheeks gradually fades in a span of 4-5 days, followed by another characteristic eruption of lacy, reticular generalized rash, which occasionally may be pruritic, and involves the trunk and extensor extremities **(Figure 6.11)**. This lasts for about 5-9 days and may recur for next few weeks to months. The rash is often precipitated by triggers such as sunlight, exercise, temperature change, bathing, and emotional stress. Appearance of lacy reticular rash on cheeks is an extremely rare finding reported in one case. Parvovirus B19 infection has also been implicated in the etiology of various dermatoses **(Table 6.6)**.

Rashes mimicking lupus erythematosus, sweet's syndrome and Henoch-Schonlein purpura are also reported as isolated findings. Tongue or pharynx may show erythema and congestion with red maculae involving buccal mucosa.

Small percentage (10%) of the patients may have arthralgias or arthritis affecting large joints. In adults, the constitutional symptoms are severe. The rash may be absent in women but may have fever, lymphadenopathy and arthritis.

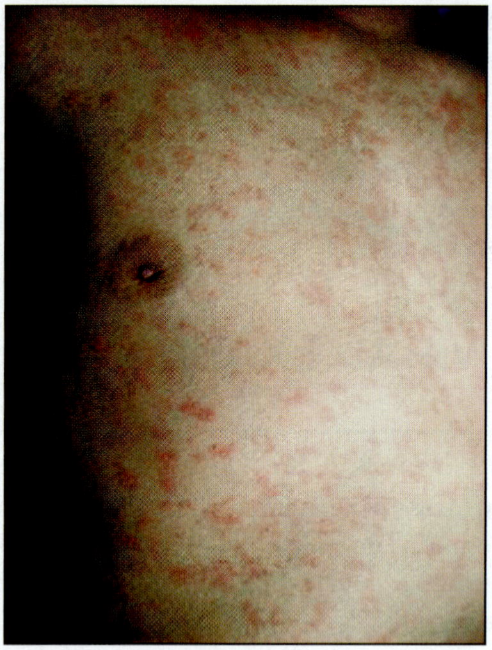

FIGURE 6.11: Diffuse maculopapular truncal eruption in a child with erythema infectiosum, with reticular pattern at places (*Courtesy:* Dr. Deepak Kotkar)

TABLE 6.6: Other unusual cutaneous findings reported due to parvovirus B19 infection

- Erythema multiforme
- Erythema nodosum
- Livedo reticularis
- Angioedema
- Pruritus without rash
- Papulo-vesicular eruptions (Gianotti-Crosti syndrome)
- Papular purpuric gloves and socks syndrome
- Vasculitis
- Purpura

Complications, Course and Prognosis

In immunocompromised individuals with HIV, congenital immunodeficiencies, acute leukemia, organ transplants, and lupus erythematosus or in infants, parvovirus B19 can cause a persistent chronic anemia due to lysis of RBC precursors resulting from active viral replication.

In the patients having chronic hemolytic anemia, EI may result in aplastic crisis with severe anemia, reticulocytopenia, and red blood cell aplasia manifesting clinically as persistent pallor, lethargy and weakness. This is often seen in patients with hereditary spherocytosis, sickle-cell disease, G6PD deficiency, pyruvate-kinase deficiency, iron deficiency, and the thalassemias.

In pregnant women, the infection may result in vertical transmission to the fetus causing infection of erythroid precursors and extensive hemolysis leading to severe anemia, tissue hypoxia, high-output heart failure, and generalized edema (hydrops fetalis) which may cause fetal loss in the first trimester of pregnancy. The rate of vertical transmission in infants (confirmed by IgG positivity in children at 1 year) is reported to be 16 percent if exposed to the infected mother during the first 20 weeks and 35 percent if exposed after 20 weeks of gestation. The risk of hydrops fetalis from hemolytic anemia is 10 percent, which tends to reduce as pregnancy progresses.

Encephalopathy, cerebellar ataxia and permanent neurological damage may result occasionally.

Treatment

The treatment of EI is symptomatic. Aplastic crisis would require fresh blood transfusions. Pregnant women with confirmed primary infection due to parvovirus B19 (IgM and rising titers of IgG) must be carefully followed for fetal complication such as hydrops fetalis. In such situation, a sophisticated care center is required for cordocentesis and fetal blood transfusion. Immunocompromised patients and those with aplastic crisis may run a risk of transmission to health care workers. Hence, due precautions to avoid droplet infection should be observed. Intravenous immunoglobulin containing pooled, neutralizing anti-B19 antibody, has been used successfully to prevent complications in immunologically compromised patients.

HAND-FOOT-MOUTH DISEASE (HFMD)

Salient features

- Highly contagious rash of older children caused by Coxsackie or enterovirus
- Painful oral ulcers and symmetrical elliptical vesicles on hands and feet
- May have serious CNS or pulmonary complication with reported fatality.

Historical Aspects

HFMD was first reported by Robinson and Rhodes in 1958 from Toronto, Canada. Aslop et al reported a similar disease from Birmingham, England in 1960 and termed the disease as HFMD.

Etiology

HFMD is caused by *enteroviruses*, members of *picorna viridae* which are single-stranded, uncapsulated RNA viruses. It is commonly associated with the infections due to Coxsackie A16 or enterovirus71. Sporadic cases are seen in association with Coxsackie A4-7, A9, 10, B1-3 and B5.

Epidemiology

The disease peculiarly affects children below 10 years of age. It rarely occurs in adults. Late summer and early fall are said to be favorable for the infection due to enteroviruses. Faeco-oral and oro-oral routes are common modes of transmission than droplet infection. Vertical spread from mother to fetus may occur. The disease is highly contagious to other family members and to other children in schools. Household contagiousness has been reported to be as high as over 80% in the siblings, particularly with enterovirus 71. Incubation period is from 3 to 6 days. Though the disease has sporadic features, the epidemics are observed to occur regularly every 3 years in USA.

Pathogenesis

Initial infection occurs within the mucosa of oral cavity and small intestine (within ileum). Later, within 24 hours the infection spreads to regional lymph nodes. Viremia follows immediately, spreading the virus to oral cavity and skin. Within a week, the virus disappears as the antibody titers in blood rise significantly.

Clinical Features

After a short incubation period, a prodrome of fever, malaise, abdominal pain, vomiting, diarrhea and anorexia occurs. Enanthem presenting as painful oral ulcers on hard palate, tongue and buccal mucosa usually precedes the onset of exanthema. It consists of symmetrical erythematous 2-8 mm maculo-papular rash on hands and feet which soon becomes vesicular with a typical erythematous halo **(Figure 6.12A)**. The oral lesions are quite sore and often disturb oral intake. These resolve within 5-10 days. Exanthem on hands is much common than on the feet. The sides of fingers and dorsa are frequently involved. The vesicles are typically elliptical with the long axes parallel to skin lines **(Figure 6.12B)**. These may be painful. The crust formation ensues within 8-10 days and heals without scarring.

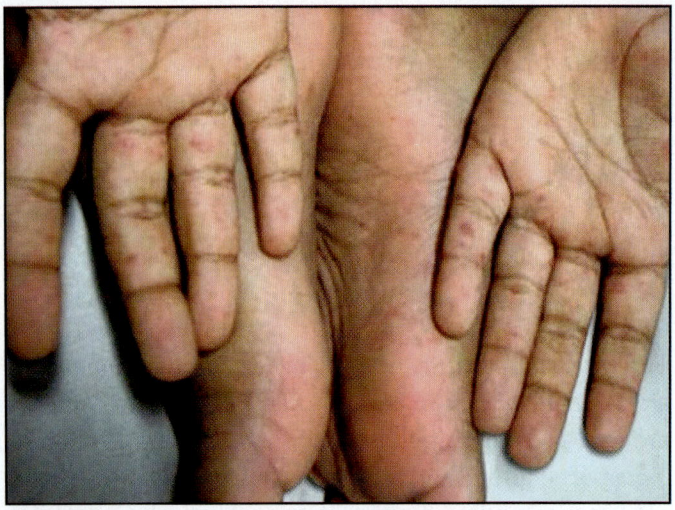

FIGURE 6.12A: Symmetrical erythematous maculopapular rash with vesiculation on palms in hand-foot-mouth disease (*Courtesy:* Dr Satish Udare, Navi Mumbai)

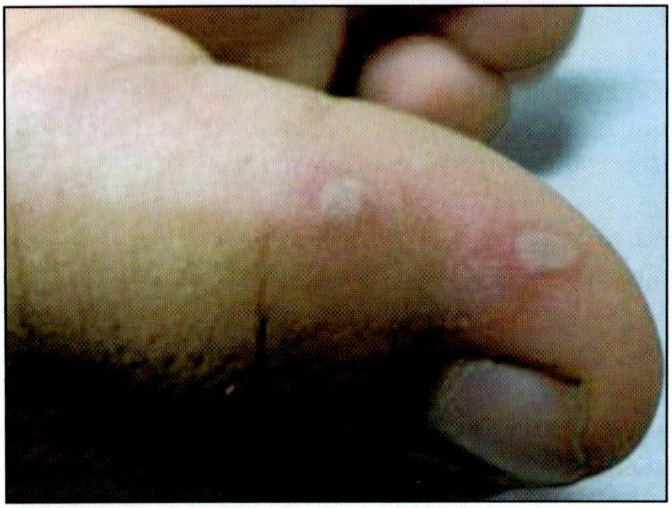

FIGURE 6.12B: Typical vesicle in hand-foot-mouth disease is elliptical, with long axis parallel to the skin lines (*Courtesy:* Dr Satish Udare, Navi Mumbai)

Diagnosis

HFMD is diagnosed by its typical clinical presentation. Paired viral serology, viral cultures from stools and PCR are helpful to clinch the diagnosis in doubtful cases.

Course and Prognosis

The disease, though dramatic in appearance, resolves spontaneously within two weeks in most of the cases. Systemic complications are uncommonly encountered.

Complications

These are rarely reported and include myocarditis, pneumonia and meningo-encephalitis. Diarrhea and arthralgia may occur occasionally. Infection in first trimester of pregnancy may result in spontaneous abortion and intra-uterine growth retardation.

Mortality is rare. However, recent epidemics due to enteroviruse 71 reported high rate of deaths resulting from complications. Neurological syndromes reported from Taiwan in 1999 include acute flaccid paralysis, aseptic meningitis, brain-stem encephalitis or rhombencephalitis. The latter present as myoclonic jerk and is associated with significant mortality. The patient should be carefully monitored for myoclonus and associated sleep disturbances, an important warning signal of early CNS involvement. Other epidemics from Taiwan and Singapore reported deaths due to pulmonary hemorrhages and pulmonary edema, and pneumonia and rhombencephalitis respectively.

Treatment

Treatment of HFMD is symptomatic. Local application of viscous lidocaine or diphenhydramine for oral lesions would reduce the pain. Systemic acyclovir 200 mg every five hours for 5 days is reported of some benefit especially in immunocompromised individuals or those with severe morbidity. Placonaril, a broad spectrum antiviral drug that inhibits attachment of enterovirus to the host cell receptors and uncoating of viral nucleic acid has demonstrated efficacy in immunocompromised patients with severe enteroviral infection in dose of 2.5-5 mg/kg for 7 days. Its efficacy specifically against HFMD is yet to be demonstrated. It might be worth using in serious neurological complications of HFMD. Isolation of the affected child from school or from other susceptible family members for about 2-3 days after the onset of enanthem or exanthem has been advised by some physicians. Routine hygienic practices are helpful in preventing faeco-oral transmission.

INFECTIOUS MONONUCLEOSIS (IM)

Salient features:

- Adolescent or young adult with fever, pharyngitis and tender cervical lymphadenopathy.
- Atypical lymphocytes and mononucleosis on peripheral smear with frequent splenomegaly
- Generalized maculopapular rash commonly triggered by beta-lactam antibiotics. May be a presenting feature if HIV seroconversion.

Syndrome: Glandular fever, Kissing disease

Historical Aspects

German physicians used to describe term 'Glandular fever' for a clinical triad of fever, pharyngitis and adenopathy. Sprunt and Evans first reported IM from USA in 1920. Causative role of EBV in IM was recognized in late 1960s.

Etiology

IM is caused by active primary infection due to EBV, a member of *gammaherpesviridae* family and genus *lymphocryptovirus* having linear DNA molecule.

Epidemiology

IM most frequently affects adolescents and young adults, though no age group is exempt. There is no specific predilection for race, sex and geographical location. The transmission of disease occurs via saliva or oropharyngeal secretions infected with EBV. Apart from close contacts of IM patients, patients with immunodeficiency predispose the individual for EBV-induced glandular fever. These include congenital immunodeficiency as well as acquired one viz. post-transplant lymphoproliferative disorder, HIV infection or those receiving immunosuppressive drugs. The incubation period is 1-2 months. Airborne transmission does not normally occur. Children with IM are potentially infectious.

Pathogenesis

Transmitted through contact with oropharyngeal secretions (therefore called, *kissing disease*), EBV infects the B cells in the oropharyngeal epithelium and affects the entire reticular endothelial system (RES), i.e. liver, spleen, and peripheral lymph nodes via circulating B cells. EBV infection of B lymphocytes induces humoral and cellular immune response. T-lymphocyte response is essential in the control of EBV infection; natural killer (NK) cells and predominantly $CD8^+$ cytotoxic T cells control proliferating B lymphocytes infected with EBV. The T-lymphocyte cellular response decides the clinical presentation of EBV infection. A rapid and efficient T-cell response results in control of the primary EBV infection and life-long suppression of EBV. Ineffective T-cell response may cause uncontrolled B-cell proliferation, resulting in B-lymphocyte malignancies such as B-cell lymphomas.

Clinical Features

Most patients infected with EBV would have no or minimal symptoms. Fatigue and malaise are usual presenting symptoms. Sore throat and low grade fever is common. Nausea and anorexia without vomiting may occur with or without arthralgia and myalgia. The fever, lymphadenopathy, rash and periorbital edema are the early signs of IM.

Exanthematous rash is of two kinds. First is a transient, asymptomatic faint maculo-papular rash occurring directly due to the viral infection and is seen in early course of disease (within 24-48 hours) **(Figure 6.13)**. The other type follows after administration of antibiotics, commonly beta-lactams viz. ampicillin or amoxicillin, but it can be seen following cephalexin, erythromycin, azithromycin or levofloxacin therapy. This type of maculo-papular eruption is profuse, often pruritic and lasts longer affecting the trunk and upper extremities. Though actual sensitization to beta-lactams may occur in IM, generally it should not be presumed that the individual is sensitive to the drug unless it is further documented.

Palatal petechiae and uvular edema, whenever present, are considered as important signs of IM. Bilateral, transient upper eyelid edema (*Hoagland sign*), though not very common, is fairly a specific sign.

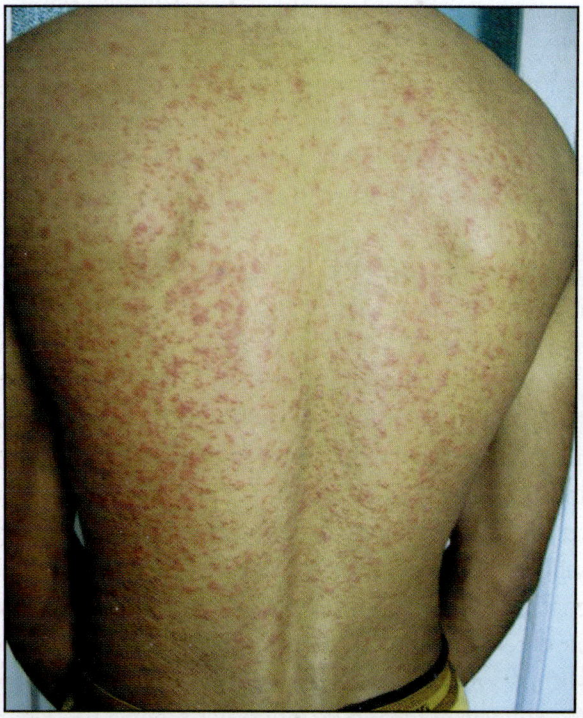

FIGURE 6.13: Diffuse erythematous, maculopapular eruptions in an adolescent boy with infectious mononucleosis

Bilateral tender posterior cervical lymphadenopathy is a common presentation of IM. Pharyngitis may be exudative or non-exudative. Severe tonsillar enlargement may occur which could result in obstruction of airway. Sinus bradycardia may occur and may be suggestive of viral myocarditis.

Systemic Complications

Splenomegaly may occur after first week, often with tenderness. Although unicteric hepatitis is frequent, jaundice is seen more often in elderly patients. Splenic rupture is an unusual but potentially life-threatening complication in 1% of patients. Other visceral manifestations include gastro-intestinal (mesenteric adenitis, acalculous cholecystitis, pancreatitis), CNS (meningoencephalitis, transverse myelitis, aseptic meningitis, cranial nerve palsies, especially facial nerve and Guillain-Barre syndrome) and renal complications (glomerulonephritis).

Differential diagnoses of febrile illness with mononucleosis include CMV, HHV6 infection, Toxoplasmosis, acute HIV infection (seroconversion illness) and viral hepatitis.

Investigation and Diagnosis

Leucocytosis is the rule in IM. Lymphocytosis with atypical lymphocytes in peripheral blood (>10%) is helpful in the diagnosis. Mononucleosis is a constant feature on peripheral smear. Thrombocytopenia may be present. Elevated ESR may be helpful in differentiating IM from streptococcal pharyngitis, which may co-exist with IM. Mild elevation of serum transaminases is frequently noticed.

The detection of antibodies against EBV antigen alone is not reliable as it can persist for years after primary infection. Up to 90% of adults are seropositive for EBV. Hence, interpretation of serology of EBV should be done carefully. Primary infection is suggested when there is positive IgM against viral capsid antigen in the absence of antibodies against EBV nuclear antigen. A very high or rising titer of IgG against viral capsid antigen in the absence of antibodies against EBV nuclear antigen is detected after at least four weeks of onset of symptoms. IgG is not likely to be detectable in the early phase of disease.

Monospot test, a latex agglutination test using horse RBCs, detects heterophile antibodies against EBV. It may not be positive until 2-6 weeks after initial symptoms. Patients may have heterophile negative IM. False negative results are seen in children below two years and false positive in toxoplasmosis, rubella, lymphoma and leukemias.

EBV-specific antibodies, IgG and IgM antibodies, against viral capsid antigen, early antigen and nuclear antigens are helpful in differentiating past and acute infections in immunocompetent patients. In those with deficient immune function, polymerase chain reaction and *in situ* hybridization are more conclusive.

Course and Prognosis

IM is generally a self-resolving disease with a potential for number of complications as enlisted above. Enlargement of spleen, if present, resolves by the end of third week. Fatality is rare and may result due to hemophagocytic syndrome.

Treatment

There is no specific therapy for IM. Short course of corticosteroids (1mg/kg/day for 3 days, gradually tapered over two weeks) should be reserved for the patients with mononucleosis induced hemolytic anemia, CNS involvement, severe tonsillar enlargement, thrombocytopenia and myocarditis. Routine use of corticosteroids should be discouraged in IM as this may trigger complications in otherwise uncomplicated IM. Positive throat cultures for group A streptococci in IM should be interpreted with caution because this often represents streptococcal colonization rather than active infection and the drug for treatment of streptococcal infection may cause drug rash. Surgical care may be needed for splenic rupture.

MEASLES (SYN: FIRST DISEASE, RUBEOLA)

Salient features:

- Young child with fever, coryza, conjunctivitis
- Generalized confluent blanching erythematous macular rash peaking with fever
- Koplik's spots in oral cavity
- Pulmonary and CNS complications may occur.

Historical Aspects

Measles is an age old exanthem known to mankind. Initial clinical descriptions date back to as early as tenth century. Thomas and Sydenham in seventeenth century gave insight into accurate clinical and epidemiologic presentations. Enders and Peebles in 1954 isolated the virus in tissue culture and they successfully attenuated it in 1960 for vaccination purpose. Measles vaccine was prepared for human use from 1963 onwards and has been proven to be of significant benefit in control of measles infection in the community.

Etiology

The causative virus of measles is paramyxovirus, genus morbillivirus, which is a single-stranded enveloped RNA virus.

Epidemiology

Most of the cases occur in infants and toddlers in urban population and in rural ones, slightly older children between 5 and 10 years of age. Winter and spring season bring most of the cases peaking in March-April. Incubation period is 10-11 days. The infection spreads through droplet infection and the initial site of infection being the respiratory epithelium of nasopharynx.

Clinical Features

After an incubation period, there is a prodrome of 1-7 days presenting with coryza, conjunctivitis, cough and high-grade rising fever corresponding to peak of rash. The barking type of cough persists after the coryzal symptoms disappear.

Erythematous blanching maculo-papular rash, usually begins behind the ears and anterior hair line, rapidly progresses to profuse coalescence involving the neck, trunk and extremities in that order within 2-4 days. The rash fades in the same order and becomes non-blanchable. Fine desquamation is often seen.

Mucosal lesions are seen as pinpoint raised lesions against red background of deeply congested pharynx for 6-7 days. Blue-gray stippling may appear on tonsils (Herman's spot). Koplik's spots, the punctate blue-white lesions surrounded by erythematous areola on buccal mucosa against second molar are pathognomonic and appear on 2-4 days of fever **(Figure 6.14)**. Similar spots may be seen on conjunctivae at the medial canthi.

Those children who received killed vaccine and subsequently are infected with natural infection present with *atypical measles*. Prodrome consists of high-grade fever, myalgia, cough, abdominal pains, headache, pleural effusion, pneumonia and hilar lymphadenopathy. Edema of extremities may occur. Maculo-papular rash beginning on hands and feet and then spreading on trunk and face often progresses to vesicular lesions and purpura.

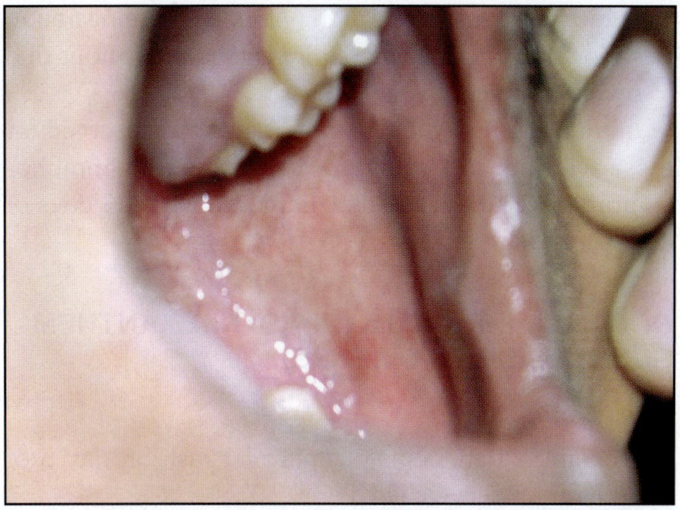

FIGURE 6.14: Koplik's spots, pathognomonic feature of measles

It needs to be differentiated from Rocky Mountain spotted fever. Milder *modified measles* may be seen in partially immune host due to prior infection, persistent maternal antibodies and routine immunization. This variant presents with less florid rash, shorter duration of illness and may be absence of Koplik's spots.

Diagnosis

Measles is diagnosed with certainty on clinical presentation. Confirmation with IgM and rising IgG antibodies is rarely necessary to establish the diagnosis.

Complications

Severe disease and complications occur frequently in very young and malnourished children. Encephalitis (1:800) is usually resolves with no sequelae but death and brain damage may occur rarely. Thrombocytopenia, purpura and lymphopenia may occur. Superadded bacterial infections result in otitis media and pneumonia. Subacute sclerosing panencephalitis (SSPE) occurs rarely (1:100000) as a delayed, serious complication, months or years after measles due to degeneration of neurons. It presents with personality changes, myoclonic seizures, coma and death. Measles during pregnancy may result in fetal loss.

Treatment

Treatment of measles is supportive. Rest, hydration, nutritional support, anti-cough preparations and respiratory isolation are necessary. Intravenous or aerosolized Ribavirin may be recommended in severely ill or immunocompromised children. Vitamin A administration has shown to decrease morbidity and complications due to severe measles.

Immune serum globulin administration is reserved for those who are too young for vaccination or immunocompromised and it should commence within 6 days of exposure.

ROSEOLA INFANTUM (RI) (SYN: EXANTHEM SUBITUM, SIXTH DISEASE)

Salient features:

- Generalized erythematous macular rash on day 5 of fever in an active child
- It completely clears within next few days.

Historical Aspects

RI is first reported by Zahorsky in 1910. Yamunishi K et al in 1988 successfully isolated Human Herpesvirus-6 (HHV-6) from the infants suffering from Roseala infantum. Hall et al reported natural history and complication of primary herpes virus infections in 1994.

Epidemiology

RI is chiefly a disease of infants and children below three years.

Etiology

HHV belongs to Betaherpesviridae family and genus Roseolovirus. HHV-6 is further subclassifed as HHV-6A and HHV-6B. Most cases of RI in infants and children are caused by HHV-6B. HHV-7 may rarely cause RI, especially in the older children.

Pathogenesis

Acquired as a droplet infection, the virus HHV-6 multiplies in salivary gland and is secreted in saliva. It remains dormant in the peripheral blood mononuclear cells and other tissues in the body for indefinite period. It is reactivated during the state of relative immunodeficiency in the host.

Clinical Features

The disease begins as acute onset of high-grade fever in a child who otherwise appears active and clinically normal. Some children may present with rhinitis, cough or diarrhea.

Ulceration or erosions at the uvulo-palatal junction may be seen in some children. On day 5 of fever appearance of generalized erythematous macules on trunk and neck is the hallmark of RI. It might involve extremities and face. The fever recedes as in the sequence of rash appearance on the body and completely clears within next 2-5 days without any residual change.

Complications

These are rare and depend on the system predominantly affected by the virus. These include otitis media, febrile convulsions, thrombocytopenia, encephalitis, Guillain-Barre syndrome and myocarditis.

Diagnosis

The diagnosis is clinical but the detection of HHV-6 DNA by polymerase chain reaction in the plasma, HHV-6 DNA in whole blood in the absence of IgG, or high HHV-6 viral DNA load in the whole blood specimen are indicative of active HHV-6 infection. Parallel testing of acute and convalescent sera indicating seroconversion is indicative of primary infection.

Treatment

The management of RI is symptomatic and supportive.

RUBELLA (SYN: THIRD DISEASE, GERMAN MEASLES)

Salient features:

- Adolescent and young adults with fever and cervical lymphadenopathy. Maculopapular rash at the onset of illness, which starts on face and neck, and spreads caudally
- Petechial enanthems
- CNS and hematological complications can occur
- Congenital rubella syndrome is a concern in pregnant women.

Historical Aspects

George Maton in 1814 first recognized that a mild illness characterized by rash, adenopathy, and little or no fever was a discrete entity. Henry Veale, in 1866, named the disease rubella. However, the disease was viewed as significant entity only when Norman Gregg in1942 noticed that first-trimester maternal rubella caused serious birth defects.

Etiology

Rubella is caused by a *togaviridae*, a single-stranded enveloped RNA virus belonging to the genus, *Rubivirus*.

Epidemiology

The distribution is world wide. Incubation period is 15-21 days, most commonly occurring during spring. Adolescents and young adults are most commonly affected. The spread occurs via droplet infection. In USA, it is thought to be commonly affecting the latin American migrant population. Adequate protection is conferred by two doses of vaccination against rubella incorporated into MMR vaccine.

Clinical Features

A prodrome of fever, headache, malaise, cough and sore throat is often present. The rash, light pink macules and papules begin usually on the first day on face and then spread caudally to trunk and extremities. It is less confluent than in measles. Enanthem of rose-pink pinpoint petechiae (*Forschimer spots*) may be seen on soft palate and uvula. Lymphadenopathy may be generalized but more remarkable in suboccipital and postauricular groups. Conjunctivitis and testalgias may occur. Neutropenia is present in some individuals.

Complications

Arthralgia and arthritis may occur in women. Encephalitis, orchitis, neuritis, thrombocytopenia and late progressive panencephalitis rarely occur. Infection during the first trimester of pregnancy runs the highest risk of causing congenital rubella syndrome. The newborn child may present with sensorineural hearing impairment, cataracts, glaucoma, retinopathy, congenital cardiac defects, and mental retardation. Neonatal thrombocytopenic purpura, hepatitis, bone lesions, meningoencephalitis, diabetes mellitus and progressive rubella panencephalitis are more recently known effects of congenital rubella infection.

Diagnosis

Clinical diagnosis sometimes needs to be supported by specific IgM and reverse-transcriptase PCR when there is a risk of transmission to fetus during pregnancy. Rubella-specific IgG serology in oral fluid is recently described with good sensitivity and specificity. Rubella has to be differentiated from other viral exanthemas and drug eruptions.

Treatment

There is no specific therapy for rubella. Management is supportive and symptomatic. Specific vigilance has to be offered to pregnant women with rubella infection. Antenatal diagnosis is possible with fetal vein sampling for RNA probes and rarely, viral culture.

NEWLY REDISCOVERED VIRAL EXANTHEMS

ASYMMETRIC PERIFLEXURAL EXANTHEM (APE)

Synonym

New papular exanthem of childhood, localized erythema of childhood with lymphadenopathy, unilateral latero-thoracic exanthem.

Salient features:

- Young children or rarely adults with asymmetric or unilateral maculopapular rash in axilla or groin with regional lymphadenopathy
- Self resolution occurs within few days.

Historical Aspects

In 1992, Bodemer C et al. reported a series of children presenting with an exanthem involving unilateral hemithorax. Immediately after that, Taieb et al. in 1993, reported a series of children with asymmetric exanthem around flexures and coined the term, "Asymmetric periflexural exanthem".

Etiology

Exact cause is unknown but the clinical and epidemiological findings support a viral etiology. Several viruses are implicated including parainfluenza 2 and 3, parvovirus B19 and adenovirus. However, none of the viruses were found to be consistently associated.

Epidemiology

APE is typically a disease of young children between 1 and 5 years. However, adult cases are reported from several countries including India. There is slight female preponderance. Winter and spring are the favored seasons for the rash to erupt, peak being in the month of September. Most cases are reported from France and Italy but the disease is prevalent world over. There is no obvious triggering factor.

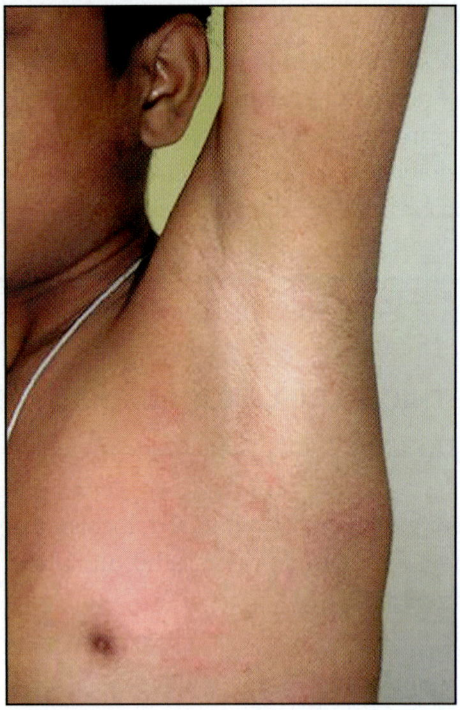

FIGURE 6.15: Erythematous, macopapular eruption of acute onset around left axilla in a child with asymmetric periflexural exanthem (*Courtesy:* Dr S Mahajan, Nashik)

Clinical Features

The rash, which can occasionally be pruritic, presents as unilateral or asymmetric bilateral eruption. Initially erythematous papular, scarlatiniform or eczematous eruptions appear in axilla or groin **(Figure 6.15)**. Later they may progress to involve trunk and extremities. There may be a short prodrome of respiratory or gastrointestinal tract, often with low-grade fever. There is often a regional lymphadenopathy confined to area of initial involvement. There are no systemic complications.

Differential Diagnoses

The differential diagnosis includes erythema multiforme, contact dermatitis, drug eruption, papular pityriasis rosea, herpes zoster in evolution. Skin biopsy is rarely required to rule out other conditions. Perisudoral infiltration is said to be fairly specific feature of APE, though it may be absent.

Course and Prognosis

Resolution within 1-3 weeks is the rule, though longer duration is reported. No significant morbidity or systemic involvement is anticipated.

Treatment

APE like other viral exanthemas is to be treated symptomatically with topical emollients or local corticosteroid creams with or without oral antihistamines.

ACUTE HEMORRHAGIC EDEMA OF INFANCY (AHEI)

Synonym

Acute infantile hemorrhagic edema, Finkelstein's disease, Seidlmeyer's syndrome, Purpura en cocarde avec edema, Cockarde purpura and edema, Post infectious cockade purpura of early childhood, acute benign cutaneous leucocytoclastic vasculitis.

Salient features:

- Rapidly progressive rash in a non-toxic child with large generalized erythematous plaques.
- Typical morphological patterns of rosettes, cockades and bands.
- Leucocytoclastic vasculitis on biopsy is diagnostic.

Historical Aspects

Snow first reported the condition from USA in 1913. Finkelstein further described its detailed clinical manifestations in 1938.

Definition

AHEI is a distinctive, cutaneous, small vessel leucocytoclastic vasculitis of unknown origin occurring in young children manifesting with dramatic, characteristic skin findings.

Etiology

The exact etiology is not established but it is most likely to be incited by an infectious agent. It is often preceded by upper respiratory infection, vaccination or drug intake. Isolated reports mention association with pulmonary tuberculosis, pneumococcal bacteremia and herpes simplex stomatitis.

Epidemiology

Typical age group affected is 4 months-4 years. However, cases have been reported in neonate as well as the older children. No racial predilection is seen. Distribution is probably worldwide, though very few cases are reported from Asian population. There is a marginal preponderance for male children. Most cases are seen in winter.

Pathogenesis

AHEI is distinct variant of leucocytoclastic vasculitis possible mediated by immune complexes. It is thought to be a variant of Henoch-Schonlein purpura by some workers but the deposition of IgA is found only in few patients and serious visceral involvement is generally not seen in AHEI. Hence, AHEI is better considered to be a separate entity.

Clinical Features

Dramatic clinical features developing rapidly in a non-toxic child is typical of AHEI. There can be a prodrome of low-grade fever but the overall health of the child remains unaffected. There is often a history of preceding upper respiratory infection treated with systemic drugs (e.g. amoxicillin).

Cutaneous findings are characteristic and consist of rapidly progressive brightly erythematous large plaques with cockade (rosette or knots), annular, or targetoid, purpuric morphology on face, ears and extremities **(Figure 6.16)**. Lesions frequently appear as large urticarial plaques of 5 cm size or more, which often become purpuric. Lesions are often pruritic. Non-tender, asymptomatic edema of hands and feet often extend proximally. Mucosal involvement as purpuric lesions is rare. Joint and abdominal pains as well as visceral involvement occur rarely and are not too distressing.

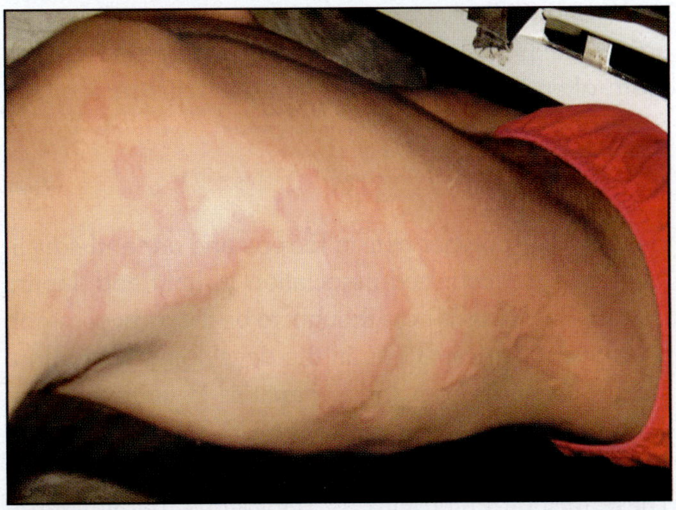

FIGURE 6.16: Rapidly enlarging, widespread, erythematous plaques with different patterns of bands, rosettes and knots in a child with acute hemorrhagic edema

Investigations

Commonly done laboratory tests are not diagnostic. Hematological findings including ESR, bleeding time, clotting time, platelet counts are normal. Skin biopsy reveals leucocytoclastic vasculitis with cellular infiltrate mainly consisting of neutrophils. The small vessels in dermis are commonly affected. There is endothelial swelling with fibrin deposition in and around the vessel walls. Perivascular neutrophilic infiltration is characteristic with evidence of scattered nuclear fragmentation (nuclear dust). Extravasation of erythrocytes around the blood vessel walls is remarkable.

The condition should be differentiated from Henoch-Scholein purpura (older children, lower leg symmetrical purpura, abdominal pains and nephritis) and menigo-coccemia.

Course and Prognosis

Self-resolution in 1-3 weeks is the rule, though longer duration is recorded. Recurrences can occur. Arthritis, nephritis, abdominal pain, gastrointestinal tract bleeding, and lethal intestinal complications are reported rarely. Long-term sequelae are not likely to occur.

Treatment

Treatment of AHEI is symptomatic. Discontinuation of antibiotic may be advisable once the culture reports are normal. Parents should be reassured of spontaneous and complete recovery. Oral antihistamines may be given for symptomatic patients.

ERUPTIVE PSEUDOANGIOMATOSIS (EP)

Synonym

Hemangioma like exanthem, cherry angioma-like exanthem.

Salient features:

- Cherry angioma-like few discrete asymptomatic eruptions
- Self-resolution within 10 days.

Historical Aspects

The condition is first reported by Cherry et al. in 1969. The term was coined by Neil Prose in 1993.

Etiology

Echoviruses were likely culprits in the initial series of Cherry. However, there was no substantiation of the same etiological agent in the further series published by the other workers. However, considering the natural course of the disease, infectious (mostly likely virus) etiology is suspected. Multifactorial viral etiology has been suggested.

Epidemiology

Majority of the cases are observed in children. However, adult cases have been reported. Cases have been reported to occur following renal transplant, lymphocytic leukemia or during the treatment of asthma and chemotherapy for cancers. Adults may have longer course. Familial occurrence is reported.

Clinical Features

The disease may have an initial prodrome of mild fever, sore throat or gastrointestinal symptoms. The rash erupts as small, discrete cherry angioma-like tiny papules surrounded by a perilesional halo on face, neck, extremities and trunk **(Figure 6.17)**. The rash completely blanches on pressure. There are usually less than 10 lesions and resolution by 10 days is the rule.

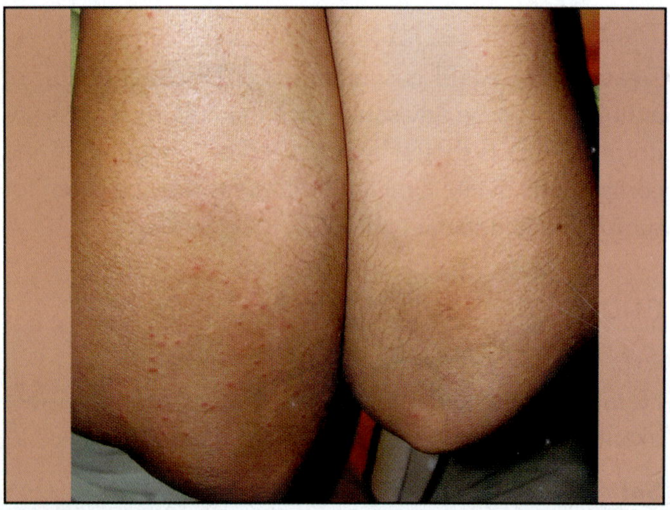

FIGURE 6.17: Multiple, erythematous, cherry angioma-like, round blanchable papules with typical perilesional halo in an adolescent patient with eruptive pseudoangioma

Diagnosis

EP may be misdiagnosed as insect bites on clinical grounds. Biopsy reveals uninvolved epidermis and dermal edema associated with dilated blood vessels with plump hobnail-shaped endothelial cells, characteristic of EP. There is no evidence of vasculitis. Perivascular infiltrates with lymphocytes and polymorphs in the superficial dermis are often found. As there was no proliferation of blood vessels, Prose et al named the disease as EP.

Course, Prognosis, Treatment

The disease is benign, self-resolving yet distinctive and lasts for short duration. Hence, treatment is not required.

GIANOTTI-CROSTI SYNDROME (GCS)

Synonym

Infantile papular acrodermatitis, papular acrodermatitis of infants, infantile lichenoid dermatitis.

Salient features:

- Monomorphic symmetric erythematous papules/ papulo-vesicles in young children
- Lymphadenopathy in 1/3 of the patients
- Association with hepatitis B and EBV infections.

Historical Aspects

Ferdinando Gianotti from Italy in 1955 observed a typical non-relapsing rash which lasted for about three weeks and was localized to face and limbs. He suspected the rash being viral in origin. This was later found to be consistently associated with hepatitis B virus infection in children.

Epidemiology

The disease appears to be worldwide though most initial cases were reported from Italy and Japan. GCS is typically a disease of children between the age group of 1 and 6 years, and 90% occur before 4 years of age. Adult cases are rare, extremely difficult to diagnose and are reported more often in women. There is no specific race or sex predisposition.

Etiology

Hepatitis B (subtypes *ayw* in Europe and *adr* and *adw* in Asia) was a recognized association in Italy and Japan. Epstein-Barr virus is now thought to be the most common causative agent especially in the developing world. In a study published from India, hepatitis B virus infection was not found to be the cause of GCS. There are several other viruses frequently implicated in the recent years. These include enteroviruses, parvovirus, parainfluenza virus, mumps virus, rotavirus, poxvirus, respiratory syncytial virus, ECHO, hepatitis A virus, hepatitis C virus, Molluscum contagiosum virus, human immunodeficiency virus and human herpes virus 6 virus (mainly 6B). Some workers suspected association of GCS with non-viral organisms such as *Mycoplasma pneumoniae, Bartonella henselae, Beta-hemolytic streptococcus and Borrelia burgdorferi*.

Many cases were reported following a history of immunization with oral polio, hepatitis B and MMR vaccines. Respiratory virus infections resulted in winter epidemics as against summer epidemics due to enteroviruses. Immunodeficient hosts may run a protracted course. Atopic background is frequently noticed in the children with GCS.

Pathogenesis

The exact pathogenesis is not well understood. Various hypotheses have been proposed for causation of cutaneous eruptions including viral infection with immunological alteration, delayed type of hypersensitivity to the viruses, circulating viruses or immune complex deposition. However, viral particles or viral antigens have not been identified on electron microscopy. Hence, it may be concluded that the rash of GCS is not directly caused by viruses but due to the stimulation of immunological system following the viral infection. Occurrence of GCS could thus be explained in atopic individuals.

Clinical Features

Acute onset of rash may precede an upper respiratory infection or diarrhea with or without minimal constitutional symptoms of fever and malaise. The commonest type of rash is pink or red papule, or papulo-vesicle of 1-10 mm size symmetrically distributed on the extensor aspect of extremities, face and buttocks **(Figure 6.18)**. Uncommonly, lichenoid dermatitis with flat-topped papules develops as the rash becomes more chronic. The rash remains at least for 10 days and may have mild to moderate pruritus. Extremes of rash duration have been identified ranging from few days to several months. Similarly, cutaneous involvement ranges from only few lesions to widespread involvement of body surface area. Involvement of trunk, palms and soles is rare. Mucosal or flexor surface involvement is only seen exceptionally as is the scaly rash. Profuse early lesions may exhibit Koebner's phenomenon.

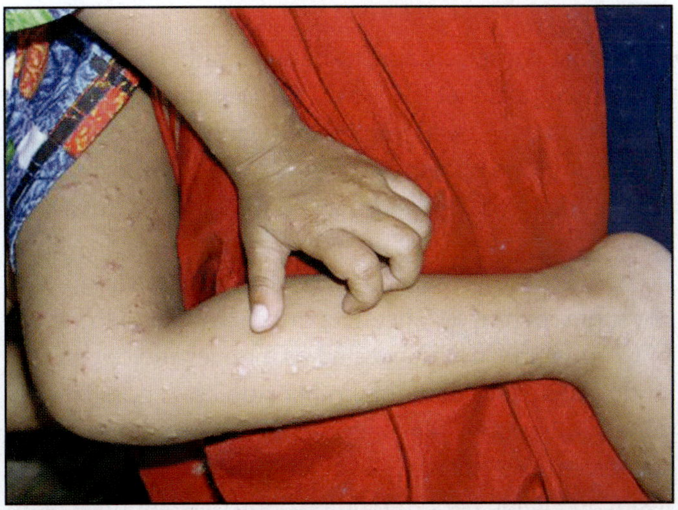

FIGURE 6.18: Monomorphic erythematous papules on legs and hands of a child with Gianotti-Crosti syndrome

Upper respiratory infection with pharyngitis and/ or tonsillitis is frequently noted. Some patients may have diarrhea, nausea or vomiting. Lymphadenopathy, though not a consistent feature, is seen in up to one-third of patients involving mainly cervical and sometimes axillary and inguinal groups. Hepatomegaly, if present, is usually anicteric as noted in the original description of Ferdinando Gianotti. Splenomegaly is observed occasionally.

Differential Diagnosis

Conditions such as papular urticaria, scabies, lichen planus or lichenoid dermatitis, erythema multiforme and atopic dermatitis are the common differential diagnoses. These can be easily differentiated clinically. In doubtful cases, a search for scabies mite, identifying the source of arthropod bite or history of antecedent drug history may clinch the diagnosis. Uncommon differential diagnoses include infectious mononucleosis and other viral exanthems, pityriasis rosea, lichen striatus, frictional lichenoid dermatitis (especially with Koebner's phenomenon), Langerhan cell histiocytosis, pityriasis lichenoides, varioliformis acuta, and Henoch- Schonlein purpura.

Laboratory Investigations

Leucocytosis with lymphocytosis or occasionally lymphopenia, remarkable monocytosis may be present indicating an active viral infection. Abnormal liver enzymes may suggest EBV or CMV infection. In the presence of clinical or laboratory evidence of hepatitis, tests for hepatitis B surface antigen, anti-hepatitis A and anti-hepatitis C antibodies should be done.

Skin biopsy is rarely required for the diagnosis. The histologic features are not diagnostic but it does help to exclude other conditions. The histologic findings in the *vesicular* type show mild acanthosis and spongiosis with intra-epidermal vesicle. Langerhans cells are present in significant number inside the vesicle. Occasional lymphocytic exocytosis is seen. Dense lymphocytic perivascular infiltrate of T cells and dendritic cells is seen in the papillary dermis. Most of the lymphocytes are CD4+ and CD8+ T cells; cytotoxic T cells are remarkable in EBV-induced GCS.

In papular variant, acanthosis, parakeratosis, hyperkeratosis with mixed lympho-histiocytic perivascular infiltrate and occasional hemorrhages may be seen.

Diagnosis

Diagnostic criteria were proposed and reported by Chuh AAT. These have been validated for the Indian children **(Table 6.7)**.

TABLE 6.7: Diagnostic criteria of Gianotti-Crosti syndrome Reprinted with permission of Cutis®2001; 68: 207-213. ©2001, Quadrant HealthCom Inc.

A patient is diagnosed as having Gianotti-Crosti syndrome (GCS) or papular acrodermatitis if:

On at least one occasion or clinical encounter, he/she exhibits all the positive clinical features, and on all occasions or clinical encounters related to the rash, he/she does not exhibit any of the negative clinical features, and none of the differential diagnoses is considered to be more likely than GCS on clinical judgment, and if lesional biopsy is performed, the findings are consistent with GCS.

The *positive* clinical features are:

- Monomorphous, flat-topped, pink-brown papules or papulovesicles 1–10 mm in diameter on at least three of the following four sites: cheeks, buttocks, extensor surfaces of the forearms, extensor surfaces of the legs.
- Being symmetrical.
- Lasting for at least 10 days.

The *negative* clinical features are:

- Extensive truncal lesions.
- Scaly lesions.

Treatment

As the disease is self-limiting, symptomatic therapy consisting of mild to moderately potent topical steroids, oral antihistamines or local anti-pruritic agents is usually enough to give good symptomatic relief. There is no specific drug therapy. Systemic steroid pulse therapy is rarely recommended for the refractory cases. Secondary infections require a course of suitable systemic antibiotics.

Course and Prognosis

Generally, the rash resolves within 2-8 weeks without scarring unless secondarily infected. Transient post-inflammatory pigmentary changes may be seen following resolution of rash. Lymphadenopathy and hepatospenomegaly, when present may require longer duration to resolve. Serious complications include chronic hepatitis especially in those positive for hepatitis B surface antigen. Parents need to be reassured that the rash is self-limiting, not likely to be contagious, has negligible complications, and usually there will not be permanent scarring.

KAWASAKI DISEASE (KD)

Synonym

Kawasaki syndrome, Muco-cutaneous lymph node syndrome.

Salient features:

- Possibly viral disease with immunological vasculitis
- An irritable child with high-grade fever, lip fissuring, conjunctivitis, cervical lymphadenopathy, truncal polymorphic non-vesicular rash, and hand and feet edema resolving with a typical distal exfoliation.
- Coronary aneurysm constitutes the serious morbidity.

Definition

Kawasaki disease or syndrome is an acute febrile illness characterized by self-limiting multisystem vasculitis of unknown etiology occurring in infants and children.

Historical Aspects

KD was first described by Tomisaku Kawasaki from Japan in 1967. This was initially thought to be a benign disease but now considered as a cause of serious cardiac disease.

Etiology

The exact cause remains to be explored. The course of events suggests that KD is an infectious disorder. Several organisms have been implicated including bacteria such as staphylococci, streptococci, *Propionibacterium, Chlamydia* and viruses such as EBV, parvovirus, and retrovirus. However, none of these have been proven to be consistently associated with KD. An association with rug shampoo has also been reported. Recently, N63 strain of Coronavirus was suggested as a novel etiology in one study but not supported by other studies. A possibility of genetic susceptibility, especially in Asian population, is suggested. Pre-existence of eczema, use of humidifiers in room and living near a standing body of water have been suggested to have added predisposition to KD.

Epidemiology

KD is regarded as a disease of children below 5 years of age. However, children older than 5 years and younger than 6 months have been reported be affected. Peak prevalence is between 18 and 24 months of age. Japanese, Korean and other Asian ethnic children are at risk of acquiring KD. Late winter to spring is the favored season for the onset of disease, when epidemics in USA and Japan have frequently occurred. The disease is most prevalent in Japanese population with occurrence of 5000 cases each year. Endemics are also reported in USA but at a lesser incidence rate epidemiologically. However, KD actually has worldwide prevalence. Male children are more affected than females (1.5:1).

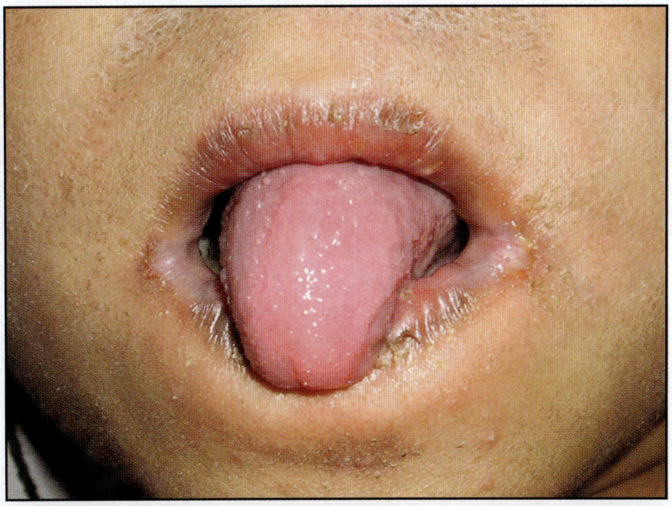

FIGURE 6.19A: Fissuring of lip and strawberry tongue in Kawasaki disease

Pathogenesis

Theories have been put forth including infectious agents and immunological alterations. Some workers consider immunologically programmed events are more important than mere infection. It has been suggested that KD may be a superantigen mediated immunological process like toxic shock syndrome caused by staphylococci. Superantigens are the infectious agents which trigger self-directed immune response by their direct interaction with T lymphocytes. Subsequent release of inflammatory mediators target small and medium sized arteries.

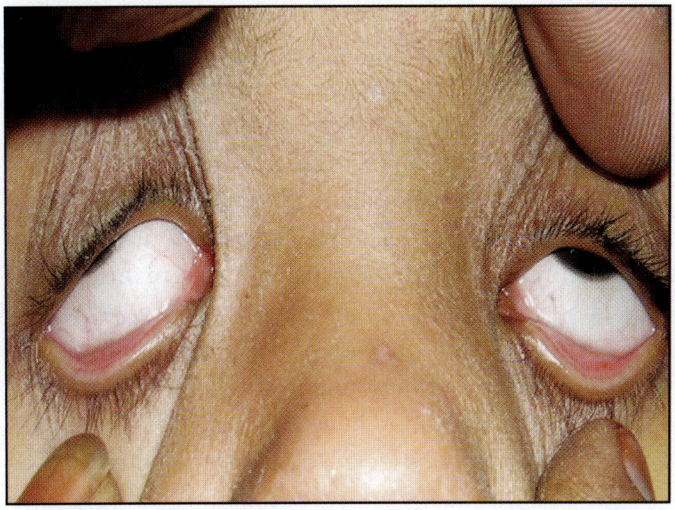

FIGURE 6.19B: Bilateral, non-exudative conjunctivitis in Kawasaki disease

Clinical Features

Acute onset of high-grade persistent fever unresponsive to antibiotic and antipyretic therapy in an irritable child should alert a clinician to look for a possibility of KD. Three distinct phases in clinical setting have been described.

1. *Acute febrile phase*: (1-11 days): It is characterized by high-grade fever (102-104°F), highly irritable child, bilateral conjunctivitis and rashes. Lips become erythematous and fissured and may bleed. Oral mucosa and tongue is swollen and erythematous with prominent papillae ("*strawberry tongue*") **(Figure 6.19A)**. Conjunctivitis is typically bilateral, bulbar and non-purulent **(Figure 6.19B)**. Hands and feet show edema and erythema, which might be painful. Polymorphic non-vesicular rash may affect trunk, extremities and face. These include non-specific diffuse erythematous maculo-papular, scarlatiniform and erythema-multiforme-like eruptions. Groin or perineal erythema and/ or desquamation and fine pustules over extensor surfaces of extremities have also been reported. Inflammation at the site of BCG vaccination is occasionally seen. Incidence of rashes noted in one Indian study was 62%. Tender lymphadenitis of cervical and less commonly of axillary and inguinal groups is often noticed. Tender, non-purulent cervical lymphadenopathy of >1.5 cm is said to be significant. Hepatic dysfunction, myocarditis and pericarditis may occur in this phase. Neck stiffness in irritable children may suggest aseptic meningitis. Acute phase reactants such as ESR, C-reactive proteins and alpha1 antitrypsin levels are high.
2. *Subacute phase*: (11-21 days): It is characterized by persistent irritability, anorexia and conjunctivitis. Fever gradually resolves (If not, may suggest a

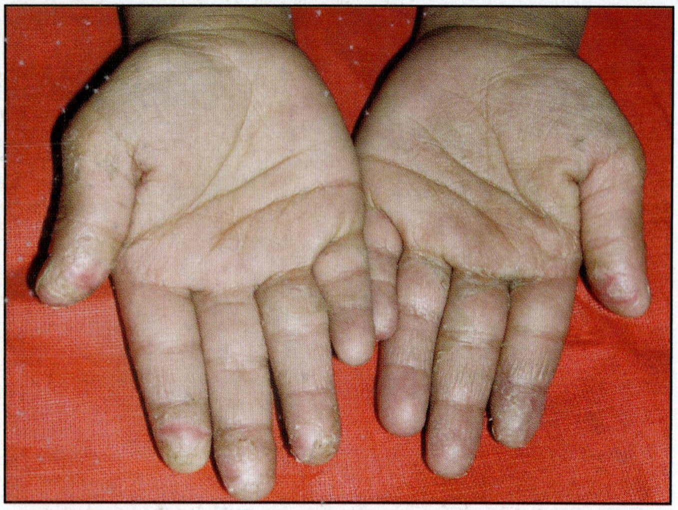

FIGURE 6.19C: Distal palmar desquamation in kawasaki disease after 8 days of illness

possibility of increased risk of cardiac complications). Thrombocytosis ensues and the platelet counts are quite high and may exceed 1 million/mm^3. Desquamation of finger and toe tips begin as the edema and erythema resolves **(Figure 6.19C)**. Beau's lines on nails may appear. Other unusual features include urethritis, arthritis or arthralgia, abdominal pain, vomiting/diarrhea, sterile pyuria, testicular swelling, hepatitis, and gallbladder distention. Coronary aneurysms may occur at this stage and child may have a risk of sudden death.

3. *Convalescent phase*: (21-60 days): All physical signs of the disease start receding and acute phase reactants begin to normalize. Coronary artery aneurysm may be recognized at this stage.

After 60 days, the child enters chronic phase of disease. It is of importance for those who demonstrated cardiac complications. The coronary dilatation or aneurysm persists indefinitely and may have risk of rupture in adulthood. Hence, a regular follow up is must in such patients.

Laboratory Investigations

These often reveal mild to moderate normochromic anemia, leucocytosis with increased band cell count, and increase in acute phase reactants such as ESR, CRP and alpha1-anti-trypsin. Blood cultures are usually negative. Platelet counts are remarkably raised in the subacute phase and may reach enormous values as high as 2 millions/mm^3. Echocardiogram is must to demonstrate the coronary aneurysm. It is ideally done on first visit, at 1-3 weeks and one month, and then every year thereafter. ECG may show conduction abnormalities and rarely myocardial infarction. Chest radiograph may detect pericardial effusion and congestive cardiac failure. Ultrasound of abdomen may show dilated gall bladder. Multislice spiral computed tomography is highly sensitive and specific for detecting coronary involvement. Electron beam computed tomography may detect coronary calcifications and may suggest necessity for vigilance for future cardiac events.

Diagnosis

There is no single diagnostic laboratory test for KD. Hence, the diagnosis is essentially clinical. Diagnostic criteria for KD put forth by American heart association are as follows:

1. High-grade, persistent fever unresponsive to antibiotics >5 days
2. Bilateral non-purulent *conjunctivitis*
3. One or more of *mucous membrane changes*: Diffuse injection of oral and pharyngeal mucosa, erythema or fissuring of the lips, strawberry tongue
4. Acute non-purulent cervical *lymphadenopathy* (>1.5 cm in atleast one node)
5. Polymorphic non-vesicular *rashes*
6. One or more of the *extremity changes*: Erythema of palms and/or soles, indurative edema of hands and/or feet, membranous desquamation of the fingertips:

   (Criterion 1 plus any 4 of 2-6, after exclusion of alternative clinical diagnosis, is diagnostic of KD.)

Incomplete or atypical cases often occur. In such situation, usually in children younger than 6 months of age, fever plus only 3 features establishes the diagnosis. Indian workers feel that KD is grossly under-diagnosed in this subcontinent and high index of suspicion is necessary for early accurate diagnosis.

KD must be differentiated from other diseases including staphylococcal scalded skin syndrome, Stevens-Johnson syndrome and other drug eruptions, other viral exanthemas (measles, enterovirus, adenovirus and EBV), toxic shock syndrome, spotted fevers, Weils' disease (leptospirosis), Still's rheumatoid arthritis and scarlet fever.

Course, Complications and Prognosis

KD is a self-limiting disease and completely resolves within 2-6 weeks. A major concern with a clinical diagnosis of KD is its ability to cause coronary aneurysm which occurs in 20-25% patients. Other cardiac complications include myocarditis, pericardial effusion, myocardial infarction, mitral valvulitis and hemopericardium. The overall mortality is 3%. Non-cardiac complications include arthritis, aseptic meningitis, pneumonitis, nephritis and peripheral gangrene. Long term follow up of the coronary arterial lesion is mandatory.

Treatment

Hospitalization is necessary. Principle of therapy is to prevent cardiac disease and provide symptomatic relief. In addition to supportive and symptomatic therapy, a full dose of intravenous gamma globulin (IVIG) at 2 g/kg is the mainstay of treatment. It is to be administered within 10 days of illness and intravenous infusion should be given slowly over 10-12 hours. Aspirin should be added to the therapy in the doses of 80-100 mg/kg/day until 36-hrs of disappearance of fever, followed by 3-5 mg/kg/day until the platelet count and ESR returns to normal or longer in the children with coronary lesion. IVIG and aspirin not only provide significant symptomatic relief to the patients but also reduces morbidity and mortality by preventing cardiac complications. Corticosteroids may be used judiciously in those who fail to respond to IVIG therapy. Thrombolytic therapy with streptokinase may be required in some patients.

Echocardiography and subsequent treatment should not be delayed in those who fail to satisfy the diagnostic criteria due to incomplete presentation, wherein there is no alternative diagnosis.

Referral to pediatric cardiologist is sought once the coronary involvement is confirmed. Cardiac catheterization, coronary artery bypass grafting and cardiac transplantation by expert pediatric cardiologist and cardiac surgeon are rarely required in certain patients.

Anticoagulation therapy with heparin or warfarin may be needed in giant coronary aneurysms (internal diameter >8 mm) with low dose aspirin. Pentoxyphylline used as an adjunct to IVIG and aspirin therapy may reduce the incidence of aneurysms. Infliximab or abciximab, cyclophosphamide, ulinastatin and plasma exchange are reserved for refractory KS.

PAPULAR PURPURIC GLOVES AND SOCKS SYNDROME (PPGSS)

Salient features:

- Sharply demarcated edema and erythema of hands and feet.
- Spontaneously resolves with exfoliation.
- Close etiological association with parvovirus B19 in many cases.
- The rash entails infectivity.
- PPGSS may be a presenting sign of HIV disease.

Historical Aspects

Halms in 1990 reported the eruption. Bagot and Ravuz in 1991 reported serological association with Parvovirus B19. This was later confirmed by Halasz et al in 1992 and Smith et al in 1997.

Etiology

At least 50% cases are caused by Parvovirus B19. Other viral association of this peculiar rash includes EBV, CMV, HHV6, HHV7, Coxsackie B6, Measles, Rubella and hepatitis B. Parvovirus B19, detected by PCR, is the only virus consistently found to be present in peripheral blood and skin biopsy specimens. A rare case caused by co-trimoxazole has been reported from Germany with classical finding of PPGSS. It has been proposed that PPGSS is a manifestation of underlying immunological mechanism induced by virus or drug antigens. The rash of PPGSS may be a presenting sign of HIV infection.

Epidemiology

PPGSS is a disease of young adults, though younger and older age groups are reported. There is seasonal propensity for spring and summer. The incubation period is about 10 days.

Clinical Features

The disease begins as asymptomatic eruption as edema and erythema of hands and feet, which soon turns out to be purpuric. There is sharp demarcation at the wrist and ankles signifying the term, "purpuric socks and gloves" **(Figures 6.20A and B)**. There may be a short prodrome of fever and fatigue. Aphthous like oral ulcerations may be present in some cases. The rash may be followed by arthralgia, myalgia, lymphadenopathy, fatigue or anorexia. The patient is clinically non-toxic. Rarely, the rash may be painful or pruritic. The condition usually resolves spontaneously within one to two weeks.

Atypical manifestation as reported in isolated cases include dysuria, vulvar erythema and edema with unilateral breast petechiae; multiple hemorrhagic bullae; resolution of purpuric lesions with superficial necrosis;

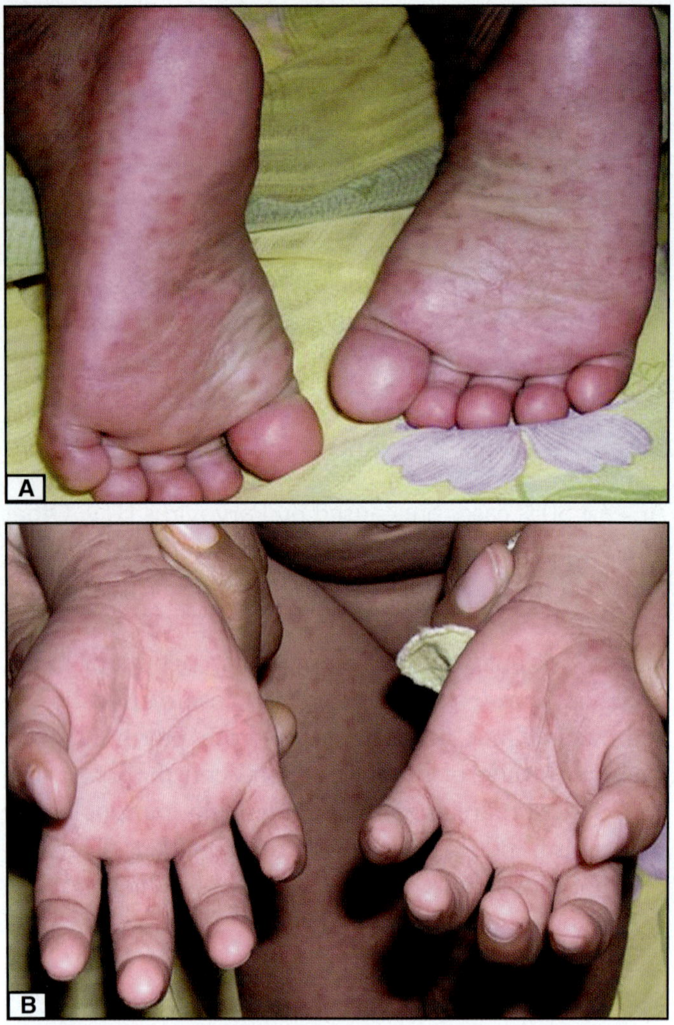

FIGURES 6.20A AND B: Papular and purpuric eruptions on palms and soles, abruptly stopping around wrists and ankles of a child with viral fever suggestive of 'papular purpuric gloves and socks syndrome'

and petechiae on palate, uvula, tongue or mucosa of lips.

The rash, in contrast with EI, is infectious as it heralds the onset of viremia. Therefore, systematic contact tracing of patients should be done especially those with evidence of parvovirus B19 infection, pregnancy, hemolytic anemia and immunosuppression.

Diagnosis

PPGSS is diagnosed clinically. Histopathological findings are non-specific. Interface dermatitis, vacuolar degeneration at the dermoepidermal junction, and a superficial perivascular lymphocytic infiltrate with occasional exocytosis has been reported.

Antibodies against parvovirus B19 were found by intracytoplasmic staining of dermal endothelial cells, keratinocytes and sweat glands. Parvovirus B19 DNA was also detectable in lesional biopsy specimens by PCR. In one reported case, PPGSS was seen concomitantly with EI in a patient with parvovirus B19 infection.

Course, Prognosis and Complications

The disease is self-resolving and the treatment is usually symptomatic with topical emollients and occasionally, systemic antihistamines.

ACKNOWLEDGMENTS

The author thanks *Cutis*® 2001; 68: 207-213. ©2001, Quadrant HealthCom Inc. for the kind permission to reproduce the **Table 6.7**, diagnostic criteria of Gianotti-Crosti syndrome.

Dr Antonio Chuh, Asso. Prof, Department of Medicine, University of Hong Kong is thankfully acknowledged for his guidance and literature support.

BIBLIOGRAPHY

1. Abzug MJ. Presentation, diagnosis, and management of enterovirus infections in neonates. Paediatr Drugs 2004; 6: 1-10.
2. Alfadley A, Aljubran A, Hainau B, Alhokail A. Papular-purpuric "gloves and socks" syndrome in a mother and daughter. J Am Acad Dermatol 2003; 48: 941-4.
3. Allen AL, Siegfried EC. What's new in Humanpapilloma virus infection. Curr opin Paediatr 2000; 12:365-9.
4. Bacelieri R, Johnson SM. Cutaneous warts:an evidence based approach to therapy. Am Fam Physician 2005;72:647-52.
5. Boer A, Herder N, Blodorn-Schlicht N, et al. Refining criteria for dignosis of cutaneous infections caused by herpes viruses through correlation of morphology with molecular pathology. Ind J Dermatol Venereol Leprol 2006;72(4): 270-5.
6. Brandt O, Abeck D, Gianotti R, Burgdorf W. Gianotti-Crosti Syndrome. J Am Acad Dermatol 2006;54:136-45.
7. Brice S. Viral diseases of skin. In: Rakel RE, Bope Et (Eds): Conn's Current therapy, 57th ed, Philadelphia. WB Saunders 2005;947-53.
8. Brown TJ, McCray M, Tyring SK. Antiviral agents:nonantiviral drugs. J Am Acad Dermatol 2002; 47:581-99.
9. Burns JC, Kushner HI, Bastian JF, Shike H, Shimizu C, Matsubara T, Turner CL. Kawasaki disease: a brief history. Pediatrics. 2000;206: E27.
10. Calza A, Saurat J. Eruptive pseudoangiomatosis: A unique childhood exanthem? J Am Acad Dermatol 1994; 31(3): 517- 8.
11. Chong CY, Chan KP, Shah VA, Ng WY, Lau G, Teo TE, Lai SH, Ling AE. Hand, foot and mouth disease in Singapore: a comparison of fatal and non-fatal cases. Acta Paediatr 2003; 92: 1163-9.
12. Chuh A, Lee A, Zawar V. The diagnostic criteria of Gianotti-Crosti syndrome: are they applicable to children in India? Pediatr Dermatol 2004;21:542-7

13. Chuh A. Pediatric viral exanthems: In Year Book of Dermatology and dermatologic Surgery 2005: Mosby publication.
14. Cohen JI, Brunnel PA, Strauss SE, Krause PR. Recent advances in varicella-zoster infection. Am Intern Med 1999; 130:920-32.
15. DeHoratius DM. Herpes zoster and varicella. In: Arndt KA, Hsu JTS, editors. Manual of dermatologic Therapeutics, Seventh edition, Philadelphia, Lippincott Williams and Wilkins 2007:103-10.
16. DeHoratius DM. Herpes zoster and varicella. In: Arndt KA, Hsu JTS, editors. Manual of Dermatologic Therapeutics, seventh edition. Philadelphia: Lippincott Williams and Wilkins 2007;102-10.
17. Diven DG. An overview of Pox viruses. J Am Acad Dermatol 2001; 44:1-14.
18. Drago F, Rebora A. The new herpes viruses. Arch Dermatol 1999;135:71-75.
19. English R. Varicella. Paediatric Rev 2003;24:372-9.
20. Frieden, I. Childhood exanthems. Curr Opin in Pediatr 1995; 7:411-4.
21. Grann JW, Whitleg RJ. Herpes zoster. N Eng J Med 2002; 347:340-6.
22. Ikediobi NI, Tyring SK. Cutaneous manifestations of Epstein-Barr virus infection. Dermatol Clin 2002; 20: 283-9.
23. Jobenputra KS, Rajpal AV, Nagpur NG. Imiquimod. Ind J Dermatol Venereol Leprol 2006;72(6):466-9.
24. Kakourou T, Theodoridou M, Mostrous G, et al. Herpes zoster in children. J Am Acad Dermatol 1998; 39:207-10.
25. Katta R. Parvovirus B19: A review: Dermatol Clin 2002:20(2): 333-42.
26. Krishnakumar P, Mathews L. Kawasaki disease is not rare in India. Ind J Ped 2006;73:544-5.
27. Mallory SB, Bree A, Chorn P. Molluscum contagiosum. In: Illustrated manual of Pediatric dermatology. First edition. UK. Taylor and Francis 2006;137-8.
28. Michael DJ. Acute hemorrhagic edema of infancy. Dermatol Online J 2006; 12(5):10.
29. Chan PKS, To KF, Zawar V, Lee A, Chuh AAT. Asymmetric periflexural exanthem in an adult. Clinical and Experimental Dermatology 2004; 29: 311–24.
30. Palit A, Inamdar A. An approach to vasculitis. Ind J Dermatol Venereal Leprol 2006;72:334-45.
31. Reed BR. Warts and molluscum contagiosum. In: Fitzpatrick JE, Morelli JG, editors. Dermatology Secrets in Color, 3rd ed, Philadelphia, Mosby 2007;213-8.
32. Renn CN, Straff W, Dorfmuller A, Al-Masaoudi T, Merk HF, Sachs B. Amoxicillin-induced exanthema in young adults with infectious mononucleosis: demonstration of drug-specific lymphocyte reactivity. Br J Dermatol 2002;147:1166-70.
33. Resnick SD. New aspects of exanthematous diseases of childhood. Dermatologic Clinics 1997;15(2):257-66.
34. Silverberg NB, Sidburg R, Mancini AJ. Childhood molluscum contagiosum:experience with cantharidin therapy in 300 patients. J Am Acad Dermatol 2000; 16:395-7.
35. Silverberg NB. Paediatric molluscum contagiosum:optimal treatment strategies. Paediatric Drugs 2003; 5:505-12.
36. Smolinski KN, Yan AC. How and when to treat molluscum contagiosum and warts in children. Paediatr Ann 2005; 34: 211-21.
37. Sterling JC. Human papilloma virus and skin cancer. J Clin Virology 2005; 32:67-71.
38. Stoeckle M. The spectrum of human herpesvirus 6 infection: from roseola infantum to adult disease. Annu Rev Med 2000; 51:423-30.
39. Thomas SL, Hall AJ. What does epidemiology tells us about risk factors for herpes zoster? Lancet Infect Dis 2004; 4:26-33.
40. Torrelo A. What's new in the treatment of viral warts in children. Paediatric Dermatol 2002;19:191-9.
41. Vazquez M, La Russa PS, Gershon AA et al. Effectiveness over time of varicella vaccine. JAMA 2004; 291:851-5.
42. Wassoner-Fountain LA, Grossman LB. Herpes simplex virus. Paediatr Rev 2004; 25:86-93.
43. Wollenberg A, Zoch C, Wetzel S, et al. Predisposing factors and clinical features of eczema herpeticum: a retrospective analysis of 100 cases. J Am Acad Dermatol 2003; 49:198-205.
44. Zawar V, Chuh A. Gianotti-Crosti syndrome in India is not associated with hepatitis B infection. Dermatology 2004; 208:87.

7

Fungal Infections

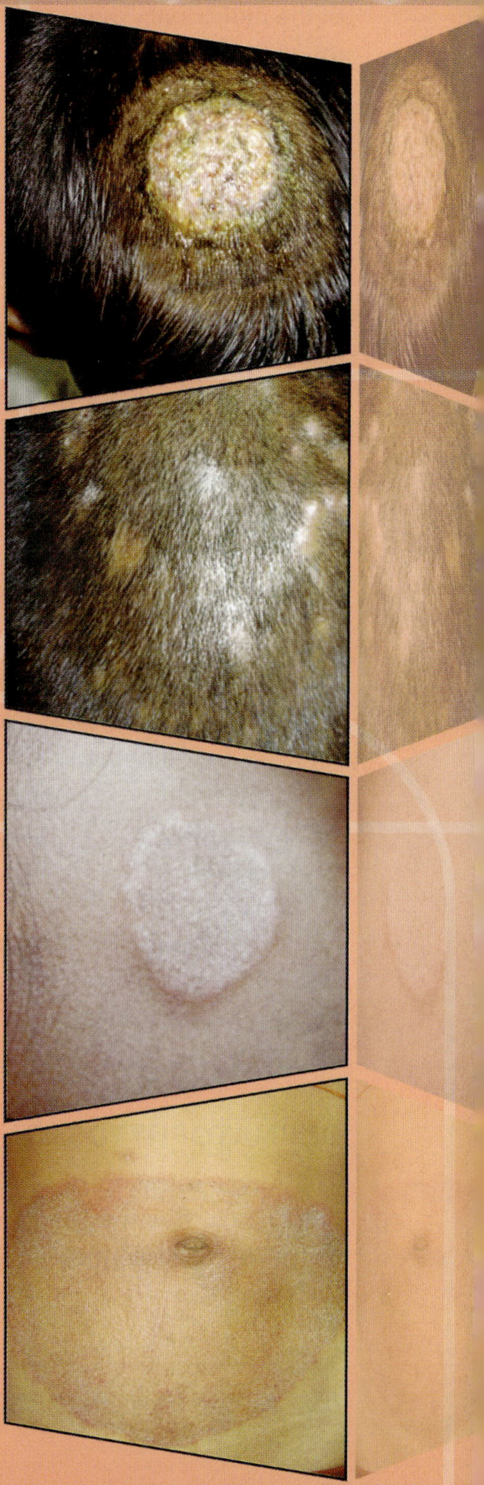

Ragunatha S, Anitha B

INTRODUCTION

Fungal infection of skin is one of the commonest dermatological conditions encountered in the dermatology clinic. The prevalence of the infection depends on the age, geographic area of residence and immunological status of the individual. The manifestations of fungal infections range from simple superficial mycoses to life-threatening disseminated or system infections. Certain fungal infections are more common in children and adolescents, though they are susceptible to develop any type of fungal infections. Fungal infections are broadly divided into two types, superficial and deep.

SUPERFICIAL FUNGAL INFECTIONS

Superficial fungal infections include superficial mycoses, dermatophytoses and candidal infections. The fungi causing these infections either thrive on the surface or invade keratinous tissue.

SUPERFICIAL MYCOSES

The fungi causing superficial mycoses do not invade deeper than superficial layers of skin (stratum corneum) or hair shaft. Therefore, these fungi do not elicit any significant inflammatory response. The diseases in this category include tinea nigra, piedras and pityriasis versicolor **(Table 7.1)**. These disorders are commonly seen in adults but can occur in children and adolescents. Some of these fungi may cause systemic infections in immunocompromised patients. M. furfur can cause systemic infection in neonates receiving intravenous lipids through a central arterial or venous catheter, though these are not necessary prerequisites for fungemia.

DERMATOPHYTOSES

The fungal infection of keratinous tissues such as skin, hair and nail is termed as dermatophytosis. The causative fungi are called dermatophytes.

Etiology

These are closely related genera of fungi that are capable of invading keratinous tissues of humans and lower animals.

Taxonomy and nomenclature: All fungi are unicellular or multicellular eukaryotic cells containing chitin and/ or cellulose in their cell walls. They generally exist as either molds or yeasts. Molds are made up of filaments (hyphae) that intertwine to form a mat-like structure called mycelium. Hyphae are further characterized by the presence or absence of cross walls as septate and aseptate hyphae, respectively. The colonies of molds typically appear as "fuzzy" or "moldy". The yeasts are unicellular that reproduce by budding. If the daughter cells do not separate from mother cell, they appear as chain of sausages, called pseudohyphae. The colonies of yeasts are pasty or mucoid. Some fungi exist as both yeasts and molds, and they are called, dimorphic fungi.

There are three anamorphs (asexual/ imperfect state) of genera, epidermophyton, microsorum and trichophyton that cause dermatophytoses. These belong to the family Arthrodermataceae of the order Onygenales. The dermatophytes capable of producing sexually (telomorphs/ perfect/ sexual state) are considered in the genus Arthroderma of the family Arthrodermataceae. Previously, the asexual states were grouped under Deuteromycota or Fungi imperfecti.

Ecology: Based on the host preference and natural habitat, the dermatophytes are grouped into three classes, geophilic, zoophilic and anthrophophilic **(Table 7.2)**. Infections caused by geophilic and zoophilic dermatophytes are usually inflammatory and show good response to treatment, whereas those caused by anthrophophilic dermatophytes are usually non inflammatory, chronic, and recurrent.

Epidemiology

The epidemiology of dermatophytoses differs in adults and children. Tinea pedis and tinea unguium are rare in children. Conversely, tinea capitis caused by both zoophilic and anthrophophilic dermatophytes is common in children. The tinea capitis is five times more likely to affect boys than girls.

The causative fungus of tinea capitis differs from one geographical region to another and also over a period of time in any geographical region. *M. canis* was the commonest cause of tinea capitis in Europe, Middle East, and some USA and Latin American cities. Now, *T. tonsurans* in USA, *T. soudanense* and *M. audouinii* in Africa, and *T. violaceum* in North Africa, Middle East and India, are the commonly isolated causative agents of tinea capitis.

TABLE 7.1: Superficial mycoses

Characteristics	Pityriasis versicolor	Tinea nigra	White piedra	Black piedra
Etiology	*M. furfur*	*P. wernickii*	*T. beigelii*	*Piedraia hortai*
Epidemiology	Humid and tropical climate	Coastal and marine climate	Temperate and subtropical climate	Tropical climate
Sites involved	Seborrheic areas	Palms and soles	Hairs on scalp, eyebrows, eyelashes, beard, axilla or pubic region	Hairs on scalp, eyebrows, eyelashes, beard, axilla or pubic region
Clinical features	Well demarcated hypopigmented or hyperpigmented macules and patches which show scales on scratching (scratch sign/ coup' de onglee)	Mottled brown to black, asymptomatic macule on the palm. It may spread with darker advancing border	Small, soft, white to cream colored nodules encircling the affected terminal hair. Nodules can be easily pulled off the shaft	Small, hard, dark colored nodules firmly adherent along the hair shaft
Differential diagnosis	Vitiligo, pityriasis alba, pityriasis rosea, erythrasma	Contact dermatitis, exogenous pigmentation, acral lentigenous melanoma	Black piedra, pediculosis, trichomycosis axillaris, hair shaft defects, scales	Pediculosis, trichorrhexis nodosa, scales
KOH preparation	Spaghetti and meat ball appearance	Olive-brown, septate, branching hyphae and elongated budding cells	Septate hyphae perpendicular to hair shaft and penetrating between the cells of cuticle	Collection of asci, each containing 2-8 crescent shaped ascospores with peripheral darkly pigmented branching hyphae
Treatment	Topical imidazoles, selenium sulfide, Terbinafine	Topical imidazoles, keratolytics	Shaving of affected hairs and topical clotrimazole or amphotericin B lotion	Shaving of affected hairs and topical keratolytics

TABLE 7.2: Grouping of dermatophytes based on host preference and natural habitat

Dermatophytes	Epidermophyton (E)	Microsporum (M)	Trichophyton (T)
Geophilic (soil)	None	*M. gypseum* *M. flavum*	None
Zoophilic (animals)	None	*M. canis* *M. equinum*	*T. verrucosum* *T. mentagrophytes var. mentagrophytes*
Anthrophophilic (human)	*E. floccosum*	*M. audouinii* *M. ferrugineum*	*T. rubrum* *T. tonsurans* *T. violaceum* *T. schoenleinii* *T. concentricum* *T. mentagrophytes var. interdigitale*

Pathogenesis

The epidemiological difference in incidence of cutaneous fungal infections in adults and children are in part due to rates of exposure and also expression of host immune response. Certain mechanisms that inhibit fungal growth such as increased proliferation of epidermal cells in response to injury to stratum corneum and reversible binding by unsaturated transferrin present in sweat and serum are not known to be affected by age. However, the composition of sebum, containing medium chain free fatty acids (FFAs) that inhibit growth of dermatophytes and promote the growth of pityrosporum yeasts, changes at puberty. The predominance of these FFAs in postpubertal sebum is responsible for rarity of tinea capitis and increased pityrosporum infections in this age group. FFAs cause direct inhibition of fungal growth and also interfere with adhesion of fungus to receptors on the keratinocytes.

Cell mediated immunity plays an important role in the pathogenesis of fungal infection. T_H1 arm of cell mediated immune response is protective against dermatophytic infections. The important steps in the pathogenesis of fungal infection include antigen reception by Langerhans' cells, activation of T-lymphocytes, production of chemotactic factors, accumulation of effector cells (neutrophils), and production of cytokines. This results in inflammation in the lesion ultimately eliminating the fungus.

Atopic individuals are susceptible to chronic dermatophytic infections due to overactivity of T_H2 lymphocytes.

Clinical Manifestations

The cutaneous infection caused by dermatophytes is commonly called as tinea infection. There are several types of tinea infections depending upon the site of involvement. The morphology of the lesions, causative agent, predisposing factors and response to treatment vary in different types of tinea infections.

Tinea capitis: Tinea capitis is the dermatophytic infection of skin and hairs of the scalp. The disease is common in children but may rarely affect infants and adults. The boys are more likely to be affected than girls. There are three microscopic types of tinea capitis, endothrix, ectothrix and favus. These types indicate the pattern of invasion into hair shaft. In endothrix the fungal hyphae segment into spores (arthroconidia) inside the hair shaft and there is no destruction of cuticle. In ectothrix the fungal hyphae segment into spores outside the hair shaft. In favus the fungal hyphae remain intact inside the hair shaft rarely showing spores.

The invasion of hair shaft occurs through stratum corneum. The dermatophytes grow downwards till the junction of nucleated cells and keratinized cells. The fungi never invade beyond nucleated cells and form a tuft of hyphae at this junction referred as Adamson's fringe. The fungus grows downwards at the same rate as the hair grows out. Therefore, hyphae are not usually found above the level of skin. The growth of fungus occurs only in anagen hairs. Once the hair enters telogen phase the growth of fungus stops. The fungal growth renders hair shaft weak and hair breakage occurs at the level of scalp.

Tinea capitis is caused by various microsporum and trichophyton species. Single fungus can produce more than one clinical type of tinea capitis **(Table 7.3)**.

Clinically there are two types of tinea capitis, inflammatory and non inflammatory. The former is commonly caused by geophilic or zoophilic fungi and the latter by anthrophophilic fungi.

1. Non inflammatory type (Figures 7.1 to 7.4)

There are several forms of non inflammatory tinea capitis. These include gray patch, seborrheic dermatitis like and black dot type. The gray patch type presents as hyperkeratotic scaly, well demarcated area of hair loss and hairs in the region appear gray and lusterless. Seborrheic dermatitis-like tinea capitis is characterized by diffuse scaling without noticeable hair loss. Black dot type presents as ill-defined area of alopecia consisting of multiple black dots resulting from break down of weakened hairs at the level of scalp.

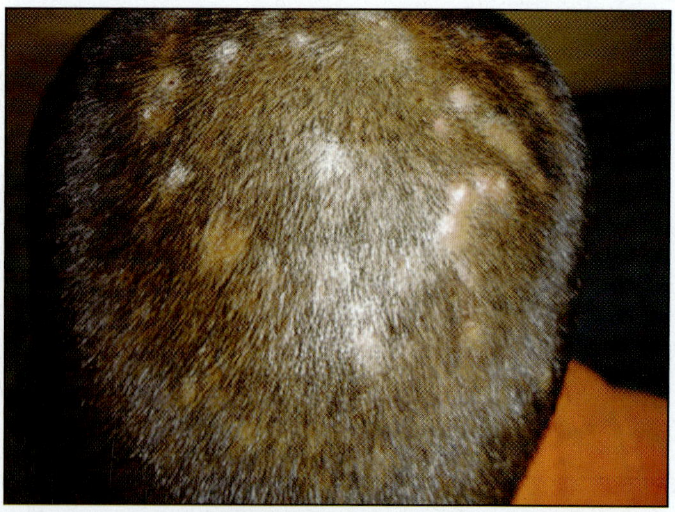

FIGURE 7.1: Tinea capitis

TABLE 7.3: Microscopic and clinical characteristics of dermatophytes causing tinea capitis

Species	Group	Microscopy	Clinical type	Wood's lamp
M. audouinii	Anthrophophilic	Ectothrix	Inflammatory, non inflammatory	Green
M. canis	Zoophilic	Ectothrix	Inflammatory, non inflammatory	Green
M. ferrugineum	Anthrophophilic	Ectothrix	Non inflammatory	Green
M. distortum	Zoophilic	Ectothrix	Inflammatory	Green
M. gypseum	Geophilic	Ectothrix	Inflammatory	No fluorescence
M. fulvum	Geophilic	Ectothrix	Inflammatory	No fluorescence
T. tonsurans	Anthrophophilic	Endothrix	Except favus	No fluorescence
T. violaceum	Anthrophophilic	Endothrix	Black dot	No fluorescence
T. verrucosum	Zoophilic	Ectothrix	Inflammatory	No fluorescence
T. mentagrophyte	Zoophilic	Ectothrix	Inflammatory	No fluorescence
T. gouvilii	Anthrophophilic	Endothrix	Non inflammatory	No fluorescence
T. rubrum	Anthrophophilic	Ectothrix	Non inflammatory	No fluorescence
T. schoenleinii	Anthrophophilic	Favus	Favus	Dull fluorescence

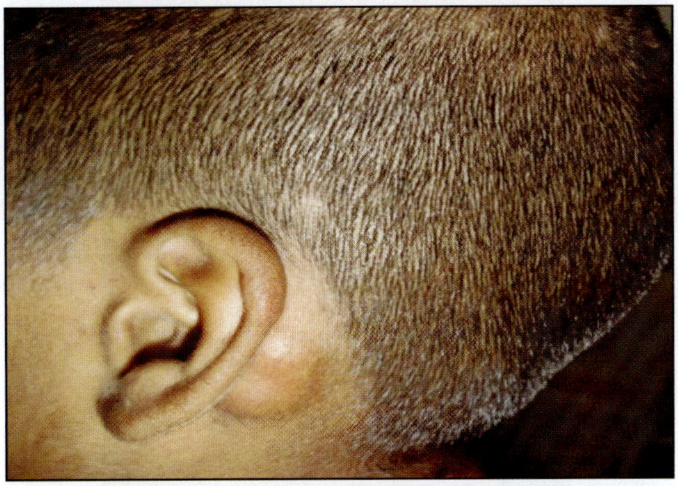

FIGURE 7.2: Tinea capitis with post-auricular lymphadenopathy

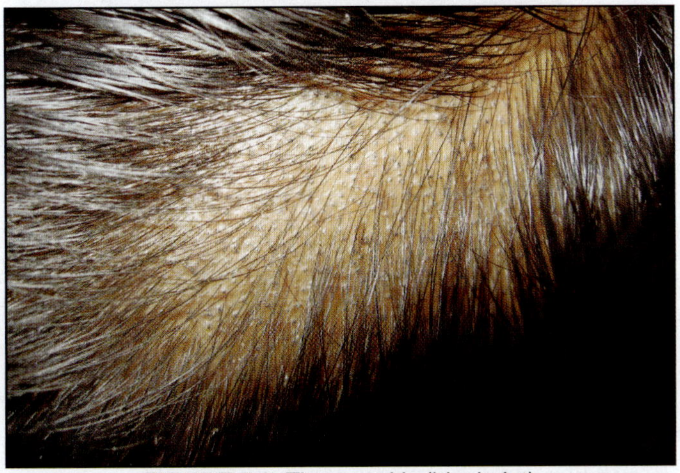

FIGURE 7.3: Tinea capitis (black dot)

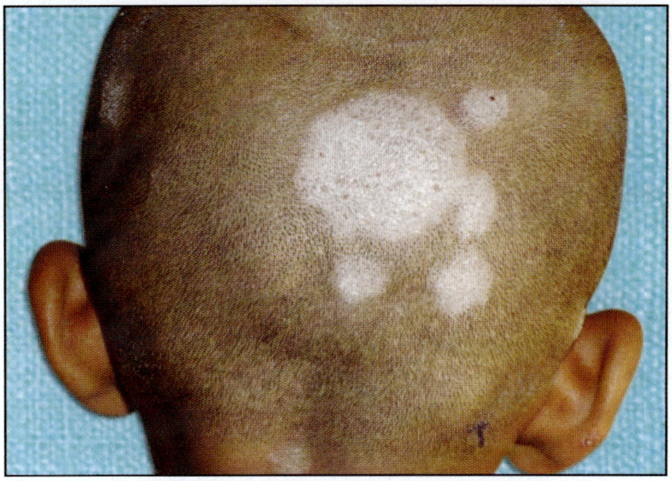

FIGURE 7.4: Tinea capitis (gray patch)

Similarly beard area can also be involved resulting in tinea barbae. The disease is common in adolescents and adults. The inflammatory type is commonly caused by zoophilic fungi such as *T. mentagrophytes, T. verrucosum* and rarely *M. canis*. Superficial less inflammatory type is caused by anthrophophilic fungi *T. violaceum* and *T. rubrum*. These two types involve hair follicles resulting in follicular papules, pustules and kerion like lesions. Easy pluckability of hair and itching are characteristics of tinea barbae. The circinate type involves facial skin and spares hair follicle resembling tinea corporis.

2. Inflammatory type

The presentation of inflammatory tinea capitis ranges from pustular folliculitis to kerion. The latter is a morphologically

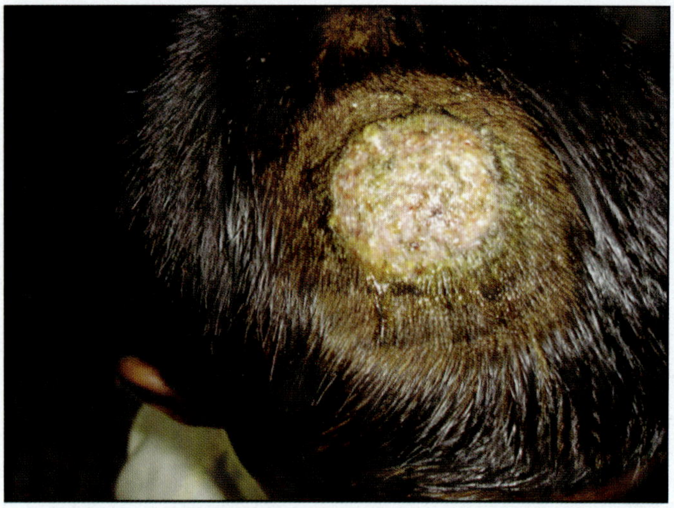

FIGURE 7.5: Tinea capitis (kerion)

distinct type presenting as boggy inflammatory swelling with multiple discharging follicular orifices **(Figure 7.5)**. The hairs are easily pluckable resulting in scarring alopecia. The lesions are associated with itching, pain and regional lymphadenopathy. Another inflammatory type is favus characterized by formation of cup shaped yellow crusts (scutula) involving multiple hairs. Sometimes it is accompanied by peculiar mousy odor.

Tinea corporis: Tinea corporis is one of the common dermatophytic infections in children. Non hairy areas (without terminal hairs) of the body are involved. The causative fungus in young children is *M. canis*. This is because of close contact with pets. *T. rubrum, T. mentagrophytes, T. verrucosum, T. tonsurans* and *E. floccosum* are common in older children. The parents with tinea pedis and tinea unguium may act as source of infection. The predisposing factors include warm humid climate, and diabetes, leukemia or immunodeficiency. Clinically tinea corporis is characterized by one or two erythematous annular plaques with peripheral scales. The margins may be vesicular, papular or pustular **(Figures 7.6A and B)**. The lesions may coalesce to form polycyclic border. Similar lesions can occur on the face resulting in tinea faciei **(Figure 7.7)**.

The common differential diagnoses are herald patch of pityriasis rosea, seborrheic dermatitis, psoriasis, nummular eczema, and annular erythemas.

Tinea imbricata: Tinea imbricata is a distinct disorder predisposing the individual to superficial fungal infection caused by *Trichophyton* concentricum. The disease is common in tropical regions of Far East, South Pacific,

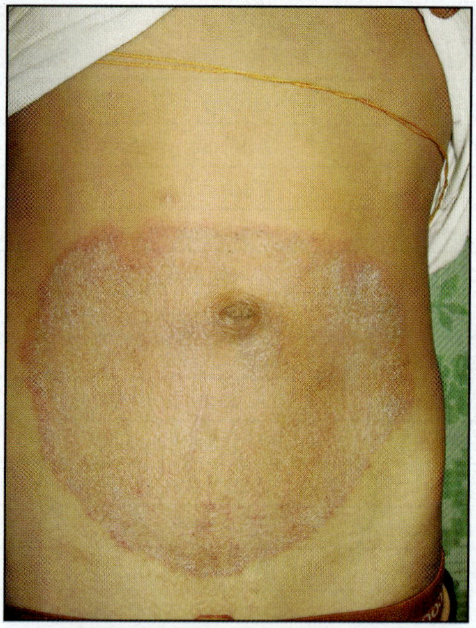

FIGURE 7.6A: Tinea corporis

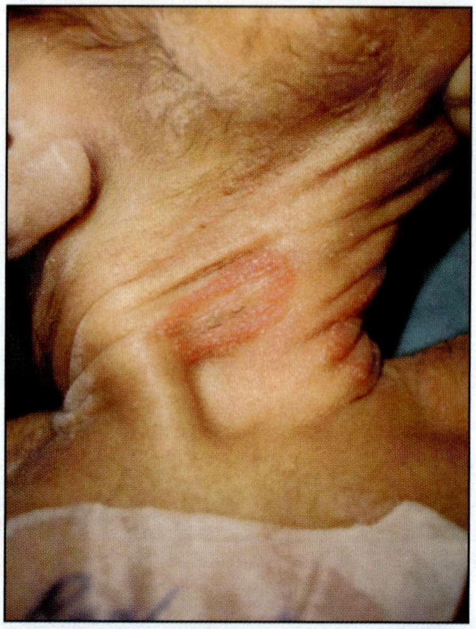

FIGURE 7.6B: Tinea corporis in a neonate

South and Central America and some parts of Africa. The infection is often life-long involving the skin or nails but not hair. The characteristic clinical manifestation is concentric rings of scaling with polycyclic border. The lesions may be extensive involving entire skin sparing scalp, axillae, palms and soles. The fully developed lesion shows parallel lines of scales overlapping each other resembling roof tiles.

Tinea cruris (Figure 7.8): Tinea cruris is common in adolescents and adults, and rare in children. *E. floccosum, T. rubrum* and *T. mentagrophyte* are the common

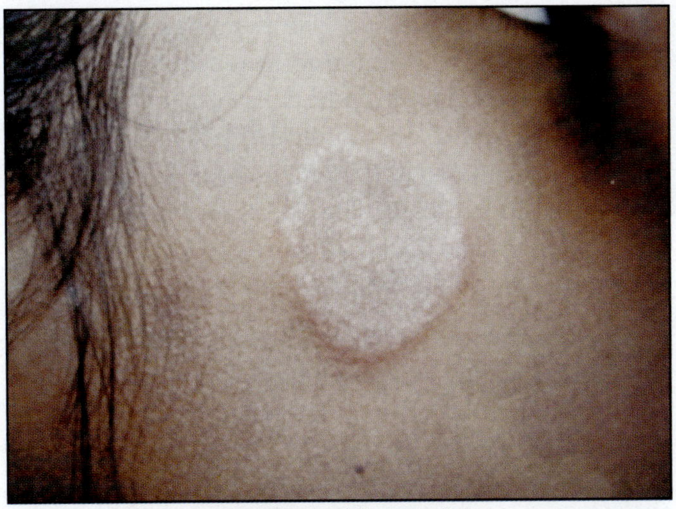

FIGURE 7.7: Tinea faciei

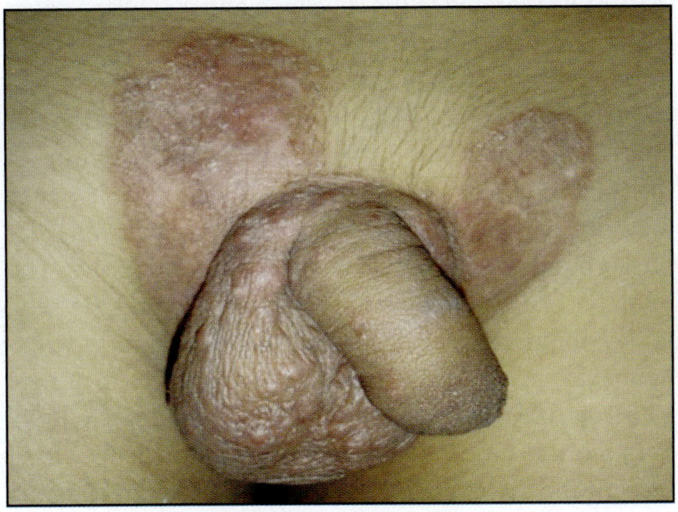

FIGURE 7.8: Tinea cruris

causative agents. The predisposing factors include hot humid climate, obesity, physical activities and tight-fitting clothes. The intertriginous folds and upper inner thighs are the commonest sites of involvement. Buttocks and perianal areas may be involved occasionally. Scrotum and penis are usually spared. Important differential diagnoses include erythrasma and candidal intertrigo. The former shows corel red fluorescence under Wood's lamp, and the latter shows satellite papules and pustules.

Tinea pedis: Tinea pedis is common in adolescents and adults, and rare in children. *T. tonsurans* infection is common in children, whereas *T. rubrum, T. mentagrophyte* or *E. floccosum* are common in adults. Three clinical types are recognized, intertriginous, vesicular and moccasin type. Intertriginous type is most common pattern characterized by erythema, maceration and scaling in the lateral toe web spaces. Vesicular type which is caused by *T. mentagrophyte* is characterized by vesicle and bullae with erythema. It is associated with vesicular id reaction involving hands, extremities and trunk. Moccasin type is characterized by diffuse erythema, scalling and hyperkeratosis of plantar surface.

The patients with tinea pedis are predisposed to cellulitis, secondary bacterial infections, id reaction and onychomycosis. Tinea pedis is usually misdiagnosed as psoriasis, juvenile plantar dermatosis, erythrasma and pompholyx.

Tinea mannum: Tinea mannum refers to dermatophytic infection of palms. The disease is common in post pubertal individuals. The causative fungi are similar to that of tinea pedis. Clinically it is characterized by hyperkeratosis of the palms, and occasionally there may be vesicular reaction or patchy erythema. Usually the involvement is unilateral which gives a clue to the diagnosis. There may be associated infection of soles. This pattern of infection is called as "Two foot one hand syndrome". The infection may extend to involve finger nails.

The differential diagnoses include psoriasis, contact dermatitis, pompholyx and id reaction.

Tinea unguium: The fungal infection of the nail caused by dermatophytes is called as tinea unguium. The disease is common in adults but can occur in children usually in association with tinea pedis or tinea mannum. The causative fungi are similar to that of tinea mannum or tinea pedis. The clinical manifestations are similar in both adults and children. The factors that are responsible for rarity of tinea unguium in children are, faster nail growth, smaller surface area of nails, and low rate of tinea pedis or tinea mannum.

The nail changes seen in tinea unguium like subungual hyperkeratosis, onycholysis and nail dystrophy should be differentiated from that of psoriasis, lichen planus, and pachyonychia congenita. Asymmetry of nail involvement and evidence of fungal infection elsewhere helps in the diagnosis of tinea unguium.

Tinea incognita and Majocchi's granuloma: The dermatophytic infection modified by the use of glucocorticoids is referred as tinea incognita. The annular pruritic papules with peripheral scaling and central clearing which are characteristics of dermatophytic infections are absent. The well demarcated border or reappearance of lesions after stopping the application of steroid preparations may aid in the diagnosis.

In Majocchi's granuloma, the fungus invades the hair follicle and enters dermis eliciting a suppurative granulomatous reaction. Trauma, friction, occlusive preparations or immunosuppression are responsible for the penetration of fungus beneath the epidermis. The disease presents as persistent follicular papules or pustules not responding to topical antifungal therapy. In such cases systemic antifungal therapy is effective.

Non-dermatophytic superficial fungal infections: Apart from dermatophytes some of the nondermatophytic molds such as Hendersonula toruloidea and Scytalidium hyalinum can also cause tinea pedis, tinea mannum and onychomycosis. The clinical features are identical to those caused by dermatophytes. However, in finger nail infection the disease starts in the lateral nail folds with associated paronychia. Onycholysis occurs without apparent thickening of nail plate. Absence of tinea infection elsewhere, failure to isolate dermatophytes, lack of response to antifungals, history of damage to nails or other nail diseases, and demonstration of septate, brown hyphae of various width aid in the diagnosis of infection. These infections are resistant to conventional antifungal therapy. Salicylic acid has been found to be effective.

Dermatophytids: Dermatophytid is a manifestation of delayed type hypersensitivity response to systemically absorbed fungal antigens. Immune reaction occurs at a site away from the primary dermatophytic infection. The reaction is usually noticed just after the initiation of systemic antifungal therapy, or during or following the peak of infection. The reaction presents as pruritic papulovesicles predominantly distributed on the trunk and extremities. On the palms and soles they mimic pompholyx. Rarely, it may present as erythema nodosum, erysipelas like lesions, erythema annular centrifugum or urticaria.

Diagnosis

The diagnostic methods include Wood's lamp examination, potassium hydroxide (KOH) preparation, and culture.

Wood's lamp: Wood's lamp examination is useful as a screening method in the diagnosis of tinea capitis. Certain dermatophytes especially those causing ectothrix infection fluoresce when exposed to ultraviolet rays (365-400 nm) filtered by Wood's filter (Barium silicate with 9% nickel oxide). Only fluorescence of hair, not the scales or skin, should be taken as positive. The examination should be conducted in the dark room to increase the efficacy of the test. Any topical preparations applied should be cleaned with wet swab to prevent flase positivity. The ectothrix infection caused by *M. audouinii* and *M. canis* show green fluorescence. The endothrix infection caused by *T. tonsurans* and *T. violaceum* show nonfluorescence. *T. schoenleinii* usually produces pale green fluorescence.

KOH preparation: KOH preparation of scales, hair and nail is used to demonstrate fungal hyphae and spores. The scales are collected by scrapping the periphery of skin lesions with blunt end of 15 no. scalpel blade. Moistening the lesion with wet swab helps to transfer the specimen easily on to the clean glass slide. A drop of 10-20% KOH is added to the specimen and carefully a cover slip is placed avoiding formation of air bubbles. The slide is then passed over the flame several times with due care to prevent boiling of KOH. The slide is examined under light microscope after 5-10 minutes. The condenser of the microscope is lowered and the light source is put to low intensity. This increases the contrast between the background and refractile fungal hyphae and spores. The addition of KOH, gentle heating, and keeping the slide for few minutes hasten the clearance of keratinocytes and epithelial debris which render clear visibility of fungal elements. If dimethyl sulfoxide (DMSO) is added to KOH then there is no need for heating the slide. DMSO itself hastens the dissolution of keratin and additional heating will dissolve fungi as well.

In case of tinea capitis, the hairs at the periphery of the lesion is cut and kept in the 10-20% KOH for 20-30 minutes. This allows complete dissolution of hard hair keratin. If hyphae and spores are present within the hairshaft, the diagnosis is endothrix **(Figure 7.9)**. If they are present outside, the diagnosis is ectothrix. In favus, air bubble like structures are seen inside the hairshaft along with hyphae.

In tinea unguium, subungual debris, nail clippings, or scrapings from the undersurface of nail plate are kept in KOH for 24 hours to dissolve the hard keratin of nail.

Under the light microscope the fungal hyphae appear as refractile, septate, and branching filaments with regular borders and uniform refractility **(Figure 7.10)**.

Calcofluor white, a fluorescent stain, which preferentially binds to cellulose and chitins present in the fungal cell wall can be used to demonstrate the fungal elements. The stain can be added to KOH preparation to increase

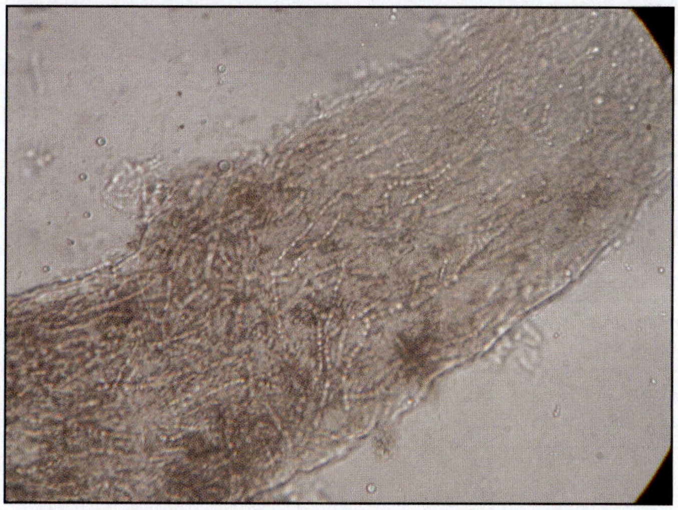

FIGURE 7.9: KOH preparation of hair showing endothrix infection

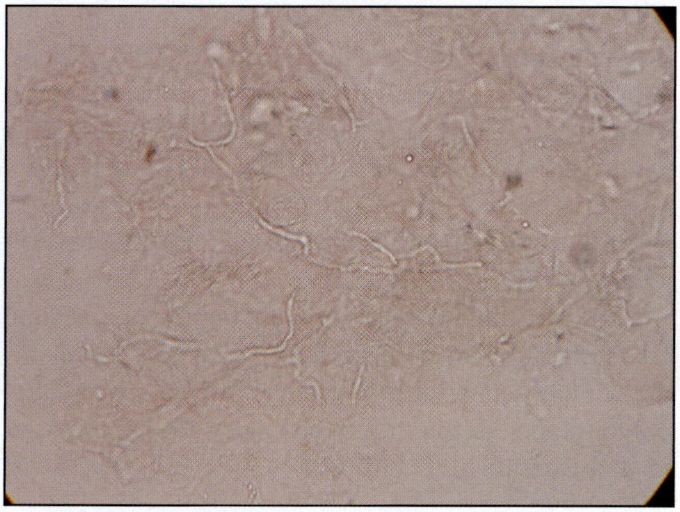

FIGURE 7.10: KOH preparation of skin scraping showing hyphae of dermatophytes

the sensitivity and specificity. When examined under fluorescent microscope the fungus appears as bright yellow-green element.

Culture methods

1. Isolation of dermatophytes

The culture media used for isolation of dermatophytes are Sabourauds Dextrose Agar (SDA) and Dermatophyte Test Medium (DTM). To inhibit bacterial growth cycloheximide is added to the former, and gentamicin and chloremphenicol is added to the latter. If non dermatophytic molds are suspected which are common in nail, palm and sole infection, cycloheximide- free medium should be used. The specimen (scales, nail clippings or hair) should be collected in a sterile Petri dish or paper cover to avoid growth of opportunistic fungi. The nail specimen should be taken from proximal part of the nail plate. The distal nail usually contains dead fungus which gives false negative result on culture.

In the DTM, color indicator is used for rapid detection (within 24-48 hours) of fungal growth. The medium turns yellow to red as a result of alkalinization caused by growth of the fungi. But DTM is not specific for dermatophytes as non dermatophytic molds and Coccidioides immitis also show positive reaction. M. canis shows false negative reaction.

Identification of Species

The colonial characteristics, microscopic morphology and certain physiological tests are employed for identification of the species of dermatophytes.

Microscopic morphology: The identification of cultured dermatophytes is based on the morphology and arrangement of conidia and hyphae **(Table 7.4)**. There are two types of conidia, microconidia and macroconidia. Apart from conidia, there are other structures such as reflexive branches, chlamydospores or nodal organs which may also help in the identification.

TABLE 7.4: Microscopic morphology of dermatophytes

Genera of dermatophytes	Microscopic morphology
Epidermophyton	Abundant broadly clavate, smooth-walled macroconidia borne singly or in cluster. Microconidia are absent
Microsporum	Spindle shaped or fusiform rough-walled macroconidia, usually numerous than microconidia which are clavate and arranged singly along the hyphae
Trichophyton	Clavate to cylindrical smooth-walled macroconidia which are often absent. Microconidia are numerous, pyriform to spherical usually arranged in clusters or singly along the hyphae

Physiologic tests for identification of dermatophytes: These tests are used to identify species of dermatophytes **(Table 7.5)**.

Treatment

Several topical and systemic antifungal agents are available for the treatment of dermatophytic infection. The choice

TABLE 7.5: Physiological tests to identify species of dermatophyte

Physiologic tests	Dermatophytes identified
In vitro hair perforation test	*M. canis, T. mentagrophytes*
Urea hydrolysis	*T. mentagrophytes, T. megninii*
Nutritional requirement using *Trichophyton* agars 1-7	Thiamine—*T. tonsurans, T. violaceum, T. verrucosum* Nicotinic acid—*T. equinum* Histidine—*T. megninii*
Growth on polished rice grains	*M. audouinii* grows poorly, resulting in brownish discoloration of rice grains
Temperature tolerance or enhancement	Growth at 37°C—*T. mentagrophytes* Stimulated growth at 37°C—*T. verrucosum*

of therapy depends on the causative agent, site of infection, extent of involvement and underlying systemic disease. The infection with anthrophophilic fungi, involvement of hair, nail, palms and soles, extensive involvement and underlying immunosuppression require systemic antifungal therapy.

Most of the topical antifungal agents that are effective against localized infection belong to imidazole group. These include clotrimazole, miconazole, ketoconazole, oxiconazole, sulconazole and econazole. Allylamines such as terbinafine and naftifine are effective when used for a short 5-15 day course. Other topical antifungals include ciclopirox (pyridoneethanolamine), tolnaftate, nystatin, and undecylenate.

Griseofulvin is a safe and effective oral antifungal agent against dermatophytes. The ultramicronized form is available with better absorption. It is used in the dosage of 7.5-10 mg/kg per day. In tinea capitis the dosage is 20 mg/kg per day which may be increased to 25 mg/kg per day if there is no response after 2-3 weeks of therapy.

Fluconazole and itraconazole have been used successfully in the treatment of dermatophytoses. However, optimum pediatric dosage has not been established yet. Fluconazole in the dosage of 8 mg/kg per week or 6 mg/kg per day and itraconazole 5 mg/kg per day can be used for the treatment of onychomycosis and tinea capitis. Itraconazole can also be given as pulse therapy, 5 mg/ kg per day × 1 week/ month. Ketoconazole is generally not recommended because of its hepatotoxicity. Terbinafine, a fungicidal agent belonging to allylamine group, is effective in the dosage of 3-6 mg/kg per day.

The duration of antifungal therapy, except for onychomycosis, is usually 4-6 weeks or for 2 weeks after clinical cure whichever is the longest. The duration of therapy for onychomycosis depends on whether finger nails or toe nails are involved. For finger nail infection the duration of therapy is shorter. The duration of treatment with griseofulvin, itraconazole, flucanozole, and terbinafine for finger nail infection is 3-9 months, 6 weeks, 12-16 weeks, and 6 weeks respectively and for toe nails it is 4-12 months, 12 weeks, 18-26 weeks, and 12 weeks respectively. Two pulses of itraconazole are effective in finger nail infection and 3 pulses are effective for toe nail infection.

Adjuvant therapies such as antibiotics or systemic corticosteroids can be used in the treatment of inflammatory types in order to prevent scarring alopecia. Oral prednisolone 0.5 mg to 1.0 mg/kg per day can be used for 2-4 weeks.

CUTANEOUS CANDIDIASIS

The infection of skin, mucus membrane and internal organs caused by yeast-like fungus belonging to the genus *Candida* is refered as candidiasis.

Etiopathogenesis

There are several species of *Candida* known to cause human infections. *Candida albicans* is the commonest cause of various types of candidiasis. Other species of *Candida* which rarely cause human infection include *C. parasilosis, C. tropicalis, C. guilliermondii, C. krusei, C. glabrata*, and *C. stellatoidea*. *C. albicans* is a commensal in various sites of the body such as oral cavity, vagina, and gastrointestinal tract. Transient colonization can occur on the fingers or body folds. Certain factors predispose to increased risk of candidiasis **(Table 7.6)**.

TABLE 7.6: Predisposing factors of candidiasis

Endocrinal disorders
Diabetes mellitus
Addison's disease
Hypothyroidism
Cushing's syndrome
Genetic disorders
Chronic mucocutaneous candidiasis
Acrodermatitis enteropathica
Down syndrome
Immunological factors
Human immunodeficiency virus infection
Leukemia
Lymphoma
Drugs
Systemic antibiotics
Systemic or inhalational corticosteroids
Immunosuppressive drugs
Local factors
Immature skin and low-birth weight (Invasive and systemic candidiasis)
Candidal vaginitis in mother (Neonatal oral thrush)
Premature labor in the presence of foreign body (Congenital candidiasis)
Moist warm conditions (Intertrigo)
Finger or thumb sucking (Chronic paronychia)
Lip licking, dental malocclusion, orthodontic prosteses (Perleche)

Clinical Features

Most cases of candidiasis are result of endogenous infection by *Candida albicans*. There are several types of clinical manifestations of candidal infection.

Oral candidiasis: Oral candidiasis commonly occurs in infants and immunosuppressed patients. Oral candidiasis is the most common secondary infection seen in AIDS patients. There are different clinical forms of oral candidiasis *viz.* acute or chronic pseudomembranous, acute or chronic erythematous, hyperplastic, and median rhomboid glossitis. The pseudomembranous form presents as creamy white easily removable membrane involving buccal mucosa, gums and palate. In severe cases tongue, pharynx, or esophagus may also be involved. Erythematous forms present with discomfort in the oral cavity upon taking foods. The mucosa appears red and glazed. Hyperplastic form usually involves cheeks and tongue as thick irregular firmly adherent white plaques. Median rhomboid glossitis is characterized by diamond-shaped plaque on the dorsum of the tongue with loss of papillae. Apart from causing oral candidiasis, the candidal infection can also complicate oral ulcerative conditions. In AIDS patient oropharynx and esophagus may also be involved.

Intertrigo: Intertrigo is characterized by intense erythema in the skin folds. This warm moist inflammatory skin leads to candidal and staphylococcal infections. The presence of satellite papules or pustules indicates candidal infection.

Candidal vulvovaginitis: Candidal vulvovaginitis is common in adults but may occur in children and adolescents. The disease accounts for 62% of all gynecological problems in children and adolescents. Erythema and edema of labia, erythema and white patches on the vaginal mucosa along with curdy white thick discharge are the typical clinical manifestations. Itching, burning and dysuria are usually present.

Perleche: Perleche is characterized by fissuring and inflammation of angles of the mouth. The collection of secretions at the angle of mouth secondary to various predisposing factors is responsible for maceration and candidal infection.

Chronic paronychia and onychomycosis: The inflammation of nail folds is referred as paronychia. The chronic paronychia is commonly caused by *C. albicans.* The disease presents with transverse ridging, loss of cuticle, and erythema and edema of nail folds.

Nail infection is always associated with paronychia. The loss of cuticle enables entry of organism through proximal nail fold. Distal and lateral subungual onychomycosis are the commonest types of candidal nail infection. The third type, total dystrophic onychomycosis usually occurs in chronic mucocutaneous candidiasis. The presence of paronychia and erosion of distal nail plate are diagnostic of candidal onychomycosis.

Neonatal candidiasis: There are two types of candidiasis that occur in newborn period; congenital form in which skin lesions present at birth; and neonatal form which is seen after the first week of life.

Congenital candidiasis is characterized by numerous erythematous macules, papules and pustules distributed over back, extensor extremities and skin folds. The diaper region is usually spared and involvement of oral cavity is uncommon. The presence of pustules on palms and soles is diagnostic of the disease. In full-term infants the congenital candidiasis resolves in 1-2 weeks. Prematurity or invasive procedures or instrumentation during delivery may result in systemic candidal infection. The important differential diagnoses include erythema toxicum neonatorum, bacterial folliculitis, bullous impetigo, and congenital varicella or herpes or syphilis.

Neonatal candidiasis is usually localized to oral cavity and diaper area. Systemic infection may occur in the presence of infected intrauterine devices or invasive procedures.

Systemic candidiasis and Invasive fungal dermatitis: Systemic candidiasis commonly follows neonatal or congenital candidiasis under certain clinical situations as described above. The presenting features include lethargy, hypotension, hyperglycemia, apnea, and temperature instability. Internal organ involvement results in septicemia, urinary tract infection, meningitis, endocarditis, septic arthritis, endophthalmos and osteomyelitis. Cutaneous lesions may or may not be present. Systemic candidiasis is associated with high mortality and permanent neurological defects in survivors.

Invasive fungal dermatitis caused by *C. albicans* is commonly seen in extremely low birth weight infants. Clinically the infection manifests as erosions and ulcers with extensive crusting. There may be vesicles, bullae or burn-like erythema. Desquamation and wide spread denudation are common.

Chronic mucocutaneous candidiasis (CMC): Chronic mucocutaneous candidiasis is a syndrome of persistent and refractory candidal infection of mucosa, skin and nails. It is commonly seen in infancy and early childhood. Many immunological defects have been reported in association with CMC. However, CMC has to be differentiated from other well-defined immunodeficiency disorders like severe combined immunodeficiency or chronic granulomatous disorders where severe candidiasis forms a minor part and is over shadowed by serious secondary infectious complications. The disease manifests in different clinical forms including autosomal recessive (AR), autosomal dominant (AD), diffuse, late onset and polyendocrinopathy associated CMC. The AR form is characterized by persistent oral and nail infections, and the general health of the child is good. The AD form is more severe and is associated with dermatophytoses. Diffuse form is severe presenting as widespread cutaneous granulomas. Late onset form is seen in adults usually with thymoma. Endocrinal abnormalities associated with CMC include hypoparathyroidism, hypothyroidism, and hypoadrenocorticalism.

Other dermatological manifestations include seborrheic dermatitis, alopecia areata, recurrent aphthous ulcers, warts and dermatophytoses.

Diagnosis

The clinical diagnosis can be confirmed by demonstration of budding yeast cells and pseudohyphae in KOH preparation and growth from the Sabouraud's dextrose agar. Gram staining of vaginal discharge detects gram positive budding cells and pseudohyphae. In systemic candidiasis the organism can be demonstrated in urine, blood and cerebrospinal fluid.

Treatment

The management of candidiasis includes identification and treatment of underlying disorders and predisposing factors. The imidazoles are the important group of topical antifungals effective against candidal infection. These include clotrimazole, ketoconazole, miconazole, terconazole, econazole, etc. The effective oral antifungal agents, fluconazole and itraconazole belong to triazole group. Other effective therapy includes amphotericin B and nystatin.

For localized disease topical antifungal agents are used. Single dose fluconazole is effective in oral thrush and candidal vulvovaginitis. In the latter, clotrimazole vaginal suppositories or tablets or cream can be used daily for 3-7 days. Systemic candidal infection requires parenteral therapy with amphotericin B 0.5-1.0 mg/ kg per day. CMC requires systemic agents such as fluconazole or itraconazole.

DEEP FUNGAL INFECTION

Unlike superficial fungal infections, certain fungi can invade skin and subcutaneous tissue and sometimes, depending upon mode of transmission, portal of entry and immune status of the host can cause systemic or disseminated infection. These deep fungal infections are divided into subcutaneous, systemic and opportunistic fungal infections.

SUBCUTANEOUS FUNGAL INFECTIONS

The subcutaneous fungal infections are common in adults and most of the infections are related to occupational exposures (soil or vegetation). These infections are prevalent in certain geographical areas. The infection is acquired by percutaneous inoculation of the causative agent. Usually the disease is localized to the site of inoculation. If not treated the disease spreads slowly to involve surrounding tissues. But the disseminated infection is very rare. The common forms of subcutaneous mycoses are sporotrichosis, mycetoma, chromoblastomycosis and rhinosporodiosis. Other uncommon forms are lobomycosis, and pheohyphomycosis.

SPOROTRICHOSIS

Sporotrichosis is a granulomatous infection of skin and subcutaneous tissue caused by a dimorphic fungus, *Sporothrix schenckii.*

Epidemiology

The disease is worldwide in distribution commonly affecting adult males. However, childhood infections can occur.

Clinical Features

Clinically three types of infections are recognized; lymphocutaneous form, fixed cutaneous form, and disseminated form. In the former two forms, the skin is affected due to direct inoculation at the site of trauma and in the latter it is due to hematogenous spread. The lymphocutaneous form is common in adults. It is characterized by erythematous, painless nodules arranged along the lymphatics starting from the site of trauma. The nodules may undergo central ulceration and heal with scarring. Regional lymphadenopathy usually occurs. The fixed cutaneous form is common in children. Variety of skin lesions can occur localized to the site of trauma, like scaly papules, verrucous or ulcerated plaques, or nodules. Lymphatics are not involved in this form. The disseminated form is seen in individual with immunodeficiency or debilitating disease. The cutaneous lesions are widespread in distribution. Other organs involved are lungs, bones, joints and central nervous system.

Differential Diagnosis

The lymphocutaneous form is to be differentiated from nocardiosis, fish tank granuloma, tularemia, and leishmaniasis. Other important differential diagnoses include mycetoma, ecthyma, chromoblastomycosis, cutaneous antrax and foreign body granuloma.

Diagnosis

The gold standard of diagnosis is fungal culture of skin biopsy specimen.

Treatment

The treatment of choice is administration of saturated solution of potassium iodide (SSKI). The dosage in infants and children is 1-2 drops per year of age three times daily and continued for 4-6 weeks after clinical cure. Newer therapeutic options for cutaneous disease include itraconazole (5 mg/ kg), terbinafine, fluconazole and local hyperthermia. For disseminated disease amphotericin B is effective.

MYCETOMA

Mycetoma is a chronic granulomatous infection of subcutaneous tissue caused by certain fungi and anaerobic bacteria resembling fungus. The disease is characterized by triad of tumefaction, nodules and grains. The latter feature is diagnostic of mycetoma. The grains of various colors are nothing but the colonies of causative organism.

Epidemiology

The disease is common in tropical and subtropical dry regions. Any age and sex can be affected. Children in rural areas are susceptible to the infection.

Etiology

Both fungi and fungus-like bacteria can cause mycetoma **(Table 7.7)**. The disease caused by the former is called eumycetoma and that by the latter is called actinomycetoma.

Clinical Feature

The common site of infection is feet followed by hands. Other parts of the body such as back, chest wall, abdomen, perinium, buttocks, thighs, neck and back of the head may be involved. The disease manifests usually several months after the inoculation of causative agent. The initial lesion is a small, firm, painless subcutaneous nodule which increases gradually in size. Subsequent evolution and progression or behavior of the infection is different in eumycetoma and actinimycetoma **(Table 7.8)**. The initial nodule softens discharing serosanguinous material. Similarly in the later stage, the swelling breaks down to form multiple discharging sinuses along with appearance of new nodules. The discharge usually contains grains, the color of which helps in identification of causative agent. The spread of infection occurs along the fascial planes involving muscles, ligaments and bones. The

TABLE 7.7: Etiology of mycetoma

Mycetoma	Genus	Species	Color of grains
Eumycetoma	*Madurella*	mycetomatis	Black
		grisea	Black
	Pyrenochaeta	romeroi	Black
	Leptosphaeria	senegalensis	Black
	Exophiala	jeanselmei	Black
	Curvularia	lunata	Black
	Pseudoallescheria	boydii	White to yellow
	Neotestudina	rosatii	White to yellow
	Acremonium spp	—	White to yellow
	Fusarium spp	—	White to yellow
Actinomycetoma	*Actinomadura*	madurae	White
		pelletieri	Red
	Nocardia	brasiliensis	White
		asteroides	White
		cavae	White
	Streptomyces	somalensis	White

TABLE 7.8: Differences between eumycetoma and actinomycetoma

Characteristics	Eumycetoma	Actinimycetoma
Etiology	Filamentous fungi	Fungus-like bacteria
Progression of disease	Slow	Rapid
Swelling	Marked in the later stage	Less well defined and merges with surrounding tissue
Tissue destruction	Marked in the later stage	Involvement of bone is earlier and extensive
Radiology (Bone cavities)	Larger and less numerous	Smaller and abundant
Grains	Dark with a coarser texture	Pale with a fine texture
Filaments	Wide and septate	Slender and non septate
Response to drugs	Unresponsive and requires radical surgical excision	Good response

tendons and nerves are resistant to invasion. The visceral involvement is rare and it is due to contagious spread from mycetoma involving chest wall or abdomen.

Differential Diagnosis

The mycetoma should be differentiated from botroyomycosis, sporotrichosis, chromoblastomycosis, chronic osteomyelitis, cutaneous tuberculosis, and atypical mycobacterial infections. Rarely, some dermatophytes cause a clinical condition similar to mycetoma called pseudomycetoma. The causative dermatophytes are *M. audouinii, M. canis, M. ferrugineum, T. mentagrophytes, T. tonsurans, T. verrucosum* and *T. violaceum*.

Laboratory Diagnosis

The clinical diagnosis is made by the presence of tumefaction, discharging nodules and grains. The diagnosis is confirmed by microscopy and culture of grains.

Microscopy: Direct examination of crushed grains after adding KOH demonstrates broad, septate filaments (fungus) or slender, non-septate filaments (bacterial). If grains are not present, removal of crust and plugging the sinus may reveal the grains on the undersurface.

Modified Z-N staining using 1% sulfuric acid can be used if nocardia infection is suspected. Gram staining of the discharge or grain reveals Gram positive slender intertwined filaments of bacteria causing actinomycetoma.

Culture: The definitive diagnosis is made by the culture of grain or tissue specimen. The causative organisms of mycetoma grow on Sabouraud's 2% dextrose agar with antibiotics at room temperature. If actinomycetoma is suspected, the specimen should be incubated in both aerobic and anaerobic culture media because the former is required for isolation of *Nocardia* and the latter for isolation of actinomadura species.

Histopathology: The lesions show suppurative inflammatory reaction with neutrophils in the subcutaneous tissue along with a granulomatous reaction comprising of epithelioid cells, plasma cells, lymphocytes and giant cells. Around the grains a refractile eosinophilic material is seen (Splendore-Hoeppli phenomenon). This phenomenon is also noticed in pseudomycetoma.

Serology: Serologic tests are only of academic value. Demonstration of precipitins in the serum may be helpful in early stages when sinus tracks are absent.

Treatment

The line of management for eumycetoma and actinomycetoma is different. Therefore, the diagnosis should be confirmed before starting the therapy.

Eumycetoma is usually unresponsive to antifungal therapy. Early diagnosis and radical surgical excision of the involved tissue successfully eradicated the infection. Initiation of treatment before the involvement of bone is essential for better therapeutic outcome. Then the treatment can be supplemented with antifungal agents. Long-term ketaconazole 3-5 mg/ kg per day appears to be the best antifungal drug to treat eumycetoma. Response to itraconazole 5-8 mg/ kg per day is variable. If the tissue destruction is extensive, amputation is advised. Amphotericin B is effective in immunocompromised children.

Actinomycetoma usually responds to antibiotics. Cotrimaxazole and sulfonamides are the treatment of choice for infection due to *Nocardia*. Other antibiotics effective against *Nocardia* include streptomycin, third generation cephalosporine, amoxacilin-clavulanate, amikacin, imipenem, minocycline, dapsone and fluoroquinolones. Parenteral penicillin is effective against infection with *Actinomyces* spp. Long duration of therapy, for 6 months to 2 years, is usually required for complete resolution of disease.

CHROMOBLASTOMYCOSIS

The skin and subcutaneous infection caused by dermataceous fungi is called chromoblastomycosis.

Epidemiology

The disease is common in tropical and subtropical regions. Adult male patients working outdoor and coming in contact with contaminated soil or wood are susceptible to the infection. However, childhood infections have been reported.

Etiology

Many dermataceous fungi such as *Phialophora verrucosa, Fonsecaea pedrosoi, F. campactum, Cladosporium carrionii and Wangiella dermatiditis* species are implicated in the etiology of the disease.

Clinical Features

The disease starts as small scaly papules developing at the site of inoculation. Later the lesions slowly expand to form nodules. The characteristic lesion is a verrucous plaque formed by the coalescence of nodules. The surface of the lesion is friable and bleeds on minor trauma. The commonest site of involvement is lower leg or foot. The adjacent skin may be involved due to autoinoculation leading to extensive infection. The lesions may wax and wane eventually leaving fibrotic scars.

Differential Diagnosis

Deep fungal infections, cutaneous tuberculosis, leishmaniasis, leprosy, tertiary syphilis and florid warts are the important differential diagnoses.

Diagnosis

The diagnosis is made by demonstrating the organism in tissue biopsy or growth from the culture. KOH preparation of the lesion demonstrates pigmented sclerotic bodies in clusters. The characteristic histopathological features are pseudoepitheliomatous hyperplasia overlying the foci of suppurative granulomatous reaction in the dermis and subcutaneous tissue. Thick walled brown cells referred as sclerotic bodies, Medlar bodies or copper pennies can be detected in giant cells or free in the tissue.

Treatment

For localized disease surgical excision is the treatment of choice. Cryotherapy, heat therapy and radiation therapy are the other modalities of treatment for localized disease. Systemic antifungal agents like itraconazole, terbinafine and 5-fluorocytosine are effective in extensive disease. Amphotericin B has been found to be less effective.

RHINOSPORIDIOSIS

Rhinosporidiosis is a chronic granulomatous disease of mucosal surfaces such as nose, eyes, and sinuses.

Epidemiology

Rhinosporidiosis is common in India and Sri Lanka. In India, the disease is prevalent in Kerala and Tamil Nadu. The disease is common in boys and men between 10 and 30 years of age. Individuals who bathe or work in stagnant water source are at increased risk of developing the infection.

Etiology

Rhinosporidiosis is caused by a fungus, *Rhinosporidium seeberi*. Earlier the organism was thought to be a protozoan parasite.

Clinical Features

The patient presents with polypoid or sessile masses in the nasal mucosa. The anterior part is frequently involved than the posterior. The lesions may be friable. There may be thin mucoid or serosanguinous discharge from the lesions.

Differential Diagnosis

Rhinosporidiosis needs to be differentiated from other nasal infections like rhinoscleroma, mucormycosis, paracoccidioidomycosis, and opportunistic infections such as aspergillosis or alternaria infections.

Diagnosis

The clinical diagnosis is confirmed by biopsy. A granulomatous reaction consisting of mixed cell granuloma, pseudoabscess, and fibrosis around the organism is seen in the biopsy specimen. Sporangia of *Rhinosporidium seeberi* containing sporangiospores at various stages of development are diagnostic of rhinosporidiosis.

Treatment

Excision of the mass using electrosurgical methods is the treatment of choice. The condition has been successfully treated by dapsone and other sulfones. Ketaconazole and clotrimazole may be effective.

SYSTEMIC MYCOSIS

The systemic fungal infections are caused by systemic and opportunistic fungal agents. The systemic mycoses share some common characteristics. The causative organisms are dimorphic fungi which shift from environmental and tissue phase at 25°C and 37°C respectively. The natural phase is a mold and tissue phase is yeast, except for *Coccidioides immitis* which forms spherules with endospores. The systemic mycoses are prevalent in certain regions of North America, South America, Central America or Africa. These are commonly seen in adults. However, childhood infections have been reported. The systemic fungi are primary pulmonary pathogens causing acute pulmonary, chronic pulmonary or disseminated disease. There may be reactivation months to years after primary infection. The inhalation of conidia into the respiratory system is the most likely portal of entry. In immunocompromised individuals there may be rapidly progressive acute disseminated infection with increased mortality rate. The diagnosis of systemic mycoses is made by demonstration of characteristic fungal elements in the tissue specimen and culture growth or by newer serological methods. The antifungal agents that are effective in the treatment of systemic mycoses are amphotericin B, itraconazole, fluconazole and ketoconazole. The duration of therapy is usually 6-12 months.

Cutaneous Manifestations of Systemic Mycoses

The cutaneous involvement is usually seen in disseminated disease. However, rarely primary cutaneous infection can occur at the site of inoculation.

Blastomycosis

Blastomycosis is caused by *Blastomyces dermatitidis*. During acute infection, rarely erythema nodosum has been reported. In disseminated infections verrucous and ulcerative lesions can occur. These lesions have distinct heaped up borders. As the lesions progress, central healing occurs with scar formation. Unlike, other systemic mycoses, blastomycosis is not common in AIDS patients. Histopathologic examination of lesions from immunocompetent patients reveals microabscesses with pseudoepitheliomatous hyperplasia.

Coccidioidomycosis

Coccidioidomycosis is caused by *Coccidioides immitis*. During acute infection erythema nodosum and erythema multiforme may develop along with arthritis. In disseminated infections, the cutaneous manifestation presents as papules, plaques, pustules, nodules, ulcers, abscesses or large warty lesions. In endemic areas, coccidioidomycosis is an AIDS defining illness.

Histoplasmosis

Histoplasmosis is caused by *Histoplasma capsulatum*. During acute infection erythema nodosum and erythema multiforme may develop along with arthritis. In disseminated infections, the cutaneous manifestations include granulomatous plaques, deep nodules, erythematous papules and plaques, pustules, papulonecrotic lesions, eczematous dermatitis and exfoliative dermatitis. In AIDS disseminated molluscum contageosum like lesions can also occur. Primary cutaneous infection has been reported in both children and adults. The histopathological features in immunocompetent patients show granulomatous reaction with intracellular budding yeasts.

Paracoccidioidomycosis

Paracoccidioidomycosis is caused by *Paracoccidioides brasiliensis*. The cutaneous lesions are common around the nose and mouth. The lesions begin as small pustules that become ulcerated acneiform papules. Ulcerative and verrucous lesions may extend and ultimately destroy the nose, lips and facies. Fistula and ulceration may develop from the underlying lymph node involvement. Subcutaneous abscess discharging dark colored pus with red to purple skin has been reported. Primary cutaneous infection is very rare. The disease is not associated with increased incidence in AIDS patients.

OPPORTUNISTIC FUNGAL INFECTIONS

Certain non pathogenic fungi cause infection in at-risk individuals. These infections are referred as opportunistic fungal infections. AIDS, cancer chemotherapy, and organ and bone marrow transplantation are the main risk factors associated with these infections.

Cryptococcosis

Cryptococcosis is an opportunistic systemic mycosis caused by dimorphic yeast *Cryptococcus neoformans*. The main source of infection is pigeon or hen droppings. The infection is transmitted through airways. Primary cutaneous infection which presents as an ulcer at the site of inoculation is rare in both immunodeficient and immunocompetent individuals. Cutaneous cryptococcosis occurs as a manifestation of neurological or disseminated disease. It presents as wide spread polymorphic lesions mimicking acne and molluscum contagiosum. Other organs involved are brain, spinal cord, lungs and bones.

The demonstration of large budding encapsulated cells on KOH or India ink preparation, and from growth on SDA confirms the diagnosis. Mucicarmine staining of skin biopsy specimen helps in the identification of *C. neoformans*.

Ketoconazole 3-5 mg/kg per day or itraconazole 5-8 mg/kg per day for 4-6 months are effective in cutaneous infection. For neurological disease fluconazole 8 mg/kg per day and maintenance dose of 5 mg/kg per day is recommended. Intravenous amphotericin B with or without fluconazole and long-term maintenance with fluconazole or itraconazole is recommended in AIDS patients.

Aspergillosis

Aspergillosis is one of the commonest opportunistic fungal infections caused by *Aspergillus fumigatus* and *A. flavus*. The infection occurs through inhalation of *Aspergillus* which is ubiquitous in the environment. Skin is affected in systemic disseminated infection, though primary cutaneous infection has been reported. The sites in contact with contaminated adhesive tapes or arm bands or catheters in immunocompromised patients are predisposed to develop cutaneous aspergillosis. A wide variety of skin lesions can occur as a manifestation of cutaneous aspergillosis. These include erythematous to violaceous indurated plaques, progressing ulceration with eschar, subcutaneous granulomas or abscesses, pustules, eruptive and suppurative papules, and vegetative plaques.

Mucormycosis, cryptococcosis and ecthyma gangrenosum are the important differential diagnoses. The diagnosis is confirmed by demonstration of the organism in the fungal culture and skin biopsy specimen. Special stains such as Gomori methenamine silver or periodic acid-Schiff are used to increase the intensity of hematoxylin and eosin staining.

Intravenous amphotericin B is the treatment of choice. Itraconazole amd flucytosine are the other antifungal agents found to be effective.

Zygomycosis

Zygomycosis is an opportunistic infection caused by fungi belonging to the class Zygomycetes. These are characterized by broad, ribbon-like hyphae with a few septation. Zygomycosis includes two forms, mucormycosis and entomophthoramycosis.

Mucormycosis

Mucormycosis is a acute, necrotic, rapidly progressive disease caused by fungi belonging to the genera, *Mucor, Rhizopus, Absidia* and *Rhizomucor*. The disease is characterized by vascular invasion and necrosis occurring in immunocompromised, diabetic or severely debilited patients. The disease occurs worldwide and can affect all age groups.

Primary cutaneous mucormycosis occurs in two forms. The first one is localized necrotic cellulitis occurring in healthy children following contact with contaminated bandages. The second form is progressive, indurated, erythematous, tender plaque of cellulitis with central necrosis. This form is seen in immunocompromised children.

Systemic zygomycosis presents as rhinocerebral and pulmonary mucormycosis. The former is seen in poorly controlled diabetic patients presenting as invasive sinusitis. Necrosis of mucosa, palate or paranasal sinuses is an early sign which rapidly spreads to retro-orbital space and brain. The latter commonly occurs in patients with leukemia, lymphoma or agranulocytosis presenting with respiratory symptoms. Disseminated infection may follow pulmonary mucormycosis particularly involving the brain.

Bacterial orbital cellulitis, aspergillosis, osteomyelitis, and atypical mycobacterial infections are the important differential diagnoses.

The diagnosis is made by demonstration of broad, ribbon like relatively aseptate hyphae branching at right angles in culture and histopathological section.

Intravenous amphotericin B with or without fluconazole is the treatment of choice. Ketoconazole, iodides, and cotrimoxazole have been used successfully when combined with surgery.

BIBLIOGRAPHY

1. Arenas R, Lavalle P. Mycetoma. In: Arenas R, Estrada R, edts. Tropical dermatology Vademecum. Georgetown: Landes Bioscience, 2001; 51- 61.
2. Arenas R. Sporotrichosis. In: Arenas R, Estrada R, edts. Tropical dermatology Vademecum. Georgetown: Landes Bioscience, 2001; 62-70.
3. Arnow PM, Houchins SG, Pugliese G. An outbreak of tinea corporis in hospital personnel caused by a patient with Trichophyton tonsurans infection. Pediatr Infect Dis 1991; 10: 355.
4. Assaf RR, Weil ML. The superficial mycoses. Dermatol Clin 1996; 14(1): 57-68.
5. Body BA. Cutaneous manifestations of Systemic mycoses. Dermatol Clin 1996; 14: 125-35.
6. Chapman RL. Candida infections in neonate. Curr Opin Pediatr 2003; 15: 91- 102.
7. Darmstadt GL, Dinulos JG, Miller Z. Congenital cutaneous candidiasis: clinical presentation, pathogenesis and management guidelines. Pediatrics 2000; 105(2): 438- 44.
8. Davis B. Sporotrichosis. Dermatol Clin 1996; 14: 69-76.
9. Dimino- Emme L, Gurevitti AW. Cutaneous manifestations of disseminated cryptococcosis. J Am Acad Dermatol 1995; 32: 844-50.
10. Elewski B. Tinea capitis. Dermatol Clin 1996; 14(1): 23- 32.
11. Elewski BE. Onychomycosis: patogenesis, diagnosis and management. Clin Microbiol Rev 1998; 11(3): 415- 29.
12. Elewski BE. Tinea capitis: A current perspective. J Am Acad Dermatol 2000; 42: 1- 20.
13. Elgart GW. Chromoblastomycosis. Dermatol Clin 1996; 14: 77- 84.
14. Elgart ML. Zygomycosis. Dermatol Clin 1996; 14: 141- 46.
15. Frieden IJ, Howard R. Tinea capitis: Epidemiology, diagnosis, treatment and control. J Am Acad Dermatology 1994; 31: S42- S46.
16. Friedlander SF, Rueda M, Chen BK, Caceres- Rios HW. Fungal, Protozoal and Helminthic infections. In: Schachner AL, Hansen CR, edts. Pediatric dermatology. 3rd edn. Edinbrgh: Mosby, 2003; 1093-140.
17. Hay RJ. Fungal skin infections. Arch Dis Child 1992; 67(9): 1065-7.
18. Hay RJ. Yeast infections. Dermatol Clin 1996; 14: 113- 24.
19. Hoppe JE. Treatment of oropharyngeal candidiasis and candidal diaper dermatitis in neonates and infants: Review and reappraisal. Pediatr Infect Dis 1997; 16: 885- 94.
20. Isaac M. Cutaneous aspergillosis. Dermatol Clin 1996; 14: 137-40.
21. Jaquiery A, Stylianopoulos A, Hogg G, Grover S. Vulvovaginitis: clinical features, etiology and microbiology of genital tract. Arch Dis Child 1998; 81(1): 64-7.
22. Jones HE. Immune response and host resistance of humans to dermatophyte infection. J Am Acad Dermatol 1993; 28: S12.
23. Karkpatrick CH. Chronic mucocutaneous candidiasis. Pediatr Infect Dis 2001; 20: 197- 206.
24. Kearse HL. Tinea pedis in prepubertal children: Does it occur?. J Am Acad Dermatol 1988; 19: 619- 22.
25. Linder N, Keller N, Huri C. Primary cutaneous mucormycosis in a premature infant. Case report and review of literature. Am J Perinatol 1998; 15: 35- 8.
26. Manns BJ, Baylis BW, Urbanski L. Paracoccidoidomycosis: case report and review. Clin Infect Dis 1996; 23: 1026-32.
27. Marakawa GJ, Harvell JP, Lubitz P. Cutaneous aspergillosis and acquired immunodeficiency syndrome. Arch Dermatol 2000; 136: 365- 9.

28. McGinnis MR. Mycetoma. Dermatol Clin 1996; 14: 97- 104.
29. Melville C, Kempley S, Graham J, Berry CL. Early onset systemic Candida infection in extremely preterm neonate. Eur J Pediatr 1996; 155: 904-6.
30. Midgley G, Moore MK. Nail infections. Dermatol Clin 1996; 14: 41-50.
31. Minotto R, Varejao C, Mallman L. Chromoblastomycosis: A review of 100 cases in the state of Rio Grande do Sul, Brazil. J Am Acad Dermatol 2001; 44: 585-92.
32. Odio CM, Navarrette M, Carrillo JM. Disseminated histoplasmosis in infants. Pediatr Infect Dis J 1999; 18: 1065- 8.
33. Ogawa H, Summerbell RC, Clemmons KV, Koga T, Ran YP, Rashid A, et al. Dermatophytes and host defence in cutaneous mycoses. Med Mycol 1998; 36: S166- S73.
34. Pappas PG, Tellez I, Deep A. Sporotrichosis in peru: Description of an area of hyperendemocity. Clin Inf Dis 2000; 30: 65-70.
35. Quimby SR, Connolly SM, Winkelmann R. Clinicopathologic spectrum of specific cutaneous lesions of disseminated coccidoidomycosis. J Am Acad Dermatol 1992; 26: 79- 85.
36. Warren NG. Taxonomy and introduction. Dermatol Clin 1996; 14(1): 1-8.
37. Weitzman I, Padhye AA. Dermatophytes: Gross and microscopy. Dermatol Clin 1996; 14(1): 9-22.

8

Protozoan and Helminthic Infections

K Ravindra

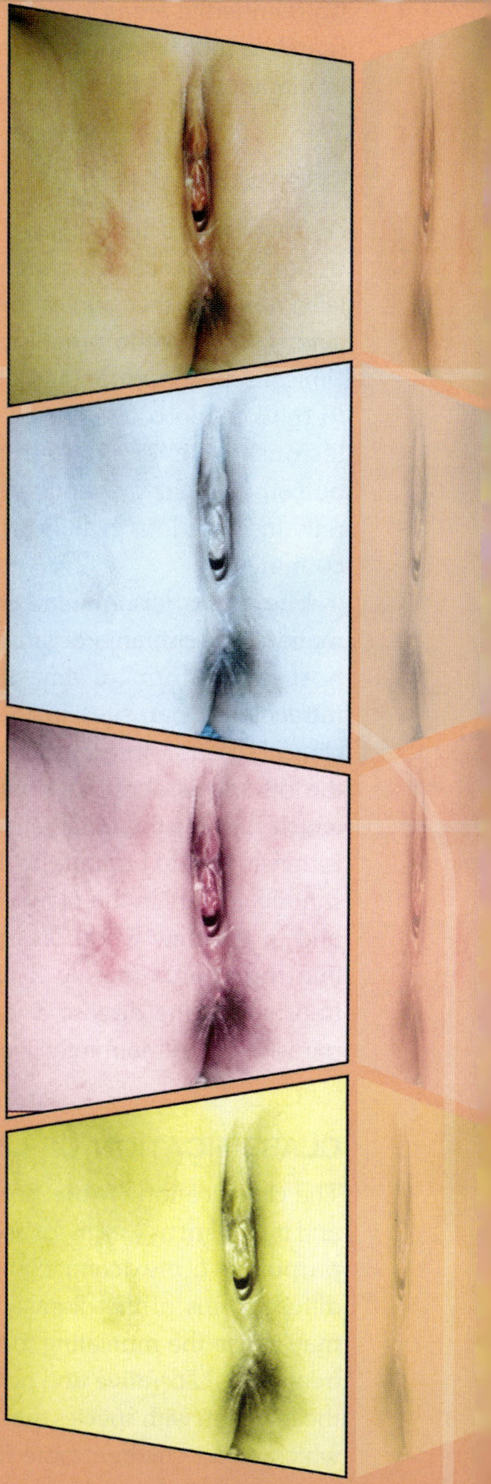

PROTOZOAN INFECTIONS

Protozoa may cause skin disease directly or may affect the skin directly. There is an increasing prevalence of protozoa infections all over the world adding considerably to mortality. Advanced travel facilities, migration of people from endemic areas to non-endemic areas especially in search of jobs has added to the prevalence of the disease in many parts of the world.

LEISHMANIASIS

A group of infections caused by a number of species of obligate intracellular parasite Leishmania comprise leishmaniasis. Invasion of the host mononuclear phagocyte system by the organism can result in a variety of clinical syndromes ranging from asymptomatic infection to self healing cutaneous or disfiguring mucocutaneous lesions to severe disseminated disease with fatal outcome. As the prevention is not effective leishmaniasis remains a serious health problem in many developing countries.

The genus leishmania belongs to family trypanosomatidae. Leishmania organisms exist in the mammalian host in the form of amastigotes which are obligate intracellular parasites in the macrophages and cause clinical disease. In endemic areas the peak incidence of the disease is about 3 months after the onset of rains which hastens the emergence of sandflies.The infection is transmitted to humans by the bite of the snand fly. The sandfly vectors in the oldworld are species phlebotomus and in the new world are species lutzomyia. Sandflies live for approximately 2 weeks and are capable of transmitting the disease 3 to 7 days after acquiring the parasite and remain infective till they die.

CLASSIFICATION OF LEISHMANIASIS

The classification **(Table 8.1)** is important for prognosis and treatment as well as for academic and epidemiological purposes. *L.mexicana* complex sometimes produces diffuse forms of the disease and *L.braziliensis* complex may cause the mutilating forms and is more resistant to treatment. Ulcerative and nodular lesions can be seen in the infection with species that cause visceral leishmaniasis which affect children more frequently.

TABLE 8.1: Classification of leishmaniasis

	Clinical form	Species
1	Cutaneous leishmaniasis [CL] Old World New World	 *L.major, L.tropica* *L.aethiopica* *L.donovani infantum* *L.braziliensis* *L.mexicana*
2	Mucocutaneous leishmaniasis (MCL)	*L.braziliensis* *L.aethiopica*
3	Diffuse cutaneous leishmaniasis(DCL)	*L.braziliensis* *L.aethiopica*
4	Visceral leishmaniasis (VL)	*L.donovani* *L.infantum*
5	Uncommon forms Leishmaniasis recidivans(LR) Post-kala azar dermal leishmaniasis (PKDL)	*L.tropica* *L.donovani*

Old World Cutaneous Leishmaniasis

[Oriental sore, Tropical sore, Bouton D'orient, Delhi boil, Aleppo boil]

Old world cutaneous leishmaniasis is due to L.major, L.aethiopica and L.donovani infantum and is endemic in central and Southern Asia, including India. Children are especially affected in endemic areas.

It is transmitted by sandflies belonging to the genus phlebotomus. The disease begins usually after 2 to 4 weeks after the bite of the sandfly. Lesions are more common over the unclothed parts of the body, i.e. the face, neck and arms. Though there is much overlap the natural history of the lesions due to the four species tends to differ due to the varied response of the host. Nodule, crusting, ulceration and healing with scar formation are a common sequence.

In cutaneous leishmaniasis caused by L.major (wet, rural or zoonotic CL) a firm, small papule develops at the site of the insect bite which grows over several weeks to months to a nodular lesions (2 cm or more) covered by fine, dry, papery scales with an infiltrated border. There will central crusting later and progresses to a large ulcer with a depressed granulomatous centre and a well defined raised margin. At the periphery of the lesions satellite papules can be seen and along the course of the lymphatics subcutaneous nodules may develop. In rare instances probably related to the host's immune response the lesions may become locally invasive and may extend to the subcutaneous tissue and muscle. Lesions are multiple (upto 100 or more), painless with a serous discharge, appear most commonly over the exposed parts and are never seen on the palms, soles and hairy scalp. After about 2 months of its onset the peripheral growth stops and remains of the same size for about 6 months and starts healing which may be complete in 6 to 12 months or leaving a depressed scar. Occasionally the ulcer last for 24 months or longer with positive smears and is called as non-healing chronic cutaneous leishmaniasis. The infection is more common in the rural areas.

In cutaneous leishmaniasis caused by L.tropica (dry, urban or anthroponotic leishmaniasis) the lesions are typically single, tend to be more inflammatory, may progress to a shallow ulcer or may not ulcerate, last longer and more difficult to treat when compared to lesions of cutaneous leishmaniasis caused by L.major the disease is common in urban areas.

In cutaneous leishmaniasis caused by L.aethiopica the lesions are single, resemble those caused by L.major but the lesions are more chronic, may not crust or ulcertate, non-inflammatory lasting several years (2-5 years) and in some patients the lesions are so widespread that they resemble lesions of lepromatous leprosy.

In cutaneous leishmaniasis caused by L.infantum the lesions are similar to those seen in infection with L.major but their duration is shorter and the disease is mild.

The differential diagnosis for old world cutaneous leishmaniasis includes insect bites, tertiary syphilis, yaws, lupus vulgarus, leprosy and pyogenic nodules.

New World Cutaneous Leishmaniasis

[Pian bois, American leishmaniasis, Uta, Chiclero ulcer]

New world cutaneous leishmaniasis is caused by L.mexicana and L.braziliensis and is transmitted by sandflies of the genus Lutzomyia. The disease is found more in Mexico, Central America. In infection due to L.mexicana the progression of the lesions is similar to those caused by the old world form. A small erythematous papule is seen at the site of the sandfly bite which gradually develops into a ulcerated nodule that heals leaving a depressed scar and lesions can develop on any part of the body. Pinna of the ear is involved in patients of Mexico and Central America (chiclero ulcer). In Peruvian and Ecuadonian children less than 10 years, more in children of less than 1 year, the lesions are round, clean and ulcerated, located over the face which heal spontaneously and are called 'Uta'.

Cutaneous lesions caused by L.braziliensis are similar to those seen in old world leishmaniasis, but some strains of L.braziliensis can invade the mucous membranes of the mouth nose, pharynx and larynx resulting mucocutaneous leishmaniasis.

Mucocutaneous Leishmaniasis (MCL)

The parasites of the L.braziliensis complex in South America and L.aethiopica in Africa cause MCL which is characterized by involvement of both skin and the upper respiratory tract. Mucosal lesions develop more frequently in those with cutaneous lesions caused by L.braziliensis whereas it is much infrequent in patients infected with L.aethiopica.

Nasopharyngeal lesions in infection caused by L.donovani have been reported in Sudan due to the extension of the cutaneous lesions to the nasal or buccal mucosa.

MCL is less common in children because mucosal manifestations appear months, years and even decades after the initial skin lesion and in those instances in more than 90% of patients in some geographic areas the scar of the previous lesion is seen.

In some patients of MCL there will be no history of previous cutaneous lesions which probably suggests the migration of the parasite from the site of inoculation in the skin to the mucosa without producing a clinical lesion or it is also possible that the initial cutaneous lesion may be discrete as to go unnoticed.

Mucosa can be involved by invasion from a contiguous cutaneous lesions located on the nose or lip.

The most frequently involved site is nasal mucosa followed by buccopharyngeal area. Rarely conjunctival and penile lesions are seen. Early symptoms include nasal blockage, rhinorrhea and epistaxis. Nasal septum will be erythematous, edematus and crusted nodular growths are seen which are followed by septal ulceration and perforation. Cartilage of the nose and columella will be destroyed resulting in caving in of the tip of the nose leading to "tapir's nose", "parrot's beak" and camel nose.

Inflammatory process can involve the floor of the mouth, soft tissues of the upper lip and cheeks producing erythema, edema and diffuse infiltration. Firm papulo-nodular lesions may involve the smooth and hard palate, uvula and pharynx. This results in halitosis, disphonia, dysphagia, secondary infections and emaciation. This disfigurement is known as "espundia". If not intervened, death results from malnutrition and acute respiratory failure.

Diffuse Cutaneous Leishmaniasis (DCL]

Diffuse cutaneous leishmaniasis is an anergic and disseminated disease caused in the old world by L.aethiopica and in South America it is attributed to L.braziliensis. It presents as papules and nodules that disseminate slowly affecting most of the skin surface with non-ulcertaing nodules found diffusely over the trunk and face resembling lepromatous leprosy but do not visceralize. It runs a protracted course and responds very poorly to treatment. The dissemination occurs anywhere from 3 months upto 11 years (average 3 years) after the appearance of first nodule. Parasites are abundant in skin smears and biopsies from DCL. Though circulating antibodies are present tests for the cell-mediated immune response, i.e. Montenegro test and lymphocyte proliferation assay are negative. Its evolution is chronic, possibly lifelong and is probably attributed to the deficiencies in host immune response rather than to the virulence of the parasite.

Visceral Leishmaniasis

The kala azar syndrome is caused by L.donovani. It is characterized by fever, Hepato spleenomegaly, pancytopenia and progressive deterioration. It is often fatal.

Post-Kalaazar Dermal Leishmaniasis (PKDL) [Dermal Leishmanoid]

Post-kala-azar dermal leishmaniasis [PKDL] occurs after several days to months after treatment especially when it is inadequate in patients suffering from visceral leishmaniasis and in a small number of people there will be no history of visceral disease. In one study, 42% were younger than 12 years. Lesions resembling PKDL present as small papules localized to the chin, cheeks, outer ear, forearms, buttocks and legs during the convalescent period are seen in Africa. The lesions heal spontaneously over a few months. But in India the lesions appear 1-2 years after recovery as hypopigmented patches resembling leparomatus leprosy which develop diffuse nodulation after a period of months to years. They progress for many years and do not heal spontaneously. PKDL is thought to represent the intraepidemic reservoir of the infection of VL in India.

DIAGNOSIS

Epidemiological and clinical criteria along with laboratory assistance are required to establish the diagnosis of leishmaniasis. History of exposure to an endemic area and sand fly bite during the previous weeks or months and high risk activities such as sleeping outdoors, jungle or desert trekking are very useful. Clinically in the above context non-healing nodules or ulcer for 4-6 weeks or longer are supportive.

Smears

Smear examination is the most effective method of detecting the parasite. The smear is stained with Wright's Giemsa or Leishman's stain. For the diagnosis of MCL nasal lesion must be sampled. With Giesma stain, the amastigotes are seen as pale blue oval bodies with a dark blue nucleus with a small point shaped kinetoplast within the cytoplasm of tissue macrophages.

Biopsy

Skin biopsy can be done when smear from the suspected lesion does not reveal amastigotes. By H and E stain intracellular amastigotes and granulomas can be seen.

In PKDL the hypopigmented macules show decreased number of pigment granules in the epidermis and the granuloma is same as in LR but there will be fibrous tissue perivascularly and the organisms are few in hypopigmented areas, more in erythematous lesions and many in the nodular lesions.

Culture

Specimen for culture can be obtained by skin biopsy and by fine needle aspiration after injecting sterile saline into the lesion. The material can be cultured on NNN blood agar (Nicolle's modification of Novy and McNeal's medium) or Schneidier's insect culture medium or rabbit blood agar. Promastigotes appear between 2 days to 2 weeks but culture should not be discarded as negative before 4 weeks.

Leishmanin (Montenegro) Test

It is a useful test in non-endemic areas but in endemic areas it is used for survey. An inflammatory halo of more than 10 mm in diameter is expressed as positive. A positivity of 90 to 98% is seen in patients of CL and MCL and is negative in patients with DCL which may become positive during treatment which indicates a better prognosis.

To identify leishmania species monoclonal antibody to surface antigen and isoenzyme analysis have been used.

TREATMENT

The treatment of leishmaniasis depends on the clinical form. Systemic treatment is indicated in patients with extensive or non-healing progressive lesions, involvement of lymphatics or invasion of mucus membranes, in all patients with L.braziliensis infection to avoid subsequent mucosal lesions and in L.amazonensis infection to avoid late disseminated disease. CL in the old world is usually self-limited and most patients do not require systemic treatment, but systemic treatment is required for extensive lesions involving the face or when there are lesions involving the deeper tissues.

Pentavalent antimonials are the drugs of choice for all the forms and remain "the best drug of a bad bunch". They are available as sodium stibogluconate (Pentostam 100 mg of antimony/ml) and meglumine antimoniate (glucantime 85 mg of antimony/ml). The dosage recommended is 20 mg/kg once daily for 20 days. If the lesions are not reduced by 75% by 6 weeks retreatment is essential. Mucocutaneous disease due to L.braziliensis and DCL will need treatment till 60-90 days. Antimonials are generally well tolerated but on occasions they can produce cephalea, malaise, vomiting, myalgia, arthralgia, abdominal discomfort, elevated hepatic transaminase levels (almost 100%) hematologic changes (decreased leukocyte count hemoglobin level and platelet count) and transient ECG changes. Sudden death rarely occurs due to cardiac toxicity with use of very high doses.

In those not responding to antimonials, amphotericin B 0.5 to 1 mg/Kg everyday or every other day for 14-20 days (total dose not exceeding 3G in adults) can be given. Liposomal amphotericin-B 3 mg/kg on days 1-5 and again on day 10 has been shown to be highly effective in children. Amphotericin may cause renal and hepatic toxicity.

Recombinant human interferon as an adjuant has been tried in refractory cases.

Miltefosine orally in a dose of 50-150 mg/day for 4-6 weeks is another alternative. Pentamedine is another effective option (especially in cases unresponsive to antimonials) given in a dose of 2-3 mg/kg every other day for 4-7 days. Ketoconazole in a dose of 400 to 600 mg once daily is well tolerated both in adults and children but is not effective in infections due to L.tropica and L.braziliensis. Allopurinol alone in a dose of 20 mg/Kg/day given in 4 divided doses is also found to be effective.

By 6 weeks after the end of treatment clinical evaluation of the patient should be done. Clinical criteria include closing of the ulcer and lack of relapse during follow-up. Search for parasites should be negative and there should not be granulomatous or plasmocytic inflammation in the biopsy specimen. Indirect IF titires must be lower than 1:16 in case of mucosal lesions in addition to the above criteria.

Local Treatment

Intralesional pentavalent antimony may be effective and is recommended in patients in whom systemic therapy is contraindicated or in patients with limited disease and is given on alternate days or weekly until resolution occurs. A combination of 15% paromomycin and 12% methylbenzethonium chloride in white paraffin applied twice daily has a cure rate of about 87% used in 30 days but paromomycin has an irritant effect.

Heat therapy has been tried in localized lesions, includes infrared radiation and therapeutic ultrasound. Using infrared radiation the skin temperature is raised to 55% and maintained for 5 minutes with good results with 2 treatments. Therapeutic ultrasound delivered at intensity of 0.5 to 3W/cm^2 two or three times weekly for a total of 10 to 15 treatments has shown good results in 5 to 10 weeks. Cryotherapy by using cryoprobe or cotton tipped applicator is of some value but better results have been obtained when combined with intralesional stibogluconate. Carbon dioxide laser, curettage, curettage with electrodessication and surgical excision are other modalities of therapy.

Though many modalities are used in adults they have been adequately evaluated in children.

AMEBIASIS

Amebiasis caused by *Entamoeba histolytica* is more prevalent in South-East Asia. Cutaneous amebiasis is a rare condition and occurs usually in the tropics or lesions are one to many and progress as sloughing or coalescing ulcers for about 2 weeks to 2 years and in the young they spread rapidly and are destructive. The lesions are found around the anus, buttocks/perineum, genitalia, trunk and legs. Amebic ulcers are oval with irregular, necrotic, ragged or verrucous borders which extend peripherally. Pain and lymphadenopathy are the common features. Skin lesions develop most frequently in patients with poor general health as a consequence of fistulous extension from gastrointestinal tract of hepatic abscess.

'Amebids' are thought to be the nonspecific hypersensitivity response to infection with E. histolytica the features of which include pruritus, urticaria, rosacea, facial melanosis, acne, eczematous dermatitis and prurigo nodules.

Microscopic examination of the fresh material taken from the edge of a cutaneous ulcer avoiding necrotic tissue by using special stains like periodic acid-schiff discloses the organism. Best test for specific diagnosis of amoebiasis in clinical settings is enzyme immunoassay (EIA) which has a sensitivity and specificity of 95%.

Metronidazole in the dose of 35-50 mg /kg/day in 3 divided dose is the drug of choice. In infants prognosis is poor in serious cases if neglected, but early diagnosis and treatment have a good prognosis.

TOXOPLASMOSIS

Toxoplasmosis is a common infection seen all over the world with a high prevalence in areas with more frequent ingestion of meat that is not cooked well and by environmental contact with the excreta of the cats. The definitive host is the cat while rodents and birds are the intermediate hosts. The infection is acquired by eating raw eggs or by ingestion of food or water contaminated with oocysts. Saliva, urine, semen, blood or blood cells are the other potential sources of infection.

The causative agent of toxoplasmosis is *Toxoplasma gondii* which is an obligate intracellular parasite that exists in 3 forms: tachyzoites characterize acute infection; bradyzoites within cysts characterize chronic latent infection and sporozoites, which develop only in the intestine of members of the cat family and are the sexual stage of the organism.

Human infection is common although 80-90% of persons affected are asymptomatic. Congenital infection can occur from immunocompetent mothers having infection for the first time or from immunocompromized mothers who have acute or chronic infection. If the infection is acquired by the foetus during the first trimester (though infrequent) it is most severe whereas infection acquired in the third trimester (though more frequent) is less severe at birth.

They can produce chorioretinitis in older children with congenitally acquired infection.

Clinical Manifestations

Congenital toxoplasmosis: Though hydrocephalus, chorioretinitis and intracranial calcification constitute the triad of clinical manifestations, congenital toxoplasmosis can present with varied manifestations. Cutaneous involvement is often seen in association with hepatic involvement in the form of jaundice that persists for several months. Petechiae and ecchymoses may progress to hemorrhagic lesions. In approximately 25% of patients erythematous to bluish macules, papules or nodules are seen. There may be subcutaneous plaques which may progress to necrosis or calcification.

Acquired toxoplasmosis: Clinical signs can develop at any stage though they are most common during childhood. In immuno competent children who acquire the disease postnatally the clinical signs of the disease may not be there. If present they are non-specific like intermittent fever, stiff neck, myalgia, bone pain, localized or generalized lymphadenopathy, hepatomegaly, hepatitis, splenomegaly, meningitis, encephalitis, confusion, malaise, pneumonia, polymyositis, pericarditis, pericardial effusion and myocarditis. Cutaneous manifestations include erythema multiforme like and roseola like lesions, purpuric, lichenoid, vegetating, vesicular or bullous lesions which may be hemorrhagic and may be accompanied by telangiectasia.

Diagnosis

Diagnosis can be established by isolation of the organism from blood or body fluids and by identification of tachyzoites in sections or preparations from tissues and body fluids, cysts in the placenta or tissues of a fetus or newborn. Serologic tests are very useful in the diagnosis but are less reliable in the first week of life and multiple serologic tests may be necessary to confirm the diagnosis of congenital or acutely acquired toxoplasmosis. They include Sabin-Feldman dye test, IgG indirect fluorescent antibody test (IgG-IFA), agglutination test, IgM indirect fluorescent anybody (IgM-IFA) test, double-sandwich ELISA, immunosorbent agglutination assay (ISAGA), Enzyme Linked Immunofiltration Assay (ELIFA), indirect hemagglutination (IHA) test and polymerase chain reaction.

Treatment

Early institution of specific treatment for congenital infection cures the manifestations including active chorioretinitis meningitis, encephalitis, hepatitis, splenomegaly and thrombocytopenia.

Pyrimethamine 0.5 to 1 mg /kg/day in two divided doses daily or on alternate days for a period of 3 to 4 weeks is the main therapeutic option. It is used in combination with sulphonamides in variable dosage for 2 to 4 months in the immuno competent and for at least 6 months in the immuno compromised patients. Spiramycin in a dose of 50 to 100 mg/kg/day admistered twice daily for 3 to 4 weeks is an alternate option. In some patients high dose trimethoprim-sulfamethoxazole twice daily in 3 week cycles has been found to be adequate. Other drugs that have been tried include roxithromycin and azithromycin. To prevent congenital transmission, pregnant women with toxoplasmosis should be treated with spiramycin for the first 17 weeks of gestation and then with pyrimethamine and sulphadiazine till delivery. Pregnant women should be counseled about the methods of transmission.

HELMINTHIC INFECTIONS

Helminthic infections occur, are more often seen in the developing and tropical countries. Because of the increased migration of people they are seen uncontrolled. Geographic factors, occupation, personal hygiene, dietary habits, living style and hobbies play important role in the causation and spread of these infections. Often the skin lesions are a clue to the diagnosis of underlying infection.

ONCHOCERCIASIS

(Blinding filariasis, river blindness, coastal erysipelas, Mal Morado, sowda, craw-craw)

The filarial nematode [round worm] Oncho-cerca vovulus is the causative agent of onchocerciasis. Infection is transmitted by Simulium fly (buffalo-gnats) which breed near flowing water, thus the name river blindness. The infection is more prevalent in children in hyper endemic areas of west Africa microfilaria are detected in up to 2% of children younger than 5 years and in 90% of children who are 15 years old. Though blindness is rare in young children, impaired vision begins to occur by second decade of life.

The larvae penetrate the skin and migrate through the connective tissue and several worms of both sexes coil together and form fibrous nodules (1 to 2 cm in diameter) most commonly over the bony prominences. Females live for up to 15 years and produce millions of microfilaria which produce the signs and symptoms and migrate from the nodule to the skin and other tissues.

Clinical Features

Most of the attacked individuals are asymptomatic but in heavily infected persons clinical manifestations are the result of localized host immune response to dead or dying microfilariae.

Apart from subcutaneous nodules major clinical manifestations are seen in the skin, lymph nodes and eye. Around 1 year after the initiation of infection skin manifestations begin. Pruritus (gale filarienne or filarial itch) and a localized eruption are the initial manifestations, can be associated with urticaria, fever and arthralgia. In children and in the earliest cases in the endemic areas there will be an infiltrated appearance of the skin giving rise to obliteration of skin markings associated with smaller, itchy papules and pustules. The early lesions are usually seen over the shoulders and around pelvis. Erysipelas de la Costa, an acute swelling on the face and cheeks with erythema and itching is seen in the acute phase more so in central Africa. In chronic onchocerciasis the skin lesions are macules and lichenoid papules varying in size from 3 to 9 mm associated with pruritus. In Arabic populations the lesions can be associated with hyperpigmentation and is called as "Sowdah" or "Sowda". Hypo and hyperpigmentaion is characteristic and is called as "Leopard skin" (depigmentation and perifollicular hyperpigmentation wth macular or minimally depressed areas). Aftrophic changes are seen more commonly over the buttocks, shoulders or lower limbs. The skin appears dry, shiny and wrinkled resembling tissue paper. The extreme form of this is referred to as "Lizard skin". Degeneration of dermal supporting tissues associated with massive inguinal adenopathy gives rise to "hanging groin" which is an apron like fold of skin containing lymphnodes. Other variants include an urticarial eruption and an inflammatory rash with hyper pigmentation called as "mal morade".

Asymptomatic onchocercial nodules (onchocercomas) containing the adult worms are seen over the bony prominences.

Eye involvement is the most serious complication. In children the early ocular changes include inflammation due to the death of microfilaria in the cornea, which causes punctate keratitis that may heal without treatment. But after years visual loss and blindness may result from sclerotic keratitis, anterior uveitis, chorioretinal lesions or optic nerve involvement.

Diagnosis

Demonstration of microfilaria in the skin by taking a skin strip is the standard method. The diagnosis can also be made by identification of adult worms by excision of the lymphnodes. If the microfilariae are present in the anterior chamber of the eye they can be detected by slit lamp examination. Inspite of a firm clinical diagnosis if all the above test are negative, a single dose of diethyl carbamazine (DEC) in a dose of 0.5-1 mg /kg can be administered to produce the Mazzotti reaction which is due to the death of microfilariae and is characterized by pruritus, maculopapular rash, fever, edema and headache. Measurement of total antifilarial IgG and IgG subclasses can be useful. Serum based ELISA and PCR have also been developed.

Treatment

Ivermectin in a single dose of 150 µg/kg is very effective and reduces the microfilaria density in the skin by 85 to 95% in 2 months, though ocular microfilaria density declines slowly. It may be repeated after 3-6 months if there are symptoms or evidence of eye infection and appears to be less effective in reducing chronic skin depigmentation and posterior ocular diseases.

DEC which was widely used before the advent of ivermectin is very rarely used and is known to cause severe exacerbation of the skin and eye disease and may even cause blindness. DEC is given in the following dosage:

Days 1 to 3—1 mg/kg body weight once daily
Days 4 to 7—2 mg/kg body weight once daily
2nd week—4 mg /kg body weight thrice daily
3rd week—4 mg /kg body weight thrice daily.

During treatment, collapse and death can occur in heavily infected patients. Before starting DEC, prednisolone in dose of 40 mg daily should be given and continued till the reaction settles.

Though suramin is a drug that kills adult worms (microfilaria), it is seldom used because of its toxicity.

Surgical excision of the nodules is recommended. Nodulectomy is usually combined with microfilaricide. Nodulectomy alone without drugs has shown to reduce the microfilarial levels by about 60% by 5 months after the surgery. Though it may reduce the burden of eye disease it cannot cure the disease or reduce transmission.

LOIASIS

[Calabar swellings, Fugitive swellings, Loa Loa filariasis, African eyeworm infection]

Loa Loa, the filarial nematode (roundworm) is the parasite that causes Loiasis. The disease is endemic in central and west Africa. It is transmitted through the bite of tabanid (horse, mangrove and deer) flies of the genus chrysops. Infection is transmitted by the fly from person to person.

Clinical Features

The clinical manifestations are pruritus, urticaria and calabar swellings (Cameroon or fugitive swelling). Calabar swellings are due to the migration of the adult worms in the subcutaneous tissue. They are erythematous and warm, 5-10 cm in diameter and may be associated with pain and pruritus, last for several days and recur many times. Though they can appear anywhere on the body they are more common over the wrist and knee. They may be associated with fatigue, myalgia, arthralgias and fever. Adult worms may be seen migrating while crossing the conjunctiva or the bridge of the nose giving the name "eye worm". At this stage there will be swelling of the face. Arthritis, lymphadenopathy, lymphedema, peripheral neuropathy, cardiomyopathy, proteinuria, hematuria and encephalopathy are the less common manifestations.

Diagnosis

Confirmation of the diagnosis is by detection of microfilariae in the peripheral blood taken during the day time or by nicking the conjunctiva and releasing the worm while traversing in the eye. Blood examination reveals eosinophilia (>3000 cells/mm^3), increased serum IgE and antifilarial antibody levels. Genus specific filarial serology by immunofluorescence or ELISA is usually positive and is useful in patients without microfilaraemia.

Treatment

Diethylcarbamazine (DEC) is the drug of choice and is given in a dose of 8-10 mg/kg/day in 3 doses for 21 days. In children with high microfilarial levels the dose of DEC should be increased gradually as follows:

1 mg /kg orally as a single dose on day 1;

1 mg/kg orally tid on day 2;

1-2 mg/kg orally tid on day 3;

6 mg/kg/24 hrs divided tid doses on days 4 to 14.

Side effects are mild and include fever, malaise, swelling of joints of arms and pruritus. In heavy infections there is risk of encephalitis with headache, giddiness, vomiting, purpura and eosinophilia, occasionally death. Elongated subcutaneous nodules indicating the presence of worms may appear after DEC therapy.

For patients not responding to DEC ivermectin in a dose of 200 μg/kg has a good response and reduces microfilaraemia. Albendazole used in a 3 week course reduces the microfilarial levels due to its embryotoxic effect on the adult worms. Surgical removal of the worm from the eye or other tissue can be done.

LYMPHATIC FILARIASIS (TROPICAL ELEPHANTIASIS)

Lymphatic filariasis is more commonly seen in people living in tropical Africa, Asia and Latin America with a clinical morbidity of up to 20%. The disease is caused by filarial worms Wuchereria bancrofti (Bancroftian filariasis), Brugia malayi (malayan filariasis) and Brugia timori. Infection due to W. bancrofti is more wide spread in Africa, Asia and Latin America accounting for up to 90% of cases of lymphatic filariasis. Mosquitoes of the genera Culex, Aedes, Mansonia and Anopheles transmit the infection by ingestion of the blood from the affected humans. After the bite, in the human the larvae pass through the peripheral lymphatics, mature and mate in the lymphatics proximal to the lymphnodes. Microfilariae are discharged principally at night. Lymphatic obstruction the main pathological feature is due to the inflammatory response to the presence of the worms. The adult worms live in the lymphatics for 5-10 years. The microfilaria entrapped in the lung causes tropical eosinophilia.

Clinical Features

The infection is asymptomatic in most of the affected. The clinical manifestations are similar in all the types. In the infected children filarial lymphadenopahy is commonly seen. The initial signs that are often seen include swelling, tenderness and erythema of the arms, legs, which are due to lymphangitis and lymphadenitis. Most patients have acute attacks of fever (filarial fever), headache and malaise, which last for 3-15 days and are accompanied by high eosinophilia and microfilaraemia.

Lymphangitis is recurrent with 6-10 episodes per year. In between the initial episodes the attested limb appears clinically normal, occasionally these may be exfoliation of the skin.

Recurrent cellulitis and edema occurring for many years result in chronic manifestations due to lymphatic obstruction and dilatation of lymph vessels by adult worms and host immune response usually after 10-15 years in endemic areas and within 2 years in non-endemic areas. In this stage in about 50% of the male patients hydrocele occurs in addition to lower leg edema and elephantiasis. In females there can be involvement of breasts and genitalia in addition to the limits. Blockage of the lymphatics around the bladder and their rupture into the urinary tract can produce chyluria (lymph causing milky urine). At this stage the microfilariae are not detectable in the blood. The skin over the affected area is hypertrophic, verrucous and fibrotic and has redundant folds. Secondary bacterial infection, fungal infection, fissures, ulceration and gangrene may occur. The elephantiasis most commonly involves the lower limb, scrotum and penis. Upper limb, breast and vulva are less commonly involved and ears, oral mucosa and periorbital area can be rarely involved. Infection due to B. malayi usually involves the lower extremities, it is not severe and genital lesions are less common.

Tropical pulmonary eosinophilia reported mostly from Asia is a syndrome of filarial aetiology in which microfilariae are found in the lungs and lymphnodes not in blood. Though children are occasionally affected it is more common in men between 20-40 years of age and occurs only in individuals who have lived in endemic areas for many years. The clinical features include paroxysmal nocturnal cough with dyspnea, fever, weight loss and fatigue. In children hepatomegaly and generalized lymphadenopathy are often seen.

Diagnosis

In endemic areas the diagnosis can be made clinically. Detection of microfilaria in peripheral blood films taken between 10 pm and 2 am is diagnostic and the three species can be distinguished morphologically. Detection of filarial antigen by filarial antigen card testing is highly sensitive and specific for W. bancrofti and avoids the need for collection of blood at night. Ultrasonography is useful in detection of the adult worms especially in children in which the movement of the worm can be seen ("Filaria dance sign").

Treatment

Diethylcarbamazine (DEC) is the drug of choice and is recommended in the dose of 6 mg/kg/day for 12 days but single dose of 6 mg/kg is also found to be effective.

In areas where lymphatic filariasis and onchocerciasis coexist DEC should be administered with special caution. Though ivermectin (400 μg/kg) is used it does not kill the adult worms.

In late stages where there will be irreversible damage to the lymphatics and elephantiasis, maintenance of good hygiene, prevention of bacterial and fungal infections, exercise, elevation of the affected part, compression stockings, prevention of trauma are the important measures. Surgical treatment may help to improve the appearance which includes debulking of the affected area, lymphnode-venous shunt. Hydroceles can be drained repeatedly or surgery can be performed.

DRACUNCULIASIS

[Dracontiasis, Guinea worm, Medina worm, Dragon worm, Dracunculosis, serpent worm]

Dracunculiasis is a chronic infection caused by the guinea worm Dracunculus medinensis. Humans are the definitive hosts and the main reservoir of infection. The disease is more common in parts of India, west, east and central Africa and is particularly intense in Ghana, on the west coast and the valley of Nile. The disease is more in rural populations where it can spread in and around communal drinking step wells and washing areas or wells.

By drinking water containing infected Cyclops the larvae enter the gastrointestinal tract and penetrate the intestine. By about one year the female worm migrates usually to the subcutaneous tissue in the lower limbs (occasionally elsewhere) causing a papule. Finally the lesion vesiculates, ruptures and a painful ulcer through which the worm can be seen is formed.

Clinical Features

Before the appearance of the worm through the skin there may be fever, pruritus, urticaria, edema, dyspnea and diarrhoea. The first sign is a papule or vesicle which expands and bursts in about 4-5 days with an induration of 2 to 7 cms. There is intense itching at the site of the emergence of the worm through the skin. The ulcer surrounding the worm is covered with slough. Often the worm is palpable. The worm may be calcified or reabsorbed. In upto 90% of cases the lower limb is the affected site but occasionally the lesions may be seen on the hands, arms and trunk. Secondary infection is the major cause of morbidity and is very common which may result in disability and can be the entry point of tetanus.

Pericardium, spinal canal, eye, broad ligament, testicle and other deep tissues are the other sites in which the worm has been found. Occasionally the worm may find its way to the joint and result in intra articular infection.

Diagnosis

Emergence of the worm through the skin is diagnostic. By applying water to the extruded segment the adult can be induced to shed larvae. Calcified worms can be detected by X-ray. During migration in the tissue eosinophilia is common.

Treatment

Removal of the worm is the main treatment which can be facilitated by giving oral metronidazole 400 mg thrice daily for 5 days or thiabendazole 50 mg per kg in divided doses twice daily for 3 days. This reduces the inflammation and allows gentle extraction of the worm. Water or ethyl chloride can be applied which induces the worm to discharge the larvae and the free end of the worm is wound to a match stick. The worm is wrapped around the stick everyday by few centimeters and finally the whole worm can be removed. Not much of tension is to be exerted because the rupture of the worm causes severe inflammatory reaction resulting in cellulitis. Hence the procedure takes several days. Additional treatment includes local antiseptics, tetanus toxoid and sometimes broad spectrum antibiotics. As the drug treatment does not affect the larvae or capable of preventing transmission providing clean drinking water, filtration of water to remove cyclops, chemical control of cyclops by using larvicides are found to be useful.

ENTEROBIASIS

[Thread worm, Pinworm, Seatworm, Oxyuriasis]

Enterobius vermicularis is the causative agent of enterobiasis. The infection is world wide and is more prevalent in cold climates and has an association with poverty and overcrowding. It most commonly affects children and females are more affected than males. Humans are the only natural hosts and the infection is acquired by ingestion of eggs. The most common mechanism appears to be direct fecal-oral spread. Transmission may also occur by ingesting infected food and drink.

Clinical Features

A large number of infected children are asymptomatic. Most common symptom is anal and perianal pruritus that is intense at night often leading to sleeplessness and irritability. Scratching may result in secondary skin changes like eczematous dermatitis, hemorrhage, and secondary bacterial infection. Foreign body granulomas involving the wall of the anal canal and ischiorectal abscess have been reported. Vulval irritation and mucoid discharge can result due to genital involvement **(Figure 8.1)**. In situations such as salpingitis, omenitis, peritonitis, and granuloma of the uterus, ovary and pelvic peritoneum, the parasite is thought to ascend the vagina and enter the peritoneal cavity through the fallopian tubes.

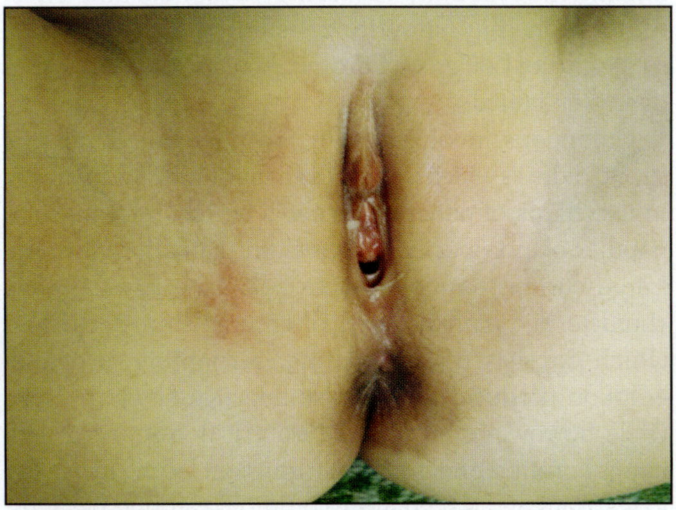

FIGURE 8.1: Vulvovaginitis due to pinworm

Diagnosis

Scotch tape test is the diagnostic test which is optimally done before the patient takes bath or defecates. Sometimes pinworms can be seen with the naked eye on the perianal area at night and resemble pieces of white thread. Worms may be found on the stool surface. Stool examination for eggs is of little value as it is positive only in about 5% of the cases, but eggs may be detected underneath the fingernails in upto 60% of the affected.

Treatment

Mebendazole is the drug of choice. Though single dose of mebendazole cures over 90% of infections, recurrence is common. Most effective dosage is 100 mg twice daily for 3 days, repeated after 2 weeks is highly effective. Alternate regimens include single dose pyrantel pamoate 10 mg/kg, piperazine citrate 65 mg/kg daily for 6 days.

Attention should be paid to cleanliness of hands after defecation and before eating. In children fingernails should be clipped short which prevents fecal-oral spread and thumb sucking should be discouraged. After each dosing, bed linen should be changed.

ANCYLOSTOMIASIS

Classic hookworm disease is caused by Ancylostoma duodenale (old world hook worm) and Necator americanus (new world hookworm) which are anthropophilic and less commonly by A. ceylanium, A. caninum and A. braziliense which are zoonotic species. The infection is more prevalent in Pakistan, China, India, Indonesia, Japan, Philippines, North America and South America. The most common mode of transmission is by exposure of unprotected skin to fecally contaminated soil harbouring the infective filariform larvae and contact of 5-10 minutes is sufficient. Infection may also be acquired when the infected filariform larvae present in the ingested raw plant food penetrate the oral or intestinal mucosa and transmission through breast milk has also been reported.

Clinical Features

In the majority of patients the infection is asymptomatic or mild. After penetration of the skin the larvae produce an immediate stinging sensation followed by skin changes within 2 days. Dermatitis known as "ground itch" or "coolie itch" develops within 2 days and is attributed to the secretions produced by the migrating larvae and to the inflammatory response of the host. Erythematous papules which last for 7-10 days are usually seen. Patients with repetitive reinfection may develop severe papulation, vesiculation, folliculitis and edema of the extremity with regional lymphadenitis, which persist for more than

2 weeks. Rarely creeping eruption may be seen. There may be associated urticaria, cough, bronchitis and pneumonitis occasionally occur during larval migration through the lungs. During the stage of larval migration over the epiglottis to the oesophagus there can be a distinct symptomatic phase with dysphagia, dysphonia, laryngitis and pharyngitis as early as 3 days after infection and may last upto 2 weeks. Although light infections do not produce abdominal symptoms heavy infections are associated with abdominal pain, anorexia, indigestion, postprandial fullness, nausea, vomiting, flatulence and gastrointestinal bleeding. Growth and developmental retardation occur in heavily infected children. Pica and geophagia may be seen. Chronic infection leads to anemia and hypoalbuminemia and the patient can present with lassitude, dyspnea on exertion, edema of the lower extremities, pallor, dizziness and anorexia. Some children with chronic hookworm disease acquire yellow-green pallor known as chlorosis. Severe anemia may contribute to high fetal and maternal mortality. Hook worm anemia may result in two distinct types of cutaneous depigmentation. The first is due to iron deficiency which is almost always present and begins to recover before the correction of anemia is complete. The second one is associated with hypoalbuminemia and is severe and resembles the one seen in kwashiorkor, primarily involving perineum, extremities and face and improves slowly with treatment. In those patients with heavy parasite burden angular stomatitis, chelosis, koilonychia, retinal hemorrhage and pallor are common.

Diagnosis

The diagnosis of hookworm infection is by identifying the typical eggs in the stool. In heavy infections ordinary direct saliva smear using 1% potassium and a small amount of feces is useful. In light infections zinc sulfate concentration technique or the formalin-ether technique are done. It is essential to remember that during the cutaneous and pulmonary phases of infection eggs will not be present. In chronic infection laboratory values reveal iron deficiency anemia, hypoalbuminemia and eosinophilia. Gross or occult blood in the stool is found. There are no satisfactory serologic and skin tests available.

Treatment

Mebendazole in a dose of 100 mg twice daily is highly effective. Alternate drugs are albendazole in a single dose of 400 mg or single dose of pyrantel pamoate 11mg/kg upto a maximum of 1G. None of these drugs are recommended in pregnancy and are reserved until after delivery. Ground itch is treated with topical corticosteroids and oral antihisamines. Pulmonary symptoms and anemia should be treated promptly.

STRONGYLOIDIOSIS

[Strongyloidal ground itch, larva currens]

Strongyloidosis is caused by intestinal nematode Strongyloides stercoralis. An uncommon cause of human strongyloidiosis is S fulleborni, a parasite of oldworld monkeys. S. stercoralis is unique by virtue of its ability to complete its lifecycle in humans without exogenous reinfection. Strongyloidiosis is more common in the tropics and subtropics. Persons who come in contact with soil in warm, moist areas contaminated with human feces are at high risk. Individuals on longterm steroids, immunosuppressive therapy, and malnutrition are more prone to infection. In mental institutions outbreaks of disease occur due to direct person to person transmission as a result of poor fecal hygiene.

Clinical Features

Cutaneous involvement is uncommon in acute stage. Gastrointestinal symptoms are more common. Pulmonary symptoms occur during larval migration through the lungs and include cough, wheezing, dyspnea and chest radiograph may show a transient, patchy infiltrate suggestive of Loffler's syndrome. Acute strongyloidiosis is often self limited.

Cutaneous involvement is the hallmark of chronic strongloidiosis which is reported in about 90% of patients. In two thirds of patients there will be recurrent maculopapular or nonspecific urticarial eruptions, pruritus ani. Larva currens ("running larva", "tracing larva") is the characteristic manifestation of chronic strongyloidiosis, which consists of a migrating, serpentine, urticarial eruption produced by a single infective filariform larva while burrowing through the skin. It is associated with intense pruritus and is typically transient lasting few hours to few days and is seen more commonly around the anus, buttocks, perineum and thighs. The advancing edge of larva currens migrates at a rate of 5-10 cms per hour. Other secondary skin changes associated with chronic strongyloidiosis include prurigo nodularis and lichen simplex chronicus.

Gastrointestinal and pulmonary manifestations similar to acute illness can be seen but are less severe.

Patients with hyperinfection and disseminated disease manifest with petichae and purpuric eruption due to massive filariform larvae dissemination to the skin and these lesions are diffuse and rapidly progressing typically involving the trunk and proximal extremities. A unique pattern of periumbilical purpura which resembles multiple thumb prints is called as "thumb print sign".

"Swollen baby syndrome" is a distinct and fulminant form of neonatal strongyloidiosis caused by S. fuelleborni. The components include protracted diarrhoea beginning in the first months of life, failure to thrive, protein malnutrition and kwashiorkor-like appearance attributable to hypoalbuminemia.

Diagnosis

Diagnosis is by examining the feces for the characteristic larvae by direct smear or concentration method such as formaldehyde-ether or Baermann test. Multiple examinations should be done. Other options include small bowel biopsy, duodenal or jejunal aspiration or the string test. In hyperinfective and disseminated disease larvae can be recovered from sputum, bronchoalveolar lavage fluid and in some cases in the cerebrospinal fluid. ELISA or IgE antibody test may be more sensitive. Serologic assays to detect subclinical infection have been designed, which help in the diagnosis in persons from endemic area presenting with unexplained eosinophilia.

Treatment

Ivermectin in a single dose of 200 μg/kg body weight to be repeated after one week is very effective and less toxic compared to thiabendazole which is given in a dose of 25 mg/kg body weight orally twice daily for 3 days and repeated after 2 and 4 weeks. However in patients with hyperinfection syndrome ivermectin has to be given for 7-10 days and repeated courses may be required. Albendazole in a dose of 400 mg/day is also effective and mebendazole can be an alternative, but is useful only in gastrointestinal disease. Fecal and jejunal samples should be examined for larvae after 3 and 6 months. Treatment of concomitant infection is an integral part of therapy.

CUTANEOUS LARVA MIGRANS

[Creeping eruption, sandworm eruption]

There are some parasites which affect the wild and domestic animals and the infective larvae of them complete their evolutionary cycle within their respective hosts. If humans, the abnormal hosts are affected by these larvae they are not able to mature or develop fully and hence they wander or migrate through the subcutaneous or viscoid tissues. When the nematodes penetrate the human skin and do not complete their lifecycles they make a tunnel in the epidermis and rarely they cross the basal layer to reach the dermis resulting in the condition called as cutaneous larva migrans (CLM). When the nematodes enter the oral route they migrate to the liver, lungs or other organs resulting in visceral larva migrans.

Primarily the animal hookworms that usually affect the dogs and cats cause CLM. A. braziliense is the most common agent. High temperature and humidity favor the transmission. Humans become infected by direct contact with soil fecally contaminated by cats or dogs. The common sites are the feet, bultocks, knees and involvement of upper extremity occurs more commonly in animal handlers and Gardener.

After penetrating the skin larvae tunnel in the epidermis and rarely cross the basal layer to reach the dermis. They migrate at a rate of few millimeters per day. It is thought that they remain confined to the epidermis because they lack the specific enzymes necessary for penetrating the basement membrane. However in their natural host they penetrate the dermis and hence the course is similar to that of A. duodenale and N. americanus in humans.

Clinical Features

A reddish pruritic papule or non-specific dermatitis develops at the site of penetration of the larva. Often there will be history of tingling or pricking sensation at the time of penetration. After several days the larva begins to migrate at a rate of upto 2 cm per day producing a linear or serpiginous trace that is slightly elevated. Often vesiculobullous lesions are seen within or around the track. Occasionally a distinct reactive eosinophilic papular folliculitis may develop in the area. The larva is located about 1-2 cm proximal to the advancing edge usually. The patient complains of intense pruritus more severe in the night which occasionally leads to excoriation and secondary bacterial infection. Swelling of the foot and pain are occasionally seen. If CLM is unrecognized or untreated, the larvae usually die in 2-8 weeks but rarely may persist upto one year. Loffler's syndrome and asthmatic reactions are reported particularly in massive infections.

Diagnosis

The diagnosis is mainly clinical because recovery of the larva from the advancing skin lesion is usually not possible and specific serologic test are not available.

Though eosinophilia and rise in total immunoglobulin E are typical they are not present in all cases.

CLM should be differentiated from larva currens produced by S. stercoralis which is usually found in the perianal area and the larvae move at a great speed of 10 cm per hour. Other diseases that mimic CLM are granuloma annulare, porokeratosis of Mibelli and erythema annulare centrifugum but can be differentiated by history, symptoms and morphology.

Treatment

Systemic thiabendazole in a dose of 25-50 mg/kg/day given twice daily for 2-3 days not exceeding a daily dose of 3G is the treatment of choice. Pruritus resolves within 48 hours and the lesions disappear in about 10 days. As soon as the treatment is begun there can be a transient worsening of the symptoms probably due to larval death and release of inflammatory products. If active lesions persist a second dose may be required. Side effects include anorexia, nausea, diarrhoea, abdominal cramps, dizziness and cutaneous rash which may be severe enough to affect compliance. Topical thiabendazole is useful in cases infected with few larvae. It is available as 10% solution containing 100 mg per ml and is applied 4-5 times per day to the affected area especially to the end of the track and is continued for 2-3 days after the disappearance of the lesions. Topical dexamethasone cream 0.1% can be overlaid and covered with an occlusive polyethylene film or it may be combined with dimethyl sulfoxide. Results are favourable without significant toxicity.

Oral thiabendazole in a single dose of 400 mg is effective but in patients with extensive lesions a 3 day course is necessary.

Ivermectin in a single dose of 200 μg/kg has been shown to be highly effective and well tolerated.

When the disease is associated with secondary bacterial infection topical or systemic antibiotics are necessary. Older topical therapeutic modalities like liquid nitrogen, dry ice and ethyl chloride are not found to be useful.

TOXOCARIASIS

[Visceral larva migrans] [VLM]

Toxocariasis is caused by Toxocara canis, T. cati most often and rarely by Baylisascaris (Bayliscaris) procyonis and lagochiloscaris minor. T. caris is the commonest agent and the infection is reported in nearly all the parts of the world, more so in temperate and tropical areas where dogs are popular pets. T. cani and T. cati resemble ascariasis lumbricoides in their life cycle, nutritional requirement and physiologic behavior but are smaller than ascaris. Humans are accidental hosts and toxocara cannot reach maturity in human hosts.

Clinical Features

Most infections are asymptomatic or not recognized. VLM is primarily seen in children below 5 years. The clinical feature includes fever, cough, dyspnoea, hepatosplenomegaly, muscle pain and failure to gain weight. Myocarditis, nephritis and central nervous system symptoms like seizures, neuropsychiatric symptoms, and encephalopathy have been described.

Though the incidence of cutaneous manifestations is not known they include generalized pruritus, urticarial and papular eruptions involving the trunk and legs are reported more often. Migratory panniculitis is rarely reported but is pathognomonic and is characterized by tender subcutaneous nodules that last for 1-2 weeks.

Ocular larva migrans (OLM) occurs usually in older children and is characterized by unilateral visual impairment due to formation of granulomas. It can also result in diffuse endophthalmitis, papillitis and secondary glaucoma.

Diagnosis

Persistent eosinophilia (> 25 × 10°L), hypergammaglobulinemia of the IgG and IgM classes are seen. Biopsy of a cutaneous nodule of liver can be confirmatory. ELISA and EIA are often useful.

Treatment

Albendazole in a dose of 10 mg/kg/day in two divided doses for 5 days is the drug of choice. Cure rates are low with thiabendazole and diethyl carbamazine. Ocular larva migrans can be treated with surgery in addition to oral medications.

GNATHOSTOMIASIS

Gnathostomiasis is a nematode infection caused by Gnathostoma spinigerum more commonly, and less commonly by G. hispidium, G. nipponium and G.doloresi. Human gnathostomiasis is more endemic in South-East Asia with greatest number of cases in Thailand.

Clinical Features

The signs and symptoms can be mild to severe and being 1 to 2 days after the ingestion of the larva which include fever, malaise, anorexia, nausea, vomiting, diarrhoea, epigastric pain and urticaria occasionally. Later intermittent migratory subcutaneous swellings associated with pain, erythema, pruritus develop which may be multiple and disappear by 4 weeks to reappear in a different location after an interval of weeks to months. The usual sites of involvement include the trunk, thighs and upper body including the orbit. There can be abscesses in the subcutaneous tissue or the muscle. Over time the episodes become less frequent, less severe, shorter in duration and may continue for years.

Other organs that may be involved include the eye, lungs, gastrointestinal tract, genito urinary tract and central nervous system. There is an increased risk of ocular involvement that may result in visual loss or central nervous system involvement which can result in fatal encephalomyelitis.

Diagnosis

Surgical extraction of the worm is confirmatory. There will be high peripheral eosinophilia and leukocytosis. Cerebrospinal fluid can be bloody or xanthochromic and may contain eosinophils when central nervous system is involved. Serological tests are available in few centres.

Treatment

The disease is typically self limited. Albendazole 400 mg/day is effective when given for 6 months. Some have found a 21 day course to be effective. Surgical excision is also very useful. The efficacy of ivermectin is not well documented.

DIROFILARIASIS

Dirofilariasis is caused by Filarial nematodes of the genus dirofilaria; dirofilaria tenuis (Raccoon), D. immitus (dog heart worm), D. repens (dog) and D.ursi (bear). Subcutaneous dirofilariasis is caused by D. tenuis, D. ursi and D. repens. D. immitus mostly causes pulmonary dirofilariasis and rarely soft tissue infection.

Clinical Features

Symptoms usually start 2-3 months after the exposure to the parasite. The lesions are 1-2 cms in diameter, tender, erythematous to skin colored nodules which are occasionally migratory. Head, neck, eyelid, breast, arm, leg and scrotum are the common sites. The parasite may involve the conjunctiva and oral cavity and present as nodules. There can be associated arthritis. Though pulmonary dirofilariasis is asymptomatic in more than 50% of the patients cough, chest pain, hemoptysis and low grade fever can be the presenting symptoms. Microfilariae are not found in the blood. The parasites occasionally survive for years and dead and calcified worms may be found many years after acquiring the disease.

Diagnosis

Definite diagnosis is by surgical excision of the nodules and identification of the worm. Though ELISA is positive in about 75% of the patients cross reaction with other helmenthic infections limits its value. In pulmonary dirofilariasis chest X-ray reveals usually a single coin shaped nodule 1-3 cms in diameter which may be calcified. There may be low grade peripheral eosinophilia.

Treatment

Treatment is by surgical removal.

TRICHINOSIS

(Trichiniasis, Trichinelliasis, Trichenellosis)

Trichinosis is caused by the intestinal nematode Trichinella spiralis. Though it is distributed world wide it is endemic in USA and more prevalent in tropical, subtropical and polar locales. The human is the host and the infection is acquired by ingestion of raw or undercooked infected meat.

Clinical Features

Clinical features following consumption of raw or undercooked meat suggest diagnosis. In the early phase serologic tests are useful because they become positive by 2 weeks and in some patients antibodies have been detected by enzyme immuno assay as early as 12 days after infection. Detection of trichinella specific DNA by polymerase chain reaction for detecting the small number of larvae in the muscles is sensitive and specific but the availability is restricted.

Diagnosis

Diagnosis in the second phase is confirmed by demonstration of larvae by biopsy from the striated muscle. The best suited muscles are gastrocnemius and deltoid and the preferable part is near the tendinous insertion in which the yield is high.

Treatment

In the early stage of infection mebendazole may reduce the number of larvae and the clinical complications. Thiabenadazole may be beneficial in the early stages (25 mg/kg twice daily for 5-7 days), corticosteroids like prednisolone can be given as an anti-inflammatory agent but can prevent Jarisch – Hexheimer reaction. Analgesics are useful which should be continued till the fever recedes.

SCHISTOSOMIASIS

(Bilharziasis, Snail fever, Katayama fever)

Trematodes of the genus schistosoma cause the disease schistosomiasis. Man and other animals are the definitive hosts and snails of the various genera are the intermediate hosts. Schistosoma affecting the man are referred to as blood flukes. Schistosoma mansoni, S. japonicum and S. hematobium are the blood flukes causing infection in the humans. S. mansoni and S. Japonicum cause gastrointestinal and hepatic disease whereas S. hematobium causes urinary tract disease. Males are affected twice compared to females.

Infection in the humans occurs through contact with water contaminated with cercariae, the free-living infective stage of the parasite.

Clinical Features

Most of the infected persons are asymptomatic and about 12-15% will have symptoms and they are the ones who are heavily infected. Schistosomal dermatitis or swimmers itch resembling cercarial dermatitis occurs 1-2 days after exposue to the larvae and the affected individuals develop a macular, papular or urticarial rash that resolves by one week in those who have been previously sensitized. In those who are exposed for the first time it resolves within hours. Acute schistosomiasis or katayma fever (Katayama syndrome, yangtse or yellow river fever) is commonly seen in upto 50% of people infected with S. japonicum and is due to hypersensitivity response to schistosomal antigens and circulating immune complex. Symptoms usually persist for 2-10 weeks and include fever, malaise, cough, wheeze, urticaria, purpura, edema of the face, extremities, genitalia and trunk, abdominal pain, anorexia and diarrhea. There may be generalized lymphadenopathy, bronchitis, pneumonia and though rare cases of fatal katayama fever are reported. Katayama fever is less commonly reported with S. mansoni and rarely with S. hematobium. During the time of deposition of eggs late hypersensitivity reaction occurs which is characterized by urticaria, localised or generalized pruritus, excoriations and lichenified papules and plaques.

Symptomatic children infected with S. hematobium usually complain of dysuria, frequency and hematuria in the chronic stage. Untreated patients may develop chronic cystitis, obstructive uropathy, bladder dysfunction, calcification and even chronic renal failure. In symptomatic children infected with S. mansoni and japonicum the eggs are deposited in the intestinal mucosa and liver. The most common signs and symptoms include abdominal discomfort, diarrhea and passage of bloody stools. Liver is enlarged, nontender without jaundice and spleen is enlarged but tender.Untreated patients may develop portal hypertension, ascites and portosystemic varices at the lower end of oesophagus, rectum and around the umbilicus. Bilharziasis cutanea tarda, the late skin involvement occurs in patients with visceral disease. The mucocutaneous manifestations are due to deposition of eggs in the skin and they are the result of granulomatous reaction incited by the parasites. S. haematobium is the commonest species that deposit eggs in the skin followed by S. mansoni and S. japonicum. The lesions appear as scattered or grouped papules that may be asymptomatic or painful or pruritic which eventually develop into nodules or tumors.

The genital lesions may develop into warty, vegetating or polypoid tumors especially in females in whom mucosal involvement is more common. In the initial stages the granuloma will be exuberant, soft and erythematous, and becomes whitish and firm later due to fibrosis. In severe cases the lesions may extend to the crural folds, perineum, labia majora and clitoris which may become thickened and result in the development of a schistosomal caruncle at the urethral meatus and there may be pseudo-elephantasis of the vulva. In the males the penis and scrotum can be affected, ulcers, fissures and sinus tracts can develop in both sexes. Lesions can develop in the perianal region and buttocks.

Extragenital cutaneous involvement occurs less frequently seen. Other than the skin the eggs may be deposited in the lungs, central nervous system, ovaries, fallopian tubes, uterus, cervix, eyes and gall bladder.

Diagnosis

Diagnosis is aided by a good history. Eosinophilia is common in the acute stage and is rare is chronic stage. A urine dipstick test may show haematuria and proteinuria. Parasitological diagnosis is by finding the eggs in the stool or urine. Stool examination is done by concentration technique. Biopsy of the affected tissue can demonstrate eggs. Ultrasound examination of the liver, kidneys, bladder and ureters may be helpful. Abdominal radiography can show bladder calcification which is referred to as "fetal head" sign. Serologic tests are not useful is endemic areas. Biopsy is diagnostic in ectopic cutaneous schistosomiasis.

Treatment

Praziquantel is the drug of choice. It is given is a dose of 40 mg/kg/day (single or two divided doses) for S. mansoni and S. hematobium infection and 60 mg/kg in three divided doses for S. japonicum. A parasitological cure rate of 80% is seen and in those who are not cured egg burden is reduced by 95 to 99%. Metrifinate is a dose of 5-15 mg/kg given at 2 week intervals for 3 divided doses is useful in S. hematobium infections. Oxamniquine in a single dose of 1.5 mg/kg is effective in S. mansoni infections. Prognosis is guarded in patients with chronic lesions such as portal hypertension, esophageal varices and hydronephrosis.

CERCARIAL DERMATITIS

(Swimmer's itch, Clam diggois itch, Sedge pool itch, Koganbyo, Sawah itch, Batner's itch, Cardiff's tropical disease)

Infestation of the skin by cercariae of non-human schistosomes for which the usual hosts are the birds and small mammals causes cercarial dermatitis.

Cercarial dermatitis is most prevalent during warmer months because of more frequent bathing in contaminated water and cercarial production within the snail is at its peak.

Clinical Features

The clinical features differ in the first and the subsequent exposures. In the primary form ie occurring in unsensitized individuals an irritant reaction characterized by a prickly eruption consisting of small macules of 1-2 mm appear 10-15 minutes after the penetration of the cercariae and persist for about 10 hours. The manifestations sometimes can be so mild that they go unnoticed. In the secondary form which occurs in sensitized individuals the lesions become strikingly larger, persist longer and are severely pruritic. After the macular stage subsides in about 12 to 24 hours pruritic papules develop which are associated with localized edema and erythema which may become pustules and painful in about 48 hours and reach their peak in 72 hours. Purpuric and urticarial lesions may be seen. Though the involution occurs in about a week pruritus persists for about 2 weeks. Blisters and eczematous changes can be seen in more severe and protracted cases and secondary infection can lead to scarring. Nausea and vomiting can occur in severe cases. Usually the lesions are 10 to 30 in number but can be over 200 in severe cases. The lesions involve the skin surfaces that are exposed to water typically sparing the areas covered by clothing.

Diagnosis

Diagnosis is based on the characteristic clinical features and the epidemiological factors. Demonstration of cercariae in the suspected water supports the clinical diagnosis.

Treatment

The treatment is symptomatic. Systemic antihistamines and antiinflammatory drugs and topical steroids are useful. In severe cases systemic steroids can be used.

ECHINOCOCCOSIS

(Hydatid disease, Hydatidosis)

Echinococcosis is due to the infection with the larval stage of cestodes of the genus echinococcus. E. granulosus causes unilocular echinococcosis or cystic hydatid disease whereas E. multilocularis causes multilocular echinococcosis or alveolar hydatid disease.

Clinical Features

Majority of the cysts occur in the liver and many never become symptomatic and regress spontaneously. In those presenting with symptoms there will be increased abdominal girth, hepatomegaly, jaundice, palpable mass, vomiting and abdominal pain. When the lungs are involved the symptoms include chest pain, cough and hemoptysis. When bones are involved there may be pathologic fractures and there can be hematuria or infertilities when the genitourinary system is involved. Cerebral involvement is characterized by seizures or signs of increased intracranial pressure of subacute onset resembling a slow-growing brain tumour and in patients with alveolar hydatid disease the neurological manifestations tend to evolve more rapidly and are more severe than in those with cystic hydatid disease. Spinal cord involvement may be associated with root pain, motor and sensory defects. Unilateral proptosis can be seen when these is orbital involvement.

Cysts may manifest as palpable, fluctuant non-tender subcutaneous or intramuscular nodules upto the size of an orange in patients with E. granulosus infection. In patients with E. multilocularis infection the clinical features include multiple supraumbilical cutaneous and subcutaneous nodules associated with ulceration, inflammation and painless fistulas, leakage of fluid from the cyst may result in wheezing, urticaria and anaphylaxis.

Diagnosis

Ultrasound, CT scan and MRI show the characteristic morphology and floating echogenic material (hydatid sand) in the liver which strongly supports the diagnosis. Though excision of the cyst and identification of the parasite is confirmatory it is very risky because spilling of the fluid during the procedure may give rise to further cysts. Serologic tests are not that useful because false negativity can be seen in upto 50% of cases. False positive reactions are common when there are other associated helmenthic infections. Molecular techniques using PCR to assess circulating antigens are being developed.

Treatment

In the earlier days surgical excision was the only option. In E. granulosus infection ultrasound or CT guided percutaneous aspiration, instillation of hypertonic saline or other scolicidal agent and reaspiration (PAIR) after 15 minutes is performed. Protoscolicidal agents like praziquantel, 95% ethanol and 0.5% cetrimide can be used perioperatively to kill any spilled protoscolices. Albendazole may be given before surgery, in the event of leakage of cystic fluid during surgery or where there is contraindication for surgery. It is given in a dose of 15 mg/kg/day in two divided doses not exceeding 800 mg daily for a period of 1-6 months with treatment free intervals of 14 days. Alveolar hydatid disease is difficult to treat by any modality but residual surgery such as partial hepatectomy, lobectomy may cure limited disease. Mortality can be upto 60% without surgical treatment.

CYSTICERCOSIS

(Larval taeniasis)

Cysticercosis is caused by larval stage of the pork tapeworm Taenia solium and is the most common helmenthic infection involving the central nervous system (CNS). Infection in the humans is caused by ingestion of eggs in the contaminated food or drink, by faeco-oral route in individuals harbouring the adult parasite in their intestine and by eating under cooked pork. Deficient disposal of human faeces, illiteracy and presence of free roaming pigs around households favours transmission.

Clinical Features

Cysticercosis can affect humans at any age, including infection by transplacental route. Incubation period is variable from months to years and cysticerces survive in humans for 10 to 15 years and the symptoms may begin or continue for long time after the death of the parasite. The condition may be asymptomatic to fatal. Clinical signs in children are different from those in adults and about 10% of cases occurs in children. Computed tomography shows an isolated cyst in the brain parenchyma surrounded by edema and inflammation. The lesion disappears by 3 months but in about one third of patients the granuloma becomes calcified after four years, remains as a permanant sequelae and the risk of seizures is high in those children. After several years epilepsy can develop, more frequently after 25 years of age. Occasionally in children, more in the adolescent girls, cysticercotic encephalitis, a severe form of central nervous system cysticercosis occurs.

Apart from the central nervous system, skeletal muscle, subcutaneous tissue and eye are the other sites affected commonly. Heart, liver, lungs and pancreas may also be involved. Muscular cysticercosis is rare both in children and adults but is more frequent in Asia. The course is benign and there will be mild muscle pain and inflamed nodules. Rarely, in massive infection, muscle shows pseudo hyper trophy. Because of the parasite burden the subcutaneous nodules may be one to hundreds in number, are 1-2 cm in diameter, rubbery, firm, rounded and painless and the condition is referred to as cysticercoides cellulose cutis.

Diagnosis

Histological demonstration of the parasite after surgical excision of a nodule is diagnostic. When the eye is involved the parasite can be visualized by fundoscopic examination. CT or MRI will show evidence of cysts showing the scolex ('hole –with-dot' image), plain radiographs show cigar-shaped calcifications in the thigh and calf muscles. Enzyme linked immunotransfer blot (EITB) has sensitivity and specificity of more than 50%.The sensitivity with ELISA and EITB is high in patients having multiple lesions.

Treatment

Subcutaneous cysts can be removed surgically or treated medically. Multiple subcutaneous cysts can be treated with albendazole or praziquantel. Albendazole is given orally in a dose of 15 mg /kg /day in a dose of 50 to100 mg/day in 3 divided doses for 30 days. Systemic corticosteroids given 2-3 days before and during therapy can ameliorate the side effects. Albendazole is less expensive than praziquantel and has 20% more cysticidal activity. If should be remembered that administration of corticosteroids concomitantly increases the plasma level of albendazole and dicreases the plasma level of praziquantel. Intraocular cysts may need surgical resection. Obstructive lesions of the brain may require placement of shunts and removal of cysts. In patients with seizures anticonvulsants have to be administered. Prognosis is bad when vital organs are involved.

BIBLIOGRAPHY

1. Addiss DG. Blood and Tissue Nematodes (Filarial worms). In : Long SS, Pickering LK, Padoes CG eds. Pediatric infectious diseases. 2nd ed. New York: Churchill Livingstone; 2003; 1347-51.
2. Al-Qurashi AR, Ghandour AM, Osman M, Al-Juma M. Dissemination in cutaneous leishmaniasis due to leishmania major in different ethnic groups in Saudi Arabia. Int J Dermatol 2000;39:832-6.
3. Bern C, Hightower AW, Chowdhury R et al. Risk factors for Kala-azar in Bangladesh. Emerg Infect Dis 2005;11:655-62.
4. Bethony J, Brooker S, Albonico M et al. Soil transmitted helminth infections : Ascariasis, trichuriasis and hookworm. Lancet 2006;367:1521-32.
5. Blackwell V, Vega-Lopez F. Cutaneous larva migrans : Clinical features and management of 44 cases presenting in the returning traveler. Bri J Dermatol 2001;145:434-7.
6. Bockarie MJ, Tisch DJ, Kastens W et al. Mass treatment to elimate filariasis in Papua New Guinea. N Engl J Med 2002;347:1841-8.
7. Boyer KM, McLeod RL. Toxoplasmosis gondii (Toxoplasmosis). In Long SS, Pickering LK, Probes CG. eds Pediatric infectious Diseases. 2nd ed Newyork: Churchill Livingstone: 2003;1303-22.
8. Brooker S, Bethony J, Hotez PJ. Human hookworm infection in the 21st century. Adv Parasitol 2004;58:197-228.
9. Brown KR, Ricci FM, Ottesen EA. Ivermectin : Effectiveness in lymphatic filariasis. Parasitology 2000;121(Suppl):S133-146.
10. Cannov SP, Vaccaro M, Guarneri F. Leishmaniasis recidiva cutis. Int J Dermatol 2000;39:205-6.
11. Caumes E, Danis M. From creeping eruption to hookworm-related cutaneous larva migrans. Lancet 2004;4:659-60.
12. Croff SL, Yardlas V. Chemotherapy of Leishmaniasis. Curr Pharm Dim 2002;8:19-42.
13. Drugs for parasitic infections. Med Lett Drug Ther 2004; 44(1189):1-12.
14. Faber WR, Oskam L, Van Gol T et al. Value of diagnostic tests for cutaneous leishamaniasis. J Am Acad Dermatol 2003;49:70-4.
15. Garcia HH, Gonalez AE, Evans CAW et al. Taenia solium cysticercosis. Lancet 2003;361:547-56.
16. Gilles HM, Hoffman PS. Treatment of intestinal parasitic infections: A review of nitazoxamide. Trends Parasitol 2002;18:95-7.
17. Haque R, Huston CD, Hughes M et al Amebiasis N Engl J Med 2003; 348:1565-73.
18. Hepburn NC. Cutaneous Leishmaniasis. Clin Exp Dermatol 2000;25:363-70.
19. Hotez PJ, Brooker S, Bethony JM et al. Hookworms infection N Engl J Med 2004;351:799-807.
20. Ito A, Nakao M, Wandro T. Human taeniasis and Cysticercosis in Asia – Lancet. 2003;362:1918-20.
21. Kafetzis DA, Mattezou HC. Visceral Leishmaniasis in pediatrics. Curr Opin Infect Dis 2002;15:289-94.
22. Kucik CJ, Martin GL, Sortor BV. Common intestinal parasites. Am Fans Physician 2004;69:1161-68.
23. Litwin CM. Pet-transmitted infections: Diagnosis by microbiologic and immunologic methods. Pediatr Infect Dis J 2003; 22:768-77.
24. Mc Leod R, Boyer K, Roizen N et al. The child with congenital toxoplasmosis. Curr Clin Trop Infect Dis 2000;20:189-208.
25. Melrose WD, Durrheim DD, Burgess GW. Update on immunological tests for lymphatic filariasis. Trend parasitol 2004;20:255-7.
26. Molyneux DH. Elimination of transmission of lymphatic filariases in Egypt. Lancet 2006;367:966-8.

27. Montoya J, Laboratory diagnosis of Toxoplasma gondii infection andToxoplasmosis. J infect Dis 2002;185 (suppl-1):573-82.
28. Montoya JG, Liesenfeld O. Toxoplasmosis. Lancet 2004, 363: 1965-76.
29. Murray HW, Berman JD, Davies CR et al. Advances in Leishmaniasis. Lancet 2005;366:1561-77.
30. Ozdemir D, Ozkan H, Akkoc N et al. Acute trichinellosis in children compared to adults. Pediatr Infct Dis J 2005;24: 897-900.
31. Remington JS, Thullez P, Montoya JG. Recent developments for diagnoses of Toxoplasmosis J Clin Microbiol 2004;42: 941-5.
32. Remme JH. Research for control: The onchocerciasis experience. Trop Med Int Health. 2004;9:243-4.
33. Sabrosa NA, Zadenweber M. Nematode infections of the eye: Toxocariasis, Onchocerciasis, diffuse unilateral subacute neuroretinitis and cysticeriosis. Ophthalmol Clin North Ans 2002;15351-6.
34. Sellman J, Bender J. Zoonotic infections in tavelers to the tropics. Prim Care 2002;29:907-29.
35. Stauffer W, Ravdin JI. Entamoeba histolytic : An update curr opin infect Dis 2003;16(5);479-85.
36. Stephen IS, Holland CV, Cooper ES. The public health significance of Trichuris trichura. Parasitology 2000;121:573-95(S73-95).
37. Vega-Lopez F. Diagnosis of cutaneous leishmaniasis. Curr Opin Infect Dis 2003;16:97-101.
38. Vincent JA, Lustigman S, Zang S, Weil GJ. A comparison of newer tests for the diagnosis of onchocerciasis. Ann Trop Med Parasitol 2000;94:253-8.
39. Witt C, Ottesen EA. Lympratic filariasis. In infection of childhood. Bull world health org 2001;6:582-06.
40. Zaha O, Hirata T, Kinjo F. Strongyloidiasis – Progress in diagnosis and treatment intern med 2000;39:695-700.
42. Zilstra EE, Musa AM, Khalil EA, El-Hassan AM. Post-Kala-azar dermal leishmaniasis. Lancet Infect Dis 2003;3:87-98.

9

Bites, Stings and Infestations

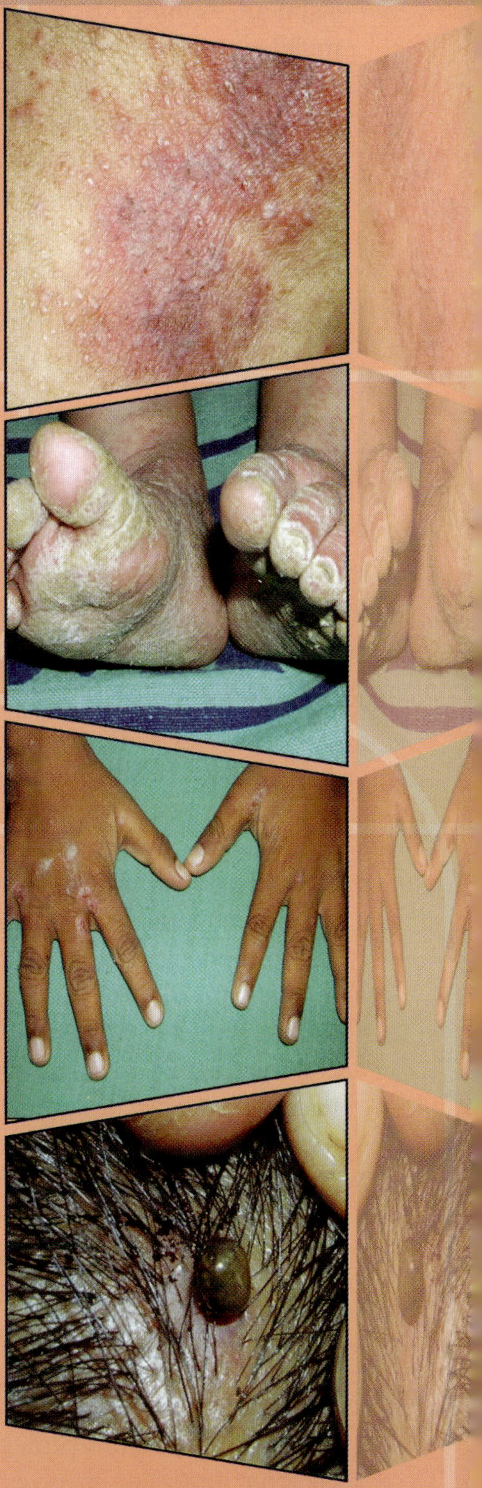

Jayadev Betkerur
Veeranna S

INTRODUCTION

Arthropoda [Gr = jointed feet] is the largest and most diverse animal phylum. Arthropods are characterized by a segmented body covered by a jointed external skeleton (exoskeleton), with paired jointed appendages on each segment. Arthropods are important in medicine for a multitude of reasons. Their bites and stings may induce allergic reactions, ranging from annoying to life-threatening. Many arthropod products are also capable of inciting allergic responses in sensitized persons.

Five of nine classes of arthropods cause local and systemic reactions associated with their bites: Arachnida, Chilopoda, Diplopoda, Crustacea and Insecta.

Arthropods that bites and stings:

1. Arachnida (four pairs of legs): mites, ticks, spiders, scorpions
   A. Acarina
      Mites: Follicle, food, fowl, harvest, murine, Sarcoptes
      Ticks
   B. Araneae: Spiders
   C. Scorpionida: Scorpions
2. Chilopoda and Diplopoda: centipedes, millipedes
3. Insecta (Three pairs of legs)
   A. Anoplura: lice
   B. Coleoptera: beetles
   C. Diptera: mosquitoes, flies, midges, gnats
   D. Hemiptera: bedbugs, kissing bugs
   E. Hymenoptera: ants, bees, wasps, hornets
   F. Lepidoptera: caterpillars, moths, butterflies
   G. Siphonaptera: fleas, chigoe

Arthropods produce their effect on the skin by a variety of mechanisms like mechanical trauma, injection of irritant, cytotoxic or pharmacologically active substances, and injection of potential allergens. Secondary bacterial infection, contact reactions, persistent granulomatous reaction to retained mouthparts and transmission of diseases also can occur.

The clinical manifestation of arthropod bites depends on the species and their biting habit. However, there are a number of common clinical features occurring in sensitized individuals, which is considered as one syndrome, papular urticaria.

Protection from insect bites is best achieved through the use of personal protection and habitat control. Personal protection involves avoiding infested habitats, wearing protective clothing, and applying insect repellents. Diethyltoluamide (DET) is the popular insect repellent used worldwide. It is available in different concentrations from 5-100%, in multiple formulation including solutions, lotions, creams, gels, aerosols and pump sprays. Preparation containing less than 10% of diethyltoluamide is recommended for use in children. Encephalopathy in children has followed repeated and extensive application of up to 20% diethyltoluamide.

SCABIES

Scabies is a common ectoparasitic infestation of human caused by an itch mite, *Sarcoptes scabiei var hominis.* This highly contagious disease is characterized by severe pruritus and typical distribution of skin lesions. The lesions in children, unlike in adults, can also occur on scalp, face, palms and soles.

ETIOLOGY

Scabies is caused by the itch mite, Sarcoptes scabiei var hominis. The scabies mite is an obligate parasite which completes its entire lifecycle on the human body. The male mite measures 0.2 × 0.15 mm and female 0.4 × 0.3 mm that cannot be visible to naked eyes. The mite is translucent, eyeless, white and oval with transverse corrugations, brown spines and bristles on the dorsal surface. Four pairs of legs are present attached to the ventral surface and the anterior two pairs bear claws **(Figure 9.1).**

After copulation the male mite dies and the gravid female burrows through the stratum corneum to the stratum granulosum at a speed of 0.5 to 5 mm per day

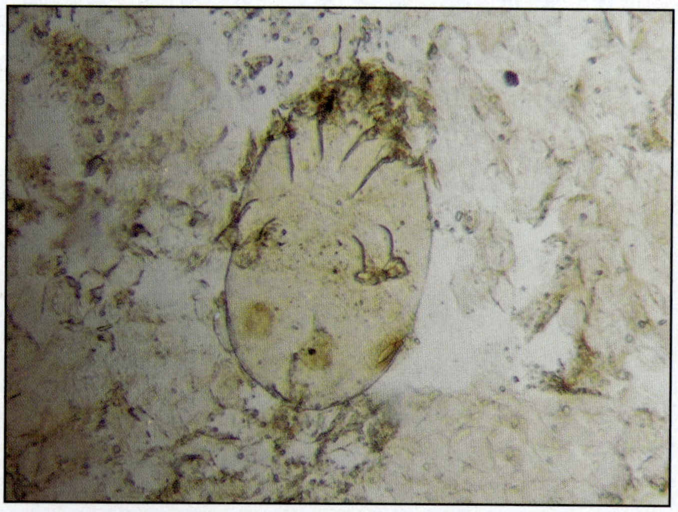

FIGURE 9.1: *Sarcoptes scabiei*–the itch mite

and lays eggs. During its life span of 5 weeks, the gravid female lays 40 eggs at a rate of 2-3 eggs per day. The eggs usually hatch larva (nymphs) after 2-3 days. After, the larvae come out of the burrow. The larva resembles adult mite but has only three pairs of leg. The larvae undergo molting three times over a period of 15 days before developing into an adult mite and the cycle repeats.

EPIDEMIOLOGY

Scabies is a disease of world wide distribution. A prevalence rate ranging from 9.44-31% has been reported. It affects all ages. Though it is common in children below 5 years of age, many authors have reported higher incidence in older children. It is more prevalent in urban areas as compared to rural areas. Close physical contact as in overcrowded schools, hugging and sleeping in crowded areas spread the disease. The role of fomites in the transmission of scabies is controversial. Scabies mite is a highly delicate organism adapted to the life style on human body and incapable of free existence. It is blind and cannot survive in the environment with humidity anything less than 100%.

CLINICAL FEATURES

Nocturnal intense itching is the main symptom. It may not be always true. In primary infestation, the onset of itching usually takes 4-6 weeks to appear whereas in re-infestation itching appears immediately.

The lesions in older children are seen on the wrists, web spaces, elbows, axilla, umbilical area, and buttocks. Papules, vesicles, pustules and crusted lesions are seen in these areas **(Figures 9.2A and B)**. Burrows are the pathognomonic lesions of scabies and are seen as grey or white serpiginous tracks **(Figure 9.3)**. These are easily visible in infants and children. An imaginary circle called the circle of Hebra covering the common areas affected- web spaces, wrists,elbows, axilla, periumbilical area and the genitals has been described.

In infants and younger children palms, soles and face are also affected **(Figures 9.4A and B)**. Vesicles and bullae are common in infants and young children. Various theories have been proposed to explain the pathogenesis of bullae in scabies. Toxins released by the mite, induction of bullous pemphigoid by the mite by altering the antigen, and id reaction have been implicated.

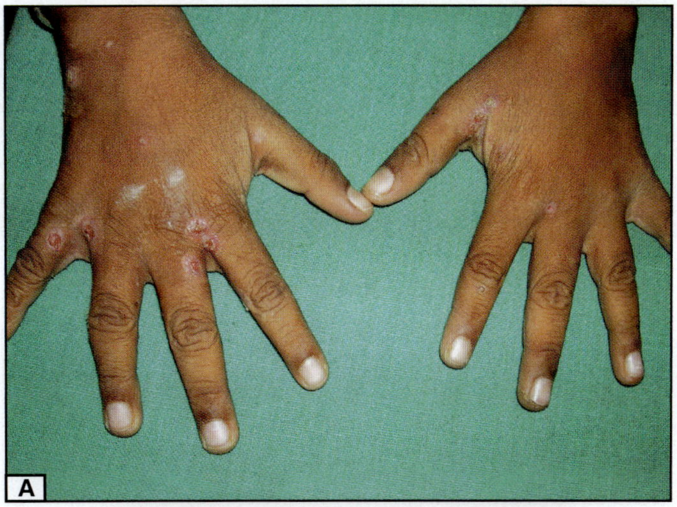

A

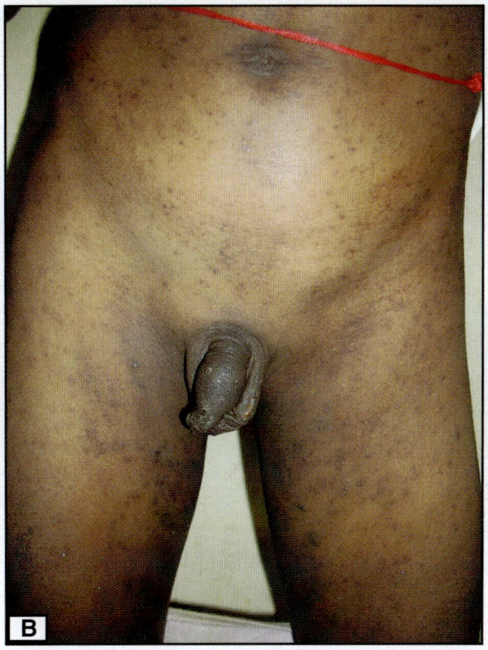

B

FIGURES 9.2A AND B: Scabies affecting web spaces and genitalia

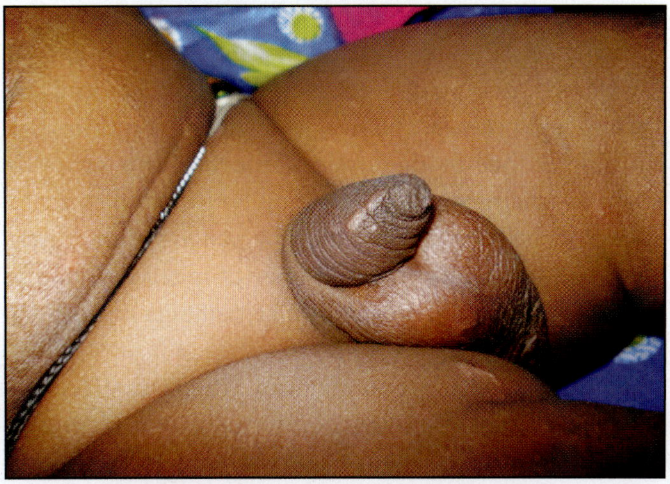

FIGURE 9.3: Burrows on genitalia and thigh

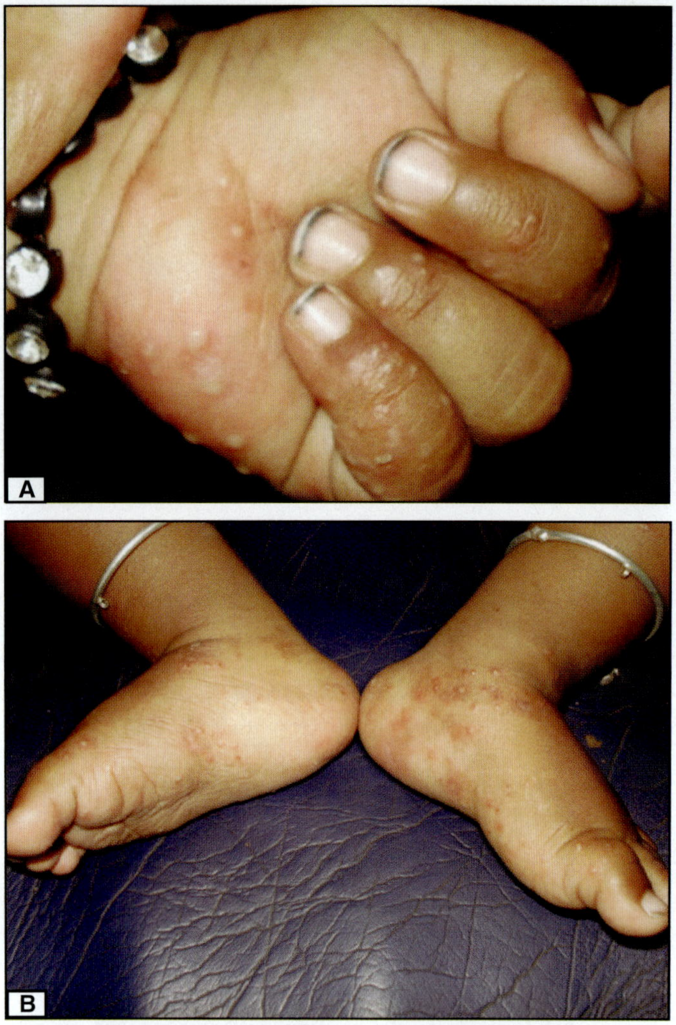

FIGURES 9.4A AND B: Scabies involving palms and soles in an infant

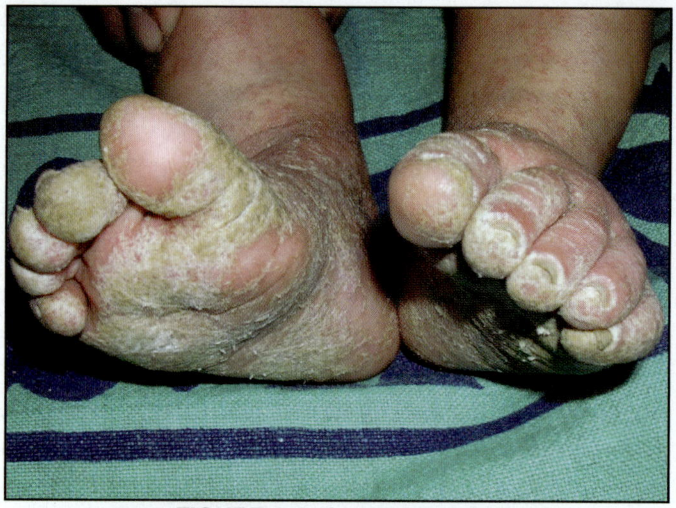

FIGURE 9.5: Crusted scabies

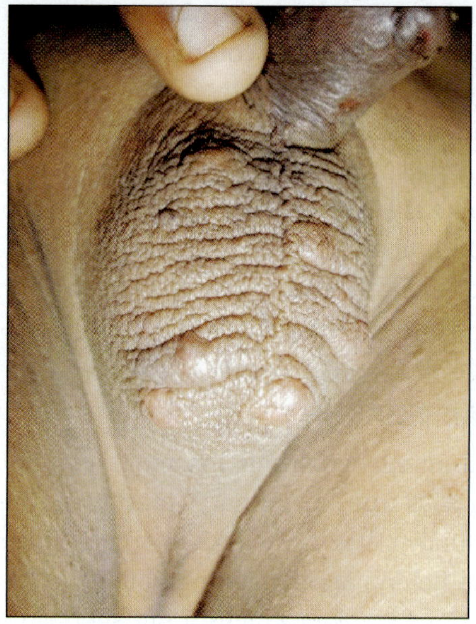

FIGURE 9.6: Nodular scabies

Special forms of scabies like nodular scabies and crusted scabies **(Figures 9.5 and 9.6)** have been described. In nodular scabies, a few violaceous pruritic nodules on the genitalia, axilla and groin persist weeks or months after treatment representing hypersensitivity reaction to mite antigens. The crusted scabies occurs commonly in immunosuppressed patients and Down's syndrome. It presents either as generalized psoriasiform eruption involving palms and soles or may be localized to scalp, face, fingers, toenails or soles. The patients with crusted scabies harbor very large number of mites resulting in outbreaks of scabies among family members and among patients in hospitals.

In infants and young children eczematization and secondary infection are common often leading to misdiagnosis and often mistreatment with steroids. It may worsen the disease leading to crusted scabies (personal observation). A thorough examination of the common sites of involvement will indicate the diagnosis.

Complications include secondary bacterial infection, eczematization and acute glomarulonephritis which is more common in children than reported.

DIFFERENTIAL DIAGNOSIS

Scabies mimicks many immunologically mediated diseases like bullous pemphigoid, urticaria, chronic lymphocytic leukemia, B-cell lymphoma with monoclonal infiltrate, CD30+ lymphoid infiltration, necrotizing vasculitis and lupus erythematosus. The crusted scabies should be differentiated from psoriasis, eczema, contact dermatitis, ichthyosis, adverse drug reaction and Darier's disease.

DIAGNOSIS

Diagnosis is usually based on clinical signs and symptoms. Demonstration of the mite from a burrow is diagnostic. Mite can be demonstrated by examining the scraping from a burrow under a light microscope using mineral oil.

Collection of specimen

Acral areas are best sites to demonstrate the mite. Gray or skin colored ridges, vesicles or non excoriated papules are selected. A drop of mineral oil is placed on the lesion or the scalpel blade and the whole lesion is scraped away.

Another method to collect specimen is Burrow ink test where the underside of a cartridge pen is rubbed on the lesion and the surface ink is wiped off using alcohol. If the burrow is present, the ink will track along the route of burrow. Similarly, tetracycline paste is smeared on the lesion and after wiping the remaining paste from the surface, the lesion is examined under Wood's light. A yellow fluorescence is seen along the burrow.

Once burrow is demonstrated, it is scrapped away as mentioned above and examined under microscope. The demonstration of adult mite or eggs or fecal pellets establishes the diagnosis of scabies. Potassium hydroxide should not be added to the slide as it dissolves fecal pellets.

In difficult to diagnosis cases skin biopsy can be done to demonstrate the mite.

Newer techniques

Epiluminescence microscopy shows the presence of characteristic small black triangular structure (pigmented anterior end of mite) and a linear segment below the base of triangular structure. Together, these two structures resemble a jet with contrail. Other non invasive techniques to demonstrate the mite in the skin are, computed dermatoscopy, and reflectance confocal videodermatoscopy. Polymerase chain reaction still at experimental stage has shown promise in diagnosis and in confirmation of clinical cure.

TREATMENT

General Considerations

1. Treat all family members to prevent ping pong effect including maid servants
2. Launder all clothes and bed linen
3. Apply scabicidal agents all over the body and wash next day
4. Repeat application after one week
5. Continue antipruritic agents for 2-3 weeks
6. Antibiotics when required

Specific Measures

Lindane (1% Gamma benzene hexa chloride) is an useful drug. Many CNS reactions like seizures, ataxia, have been reported. These are more common in infants and children with wasting and chronic illness. Systemic absorption can occur in patients with eczematization and secondary infection. Significant blood levels of GBHC have been found in normal cases also. It is of use in older children. The contact period of at least 6 hours is necessary to achieve a cure rate of 96%.

Permethrin 5% cream applied overnight (8-12 hours) is a very effective agent. It is safe in infants and children. Though 5 day application of crotamiton has been found to be useful, many authors disagree with this. The antipruritic effect may be of help. Sulphur (2.5% or 5%) ointment in soft paraffin is effective, but not prefer red for its smell and staining.

Ivermectin, a macrocyclin lactone, is an effective scabicidal. Though it is not recommended for use in children less than 5 years of age or less than 15 kgs, some have used it safely in children as young as 14 months. The dosage is 200 μg/kg single doseage repeated after 10days. Topical ivermectin is also used. Fever, pruritus, dizziness, mydriasis, depressed motor activity is some of the adverse events reported with ivermectin. Our experience suggests that a combination of GBHC with ivermectin is more effective in school children than the individual agents for mass treatment (unpublished data).

PEDICULOSIS

There are three types of pediculosis- pediculosis capitis caused by Pediculus humanus var capitis, pediculosis corporis by Pediculus humanus var corporis and pediculosis pubis by Phthirus pubis.

ETIOLOGY

Pediculosis species are obligatory ectoparasites of human hair. Both head and body louse have three body segments and six legs. The abdomen is elongated and the head is small with anterior piercing mouth parts. In contrast, the body of pubic louse is wide with two large crab-like claws.

The nits are translucent and firmly cemented to the hairs (head and pubic louse) or cloth fibers (body louse) at an acute angle.

EPIDEMIOLOGY

Pediculosis is a disease of worldwide distribution. The disease is common in school age children (5-12 years). The prevalence varies from 4-50%. Girls are more commonly affected than boys. This female bias was reported in 1898 and still holds good. The long hair, poor grooming and sharing of combs are the probable factors for this. Whether the length of hair has a role is debatable. School environment, prolonged close contact, overcrowding, and large family are the reasons for its high incidence among children. All socioeconomic groups are equally affected. Pediculosis capitis never occurs in African Americans because of physical structure of their hair. Pediculosis pubis is transmitted through sexual contact.

Body louse is a vector for many diseases like epidemic typhus (Rickettsia prowazakii), trench fever (Bartonella quintana) and relapsing fever (Bartonella recurentis). The identification of Bartonella quintans by PCR suggests that head lice may have a role in transmission of trench fever.

CLINICAL FEATURES

Intense itching is the hallmark of the disease. Scratching or excoriation leads to secondary infection. Crusting, oozing and eczematization are commonly seen. Cervical lymphadenopathy may be the presenting sign of pediculosis capitis in children.

The lice are densely present in the sub occipital and postauricular area. The suboccipital depression is called the louse pit. The eggs or nits are found firmly adherent to the hair shaft. Adult lice are hard to find as they are fast moving and less in number. The nits found at the distal part of the hair are non-viable. The duration of the infestation can be estimated by the distance of nits from the surface of scalp. Pediculid—an erythmatous maculopapular rash over trunk can occur and could be mistaken for exanthema or pityriasis rosea. In pediculosis corporis, pruritus may be the only symptom. In some cases, erythematous papules may be present under the arms, on the upper part of shoulder, the flank and the neck. The patients may present with hemorrhagic puncta, linear excoriations and hyperpigmentation on the trunk secondary to chronic scratching. Macula ceruleae, characteristic lesions of pubic louse infestation may also be found on the body.

Pubic louse infestation is usually limited to the pubic region. However, other small curly hair bearing areas such as eye brows, eye lashes or hair at the scalp line may also be involved. The eyelash infestation is called pediculosis ciliaris. Macula ceruleae are the characteristic lesions of pediculosis pubis distributed over pubic and adjacent areas. These are bluish brown hemosiderin-laden macules. Pruritus usually manifests 30 days after the infestation.

In children with malnourishment and mild iron deficiency, heavy infestation of the scalp may lead to anemia as it is estimated that a person looses 0.7 ml of blood daily due to sucking of blood by the louse.

DIFFERENTIAL DIAGNOSIS

Pediculosis capitis should be differentiated from psocids (lice-like insects) infestation and hair casts. The former is commonly found on the moist decaying paper or vegetable matter. The human scalp infestation by psocids can be differentiated by their large head, large chewing mouth parts, large hind legs and large antennae. The latter is opaque amorphous remnants of inner root sheath of the hair follicle. In contrast to nits, hair casts are freely moveable along the hair shaft and under the microscope they appear as opaque bodies encircling the hair shaft.

Rarely, the scales of papulosquamous disorders may be mistaken for nits. The scales are flat and not attached to the hair shaft. Under the Wood's light, the parakeratotic scales appears bluish white specks whereas nits appear yellow green.

DIAGNOSIS

Demonstration of nits, nymphs or adults is diagnostic **(Figure 9.7)**. Dermascopic examination is useful in diagnosis and also to evaluate efficacy of treatment.

TREATMENT

Many pediculicides have been used in the treatment of head lice. 1% permethrin applied overnight after shampooing and drying is found to be very effective. Drying of hair prevents the dilution of permethrin. Resistance to Permethrin was reported in 1994. This is due to mutation at T929I and L932F genes. This is a knock down resistance

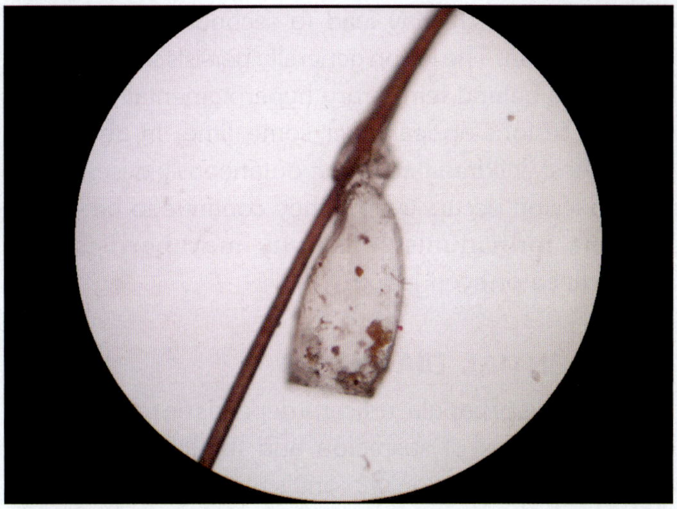

FIGURE 9.7: Empty egg-case of hair louse attached to hair shaft (under microscope)

(KDR).There is cross resistance to other Pyrethroids. Permethrin resistance is more common in America. It could be due to overuse, change in packaging and change in usage instructions. The available pediculicides are ineffective against immature nits which lack nervous system. Therefore, the treatment should be repeated after 7-10 days to kill newly hatched lice.

Some authors recommend 5% permethrin for the treatment of pubic louse infestation. For the treatment of eyelash infestation only occlusive substances like petrolatum for 10 days have been used.

Malathion 0.5% is an effective pediculicide. Twenty minute application has been found to be effective. This also reduces the chance of resistance and irritation. Malathion resistance has been reported from UK.

Ivermectin 200 μg/kg has been used successfully in the treatment of head lice. A second dose at day 10 is advisable. This could become the drug of choice in near future.

Co-trimoxazole is effective as a treatment for pyoderma and it also kills the lice. Many other agents like Levamisole, Thiabendazole, and Albendazole have been used.

Physical methods like shaving of scalp, manual removal, mineral oil, kerosene and hot air are not so effective treatment for head lice but can be used as adjuvants.

The treatment failure could be due to resistance, non compliance or re-infestation. Good public health measure, avoidance of sharing of hats, comb and scarves during outbreaks is useful. Treatment of entire household is effective in preventing outbreaks and treatment failures. Complications like secondary infection and eczematization should be treated accordingly.

PAPULAR URTICARIA

Syn: Lichen urticatus, prurigo simplex acuta of Brocq, strophulus.

Papular urticaria was originally described in 1813 by Bateman. Papular urticaria is a term used to describe a chronic or recurrent eruption of pruritic papules, often grouped in irregular clusters, frequently seasonal in incidence, and affecting predominantly children between 2-7 years. Papular urticaria constituted 5.27% of pediatric dermatoses in a referral center in South India.

ETIOLOGY

Many causes were attributed to papular urticaria in the late 19th and early to mid 20th century.The role of arthropods gradually gained support because of several observations: the lesions usually appeared in the summer months; the disease was more common among households with pets; the disease was cured simply by admission to hospital; the histologic features were identical to that of persistence insect bite reaction.

It is clear that papular urticaria can be produced by many different parasites. Which particular insect is the cause varies with geographic location.The most commonly implicated are the cat flea, dog flea, human flea, mosquitoes, bed bugs and various species of mites.

In clinical settings and experimental models, continuous exposure to biting arthropods will produce five stages of reactivity

Stage 1	Bite is non-reactive
Stage 2	Delayed red papule develop 24 hours after the bite
Stage 3	An immediate wheal after a bite, followed by the delayed papule
Stage 4	Immediate wheal only
Stage 5	Immunologic tolerance and no reaction

Clinical manifestations of papular urticaria are mediated by a complex immune response involving more than one mechanism, with evidence for both an IgE response and a cell-mediated type IV response. Children eventually "outgrow" this disease, probably through desensitization after multiple arthropod exposures. There is an increased susceptibility to mosquito bites in patients with HIV infection.

HISTOPATHOLOGY

The histopathologic features of papular urticaria are inadequately documented. In the early lesions there is mild spongiosis, exocytosis in the epidermis, and localized perivascular infiltrate with lymphocytes, histocytes, eosinophils and mast cells in the upper dermis. Older excoriated lesions show epidermal necrosis and a dermal infiltrate with neutrophils and more abundant lymphocytes. Bullae can form secondary to marked edema, especially in children. Chronic lesions can present diagnostic problems when they take on a pseudolymphomatous appearance. In a histopathologic study of 30 cases, immunohistochemistry showed T-lymphocytes (CD45RO, CD3) and macrophages (CD68) in all cases. B-lymphocytes (CD20) and dendritic antigen-presenting cells (S100) were absent. IgA, IgG, IgM, C3, and fibrin could not be demonstrated by direct immunofluorescence. The histopathologic differential diagnosis of papular urticaria includes other spongiotic dermatosis, pityriasis lichenoides et varioliformis acuta, the pruritic papular eruption of human immunodeficiency virus disease, and papulonecrotic tuberculid.

CLINICAL FEATURES

The condition consists of small, 3-10 mm diameter, pruritic urticarial papules **(Figure 9.8)**, sometimes surmounted by a vesicle. The lesions are often grouped in clusters and develop in crops at regular interval. Extensor surface of the extremities are commonly involved though the number and distribution of skin lesion depends on the type of exposure and the feeding habit of the arthropod involved. Scratching results in excoriations which may lead to secondary infection or eczematization. The lesion generally persists for 2-10 days and leaves behind temporary hyperpigmentation. Fresh crops of lesions appear after some time. In about 4-5 years, most children become spontaneously desensitized and no lesion occurs even if they continue to be bitten. In some individuals sensitivity may persists into adolescence or even longer.

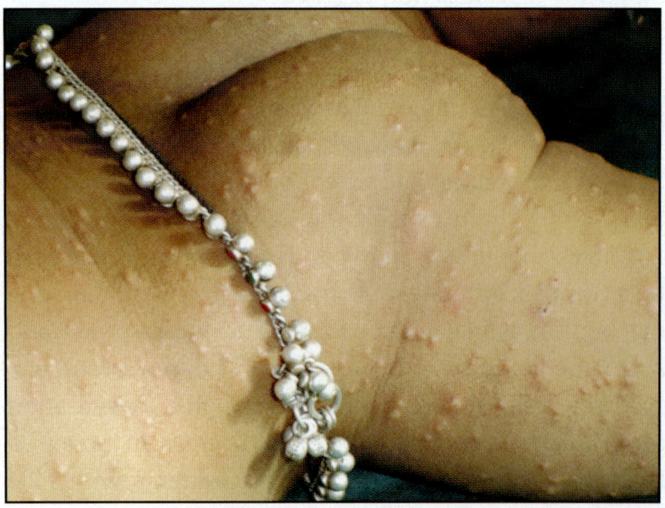

FIGURE 9.8: Papular urticaria

DIFFERENTIAL DIAGNOSIS

The diagnosis of papular urticaria depends on maintenance of a high index of suspicion and familiarity with the arthropod fauna not only in one's region of practice, but also in the travel regions of one's patients. Papular urticaria may be mistaken for varicella, scabies, 'true' urticaria, atopic dermatitis, drug rashes, miliaria rubra, polymorphic light eruption and allergic contact dermatitis.

TREATMENT

The ideal treatment is to identify and remove the cause.The patient's pet animals should be examined if possible for the signs of infestation. Calamine lotion, mild topical steroids, and systemic antihistamines helps to control the symptoms. Oral antibiotic can be recommended if secondary infection is present. Disinfection of all pets,along with fumigation of the home may produce dramatic cure. Use of passive measures like screen, nets, and application of insect repellents helps in prevention of recurrences.

OTHER REACTION TO ARTHROPOD BITE AND STINGS

ORDER DIPTERA

The order Diptera is one of the largest of the insect orders and includes mosquitoes, flies, gnats and midges. Diptera are important as biting insects and as the cause of myiasis, in addition to their capacity to transmit disease. The clinical features of this large and diverse order are variable and depend on the substance injected and the degree of allergic sensitivity to the antigenic substance in the saliva.

Mosquitoes may be found all over the world except Antarctica. Members of the genera Anopheles, Culex and Aedes commonly bite humans. Mosquitoes are attracted by the warmth, scent, bright color, carbon dioxide, estrogen and L-lactic acid in the sweat.

TABLE 9.1: Arthropod –borne infections and infestations

Arthropod	Associated illness
1. Insecta	
Lice	Pediculosis, typhus, trench fever, relapsing fever
Fleas	PU, Bubonic plague, typhus, tungiasis
Bedbugs	PU, possibility of HBV transmission
Flies	PU, myiasis,onchocerciasis, leishmaniasis, trypanosomiasis
Mosquitoes	PU, malaria, encephalitis, yellow fever, dengue fever, filariasis
Bees,wasps and ants	Anaphylaxis, local reaction
Reduvid bugs	Chagas disease, anaphylaxis
2. Arachnida	
Spiders	Necrotic arachnidism,paralysis
Scorpions	Local tissue damage, neurotoxicity Cardio respiratory collapse
Ticks	Lyme boreliosis, Rocky mountain Spotted fever, tick paralysis, babesiosis, Q fever Tularemia, ehrlichiosis
Mites	PU, Scabies, scrub typhus

PU: Papular urticaria, HBV: Hepatitis B virus

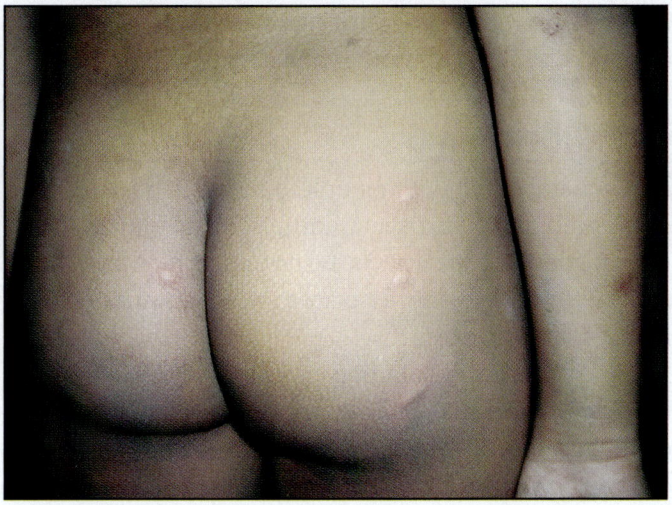

FIGURE 9.9: Immediate wheals to mosquito bite

CLINICAL FEATURES

Early pruritic wheals and late papular lesions form in response to irritating salivary secretions. Depending on the sensitivity of the victim, mosquito bites may have an urticarial, vesicular, eczematoid or granulomatous appearance **(Figure 9.9)**. Rare presentations like anaphylaxis or serum sickness like reactions has been reported. Many cases of triad of hypersensitivity to mosquito bites, chronic Epstein-Barr virus infection and NKcell leukemia/lymphoma occurring in the first two decades of life has been reported from Japan.

Phlebotomine sand flies are of dermatological importance as they transmit diseases like leishmaniasis and bartonellosis. Multiple sand fly bites are responsible for the syndrome known as harara (urticaria multiformis endemica) in highly sensitive individuals who travel to endemic areas.

Black flies also known as buffalo flies, transmit onchocerciasis. The bites of blackfly are very painful and produce local swelling, vesicles and crusted plaques.

TREATMENT

The treatment of Diptera bites requires meticulous attention to wound care by cleansing with soap or other antiseptics to avoid secondary infection. Local application of steroid ointment and systemic treatment with antihistamines will reduce itching and redness. Scents and bright colors which attract the mosquitoes are best avoided. Insect repellent like diethyltoluamide in concentration less than 10% should be used in children. Antihistamines like cetirizine and ebastine, administered prophylactically can decrease the wheal formation and pruritus.

MYIASIS

Myiasis is the infestation of body tissue of human and animals by the larvae of dipterous flies. Larvae penetrate the skin or may be deposited onto open wounds to cause cutaneous myiasis. These larvae may be divided into three broad groups as obligatory, facultative, and accidental parasites. Myiasis in humans is commonly caused by Musca domestica (housefly), Dermatobia homonis (human bot fly) and Cordylobia anthropophaga (tumbu fly). Gastrophilus (horse botfly) causes a form of migratory cutaneous myiasis known as 'creeping eruption'.

Clinical Features

Clinically, myiasis can be classified according to the part of the body involved like cutaneous myiasis, nasopharyngeal myiasis, ophthalmic myiasis, intestinal myiasis and urogenital myiasis.

Cutaneous myiasis is classified into three forms; furuncular, creeping and wound myiasis. Furuncular myiasis presents as boil like painful lesion on the exposed skin. Each lesion has central punctum through which the posterior end of the larva is visible. The second form is a creeping eruption which presents as tortuous, thread like red line with a terminal vesicle.

Wound myiasis is seen in neglected ulcers or wounds. The characteristic larvae, the maggots are seen in large number in the suppurating tissue.

Treatment

Treatment include mechanical removal of the larvae with the forceps in wound myiasis. If the larvae have burrowed in to the deeper tissue, they can be made to come out by applying gauze soaked in turpentine. Irrigation of the ulcer with ether or chloroform will anesthetize the larvae, which can be removed with the forceps. In furuncular form occluding the punctum with mineral oil or petrolatum or injection of lidocaine around the nodule may be sufficient to push the larva out. In creeping form, the larva can be extracted with a needle or killed in situ by freezing with ethyl chloride spray.

FLEAS

Fleas are small (1-8 mm), wingless, laterally compressed insects. Fleas has a unique body shape that is flattened laterally rather than dorsoventrally. Their ability to jump to a height of 18 cm aids in their movement from host to host. All species bite humans since host specificity is relatively low; severe attacks may occur where the fleas that predominantly bite domestic cats (*Ctenocephalides felis*), dogs (*Ct. Canus*) and birds (*Ceratophyllus gallinae, C. columbae*) have recently resided. Survival of adult fleas for months in the absence of host animals makes flea-borne epidemics difficult to detect and eradicate.

Clinical Features

Flea bite usually provokes typical papular urticaria in a sensitized individuals. The lesions are commonly seen on the legs. Occasionally reaction is more severe in the form of blisters; even erythema multiforme like lesions may be seen. Usually the bite of the human flea (*Pulex irritans*) causes minimal irritation in a non sensitized person and produces typically linear or clustered urticarial papules.

A tropical species called Tunga penetrans (sand flea) is the etiologic agent of tungiasis, an infestation caused by the penetration of the adult flea into the skin of feet, leading to pain, pruritus, bacterial infection, and sometimes auto amputation of the toes.

Treatment

Treatment should be directed at the household as well as infected animal.Skin lesions are treated with topical calamine, steroids and oral antihistmines.

HYMENOPTERA

The general family Hymenoptera includes bees (Apidae and Bombidae), wasps and hornets (Vespidae), and ants (Formicidae). These insects are notorious for their painful stings, which may be associated with an anaphylactic reaction and/or death.

Stings by the female bee, hornet, or wasp from the modified ovipositor (stinger apparatus) produce immediate burning and pain followed by an intense, local, erythematous reaction with swelling and urticaria. Severe systemic reactions occur in 0.4 to 0.8 percent of patients and are divided into three categories: angioedema or generalized urticaria; respiratory insufficiency from laryngeal edema or bronchospasm; and shock. The cumulative effect of large number of stings may be fatal particularly in children.

The treatment of Hymenoptera stings is based on the severity of patient response. Cutaneous reactions may be managed by application of ice and local injection of lidocaine to relieve pain. Hypotension and respiratory failure must obviously be treated vigorously. Systemic reactions require administration of subcutaneous epinephrine, while glucocorticoids and antihistamines may be helpful for urticaria or edema. If a patient experiences an anaphylactic reaction and has a positive skin test, desensitization should be strongly considered.

HEMIPTERA

The Cimicidae (bed bugs) and Reduviidae (kissing bugs) families commonly feed on animals including humans.

Bedbugs are characteristically very flat dorsoventrally and have broad bodies. Bedbugs are nocturnal feeders. Epidemiologically, it has been shown that bedbug is a good incubator for Leishmania donovanii, L. tropica, and Rickettsia burnetii (epidemic typhus). Bites by these bloodsuckers are usually not noticed immediately unless large numbers of bugs are present. The lesions are commonly seen on the face, neck, hands and arms. Only purpuric macules are seen if the person is not sensitized early. In sensitized individuals, intensly irritating wheals or papules are seen. The bites are usually painless and multiple, arranged in an irregular linear pattern. Bites that occur in rows of three are usually referred as "breakfast, lunch, dinner". Other less common type of lesions produced by bedbug bites are, papules with central hemorrhagic puncta, papular urticaria and bullae. Topical treatment with calamine lotion, steroids and oral antihistamines will control the symptoms.

COLEOPTERA (BEETLES)

There are over 370,000 species of beetles in the Coleoptera order. The Spanish fly, *Lytta vesicatoria* (family Meloidae), is the most famous of the "blister beetles." Although these beetles neither bite nor sting, they produce blisters because of the chemical cantharidin contained in their bodies. This chemical may be emitted by the beetle, but it is most often encountered when the beetle is crushed against the skin. Several other beetle species, which contain chemicals similar to cantharidin, may be the cause of blisters in various geographic areas. Rove beetles (genus *Paederus*) contain the vesicant paederin. These beetles have been associated with a blistering dermatitis, or *Paederus* dermatitis, in various areas of the world. The species commonly causing Paederus dermatitis are *Paederus melampus* in India.

Clinical Features

Paederus dermatitis, also known as dermatitis linearis or blister beetle dermatitis is a peculiar irritant contact dermatitis characterized by erythematous and bullous lesions of sudden onset on exposed areas of the body **(Figure 9.10)**. A characteristic clinical feature of blisters from beetles is "kissing" or touching lesions, which may produce infection and ulceration. The lesions are erythematous and edematous which may be linear, giving a whiplash appearance. Complications include post inflammatory hyperpigmentation, secondary infections, and extensive exfoliating and ulcerating dermatitis requiring hospitalization.

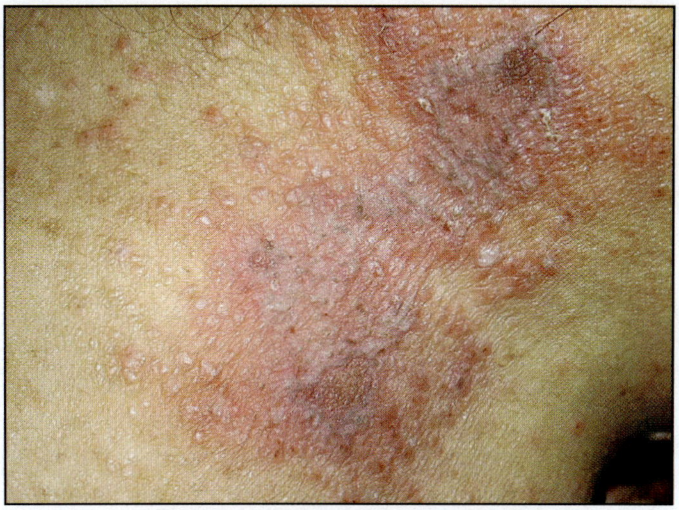

FIGURE 9.10: Blister beetle dermatitis

Histopathological changes include intraepidermal and subepidermal blistering, epidermal necrosis and acantholysis.

Clinical appearance of paederus dermatitis may be confused with herpes simplex, herpes zoster, liquid burns, acute allergic or irritant contact dermatitis, millipede dermatitis and phytophotodermatitis.

Treatment with wet compresses and topical or systemic glucocorticoids may be needed.

LEPIDOPTERA (BUTTERFLIES AND MOTHS)

The Lepidoptera order is medically important solely because of the irritant and allergenic properties of the hairs (setae) from caterpillars, moths and butterflies. Lepidopterism describes the aggregate of medical effects caused by these insects. Skin lesions typically appear as papular urticaria, which can become generalized in severe cases. Systemic reactions to some species have been reported. Treatment of acute disease is largely symptomatic with topical menthol and camphor, topical steroids and systemic antihistamines.

CLASS ARACHNIDA

Three of seven orders of Arachnida are of medical importance:

1. Araneae (spiders)
2. Scorpions (scorpions)
3. Acari (ticks and mites)

SPIDERS

Of the many species of spiders only few are capable of causing significant morbidity or mortality. The genera *Loxosceles, Latrodectus*, and Tegenaria are the species whose venom produces significant toxic effects in humans. The clinical syndrome following the bite of spider is known as arachnidism. The form of arachnidism caused by Loxoscelidae is known as loxoscelism and that by widow spider (Latrodectus) latrodectism.

Latrodectism

Genus Latrodectus are widely distributed throughout the world. Latrodectus mactans, the black widow spider, occurs throughout tropical and subtropical regions. Its venom is considered as the most toxic, exceeding that of snake venoms.

Clinical features

Spider bites may be sensed as a pinprick or sharp pinch. Skin manifestations are limited to slight erythema, local piloerection, mild edema or urticaria, and possibly lymphangitis. Systemic symptoms peak at 1 to 8 h after the bite and may last 24 to 48 hours. Severe pain in local muscle groups may spreads to regional muscle groups. The characteristic crampy abdominal and chest pain may lead to confusion with acute appendicitis, renal colic, or acute myocardial infarction. Headache, restlessness, anxiety, fatigue, insomnia, salivation, lacrimation, diaphoresis, tremors, tachycardia, bradycardia, hypertension, shock, and coma have all been associated with latrodectism. The bite may be fatal in young children.

Treatment

Treatment of most cases of latrodectism is supportive and generally does not require hospitalization. Exceptions to this rule include the very young and the very old and persons with cardiovascular disease, who are at greater risk for complications. Traditional treatment with intravenous calcium gluconate (10%) and muscle relaxants has proved effective in most patients. Relief of pain with narcotics may reduce the severity of symptoms and muscle spasms.

Loxoscelism

The brown recluse spider, *L. reclusa*, is the most notorious of the genera *Loxosceles*. It is also known as 'violin' or 'fiddle back' spider.

Clinical Features

The bite itself is generally painless. Later sever pain accompanied by erythema, edema and a central bulla develops at the site. In severe cases, a target lesion is seen – central blue/purple discoloration surrounded by an ischaemic halo and an outer ring of erythema (the 'red, white and blue' sign. After 3 or 4 days, the central area becomes necrotic, and an eschar develops. This response may be associated with a maculopapular exanthema, fever, headache, malaise, arthralgias, nausea, and vomiting.

Treatment

Ice and elevation are useful in reducing erythema and swelling. Glucocorticoids have not proved useful for the local wound but should be considered for patients with significant systemic symptoms such as hemolysis. Antibiotics are useful in reducing the incidence of abscess formation and secondary infection in large lesions. Although dapsone is said to be beneficial its use is controversial.

SCORPIONS

Scorpions are widely distributed in the tropics and subtropics. Their venom contains neurotoxins, histamine, 5-HT and kinins.

Clinical Features

Scorpion stings can produce both local and systemic effects. Most stings occur on the limbs, head, or neck. The local effects are severe burning pain and swelling. Systemic symptoms involve primarily the neurological, cardiopulmonary, and pancreatic systems. Neurologically; these symptoms may include convulsions, coma, hemiplegia, hyper- or hypothermia, tremor, restlessness, and irritability. Deaths are most commonly related to cardiopulmonary abnormalities, particularly in children. Hypertension, arrhythmias, and pulmonary edema are seen frequently.

Treatment

In milder cases with only local effects, therapy is largely supportive and includes local wound care, applications of ice packs, and antihistamines to control inflammation. Local injections of anesthetics may also help to control pain. Specific antivenoms are also available.

TICKS

Ticks are the largest members of the order Acarina. They are important worldwide as vectors of many systemic diseases like Rickettsial infection, Lyme disease, viral encephalitis, Ehrlichiosis and Babesiosis. Reactions to tick bites include foreign body reactions, reactions to salivary secretions, reactions to injected toxins, and hypersensitivity reactions. Ticks are divided into the Argasidae (soft tick) and Ixodidae (hard tick) families. Tick bites occur most commonly in the spring and summer, coinciding with the life cycle of the tick.

Clinical Features

Most bites are not painful as an anesthetic and anticoagulant is introduced. Ticks are often seen or felt by the patients. In many instances, victims are not even aware that they have been bitten and there may be only a red papule at the bite site. This papule can progress to local swelling and erythema. Blistering, severe pruritus, and ecchymoses can be seen **(Figure 9.11)**. Granulomatous foreign body reaction occurs when mouth parts are retained in the skin. Non dermatological manifestation of tick bite includes anaphylaxis and tick paralysis.

Tick paralysis often affects children. The paralysis is an acute ascending lower motor neuron paralysis. If the tick is found and removed, symptoms disappear rapidly. Severe cases may require respiratory support.

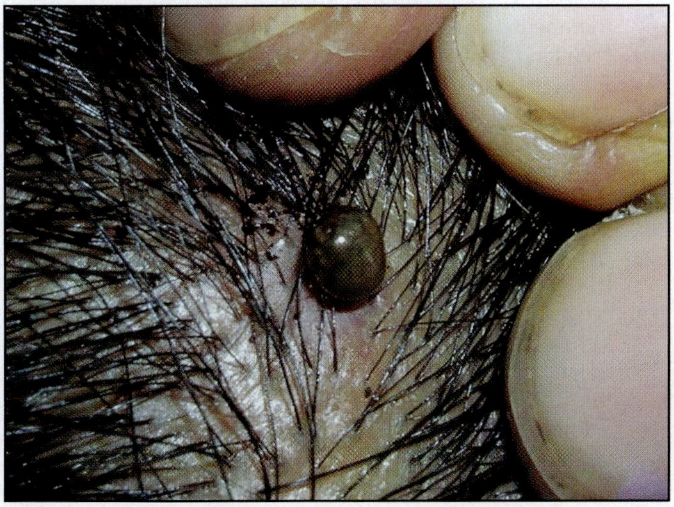

FIGURE 9.11: Tick bite on the scalp

Dermatologic manifestations of Lyme disease include erythema migrans, lymphocytoma, acrodermatitis chronicum atrophicans, morphea and other sclerotic skin disorder. Skin lesions of Tularemia include ulceroglandular lesions, erythema nodosum, erythema multiforme and papulovesicular lesions.

Treatment of Tick Bite

Avoiding tick habitat,use of diethyl toluamide on skin and permethrine on cloths is effective in preventing the tick bite. Early removal of the tick reduces the spread of the infectious organism.Gentle traction after holding the tick with forceps usually succeeds in removing it. Clean the bite site after removal.Topical steroids and oral antihistamines can be used to control pruritus.

CHILOPODA AND DIPLOPODA (CENTIPEDES AND MILLIPEDES)

Centipedes are distinguished from millipedes in that the former have one pair of legs per body segment and the latter have two. Centipedes produce painful wounds by discharging neurotoxic venom through their claws as they grip the victim. In addition to severe pain and paresthesia, localized sweating, large surrounding zone of erythema and edema, hemorrhagic vesicles, necrosis of the site, secondary infection, and ulceration may be seen. The accidental ingestion of centipede by children results in systemic toxicity, and bites can rarely result in rhabdomyolysis with renal failure.

Millipedes are generally harmless but when disturbed or threatened they emit a toxic substance from glands on each side of each segment. This fluid may produce burning, blistering, and pigmentation of the skin. Children often try to pick up millipedes and are therefore at most risk of millipede burns. If introduced into the eye, it may cause severe inflammation.Skin lesions should be washed with water. Blisters should be treated with topical antiseptics.

OTHER NOXIOUS AND VENOMOUS STINGS

LEECHES (HIRUDINEA)

Although freshwater leeches are capable of attaching painlessly to their human host, saltwater leeches produce pain similar to a bee sting. Leeches inject a powerful anticoagulant, hirudin, into the wound, as well as other antigenic substances that are capable of eliciting allergic reactions (including anaphylaxis) in sensitized individuals. Local symptoms of leech bites include bleeding from the puncture sites, pain, swelling, redness, and severe pruritus; urticarial, bullous, or necrotic reactions may occur in sensitized persons. Leeches must therefore be removed carefully by inducing them to fall off by applying a noxious agent (such as alcohol, vinegar, brine, or a match flame) to their site of attachment. After the leech has been removed, the wound should be carefully cleansed and minor bleeding controlled. Secondary infections may be prevented by cleansing the bite site for several days with antiseptic solutions.

Leeches are being employed in microvascular surgery and also for drainage of large hematoma.Unfortunately the use of leeches carries the risk of introducing wound infection, most frequently with Aeromonas hydrophilia.

INJURIES CAUSED BY JELLYFISH, PORTUGUESE MAN-OF-WAR, SEA ANEMONES, AND CORALS

All these aquatic creatures belong to the phylum Cnidaria.Cnidarian stings may range from mild, self-limited irritations to extremely painful and serious injuries, depending on the toxin of the species involved and the magnitude of the envenomation. In certain species such as the cubomedusae, or box jellyfish, stings can be fatal. In most cases, jellyfish stings elicit toxic rather than allergic types of reactions.

INJURIES DUE TO ECHINODERMS: SEA URCHINS, STARFISH, AND SEA CUCUMBERS

Sea urchins have calcareous spines, which can break off in skin following a puncture wound. In certain species spines are venomous, causing excruciating pain. Envenomation by sea urchins produce immediate burning pain, edema and paresthesia. Delayed granulomatous reactions usually develop several months after the injury and presents as bluish papules or nodules. Careful removal of spines and immersion of affected part in hot water will provide pain relief. Granulomatous lesions may be treated with intralesional steroid.

Starfish injuries are similar to that of sea urchin. Sea cucumbers can cause a papular contact dermatitis.

OTHER ANIMAL AND HUMAN BITES

Dogs and cats are responsible for most of the animal bites that occur in children. Human bites occur in children involved in fist fight.

Animal bites range from small scratches to severe lacerations involving muscle and tendon. These bites can become infected with a complex group of pathogens including Pasteurella sp.

The wound should be washed thoroughly. Primary closure of the wound should be avoided. Tetanus toxoid should be updated and post exposure rabies prophylaxis should be considered.

BIBLIOGRAPHY

1. Akisu C, Delibas SB,Aksoy V.Albendazole single or combination therapy with Permethrin against P. Capitis. Pediatr Dermatol 2006;23(2):179-82.
2. Biswas A, Chakraborthy S, Datta PK. Seizure following topical GBHC therapy. Indian J Dermatol Venereol Leprol 2002;47(1):33-35.
3. Chosidow O. Scabies. N Engl J Med 2006; 354 (16): 1718-27.
4. Daniel E, McGinley-Smith. Dermatoses from ticks. J Am Acad Dermatol.2003; 49(3):363-84.
5. Das S, Chattergee J, Banerji G, Biswas I. Evaluation of the commonest site, demographic profile & most effective therapy in scabies. Indian J Dermatol Venereol Leprol 2006;51: 186-8.
6. Di Stefani et al. Dermascopy for diagnosis and treatment of pediculosis capitis. J Am Acad Dermatol 2006;54(5)909-11.
7. Garcia E, Halpert E, Rodriguez A, Andrade R, Fiorentino S, Garcia C. Immune and histopathologic examination of flea bite-induced papular urticaria. Ann Allergy Asthma Immuno 2004;92(4)446-52.
8. Goates BM, et al. An effective non chemical treatment for head Lice: A lot of hot air. Pediatrics 2006;118(5):1962-70.
9. Malcom C, Bergman JN. Trying to keep ahead of Lice: A therapeutic challenge. Skin Therapy Lett 2006;11(10):1-6.
10. Meinking TL, Clinical updates on resistance and treatment of P Capitis. Am J Manag care 2004;10:S264-8.
11. Moon TD, Oberhelman RA. Anti Parasitic Therapy in Children. Pediatr Clin N Am 2005;52:917-48.
12. Pavithran K. Scabies. Indian J Dermatol Venereol Leprol 2002;68:283.
13. Shah H,Mehta A, Shah K Trivedi A. Scabies with bullous pemphigoid like eruption. Indian J Dermatol Venereol Leprol 2003;69:9-10.
14. Singh G, Yousuf Ali S. Paederus dermatitis. Indian J Dermatol Venereol Leprol 2007; 73:13-5.
15. Steen CJ, Carbonaro PA, Schwartz RA. Arthropods in dermatology. J Am Acad Dermatol. 2004 Jun; 50(6):819-42.
16. Stibich AS, Schwartz RA. Papular urticaria. Cutis 2001; 68(2):89-91.
17. Yoon KS et al. Permethrin resistant human head lice- P Capitis and their treatment. Arch Dermatol 2003;139:994-1000.

10

Sexually Transmitted Infections Including HIV Infection

Hemanta Kumar Kar

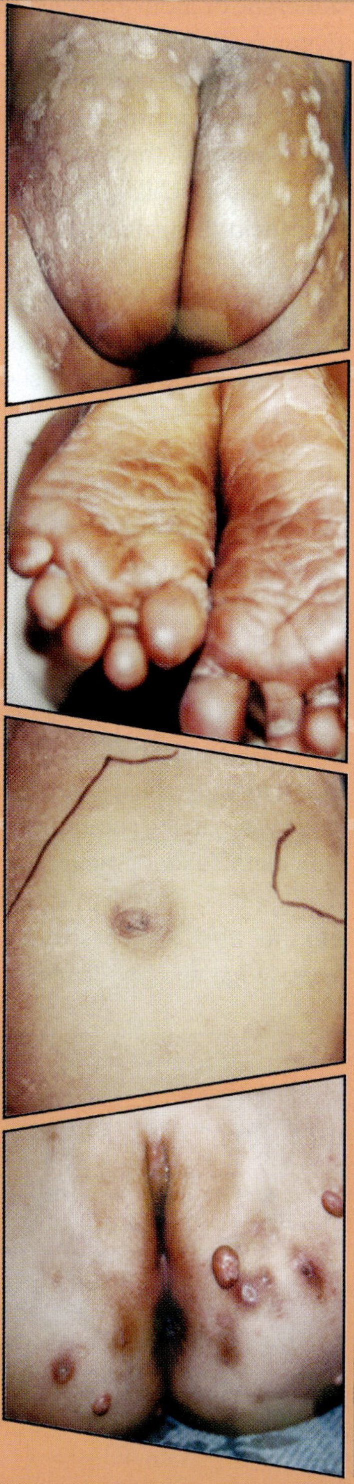

INTRODUCTION

Sexually transmitted diseases (STDs) or infections (STIs) primarily affect the sexually active population in the reproductive age group and largely acquired by sexual route. In children, the acquisition of an STD can be venereal or nonvenereal. The pattern of transmission depends on the age of the child.

1. Transplacental transmission (intrauterine), intrapartum transmission (during labor and delivery) and postnatal (breast feeding) transmission are more likely in children aged less than two years. These include syphilis, human immunodeficiency virus (HIV) infection, cytomegalovirus (CMV) infection, human papilloma virus (HPV) infection, gonococcal and chlamydial infections.
2. Sexual transmission should possibly be considered as the primary mode of infection for children between 2 and 10 years of age and sexual abuse as a definite possibility in such cases.
3. In adolescents, voluntary sexual activity and to a certain extent sexual abuse are the main modes of transmission.

Rare cases of STD in children, due to accidental infection from mother or nurse, through wet towels, bedding and sharing toilet seats have been reported.

A child with STD is unique because, not only it is reflective of the pattern of STDs among the adult population in the community, but also of the social milieu, prevalent sexual practices and psycho-sexual disorders. The treating physician should consider the possibility of sexual abuse and should be conversant with the knowledge and application of professional laws.

By definition, child abuse is the use of a child as an object of gratification for adult sexual needs or desires. Sexual abuse ranges in severity from gentle fondling to forcible rape resulting in physical injury. The common sexual abuses encountered by girls are genital contact, masturbation, vaginal, oral, or anal intercourse by a male perpetrator, while boys are subjected to fellatio and anal intercourse. The psychological morbidity caused by the traumatic childhood experience of sexual abuse may affect the normal growth and development afterwards. Hence, these children need prompt attention for the holistic management of the STDs including counseling accompanied by parents.

PREVALENCE

It is difficult to assess the exact prevalence of STDs in children as they frequently go unnoticed and remain undiagnosed. A retrospective hospital based report from a STD clinic in Delhi, India, shows that 2.5% cases of STDs are among children (52.9 boys and 47.1% girls).

The prevalence of different STDs in children from southern and northern zones of India is depicted in **Table 10.1**.

In two studies, conducted in an institution (specific for women and child care) at different time, a declining trend of prevalence of congenital syphilis was observed (from 57 to 11.5%). This is reflective of better antenatal health care for the pregnant women compared to earlier. On the contrary, western world has been experiencing an increase in the incidence of congenital syphilis in last two decades.

TABLE 10.1: Prevalence of STDs in children in India

Diseases	Garg et al 1985 n = 30 (%)	Pandhi et al 1995 n = 58 (%)	Mendiratta et al 2004 n = 17 (%)
Syphilis			
Primary	-	3 (5.1)	1 (5.6)
Secondary	9 (30, 0)	11(19.1)	5 (29.4)
Congenital	10 (33.3)	2(3.5)	2(11.5)
Chancroid	-	13(22.4)	1(5.6)
Herpes progenitalis	2(6.2)	4(6.9)	1(5.6)
Gonorrhea	4(12.6)	14(24.1)	1(5.6)
Non-gonococcal			
Urethritis	-	1(1.7)	-
Candidiasis	-	6(10.3)	-
Condyloma acuminata	-	-	6(35.2)

The prevalence rates of various STDs in prepubertal children, evaluated for suspected sexual abuse in different studies were gonococcal infection (5–14.8%), syphilis (0.1–6%), Chlamydial infection (1.2–6%), trichomoniasis (2–18%) and condylomata acuminata (2–5.6%). In one study from an orphanage in India, 53 of the 95 abused girls were infected with gonococcus.

India has an estimated 2,02,000 children infected by HIV/AIDS (UNAIDS, 2004).

Using a conservative vertical transmission rate of 30%, a new cohort of approximately 56,700 HIV infected infants is added every year (NACO, 2005).

BACTERIAL STD

SYPHILIS

Syphilis is a STI caused by *T. pallidum*. The transmission occurs either transplacentally (congenital) or postnatally (acquired). Congenital syphilis is always caused by maternal syphilis and the acquired syphilis is due to sexual contact.

CONGENITAL SYPHILIS

Congenital syphilis may occur when an infected woman becomes pregnant or when a pregnant woman becomes infected. Syphilis does not seem to cause abortion in the first four months of pregnancy. It is thought that the Langhans cell layer provides a barrier against spread of infection to the fetus.

Outcome of Pregnancy with Syphilis

The following may be the outcomes of untreated syphilis in pregnancy:

1. Miscarriage may occur any time beyond 12-16 weeks, following the formation of placenta.
2. In 30% cases, the fetus may die *in utero* late in pregnancy resulting in a still birth/macerated fetus.
3. In few cases, the neonate is born apparently normal, but develops signs of early congenital syphilis during first few weeks or months (Profeta's law).
4. In some cases, the neonate is born with signs of congenital syphilis.
5. The infant with early congenital syphilis may or may not develop signs of late congenital syphilis later on.
6. The child may not develop clinical features of early congenital syphilis but may develop late congenital syphilis in later years.
7. The fetus may escape the infection. This probability increases with longer duration of the disease in expectant mother.

Kassowitz's or Diday's law: The untreated syphilitic mother tends to improve on past performances; that is to have later and later miscarriages, then syphilitic and finally non-syphilitic children.

Pathology

Gross placental changes are seen only when pregnancy ends in still birth. Survival of the fetus is possible only with minimal placental involvement. Diseased placenta is bulky, heavy, pale and greasy. Syphilitic endarteritis produces alterations in the chorionic villi resulting in decrease in the blood vessels, increased connective tissue and infarcts. The diagnosis is confirmed by demonstration of *Treponema pallidum* in the placenta.

After entry of the *T pallidum* into fetal circulation, dissemination occurs to all tissues with characteristic cellular inflammatory response of small lymphocytes and plasma cells. The fetus may die due to severe infection. The stillborn fetus may be macerated with collapse of the skull and protuberant abdomen. The skin may be livid red in color with hemorrhagic bullae. The liver and spleen are enlarged with cellular inflammatory response in other organs including bones. Placental histopathology may show necrotizing funisitis, vellous enlargement and acute villitis. If the fetus survives, the infection may still interfere with normal development at various stages of intrauterine and extra uterine life. Certain manifestations at a later life, such as interstitial keratitis and Clutton's joints, are possibly not due to direct Treponemal effects, but believed to be a phenomenon of hypersensitivity.

Clinical Manifestations

Congenital syphilis has been classified into:

I. Early congenital syphilis (first two years of life)
II. Late congenital syphilis
III. Stigmata of congenital syphilis

Early Congenital Syphilis

There is usually no sign of the disease at birth. Presence of hemorrhagic bullae and muco-cutaneous lesions at the time of birth indicates severe infection. Usually after a 2-6 weeks period after birth, early congenital syphilis manifests. By the time the skin lesions appear, the serological tests for syphilis are already positive.

There is no primary stage. The first signs developed are similar to those of secondary stage of acquired syphilis. If at all there is a lesion resembling primary chancre in an infant, it might have been acquired from the genital lesion of a very recent infection in the mother.

Clinical Features

General:

1. Marasmus and old-man look
2. Failure to regain birth weight

Cutaneous: There is no primary lesion, only secondary lesions are observed **(Figures 10.1A to C)**.

1. Symmetrical, bullous rash on palms and soles or occasionally on other parts is the earliest manifestation noticed at the time of birth.
2. Some weeks later, other rashes similar to that of acquired secondary syphilis develop.
3. Confluence of rashes near lower part of the face.
4. Movement of the lips produces radiating fissures at the angle of the mouth, which when secondarily infected produces linear scars (rhagades).
5. Brittle and sparse hair and infantile alopecia of eyebrows.
6. Paronychia of fourth and fifth digits leading to narrow atrophic nails and claw nail deformity.

Mucous membrane

1. Syphilitic rhinitis gives rise to a highly infectious nasal discharge (snuffles). It is initially watery, later becomes thick, purulent and sometimes bloody. It may result in ulceration and perforation of the septum with collapse of the bridge of nose leading to saddle nose deformity. There may be difficulty in breathing and suckling.
2. Pharyngitis and laryngitis lead to cough and hoarse cry.

Bone lesions

A. First six months:

1. Osteochondritis of rapidly growing long bones and periosteal reaction with sub-periosteal, cortical deposition of new bones leads to loss of movement of the affected limb (syphilitic pseudo paralysis). Upper end of tibia and distal end of radius and ulna are most commonly affected.
2. Wimberger's sign: Loss of density on the medial side of the upper end of tibia, seen radiologically, is characteristic of congenital syphilis.

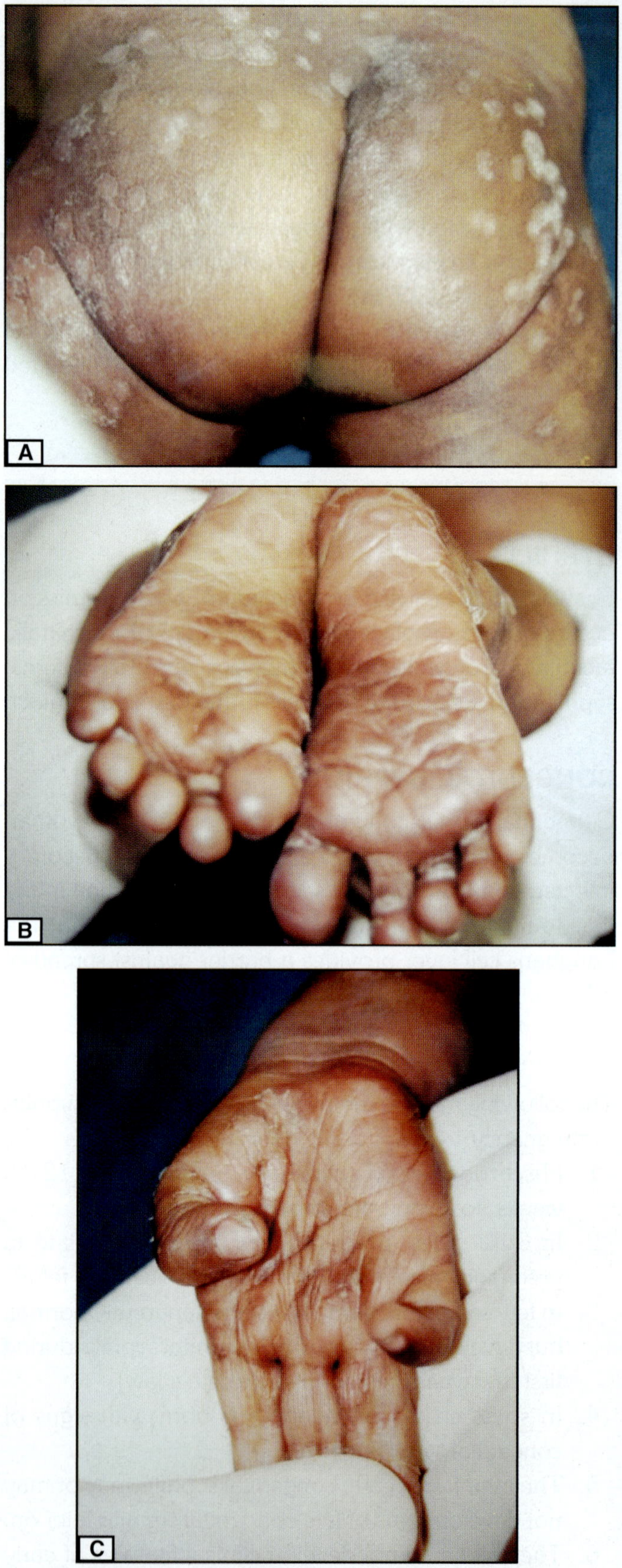

FIGURES 10.1A TO C: Papulo-squamous rash of early congenital syphilis

B. Next sixth months:
1. Osteochondritis disappears, but periosteitis persists (onion- peel periosteum on radiographic examination)

C. Second year:
1. Oseochondritis of phalanges (syphilitic dactylitis), proximal phalanges are more commonly affected, and involvement of fingers is more frequent than toes. One or several digits may be affected, with painless and fusiform swelling.

Lymph Nodes:
1. Generalized lymphadenopathy is seen in 20 to 50% cases.
2. Nodes are firm, discrete, rubbery, and non-tender.
3. Epitrochlear gland enlargement is a finding in 20% cases.

Liver and Spleen **(Figure 10.2)***:*
1. Hepatospenomegaly with protuberant abdomen.
2. Mild icterus.

Kidney:
1. Proliferative or membranous glomerulonephritis may be present in some cases, giving rise to albuminuria and few to many hyaline and granular casts in urine.

Lungs:
1. White pneumonitis due to widespread infiltration of the lungs leading to early death in some cases.

Eyes:
1. Choroidoretinitis, glaucoma, and uveitis

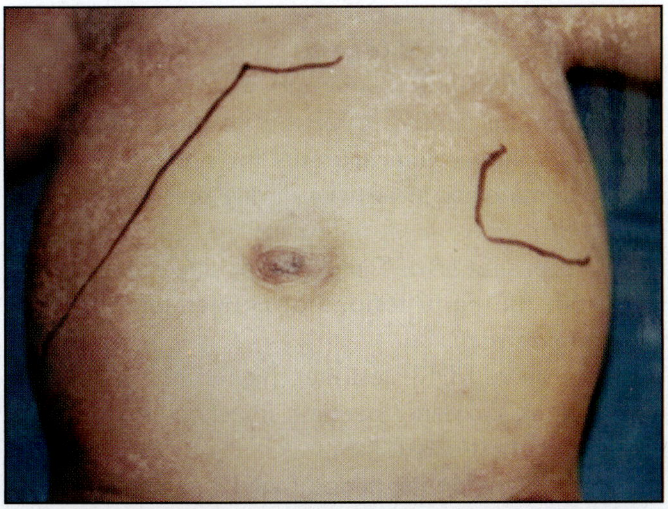

FIGURE 10.2: Pot-belly due to hepatosplenomegaly in early congenital syphilis

Central Nervous System:
1. Asymptomatic neurosyphilis, abnormal CSF findings with clinical involvement are seen in 40 to 60% of infected infants
2. Meningitis or meningoencephalitis presenting with convulsions, bulging fontanelles, stiffness of neck and hydrocephalus.

Late Congenital Syphilis

1. Beyond 2nd year of life.
2. Early stage remains unnoticed in 80% cases.
3. Late manifestations correspond to tertiary phase of acquired syphilis.
4. Rare due to concomitant antibiotic treatment for other infections.

Clinical features

Clinical features develop as a result of hypersensitivity reaction to *T. pallidum*. The main features/organ involvements are as follows:

A. *Interstitial Keratitis:*
1. Commonest late manifestation.
2. More common in females
3. Initially circumcorneal vascularization, followed by extension into the deep layers of the cornea and cellular exudation into deep corneal structures.
4. Starts in one eye, but the other eye is likely to be affected, irrespective of the antisyphilitic treatment.
5. It has a limited or self-limiting course, but ends with corneal ground glass appearance. A dull pink patch (salmon patch) may be seen at the periphery of the cornea.

B. *Iridocyclitis:*
1. Photophobia.
2. Pain and excessive watering.
3. Blurring of vision.

C. *Teeth:*
1. Hutchinson's teeth: It appears at the age of 6 years or thereafter. The permanent upper central incisors are shorter than the lateral incisors and widely spaced. The biting edge may be notched due to defective enamel formation assuming a barrel or peg shape.
2. Mulberry or Moon's molars: The first molar tooth is dystrophic. The biting surface looks dome

shaped, with small, poorly developed cusps. It is prone to develop caries and cavitations and destroyed early due to poor development of the enamel.

D. *Neural Deafness:*
   1. The primary lesion is osteochondritis affecting the otic capsule leading to cochlear degeneration.
   2. Nerve deafness generally develops irrespective of antisyphilitic treatment, but can be modified with steroid therapy.

E. *Neurosyphilis:*
   1. Either asymptomatic or symptomatic.
   2. Juvenile paresis is more frequent than juvenile tabes.

F. *Hutchinson's Triad:*
   A definite sign of late congenital syphilis, consists of:
   1. Interstitial keratitis
   2. Hutchinson's teeth
   3. Eighth nerve deafness

G. *Skin and mucous membrane:*
   1. Gumma leads to nasal septal and palatal perforations
   2. Nasal intonation and regurgitation of food

H. *Bony lesions:*
   1. There is sclerosis and new bone formation.
   2. Destructive lesions in palate and nasal septum.
   3. Thickening of the middle third of tibia.
   4. Localized osteo-periostitis of the bones of the vault of skull leading to globular, bony swelling called "Parrot's nodes".
   5. Thickening of the inner end of the clavicle (Higoumenaki'sign).
   6. Occasional dactylitis.

I. *Clutton's joint:*
   1. Perisynovitis results in hydro-arthrosis, usually involving both knee joints. Rarely elbow joints are involved. It runs a chronic course.
   2. The condition is painless, with little impairment of function of joints.
   3. X-ray shows enlargement of the joint space without bony changes.
   4. Unresponsive to antisyphilitic treatments as *T. pallidum* is always absent in the tissues or joint fluid.

J. *Paroxysmal cold hemoglobinuria:*
   1. On exposure to cold, there will be sudden chills, fever, malaise, headache, pain in the back and urticaria.
   2. The urine collected just after the attack is red or brown.
   3. The serum contains a hemolysin, which along with complement, sensitizes the red cells during chilling, thereafter hemolysis occurs when the body temperature returns to normal. This is called as "Donath-Landsteiner reaction", which can be used as a diagnostic test.
   4. Antisyphilitic treatment cures the condition

K. Cardiovascular and hepatic involvements are rare in late congenital syphilis.

Stigmata

The stigmata are the diagnostic of congenital syphilis with positive serological tests. These are:

1. Saddle nose,
2. Frontal and parietal bossing,
3. Short maxillae,
4. Bulldog jaws,
5. High arched palate,
6. Sabre tibia,
7. Scaphoid scapulae,
8. Hutchinson's teeth,
9. Moon's molar,
10. Corneal opacities, salt and pepper fundus, optic atrophy,
11. Eighth nerve deafness
12. Rhagades

Diagnosis

1. All women should undergo serological screening for syphilis during early stage of pregnancy. In communities with high prevalence of syphilis or for high-risk patients, twice screening is recommended, once at 28 to 32 weeks of gestation and again at delivery (CDC-2006).
2. No infant should leave the hospital without the maternal serological status for syphilis has been determined at least once during pregnancy (CDC-2006).
3. Demonstration of *T. pallidum* by direct examination from the early lesions of congenital syphilis is confirmatory.
4. A positive VDRL test titer, higher than that of the mother, suggests a perinatal infection and the infant should be treated.
5. After the neonatal period (aged 1 month or more), children with syphilis should have a CSF examination to detect asymptomatic neurosyphilis (CDC-2006).

TABLE 10.2: Treatment of neonatal syphilis (first month of life) (WHO - 2005)

	Mother's RPR/VDRL status		
	Reactive	**Unknown**	**Non-reactive**
Infant with signs of congenital syphilis*	Treatment 1 or 2	Test mother Start treatment 1 or 2 while awaiting results (if delay expected) a. If reactive, continue treatment b. If negative, investigate for other causes and modify treatment accordingly	Repeat test
Infant without signs of congenital syphilis	Treatment 3 Single injection	Test mother	No treatment

(**Treatment 1:** Injection aqueous benzyl penicillin 100,000–150,000 IU/kg/day administered as 50,000 IU/kg/dose IV every 12 hours, during the first 7 days of life and every 8 hours thereafter, for a total of 10 days

or

Injection procaine benzyl penicillin, 50,000 IU/kg by intramuscular/intravenous route, every 12 hours during the first 7 days of life and every 8 hours thereafter for a total of 10 days.

Treatment 2: Procaine benzyl penicillin 50,000 units/kg body weight, intramuscularly, in a single dose for 10 days.

Treatment 3: Benzathine benzyl penicillin 50,000 units/kg body weight, intramuscularly, in a single dose)

* (Signs of congenital syphilis: vesicular eruptions on palms or soles, hepatosplenomegaly, pseudo paralysis, edema/ascitis, fever (in first week of life), prolonged or conjugated hyperbilirubinemia, petechiae, bleeding, syphilitic facies. Infants are often asymptomatic at birth.)

Prevention

Congenital syphilis is mainly a consequence of lack of antenatal care and control of STIs. The mainstay of prevention is identification and adequate treatment of infected mothers during pregnancy. If possible, serological tests should be repeated in late pregnancy, to identify women infected during pregnancy; all women should be tested at least once during each pregnancy, and all women with reactive serology and their sexual partners with reactive serology should receive treatment (STI guidelines, WHO 2005).

TREATMENT SCHEDULES

Congenital Syphilis

See **Table 10.2**.

Early Congenital Syphilis (up to 2 years of age) and Infants with Abnormal CSF

Recommended regimen (WHO-2003) is as follows - Injection aqueous benzyl penicillin 100,000–150,000 IU/kg/day administered as 50,000 IU/ kg/dose IV every 12 hours, during the first 7 days of life and every 8 hours thereafter for a total of 10 days,

or

Injection procaine benzyl penicillin 50,000 IU/ kg by intramuscular injection, as a single daily dose for 10 days.

Some experts prefer to treat all infants with congenital syphilis as if the CSF findings were abnormal. Antimicrobials other than penicillin (e.g. erythromycin) are not recommended for congenital syphilis except in cases of allergy to penicillin. Tetracycline should not be used in young children.

Congenital Syphilis of 2 or More Years

Recommended regimen (WHO-2003) is as follows - Injection aqueous benzyl penicillin, 200,000 – 300,000 IU/kg/day by intravenous or intramuscular route, administered as 50,000 IU/kg/dose every 4-6 hours for 10-14 days. In patients allergic to penicillin, after the first month of life, erythromycin, 7.5-12.5 mg/kg orally, 4 times daily can be given for 30 days.

Acquired Syphilis in Children

Children can acquire syphilis following sexual abuse by an infected individual, or through breast feeding and rarely due to contact with extra genital primary chancre.

Clinical features in this age group are similar as in adult;

a. Primary chancre,
b. Secondary stage,
c. Latent stage,
d. Tertiary syphilis.

After incubation period of 9 to 90 days, primary chancre develops. Usual sites are vulva or anus, and the lesions are smaller in size and difficult to recognize. After a gap of 2 weeks to 6 months, skin lesions of secondary stage develop. All classical features like, erythematous, papular or papulosquamous rashes with involvement of palms and soles, moist verrucous plaques in and around the genitalia (**Figure 10.3)** and mucous patches are seen.

Diagnosis is made by demonstration of *T.pallidum* under dark ground microscopy, non-treponemal tests (VDRL, RPR) and treponemal tests (TPHA, FTA-ABS, MHA-TP), IgG and IgM enzyme immunoassays and PCR.

For treatment of acquired primary, secondary and early latent syphilis, injection benzathine penicillin G, 50,000 units/kg IM, up to the adult dose of 2.4 million units administered in a single dose. In late latent or latent syphilis of unknown duration, injection benzathine penicillin G, 50,000 units/kg IM is administered as three doses at 1 week intervals.

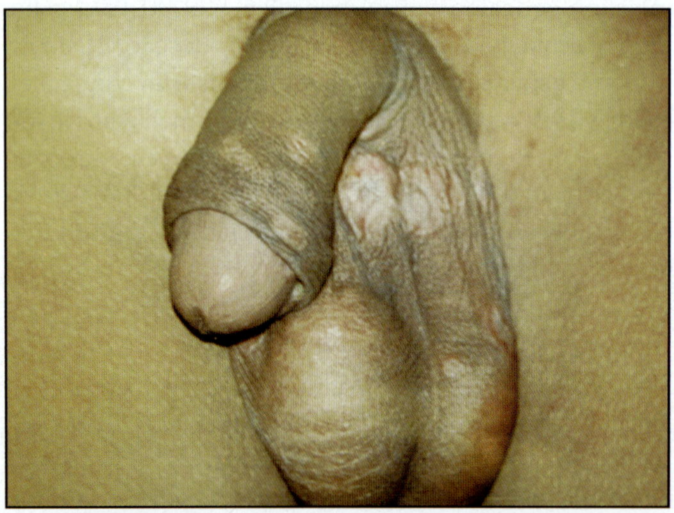

FIGURE 10.3: Lesions of secondary syphilis in an adolescent boy

GONORRHEA

In children, gonococcal infection can be acquired in the following ways:

1. Perinatal
2. Intimate contact
3. Sexual abuse

Neonates are infected by direct contact with the secretions while passage through the birth canal of an infected mother during vaginal delivery. Clinical presentations are gonococcal conjunctivitis (42%), orogastric contamination (7%) and disseminated infection (<1%).

Among children below 12 years of age, the prevalence of gonococcal infection due to sexual abuse or adolescent sexual activity has been reported to be 2.8 to 20% in various surveys. Among prepubertal girls the most common manifestation of gonococcal infection is vaginitis (75%) because of the low estrogen level and alkaline pH of the vaginal mucosa. There is profuse purulent vaginal discharge, vulval edema, urethritis and pruritus. Rectal infection is commoner in girls, either due to spread of infection through the profuse vaginal discharge or rectal intercourse. Rarely there can be an ascending infection leading to salpingitis and peritonitis. Among boys, the chances of infection is less. It presents with pyuria, urethral discharge, penile edema, epididymitis, testicular swelling and conjunctivitis. Pharyngeal and rectal infections are common in both the sexes, but mostly asymptomatic.

Dissemination of gonorrhea in infants and children is rare, often preceded by asymptomatic genitourinary tract infection. It is characterized by polyarthralgia (involving joints like knees, ankles, wrists and hands), meningitis, neonatal sepsis and pseudo paresis of involved joints.

Gonococcal arthritis in older children is characterized by suppurative arthritis, inflammation of periarticular surface and tenosynovitis of joints. It may be associated with cutaneous manifestations and osteomyelitis.

Chlamydial Infection

Chlamydial infection was more prevalent than gonococcal infection in children from developed countries, but, no such data are available in India. The source of infection and the clinical features are as follows:

1. During vaginal delivery, approximately 50-70% infants acquire the infection from infected mother and clinical manifestations may be in the following forms:
   a. Conjuctival infection (accounts for 30-50% of neonatal chlamydial infection)
   b. Nasopharyngeal infection and otitis media
   c. Chlamydial pneumonia
   d. Rectal infection
   e. Vaginal infection
   f. Asymptomatic shedding till the age of 3 years.

2. In children with chlamydial infection after 3 years of age, possibility of sexual abuse should be thought of. The clinical manifestations are:
   a. Proctitis
   b. Pharyngeal infection in both sexes
   c. Vaginitis in female child
   d. Urethritis in boys
   e. Salpingitis and pelvic inflammatory disease (PID), mostly among adolescents.

Treatment

Recommended regimen for neonatal conjunctivitis (see below) and pneumonia: Erythromycin base or ethyl succinate 50 mg/kg /day orally in four divided doses for 14 days. In children with body weight less than 45 kg, the dose is same as above. For those above 45 kg, but less than 8 years of age, azithromycin 1g orally in a single dose is recommended, and in children above 8 years, either azithromycin 1 g orally single dose or doxycycline 100 mg twice daily for 7 days is recommended.

OPHTHALMIA NEONATORUM

Ophthalmic inflammation associated with discharge in an infant within 21 days of birth is known as ophthalmia neonatorum.

The causes of ophthalmia neonatorum include:

a. *N. gonorrheae*
b. *Chlamydia*
c. Nonspecific organisms like *streptococcus*, diphtheroids, moraxenfield bacilli
d. Chemicals instilled into the eyes.

Clinical features include profuse mucopurulent discharge and congested and edematous conjunctiva. Smear and culture from the discharge should be done to reach a diagnosis.

Treatment (WHO-2003)

a. For gonococcal infection, injection ceftriaxone, 50 mg/kg IM as a single dose, to a maximum of 125 mg.
b. For chlamydial infection, syrup erythromycin, 50 mg/kg/day orally, in 4 divided doses for 14 days.
c. In syndromic approach, where facilities for laboratory diagnosis are not available both treatments should be given to cover both the infections.

Prevention (WHO-2005): Neonatal eye prophylaxis, regardless of maternal signs and symptoms of either infection should be provided to all neonates to prevent ophthalmia neonatorum. One drop of the following should be administered in each eye within one hour of birth:

1. Tetracycline ophthalmic ointment (1%) as single application

or

2. Iodine drops 2.5% as single application

or

3. Freshly prepared aqueous solution of silver nitrate (1%), as single application

BACTERIAL VAGINOSIS (BV)

In prepubertal girls, incidence of bacterial vaginosis is low. Causative organisms are *Gardnerella vaginalis*, *Mobiluncus sp.*, bacteroides, and peptostreptococcus. However, evidence of sexual abuse as a cause of BV in prepubertal girls is often inconclusive. Perinatal transmission of BV during vaginal delivery is not known. The children present with grayish white to yellow vaginal discharge with malodor. Determination of vaginal pH for diagnosing BV is not useful in prepubertal girls, because of the normally occurring alkaline pH of the vaginal mucosa at this age group.

The differential diagnosis includes vulvovaginitis due to non-venereal causes like enterobius vermicularis infestation, candidial infection, poor hygiene, or foreign bodies in the vagina.

OTHER BACTERIAL STIs

Chancroid, donovanosis and *Mycoplasma* infections are very rarely reported in children. Painful chancroid lesions in female children can give rise to acute urinary retention with dysuria and may present as an acute emergency in pediatric surgery department.

Trichomonal Infection

Trichomonal infection in children more than 1 year of age is mostly due to sexual contact. The rate of perinatal transmission is 0-0.6% and the reported rate in probable cases of sexual abuse is 0.4%.

In infant, the sites of infection are nose, throat and vagina. It may be asymptomatic, but transient vulvovaginitis is observed in prepubertal children. They present with vulvar excoriations, dermatitis and greenish-white, frothy and offensive vaginal discharge. Diagnosis is confirmed by demonstration of *Trichomonas vaginalis* by wet mount preparation of the discharge, examined under high power objective of a light microscope

Treatment includes syrup/tablet metronidazole, 30 mg/kg/day in three divided doses for 7 days.

VIRAL STI

Viral STIs in children include:

1. Herpes virus infection
2. Human papilloma virus infection
3. Molluscum contagiosum
4. HIV infection

HERPES VIRUS INFECTION

a. Cytomegalovirus (CMV)
b. Herpes simplex virus type 2 (HSV-2)

CMV

The infection is usually sub-clinical in 90% cases. The children get the infection from the infected mother *in utero* or perinatally. Primary CMV infection due to sexual abuse in children has not been reported from India. Symptomatic infection manifests as hepatosplenomegaly, microcephaly, jaundice, and petechiae.

HSV-2

The infection is common in children due to sexual abuse However, it is rarely reported even in presence of active maternal infection. This may be either due to non-recognition, lack of diagnostic facilities or passive transfer of maternal antibodies, thereby offering protection to the baby.

Clinical features: In neonatal HSV infection, symptoms appear within first week.

Skin and mouth shows clusters of vesicles on erythematous base, initially appearing on the presenting part that was in direct contact with the virus during birth, gradually progressing to other areas. Vesicular lesions may progress to bullous lesions.

Ocular manifestations include keratoconjuctivitis associated with microphthalmia which may lead to chorioretinitis, cataract and retinal detachment. Systemic involvement is frequently lethal, affecting liver, brain and adrenal glands. The dissemination of the virus is marked by constitutional signs and symptoms including irritability, respiratory distress, jaundice, bleeding diathesis and shock along with exanthemas. The child may present with irritability, tremors, poor feeding, unstable temperature, bulging fontanelle and pyramidal tract signs as manifestations of encephalitis.

Laboratory investigations show elevated serum transaminases, GGT, conjugated bilirubin, neutropenia and thrombocytopenia. CSF analysis shows pleocytosis and elevated protein level (as high as 500 to 1000 mg/dl). CSF culture grows HSV in 25 to 40% cases.

Preventive measures include examination of the expectant mothers for lesions of herpes genitalis. If a pregnant woman has skin lesions suggestive of herpes genitalis (primary or recurrent) in and around genitalia after 32 weeks of gestation, cesarean section is the ideal mode of delivery to prevent neonatal infection. Women without symptoms and signs of genital herpes or its prodrome can be delivered vaginally. Acyclovir may be administered orally to pregnant women with first episode or severe recurrent episode of herpes genitalis (WHO-2003, NACO-2007).

Treatment of neonatal HSV infection includes injection acyclovir 20 mg/kg intravenously, 8 hourly for 21 days in patients with central nervous system and disseminated disease or for 14 days for disease limited to the skin and mucous membrane.

HUMAN PAPILLOMA VIRUS INFECTION (HPV)

Children may acquire genital warts in different ways. It may be from the maternal genital tract during birth, autoinoculation from digital warts, and non-sexual transmission through contact from family members or carriers. The prevalence of genital warts among the children with STDs following sexual abuse was 10% in an Indian study. In a retrospective, hospital-based study from Delhi, India, condyloma acuminata was found to be the commonest (35.2%) infection among children with STDs. Maternal genital warts present during delivery are associated with a risk (1 in 400) of the infant developing juvenile laryngeal papillomatosis. Whether treatment of pregnant women with genital warts diminishes this risk is yet uncertain, but reduction of viral burden may be possible.

Common sites of occurrence include anogenital area, perineum, labia, around vaginal orifice, anus and in the rectum. It is found rarely in intravaginal location in young girls. Often the lesions are present around the mouth and between the toes.

Treatment of children above 2 years of age includes chemical cauterization with 25% podophyllin solution. Below 2 years, cryosurgery is the treatment of choice in order to avoid the possibility of neurotoxicity associated with podophyllin.

MOLLUSCUM CONTAGIOSUM

Molluscum contagiosum may occur in children due to sexual abuse and the clinical features and treatment do not differ from adults.

HIV INFECTION (NACO-2006)

Mother to child transmission (MTCT) is by far the most significant route of transmission of HIV infection in children below the age of 15 years. HIV can be transmitted during pregnancy, childbirth, or breast-feeding **(Table 10.3)**. Without intervention, the risk of transmission from an infected mother to her child ranges from 25% to 45% in developing countries and 15% to 25% in developed countries.

With approximately 27 million pregnancies/year and an overall HIV-prevalence rate of 0.7% among pregnant women, an estimated 1,89,000 HIV infected women are being delivered every year in India. However, with the current uptake coverage of HIV testing among pregnant women in India, the HIV status of over 90% of these exposed infants remain unknown.

DIAGNOSIS OF HIV INFECTION IN CHILDREN

There is passive transplacental transfer of maternal HIV antibody to the fetus during pregnancy and this is detectable in children born to HIV-infected mothers till 18 months. Hence, interpretation of positive HIV antibody test results is difficult in children below this age. Moreover, breastfed children have ongoing risk of acquisition of HIV infection. Hence, HIV infection can only be excluded after breast-feeding is stopped for more than 6 weeks.

TABLE 10.3: Estimated risk and timing of MTCT in the absence of intervention

During pregnancy	5-10%
During labor and delivery	10-15%
During breast-feeding	5-20%
Overall without breast-feeding	15-25%
Overall with breast-feeding to 6 months	20-35%
Overall with breast-feeding to 18 to 24 months	30-45%

1. In India, antibody tests and ELISA can be performed for infants more than 18 months as in adults. If the infant is positive at 12 months, a confirmation with a second HIV test should be done at 18 months of age to exclude a positive test result due to passively transferred maternal antibodies. Two positive HIV antibody test results (done sequentially) in a clinically symptomatic child (suggestive of HIV infection) more than 18 months old, indicate HIV infection in that child.
2. For infants less than 18 months, DNA PCR is done using dried blood spots (DBS). As per NACO recommendation, the first DNA PCR shall be conducted at 6 weeks of age. If the PCR test is positive, it has to be repeated immediately (or as early as possible) for confirmation. If PCR is negative in a non-breast-fed baby, confirmation with a second PCR test at 6 months is recommended. In a breast-fed baby, PCR should be repeated at 6-8 weeks after cessation of breast feeding to rule out HIV infection.
3. If testing facility (DNA PCR) is not available for infants less than 18 months, then diagnosis is made clinically, using presumptive diagnostic methods as follows:
   - The infant is confirmed HIV antibody positive

     and
   - Diagnosis of any AIDS-indicator condition(s) can be made

     or
   - The infant is symptomatic with two or more of the following:
     a. Oral thrush; creamy white to yellow, soft, small plaques on erythematous or normal-looking mucosa which can often be scraped off (pseudo membrane), or red patches on tongue, palate or lining of mouth, usually painful or tender, and not responding to topical antifungal treatment.
     b. Severe pneumonia; cough or difficult breathing in a child with indrawn chest, stridor or any other danger signs like lethargy or unconsciousness, inability to drink or breastfeed, vomiting, and presence or history of convulsions during current illness; not responding to antibiotics.
     c. Severe sepsis; fever or low body temperature in a young infant with any ominous sign such as fast breathing, indrawn chest, bulging fontanelle, lethargy, reduced movement, not feeding or sucking breast milk, convulsions, etc.

CLINICAL EVENTS IN INFANT AND CHILDREN WITH CONFIRMED HIV INFECTION

Primary HIV Infection

The affected infant is either asymptomatic or suffer from acute febrile illness 2-4 weeks post exposure, often associated with lymphadenopathy, pharyngitis and skin rashes. A positive virological test for HIV virus or its components [RNA or DNA or ICD (Immune-Complex Dissociated) HIV p24 antigen] confirmed by a second virological test obtained from a separate determination is required for confirmation in children below 18 months and positive HIV antibody test in children aged 18 months and over.

TABLE 10.4: WHO classification of HIV–associated clinical disease

Classification of HIV—associated clinical disease	WHO clinical stage
Asymptomatic	1
Mild	2
Advanced	3
Severe	4

WHO clinical stage 1:

The child is either asymptomatic or present with persistent generalized lymphadenopathy (PGL) characterized by swollen or enlarged lymph nodes > 1cm at two or more non-contiguous sites, without known cause.

WHO clinical stage 2:

1. Unexplained persistent hepatosplenomegaly.
2. Papular pruritic eruptions (scabies and insect bite have to be excluded).
3. Fungal nail infection; paronychia, onycholysis, proximal subungual white onychomycosis is specific for immunodeficiency.
4. Angular cheilitis; splits or cracks at the angle of the mouth with depigmentation, usually responding to antifungal treatment, but may be recurrent.
5. Linear gingival erythema (LGE); erythematous band that follows the contour of the free gingival line; may be associated with bleeding.
6. Extensive warts; characteristic warty lesions; small, fleshy, grain-like lesions, bumps, often rough, flat on the sole (plantar warts); facial, more than 5% of body surface area involvement.
7. Extensive molluscum contagiosum; small, flesh-colored or pearly-white, dome-shaped, umbilicated papules, may be inflamed or red; facial, more than 5% of body surface area involvement or disfiguring lesions **(Figure 10.4)**.

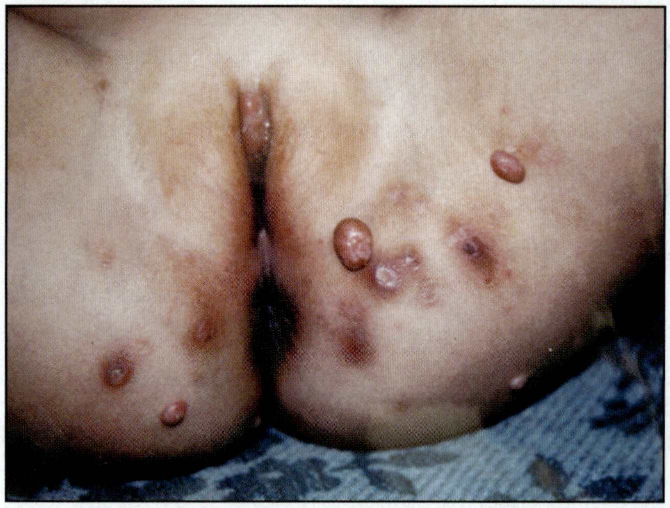

FIGURE 10.4: Multiple mollusca contagiosa in an HIV-infected child.

8. Recurrent oral ulcerations (2 or more in 6 months); aphthous ulceration, typically with a halo of inflammation and yellow-grey pseudo-membrane.
9. Unexplained parotid enlargement; asymptomatic bilateral swelling that may spontaneously resolve and recur.
10. Herpes zoster.
11. Recurrent upper respiratory tract infection (URTI).

WHO clinical stage 3:

1. Unexplained moderate malnutrition; weight loss-for-age, up to 2 standard deviations (SDs), not explained by poor or inadequate feeding and other infections, and not adequately responding to standard management.
2. Unexplained persistent diarrhea; for 14 days or more, loose or watery, three or more times daily, not responding to standard treatment.
3. Unexplained persistent fever; for more than one month, either intermittent or constant with no response to antibiotics and antimalarials.
4. Oral candidiasis; persistent or recurrent, creamy white to yellowish, soft, small plaques which can be scraped off (pseudo membranous) or red patches on tongue, palate or lining of mouth, usually painful (erythematous form), confirmed by microscopy and culture.
5. Oral hairy leukoplakia; fine small linear patches on lateral borders of tongue, generally bilateral, which cannot be scraped off.

TABLE 10.5: Revised classification of immune suppression in children (CD4 levels in relation to severity of immune suppression)

Classification of HIV-associated immune-deficiency	Age-related CD4 cell values			
	< 11 months (%)	12 – 35 months (%)	36 -59 months (%)	> 5years
Not significant (Normal CD4 cells)	>35	>30	>25	>500
Mild	30 - 35	25 - 30	20 - 25	350 - 499
Advanced	25 - 30	20 - 25	15 - 20	200 - 349
Severe	<25% or <1500 cells/mm^3	<20 or <750 cells/mm^3	< 15 or <350 cells/mm^3	<15% or < 200 cells/mm^3

Notes:

- CD4 count is the best measurement for assessing immune deficiency.
- CD4 count should be used in conjunction with clinical assessment; however, estimation of CD4 count allows an earlier detection of worsening of HIV disease as decline of CD4 count usually occurs prior to the clinical progression of the disease.
- CD4 count monitoring can aid in the decision to initiate antiretroviral therapy (ART).
- Younger children normally have higher CD4 count than older children and adults.
- Percentage (%) of CD4 cells is less variable in children < 6 years old and is the preferred method.
- At age $\geq$ 6 years, either % CD4 and /or absolute CD4 count can be used.
- The threshold CD4 cell levels for severely immunodeficient children aged $\geq$1 year corresponds with a 12-months mortality risk of $\leq$ 5%. In children younger than 1 year and especially < 6 months, CD4 is less predictive of mortality and there is high risk for death even if the % CD4 is high.
- Normal CD4 count/percentage in children are:
  a. <12 months: >1500 cells/mm^3 ($\geq$ 25%), b. 1- 5 years: >1000 cells/mm^3 ($\geq$ 25%), c. >6 years: >500 cells/mm^3

6. Lymph node tuberculosis; non-acute, painless (cold) enlargement of lymph nodes, usually matted, localized to one region, may have draining sinuses. Diagnosis is confirmed by histology or fine needle aspiration cytology stained by Ziehl Neelsen stain and culture.
7. Pulmonary tuberculosis confirmed by chest X-ray and positive sputum smear or culture.
8. Severe, recurrent, presumed bacterial pneumonia, confirmed by bacteria isolation from sputum, BAL, lung aspirate.
9. Acute necrotizing ulcerative gingivitis or stomatitis, or acute necrotizing ulcerative periodontitis.
10. Symptomatic lymphocytic interstitial pneumonia (LIP).
11. Chronic HIV associated lung disease.
12. Unexplained anemia (<8g/dl).

WHO clinical stage 4:

1. Unexplained severe wasting, stunting or severe malnutrition not adequately responding to standard therapy.
2. *Pneumocystis* pneumonia (PCP); dry cough, progressive difficulty in breathing, tachypnea and fever. Diagnosis is confirmed by typical chest X-ray finding of bilateral diffuse infiltrate, microscopy of induced sputum or broncho-alveolar lavage or NPA, or histopathology of lung tissue.
3. Recurrent, severe, presumed bacterial infection like, empyema, pyomyositis, bone or joint infection, meningitis.
4. Chronic herpes simplex infection (painful, orolabial, genital, or anorectal lesions caused by HSV infection present for more than one month duration or visceral at any site.
5. Esophageal candidiasis (or candidiasis of trachea, bronchi or lungs) characterized by dysphagia, odynophagia or retrosternal pain while swallowing.
6. Extra pulmonary/disseminated tuberculosis; systemic illness with fever, night sweat, weight loss, sterile pyuria, pericarditis, ascites, pleural effusion, meningitis, arthritis, orchitis, all responding to anti-tuberculosis therapy.

MANAGEMENT

Comprehensive care of HIV-infected children include:

1. Early diagnosis of HIV infection in children.
2. Early diagnosis of opportunistic infections (OI).

3. Effective prevention and management of OI.
4. Early initiation of ART to prevent OI.
5. Cotrimoxazole (CTX) prophylaxis for prevention of OI.
6. Immunization for vaccine preventable diseases.
7. General prevention advice for caregivers, such as hand washing, drinking clean water, washing of raw fruits and vegetables before consumption.
8. Nutritional counseling and ensuring good diet.
9. Psycho-social support and counseling support to ensure adherence.
10. Involvement of family and gradual disclosure to the child as appropriate to maturity and understanding.
11. Continuum of care and support for children and infants not yet requiring ART.

Assessment and management after confirmed HIV diagnosis:

1. Assess growth and nutritional status, and intervention needs.
2. Assess immunization status and provide appropriate immunization.
3. Assess for signs and symptoms of opportunistic infections and risk behaviour exposure. If OI is suspected, diagnosis and treatment of OIs take priority over initiation of ART. Discussion of management of all OIs is beyond the scope of this chapter.
4. Ensure that the child is on co-trimoxazole prophylaxis. It protects the child from PCP, toxoplasmosis, and other bacterial infections, thereby reducing the mortality and morbidity of children less than five years of age. The recommended prophylaxis is 5 mg/kg/day as a single dose.
5. Ensure any concomitant medication use that may have drug interactions with ART.
6. Perform CD4 count (% CD4 is preferred in children less than 5 years and CD4 count in children above 5 years of age)
7. Assess criteria for starting ART.
8. Assess family situation including financial status, their current health/treatment status and availability of primary care giver.

Management of some common mucocutaneous opportunistic infections:
See **Table 10.6**.

Antiretroviral Therapy (ART)

When to start ART?

Under the national programme, CD4 count or CD4 % will be done to determine the child's eligibility for starting ART. However, when these investigations are not available, there should not be any delay in offering ART based on the clinical staging as presented in **Table 10.7**.

What to start?

In the 2006 WHO guidelines for treatment of infants and children, several drugs have been recommended for use, based on evidence –

- Nucleoside reverse transcriptase inhibitors (NRTI) like d4T (stavudine), 3TC (lamivudine), AZT (zidovudine), ABC (abacavir)
- Non-nucleoside reverse transcriptase inhibitors (NNRTI) like NVP (nevirapine), EFV (efavirenz),
- Protease inhibitors (PI) like LPV/r (lopinavir/ritonavir), NFV (nelfinavir), and SQV (saquinavir).

There are little data on other antiretroviral (ARV) drugs for use in children. The recommended preferred first-line ARV regimens for infants and children are:

Regimen of 2 NRTI plus 1 NNRTI -
1. AZT* + 3TC + NVP or EFV**
2. D4T + 3TC + NVP or EFV**

* AZT should not be given in combination with D4T.

** EFV is not currently recommended for children below 3 years of age or less than 10 kg and should be avoided in post-pubertal adolescent girls who are either in 1st trimester of pregnancy or are sexually active and not receiving adequate contraception. EFV is used to substitute NPV when anti-tuberculous treatment has to be provided concomitantly. However, after 2 weeks of completion of ATT, EFV should be switched back to NVP.

*** ABC + 3TC + NVP or EFV is an alternative, however, in national programme – ABC is not available and is still costly.

Dosage of anti-retroviral drugs in children has been presented in **Table 10.8.**

Immune Reconstitution Inflammatory Syndrome with HIV Treatment

Immune reconstitution inflammatory syndrome (IRIS), also referred to as "Immune restoration disease" occurs weeks to months after the commencement of ART or HAART (highly active antiretroviral therapy). It represents

TABLE 10.6: Management of some common mucocutaneous opportunistic infections

Opportunistic infection	Diagnosis	Treatment
Candidiasis	Oral candidiasis: KOH preparation demonstrates budding yeast cells. Esophageal candidiasis: Barium swallow shows cobblestone appearance. Endoscopy shows small white raised plaques with hyperemia and extensive ulceration.	Oral fluconazole 3-6 mg/kg once daily 7-14 days for oral candidiasis and 14 to 21 days for esophageal candidiasis
Penicilliosis	1.Translucent umbilicated papules resembling molluscum contagiosum along with fever, anemia, hepatosplenomegaly & generalized lymphadenopathy. 2.Wright stain of skin scraping shows basophilic, spherical or oval yeast-like organisms with clear central septa.	**Induction therapy:** Amphotericin B (0.7-1.5 mg/kg/day) for 2 weeks **Consolidation therapy**: Itraconazole 5-6 mg/kg/dose twice daily for 8 weeks **Maintenance therapy**: Itraconazole 3-6 mg/kg/day
Cryptococcosis	**Meningoencephalitis:** Fever, headache, altered mental status. India ink stain of CSF shows budding yeast and cryptococcal antigen can be detected in CSF or serum by latex agglutination test. **Disseminated manifestations:** Translucent umbilicated papules resembling molluscum contagiosum. Wright stain of skin scraping shows budding yeast.	**Induction therapy:** Amphotericin B (0.7-1.5 mg/kg/day) plus flucytosine (25 mg/kg/dose four times daily) for 2 weeks. **Consolidation therapy**: Fluconazole 5-6 mg/kg/dose twice daily for 8 weeks. Maintenance therapy: Fluconazole 3-6 mg/kg/day.
Herpes simplex virus	**HSV gingivostomatitis:** Fever, irritability, superficial painful ulcers in the gingival, oral mucosa and perioral area. **HSV encephalitis**: Fever, altered consciousness, abnormal behavior, detection of HSV DNA in CSF.	**HSV gingivostomatitis:** Oral acyclovir 20 mg/kg/dose three times daily Or IV acyclovir 5-10 mg/kg/dose three times daily for 7-14 days. **Disseminated HSV or encephalitis:** IV acyclovir 10 mg/m^2/dose three times daily for 21 days.
Herpes zoster virus (VZV)	**Primary varicella infection:** Generalized pruritic vesiculobullous lesions/rash. **Herpes zoster:** Painful vesiculobullous lesions/ rash in unilateral dermatomal distribution. Tzanck preparation with Giemsa staining of cell scrapings from the lesion shows multinucleated giant cells suggestive of VZV.	**Primary varicella infection:** IV acyclovir 10 mg/kg/dose or 500 mg/m^2/dose three times daily for 7 days in children with moderate to severe immune-suppression. Oral formulation to be used with mild immune-suppression. **Herpes Zoster**: Oral acyclovir 20 mg/kg/dose four times daily (max. 800 mg/dose) for 7 days.

a restoration of both number and function of CD4 positive T lymphocytes and manifests with a flaring or reactivation of either inflammatory conditions or immune response to opportunistic infections like herpes zoster. Tangsinmankong and colleagues presented a historical cohort study where they followed up 61 perinatally acquired HIV-infected children for a period of more than 6 months. Seven cases of IRIS, in the form of herpes zoster within 6 months of commencing HAART were detected. Herpes zoster occurred only in those who experienced virologic success, (defined as a decrease of more than 2 log viral RNA in plasma or achieving a plasma RNA level lower than 400 copies/ml) and immunologic success (defined as an increase in CD4-positive cells of more than 5% from the baseline or a total CD4-positive cell count higher than 250 cells/ml within 6 months of

TABLE 10.7: Clinical and immunological criteria for starting ART

WHO Pediatric stage	Availability of CD4 cell measurement	Age-specific treatment recommendation <12 months	>12 months
4	CD4 No CD4	Treat all	
3	CD4	Treat all	Treat all, CD4 guided In those children with TB, LIP, OHL, Thrombocytopenia
	No CD4		Treat all
2	CD4 No CD4		CD4 guided [d] Don't treat
1	CD4 No CD4		CD4 guided Don't treat

Notes:

- Stabilize any opportunistic infection prior to initiation of ARV therapy
- Baseline CD4 estimation is useful to monitor ART even if it is not required to initiate ART.
- In children with pulmonary or lymph node tuberculosis, the CD4 level and clinical status should be used to determine the need for and timing of initiation of ART in relation to tuberculosis treatment
- For CD4 count %, refer to **Table 10.5.**

TABLE 10.8: Formulation of fixed drug combinations (FDCs) for pediatric HIV use in India

Formulation	Stavudine (d4T)	Lamivudine (3TC)	Nevirapine (NVP)
FDC 6 (baby tablet)	6 mg	30 mg	50 mg
FDC 10 (tablet)	10 mg	40 mg	70 mg
FDC 12 (junior tablet)	12 mg	60 mg	100 mg
FDC 30 d4T (adult tablet)	30 mg	150 mg	200 mg
FDC -30 AZT (adult tablet)	300 mg	150 mg	200 mg

starting HAART). Furthermore, children who had a prior history of varicella had a greater risk of developing zoster if they had not achieved a protective level of varicella-specific IgG.

SUMMARY

A team effort of health care personnel, caregiver and child is required to ensure long term adherence and good response to ART. Malnutrition is a common condition in HIV-infected children and is a major contributor to mortality. Nutritional assessment and support should be the integral part of the care plan of HIV- infected children. Essential components in palliative care for children includes prevention of opportunistic infections (cotrimoxazole prophylaxis), relief of symptoms and management of pain and establishing a mutual trusting relationship between the child and family with the clinical team (counselor/pediatrician/dermatologist/nurse/NGO/volunteer).

BIBLIOGRAPHY

1. Ahmed HJ, Ilard I, Antognoli A, et al. An epidemic of Neisseria gonorrheae from infants and children. Pediatr Infect Dis 1988;7:32.
2. Chacko RM, Wood Jr CR. Gynecological infections in children and adolescent. In: Feigin RD, Cherry JD, Eds.Textbook of Paediatrics Infection. 4th Edn. Philadelphia: WB Saunders; 1998. p 509-547.
3. Garg BR, Mohammed AS, Baruah MC. Sexually transmitted diseases in children. Indian J Sex Transm Dis 1986; 7:11-13.
4. Guidelines for HIV care and treatment in infants and children, November 2006, prepared by Indian Academy of Paediatrics and National AIDS Control Organisation with support from Clinton Foundation. UNICEF. WHO.
5. Guidelines for HIV care and Treatment in infants and children, November 2006, NACO and Indian Academy of Paediatrics,

6. Gutman LT. Gonococcal diseases in infants and children. In: Holmes KK. Mardh PA, Sparling PF, et al. Eds. Sexually transmitted diseases. 3rd Edn. New York: Mc Graw Hill; 1999;1145-53.
7. Haldich SF, Kohl PK, Sexually transmitted diseases in children- a practical approach. Dermatol clinics (sexually transmitted diseases) Vol.16, No, 4 Oct.1998, 859-61.
8. Mendiratta Vibhu, Harjal Bhawna, Koranne Ravindra V. Profile of STDs in children. Indian J Sex Dis 2004; 25:67-69.
9. Mendiratta Vibhu, Kumar V, Sharma RC et al. STD profile in children. Indian J Sex Dis 1996; 17:1-3.
10. Mohan Kumar V, Sathish Kumar A, Arun Kumar, Venkateswaran, Balasubramaniam MP. Sexually transmitted infection in child sexual abuse. Indian J Sex Transm Dis 2001;22:75-78.
11. Murugan S, Raman LG, Solomon PJ, Kumarasamy.Morbidity pattern of STD in children of south Tamil Nadu. Indian J Sex Transm Dis 1987; 8:47-50.
12. Pandhi RK, Khanna N, Sekhri R, Sexually transmitted diseases in children. Indian J Sex Transm Dis 1995; 32:27-30.
13. Sheffield JS, Sanche PJ, Wendel GD Jr, et al. Placental histopathology of congenital syphilis. Obstet Gynecol 2002;100:126-33.
14. Singh O P. Congenital Syphilis In: Sharma Vinod K Eds. Sexually Transmitted Diseases and AIDS. 1st Edn. New Delhi:Viva Books Private Ltd 2003;183-91.
15. Singh OP, Bhargava NC, Jaisal NL, STDs in children. Ind J Dermatol Leprol 1977; 43:155-57.
16. Tangsinmankong N, Kamchaisa tian W, Lujan Zilbermann J, et al. Varicella zoster as a manifestation of immune restoration disease in HIV-infected children. J Allergy Clin Immunol 2004;113:742-46.
17. Thappa DM, Senthikumar M, Laxmisha Chandrashekar. Anogenital warts—an overview 2004;25:55-66.
18. Von Krogh G, Lacey CJN, Gross G, Barrasso R, Schneider A. European course on HPV associated pathology; guielines for primary care physician for the diagnosis and management of anogenital warts.Sex Trans Infect 2000;76:162-168.
19. Walker DG, Walker GJ. Forgotten but not gone:The continuing scourge of congenital syphilis. Lancet Infect Dis 2002;2:432-36.

11

Cutaneous Mycobacterial Infections

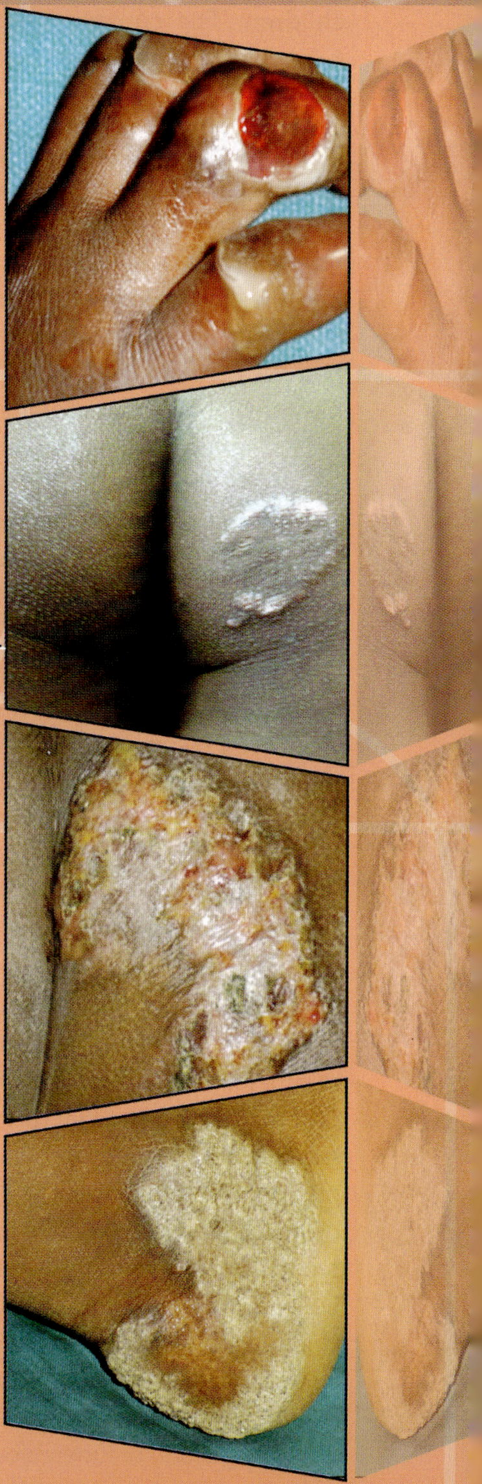

Cutaneous Tuberculosis
V Ramesh, M Ramam

Nontuberculous Mycobacterial Infections
Ragunatha S

Leprosy
PVS Prasad

CUTANEOUS TUBERCULOSIS

Tuberculosis is an important infection prevalent in communities throughout the world and children form a vulnerable group. Like in adults, tuberculous skin infections can present with varied manifestations in children. The causative organism is *Mycobacterium tuberculosis*, human and rarely the bovine strains.

OVERVIEW

Using surveillance figures to update estimates of incidence, the global data was summarized in the WHO tuberculosis report of 2005, which calculated that there were 8.9 million new cases of tuberculosis in 2004. More than 80% of all new patients are in the African, South-East Asia and Western Pacific regions (WHO report 2006). India has the highest burden of tuberculosis with an incidence of 1.8 million cases per annum. Primary multidrug resistant tuberculosis is 2.4% and in previously treated cases multidrug resistant tuberculosis is estimated at 25% (WHO 2006). It is a major cause of childhood morbidity and mortality. It is estimated that about 6-8% of all new cases are in the pediatric age group, particularly in those <5 years, who have less immunity to resist the development of the disease [Revised National Tuberculosis Control Programme (RNTCP), 2007]. Childhood tuberculosis is a reflection of the prevalence of sputum smear-positive pulmonary tuberculosis in the community and the extent of transmission in the population.

Although pulmonary tuberculosis has a very wide distribution and affects a large number of people throughout the world particularly after the advent of HIV, the picture is not the same with cutaneous tuberculosis. Even in the past when death rates in US were high due to tuberculosis, cutaneous tuberculosis was uncommon, probably suggesting that racial factors may have a role in susceptibility. Lupus vulgaris was endemic in Europe in the nineteenth century and has been almost eradicated by good improvement in living standards. Now and then reports appear from the south and eastern countries of Europe like Spain and Turkey, but few of these are in children. Tuberculous skin infections have also been seen to be rare in Africa but frequent in Latin American and Asian countries such as India and China which already have a high load of tuberculosis. In a tertiary care hospital in India cutaneous tuberculosis accounted for 0.1% of the total dermatology out-patient attendance and in a similar institution where only children with skin ailments were seen, it was 0.36%. In most centers cutaneous tuberculosis in children is seen in a quarter of the total number of patients with cutaneous tuberculosis. This is also evident from a large recent study from South India. These figures are in sharp contrast to Hong Kong, where cutaneous tuberculosis represented 0.066% of all new skin patients. Most of these patients had erythema induratum which is far less common in children, indicating that improvement in general standards of living are more important than treatment alone in decreasing the incidence of cutaneous tuberculosis. In the English language reports, India would perhaps account for the largest number of cutaneous tuberculosis seen among children.

CLASSIFICATION AND CLINICAL FEATURES

A number of clinical manifestations of cutaneous tuberculosis have given rise to many classification systems indicating attempts to make it as meaningful as possible. Some have used the modes of acquisition of infection namely exogenous or endogenous routes and others have tried to devise a microbiological classification based on the species of mycobacterium isolated. Both these are not satisfactory since the organisms are often not isolated on culture. In most studies, an active focus of tuberculosis or a history of this infection is obtained scarcely making it difficult to comprehend whether it was truly exogenous or due to endogenous dissemination. Often the lesion is solitary and to attribute it to dissemination sounds far fetched. Occasionally both reactivation of a latent focus and exogenous inoculation have been suggested to explain the clinical picture. To evolve a universally acceptable classification system, as stated much earlier, it is somewhat logical to accommodate the various types in a classification based on the host response determined by previous exposure to the mycobacterium.

It is important to note that, though the clinical types of cutaneous tuberculosis are same in children and adults, some differences exist. The primary forms are commoner in children, lymph node involvement is more, lesions are more extensive compared to adults, and some forms of tuberculids like erythema induratum are almost never encountered in children. Tuberculosis cutis orificialis, which is secondary to advanced visceral tuberculosis, is a disease of the elderly. The mode of acquisition of the infection may also differ. Inoculation tuberculosis, seen in butchers and laboratory workers, is a disease of adults rather than children.

A working classification of cutaneous tuberculosis in children has been presented in **Table 11.1**.

TABLE 11.1: Classification of cutaneous tuberculosis

A. Primary cutaneous tuberculosis in the nonsensitized or without previous exposure
- Miliary tuberculosis
- Tuberculous chancre

B. Secondary cutaneous tuberculosis in sensitized children with previous exposure
- Lupus vulgaris
- Scrofuloderma
- Tuberculosis verrucosa cutis
- Unusual forms of tuberculosis

C. Tuberculids
- Lichen scrofulosorum
- Papulonecrotic tuberculid
- Erythema nodosum

D. Dermatological complications of BCG vaccination

Miliary Tuberculosis of the Skin

Miliary cutaneous tuberculosis is a rare acute condition, occurring as a part of fulminant infection resulting from hematogenous spread of mycobacteria to multiple organs including the skin. The initial infection is usually pulmonary or meningeal. This clinical pattern is mainly seen in children and may be coincident with other infections like measles. Tuberculin sensitivity is absent, and bacillary load is significant. The condition presents often on the trunk as small red macules and papules. Purpura, vesicles and central necrosis are common. Children are gravely ill with a poor prognosis and often succumb rapidly before being investigated. Acute miliary tuberculosis has been reported in a malnourished infant with thrush, and an ulcerative rash has been seen in a malnourished 3-year-old girl with miliary pulmonary tuberculosis, indicating that poor nutrition may play an important role in cutaneous dissemination of the disease.

The possibility that cases of miliary cutaneous tuberculosis would be on the rise is evident from a recent report, in which, almost every organ was seen to be involved in patients with HIV infection.

Tuberculous Chancre

A chancre results due to entry of bacilli through the skin or mucosa of a nonsensitized child. Since mycobacteria cannot penetrate intact skin, it may be seen after BCG vaccination. Such children are usually malnourished or premature neonates, but this can also result following trauma, ritual circumcision and cosmetic procedures like ear piercing. The lesion starts as a papulo-nodule that ulcerates with associated regional lymphadenopathy. If the host immune response improves as seen by development of epithelioid cell granuloma on histopathology, the lesion heals with scarring within 3 months. If not, the bacterial load increases with necrosis of skin and healing is much delayed necessitating treatment. The lymph nodes may break down giving rise to scrofuloderma. Latent focus of infection remains at the site and progress to lupus vulgaris. The tuberculin reaction is negative initially but becomes positive later.

Secondary Cutaneous Tuberculosis in Sensitized / those Exposed to Tuberculous Infection

Large number of children above 5 years of age with cutaneous tuberculosis belongs to this group. Unlike in adults, the proportion of scrofuloderma is slightly higher than lupus vulgaris, and girls are more commonly affected than boys. It may reflect the poor nutritional status of the girls compared to boys or the fact that remaining confined to their homes without being sent to school, they are in closer contact with tuberculosis patients in the family or neighborhood. All children should be investigated to exclude systemic infection. If scrofuloderma resulting from bone and joint tuberculosis are excluded, a systemic tuberculous focus is found in <20% of children.

Lupus Vulgaris

This is the commonest form of cutaneous tuberculosis but its incidence in children may be next to scrofuloderma, and this may be attributed to the higher incidence of lymph node affection at this age group. Lesions start as solitary, red-brown, soft papules which evolve to larger plaques. Atrophy and peripheral extension is the rule. On diascopy, these early papules show the appearance of apple-jelly, but this may be seen in many unrelated conditions with a similar presentation. More lesions may appear and hyperkeratotic changes occur in the course of time. Unlike adults, many children show regional lymphadenopathy. Lower half of the body is often the preferred site of occurrence of lesions. This may be due to the custom of scant clothing and living in open spaces in the Indian set-up, which facilitates acquiring infection from any form of infective material present on the ground. Thus lupus vulgaris may occur on the buttocks, thighs

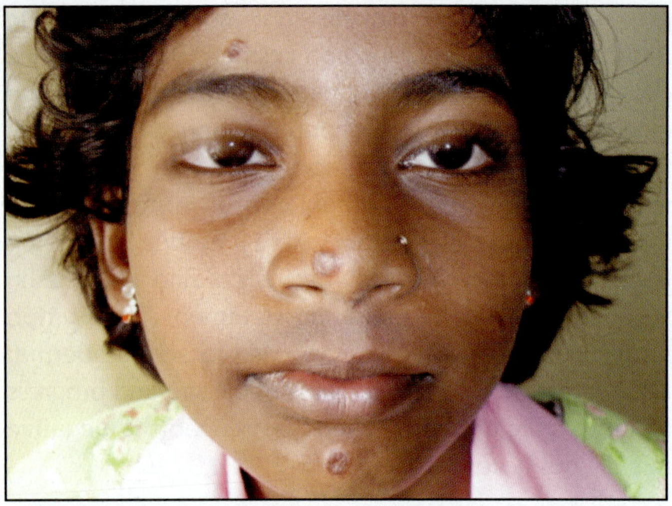

FIGURE 11.1: Multiple lesions of lupus vulgaris on the face

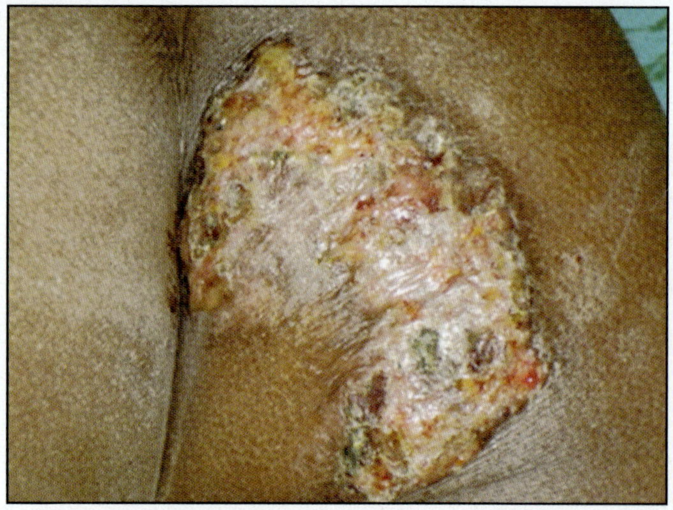

FIGURE 11.2B: Lupus vulgaris (ulcerative)

and knees. The upper limbs and face are also common sites of involvement. Extensive lesions can be seen in neglected children **(Figure 11.1)** and lesions overlying the joints may give rise to contractures. The lack of constitutional symptoms or pain in the lesions leads to long delays before these children are examined by a dermatologist. The clinical forms vary depending on the evolution of the lesion;

- Plaque, keratotic or hypertrophic variety, commonest type, with crusts covering the lesion **(Figure 11.2A)**,
- Ulcerated form, in which the deeper tissues are affected, **(Figure 11.2B)**
- Mutilating form in which there is destruction of structures like the ears and nose or severe contracture of the joints like knees and elbows.

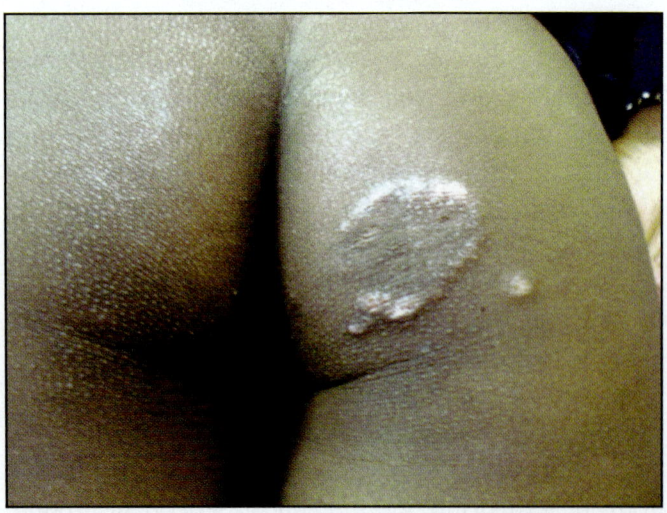

FIGURE 11.2A: Lupus vulgaris (plaque)

In all forms of lupus vulgaris, the tuberculin test is strongly positive. Rarely, in a malnourished child with few lesions, sudden dissemination of lesions all over the body may occur following an episode of exanthematous illness. A severe attack of measles or varicella temporarily depresses the immune system; however the lesions show signs of clearing when the attack subsides. Lupus vulgaris of the mucous membranes is rarely seen alone; it is often an extension from the surrounding skin, either on the face or the genital area. Hideous contractures of the genital area can result if the disease is left untreated. Interestingly, squamous cell carcinoma arising from the scar of healed lupus vulgaris, usually seen in elderly persons has been observed in the knee of a teen aged boy for which repeated trauma might have been the provocative factor. Total surgical excision of the lesion followed by anti-tubercular therapy was curative without any relapse.

Scrofuloderma

Scrofuloderma is the commonest form of cutaneous tuberculosis encountered in children. It is also termed as tuberculosis colliquativa cutis. Almost always it results from enlarged cervical lymph nodes, which in the older days was likened to a breeding sow, called *'scrofula'* in Latin. When the overlying skin is involved by breakdown of the lymph nodes, it is known as scrofuloderma. Currently the term refers to any underlying focus of tuberculosis, including bones, joints or viscera, which break down to involve the overlying skin. Lymph nodes remain the commonest source of infection in scrofuloderma. Multiple bone involvement is common in children. Irrespective of

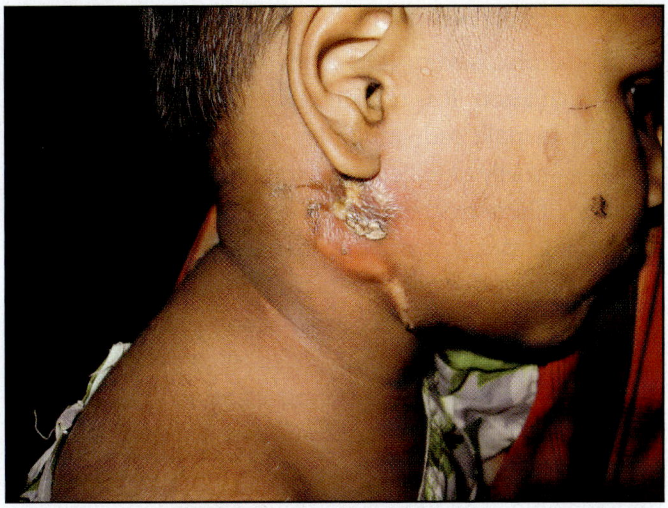

FIGURE 11.3: Scrofuloderma

the underlying structure affected, scrofuloderma manifests as chronic sinuses or necrotic ulcers with unhealthy ragged margins, intermittently discharging caseous material and may give rise to irregular, ugly scars **(Figure 11.3).** It involves the contiguous tissues and spreads slowly with discharge, crusting, destruction, fibrotic bands and contractures. Severe fibrotic process involving draining lymph nodes may cause elephantiasis of a limb or the genitalia. Constitutional symptoms like fever, night sweat and weight loss may be present when several groups of lymph nodes are affected. At times scrofuloderma may give rise to gummatous lesions called scrofulous or tuberculous gumma, in which the infection breaks out from the subcutaneous tissue. These are metastatic lesions seen initially as subcutaneous swellings. Spread and behavior of these lesions is similar to scrofuloderma. The Mantoux test is positive but in malnourished patients with extensive scrofuloderma it may be weakly positive or negative.

Tuberculosis Verrucosa Cutis

This is a quite common type seen among children and when present on the palms or soles, it may be deceptive as a wart. With increase in size, the lesions become more verrucous with fissuring and secondary infection resulting in big warty excrescence **(Figures 11.4A and B)**. The regional lymph nodes are not affected in most of the cases. At times the keratotic material may become very hard. Since there is little to differentiate it from hypertrophic lupus vulgaris, tuberculosis verrucosa cutis can well be regarded as a variant of this entity. The lesions can also present at other trauma-prone sites like heel, knee and elbow. The tuberculin test is strongly positive.

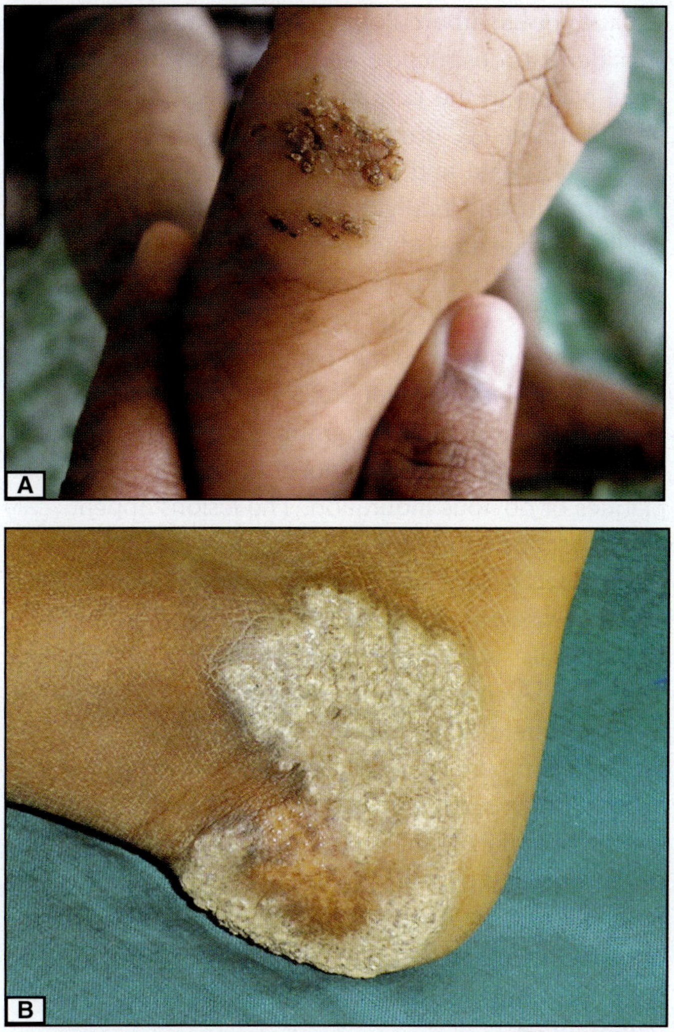

FIGURES 11.4A AND B: Tuberculosis verrucosa cutis

Unusual Presentations

Some forms of cutaneous tuberculosis have distinct morphology but are rare and may be misleading. These may go unsuspected for long before being recognized as this infection.

Sporotrichoid form refers to multiple, linearly arranged lesions simulating sporotrichosis. The limbs are often affected and the infection spreads along the lymphatics. This presentation is well-known with atypical mycobacteria but may also be caused by *M. tuberculosis*. Both lupus vulgaris and scrofuloderma can present in this pattern. Sometimes multiple gummas may be seen in the buttocks or thighs of older children arranged horizontally in a linear distribution, though this is not a typical sporotrichoid pattern.

Cutaneous tuberculosis involving face can cause considerable destruction and mutilation. It starts as a small plaque in the perioral area, or as a firm swelling on the upper lip, gradually spreading to the mucosa including tongue and nose. Vegetative plaques around the mouth have been described. Extension into the palate, nasolacrimal duct and nasal septum can cause profound local destruction and may even lead to middle ear disease.

Flat and erosive or scaly plaque on the sole is one of the most elusive presentations of cutaneous tuberculosis. It can be seen in any age group. Constant friction and pressure on the soles prevent the formation of raised plaques or obvious induration. The lesions appear scaly and eroded, and notoriously persistent with little symptoms. Such lesions are normally mistaken for eczema, Bowen's disease or psoriasis and the diagnosis becomes evident only when skin biopsy reveals a granulomatous pathology. A chronic ulcer on the sole should also raise the suspicion of tuberculosis.

Orificial tuberculosis results from seeding of the skin around body orifices by mycobacteria derived from an affected internal organ. Small, painful, necrotic ulcers may be seen around mouth or in the perianal area in patients with pulmonary or gastrointestinal tract tuberculosis respectively.

Tuberculids

Tuberculids are eruptions resulting from hypersensitivity to some mycobacterial products. The patients are in average or good health. These patients show the following features:

- Positive tuberculin reaction.
- A focus of tuberculosis involving viscera or lymph nodes.
- Absence of AFB in the affected skin and a negative culture.
- Spontaneous remission and relapse, or remission following treatment.

In the past, a number of terminologies had been used for these eruptions resulting in an uncharted forest of names. Even the existence of tuberculids as an entity was doubtful. Currently, with the advent of better diagnostic techniques like PCR, mycobacterial DNA has been detected in these lesions on some occasions and these are definitely considered as tuberculids.

Lichen Scrofulosorum

Lichen scrofulosorum (LS) is the commonest tuberculid seen in children. It is recognized as asymptomatic, skin-colored to pale red, multiple, grouped, pin-head size papules, mostly at follicular or sometimes at perifollicular location. There may be scaling and crusting. The lesions are mostly present on the trunk but can be present elsewhere including the genitalia. A high index of suspicion is needed at times to recognize lichen scrofulosorum as these are asymptomatic and regress spontaneously to reappear in crops over a period of time. Lymph nodes or the lungs remain the commonest focus of infection followed by the bones. Occasionally focus of infection is undetectable. The tuberculin test is strongly positive.

Papulonecrotic Tuberculid

Papulonecrotic tuberculids are not as common as lichen scrofulosorum but have been reported in few children from India. A larger number has been reported from South Africa.The individual lesion starts as an inflammatory papule or papulo-pustule and grows up to 0.5 cm in size. Necrosis results in a crusted top and ulcers may be formed. The distribution is similar as in adults; the extensor aspects of the limbs are mainly involved followed by the trunk. The lesions appear in crops leaving varioliform scars. The face and genitalia are usually spared. The Mantoux test is strongly positive. A vasculitic form with extensive involvement of the flexor surfaces of limbs, trunk, perineum and vulva has been reported in a 2-year-old girl.

Erythema Nodosum

Of all the tuberculids, erythema nodosum is the non-specific one, as it can be seen in association with other infections, notably streptococcal diseases and drug reactions. The histopathology shows septal panniculitis, and granuloma may be present. In India and other developing countries tuberculosis still remains an important cause of erythema nodosum but children are very rarely affected. It is characterized by sudden eruption of large, painful, subcutaneous nodules over the limbs. These may be accompanied by fever and disappear within 1 to 2 weeks, even without treatment, leaving slight discoloration. The tuberculin test is of great help when no focus of tuberculosis is detectable. If negative, the possibility of tuberculosis may be ruled out.

At times, uncommon and previously undocumented skin lesions have been described with visceral or cutaneous tuberculosis and these have subsided with anti-tubercular therapy. These include recurrent papular eruptions of the palms associated with tuberculoma of the brain, and a condition termed nodular tuberculid, which simulates erythema nodosum clinically with a strong tuberculin reaction and granulomatous vasculitis in histopathology. In association with skin lesions, conjunctiva has also been affected in some children. Lesions resembling perforating dermatosis both clinically and histopathologically have been seen. Pityriasis lichenoides et varioliformis acuta (PLEVA)-like tuberculid, in association with exogenously acquired cutaneous tuberculosis, which resolved after anti-tubercular therapy has been described.

More than one form of secondary cutaneous tuberculosis, with or without tuberculids may be seen in the same patient and this is more common among children. Isolated reports of lupus vulgaris, tuberculosis verrucosa cutis and scrofuloderma over widespread or localized body areas and a variety of clinical lesions with tuberculids present in profusion over the lower limbs has been reported.

DERMATOLOGICAL COMPLICATIONS DUE TO BCG VACCINATION

Bacille Calmette Guerin (BCG), an attenuated strain of bovine tubercle bacilli has been used extensively for vaccination of human beings against tuberculosis, since the early part of 20th century. It was initially used in the Scandinavian countries and thereafter throughout most part of the rest of the world. Normally the cutaneous reaction at the vaccine site is self-healing and the vaccination imparts some immunity to the recipient against tuberculous infection. However, some other dermatological manifestations **(Table 11.2)** are symptomatic and require anti-tubercular treatment.

Sometimes clinical examination in a vaccinated child would be normal and ultrasound examination may reveal regional lymph node involvement. Clinically and histopathologically the lesions are indistinguishable from the spontaneously acquired forms of cutaneous tuberculosis but are said to run a milder course. The important observations of workers from all over the world taken together, it has been concluded that BCG protects children from the severe forms of tuberculosis. It is time-tested, economical, rarely causing complications, and its use in neonates should be continued.

INVESTIGATIONS

The Mantoux or tuberculin test is an invaluable aid in the diagnosis of cutaneous tuberculosis. It is performed by intradermal injection of 0.1 ml of PPD (containing 5 TU) on the volar surface of the forearm. The reaction is read after 48-72 hours. It is considered positive if the induration is >10 mm. In general, it can be taken as a very good indicator of infection when there is a typical clinical picture and histopathology reveals a granulomatous inflammation. Strong or vesicular reactions mostly favor an active focus of tuberculosis. This has also been the opinion of those treating other extrapulmonary forms like

TABLE 11.2: Cutaneous complications due to BCG vaccination

Nonspecific	Inoculated site	Eczema Infection Hypertrophic scar and keloid Basal cell carcinoma
	Nonvaccinated area	Erythema nodosum Maculopapular rash Erythema multiforme
Specific	Inoculated site	Poor healing, ulcers, abscesses and suppurative lymphadenitis Koch's phenomenon Lupus vulgaris Verrucous tuberculosis
	Nonvaccinated area	Papular tuberculids Organ BCG itis (lymph node, bone and skin) Disseminated BCG infection

osteoarticular tuberculosis, where demonstration or isolation of organisms is futile.

There are occasions where lupus vulgaris or scrofuloderma were 'caught red handed' by positive tuberculin reaction and misdiagnosis of well known mimickers, like fixed sporotrichosis, porokeratosis and pyogenic abscess could have been avoided if this simple test would have been performed along with other investigations. Unique presentations of cutaneous tuberculosis in immigrant children from the west might not have gone unsuspected, if this test would have been done. A negative Mantoux test is more significant than positive as it suggests an etiology other than tuberculosis. In our experience, this can be encountered in about 15% of the patients with cutaneous tuberculosis, the reasons for which are not always clear.

Culture of *M. tuberculosis* from skin tissue or the lesional aspirate is conventionally done in Lowenstein-Jensen medium which takes 4-8 weeks to grow. Better media like Middlebrooks and Bactec can be used which give results in a shorter time but does not increase the chance of positivity and care should be taken to avoid contamination. It is generally believed that culture of skin biopsy is unrewarding, but a recent study from Chennai showed a positivity rate of 55%. The high success rate was ascribed to preservation of the tissue in Kirchner's liquid medium before processing and the use of multiple media.

Skin biopsy is an important investigation in the diagnosis of cutaneous tuberculosis. In patients who have ulcers and sinuses, it is best to avoid the eroded area and take biopsy from the adjacent, nonulcerated skin. In lesions with prominent scarring, the biopsy should be from the active portion of the plaque avoiding scarred area. Hyperkeratotic lesions may be pared before biopsy to ensure that the deeper tissues are also included; otherwise, the biopsy material taken with punch consists only of the keratotic component which is of little diagnostic value. Acid fast bacilli are difficult to demonstrate in skin biopsy.

Broadly, two histopathological patterns are seen in biopsies from secondary tuberculosis. A dense, mixed infiltrate is seen in some specimens.The infiltrate is composed of lymphocytes, histiocytes, plasma cells, neutrophils and less frequently, eosinophils. Epithelioid cells and giant cells may form discrete granulomas or remain admixed in the infiltrate. There are areas of edema, hemorrhage and necrosis, and dermal fibrosis. This pattern is observed in biopsies from scrofuloderma or tuberculous gumma. The second pattern consists of epithelioid cell granulomas with giant cells, lymphocytes and histiocytes, typically present in upper dermis but may also involve the entire dermis. Necrosis is not a prominent finding and focal areas of necrosis may be present in some granulomas. Dermal fibrosis is frequent. The overlying epidermis is usually acanthotic and may show follicular plugging. The infiltrate impinges on the epidermis with damage to the basal cells. Parakeratotic follicular plugs enclosed within acanthotic epidermis with basal cell damage and underlying lichenoid infiltrate are distinctive findings in some biopsies. This histopathological pattern is usual in lupus vulgaris.

Though usually distinct, the clinical and histopathological patterns may show overlap in some cases. The histopathological picture of tuberculosis verrucosa cutis is dominated by the epidermal changes. There is marked hyperkeratosis, papillomatosis and acanthosis. There is a band-like papillary dermal infiltrate composed predominantly of lymphocytes and histiocytes. Nests of epithelioid cells and giant cells are found in the infiltrate but the granulomas are small and may require multiple sections to demonstrate.

Lichen scrofulosorum reveals small epithelioid cell granulomas centered on hair follicles and/or sweat glands. Since the clinical lesions are small, multiple sections should be examined to ensure that the diagnostic changes are not missed. Papulonecrotic tuberculids show a wedge-shaped dermal infiltrate beneath epidermal necrosis. The infiltrate is composed of lymphocytes and histiocytes, and may be accompanied by epithelioid cell granulomas. Leucocytoclastic vasculitis has been described in a severe form of papulonecrotic tuberculid. Erythema induratum demonstrates a granulomatous lobular panniculitis with vasculitis of medium-size vessels in the subcutaneous fat. Erythema nodosum reveals a septal panniculitis with histiocytes and giant cells without vasculitis.

Fine needle aspiration cytology of the enlarged lymph nodes should be carried out. This method of demonstration of acid fast bacilli has been shown to be much more successful than histopathology, particularly in scrofuloderma.

Polymerase chain reaction (PCR) is the latest investigation being employed to improve the diagnostic accuracy in cutaneous tuberculosis. It is a method where target DNA is amplified several million times using the enzyme Taq polymerase obtained from Thermos aquaticus. The procedure is performed manually in the thermocycler or can be automated using real time PCR systems. However, reports of sensitivity in patients with cutaneous tuberculosis as of now show great variation in the hands of researchers. In occasional instances it has been proved to be truly useful. However, the sensitivity and specificity being only around 50%, or even lower, it cannot be accepted unequivocally to exclude cutaneous tuberculosis. In a comparative study of various diagnostic methods used to diagnose cutaneous tuberculosis, it was found that PCR and histopathology had similar sensitivity.

Sometimes, even after investigating a case adequately, it may not be possible to make a conclusive diagnosis of cutaneous tuberculosis. In such difficult situations, therapeutic trial may be undertaken as a test of diagnosis. Recent studies have shown that response to therapy is demonstrable early in cutaneous tuberculosis and nearly all patients show some response within a month of initiating treatment. This has led to the recommendation that when a therapeutic trial is conducted, 6 weeks of therapy is adequate to prove or exclude the diagnosis. In patients who have not shown response, continuing treatment beyond 6 weeks is not helpful and an alternative diagnosis should be considered.

Investigations should be done to rule out systemic tuberculous infection. These include X-ray of the chest and other possible sites of affection, if required. Family history of tuberculosis must also be elicited and family members are investigated when necessary. In a fair percentage of cases there would be a source of infection in the family.

TREATMENT

Treatment of cutaneous tuberculosis is the same as recommended for pulmonary tuberculosis from time to time. Monotherapy should never be given with the rising incidence of resistance, and to those coinfected with HIV. Either 3 or 4 drugs must be used in adequate dosage in all forms of cutaneous tuberculosis in children. These include rifampicin (10-20 mg/kg), INH (3-5 mg/kg), pyrazinamide (20-30 mg/kg) and ethambutol (15-20 mg/kg). Rifampicin and INH being bactericidal are always given in the regimen. The other two are bacteriostatic drugs. In a given patient the disease responds dramatically within a month which leads to discontinuation of the therapy, but it is important to counsel the parents repeatedly to adhere to the full course of treatment, which is for 6 months duration. It is possible that some patients with extensive skin disease or those with visceral tuberculosis may need a longer period of therapy. Regular intake of the drugs and monitoring for side-effects are important to ensure success of therapy. The fear of using ethambutol in children below 6 years had been overemphasized in the past and currently, it can be used in them with proper monitoring.

Today the treatment of tuberculosis is by the DOTS (directly observed treatment, short-course) strategy implemented by the WHO and has been fully adopted by the RNTCP, Government of India. The DOTS strategy is said to be cost-effective and is the international standard for tuberculosis control. More than 180 countries are implementing this strategy and India is one of them. Cutaneous tuberculosis is placed among less severe form of extrapulmonary tuberculosis in Category III. A large study in children has also shown that, all categories as classified by the WHO, are well suited for DOTS therapy. To ensure uninterrupted supply of drugs, the program has introduced patient-wise boxes (PWBs) wherein the complete course of medicine is earmarked the day the patient is registered for treatment. The drugs are given under direct observation of a DOT provider, who is accessible and accountable to the system. In most cases, category III treatment would mean giving 3 drugs, rifampicin, INH and pyrazinamide 3 days a week for the first 2 months followed by rifampicin and INH for 4 months. When the lesions are extensive or when more than one group of lymph nodes are affected in scrofuloderma, category I can be given in which ethambutol is added to the regimen which means 4 drugs for the first 2 months followed by rifampicin and INH for the following 4 months. The RNTCP, in consultation with the Indian Academy of Pediatrics, has taken steps to make pediatric drugs available in PWBs similar to that supplied for adult patients. The boxes are designed according to the dosages used for different weight bands given in **Table 11.3**. With the availability of these, training would be imparted to the RNTCP staff in all states to use these boxes. Children with risk of development of complications, particularly contractures, must be regularly supervised to exercise the limb to prevent limitation of mobility.

TABLE 11.3: Pediatric Dosage and Weight Bands (New Delhi 2007)

Drugs	Dosage (mg/kg)	Dosage in mg for weight bands in kg			
		6-10 kg	11-17 kg	18-25 kg	26-30 kg
Isoniazid	10-15	75	150	225	300
Rifampicin	10	75	150	225	300
Pyrazinamide	30-35	250	500	750	1250
Ethambutol	30	200	400	600	1000
Streptomycin	15	-	-	-	-

NONTUBERCULOUS MYCOBACTERIAL INFECTIONS

Nontuberculous mycobacteria (NTM) are a large number of mycobacterial species frequently found in environmental habitats that may colonize and occasionally cause infections in humans and animals. There has been a rise in the incidence of infections caused by NTM because of increase in the immunosuppression and surgical procedures during the last few decades. NTM usually cause systemic infections, but may present with an assortment of cutaneous findings. NTM are often overlooked as cause of skin and soft tissue infections. One should have a high index of suspicion for NTM infection when evaluating any persistently draining nodules, plaques, or area of chronic panniculitis or cellulitis, especially in patients with a history of preceding trauma, surgery or immunosuppression.

HISTORY

NTM were first observed soon after Koch's discovery of tuberculous bacillus, but they were recognized as human pathogens only in 1950s. *M. ulcerans* was identified as the cause of an ulcerating skin condition in Australia in 1948 and in the Buruli district of Uganda in 1958. *M. marinum* which has been known since 1926 was isolated from patients with swimming pool granuloma in 1954. The rapid growers have been known as human pathogens since 1938 when *M. fortuitum* was isolated from a postinjection abscess.

GENERAL CHARACTERISTICS AND CLASSIFICATION OF NTM

NTM, like tuberculous bacilli are non-motile, non-sporing, weakly gram positive, acid- fast, aerobic or micro-aerophilic, straight or slightly curved rod shaped bacteria. Some mycobacteria show coccobacillary, filamentous or branching forms and some produce yellow to orange pigment in dark or after exposure to light.

Runyon originally classified NTM according to colony pigmentation and growth rate as:

I. *Photochromogens:* Produce yellow pigment only when exposed to light and form visible colonies in 2-3 weeks. e.g. *M. marinum, M. kansasii.*
II. *Scotochromogens:* Produce yellow-orange pigment both in dark and light, and form visible colonies in 2-3 weeks. e.g. *M. scrofulaceum.*
III. *Nonchromogens:* Form visible colonies in 2-3 weeks and do not produce pigment. e.g. *M. avium-intracellulare* (MAC), *M. ulcerans* and *M. hemophilum.*
IV. Rapid growers (RPG): Form visible colonies within 7 days (2-5 days). e.g. *M. fortuitum. M. cheloni, M. abscessus.*

This classification is of little importance from a clinical point of view as it is based on cultural characteristics. The classification of NTM based on primary involvement of organ system like lung, lymph node, skin and soft tissue is more useful to clinician.

EPIDEMIOLOGY

The incidence of NTM infection dramatically increased since last two decades as a consequence of decrease in prevalence of tuberculosis, AIDS epidemic and increased use of immunosuppressive drugs. Among the isolates of mycobacteria, the NTM has been reported to account for 15%. NTM are ubiquitous in the environment and have been isolated from water, soil, dust, domestic and wild animals, milk and food. However, there is a great variability in geographical distribution of NTM. Therefore, the clinical implication of an NTM isolate is not always clear. The characteristics of NTM that are responsible for their survival in various environmental habitats are high innate chlorine and biocide resistance; capacity to form biofilm in water flowing system (*M. fortuitum*, *M. chelonei*, *M. avium*); tolerance to extreme temperatures (MAC, *M.chelonei*); ability to survive in low nutrient levels (*M. intracellulare*); adaptation to acidic and microaerobic conditions (MAC).

Skin and soft tissue infections in immunocompetent patients are consequence of direct exposure to contaminated water sources through inoculation after accidental trauma, surgery or injection. There is no firm evidence of human to human or animal to human transmission of NTM infection. There is an inverse relationship between tuberculosis (TB) and diseases caused by NTM. Where TB is endemic, the opportunist NTM infection is rare and vice versa. Exposure to environmental mycobacteria has been suggested to influence immune responsiveness to the pathogenic mycobacteria and to sensitize individuals to skin test agents. There has been a species shift in mycobacteria causing cervical lymphadenitis from *M. scrofulaceum* (10-20%) to MAC (80%) during last 3 decades.

PATHOGENESIS

NTM are essentially environmental saprophytes and can elicit an immune response in man without causing overt infection. Some may produce a state of disease depending upon the species; the degree of exposure; and the state of immunity of the host.

The mycobacterial cell wall, composed of glycopeptidolipids, is probably a key element responsible for survival and multiplication of NTM within the hostile intracellular environment of macrophages. The interaction between mycobacteria and macrophage is a critical factor that determines whether the infection is established or not. Once organisms are engulfed and taken into intracellular vacuoles, a cell mediated immune response including CD4+ T cells and natural killer (NK) lymphocytes is triggered. The interleukin (IL) -12 produced by infected macrophages activates CD4+ T cells and natural killer (NK) lymphocytes. These activated cells release interferon (INF) - γ which stimulates macrophages to secrete tumor necrosis factor (TNF)-α; kill mycobacteria; and produce more IL- 12.

Usually mycobacteria are avirulent and do not produce toxins. However, *M. ulcerans* produces a macrolide toxin, mycolactone that is responsible for coagulative necrosis of subcutaneous tissue.

CLINICAL FEATURES

NTM infections usually present as four clinical syndromes, *viz*, pulmonary disease, lymphadenitis, disseminated disease and skin or soft tissue infections. Cutaneous involvement can be primary or part of disseminated infection. Lymphadenitis is the common disease caused by NTM in children followed by skin and soft tissue infections. The clinical manifestation depends on various factors; immune status of the host (presence or absence of internal organ involvement); distribution of lesions (localized or disseminated); morphological pattern (lymphocutaneous or nonlymphocutaneous); and source of infection (aquagenic or nonaquagenic) **(Table 11.4)**.

Buruli ulcer in Africa or Bairnsdale ulcer in Australia is most common in children aged 5-8 years. During active stage (nodular and ulcerative) of the disease lymphadenopathy is typically absent and Burulin skin reagent test is nonreactive. There has been no epidemiologic association of Buruli ulcer with Human Immunodeficiency Virus (HIV) infection.

Apart from NTM mentioned in **Table 11.4**, other species can also cause infections in children. *M. kansasii* is a primary pulmonary pathogen. However, rarely primary cutaneous infection presenting as crops of erythematous, crusted papules and plaques over elbows in an immunocompetent child has been reported. *M. hemophilum* in immunocompetent children causes lymphadenitis similar to MAC infection.

Though commonly causes lymphadenitis in children aged 6 months to 2 years, *M. scrofulaceum* and MAC can also manifest with primary cutaneous infections. The former presented as localized asymptomatic ulcerated red nodule in an immunocompetent child. The latter manifesting as familial cluster of primary cutaneous infection has been reported. The source of infection was a circulating, constantly heated (40°C) bath water system. The affected children presented with localized single ulcerated inflammatory nodule, and combination of nodules and indolent ulcers on extremities, and abscesses on the trunk. Similar clinical manifestations caused by MAC have been reported in children aged 2-10 years

TABLE 11.4: Clinical manifestations of common NTM infections

Species/IP	Source of infection	Clinical manifestations		Common Site
		Normal host	Immunosuppression[a]	
M. marinum (Swimming pool / fish tank granuloma)/ 2-6 weeks	Aquagenic[b]	Single bluish-red inflammatory nodule and Sporotricoid lesions,	Disseminated papules, nodules or ulcerations (rare)	Upper limbs
M. ulcerans (Buruli ulcer)/ 3 months	Aquagenic[b]	Shallow, painless, necrotic ulcer with undermined edge	—	Lower limbs
M. scrofulaceum	Ingestion of contaminated milk/ water	Lymphadenitis	Cutaneous nodules and abscesses	Unilateral Submandibular, submaxillary lymphnodes
MAC	Ingestion of contaminated water	Lymphadenitis	Disseminated maculopapules, painful subcutaneous nodules, ulcers, panniculitis	Lymphnodes (as above). Extremities and trunk (cutaneous lesions)
M. fortuitum / 1-2 months	Nonaquagenic[c]	Localized painful nodules, ulcers, sinuses or cellulitis	Multiple episodes of generalized morbiliform eruption, nodules, or multiple abscesses	Extremities (site of inoculation)
M. chelonei / 4-6 weeks	Nonaquagenic[c]	Localized cellulitis or subcutaneous abscesses	Disseminated erythematous nodules with multiple draining fistulas	Extremities (site of inoculation)
M. abscessus / 4-6 weeks	Nonaquagenic[c]	Localized erythematous, violaceous nodules or abscesses	Disseminated cutaneous nodules or abscesses	Site of trauma

Note: IP, incubation period; M, Mycobacterium; MAC, *M. avium* complex; NTM, Nontuberculous mycobacteria

[a] Acquired immunodeficiency syndrome, immunosuppressive drugs of > 6 months duration, lymphoma and leukemia, and organ transplantation (not related to water exposure or trauma)

[b] Exposure of injured body surface to tropical fish or swimming pool (*M. marinum*) and rivers and streams (*M. ulcerans*)

[c] Inoculation through accidental injuries, medical procedures (surgeries, injections, catheters), and medical and paramedical cosmetic procedures (pedicures, mesotherapy, botox injection, depilation)

without any history of prior trauma or underlying systemic disease.

HISTOPATHOLOGY

Several histopathological patterns have been reported: tuberculoid, suppurative, palisading and sarcoidal granulomas, abscesses, histiocytic cell infiltration, panniculitis, nonspecific inflammation and folliculitis. The lesions in immunocompetent patients usually show granulomatous inflammatory reaction, whereas in immunocompromised patients suppurative inflammatory reaction with numerous acid-fast bacilli (AFB) predominates.

DIAGNOSIS

The laboratory diagnosis is established by culture of NTM from skin biopsy specimen or from discharge or from aspiration of abscess. Currently, three culture media are routinely used, Lowenstein-Jensen medium, Middlebrook 7H 10 and 7H 11, and Middlebrook 7H 9 liquid medium. The inoculated media for primary isolation should be incubated in an atmosphere of 10% carbon dioxide to obtain optimal growth. The optimal temperature for growth is 35-37°C. However, if the specimen was obtained from skin or a superficial lesion suspected to contain *M. marinum*, *M. ulcerans* or *M. hemophilum*, the incubation should be at 25-33°C. Similarly, specimen suspected to contain *M. avium* or *M. xenopi* should be incubated at 40-42°C. The optimum pH for growth is 6.0-6.5 but this may vary from species to species.

Rapid diagnostic methods with high sensitivity and specificity are also available. These include high performance liquid chromatography, DNA probes, polymerase chain reaction and restriction fragment length polymorphism. However, conventional biochemical tests like, pigment production, niacin accumulation, reduction of nitrates, catalase activity, urease activity, etc. are gold standard for identification of NTM species from primary isolates.

A variety of intradermal test antigens have been prepared from various species of NTM including PPD-A and PPD-B from *M. avium* and *M. intracellulare*, respectively. However, these are nonspecific and are not useful in the diagnosis.

DIFFERENTIAL DIAGNOSIS

NTM infections present with different clinical patterns mimicking various dermatological conditions. History of preceding trauma, exposure to contaminated source, distribution of lesions, unresponsiveness to conventional antibiotic therapy, cultural characteristics and histopathology will help in the diagnosis of NTM infection. Swimming pool or fish tank granuloma should be differentiated from sporotrichosis, leishmaniasis, tuberculosis verrucosa cutis and lupus vulgaris. Buruli ulcer during nodular stage has to be differentiated from panniculitis, nodular vasculitis and foreign body granuloma. The ulcerative stage should be differentiated from deep fungal infections, pyoderma gangrenosum and suppurative panniculitis. Lymphadenitis caused by *M. scrofulaceum* and *M. avium* complex usually involve submandibular and submaxillary nodes situated high in the neck compared to tonsillar and anterior cervical nodes affected in tubercular lymphadenitis. Sometimes NTM infections may present as sporotrichoid pattern which is also seen in other dermatological conditions **(Table 11.5)**.

TABLE 11.5: Differential diagnosis of sporotrichoid (lymphocutaneous) lesions

Nontuberculous mycobacteria
M. arinum, M. kansasii, M. scrofulaceum, M. avium complex, M. chelonei
Bacteria
Nocardia brasiliensis, Francisella tularensis, Staphylococcus aureus, Streptococcus pyogenes
Fungus
Sporothrix schenkii
Virus
Herpes simplex, Cowpox virus
Protozoa
Leishmania donovanii

TREATMENT

In general, like in other mycobacterial infections, the treatment with multiple antimicrobial agents is necessary to prevent emergence of resistance and to get a synergistic effect. The therapy should be given over a period of months or even longer in case of immunosuppression. Most of NTM are not susceptible to conventional antitubercular drugs. Therefore, antibiotic sensitivity testing is invaluable in the management of NTM infections. The newer antimicrobials like clarithromycin, azithromycin, amikacin, imipenem, cefoxitin and rifabutin have considerably improved the prognosis of NTM infections **(Table 11.6)**. Surgical intervention is required in the presence of deeper infections or persisting pain or discharging sinus tracts. Sometimes local heat therapy with a lamp or hot water may be helpful in *M. marinum* infection. Hyperbaric oxygen may be useful in *M. ulcerans* infection.

COMPLICATIONS, COURSE AND PROGNOSIS

M. marinum infection sometimes involves deeper structures leading to tenosynovitis and osteomyelitis with pathological fractures in the infected bones. If untreated cutaneous lesions heal spontaneously within few months often with scarring.

Buruli ulcer generally follow a prolonged course persisting for months to years before healing spontaneously with disabling scarring, contractures, deformity and lymphedema.

LEPROSY

Leprosy is a chronic infectious disease caused by *Mycobacterium leprae*. Disease manifestation occurs in a

TABLE 11.6: Recommended treatment of common cutaneous NTM infections

NTM	Recommended Treatment[a]	Duration of therapy
M. marinum	Clarithromycin + Minocycline/ Doxycycline + Cotrimoxazole	12-24 weeks (including 4-8 weeks of therapy after clinical cure)
M. ulcerans	Wide surgical excision and debridement	——
M. scofulaceum	Total excision of involved lymphnodes Isoniazid + Rifampicin (if excision not possible)	9 months
MAC	Clarithromycin + Ethambutol + Rifampicin/ Rifabutin	Continued for 4-8 weeks after clinical cure
M. fortuitum	Surgical debridement and Amikacin + Ciprofloxacin + Sulfonamides **or** Amikacin + Cefoxitin/ Imipenem/ Clarithromycin/ Doxycycline	Maintenance therapy for 2-6 months (in severe cases)
M. chelonei	Surgical debridement and Tobramycin/ Imipenem **or** Clarithromycin + Ciprofloxacin/ Doxycycline	Continued for at least 6 months after clinical cure
M. abscesses	Surgical debridement and Clarithromycin + Cefoxitin/ Amikacin	3-6 months (localized infection) At least 6 months (disseminated infection)
M. hemophilum	Surgical excision of affected lymphnodes (in immunocompetent children) Rifampicin/ Rifabutin + Clarithromycin ± Amikacin	6-9 months (may be indefinite in immunocompromized)

Note: M, Mycobacterium; MAC, *M. avium* complex; NTM, Non tuberculous mycobacteria
[a] Doxyxycline and minocycline are indicated in children aged < 8 years

small proportion of infected individuals. Leprosy has world wide prevalence and is endemic in some countries including India. It has a long incubation period ranging from 9 months to 20 years and affects all age groups. Its potential to cause deformities deserves special medical attention. Moreover, the obvious deformities carry significant social stigma. Though the total number of cases have reduced considerably after the advent of multidrug therapy, the number of new cases is alarming.

India harbors one third of the leprosy cases worldwide. In different Indian studies, children constituted a considerable proportion of these patients, though the percentage is variable. This chapter deals with the diagnosis and management of leprosy in children.

ETIOLOGY

In his annual report (1874) on the "causes of leprosy", Gerhard Henrik Armeur Hansen opined that leprosy is caused by *Mycobacterium leprae*. The reasons for his strong belief were: (i) constant presence of bacillus in leprosy lesions, (ii) characteristic cellular reactions provoked by *M.leprae* or its chemical fractions and (iii) absence of *M.leprae* in healthy individuals.

M.leprae belongs to the family *Mycobacteriaceae*. It is a straight or slightly curved slender, capsulated, non motile, non-sporing, acid fast, rod ranging from 1-8 μ in length and 0.2 to 0.5 μ in width. The ends are rounded or blunt but may be pointed. *M.leprae* divides by binary fission, is Gram positive and strongly acid fast following staining with carbol fuschin. The bacteria stain homogenously or may appear fragmented or beaded.

M. leprae is noncultivable but is capable of limited multiplication in the footpad of mice after local inoculation. It possesses the enzyme phenol oxidase. It is an obligate intracellular organism seen predominantly inside macrophages. It frequently appears in clumps termed as globi, which simulate tightly packed cigar-bundles. The globi are colonies growing within an unidentified membrane and appear to be bound together by a lipid like substance, the glia. *M.leprae* appears as both intra and extracellular glial masses which suggests that they are enclosed in a capsular membrane. Globi are seen in lepromatous leprosy. Morphological variations can occur, which include short forms, broken forms, coccoid and granular forms. It is the only *Mycobacterium* which infects peripheral nerves.

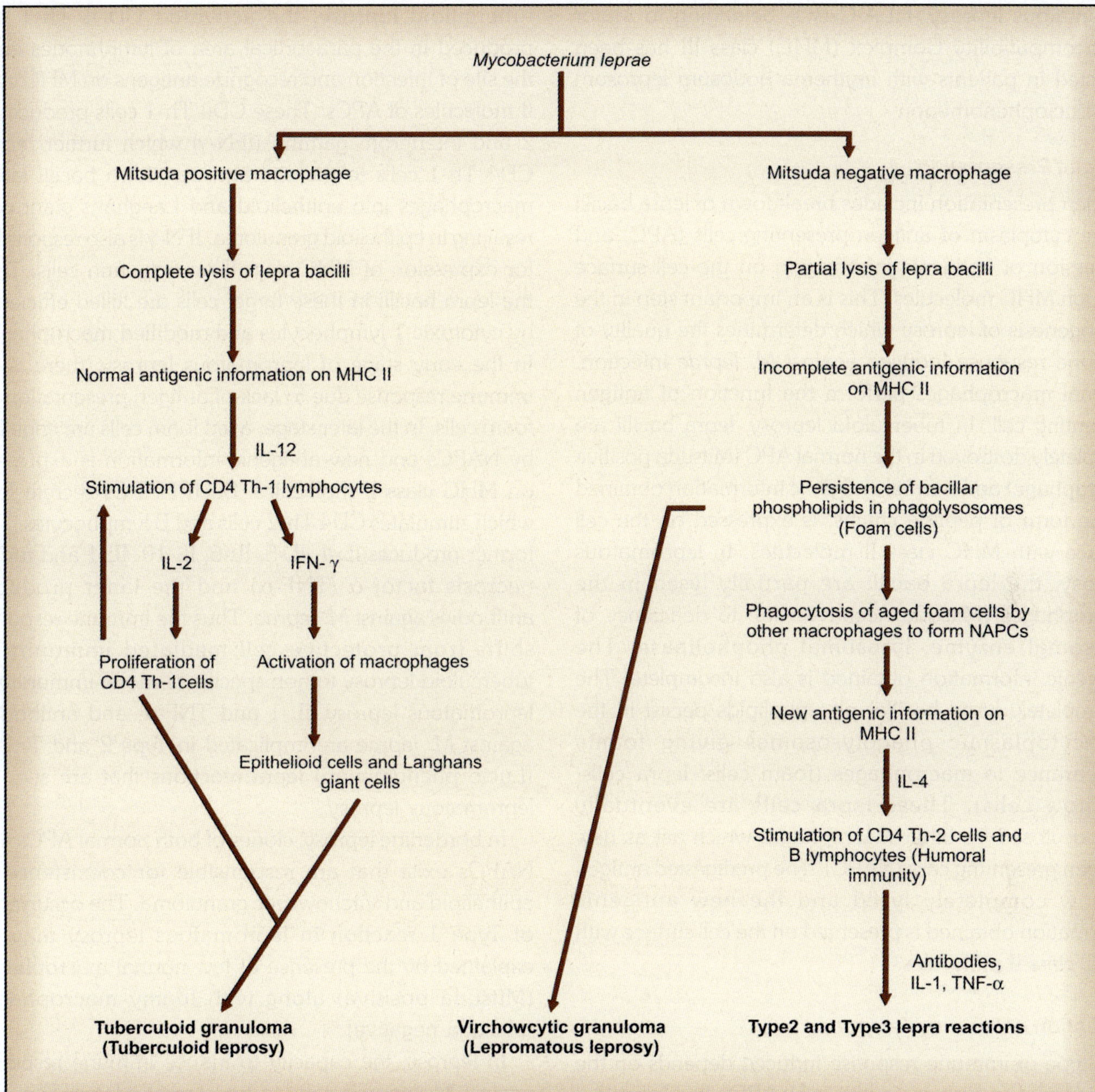

Flow Chart 11.1: Pathogenesis of leprosy

Note: IFN—Interferon; IL—Interleukin; MHC—Major histocompatibility complex; NAPC—New antigen presenting cell; Th—T helper; TNF—Tumor necrosis factor

PATHOGENESIS OF LEPROSY (FLOW CHART 11.1)

The presentation of leprosy as various clinico-pathological forms depends on the induction and expression of cell mediated immunity. Immune response against *M. leprae* includes human leukocyte antigen (HLA) susceptibility, antigen presentation, and induction and expression of immune response.

Human Leukocyte Antigen (HLA) Susceptibility

HLA controls the manner in which antigens are presented to lymphocytes and thereby induction of cell mediated immunity. Therefore, to some extent, HLA determines the outcome of an infection and also development of disease into different clinical patterns. In relation to leprosy, HLA studies have revealed predominance of $HLA\text{-}DR_3$ in tuberculoid leprosy and $HLA\text{-}DQw_1$ in lepromatous leprosy. HLA-C_4BQ_0 belonging to Major Histocompatibility Complex (MHC) class III has been detected in patients with erythema nodosum leprosum and Luciophenomenon.

Antigen Presentation

Antigen presentation includes breakdown of lepra bacilli in the cytoplasm of antigen presenting cells (APC) and expression of antigenic information on the cell surface through MHC molecules. This is an important step in the pathogenesis of leprosy which determines the quality of immune response induced against *M. leprae* infection. Normal macrophages perform the function of antigen presenting cell. In tuberculoid leprosy, lepra bacilli are completely destroyed in the normal APC (Mitsuda positive macrophage) and normal antigenic information obtained in the form of peptide chains, is expressed on the cell surface with MHC class II molecules. In lepromatous leprosy, the lepra bacilli are partially lysed in the macrophages (Mitsuda negative) due to deficiency of lysosomal enzyme, lysosomal phopholipase. The antigenic information obtained is also incomplete. The incompletely lysed bacillar phospholipids persist in the intracytoplasmic phagolysosomes giving foamy appearance to macrophages (foam cells/ lepra cells/ Virchow cells). These lepra cells are eventually phagocytosed by other macrophages which act as new antigen presenting cells (NAPC). The predigested antigen is now completely lysed and the new antigenic information obtained is presented on the cell surface with MHC class II molecules.

Induction of Immune Response

The type of immune response induced depends on the efficiency of antigen presentation by APCs. In tuberculoid leprosy, the APCs produce interleukin 12 (IL-12) which in turn stimulates CD 4 Th 1 (helper 1) lymphocytes resulting in cell mediated immune response. In lepromatous leprosy, the NAPCs produce IL-4 which in turn stimulates CD 4 Th 2 lymphocytes resulting in humoral immune response.

Expression of Immune Response

The protective immunity against infection with intracellular organisms like *M. leprae* is cell mediated immunity because antibodies do not penetrate the host cells. In tuberculoid leprosy, the activated CD 4 Th-1 cell produced in the paracortical area of lymphnodes enter the site of infection and recognize antigens on MHC class II molecules of APCs. These CD4 Th-1 cells produce IL-2 and interferon- gamma (IFN-γ) which further recruit CD4 Th-1 cells to the site and transform bacilli laden macrophages into epithelioid and Langhans giant cells resulting in epithelioid granuloma. IFN-γ is also responsible for expression of MHC class II on Schwann cells. Thus the lepra bacilli in these target cells are killed efficiently by cytotoxic T lymphocytes and modified macrophages. In the early stage of lepromatous leprosy, there is no immune response due to lack of antigen presentation by foam cells. In the later stage, aged foam cells are engulfed by NAPCs and new antigenic information is expressed on MHC class II molecules. Such NAPCs secrete IL-4 which stimulates CD4 Th-2 cells and B lymphocytes. The former produces IL-4, IL-5, IL-6, IL-10, IL-1 and tumor necrosis factor-α (TNF-α) and the latter produces antibodies against *M. leprae*. Thus the immune response shifts from protective cell mediated immunity in tuberculoid leprosy to non specific humoral immunity in lepromatous leprosy. IL-1 and TNF-α, and antibodies against *M. leprae* are implicated in Type 2 and Type 3 (Lucio phenomenon) lepra reactions that are seen in lepromatous leprosy.

In borderline leprosy, clones of both normal APCs and NAPCs exist that are responsible for coexistence of epithelioid and Virchowcytic granuloma. The occurrence of Type 1 reaction in lepromatous leprosy may be explained by the presence of few normal macrophages (Mitsuda positive) along with foamy macrophages (Mitsuda negative).

In leprosy, the capacity to induce immune response against *M. leprae* seems to be normal. However, it has been proposed that the mitochondrial dysfunction of APCs in lepromatous leprosy patients may lead to overproduction of free radicals causing deficiency of lysosomal phospholipase enzyme. The antioxidant property of sulfones results in neutralization of free radicals and restoration of lysosomal phospholipase enzyme function. Clofazimine is also effective by promoting the synthesis of phospholipase A_2 enzyme. Rifampicin is effective for neural bacilli and also in cases of bacillemia. Therefore, dapsone though a bacteriostatic drug, is an integral part of any antileprosy regimen.

CLASSIFICATION OF LEPROSY

Classification of leprosy helps the physicians involved in management of these patients. Classification should also differentiate infective from noninfective patients and predict outcomes based on prognosis and complications of the disease. Complete examination of the patient is mandatory to categorize them into different groups. Results of skin smears will also ultimately help in the classification and hence the treatment.

There are different classification systems proposed since 1870. Here, the most important classifications are highlighted.

Indian Association of Leprologists (IAL) Classification (1955)

This is a simpler and complete classification which suits the Indian leprologists. The different groups are:

a. Indeterminate (I)
b. Maculoanesthetic (MA)
c. Tuberculoid (T)
d. Borderline (B)
e. Lepromatous (L)
f. Neuritic (N)

In indeterminate leprosy, few macular lesions are seen. Anesthesia is difficult to elicit or absent. Bacilli are absent and lepromin test is weakly positive or negative.

In maculoanesthetic leprosy, macules are seen. Lepromin test is moderately or strongly positive. In tuberculoid leprosy, infiltrated lesions are observed with strongly positive lepromin reaction.

In borderline leprosy, infiltrated lesions are seen with variable lepromin reactions but it is never strongly positive.

Lesions in lepromatous leprosy may be macular, infiltrated or nodular. Lepromin reaction is negative.

In neuritic leprosy, anesthetic areas are present in the distribution of peripheral nerves, without cutaneous lesions. Primary neuritic leprosy may be mono or poly neuritic with one or more groups of nerves affected. Lepromin reaction is variable.

Revised IAL Classification (1981)

IAL in 1981 presented a revised classification system, which is as follows:

a. Tuberculoid
b. Borderline
c. Lepromatous
d. Indeterminate
e. Neuritic

In this classification maculo anesthetic type was merged with tuberculoid leprosy.

Ridley and Jopling Classification (1962)

Ridley and Jopling recommended a five grade classification system based on clinical, bacteriological and immunological patterns of leprosy. The objective of this classification was to assess the prognosis and response to treatment. The types are:

a. Tuberculoid (TT)
b. Borderline Tuberculoid (BT)
c. Borderline Borderline (BB)
d. Borderline Lepromatous (BL)
e. Lepromatous (LL)

The spectrum of tuberculoid to lepromatous leprosy transits from one to another through intervening sub-stages where clinical overlap may be observed. Skin lesions of borderline leprosy have intermediate characteristics between few, asymmetric, irregular, well-defined, dry, large lesions of tuberculoid leprosy and symmetric, numerous, ill-defined, small, shiny, smooth lesions of lepromatous leprosy. Annular lesions are common in borderline spectrum. Unlike lepromatous disease, where lesional sensation is almost preserved, borderline skin lesions show definite loss of sensation, which is not as complete as in tuberculoid lesions.

The application of this classification is strictly limited for clinicians' use. It is imperative for assessing individual patient's immune status. However, it is difficult for field workers to adopt it while taking rapid decision on therapy. Hence, this classification has more of scientific value. Later, sub polar tuberculoid and sub polar lepromatous groups were added to it. Hence the complete classification is as follows; TTp, TTs, BT, BB, BL, LLs, LLp. The sub polar types are indicative of good immune status of the patient at one time.

WHO Classification (Table 11.7)

This is the simplest classification system recommended for field workers. This includes two types:

a. Paucibacillary (PB)
b. Multibacillary (MB)

Paucibacillary includes TT and BT leprosy. MB spectrum includes BB, BL and LL. The cases are also classified according to skin smears. Smear negative cases are included under PB and smear positive cases are included under MB. Similarly if the number of skin lesions are ≤ 5, it is paucibacillary and if ≥ 5 they are categorized as multibacillary.

The constant revisions in the classification of leprosy were undertaken in order to simplify and justify the treatment at all levels.

WHO added single lesion paucibacillary (SLPB) as a separate entity in 1995 **(Table 11.8)**. The purpose of this delineation was to differentiate patients of leprosy with good immunity and to initiate a separate single dose regimen for them.

TABLE 11.7: WHO classification of leprosy

	SLPB	PB	MB
Skin	Single patch only	2-5 patches	6 and more
Nerve	No nerve	No/1 nerve trunk.	No/1/more nerve trunk(s)

TABLE 11.8: Comparison of various classifications

Indian	WHO	Ridley Jopling
Indeterminate	SLPB	TT polar
Tuberculoid	PB	TT subpolar
Borderline	MB	BT
Lepromatous		BB
Pureneuritic		BL
		LL subpolar
		LL polar

EPIDEMIOLOGY

Leprosy is known to occur at all ages ranging from early infancy to very old age. The youngest age reported for occurrence of leprosy is 3 weeks in Martinique. There is a clear peak at ages 10-14 years followed by a depression, which in turn is followed by a rise and a plateau covering the ages 30-60 years. Approximately 300,000 new cases of leprosy are detected in India every year and 15% of these are children. There are some difficulties in the diagnosis of leprosy in children. Often, the site of lesion (especially on the face) may be such that sensory deficit may not be apparent. Over and under diagnosis is possible in such cases.

Studies from other endemic countries and India showed that childhood leprosy is not an uncommon entity. We detected 66 cases of childhood leprosy in Rajah Muthiah Medical College and Hospital, Annamalainagar (Tamilnadu, India) during 1991-'95. This group comprised of 7.2% of the total leprosy cases detected during that period. Male to female ratio was 2:1. There were 62 PB and 4 MB cases. Deformities were seen in 2 cases. No patient developed reactions. Relapse rate was 7.1%.

In a study from north India, 132 cases of childhood leprosy were detected, of whom 7.6% were TT, 59% were BT, and 3.8% were indeterminate. SLPB was diagnosed in 43.9% of childhood leprosy cases. Nerve involvement was seen in 66.6%. Family history of contact was obtained in 20%.

Another large study from Hyderabad, South India, reported 306 childhood leprosy cases with similar observations. The youngest patient recorded in this study was of nine months age and single patches were observed in 3% of cases.

An earlier Indian study had shown that, the extent of spontaneous regression of leprosy lesions among children was about 90% over a period of 20 years.

The two portals of exit of *M. Leprae* often described are skin and nasal mucosa and portals of entry are the skin and upper respiratory tract. Incubation period ranges from few weeks to thirty years (mean approximately 4.4 years). In general, the longer the exposure to contacts, greater is the chance of getting the disease.

From the studies on household contacts of leprosy patients, it was apparent that segregation of PB cases is needless as the risk of transmission is 4-5 times lower than in MB cases. Attack rate among household contacts are not significantly different from others in the community. Segregation of MB cases for a long period is also unnecessary since most bacilli become nonviable very quickly with MDT. Children of treated mothers have much lower risk of contacting the disease when compared to those of untreated. Short-term hospitalization of infective parents may be considered. Segregation of neonates at birth from mothers suffering from lepromatous disease is not recommended. The risk of transmission is not so high in such cases, reaching approximately 20% over an 8 years period, 75% of whom presented subsequently with single lesion which healed spontaneously.

Until now, the most reliable method of assessment of the burden of leprosy in an area is random sample prevalence survey. But conducting such surveys routinely becomes costly. Studies suggest that presence of IgM antibodies to phenolic glycolipid (PGL-1) of *M. leprae*

TABLE 11.9: Childhood leprosy cases (NLEP, Tamilnadu)

Year	MB child	PB child	Total	Percentage (%)
2003-4	-	3493	3493	21.8
2002-3	-	4419	4419	17.8
2001-2	332	6910	7242	22.5
1999-2000	524	19341	19865	31.6
1998-9	372	14196	14568	31.8
1997-8	296	11061	11357	27.1
1996-7	252	16929	17181	27
1995-6	307	23754	24061	39.6
1994-5	259	27746	28005	42.1
1993-4	320	21932	22252	36.5

may be indicative of past or present infection. High prevalence of anti PGL-1 IgM antibodies among children may be indicative of active transmission of *M leprae* in their surroundings.

National Leprosy Control Programme, Tamilnadu, provides a sample data for childhood leprosy **(Table 11.9).**

CLINICAL LEPROSY

No other human infection shows as varied manifestations as leprosy. No organ is spared in leprosy except the brain, spinal cord and lungs where the organisms cannot survive.

M.leprae enters through the abraded skin or nasal mucosa. Thereafter it lodges in the Schwann cells. Nerve damage in leprosy is universal; early neuritis is microscopic, evident only in histopathological specimens or there is clinical evidence as thickened, palpable peripheral or cutaneous nerves.

Lepromatous leprosy is considered as a postprimary infection like tuberculosis and affects the adults most commonly. In our series of childhood leprosy cases we have encountered with only one patient (13- year-old) of lepromatous leprosy. When the host's immunological functions are good, localized forms of the disease (indeterminate or tuberculoid leprosy) occur, which is true for children.

The initial symptoms may be in the form of ant-crawling sensation under the skin. Pain in one of the major nerve trunks may also be the presenting feature. If skin lesion appears at this stage, the diagnosis becomes obvious. However, skin lesions may appear after many years of hypoesthesia. A single vague hypopigmented patch may evolve into multiple skin lesions in due course of time.

The child has to be examined thoroughly, including the gluteal region, in good daylight.

In eliciting the history of the patient importance is given to the following facts.

1. History of residence in an endemic area.
2. Familial contact of leprosy.
3. Other diseases which may present with enlarged nerves during childhood.

The three cardinal signs of leprosy are:

1. Anesthetic/hypoesthetic skin lesions
2. Enlarged nerves, with loss of sensation in its distribution.
3. Demonstration of *M. leprae* from the lesions

Anesthetic skin lesions may vary from a single vague hypopigmented macule or a patch to multiple well defined small macules or patches, or infiltrated macules, papules or nodules. In leprosy, all modalities of sensation must be tested, as, in the initial stages, only the temperature sensation may be impaired. Pain must be tested with a needle or a pin. Touch sensation must be tested with the index finger of examiner's hand or with a wisp of cotton wool. While interpreting the results the normal variations must be considered which may be variable up to five centimeters, known as misreference. While examining sensations in children, due care should be taken not to scare them. As an alternative, the parents may be taught to test the sensations and inform the results of sensory testing **(Table 11.10)**.

TABLE 11.10: Salient steps of sensory testing

Points to remember
Choose the right environment
Use standard instrument (pin)
Explain to the patient
Trial test – demonstrate with the patient's eyes open
Real test – do the test with the patient's eyes closed
Pin perpendicular to the skin, gently place it, from normal to affected area; never stroke; no repeated stimuli.
Do not ask the patient, "can you feel it?"
Ask the patient to show the spot touched, with index finger (accessible part of body)
Ask the patient to count in case of inaccessible body parts

Apart from eliciting hypoesthesia or anesthesia, the skin lesions are to be examined for number, size, shape, margin, borders, dryness, hair loss, symmetry and enlarged cutaneous nerve over a patch.

Leprosy is one of the most important causes of nerve thickening in children apart from neurofibromatosis. Appreciation of thickened nerve is an art which can be learnt by constant practice. Peripheral nerves like supra orbital, supra trochlear, great auricular, ulnar, median, radial, common peroneal, posterior tibial and cutaneous nerves like ulnar cutaneous, radial cutaneous, cutaneous branch of common peroneal or sural nerves may all be palpated as these lie in a superficial location. Once the nerve or nerves are significantly thickened, additional features like the number, uniform thickening, nodularity, abscess formation and symmetry are all to be noted, as these points are useful to categorize the patient according to Ridley and Jopling classification. Thorough examination of the patient gives us more information on the complications like impending paralysis. Early diagnosis of nerve damage is the mainstay of preventing paralysis and deformities in childhood leprosy.

Apart from examination of skin and nerve, other features of leprosy are also to be noted, like super ciliary madarosis, ear lobe infiltration, leonine facies, bilateral gynecomastia, and testicular atrophy. However these features are seen only in late cases of lepromatous leprosy, which is uncommon in childhood. Following this, evidence of deformity and reactions are to be noted, which gives the complete picture of leprosy.

TYPES OF CHILDHOOD LEPROSY

Indeterminate Leprosy

Indeterminate leprosy is a common presentation (20 to 80%) in children. The first sign of leprosy is seen before the host develops immune response to *M. leprae*. This type of leprosy finds a separate place only in Indian classification. It represents early growth of the bacilli, recognized only by nonspecific immune mechanisms. The signs are minimal at this stage. All types of leprosy start as indeterminate stage. If the host response is good the lesions heal without forming any sequelae.

The skin lesions consist of flat macules, usually hypopigmented or sometimes erythematous, which vary in number, size and location **(Figure 11.5)**. Size of the lesions varies from less than 1 cm, up to 5 cm in diameter.

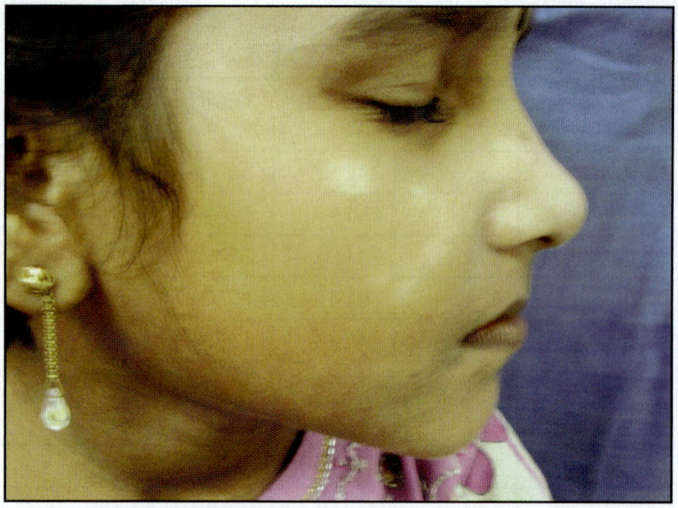

FIGURE 11.5: Indeterminate leprosy

Sensory loss may be minimal. The surface is even but not dry. Margin is vague and indefinite. Thickening of the margins is indicative of progression to next stage.

Clinician should be careful to make a diagnosis of indeterminate leprosy in children. Doubtful cases have to be confirmed by skin biopsy, which shows perineural and peri adnexal lymphocytic infiltrate. With treatment, the lesions may subside completely without any sequlae. In the absence of treatment, the patient passes onto tuberculoid or lepromatous spectrum after a variable period of time.

Tuberculoid Leprosy

The World Health Organization expert committee defined tuberculoid leprosy as "*a benign form, relatively stable, infrequently positive on bacteriological examination, presenting as erythematous skin lesions which are elevated, marginally or more extensively and almost always positive to lepromin test. In a limited proportion of cases complications arise which are due to peripheral nerve involvement. This frequently appears to occur as a result of extension from or through cutaneous nerve branches rather than systemic dissemination, and characteristically it is often asymmetrical and unilateral*".

The skin lesions may be in the form of macules or infiltrated plaques. The lesions are large, single or up to four in number, hypopigmented, asymmetrical in distribution and still confined to one region of body. The edges are definite and there is loss of sensation. The macules are to be differentiated from macules of lerpomatous leprosy which are usually not anesthetic.

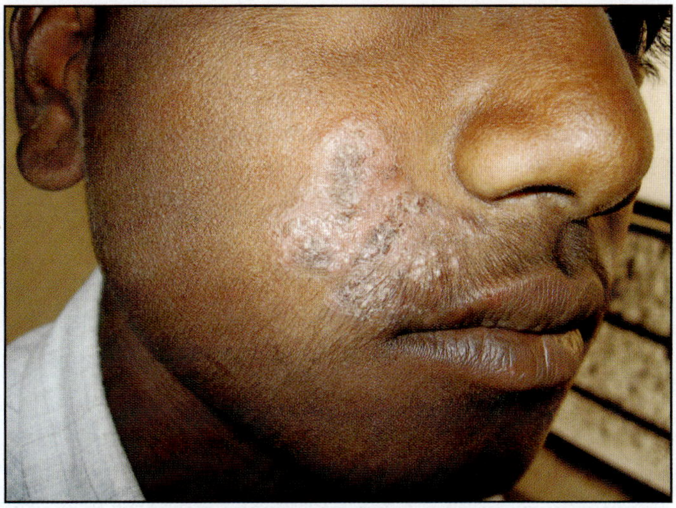

FIGURE 11.6: TT lesion on face

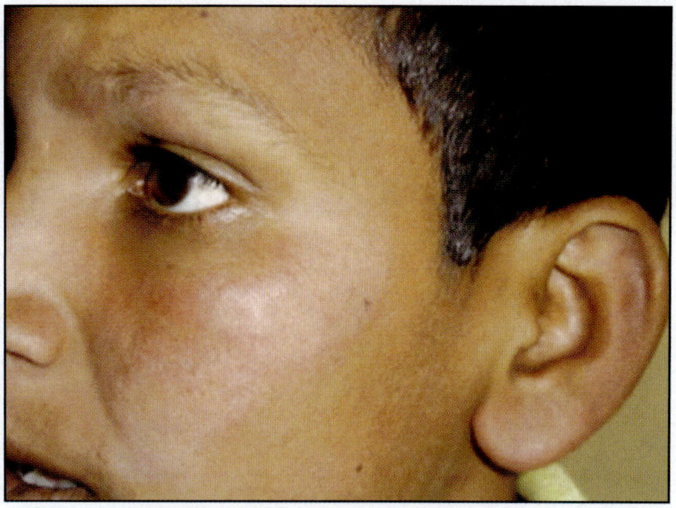

FIGURE 11.7A: Dry patch of BT leprosy

Two types of infiltrated lesions were described previously, namely the minor tuberculoid and major tuberculoid. In the minor tuberculoid, the lesions are moderately elevated, showing characteristic papules at the periphery, known as "pebbling" **(Figure 11.6)**. Major tuberculoid lesions are markedly elevated, infiltrated plaques showing well-defined edges. Central clearing of the plaque may give an annular appearance. The surface is dry and sweating is lost over the lesion. Lesions may have complete loss of sensation to temperature, touch and pain.

At this stage, histopathology of the skin lesion shows well-defined tuberculoid granuloma with complete destruction of the nerve fibers. This feature indeed explains the complete absence of sensation over the lesion. Mitsuda lepromin test is strongly positive, indicating that the patient has well preserved cell mediated immunity against the pathogen.

Tuberculoid leprosy may heal on its own even without treatment. In a large study conducted in pre sulfone era at Chennai, India, it was evident that, in 88% of tuberculoid patients the skin lesions heal by itself. There are two forms of tuberculoid leprosy according to Ridley and Jopling classification. Polar tuberculoid lesions are stable and do not change, whereas in sub polar variant, in absence of treatment, the skin lesions may downgrade in to borderline tuberculoid leprosy.

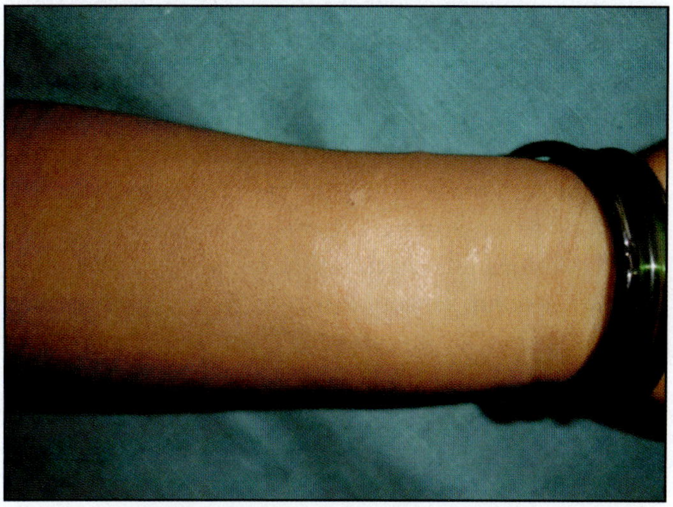

FIGURE 11.7B: Single lesion BT leprosy

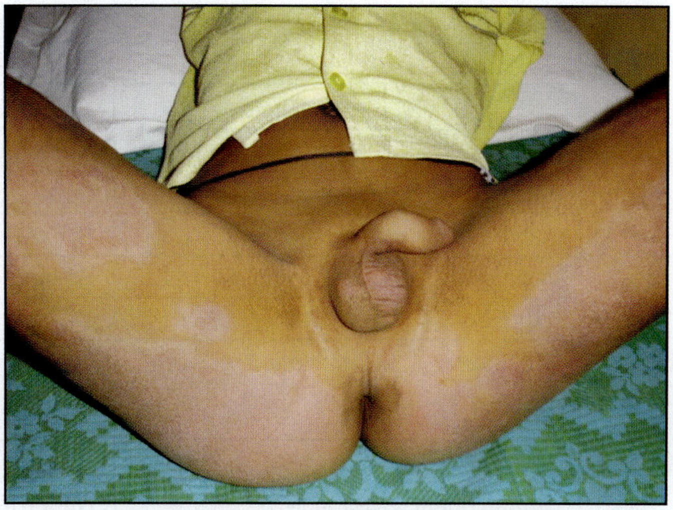

FIGURE 11.8: Large lesions of BT leprosy

Borderline Tuberculoid Leprosy (Figures 11.7A to 11.9)

Borderline leprosy was earlier designated as dimorphous leprosy because of its variable features. The skin lesions

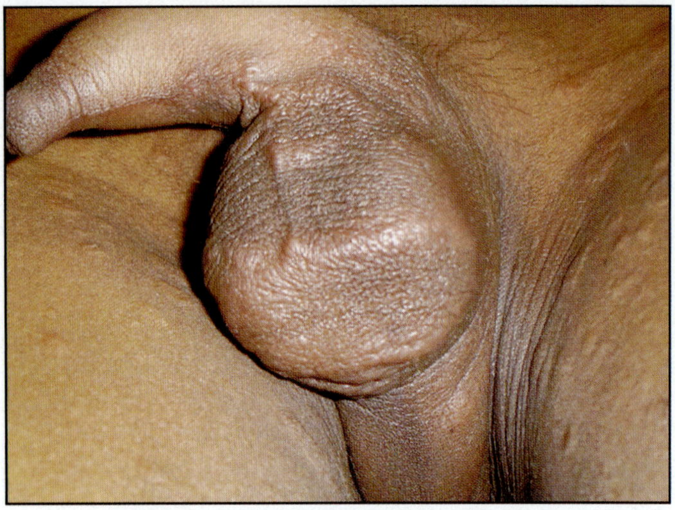

FIGURE 11.9: Genital lesion in BT leprosy

may show features of either tuberculoid or lepromatous leprosy. The skin lesions are mostly macules, the number of which is variable between tuberculoid and lepromatous spectrum. Pebbling is not seen at the borders of raised lesions. Instability is the predominant feature of this spectrum of disease. The number of skin lesions may extend up to ten and the size may as large as 10-15 cm. Satellite lesions are characteristic feature of this type of leprosy. Lesional sensory loss may be complete at one end and partial at the other. BT skin lesion with large hypopigmented patch was originally known as maculoanesthetic leprosy. It is also known as low resistant tuberculoid and is prone to develop frequent reactions.

The lesions are asymmetrical, dry with loss of hair. Nerves are severely involved in this type of disease. Various deformities may result from repeated episodes of reactions or due to silent paralysis. Nodular thickening may occur in the course of nerve which leads to abscess formation. Reactions may manifest as lesional erythema and edema or as neuritis, impending paralysis and deformity. Lepromin test is weakly positive and histopathology shows tuberculoid granulomas with moderate lymphocytic infiltration.

The other types of leprosy like mid borderline, borderline lepromatous and lepromatous leprosy are uncommon in children and hence not detailed here.

Pure Neuritic Leprosy

Pure neuritic leprosy is also included in the Indian classification. In this form of leprosy nerve is the only structure which is involved. Patients present with thick nerve and loss of sensation in an area corresponding to the nerve supply. Muscle wasting may also occur with trophic changes or trophic ulcers.

Comparison of skin lesions of various forms of leprosy has been presented in **Table 11.11**.

REACTIONS IN LEPROSY

Leprosy is a chronic disease, with long term activity. In several patients there are bouts of acute exacerbations during the long course of the disease. These can occur in lepromatous, borderline and tuberculoid spectra of the disease in that order of frequency. The word reaction in leprosy is used to describe only an episode in a major disease. The old concepts like tuberculoid reaction, reactional tuberculoid and lepra fever have been replaced by Type-1 and Type-2 reactions.

TABLE 11.11: Comparison of skin lesions in various forms of leprosy

	Tuberculoid	Lepromatous	Borderline
Number	Up to four	Numerous	Many
Size	Large	Small	Initially large, subsequently small
Distribution	Asymmetrical	Symmetrical	Usually symmetrical
Texture	Rough and dry	Smooth and shiny	Rough and wrinkled
Periphery	Definite	Vague	Variable
Sensation	Complete anesthesia	Little or no loss of sensation	Larger lesion are anesthetic, smaller lesions hypoesthetic / sensation preserved.
Bacilli	Negative	Positive	Variable
Lepromin test	Strongly positive	Negative	Variable

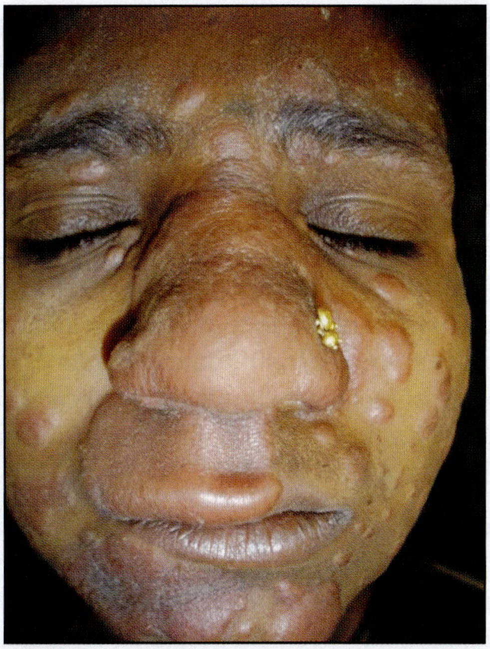
FIGURE 11.10: BL leprosy with type 1 reaction

Type-1 Reaction

Type-1 reaction occurs in borderline spectrum of the disease. The patient complains of sudden increase in the size of the lesions. There is edema of the existing patch **(Figure 11.10)**. Nerve trunks may be enlarged and tender. Nerve damage occurs frequently followed by paralysis. There are no constitutional symptoms associated with this type of reaction.

Type-1 reaction may be upgrading or downgrading. Upgrading reaction occurs in BT spectrum when the patient's immunological status improves. Down grading reaction occurs in untreated BT patients and there is a shift towards BL spectrum with increase in the number of skin lesions and newer nerve involvements.

Type-1 reaction is also known as reversal reaction in leprosy. Reversal reaction usually occurs within six months of completion of treatment. This has to be differentiated from relapse which occurs after six months of stopping treatment. The high risk patients belonged to borderline group with more than ten skin lesions and more than three nerve involvements.

Histopathological examination of skin lesion reveals the following:

1. Diffuse edema in and around granuloma
2. Rapid influx of lymphocytes and diffuse proliferation of fibroblasts.
3. Presence of foreign body giant cells.
4. A patch of fibrin necrosis in upgrading reaction and
5. Loss of localization of granulomas in down grading reactions

Type-2 Reaction

Type-2 reaction is also called as erythema nodosum leprosum. This occurs in BL and LL spectra of the disease which are uncommon in children. Type-2 reaction manifests as sudden onset of crops of multiple painful erythematous nodules with generalized distribution, fever, arthralgia, myalgia, episcleritis, iritis, iridocyclitis and testicular swelling. Investigations reveal neutrophilia, leukocytosis, and albuminuria.

DEFORMITIES

Leprosy was once considered as the most benign and baneful of all diseases. Except the deformities in a small percentage of patients, leprosy can be considered as an innocuous infection. Deformities present in certain patients at the time of diagnosis are because of late detection. Occasionally neuritis can occur in patients on treatment or released from treatment, which may go undetected, resulting in residual nerve paralysis and consequent deformity. The ideal way to deal with deformities is to adopt measures which would prevent its occurrence, namely, early detection and prompt treatment of disease and associated neuritis. Leprosy is on the decline but the same is not true for the disabilities associated with it. Deformity and disability can be differentiated by the visibility in the former, whereas the later is experienced by the patient alone. For example, anesthetic extremity is a disability whereas trophic ulcer is a deformity. In a study conducted by the urban leprosy project it was found that 7% of children were suffering from deformities.

Claw Hand (Figures 11.11 and 11.12)

Claw hand may result from isolated ulnar nerve palsy, which affects little and ring fingers only (ulnar claw hand). In the combined median and ulnar palsy all the four fingers are involved (total claw hand). Grasp is affected in claw hand. In a normal hand grasping of an object starts with the flexion of the metacarpophalangeal joint followed by the flexion of the interphalangeal joints. This order gets reversed in claw hand making it difficult for the fingers to close around a large object. Moreover, the integrity of the metacarpal arch, essential for grasp, gets distorted in claw hand. While grasping small objects the fingertips exert excessive pressure getting ulcerations in due course.

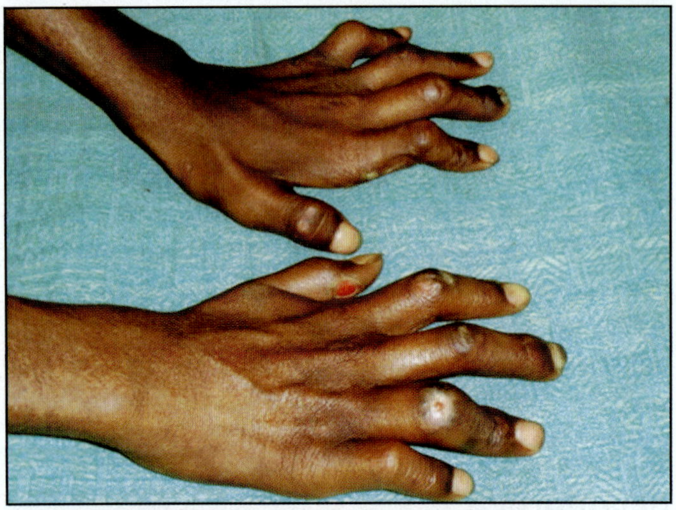

FIGURE 11.11: Bilateral complete claw hands

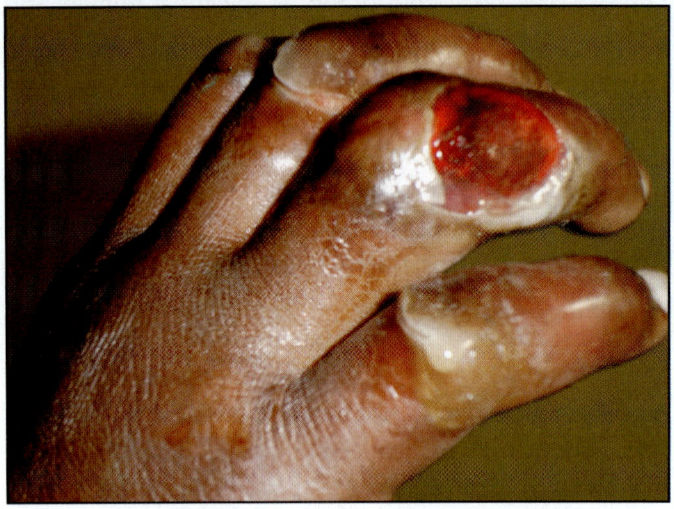

FIGURE 11.12: Claw hand with dactylitis

Lumbricals are the primary flexors of the metacarpophalangeal joints, but interossei also contribute as accessory flexors. Hence a claw hand manifests only when there is paralysis of both lumbricals and interossei. In isolated median nerve paralysis, the two radial lumbricals are paralyzed. Since interossei are intact, the claw hand does not manifest, but the grasp becomes weak.

Treatment of claw hand is based on the principle of ensuring metacarpophalangeal joint flexon either actively or passively. This restores the normal order of flexion of joints during grasp.

The following procedures are done:

1. The sublimis transfer (Stiles-Bunnel)
2. The extensor to flexor four tailed graft
3. Palmaris longus many tailed graft
4. Extensor indices transfer

In the lower limb the common peroneal and the tibial nerves are affected frequently. The paralysis of muscles combined with loss of sensation affects the foot in various ways.

Foot Drop

Foot drop occurs due to paralysis of the common peroneal nerve. There is loss of dorsiflexion of the foot at the ankle joint and eversion of the foot at the subtalar joint. This predisposes to ulceration at the lateral border of foot and at the region of metatarsal heads. The patient displays a typical gait while he lifts his foot high up before placing it on ground.

Treatment: Spontaneous recovery occurs in many cases after several weeks. Hence surgery is deferred for one year, when conservative therapy is continued. If there is no spontaneous improvement even after one year, tibialis posterior tendon transfer is undertaken.

DIFFERENTIAL DIAGNOSIS

Hypopigmented Macules

Pityriasis versicolor: Pityriasis versicolor may be easily distinguished from leprosy as it shows numerous macules on the upper half of the body with fine, branny scales. Patients may complain of mild itching or burning sensation on exposure to sunlight. Wood's light examination shows greenish yellow fluorescence and KOH examination shows the presence of short thick hyphae and bunches of spores which can confirm the diagnosis. Atypical pityriasis versicolor, which may present with a single patch at an unusual site, has to be differentiated from leprosy. In such doubtful cases, histopathological examination confirms the diagnosis of leprosy. If the lesions are seen on face, where biopsy is avoided for fear of postoperative scars, a trial of anti-fungal therapy may be administered for one month and the patient reviewed.

Early vitiligo: Vitiligo presents as depigmented macule or patch with leukotrichia. Repigmentation occurs at the perifollicular regions or at the margin of the lesions. Pre vitiligo is a stage in the evolution of the disease, where only hypopigmented macules are seen for a few months prior to development of full clinical features of vitiligo. This condition mimics lesions of indeterminate leprosy. Testing for sensory loss and signs of autonomic nerve damage may differentiate these two conditions.

Postinflammatory hypopigmentation: Postinflammatory hypopigmentation occurs in many conditions including pityriasis rosea. In pityriasis rosea the lesions show "Christmas tree" pattern and is usually situated on the trunk.

Nevus anemicus: Nevus anemicus is a developmental anomaly. It presents as a circular patch of pale skin of normal texture. On diascopy, it is indistinguishable from the blanched surrounding normal skin. Intradermal injection of histamine produces a flare. In leprosy the flare is delayed, feeble or entirely absent.

Nevus achromicus: Nevus achromicus is a birth mark and has to be differentiated from leprosy. Diascopy does not show any change of color in this condition. There is erythema on stroking. Histopathology reveals decreased number of melanocytes.

Pityriasis simplex (alba): This is the most common condition which has to be differentiated from indeterminate leprosy in children. It is considered as a milder form atopic dermatitis. Pityriasis alba presents as hypopigmented macule or a patch with mild branny scales. This condition shows a seasonal variation and is aggravated in summer season. In doubtful cases, hydrocortisone cream may be given for a month and the case may be reviewed. If the patch persists, a punch biopsy to confirm the diagnosis is ideal.

Polymorphic light eruption (PMLE): PMLE is bilaterally symmetrical on the face. It produces few hypo pigmented patches normally seen on the outer aspect of the face or cheeks. There is history of sun exposure in children during their outdoor activities and hence it commonly affects this age group. There may be history of itching and burning sensation on sun exposure. In doubtful cases, combination of topical sunscreens in the day time and application of mild corticosteroids like hydrocortisone for a month may be useful before attempting a biopsy.

CHEMOTHERAPY

Multidrug Therapy, Paucibacillary Regimen (PB-MDT)

WHO in 1981 defined PB as patients with a bacterial index of less than 2. Subsequently (1990), this was redefined as all patients with negative bacterial index. This group includes indeterminate, TT and BT leprosy. PB patients have lower bacillary load and the problem of drug resistant mutant bacilli is insignificant.

Rifampicin is included in the regimen as the monthly pulse dose **(Table 11.12)**. It is the anchoring drug in leprosy control. It decreases the incidence of primary dapsone resistance and ensures patient compliance by providing a cost effective therapeutic regimen of shorter duration.

TABLE 11.12: PB-MDT regimen

	Child 5-14 years	Adult >14 years
Monthly treatment	Rifampicin 450 mg	Rifampicin 600 mg
Daily treatment	Dapsone 50 mg	Dapsone 100 mg
Duration	6 pulses to be completed in 9 months time	6 pulses to be completed in 9 months time

In contrast to smear positive patients, the outcome or the end point of treatment in smear negative cases is difficult to define. Though the overall results are good, there are few practical problems. Presence of disease activity at the end of 6 pulses has been found to be 10 to 67 % in different studies. However, it has also been found that in 80% of these patients the disease activity wanes away even without further treatment. In the remaining, the disease continues to be active even beyond 18 months.

The results of MB treatment have been encouraging. MB patients who were treated for 12 months responded well with rare incidence of relapse **(Table 11.13)**. However, despite adequate treatment 10% of patients continue to harbor viable persisters which are difficult to

TABLE 11.13: MB-MDT regimen

	Children 6-9 years	Children 10-14 years	Adult >14 years
Monthly treatment	Rifampicin 300 mg and Clofazimine 100 mg	Rifampicin 450 mg and Clofazimine 150 mg	Rifampicin 600 mg and Clofazimine 300 mg
Daily treatment	Dapsone 25 mg	Dapsone 50 mg	Dapsone 100 mg
	Clofazimine 50 mg twice a week	Clofazimine 50 mg on alternate days	Clofazimine 50 mg daily

treat. In addition, patients with LL lack the specific CMI to deal with these remaining organisms. The relapse rate among MB patients varied from 0-1.6%. Bacteriological relapse occur earlier than clinical relapse. On the contrary, in a study done on defaulters, who had discontinued treatment for approximately six to eleven months, majority of the patients were found to be improved without any further treatment. Hence, shortening of the duration of MB-MDT is being considered.

Twelve monthly pulses of treatment are to be completed within a time span of 18 months in all categories **(Table 11.14)**.

TABLE 11.14: SL-PB regimen

	Children 5-14 years	Adult > 14 years
Single dose	Rifampicin 300 mg	Rifamipicin 600 mg
Single dose	Ofloxacin 200	Ofloxacin 400 mg mg
Single dose	Minocyclin 50 mg	Minocyclin 100 mg

Even though field trials with ROM therapy have been encouraging, institutional studies raised some controversies. These are:

1. Recommendation of a single dose therapy for a chronic infectious disease has been questioned by many authorities as it is not being done for other such infections.
2. Only a few bacilli are expected to be in the multiplication phase when there is adequate blood level of the drugs following the single dosage. The bacilli, which are not multiplying are likely to escape the effect of the drugs and may result in relapse latter.
3. The diagnosis of single lesion leprosy may sometimes be difficult in the field set-up. In a recent study from Brazil it was observed that 3-4% of single lesion leprosy cases were histopathologically multibacillary. Another 4% were diagnosed wrongly.

If patient develops a reaction to dapsone in MDT-PB regimen it is substituted with clofazimine. In MDT-MB, dapsone is stopped and the other two drugs are continued.

If patient develops reaction to rifampicin, it is substituted with ofloxacin 400 mg with minocyclin 100 mg for six months and thereafter only ofloxacin or minocyclin alone for the rest of the period.

If clofazimine is unacceptable because of its pigmentation, ofloxacin 400 mg daily may be substituted.

TREATMENT OF REACTIONS IN LEPROSY

Drugs used in Reactions

Corticosteroids constitute the most powerful weapon in the management of severe reactions where they bring dramatic response by antipyretic, anti-inflammatory and mood elevating properties **(Table 11.15)**. However, once started, it may become difficult to taper off the drug because of frequent relapse of symptoms. Corticosteroids are used both in type-1 and type-2 reactions. In type-1 reaction prompt treatment with steroid is necessary to prevent paralysis and consequent disability. The recommended dose of prednisolone is as follows:

40 mg once daily for 2 weeks
30 mg once daily for 2 weeks
20 mg once daily for 2 weeks
15 mg once daily for 2 weeks

TABLE 11.15: Common side effects of drugs used in leprosy

Drugs	Side effects
Dapsone	Anemia, methhemoglobinemia, hemolytic anemia, neutropenia, thrombocytopenia, lymphopenia, pseudo leukemoid like picture, maculopapular rash, urticaria, fixed drug eruption, erythema multiforme, Steven-Johnson syndrome, toxic epidermal necrolysis, photo sensitivity, exfoliative dermatitis, dapsone syndrome, gastritis, jaundice, peripheral neuropathy, psychosis and renal failure.
Rifampicin	Discoloration of urine, sweat and feces, hepatitis and flu like syndrome.
Clofazimine	Discoloration of skin and sweat, ichthyosis, conjunctival xerosis, and abdominal symptoms including acute abdomen.
Ofloxacin	Abdominal and CNS symptoms.
Minocyclin	Discoloration of teeth in children, pigmentation of skin, dizziness and abdominal pain.

10 mg once daily for 2 weeks and
5 mg once daily for 2 weeks

If type-1 reaction occurs during the course of treatment, the other antileprosy drugs should be continued. If reaction occurs after completion of treatment there is no need to restart the antileprosy drugs beyond the recommended period.

In type-2 reactions, corticosteroids are started at a lower dosage of 30 mg/day for adults. However type-2 reactions are rare in children as multibacillary leprosy itself is uncommon at this age group.

Steroid produces many side effects in children like frequent infections, weight gain, cushingoid features, striae, acne, stunted growth and irregular menstrual periods.

Chloroquin in the dosage of 250 mg/ day is the other drug which may be used for mild type of reactions without much of neuritis. Ocular side effects like double vision and visual halo may occur as the earliest complication. Regular ophthalmologic check-up is required if the treatment is continued beyond 4 to 6 weeks.

VACCINES IN LEPROSY

Various forms of immunological interventions have been tried in leprosy. These are known as immuno-prophylaxis and immuno-therapy. Immuno-prophylaxis is aimed to induce protective immunity in unaffected population. This helps to enhance the ability to limit mycobacterial multiplication and reduce the chances of evolution to clinical disease after infection. Immunotherapy is administered to patients who have already established disease. The procedures for these modalities are almost similar. Immuno-prophylaxis is of value in patients with positive 'fluorescent leprosy antibody absorption test' and negative lepromin test.

BCG vaccination is an example of cross reacting *Mycobacterium* used to induce protective immunity against another mycobacterial disease. Large scale studies on efficacy of BCG vaccination in prevention of leprosy were conducted in various countries including south India and it was found to vary from 25 to 85%.

The other first generation leprosy vaccines used are:

1. Live *M. leprae*
2. Killed *M.leprae*
3. Killed *M.leprae* with an adjuvant
4. Killed cross reacting mycobacterium

The second generation vaccines are based on recombinant DNA technology with *M.leprae* specific monoclonal antibody. These vaccines appear to be useful in patients with high bacillary load, who do not show bacterial clearance at the usual pace. It is also useful in killing persisters and in patients with relapse.

Immunotherapy

In immunotherapy the following are used:

1. IV injection of peripheral blood lymphocytes collected from TT patients or from healthy donors.
2. IV injection of transfer factor
3. Levamisole for six weeks
4. Injection of gamma interferon
5. Injection of interleukin-2.
6. Addition of zinc

Leprosy in Children Born to Mothers with Leprosy

Duncan, in his study on historical and clinical review of the interaction of leprosy and pregnancy, found that, up to 20% of children born to mothers affected with leprosy may develop the disease by puberty. Early leprosy in young children is self healing. However, if the daughters of mothers affected with leprosy are subjected to early marriage and pregnancy, they may experience the adverse influences of pregnancy on leprosy. He also observed that weight gain of the children of mothers with leprosy by 2 years of age was less compared to those of healthy mothers; the placental weights and coefficients followed the same trend. The growth rate of such children was slow and this was more obvious in mothers with lepromatous leprosy. There is no prospective controlled study to document the effect of multidrug therapy in the pregnancy outcome of women with leprosy.

LEPROSY ELIMINATION

In the month of January 2006, India was declared to have eliminated leprosy. The elimination of leprosy as a public health problem is defined as attaining a prevalence rate of less than one case per 10,000 population. With this the vertical program comes to an end and the leprosy control program has been integrated with general health services. In the postelimination era, the diagnosis, treatment and care of leprosy patient shifts from general physicians to dermatologists. New leprosy cases, though lesser in number, continue to report at all levels of health care due to lack of active case detection, surveillance, and trained staff. The delay in diagnosis due to inexperienced staff at primary care level results in increased number of MB cases. The childhood leprosy is an indicator of transmission of leprosy and hence, presence of MB cases in the community. In the post-elimination era, dermatologists have to play a major role not only in patient care but also in teaching and training of students, medical officers and practitioners to achieve a new target, eradication of leprosy.

The diagnosis of leprosy in a child causes intense psychological distress to the child and the family members. One should be careful in confirming leprosy in children. Childhood leprosy is clinically challenging, epidemiologically significant and socially consequential. It is also the barometer for effective intervention by WHO.

BIBLIOGRAPHY

1. Amladi S, Jerajani HR, Rupani S. Unusual cutaneous ulcers in a case of miliary tuberculosis. Indian J Dermatol Venereol Leprol 1993;59:24-26.
2. Anandam K, Seethamma K, Venkateshwarlu K, Sharma KMA. Varied forms of lupus vulgaris. Indian J Dermatol Venereol Leprol 1998;64:183-84.
3. Arya L, Koranne RV, Deb M. Cutaneous tuberculosis in children. A clinicomicrobiological study. Indian J Dermatol Venereol Leprol 1999;65:137-39.
4. Bartralot R, Garcia-Patos V, Sitjas D, Rodriguez-Cano L, Mollet J, Martin- Casabona N, et al. Clinical patterns of cutaneous nontuberculous mycobacterial infections. Br J Dermatol 2005; 152: 727-34.
5. Beena KR, Ramesh V, Mukherjee A. Lichen scrofulosorum – a series of eight cases. Dermatology 2000;201:272-74.
6. Bryceson A and Pfaltzgraff RE: Leprosy, 3rd edn. Churchchill Livingstone, Edinburgh 1990.
7. Chatterjee G, Kundu AK, Das S. Vulval tuberculosis. Ind J Dermatol 1999;44:193-94.
8. Chaves A, Torrelo A, Mediero IG, Menedez- Revas M, Ortega-Calderon A, Zambrano A. Primary cutaneous M. kansasii infection in a child. Pediatr Dermatol 2001; 18 (2): 131-34.
9. Consensus Statement of IAP Working Group: Status Report on Diagnosis of Childhood Tuberculosis. Ind Pediatr 2004;41:146-55.
10. Dhillon GPS. NLWP- Current situation and strategy during the 11th plan (2007-12) J Indian Med Assoc 2006;104: 671-2.
11. Ebenezer L, Arunthathi S, and Kurian N. Profile of leprosy in children: Past and present Ind J Lepr 1997:69: 255-59.
12. Gangopadhyay AK. Scrofuloderma—An unusual complication of BCG vaccination. Ind J Dermatol 1997;42:249-250.
13. Global Tuberculosis Control. Annexure 1-Profile of High Burden Countries. WHO Report 2006;92-94.
14. Guptae MD. South India immunoprophylaxis trial against leprosy: relevance of findings in the context of leprosy trends. Int J Lepr 2001:69: S10-3.
15. Jain S, Reddy RG, Osmani N, Lockwood DNJ and Suneetha S. Childhood leprosy in urban clinic, Hyderabad India: clinical presentation and role of household contacts. Lepr Rev 2002: 73:248-53.
16. Jang HS, Jo JH, Oh CK, Kim MB, Lee JB, Cheng CL, et al. Successful treatment of cutaneous infection caused by M. scrofulaceum with clarithromycin. Pediatr Dermatol 2005; 22 (5): 476-9.
17. Jopling EH: Hand book of Leprosy. 3rd edn. William Heinmann Medical Books Ltd, London 1984.
18. Jordaan HF, Schneider JW, Abdulla EA. Nodular tuberculid: a report of four patients. Pediatr Dermatol 2000;17:183-8.
19. Kabra SK, Lodha R, Seth V. Category based treatment of tuberculosis in children. Ind Pediatr 2004;41:927-37.
20. Kar. H.K. Leprosy free India: clinical perspectives and challenges ahead. Lepr Rev 2007; 78: 38-9.
21. Krishnamurthy P. Diagnosis of leprosy. J Indian Med Assoc 2006: 104:680-1.
22. Kumar B, Rai R, Kaur I, Sahoo B, Muralidhar S, Radotra BD. Childhood cutaneous tuberculosis: a study over 25 years from northern India. Int J Dermatol 2001;40:26-32.
23. Mahajan M, Jogaikar DG, Mehta JM. Study of deformities in children with leprosy: An urban experience. Ind J Lepr 1995: 67:405-09.
24. Maniar JK, Kamath RK, Mandalia S, Shah K, Maniar A. HIV and tuberculosis: partners in crime. Indian J Dermatol Venereol Leprol 2006;72:276-82.
25. NLEP- Current leprosy situation in India, Director General of health services, Leprosy division, New Delhi, April 2006.
26. Norman G, Joseph GA, Udyasuriyan P, Samuel P and Venugopal M. Leprosy case detection among school children Lep Rev 2004: 75: 34-9.
27. Padmavathy L, Rao LL. Ulcerative lupus vulgaris. Indian J Dermatol Venereol Leprol 2005;71:134-5.
28. Pandhi D, Reddy BSN, Chowdhary S, Khurana. Cutaneous tuberculosis in Indian children: the importance of screening for involvement of internal organs. J Eur Acad Dermatol Venereol 2004;18:546-51.
29. Prasad PVS. All about Leprosy, JayPee Brothers New Delhi. 2005.
30. Prasad PVS. Childhood leprosy in a rural hospital. Ind J Pediatr 1998;65:751-4.
31. Primm TP, Lucero CA, Falkinham III JO. Health impacts of environmental mycobacteria. Clin Microbio Rev 2004; 17 (1): 98-106.
32. Ramam M, Mittal R, Ramesh V. How soon does cutaneous tuberculosis respond to treatment? Implications for a therapeutic test of diagnosis. Indian J Dermatol 2005;44: 121-4.
33. Ramam M, Tejasvi T, Manchanda Y, Sharma S, Mittal R. What is the appropriate duration of a therapeutic trial in cutaneous tuberculosis? Further observations. Ind J Dermatol Venereol Leprol 2007. In Press.
34. Ramesh V, Misra RS, Beena KR, Mukherjee A. A study of skin tubercuolosis in children. Pediatr Dermatol 1999;16:264-9.
35. Ramesh V. Sporotrichoid cutaneous tuberculosis. Clin Exper Dermatol 2007 (in press).
36. Raut WK, Sawaitu VK, Bobhate SK, Fule RP, Salodkar AD. Acute miliary tuberculosis of skin- a case report and review of literature. Ind J Dermatol 2002;47:57-59.
37. Sarveshwari KN, Swamikannu M, Ramakrishnan S. An aetiological analysis of erythema nodosum in a community hospital. Indian J Dermatol Venereol Leprol 2001;67:287-9.
38. Sehgal VN. Lichen scrofulosorum – current status. Indian J Dermatol 2005;44:521-3.

39. Selvakumar A, Geetha J, Nisha K, Manimozhi N, Jesudasan K and Rao PSS. Childhood leprosy in an endemic area. Lepr Rev 1999; 70: 21-7.
40. Sethuraman G, Kaur J, Nag HL, Khaitan BK, Sharma VK, Singh MK. Symmetrical scrofuloderma with tuberculosis verrucosa cutis. Clin Exp Dermatol 2006;31:1-3.
41. Singal A, Aggarwal P, Pandhi D, Rohatgi J. Cutaneous tuberculosis and phlyctenular conjunctivitis: a forgotten association. Indian J Dermatol Venereol Leprol 2006;72:290-2.
42. Singal A, Bhattacharya SN. Lichen scrofulosorum: a prospective study of 39 patients. Int J Dermatol 2005;44:489-93.
43. TB: Burden of the disease in India. Revised National Tuberculosis Control Programme, Central Tuberculosis Division, Directorate General of Health Services, Ministry of Health and Family Welfare, Govt of India, New Delhi, 2007.
44. The final push strategy to eliminate leprosy as a public health problem. Questions and Answers. 2nd edn. WHO, Geneva 2003.
45. Vashisht P, Sahoo B, Khurana N, Reddy BSN. Cutaneous tuberculosis in children and adolescents: a clinicohistological study. J Eur Acad Dermatol Venereol 2007;21:40-47.
46. WHO Report 2006. Global Tuberculosis Control – Surveillance, Planning, Financing, Geneva, Switzerland.
47. Wietzul S, Eicchorn PJ, Pandya AG. Nontuberculous mycobacterial infections of the skin. Dermatol Clin 2000;18 (2): 359-77.

12

Diseases of the Mucous Membrane

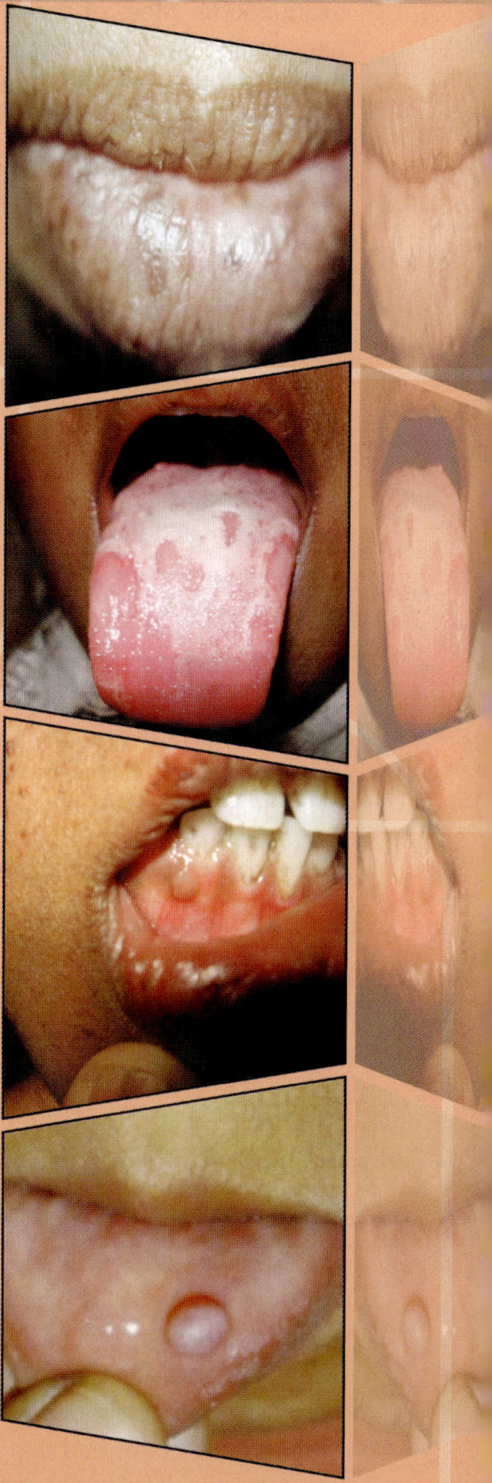

Anandan S, Rashmi Mittal

INTRODUCTION

Lesions of the oral mucosa may occur in isolation as a specific disease entity or as a manifestation of a systemic disease process. Mucosal lesions may occasionally be correctly diagnosed from a brief history and rapid clinical examination. Most of the diseases of the oral mucosa have a similar clinical appearance due to the fact that oral mucosa being thin causes vesicles and bullae to rupture rapidly into ulcers. These ulcers are rapidly traumatized by teeth and food and get secondarily infected by oral flora. History taking, if correctly performed gives as much information as does the clinical examination. It is beyond the scope of this chapter to discuss all the conditions mentioned in great detail. It is divided into sections, depending upon the most likely presenting signs and symptoms.

1. Mouth ulcers
2. White patches
3. Red and pigmented lesions
4. Swellings /Lumps
5. Tongue lesions

MOUTH ULCERS

Recurring oral ulcers are the most common problems encountered by clinicians who manage diseases of the oral cavity.

RECURRENT APHTHOUS STOMATITIS (RAS)

It is a disorder characterized by recurring ulcers confined to the oral mucosa in patients with no other signs of disease. It heals and recurs at fairly regular intervals. RAS affects approximately 20% of the general population.

Etiology

The etiology of RAS is not exactly known. The current concept is that it is a clinical syndrome with several possible causes. The major factors include heredity, hematologic deficiencies and immunologic abnormalities. The best documented factor is heredity. These patients have an increased frequency of HLA-A2, HLA-11, HLA-B12, and HLA-DR2. It was once assumed that RAS was a form of recurrent herpes simplex virus infection (HSV). Many studies have confirmed that RAS is not caused by HSV. Hematologic deficiency, particularly of serum iron, folate, and vitamin B_{12} appears to be an etiologic factor in a subset of patients with RAS2.In cases of refractory disease, Hay and Reade reported the benefit of an elimination diet in some patients with suspected or proven allergy to foods such as milk, cheese, wheat and flour. RAS – like ulceration has also been described in association with HIV infection, Behcet's syndrome, Sweet's syndrome and other malabsorption diseases like Crohn's disease.

RAS can be divided into 3 clinical types which are summarized in **Table 12.1**.

TABLE 12.1: Clinical features of clinical types of RAS

	Minor	Major	Herpetiform
Synonym	Mikulicz ulcer	Sutton's ulcer	
Incidence	80%	10%	10%
Age (years)	10-19	10-19	20-29
Sex(F:M)	1.3:1	0.8:1	2.6:1
Site	Non-keratinized mucous membrane	Anywhere	Anywhere
Number	1-5	1-10	10-100
Size	<10mm	>10mm	1-2mm
Duration (days)	7-10	>20	7-10
Scarring	8%	64%	32%
Recurrence	1-4months	<1month	>1 month
Duration of disease (years)	<5	>15	>5

Treatment

Medication prescribed should relate to the severity of the disease. In mild cases, use of a protective emollient such as orabase is all that is necessary. Pain relief of minor lesions can be obtained with topical anesthetic gels. Chlorhexidine gluconate (0.2%) mouthwashes are a good starting point and often give good symptomatic relief. Topical steroid such as triamcinolone acetonide in carboxymethylcellulose applied to the ulcers four times daily is often beneficial. The gel can be carefully applied directly to the lesions after meals and at bedtime two to three times a day. It should be emphasized that no available topical therapy decreases the onset of new lesions. In patients with major aphthae or severe cases of multiple minor aphthae not responding to topical therapy, use of systemic therapy should be considered. Drugs that have been reported to reduce the number of ulcers in selected cases are colchicine, dapsone, short bursts of oral corticosteroids, thalidomide, immunosuppressants like azathioprine and cyclosporine. Their use in children must be carefully monitored and they should be used only as a last resort.

BEHCET'S SYNDROME

Described by the Turkish dermatologist Hulusi Behcet, was classically described as a triad of symptoms including recurring oral ulcers, genital ulcers and eye lesions. The concept has been changed from a triad of signs and symptoms to a multisystem disorder. Behcet's syndrome in children most frequently presents between the ages of 9 and 10 years. Oral ulcers are a more common sign and uveitis is less common as compared to the adults. A variant of Behcet's syndrome, MAGIC syndrome, characterized by mouth and genital ulcers with inflamed cartilage has been described.

Etiology

There is considerable evidence to suggest an immunological etiology. HLA-B5, HLA-BW51, HLA-DR7 appear to be associated with Behcet's syndrome.

Clinical Features

Five different sets of criteria have been in use for the past 20 years. In 1990, an international study group reviewed data from 914 patients from seven countries. A new set of diagnostic criteria was developed that includes recurrent oral ulceration occurring at least three times in one 12-month period plus two of the following four manifestations:

1. Recurrent genital ulceration
2. Uveitis or retinal vasculitis
3. Skin lesions including erythema nodosum, pseudofolliculitis, papulopustular lesion, acneiform nodules in adolescent patients not receiving corticosteroids
4. A positive pathergy test

A positive pathergy is defined as an inflammatory reaction forming within 24 hours of a needle puncture, scratch or saline injection.

Treatment

The management of Behcet's syndrome depends on the severity and the sites of involvement. Azathioprine, cyclosporine, colchicine in combination with systemic corticosteroids has been shown to be useful in severe disease. Systemic corticosteroids remain the mainstay of treatment and are particularly useful in rapidly controlling the disease until immunosuppressive agents begin to work. Thalidomide may be required in cases of recalcitrant orogenital ulceration but requires extreme caution as it is teratogenic.

TRAUMATIC ULCERATION

Trauma to the oral mucosa is common and may cause localized ulceration. The trauma may be physical, thermal or chemical. It may be self-inflicted in disorders such as congenital insensitivity to pain, Lesch-Nyhan syndrome, epilepsy, athetosis and mental retardation. Oral ulceration may also be caused by non-accidental injury.

INFECTIONS

Infections whish cause oral ulcers are: Viral, bacterial, fungal.

Viral

Herpes simplex virus type 1 and increasingly type 2 cause primary herpetic gingivostomatitis. Following primary infection, the virus remains latent in the trigeminal ganglion. About one-third of patients experience recurrent herpes infections, the most common of which is herpes labialis (cold sore). Typical triggering events include exposure to sunlight, infections such as common cold, stress and trauma. The lesions consist of vesicles which may rupture to form painful, circular, sharply defined shallow ulcers with a yellowish grey floor and erythematous margin. There is often associated cervical lymphadenopathy, pyrexia and malaise. Severely immunocompromised children, such as those undergoing bone marrow transplantation, may develop acyclovir resistant herpes simplex infection. The lesions present as well defined oral ulcers with a characteristic adherent greyish – white slough, which has a leathery texture.

Treatment in majority of case is supportive, with antipyretic analgesics, bed rest and adequate fluid intake. Systemic acyclovir hastens recovery but is only really useful if used in the first three days of onset. In acyclovir-resistant cases, valacyclovir, ganciclovir, cidofir and foscarnet are alternative treatments.

Other viral infections which can cause oral ulcers in children are chicken pox, herpes zoster (immunocompromised), herpangina, hand, foot and mouth disease, infectious mononucleosis, cytomegalovirus, human immunodeficiency virus.

Fungal

Deep fungal infections may give rise to oral ulcers particularly in immunocompromised children, those undergoing cytotoxic chemotherapy or bone marrow transplantation, or in patients with acquired immunodeficiency syndrome. Aspergillosis may cause black necrotic ulceration of the palate. The infection originated from the maxillary sinuses. Mucormycosis may give rise to a similar picture of aspergillosis. It has been associated with diabetes mellitus. Histoplasmosis oral lesions present as an ulcer or a lump.

Bacterial

The causative organisms are a proliferation of two normal oral commensals, the gram-negative anerobes *Borrelia vincentii* and *Fusobacterium nucleatum.* It causes Acute Ulcerative Gingivitis . This disease classically begins in the tips of the interdental papillae, causing intense pain and halitosis. There is ulceration which is far more destructive in an immunocompromised child. This condition responds very well to oral metronidazole.

NEOPLASIA

This is very rare in children. It may be the presenting feature of lymphoma, histiocytosis.

SYSTEMIC DISEASE

This section includes hematological diseases, gastrointestinal diseases like celiac disease, Crohn's disease, ulcerative colitis.

DERMATOLOGICAL DISEASES

Dermatological disorders rarely cause mouth ulcers in childhood; if they occur, skin lesions can aid in diagnosis.

Lichen Planus/Lichenoid Reactions

This is rare in childhood. Reticular lesions are usually asymptomatic and distributed on the buccal mucosa and lateral borders of the tongue. Atrophic or ulcerative lichen planus is symptomatic. It may occur in association with graft versus host disease. Treatment with topical and systemic corticosteroids is in the same way as in RAS. Immunosuppressive therapy is helpful particularly in GVHD.

Vesiculobullous Diseases

The major diseases in this group are, pemphigus vulgaris, benign mucous membrane pemphigoid, epidermolysis bullosa, dermatitis herpetiformis, chronic bullous disease of childhood and erythema multiforme.

Pemphigus vulgaris: Eighty to ninety percent of patients with pemphigus vulgaris develop oral ulcers and in 60% oral lesions are the first sign. The lesions begin as classical bullae but evident as shallow irregular ulcers thereafter. The ulcers extend peripherally to involve large portions of the oral mucosa. Common sites of involvement are buccal mucosa, palate and gingival.

Benign mucous membrane pemphigoid primarily affects patients over the age of 50 years.

Epidermolysis bullosa is a mechano-bullous disorder where bullae formation in the oral mucosa may be precipitated by suckling in infancy. These break down to form ulcers which heal with scarring. Oral hygiene is usually poor and the incidence of caries and periodontal disease is high.

Dermatitis herpetiformis may occur in childhood and is associated with gluten enteropathy. Oral lesions may occur in the form of erythematous papules, macules, petechiae, vesicles, bullae and erosions.

Chronic bullous disease of childhood: It is another blistering disorder, which chiefly affects children below the age of 5 years. Oral mucosal involvement is present in upto 50% of the cases.

Erythema multiforme: Oral lesions may occur in isolation or with a skin rash, which characteristically consists of 'target lesion' and ocular involvement. Hemorrhagic crusting of lips may be associated.

CONNECTIVE TISSUE DISORDERS

These include discoid and systemic lupus erythematosus (SLE). Discoid lesions may involve lips or oral mucous membrane. Asymptomatic oral ulcers may be present in SLE and commonest site of occurrence is posterior part of hard palate.

WHITE LESIONS

The term 'leukoplakia' is often used clinically to describe a chronic white lesion of the oral mucosa. It is usually restricted to those white lesions where there is no identifiable cause or underlying disease process.

NORMAL ANATOMICAL VARIATIONS

Fordyce's Spots

They are ectopic sebaceous glands present in the oral mucosa and become clinically apparent only after puberty. These appear as asymptomatic, slightly raised yellowish papules on the buccal or labial and retromolar mucosa.

Epstein's Pearls and Bohn's Nodules

These are gingival cysts seen in the newborn. They may rupture spontaneously or involute and are rarely apparent after 3 months of age. Bohn's nodules occur on the crest of the alveolar ridge and Epstein's pearls on the midline of the palate.

CONGENITAL LESIONS

White Sponge Nevus

It is a rare autosomal dominant disorder. Lesions may be present at birth or may first manifest during puberty. It presents as bilateral, symmetric, asymptomatic, white, spongy or velvety plaques on the buccal mucosa. Other sites involved are the ventral tongue, floor of the mouth, labial mucosa, soft palate and alveolar mucosa.

Hereditary Benign Intraepithelial Dyskeratosis

It is a rare autosomal dominant condition in which oral lesions occur in childhood and become more obvious in adolescence. It is characterized by oral lesions and bilateral limbal conjunctival plaques. The ocular findings are seen in the first year and are the most characteristic feature.

Darier's Disease

It is an autosomal dominant disorder of keratinization. Oral involvement is seen in 50% of patients. Clinically, the oral lesions consist of erythematous papules which coalesce to give a cobblestone appearance, mainly seen on the palate or tongue and gingiva.

Pachyonychia Congenita

Oral involvement is seen in 60% of patients. The lesions occur in the form of generalized grayish-white thickening of the oral mucosa. Natal or neonatal teeth may be present in 16% of individuals. There is an increased risk of oral candidiasis in this group.

Dyskeratosis Congenita

This is a rare sex linked recessive disorder. Oral lesions occur between the ages of 5 and 10 years. Lesions usually consist of white patches affecting the palate or tongue which may be preceded by vesicles or erosions.

ACQUIRED CAUSES

Frictional (traumatic) Keratosis

It presents as a white plaque with a rough and frayed surface caused by an identifiable source of mechanical irritation like a sharp tooth or habits of cheek biting. It usually resolves on elimination of the irritant.

Chemical Injuries

Transient white lesions of the oral mucosa may be attributed to the formation of a psuedomembrane composed of necrotic surface tissue and an inflammatory exudate. This may be caused due to chemical trauma following ingestion of caustic or acidic agents, e.g. household cleansing agents which cause an epithelial cell death. Aspirin burns may occur due to the tablet being placed next to a painful tooth.

Koplik's Spot

This is oral manifestation of measles seen on the buccal mucosa and precedes the skin rash by 1–2 days.

Candidiasis

Candida sp. can be isolated in about 50% of the population as a normal oral commensal. The commonest species isolated are *Candida albicans, C. krusei, C. guilliermondii, C. tropicalis* and *C. parapsilosis*. In case of disturbed oral environment as in presence of systemic infection, depressed cell mediated immunity, iron deficiency, etc., the commensal candidal organisms may proliferate giving rise to the infection. These may attain one of the following clinical patterns:

Thrush—typically seen in the neonatal period when the immune mechanisms have not fully developed. Lesions are asymptomatic and manifest as thick, creamy plaques which are easily wiped off leaving an erythematous mucosa.

Erythematous candidiasis—Patchy erythematous lesions may occur and is associated with HIV infection.

Chronic atrophic candidiasis—It is bright red in color and is seen under a removable orthodontic appliance.

Angular stomatitis—It is an inflammatory lesion at the angles of the mouth. It may be asymptomatic or painful.

Chronic hyperplastic candidiasis—Oral lesions are white, tough and firmly adherent to the underlying mucous membrane. It is seen in congenital immunodeficiencies and AIDS.

Hairy Leucoplakia

It is caused by *Epstein Barr* virus and may be a feature of immunodeficient children, particularly in presence HIV infection.

RED AND PIGMENTED LESIONS

a. Amalgam tattoo—They are the most common cause of localized oral pigmentation. It may result from minor trauma to the oral mucosa during extraction of a tooth containing an amalgam restoration.
b. Racial pigmentation
c. Drug induced pigmentation—Anticonvulsants, cytotoxic agents, ACTH replacement and anti-malarials may result in oral pigmentation.
d. Melanocytic nevi
e. Peutz Jegher's syndrome—Oral pigmentation is confined to the lower lip and buccal mucosa **(Figure 12.1)**. It is an autosomal dominant condition with associated intestinal polyposis and melanotic pigmentation of the face and mouth.
f. Hemangiomas—These may occur as purple/ bluish macule on lips, palate and buccal mucosa.
g. Gingivitis—It usually occurs in older children and is concurrent with poor oral hygiene. It presents as redness of the gingiva surrounding the teeth. There may be bleeding from the gingiva on brushing the teeth.
h. Addison's disease, Albright's syndrome.

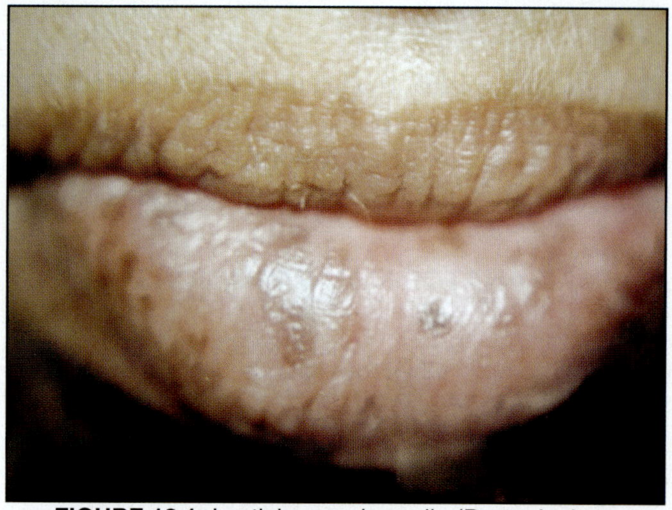

FIGURE 12.1: Lentigines on lower lip (Peutz-Jeghers syndrome)

i. Hereditary hemorrhagic telangiectasia(Osler-Weber-Rendu disease): It is an autosomal dominant disorder characterized by multiple telangiectasia of the skin and mucous membrane.

SWELLINGS/LUMPS

a. Soft tissue swellings
b. Bony swellings
c. Gingival swelling
d. Salivary gland swelling

SOFT TISSUE SWELLING

i. Congenital granular cell epulis of the newborn
ii. Eruption cyst
iii. Lymphangioma
iv. Hemangioma
v. Neurofibromatosis
vi. Tuberous sclerosis **(Figures 12.2A and B)**.
vii. Fibroepithelial polyp
viii. Granuloma pyogenicum
ix. Molluscum contagiosum
x. Burkitt's lymphoma
xi. Sarcomas
xii. Squamous papilloma

BONY SWELLINGS

i. Tori: These are slow growing exostoses, thought to be inherited as autosomal dominant trait. Torus palatinus occurs in the midline of the hard palate.

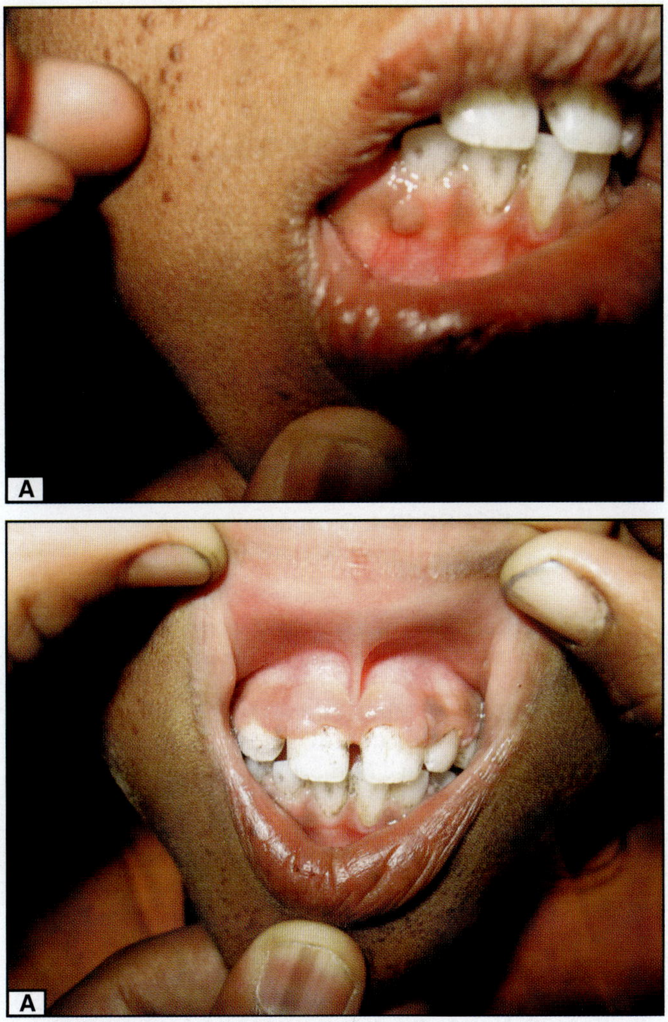

FIGURES 12.2A AND B: Gingival fibroma in tuberous sclerosis

Torus mandibularis occurs in the premolar area of the mandible.

ii. Fibrous dysplasia
iii. Odontogenic cysts
iv. Juvenile active ossifying fibroma

GINGIVAL SWELLING

i. Hereditary gingival fibromatosis: This is an autosomal dominant condition with fibrous gingival enlargement, hypertrichosis and coarse facial features.
ii. Gingival hyperplasia: It may be caused by certain drugs like phenytoin, cyclosporine, calcium channel blockers. It is aggravated by poor oral hygiene.
iii. Acute leukemia: It is usually seen in acute myeloid leukemia but may also be associated with acute lymphoblastic leukemia.

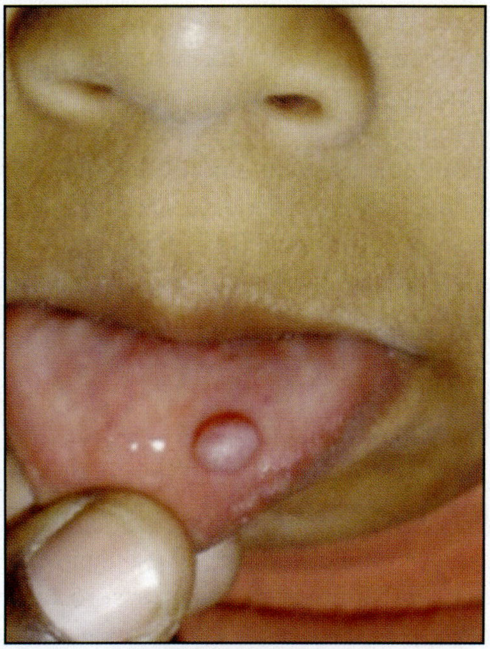

FIGURE 12.3: Mucocoele

SALIVARY GLAND SWELLING

i. Infections—Mumps is the most common cause of salivary gland swelling. Other viral infections causing salivary gland enlargement are Coxsackie A, echovirus, parainfluenza, *Epstein Barr* virus and cytomegalovirus.
ii. Mucocele/ranula—The most common sites are the lower lip, palate, upper lip and buccal mucosa **(Figure 12.3)**.
iii. Cystic fibrosis
iv. Sarcoidosis

Salivary gland malignancy is rare in childhood.

LESIONS OF THE TONGUE

CONGENITAL LESIONS

a. Macroglossia: It may be seen in syndromes like Down's syndrome, Beckwith Wiedmann syndrome, Hurler's syndrome and cretinism. In these conditions the macroglossia is due to tongue muscle hypertrophy. It may also be caused by tumor or hamartoma of tongue, most commonly lymphangioma in childhood.

b. Microglossia: It is a rare congenital anomaly and causes difficulty in talking and eating.

c. Ankylogossia: It affects 1.7% of children and is usually caused by a short lingual faenum.

d. Fissured/scrotal tongue: Multiple small fissures or grooves are seen on the dorsal surface of the tongue. It is rarely seen before the age of 4 years. It is a developmental anomaly affecting about 1% of children. It is frequent among children with mental retardation, such as Down's syndrome. It is also a feature of Melkersson-Rosenthal syndrome which has additional features of labial swelling and facial palsy.
e. Lingual thyroid
f. Lingual tonsil
g. Sublingual dermoid cyst

ACQUIRED LESIONS

a. Glossitis: Nutritional deficiency (vitamin B_{12}, ferritin, and folate) may give rise to a sore tongue and atrophic glossitis. Beefy tongue is a feature of vitamin B_{12} deficiency.
b. Infections: Scarlet fever and Kawasaki disease may both cause a 'strawberry tongue'. There is furring of the tongue and prominence of the fungiform papillae. In scarlet fever, the coating on the tongue rapidly subsides and the tongue looks smooth and deep red in color (raspberry tongue).
c. Erythema migrans (geographic tongue): It is a benign condition which gives rise to a well-defined area of depapillation of the tongue.
d. The presenting symptom is soreness of the tongue which is usually aggravated by salted and spicy foods **(Figure 12.4)**.
e. Hairy tongue: This results from excessive elongation of the filiform papillae on the posterior part of the tongue, caused by chronic irritation. In young children it is usually idiopathic.

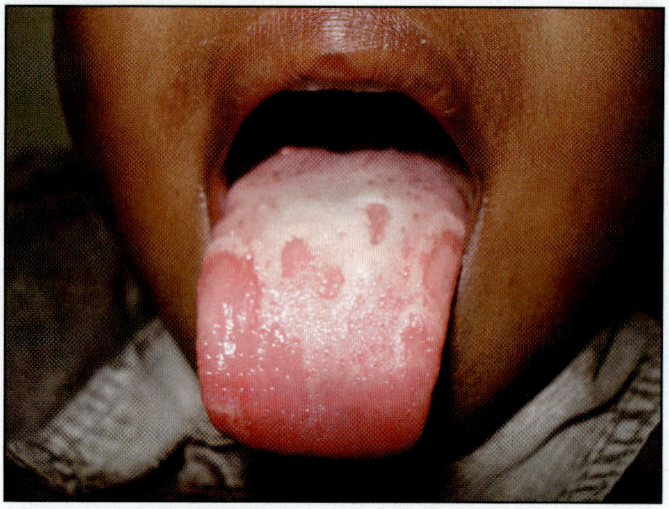

FIGURE 12.4: Geographic tongue

BIBLIOGRAPHY

1. Baker SR, Malone B. Salivary gland malignancies in children. Cancer 1985; 55:1730-6.
2. Hay KD, Reade PC. The use of elimination diet in the treatment of recurrent aphthous ulceration in the oral cavity. Oral Surg 1984;57;504.
3. Imai H, Motegi M, Mizuki N,et al. Mouth and genital ulcers with inflamed cartilage(MAGIC syndrome): A case report and literature review. Am J Med Sci 1997; 314: 330-2.
4. International study group. Criteria for diagnosis of Behcet's disease. Lancet 1990;335:1078.
5. Jacobson JM, Greenspan J, Spritzler N, et al. Thalidomide for the treatment of oral aphthous ulcers in patients with human immunodeficiency virus infection. N Eng J Med 1997;336:1487-93.
6. Katz j, Langeritz P, Shemer J. Prevention of RAS with colchicines: an open trial. J Am Acad Dermatol 1995;35:680.
7. Krause I, Uziel Y, Guedj D, et al. Mode of presentation and multisystem involvement in Behcet's disease: The influence of sex and age of disease onset. J Rheumatol 1998;25:1566-9.
8. Lamey PJ, Rees TD, Binnie WH, et al . Oral presentation of pemphigus vulgaris and its response to systemic steroid therapy. Oral Surg 1992;74:54.
9. Masuda K, Nakajima A, Urayama A. Double masked trial of cyclosporine versus colchicines and long term open study of cyclosporine in Behcet's disease. Lancet 1989; 1:1093.
10. O'Duffy JD. Behcet's syndrome. N engl J Med 1990;322:326.
11. ScullyC, Porter SR. Recurrent aphthous stomatitis:current concepts of aetiology, pathogenesis and management. J Oral Pathol Med 1989;18:21-27.

13

Disorders of Hair

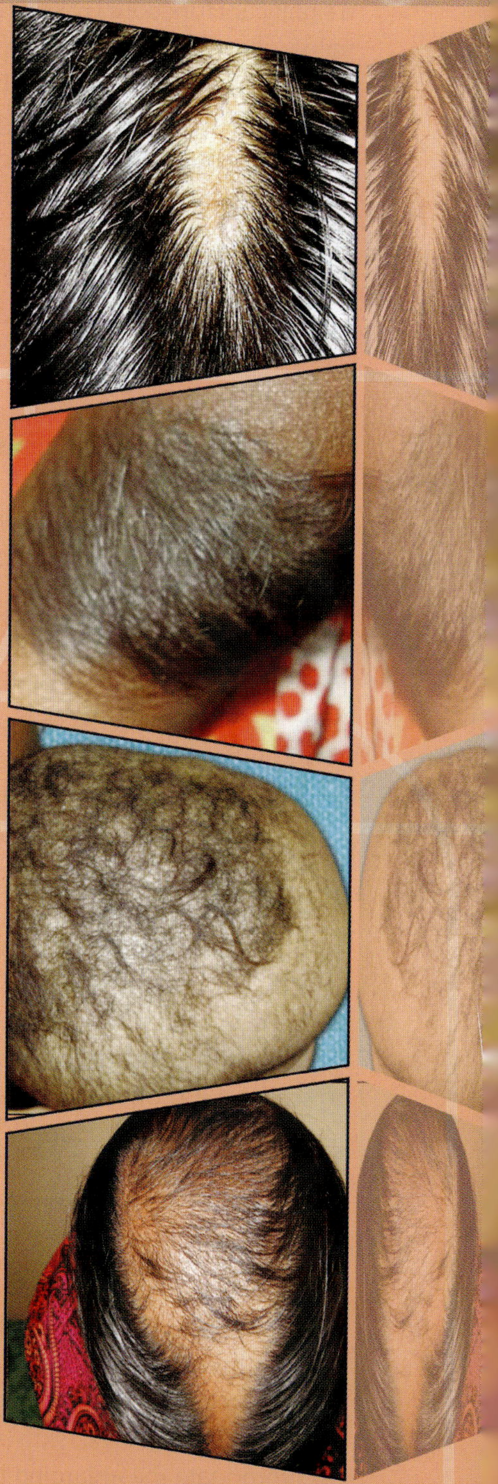

Anitha B, Ragunatha S

INTRODUCTION

Hair is a keratinized structure arising from the hair follicle distributed all over the body surface sparing palms, soles, lips, glans and shaft of the penis, sides of fingers and toes, and distal phalanges. Although hair does not have a significant functional role in humans except the cosmetic value, disorders of hair have a profound psychological impact on children and their parents causing a great concern. Therefore, knowledge of hair structure and the factors regulating the hair growth cycle is necessary for the understanding and efficient management of hair disorders.

NORMAL HAIR

DEVELOPMENT

The formation of hair begins around 8-12th week of fetal life with the appearance of bud in the basal layer of epidermis. This hair germ first appears in the scalp and proceeds cephalo-caudaly (refer chapter 1 for details).

TYPES OF HAIR

Depending upon the length, texture and pigmentation, hairs can be classified as lanugo, vellus and terminal hairs.

- **Lanugo hairs:** These are long, fine, soft, non medullated and poorly pigmented. They cover entire fetal surface and shed after birth except in the rare hereditary syndrome, hypertrichosis lanuginosa.
- **Vellus hairs:** These are short, fine and lightly pigmented hairs seen on the arms and face of children and face of women.
- **Terminal hairs:** These are long, thick, mature, medullated and darkly pigmented hairs seen on the scalp, eye brows, eye lashes and areas of secondary sexual hair distribution.

DENSITY, DISTRIBUTION AND GROWTH RATE OF HAIR

The density and distribution of hair follicles are genetically determined and new hair follicles do not develop after birth in most circumstances. Follicular density varies in different regions of the body, being highest on the scalp. As the infant grows, skin surface area increases to accommodate the enlarging body and the density of the hair follicles progressively decreases. The average density of scalp hair at birth is reported as 1135/cm^2, diminishing to 795/cm^2 by the end of the 1st year and 615/cm^2 by third decade.

The rate of hair growth varies in different body regions. Scalp hairs grow about 0.4 mm/day and can reach a length of more than 1 m. Eyebrows and eyelashes grow at a rate of 0.16 mm/day, axillary hair at a rate of 0.3 mm/day and hair on lower limbs at a rate of 0.2 mm/day.

STRUCTURE OF HAIR

A mature hair follicle is divided into two segments:

- The upper permanent segment
- The lower dynamic segment which reforms itself over the cycle.

Upper segment is composed of infundibulum that extends from the ostium of the follicle above to the sebaceous duct entrance below, and isthmus that extends from sebaceous duct entrance above to the attachment of arrector pili muscle below.

Lower segment is composed of stem that extends from the attachment of arrector pili muscle above to Adamson's fringe below, and hair bulb that extends from Adamson's fringe above to the base of the follicle.

The Hair bulb, the deep bulbous portion of hair follicle that surrounds dermal papilla, contains the hair matrix which produces hair shaft, and its outer and inner root sheaths. The outer root sheath is composed of pale and clear cells with abundant glycogen and extends from base of the bulb to the infundibulum. The inner root sheath is composed of 3 layers- Henle's layer, Huxley's layer and cuticle from outside inward. It extends from the upper half of bulb to the isthmus. The hair shaft is made up of 3 structures namely the cuticle, the cortex and the medulla from outside inward. The hair shaft cuticle interdigitates with the inner root sheath cuticle.

HAIR CYCLE

The growth of hair is cyclical consisting of three phases.

Anagen

This is a phase of hair growth where hair is formed through continued proliferation and differentiation of matrix cells at the follicle base. The cell cycle length of matrix cells is approximately 18 hours. The proliferating cells move upwards to differentiate into one of the layers of inner root sheath and hair shaft. This phase is the longest of hair cycle and its duration determines the length of hair shaft. Duration of anagen is different in different body areas. It is longest in scalp (2-6 years) and shortest in eyebrows, eyelashes and thighs (1-2 months). Over the chin, legs, axillae and arms it is 1 year, 4-6 months, 4 months and 3 months respectively. The anagen phase is very sensitive to noxious insults [e.g. chemotherapeutic agents] because of its high mitotic index.

Catagen

This is a transitional phase lasting for 2-3 weeks and is characterized by degeneration of the lower dynamic portion of the follicle in a process that includes cessation of melanin production, apoptosis of the matrix cells and cessation of hair shaft differentiation. The bottom of the hair shaft seals off into a rounded structure called a club, which moves upwards to reach the non-cycling, permanent upper segment in mid dermis. As the lower segment recedes, a temporary structure forms- the epithelial strand- which connects the dermal papilla to the upper segment of the follicle. It contains many apoptotic cells and is completely eliminated by the time the dermal papilla reaches the cells that surround the remnant club hair.

Telogen

This is the resting phase during which the follicles lie dormant. Telogen phase, in the scalp follicles, lasts about 3 months but it is considerably longer in other body regions such as lower limbs. The hair shaft remains anchored to the follicle during telogen. Hair shedding (teloptosis/ exogen) usually occurs when the follicle re-enters a new anagen phase. This transition from telogen to anagen occurs when one or two quiescent multipotent epithelial stem cells at the lowest permanent portion of the hair follicle- the bulge, are activated to produce a new hair shaft.

The follicular stem cells repopulate the hair matrix at each cycle. Destruction of follicular stem cells results in scarring alopecia. Programmed cell death of these stem cells might play a role in the physiologic, slowly progressing loss of hair follicles in aging human scalp or during the final stages of androgenetic alopecia. Apoptosis of melanocytic stem cells might be an important factor for hair greying.

Factors that regulate the hair growth cycle are not completely known. Several cytokines and growth factors like insulin- like growth factor, hepatocyte growth factor, fibroblast growth factor, parathyroid hormone related peptide, calcineurin, transforming growth factor β, neurotrophins and vascular endothelial growth factor are possibly involved.

NEONATAL HAIR

At birth, the terminal scalp hairs are in the anagen phase. Majority of the hairs are 5 to 6 months old. Within few days, a physiologic anagen to telogen transition occurs resulting in loss of high proportion of scalp hairs. This is known as telogen effluvium of the newborn. The hair loss may be sudden leading to complete alopecia or may be gradual and perceptible. Whether sudden or gradual, replacement of the first terminal hairs is completed within 6 months of life. In neonates, the frontal hairline extends along the forehead and temples to the lateral margin of the eyebrows. These terminal hairs are gradually converted to vellus hairs during first year of life.

DISORDERS OF HAIR

Hair reacts to both local and systemic insults in different ways such as change in hair growth density and pattern, and alteration in its texture and color. The severity of hair disorders depending on the type of insult, segment of hair and phase of hair growth cycle involved, range from physiological hair loss (e.g. pregnancy) to irreversible hair loss (e.g. scarring alopecia).

Disorders of hair can be broadly classified as:

- Congenital or early onset alopecia
- Nonscarring alopecia
- Scarring alopecia
- Hypertrichosis: Diffuse and Localized
- Hirsutism
- Eruptive vellus hair cysts
- Pigmentary changes of hair: Premature greying, green discoloration
- Disorders of follicular plugging: Keratosis pilaris, keratosis pilaris atrophicans

CONGENITAL OR EARLY ONSET ALOPECIA

Alopecia that is present at birth or in the early months of life may be diffuse or localized.

CONGENITAL DIFFUSE ALOPECIA

Diffuse congenital alopecia may be partial (hypotrichosis) or complete (atrichia). It may occur alone, with other minor cutaneous abnormalities, as a part of a variety of syndromes or in some of the genetic hair shaft abnormalities.

Hypotrichosis Occurring Alone or with other Minor Abnormalities

Isolated congenital atrichia or hypotrichosis: Several genotypes occur in this group with recessive, dominant and X-linked inheritance patterns. Recessively inherited ones are most severe and are of congenital onset. Total absence of hair or extremely sparse hair involving scalp, eyebrows, eyelashes and general body hair occur.

Marie unna hypotrichosis: This is an autosomal dominant disorder presenting with sparse hair or complete absence of hair at birth. During early childhood, characteristic coarse and wiry hair appears. Microscopic examination of hair reveals irregularly distributed twisting and longitudinal ridging.

Atrichia with papular lesions: In this disorder, normal neonatal hair is shed in first 3 months of life and is never replaced. Small, white papular lesions, which represent keratin-filled follicular cysts histopathologically, occur diffusely but predominate on face and scalp.

Congenital hypotrichosis and milia: This is an X-linked dominant disorder characterized by hypotrichosis with sparse, coarse hair and multiple milia, present at birth, on the face and sometimes also on limbs and trunk.

Hypotrichosis with Ectodermal Dysplasias

Hypotrichosis is an important feature in many of the ectodermal dysplasia (ED) syndromes but often becomes obvious only after the neonatal period **(Figure 13.1)**. These conditions include Hidrotic ED, Hypohidrotic ED, AEC (Ankyloblepharon, ED and clefting syndrome), Rapp-Hodgkin syndrome, and Bazex-Dupre-Christol syndrome.

Hypotrichosis with Ichthyoses

Lamellar Ichthyosis: This ichthyosis presenting as the "collodion baby" phenotype is characterized by alopecia which often occurs as a result of hair being caught up in and shed with the large plates of scale which exfoliate from the scalp, or due to secondary bacterial infection.

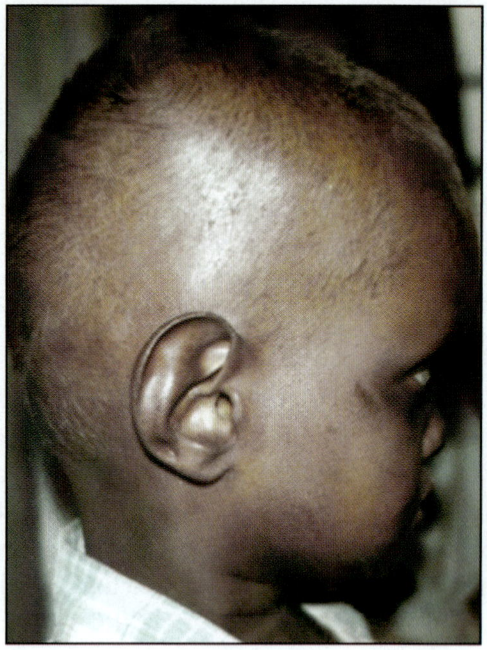

FIGURE 13.1: Hypotrichosis in hypohidrotic ectodermal dysplasia

Ichthyosis follicularis, congenital atrichia and photophobia (IFAP): This is an X-linked trait characterized by atrichia or severe hypotrichosis, keratotic follicular papules and photophobia since birth. Other features include periorificial erosions and keratotic plaques, nail dystrophy, gingival erythema and recurrent infections.

Peeling skin syndrome: There is a single case report of a child with the inflammatory variant of the peeling skin syndrome who in addition had hair abnormality like trichorrhexis invaginata-like changes, irregular twisting of the hair and areas of hair shaft narrowing.

Keratitis, Ichthyosis and Deafness syndrome: Severe hypotrichosis of scalp, eyebrows and eyelashes may be evident at birth and persists throughout life along with spiny follicular plugging, widespread thickened erythematous plaques, perioral furrowing, reticulate hyperkeratosis of palms and soles, keratitis and hearing loss.

Congenital ichthyosis, follicular atrophoderma, hypotrichosis and hypohidrosis: This combination of traits has been described as a new autosomal recessive genodermatosis and all the features are present from neonatal period.

Hypotrichosis with premature aging syndromes: Hypotrichosis is evident in early infancy in cases of

Hutchison-Gilford Progeria, Rothmund-Thomson syndrome and Cockayne syndrome.

Hypotrichosis with immunodeficiency syndromes: Severe combined immunodeficiency-associated congenital graft-versus-host disease and Omenn syndrome present in early infancy with alopecia, erythroderma, failure to thrive and diarrhea. Sparsity of scalp, eyebrow and eyelash hair is evident in neonatal period in cartilage hair hypoplasia syndrome.

Hypotrichosis with genetic disorders of the hair shaft: Increased fragility of hair in many genetic disorders of hair shaft leads to early alopecia which will be discussed later in this chapter.

CONGENITAL LOCALIZED ALOPECIA

Neonatal Occipital Alopecia

Alopecia that occurs in occipital area in neonates has been earlier attributed entirely to rubbing of occipital region of scalp on the bedding. But, now it is attributed to the patterns of hair cycle evolution in fetal and early neonatal life **(Figure 13.2)**.

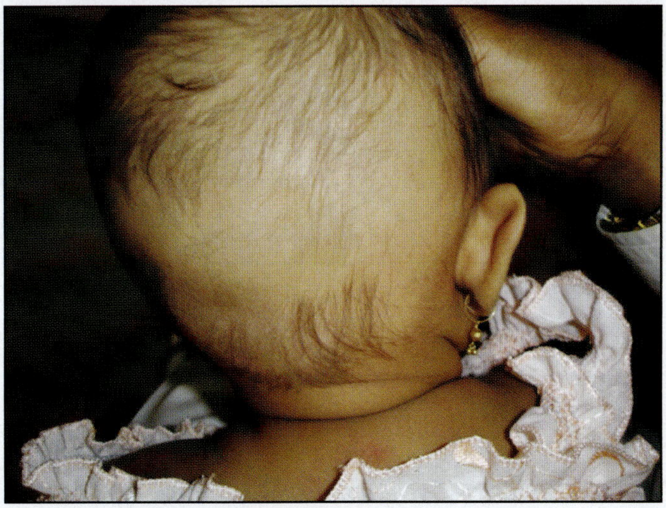

Figure 13.2: Neonatal occipital alopecia

Scalp Injury

During the process of delivery, temporary alopecia may occur in areas of scalp damaged by instrumentation such as forceps, vacuum extractor or scalp monitors and also over cephalhematomas.

Temporal Triangular Alopecia

Well-circumscribed triangular or lance-shaped area of non scarring alopecia occurs in fronto-temporal area with vellus hairs seen in the affected area and occasionally a few terminal hairs are retained. It is unilateral in 80% cases. This condition may be congenital and may be noted in neonatal period which is often attributed to forceps trauma. It is more often first noted in early childhood and adult onset has been reported.

Localized Alopecia Associated with other Nevoid Conditions

Congenital melanocytic nevus: These are usually associated with hypertrichosis but large folded lesions causing a cutis verticis gyrata appearance may have sparse covering hair or even complete absence of hair.

Sebaceous nevus: These nevi are characteristically hairless **(Figure 13.3)**.

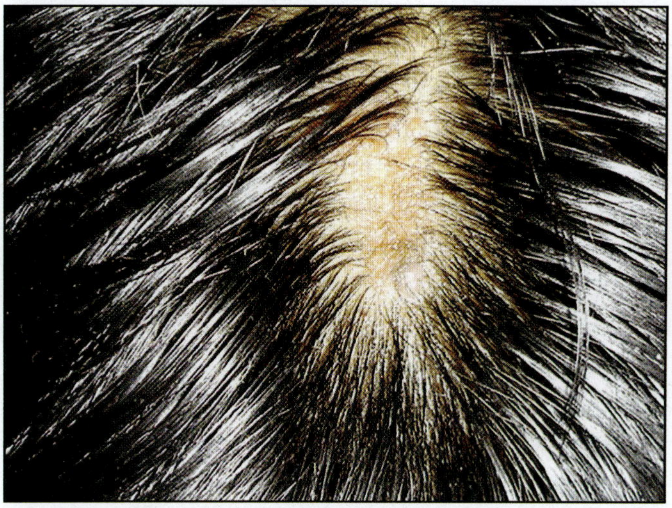

FIGURE 13.3: Localized alopecia due to nevus sebaceous

Aplastic nevus (minus nevus): This is a nevoid condition in which there is complete absence of skin appendages in an area of otherwise normal skin.

Aplasia cutis: Aplasia cutis congenita is characterized by irregularly shaped erosion which eventually heals with hypertropic scarring and alopecia. Membranous aplasia cutis is characterized by oval or round, hairless area covered by a smooth membrane and occasionally surrounded by a hair collar. Aplasia cutis producing a localized congenital alopecia may be a feature of a number of syndromes including Adams-Oliver syndrome and Toriello oculoectodermal syndrome.

Cranial meningoceles, encephaloceles and heterotopic meningeal or brain tissue: These lesions are either hairless or have sparse overlying hair often with a "hair collar sign".

Hypotrichosis with Congenital Forms of Cutis Verticis Gyrata

It may occur as a feature of certain syndromes like Turner syndrome, Beare Stevenson syndrome, Michelin-tire baby syndrome, Shau Pai dog syndrome.

Localized Alopecia Associated with Syndromes

Hallermann-Streiff syndrome: Hair may be normal at birth but in some cases the typical alopecia, located in frontal and parietal areas over the cranial sutures, may be evident in early months, together with atrophic facial skin and multiple craniofacial and ocular abnormalities.

X-linked dominant conditions: Certain conditions like focal dermal hypoplasia (Goltz syndrome), incontinentia pigmenti, oral facial digital syndrome and X-linked dominant chondrodysplasia punctata are characterized by patchy alopecia, sometimes obviously linear or spiral as it follows the lines of Blaschko. The X-linked dominant genes responsible for these conditions interfere with hair growth and produce a mosaic pattern of alopecia in affected females as a result of functional X-chromosome mosaicism. The hemizygous males with these conditions rarely survive.

NONSCARRING ALOPECIA

Nonscarring alopecia results from causes like alteration of the hair growth cycle, structural abnormalities of the hair and inflammatory cutaneous diseases **(Flow Chart 13.1)**.

TELOGEN EFFLUVIUM

The human hair follicle growth is cyclical consisting of 3 phases: anagen (growth phase), catagen (transitional phase) and telogen (resting phase). Human scalp contains 1, 00,000 hairs on an average, with an average growth rate of terminal hair being 2.5 mm/week, approximately. In an healthy individual, normally 50 to 100 hairs are shed and simultaneously replaced each day.

The normal cyclic pattern may be interrupted by a variety of stimuli and may lead to excessive generalized shedding of normal telogen club hairs **(Table 13.1)**. This condition is termed as telogen effluvium which is the most common type of alopecia being second in incidence only to male pattern baldness.

Depending upon the abnormality of hair cycle, the telogen effluvium is divided into 5 types. These include premature termination of anagen, prolongation of anagen (postpartum), reduced anagen (in androgenetic alopecia patients), immediate telogen release, and delayed telogen

TABLE 13.1: Causes of telogen effluvium

- Childbirth
- Severe infection
- Severe chronic illness
- Severe psychological stress
- Surgical shock
- Crash diets
- Hypothyroidism/hyperthyroidism
- Iron deficiency anemia
- Anticoagulant drugs
- Excessive ingestion of vitamin A (hypervitaminosis A)

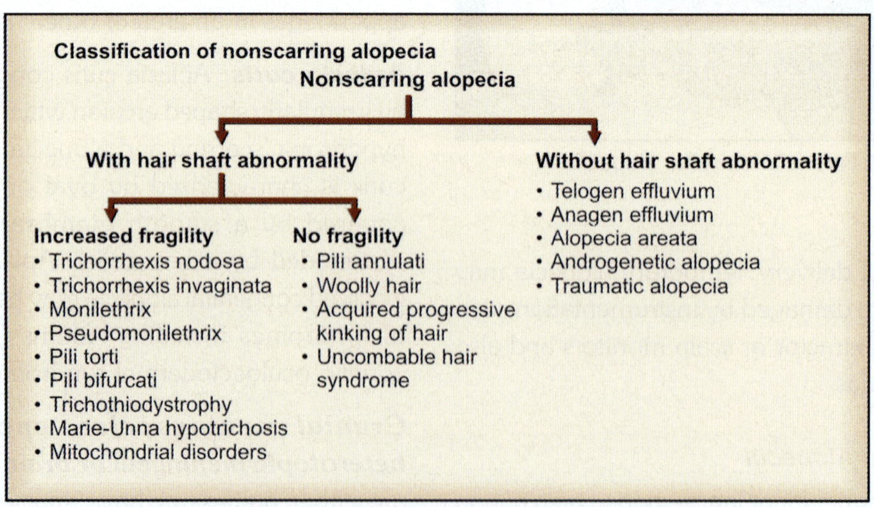

Flow Chart 13.1: Classification of nonscarring alopecia

release (scalp psoriasis). The proportion of follicles affected and the severity of the alopecia depends on the duration and severity of the stress and individual variations in susceptibility. These stimuli induce hair loss by abruptly shifting hair follicles from anagen to telogen phase, thereby affecting the anagen-telogen ratio. Hair loss does not actually occur until 2-4 months after the period of initial stress, since hair shafts are usually not shed until 2-4 months after entering the telogen phase. Therefore, the shedding seen in telogen effluvium actually marks the end, not the beginning of this disorder.

A detailed history about any stressful event, severe diet restriction, drugs, vitamin A supplements, and thyroid symptoms preceding the onset of alopecia by 2-4 months suggests the diagnosis of telogen effluvium and can be confirmed by certain tests like hair pull test, daily hair counts and hair pluck test.

Hair Pull Test

Approximately 50-60 hairs from the patient's temporo parietal scalp are firmly grasped between thumb and forefinger, and gently pulled with a slow constant traction. In normal adults, 2-5 telogen hairs will be obtained in this manner, whereas in telogen effluvium, more than 6 club hairs will be extracted.

Daily Hair Count

Patient is instructed to collect the hair lost in the first morning combing and those lost during washing for 14 days, saving them in clear plastic bags. Patient is asked to count the hairs and record the number on the bags. The hair bulbs are examined under microscope to determine if they are anagen or telogen. It is normal to lose up to 100 hairs daily and 200 to 250 hairs on the day of shampooing. In telogen effluvium, more than 100 telogen hairs are lost daily.

Hair Pluck Test (trichogram)

Approximately 50 hairs from the patient's temporo-parietal scalp are clamped about 1 cm from the skin surface with a hemostat (the jaws of which should be covered by rubber tubing to prevent trauma to the hair shafts), followed by a gentle and short tug. Hairs thus obtained are float onto a wet microscope slide and are examined under low power. Anagen bulbs are recognized by the presence of intact outer and inner root sheaths with/ without a portion of the dermal papilla adherent to the root tip. Telogen bulbs are identified by their uniform shaft diameter and club shaped root tip containing no pigment. They resemble tip of cotton tipped applicator. A simple method of identifying anagen hairs is by adding anagen hair dye (4-dimethylamino-cinnamaldehyde, DACA) to the hair pluck preparation and moving the hairs gently from side to side for 15-20 seconds to allow penetration of the dye. DACA reacts with citrulline; an amino acid found only in the inner root sheath and stains the anagen hairs, leaving behind the telogen hairs unstained as they do not contain an inner root sheath.

The ratio of telogen to anagen hairs is determined. A telogen count of 25% or more is considered to be diagnostic of telogen effluvium.

There is no effective treatment for telogen effluvium. Replacement therapy has been reported to result in decreased hair shedding, but there are no controlled studies regarding the efficacy of iron supplementation in pre anemic or anemic patients, nor on thyroid hormone supplementation on the outcome of telogen effluvium. Spontaneous regrowth is characteristic of this disorder and unless the stressful event or stimuli is repeated, complete regrowth takes place almost invariably within about 6 months. However, in conditions like exceptionally prolonged illness with high fever, some follicles may be completely destroyed resulting in only partial recovery in such cases. The patient should be explained about the cause of this disorder and its favorable prognosis, and should be instructed to avoid manipulation such as vigorous shampooing, combing and brushing until new growth has occurred.

ANAGEN EFFLUVIUM

Anagen effluvium is a condition characterized by abrupt loss of hair from follicles that are in their growing phase. It occurs as a result of an abrupt insult to the metabolic and follicular reproductive apparatus of the hair follicle. This is a far less common disorder of hair loss. The causes of anagen effluvium are mentioned in the **Table 13.2.**

The insult affects the rapidly dividing cells of the matrix and cortex, changing the rate of hair growth, but does not convert the follicle to a different growth phase, as occurs in telogen effluvium.

The clinical features of anagen effluvium depend on the degree of toxicity created by the causative agent. High concentrations of antimetabolites or radiation bring the

TABLE 13.2: Causes of anagen effluvium

Cancer chemotherapeutic agents
Folic acid antagonists (aminopterin, amethopterin)
Purine antagonists (6-mercaptopurine)
Alkylating agents (cyclophosphamide, nitrogen mustard)
Natural alkaloids (vincristine)
Poisoning
Lead
Thallium (rat poison)
Arsenic
Bismuth
Coumadin
Scalp radiation therapy

entire metabolic process to an abrupt halt and the entire hair and hair roots are shed intact. Less intensity insults slow down the mitotic rate of the bulb and cortex cells, causing bulb deformity and narrowing of the lower hair shaft. Narrow, weakened hair shafts are easily broken and shed without bulbs. Since an average of 85% of scalp hairs are in anagen phase at a given time, severe toxicity may result in profound hair loss, leaving behind only the telogen hairs on the scalp.

There is no effective treatment for anagen effluvium except removal of the precipitating cause. Cessation of the responsible drug generally results in regrowth of hair. However, there are remedies to prevent this disorder in some situations like use of a specially designed scalp tourniquet placed around the head just above the ears and inflated to 10 mm of Hg above systolic pressure immediately before intravenous vincristine. This technique helps to minimize the toxic effects of vincristine on the hair follicles of the scalp.

Comparison between telogen effluvium and anagen effluvium is given in **Table 13.3.**

ALOPECIA AREATA

Alopecia areata (AA) is a common asymptomatic hair disorder characterized by the sudden appearance of sharply defined round or oval patches of hair loss. Incidence of this disease is 17.2 per 100000 population, affecting 1:1000 individuals at any one time. There is a history of familial occurrence in 10 to 20 % of affected individuals. It affects all age groups and the first attack usually appears in patients younger than 25 years of age.

Etiopathogenesis

The exact etiology of AA remains unknown, but various causes have been proposed. It is generally believed to be an autoimmune disease. CD4+ T-lymphocytes mediate the perifollicular immune attack against the antigen which may be present in the follicular keratinocyte, melanocyte or dermal papilla, by triggering a cascade of events via cytokine production. Cytokines such as INF γ, IL 2 and IL 1β have been found in the affected areas of the scalp. Calcitonin gene related peptide, which has potent anti-inflammatory actions and substance P, which is capable of inducing hair growth, are found to be decreased in the scalp of AA patients.

AA is associated with classic autoimmune disorders like thyroid diseases especially Hashimoto's thyroiditis, vitiligo, pernicious anemia, Addison's disease, diabetes mellitus, lupus erythematosus, rheumatoid arthritis and myasthenia gravis. An increased incidence has also been noted in patients with Down's syndrome and atopy.

A recent study concludes that there is little evidence that emotional stress plays a significant role in the pathogenesis of this hair disorder. AA appears to progress as a wave of follicles prematurely entering telogen. The event weakens or narrows the hair shaft, which continues to grow before the telogen phase is complete. Most weakened hairs fracture when they reach the surface. The affected hairs that are found at the periphery of the lesions have a normal upper shaft and a narrowed base – "exclamation point" hair.

TABLE 13.3: Comparison between telogen effluvium and anagen effluvium

Clinical features	Telogen effluvium	Anagen effluvium
i) Time interval between insult and onset of hair loss	2 to 4 months	1 to 4 weeks
ii) Severity of hair loss	Less severe (20-50% hair loss)	More severe (80-90% hair loss)
iii) Type of hair shed	Normal club hair (nonpigmented white bulb)	Anagen hair (pigmented bulb)
iv) Hair shaft	Normal	Narrowed or fractured
v) Conversion of the follicular growth phase	Occurs	Does not occur
vi) Change in rate of hair growth	Does not occur	Occurs

Clinical Features

AA typically presents with sudden appearance of one or more round or oval well defined patches of hair loss. The hair loss may occur overnight or over a period of several days. In some children, the initial patch may not be well defined and may show scattered long hairs within the bald area. Occasionally, the initial loss may be diffuse and the patches of baldness may be apparent only after 1 or 2 weeks **(Figures 13.4A and B)**. The primary patch is usually seen on scalp. Rarely, eyebrows, beard and other parts of the body may be involved. Skin over the bald patch is smooth, soft and almost totally devoid of hair. Occasionally slight erythema and edema may be found in early stage. At the margins of patches of alopecia, the pathognomonic "exclamation- mark" hairs may be detected. These loose hairs, with attenuated bulbs and short stumps are easily plucked out of the scalp, and when examined under a low power microscope reveals an irregularity in diameter and a poorly pigmented hair shaft that tapers to an attenuated bulb. The telogen bulb represents the dot of the exclamation point. Hair regrowth in alopecia areata may occur as depigmented hairs which may repigment with time or may remain white.

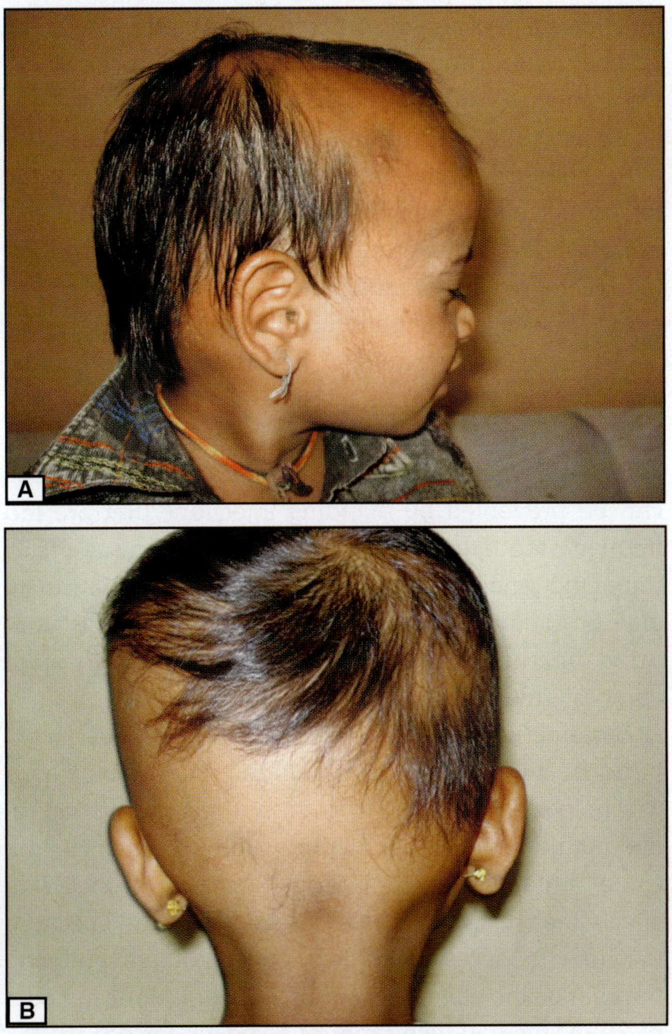

FIGURES 13.4A AND B: Alopecia areata

An unusual clinical form of alopecia known as *ophiasis* can occur, particularly in children. Here, a bald patch develops initially over the occiput and later extends anteriorly and bilaterally as a 1-2 inch wide band above the ears, sometimes extending to meet on the anterior aspect of scalp. Ophiasis generally has a poor prognosis.

Some cases of partial alopecia (around 5-10% cases) can progress slowly to involve the entire scalp with total loss of all scalp hair. This is referred to as *alopecia totalis.* Progression to the totalis form occurs more slowly, but more frequently in children than in adults. Very rarely, about 1% of cases develop *alopecia universalis*, with complete or virtually complete loss of all body hair including eyebrows and eyelashes.

Nail involvement is seen in about 10-20% cases. The most characteristic nail abnormality is a fine grid-like stippling, regularly arranged in horizontal or vertical rows or both, with pits smaller and shallower than those seen in patients with psoriasis. Onychomadesis, longitudinal ridging, opacification, serration of the free edges and severe dystrophy may be seen in patients with alopecia totalis and universalis. Although, the possibility and severity of nail involvement is more likely in severe cases of AA, some patients may have gross nail dystrophy with little hair change.

Diagnosis and Differential Diagnosis

The diagnosis of AA is made based on its clinical presentation. Sudden appearance of circumscribed nonscarring patterned nature of hair loss is the typical presentation of AA. Clinically, the differential diagnosis includes tinea capitis, trichotillomania, telogen effluvium, androgenetic alopecia and secondary syphilis. Absence of signs of inflammation, scaling and lymphadenopathy help in distinguishing AA from tinea capitis. In trichotillomania, bizarre, irregular patches of hair loss, with areas of twisted and broken hairs of different lengths are seen. Alopecia in secondary syphilis is recognized by its moth-eaten appearance, irregular borders, incomplete hair loss within individual patches and a predilection for the posterior scalp. Patients with androgenetic alopecia usually demonstrate typical pattern of balding with bitemporal recession of the frontal hair line followed by thinning over the vertex and shedding is not very prominent. When the diagnosis is in doubt, microscopic examination of hairs with potassium hydroxide, fungal cultures, serologic testing and cutaneous punch biopsy will help to establish the proper diagnosis.

In newly formed patches of AA, hair pull test will show an increased number of telogen hairs and dystrophic anagen hairs. At a later stage, most hairs will be in anagen phase. Histopathologic examination of the affected area in AA shows a characteristic feature consisting of peribulbar lymphocytic infiltrate which is described as "swarm of bees". Other features include a reduction in anagen-telogen ratio, miniaturized dystrophic hairs, fibrous tracts, pigment incontinence and the presence of eosinophils.

Course and Prognosis

The course of AA is variable and difficult to predict. There may be extension of the bald patches over a few weeks and new patches may appear within 4 to 6 weeks. Occasionally, spontaneous regrowth may occur after 4-10 months. So the natural history of AA includes frequent spontaneous remissions and recurrences.

When the process is limited to a few patches, the prognosis is good, with complete regrowth occurring within one year in 95% of children. It is estimated that 7-10% of patients can eventually develop the severe chronic form of the condition. When the disorder is extensive or total, the possibility of complete and permanent recovery is poor, and about 30% of patients will have future episodes of AA. Indicators of poor prognosis are atopy, presence of other autoimmune diseases, family history of AA, an early age of onset, extensive hair loss, ophiasis and nail dystrophy.

Management

The treatment available for AA at present can only control the problem and do not cure the condition **(Table 13.4)**. Local treatment may help the treated areas but do not prevent further spread of the condition. Any mode of treatment should be used for long periods because of the chronic nature of AA. Any therapy should be tried for a minimum period of 3-6 months before considering it to have failed because of the long period before regrowth.

TABLE 13.4: Treatment of alopecia areata

1. Corticosteroids
   a. Topical
   b. Intralesional
   c. Systemic
2. Immunotherapy
3. Anthralin
4. Minoxidil
5. Photochemotherapy (PUVA)

The first and most important step in the management of AA is to give psychological support, and counseling. A hairstyle change, caps, hats, head bands and wigs may be required for adequate camouflage. As a high percentage of AA will spontaneously remit in one year, prescribing no medical therapy is a valid way to manage classic AA in some children.

Topical ***corticosteroid*** therapy is used frequently in children with AA. Immunosuppression is the main mechanism of action of corticosteroids. Moderate to high potency steroids applied twice daily to the patch of AA will sometimes show response in 1-2 months.

Intralesional corticosteroids are appropriate only for older children (above 6 years) because of pain at the injection sites. Triamcinolone acetonide 2.5-10 mg/ml is administered intradermally with a 30 gauge needle, 0.1-0.3 ml per site at multiple sites, approximately 1 cm apart. Weaker concentration of 2.5 mg/ml is used for the beard area and eyebrows. A maximum of 3 ml can be used on the scalp in one visit and the injections are repeated at an interval of 4-6 weeks. Side effects include transient atrophy, telangiectasia and folliculitis. Atrophy can be prevented by avoiding injections that are too frequent, too large in volume per site, or too superficial (intraepidermal). If there is no response to treatment even after 6 months, intralesional steroids should be discontinued because these patients may lack adequate corticosteroid receptors in the scalp.

Systemic steroids may be considered only for selected patients with severe involvement or an associated psychological handicap who do not respond to topical and intralesional steroid therapy. Although effective, the use of systemic steroids is limited because of their side effects, their relapse rate after dose reduction, and because they may be necessary for long periods of time and may not change the ultimate prognosis. Prednisolone in doses of 20-40 mg/day with taper of 5 mg/wk for 4-6 weeks, followed by alternate day therapy may be administered with relatively few significant side effects.

Anthralin, in the concentrations of 0.25% to1% cream is used in the treatment of AA as it may have a nonspecific immunomodulating effect eliciting hair regrowth. It can be applied overnight or as short contact therapy, initially for 30 minutes and gradually to one hour. Cosmetically acceptable hair regrowth has been reported to occur in 25% of patients. A mild dermatitis is desired for therapeutic effect. Response is seen with in 3-6 months. It can be applied simultaneously with twice daily topical steroid therapy. Scalp irritation and staining of skin and clothes are the drawbacks to its use.

Minoxidil is a biologic response modifier that enhances hair growth. Its mechanism of action in AA is unknown, but it is known to stimulate follicular DNA synthesis, has a direct effect on the proliferation and differentiation of follicular keratinocytes *in vitro* and regulates hair physiology independently of blood flow. Topical minoxidil is applied twice daily to the affected area. Response is usually seen in 2 months. 20-45% cases have shown good response to this treatment. More successful results are seen in less severe cases and this treatment is not suitable for alopecia totalis/ universalis. Efficacy of minoxidil solution can be enhanced with anthralin or topical corticosteroid. Anthralin is applied 2 hours after second minoxidil application. Topical steroid cream is applied twice daily 30 minutes after each use of minoxidil. Side effects of minoxidil include local irritation, allergic contact dermatitis and facial hair growth. These are rare in occurrence. Systemic absorption is minimal.

Topical ***immunotherapy*** is an accepted therapeutic modality in the treatment of chronic severe AA. The principle of this treatment is to create antigenic competition with putative hair follicle antigens by provoking contact eczema on the scalp. This theory presumes that the generation of T- suppressor cells into the area may exert a nonspecific inhibitory effect on the autoimmune reaction to the hair-associated antigen and thus allow hair to regrow. The first step is sensitization by means of a patch test and then application of increasing concentration of the allergen after 2 weeks. The aim is to maintain a low-grade tolerable erythema, scaling and pruritus without causing too much discomfort for the patient.

The contact sensitizers that have been used in AA are dinitrochlorobenzene (DNCB), squaric acid dibutyl ester (SADBE) and diphenylcyclopropenone (DPCP). DNCB was the first agent used but was found to be mutagenic and is not frequently used. SADBE is found to be effective in 29-87% of patients with AA. It can be effective for relapses too. First, sensitization is achieved with 2% SADBE in acetone applied to a small area on scalp, later starting with low concentration (0.0001 to 0.001%) the applications are performed once a week. Doses are increased every month according to individual tolerance. Side effects include local lymphadenopathy, vesiculation, staining of skin and clothing, and skin dryness. DPCP has been effective in 48%-85% of cases. Sensitization is first achieved with 2% DPCP solution in acetone, later starting with low concentration, 0.001% solution is applied to scalp and left for 48 hours before being washed off. Application is repeated every week, increasing the concentration every month up to 1% according to individual tolerance. Response is usually seen in 12-24 weeks. Patient should be advised to protect the scalp from light because DPCP is degraded when exposed to light. Side effects include eczematous reactions, extension of contact dermatitis to other body areas, itching, edema of the scalp/face, cervical and post auricular lymphadenopathy, post inflammatory hyper- or hypopigmentation.

PUVA has also been effective in treating AA. Response rate varies from 20-53%. The mechanism of action of PUVA on AA is believed to be a photoimmunologic action. It may affect T-cell function and antigen presentation, and possibly inhibit local immunologic attack against the hair follicle by depleting langerhans cells. The psoralens are administered either topically or orally and followed 2 hours later by UVA exposure. Treatment is administered 2-3 times a week with gradual increase in UVA dosage. Though a good response is seen with PUVA treatment, there is a high relapse rate after PUVA is tapered and it is not recommended for use in young (less than 10 years of age) children.

ANDROGENETIC ALOPECIA

Androgenetic alopecia (AGA) or male-pattern baldness is an androgenetically induced disorder which appears to be inherited as an autosomal dominant trait with variable expression. It occurs both in men and women. The onset of this disorder can be as early as 14 years of age, the earlier the onset, the more profound the subsequent alopecia.

In males, the mildest form of AGA begins as a symmetrical triangular recession of the hairline in the frontoparietal and occasionally frontal scalp margins. Uniform recession of the frontal hairline is seen during adolescence in 96% of males and in about 80% of females. It is generally not until the 3rd or 4th decade that the incidence of this pattern increases and in association with some loss of hair in the crown of the scalp. In females, AGA is generally less severe than seen in males. The frontal hairline is relatively unaffected with only slight recession. The process may become apparent at any time after puberty (during the 2nd or 4th decade); progress is slow and male type baldness is rare. Although genetic susceptibility and androgenetic stimulation are essential factors in the pathogenesis of female AGA, females may be endocrinologically normal or may have abnormal androgen metabolism. Hence, in females with severe forms of AGA, especially if there is evidence of hirsutism, acne, menstrual disturbance, or other evidence of virilization, evaluation for possible elevation of dehydroepiandrosterone sulfate, free plasma testosterone, and testosterone-binding globulin levels is recommended.

Topical minoxidil solution (2% or 5%) application is the currently recommended treatment. The response rate for cosmetically acceptable hair with this treatment appears to be 15 to 25%. With good response, the treatment has to be continued throughout the patient's lifetime. If the balding history is of less than 5 years duration and the area of baldness on vertex measures less than 10 cms in diameter, a good response to the treatment has been observed. Other treatment modalities like hair transplantation, implantation of nylon filaments may be considered if no response is seen with medical line of treatment for duration of 6 months to 1 year. In females, if endocrinologic abnormality is present, hormone therapy with dexamethasone and spironolactone is indicated.

TRAUMATIC ALOPECIA

Traumatic alopecia is a type of alopecia resulting from forceful extraction of hair or breaking of hair shafts by friction, traction or other physical trauma. The various causes for traumatic alopecia include:

- Cosmetic practices such as tight braiding or ponytail, use of tight rollers, barrettes or head bands, hair straightening practices, frequent brushing with nylon bristles or use of hot combs.
- Trichotillomania.
- Due to pressure as seen on occiput of infants who lie on their back or are in the habit of "head-banging."
- Pressure on a particular area of scalp due to prolonged bed rest in one position as seen in chronically ill patients.
- Postoperative alopecia as a result of pressure induced ischemia during long surgical procedures.
- Thermal or electric burns.
- Repeated vigorous massage.
- Severe blow to the scalp
- Occipito-parietal alopecia may be induced by spinning on the crown of the head during "break-dancing".
- Prolonged use of wide-strapped heavy head phones.

Traction Alopecia

Traction alopecia occurs as a result of a constant pulling tension on the hair follicles causing damage, fracture of hair shafts with possible loss of hair follicles, and subsequent alopecia. Unlike trichotillomania, it is unintentionally induced hair loss secondary to grooming styles and techniques such as tight braiding, wearing of tight ponytails commonly in female athletes or using hot combs to straighten hair.

Clinically, patients present with patchy (oval or linear) hair loss with scaling and perifollicular erythema, at the margins of the hairline, along the part, or scattered through the scalp, depending on the type of traction or trauma. Performing the 'hair pull test' results in extraction of more than 6 telogen hairs.

Treatment involves preventing the cause and changing the styling techniques. In the early stages, hair loss is reversible by discontinuing any practices that exert traction on the hair, but failure to do so can result in permanent alopecia and other hair-growth promoters may be needed in such end-stage disease.

Trichotillomania

Trichotillomania is a self-inflected form of alopecia caused by a person's compulsion or tic to pull or twist hairs leading to fracture of hair shafts, extraction of hairs or localized forms of telogen effluvium. It is more commonly found in children than adults. The mean age of onset is 8 years in boys and 12 years in girls, and it is the most common cause of childhood alopecia. The most common site of involvement is scalp, although the eyebrows and eyelashes may also be affected.

The child usually practices plucking, twirling or rubbing the hair bearing areas in bed before falling asleep or while watching television or reading or writing. This condition is frequently associated with thumb or finger sucking.

Trichotillomania is a psychiatric impulse-control disorder seen in patients with severe psychological problems or in individuals who are merely under varying degrees of emotional stress or have developed a habit that can be managed by a sympathetic physician and understanding parent.

The hair loss usually begins insidiously and often follows a bizarre pattern with areas of partial clearing but never complete loss **(Figure 13.5)**. The affected area is usually single and located on the frontal or frontoparietal or frontotemporal region of the scalp, frequently on the contralateral side of the right or left-handed individual. Hair in the involved area is short or stubbly and of varying lengths. The scalp may appear normal or have areas of erythema and pustule formation. Patients also may eat the plucked hairs (trichophagy), causing intestinal complications such as bowel obstruction.

The diagnosis is made by careful assessment, characteristic configuration and distribution of hair loss and by exclusion of other causes like traction alopecia, tinea and alopecia areata. A further clue to the diagnosis of trichotillomania is eyelash or eyebrow involvement. Occasionally wads of hair may be seen under the pillow or bed and the habit might be observed by the parents or teacher or the physician which confirms the diagnosis. Regrowth of hair in a carefully shaved or occluded patch of scalp in the involved area will also confirm the diagnosis. If the diagnosis still remains in doubt, scalp biopsy from the affected area will be helpful. Histopathologic features consist of normal follicular unit architecture, melanin casts and trichomalacia, about 20% to 30% of catagen and telogen follicles, presence of keratin plugs and dilated follicular infundibula, excoriation with variable necrosis and spongiosis in overlying epidermis associated with superficial dermal inflammation, replacement of hair follicles by fibrosis, absence of significant inflammation or scarring, and disruption of follicle with adjacent microhemmorhage (rare).

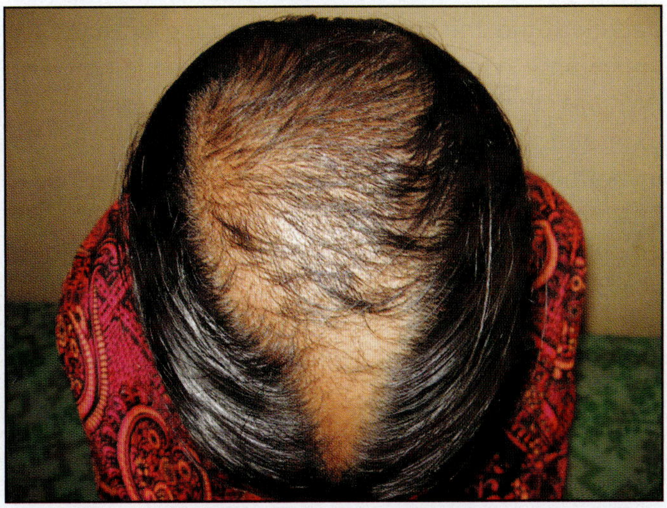

FIGURE 13.5: Trichotillomania

Since these patients often have psychological problems, treatment is difficult and requires a strong doctor, patient, and parent relationship. The mainstays of treatment are counseling, behavior modification techniques and hypnosis. Patients should be reassured and given an opportunity to express their emotional needs. Sometimes mild shampoo and scalp lotion (Hydrocortisone in 1% concentration as a placebo or to 'relieve pruritus or possible irritation') may be helpful to the patient. In cases of persistent or severe obsessive-compulsive or emotional problems, anti-depressants such as clomipramine or fluoxetine should be considered.

LOOSE ANAGEN HAIR

Loose anagen hairs occur sporadically on normal scalps, as a part of the loose anagen hair syndrome (with no associated abnormalities), or in association with a syndrome with other developmental defects (e.g. Noonan's syndrome, nail-patella syndrome, ectodermal dysplasia)

Loose anagen syndrome (short anagen syndrome) is predominantly a disease of childhood showing autosomal dominant inheritance with variable expression and incomplete penetrance, characterized by actively growing anagen hairs on the scalp that can be pulled out easily and painlessly. This disease can be sporadic or familial. The condition is due to defective anchoring of the hair shaft to the follicle, which enables the anagen hairs to be separated from the inner root sheath and released from the follicle with minimal traction.

Loose anagen hair syndrome typically is diagnosed in childhood, usually in children younger than 2 years of age, with the mean age of patients being 6 years. Adult cases have occasionally been described, mostly in parents of affected children. The hair grows only up to a short length, seldom requires haircuts, may be sparse but covers the scalp adequately, leading to complaints that "they do not grow".

The diagnosis of loose anagen hair syndrome is based on the microscopic evaluation of the hair, which shows heavily pigmented misshapen bulb and a ruffled cuticle on the proximal portion of the hair. A scalp biopsy, which is unnecessary for diagnosis, may show premature and abnormal keratinization of the inner root sheath, with clefts between the inner and outer sheath and the hair shaft.

Although there is no treatment for this disorder, the hair loss may improve with age and gentle handling decreases shedding.

HAIR SHAFT DISORDERS

Hair shaft disorders or abnormalities can be congenital or acquired. Congenital hair shaft disorders usually manifest at birth or within first few months of life. The abnormalities are usually limited to scalp, but may involve other terminal hair and rarely body hair. Acquired hair shaft disorders are most commonly caused by mechanical, physical or chemical traumas.

Hair shaft disorders may be classified into two main groups:

i. Hair shaft disorders causing increased fragility and therefore hair breakage with patchy or diffuse alopecia.
ii. Hair shaft disorders without hair fragility, which may interfere with hair texture and luster, rather than resulting in alopecia.

HAIR SHAFT ABNORMALITIES WITH INCREASED FRAGILITY

Defect in the structure of hair with increased fragility results in easy breakage of the hair shaft. Hair shaft abnormalities occur commonly and sometimes may be associated with other pathologic abnormalities. All hair shaft abnormalities, except monilethrix, pili annulati and pili bifurcati, may be seen sporadically even in normal hair and hair shaft abnormalities should be considered significant only if found consistently in samples from different sites. Distinctive morphology of each hair shaft defect helps in easily diagnosing the condition by microscopic examination of the hair. Hairs for the microscopic examination should be preferably snipped rather than pulled.

Monilethrix

Monilethrix (necklace hair) is an autosomal dominantly transmitted trait with variable expressivity and high penetrance, affecting both sexes equally. Mutation in the hair keratin type I controlling genes on chromosome 12q, resulting in defective cortical keratinization, is the probable mechanism for hair constrictions and breakage seen in this disorder. It is characterized by variation in hair shaft thickness, with small node like deformities that produce a beaded appearance, internodal fragility, breakage and partial alopecia.

At birth, normal lanugo hairs may be seen, which are shed in few weeks and the subsequent hair growth, generally at about second month of life, becomes dry, lusterless and brittle failing to grow to any appreciable length. Some of the broken hair stubs project from keratotic follicular papules. In severe cases, the infant may appear bald. Body hairs may also be affected in some cases. Sometimes, the disorder may not be evident in infancy and become evident later in childhood or adult life. Monilethrix may be associated with trichorrhexis nodosa, keratosis pilaris, syndactyly, brittle nails, cataracts, dental abnormalities or physical retardation.

There is no definite treatment for this condition, although avoidance of mechanical and chemical trauma may be helpful. Spontaneous remission may be seen at puberty or pregnancy, or the disease may persist unchanged throughout adulthood.

Pseudomoniletrix

Pseudomoniletrix is an autosomal dominant disorder. Unlike monilethrix, this disorder manifests only at a later age (8 years or older). The hair shaft shows irregular flattened and thickened areas that give an indented appearance. Here follicular hyperkeratosis is not seen. At times, there may be twisting along the longitudinal axis and distal fractures similar to those seen in trichorrhexis nodosa. Mechanical trauma due to combing, brushing and massaging can result in breakage of hairs. Treatment of this condition includes reassurance and avoidance of mechanical trauma.

Trichorrhexis Nodosa

Trichorrhexis nodosa (TN) is the commonest hair shaft anomaly leading to hair breakage. It is manifested by increased hair fragility due to the presence of grayish white nodules along the shaft where the cuticle is lost, which under a light microscope, gives the appearance of two interlocking paint brushes or brooms due to segmental longitudinal splitting of fibers without complete fracture, and eventual separation and fraying of the exposed cortical fibers.

TN is characterized by dry lusterless short hair that is easily fractured and leaves short stubbly broken ends and areas of partial alopecia. It mainly affects the scalp hair. Uncommonly, it may affect the beard, moustache, eyebrows, eyelashes, axillary or pubic region.

TN may be congenital or acquired.

Congenital: Congenital TN may be present at birth or may appear within the first few months of life. Although it may occur as an isolated defect or rarely with follicular hyperkeratosis or, teeth or nail abnormality, the occurrence of congenital TN should lead to a search for an underlying metabolic disorder like arginosuccinic aciduria, citrullinemia, Menkes' syndrome or trichothiodystrophy.

Acquired: Acquired TN is seen in two clinical varieties, proximal TN (commonly seen in Blacks) and distal TN (commonly seen in Whites and Asians). Proximal TN appears to be associated with a genetic predisposition and trauma from hot-comb hair straightening, tight caps, harsh brushing or combing techniques. Distal TN occurs in otherwise normal hair as a result of cumulative cuticular damage due to vigorous brushing and combing, repeated salt water bathing, prolonged sun exposure, dyeing and frequent shampooing.

Treatment of TN, congenital or acquired, is by avoidance of physical, chemical and thermal trauma to the hair. Cream rinses with protein conditioners may be helpful. With the avoidance of trauma, the acquired forms of TN generally improve within 2 to 4 years.

Trichorrhexis Invaginata

Trichorrhexis invaginata (Bamboo hair) is a distinctive hair shaft abnormality characterizes by multiple nodules caused by abnormal intussusception or telescope-like invagination along the hair shaft, which under a light microscope resemble the "ball and cup" joints of bamboo.

The primary defect appears to be abnormal keratinization of the hair shaft at the keratogenous zone resulting from incomplete conversion of sulfhydril groups into disulphide bonds in cortical fibers. This leads to softening of the hair cortex and allows intussusception of the fully keratinized and hard distal shaft into the incompletely keratinized and soft proximal shaft.

This disorder may occur sporadically, either in normal hair or other hair shaft abnormalities, or regularly as a marker of Netherton's syndrome which is an autosomal recessive genodermatosis consisting of a triad of trichorrhexis invaginata, ichthyosis and atopic diathesis. Trichorrhexis invaginata is more common in females than in males and may involve all body hairs. Beginning in infancy, this disorder is clinically characterized by dry, lusterless, easily fractured, sparse and short hair.

There is no specific therapy for this hair abnormality. Although spontaneous remission of the hair defect can occur between 6 and 15 years of age, many cases will persist into adulthood.

Pili Torti

Pili torti (twisted hair) is an autosomal dominant congenital hair shaft abnormality of variable expression characterized by dry, fragile, twisted hairs.

Pili torti is more common among females than males. At birth, the affected child will have normal hair. Later during infancy or by 2 or 3 years of age, it is replaced by brittle hair, ultimately leading to patchy alopecia with coarse stubble or longer broken hair or diffuse hair loss. In this disorder, the hair shaft is flattened and twisted at angles of about 180 degrees with 4 to 5 twists at irregular intervals. The affected hairs are unable to resist stretching forces and break at the twists. The hair shimmers in reflected light with a "spangled" (glittering piece of metal) appearance owing to the twisted feature of this disorder.

Pili torti can be seen in normal individuals and also in association with

- Hypohidrotic ectodermal dysplasia
- Keratosis pilaris
- Ichthyosis
- Nail dystrophy
- Widely spaced teeth
- Enamel hypoplasia
- Corneal opacities
- Congenital sensorineural deafness
- Citrullinemia
- Arginine deficiency
- Bjornstad's syndrome
- Basex syndrome
- Crandall's syndrome

- Pseudomonilethrix
- Menkes' syndrome

The hair abnormality may improve with time and the cosmetic appearance may be normal by puberty, although twisted hairs can still be found in the adult scalp. Those who do not show any improvement by puberty are unlikely to improve with age. Other than reduction of trauma to reduce breakage, there is no effective treatment for this disorder.

Pili Bifurcati

Pili bifurcati is an uncommon disorder of hair growth, characterized by intermittent longitudinal splitting of the hair shaft along its length. The affected hairs divide into two separate shafts with their own cuticle and again become rejoined along the hair shaft. This bifurcation is repeated at regular intervals. This hair shaft defect appears to be transitory, with only a small percentage of hair exhibiting the bifurcation.

Menkes' Kinky Hair Syndrome

Menkes' kinky hair syndrome (Trichopoliodystrophy) is a rare, X-linked recessive neurodegenerative disorder that affects male infants and is characterized by coarse expressionless facies, pili torti, temperature instability, seizures, psychomotor retardation, arterial intimal changes, low or absent plasma copper and ceruloplasmin levels, growth failure, increased susceptibility to infection and death, generally by the age of 3 or 4 years.

In this disorder, there is defective copper metabolism resulting in the alteration of keratinization as well as pigmentation of hair, as copper is required in the formation of both melanin and cystine. The defective gene which maps to X $_{q}$13.3, encodes a copper translocating membrane protein ATPase that prevents effective copper transport and leads to accumulation of intracellular copper in some tissues. The excess intracellular copper triggers the synthesis of metallothionein, whose normal function is to chelate copper to prevent cellular toxicity. This further deprives the copper requiring enzyme needed for the normal function.

Clinical features often include premature birth, hypothermia and relatively normal development until 2 to 6 months of age, when drowsiness and lethargy are noted, intractable seizures begin, and growth and development cease. The hair is normal at birth, but after the shedding of first hair in infancy, the new hair that grow is silver or white colored, twisted and fragile, sparse; it stands on end, looks and feels like steel wool. Pili torti is generally a prominent feature of this disorder, sometimes monilethrix and trichorrhexis nodosa may also be seen. Additional features include tortuous cerebral and other medium-sized arteries; osteoporosis; frequent subdural hematomas; widening of the metaphyses, with spurring; and frequent fractures, at times simulating the radiologic findings characteristic of patients with the battered child syndrome.

The combination of clinical features, bone abnormality, and low plasma copper and ceruloplasmin levels establishes the correct diagnosis in these patients. Parenteral copper and ceruloplasmin therapy has not been very effective in the treatment of this disorder but copper – histidine given immediately within the first month of life may prevent or ameliorate the severe neuro-degeneration.

Trichothiodystrophy

Trichothiodystrophy (TTD) is a rare autosomal recessive disorder characterized by sulfur – deficient, sparse, short, dry, brittle, unruly, transversely broken hairs (trichoschisis) **(Figure 13.6)**, variable degrees of alopecia, physical and mental retardation, and a wide spectrum of other developmental defects.

The hairs break with a clean transverse fracture through the entire hair shaft at a location where there is a focal absence of cuticle. This breakage is due to a reduction in the sulfur and cystine content of the hair, which is necessary for the normal tensile strength. Along with scalp

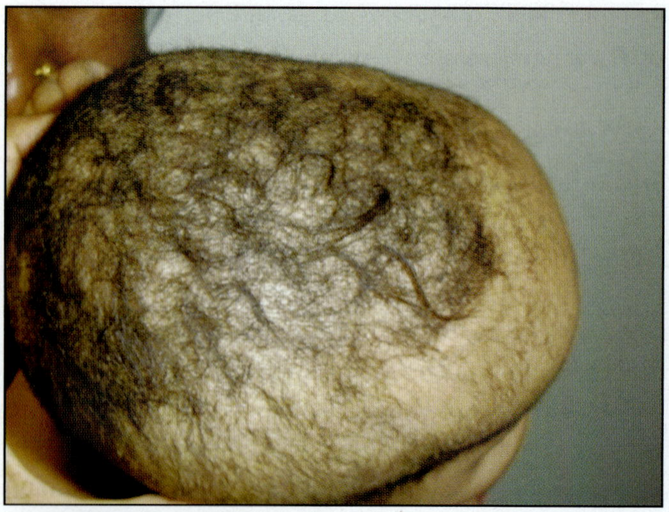

FIGURE 13.6: Sparse, brittle hair in trichothiodystrophy.

hairs, eyebrows and eyelashes can also be affected. Brittle nails are often associated. Examination of the affected hairs under polarizing microscopy shows a typical tiger tail appearance with alternating dark and light bands, presumably secondary to variations in sulfur content.

TTD is associated with various syndromes like

i. BIDS syndrome, a disorder characterized by brittle hair, impaired intelligence, decreased fertility and short stature.
ii. IBIDS or Tay syndrome, a similar disorder with additional ichthyosis.
iii. PIBIDS syndrome, with additional photosensitivity.
iv. Marinesco Sjogren syndrome, characterized by cerebellar ataxia; dysarthria; cataracts; physical and mental retardation; abnormal teeth; flat, thin and fragile nails; fine, light, brittle and unruly hair.

Patients with TTD, particularly the 50% with associated photosensitivity, may have a defect in DNA excision repair of UV damage but without an increased risk of skin cancer.

Trichoschisis is not diagnostic of TTD; the diagnosis needs to be established by polarizing microscopy and cystine and sulfur analysis of hair which reveals a 50% decrease in cystine and sulfur content. No treatment is currently available for this disorder. Although, avoidance of cosmetic trauma and the use of hair conditioners are sometimes helpful. Its course and prognosis depends on other physical features of its variants.

HAIR SHAFT ABNORMALITIES WITHOUT INCREASED HAIR FRAGILITY

Fragilitas Crinium

Fragilitas crinium (trichoptilosis, split hair) is a common condition occurring particularly in girls and women who subject their hair to various chemical and mechanical trauma resulting in a longitudinal split of the hair shaft towards the tip (split ends). Central trichoptilosis can also occur. The bifurcated hair shaft is not surrounded by cuticle. Other effects of trauma like trichorrhexis nodosa and weathering may coexist.

Treatment of this disorder consists of gentle grooming techniques and application of oils or cream rinses.

Pili Annulati

Pili annulati (ringed hair) is a rare autosomal dominant disorder with variable expression, characterized by alternating light and dark bands of hair both clinically and under light microscopy. The banding is secondary to air filled spaces in the cortex of hair shaft (due to defect in keratin synthesis) which appear lighter by reflected light and darker by transmitted light. This disorder manifests shortly after birth and has equal sex distribution. The hair shaft is structurally strong and bright rings tend to produce an attractive shiny spangled appearance.

Pseudopili annulati is an unusual variant of normal hair with similar banded appearance seen under light microscopy but it is non hereditary and is not associated with any hair shaft cortex abnormality. The reason for banding in this condition is periodic flattening and slight twisting of the hair shaft that causes light to be reflected as bright bands.

Both conditions appear more evidently on blond hair and are not associated with hair breakage. With transverse illumination, the banding in pili annulati is seen in whatever way light strikes the hair, but pseudopili annulati is seen only when hair is rotated into certain positions. Both the conditions are generally an attractive phenomenon with no associated defects and do not require therapy.

Woolly Hair

Woolly hair is unruly scalp hair that curls readily in spirals but does not form locks or lie down flat on the scalp and is difficult to comb or brush **(Figure 13.7)**. The hair shows a slow twist on its long axis. Hair shafts are usually ovoid in cross section and shaft diameter may at times be reduced.

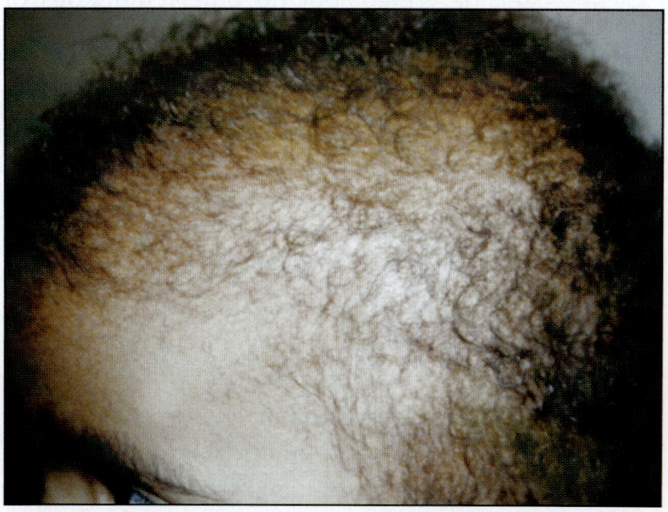

FIGURE 13.7: Wooly hair

Three types of woolly hair can be distinguished according to clinical features and inheritance:

a. Hereditary woolly hair: It is an autosomal dominant hair disorder, not associated with hair fragility. The scalp hairs are fine, dry, light colored and corrugated at intervals resembling the crimp found in the wool of the sheep. It is present at birth and improves with age. It may be associated with palmoplantar keratoderma and cardiac abnormalities.
b. Familial woolly hair: It is autosomal recessively inherited and is associated with hair thinning. The hair is sparse, thin and short. The hairs are short probably due to a shortened growth cycle rather than due to an increased fragility. Severe alopecia is common. It may be associated with congenital ichthyosis and follicular atrophoderma.
c. Woolly hair nevus: It is a rare condition usually present at birth without familial correlation. It occurs on scalp as one or more patches of unruly hair that are different in color, shape and consistency from the normal surrounding scalp hair. The hairs on the affected area are smaller in diameter, lighter in color and appear sparse than those on rest of the scalp. The majority of reported cases of woolly hair nevus have been recognized during the first few months of life but some have appeared in young adulthood. The cause for this disorder is unknown and there is no known treatment. In about 50% of cases, woolly hair nevus is associated with linear epidermal nevus in the same area or on the neck or arm. Ocular involvement has been described as an associated feature, and a persistent papillary membrane has been described, but no other cutaneous or systemic disorders have been associated with this condition.

Uncombable Hair Syndrome

Uncombable hair syndrome (pili trianguli et canaliculi, spun glass hair syndrome) is an autosomal dominant disorder characterized by very pale, silvery, blond or straw colored hair that is dry, frizzy, and unruly, and does not lie flat on the scalp, thus making combing impossible but not unduly fragile.

Under light microscopy, the hair shows a longitudinal groove or ribbon like flattening. Scanning electron microscopy confirms a longitudinal groove and on cross section the hair appears triangular or kidney bean shaped with a groove, instead of the usual oval shape. At least 50% of the scalp hairs are affected. Eyebrows and eyelashes are unaffected. This disorder affects children aged between 3 and 12 years.

The defect is probably due to distorted papilla which in turn alters the shape of the inner root sheath and the hair. This condition may be associated with ectodermal dysplasia, juvenile cataract, retinal dystrophy, digit abnormality, dental abnormality, phalangoepiphyseal dysplasia or mental retardation.

Although there is no definitive treatment, the unruly characteristic of the hair generally resolves with age and biotin (0.3 mg, three times a day) has been reported to show some improvement in this disorder.

Acquired Progressive Kinking of the Hair

Acquired progressive kinking of the hair is a rare disorder of scalp hair, with onset in adolescence or young adulthood. It is common in males. It is characterized by rapid onset of extreme curliness of the hair (mainly on frontoparietal region of the scalp and vertex) resembling pubic hair; often in association with increased coarse texture, diminished luster and striking unruliness. The hair may become darker or remain unaltered in color. The hair growth rate may be decreased or unchanged. The exact etiology of this condition is not known. It has been suggested that androgenic hormonal changes at puberty may be associated with its pathogenesis. Retinoid (Isotretinoin or Etretinate) therapy may also lead to this condition.

Under light microscopy, the affected hairs show alterations in hair shaft diameter with partial twisting along its longitudinal axis resulting in a beaded appearance. Cross section reveals an elliptical or irregular configuration with partial twists and sporadic canalicular grooves that extend for variable lengths along the hair shaft.

There is no effective therapy for this disorder. Although the condition may persist for many years, spontaneous reversion to normal hair has been reported in some individuals.

Felted Hair Syndrome

Felted hair (bird's nest hair) is a rare condition characterized by sudden and severe tangling of scalp hair. Although its cause is unknown, this disorder appears to be associated with shampooing, chemical treatments and damaged hair. The best remedy for this disorder is cutting out the hair in affected areas. Separation of the tangled hairs, although long and laborious, can also be used as an alternative option for patients unwilling to cut out the hair in affected area and allow the hair to regrow normally.

SCARRING ALOPECIA

Scarring alopecia or cicatricial alopecia represents a group of disorders characterized by permanent and pathologic destruction of the hair follicle, as an end result of a wide number of inflammatory processes in and about the pilosebaceous units, leading to irreversible hair loss in the affected areas **(Figure 13.8)**. The hair follicle can be destroyed by a primary process aimed directly at the follicle (primary cicatricial alopecia) or due to a non follicular process in diseases that affect the dermis and secondarily cause follicular destruction (secondary cicatricial alopecia). Cicatricial alopecia occurs due to stem cell failure at the base of the follicles, which inhibits follicular recovery from the telogen phase. The scarring alopecias are differentiated from the non-scarring ones, by the absence of follicular openings, increased wrinkling and thin, shiny, dry, depressed skin covered with telangiectases. Towards the periphery of the hairless area, the hair may be twisted and standing on end due to the fibrotic process in the dermis. Another characteristic finding in active areas of cicatricial alopecia is the positive pull test with anagen bulbs on the hair mount. A biopsy is necessary to establish an accurate diagnosis. Scarring alopecias are considered true trichologic emergencies, as hair loss is irreversible once hair follicles are scarred. Prompt appropriate therapy is crucial.

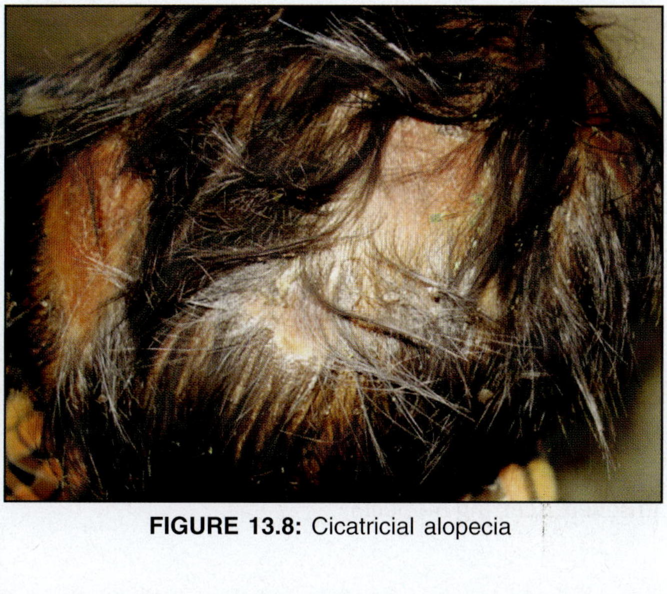

FIGURE 13.8: Cicatricial alopecia

The scarring may be the result of:

1. Developmental defects (aplasia cutis).
2. Inflammatory changes of infective origin such as severe bacterial, viral or fungal infection.
3. Physical trauma (irradiation, trichotillomania practiced over a long period of time, thermal or caustic burns).
4. Neoplastic disorders (primary and metastatic carcinoma).
5. Various dermatoses (lichen planus, lupus erythematosus, localized or systemic scleroderma).
6. Various dermatologic disorders (keratosis pilaris atrophicans, folliculitis decalvans, dissecting cellulitis of the scalp, acne keloidalis, pseudopelade, alopecia mucinosa).

Some of these conditions are discussed in Table 13.5.

TABLE 13.5: Etiology of cicatricial alopecia

Primary cicatricial alopecia (follicular disease)	Lichen plano pilaris Frontal fibrosing alopecia Fibrosing alopecia in a pattern distribution Discoid lupus erythematosus Keratosis follicularis spinulosa decalvans Folliculitis decalvans Traction alopecia
Secondary cicatricial alopecia (dermal fibrosis)	Localized scleroderma Radiation Pemphigoid Chemical or physical injuries Bacterial, viral, fungal infection

KERATOSIS PILARIS ATROPHICANS

This term is used for many dominantly inherited conditions characterized by inflammatory keratotic follicular papules that are followed by permanent follicular destruction and atrophy. These disorders occur sporadically and are presumed to be the result of inborn defects. The major histologic features include plugging and distention of hair follicles, dilatation of dermal vessels, perifollicular and perivascular lymphocytic infiltration, dermal atrophy and horn cysts. Three categories of keratosis pilaris atrophicans are generally accepted;

- The more localized entities of keratosis pilaris atrophicans faciei and atrophoderma vermiculatum
- The more generalized keratosis follicularis spinulosa decalvans of Siemens.

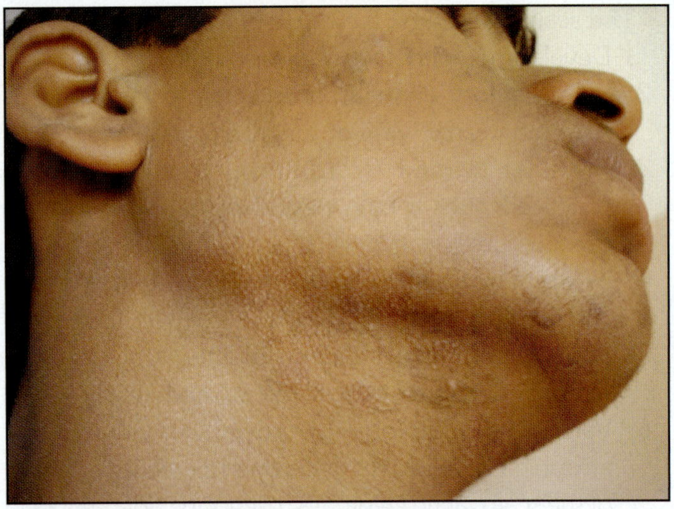

FIGURE 13.9: Keratosis pilaris atrophicans faciei (Ulerythema ophryogenes)

Keratosis Pilaris Atrophicans Faciei (Ulerythema ophryogenes)

It is a disorder primarily affecting infants, boys and young men, characterized by persistent reticular erythema, small horny papules, atrophy and permanent loss of involved hairs. The process begins in the lateral third of the eyebrows and may occasionally extend to include adjacent skin, adjacent scalp and cheeks **(Figure 13.9)**. There is no effective therapy for this disorder.

Atrophoderma Vermiculatum

This variant of keratosis pilaris atrophicans has a later age of onset (between 5 and 12 years of age and occasionally at puberty or in adulthood). It is characterized by numerous tiny scars like atrophic pits, at times erythematous, on the cheeks, and occasionally the forehead and eyebrows. These pits are irregular in shape- approximately 1 mm in depth and 2 mm across, and are separated from each other by narrow epidermal ridges with a reticulate "honeycomb-like" or "worm-eaten" appearance. There is no effective treatment for this disorder. Dermabrasion may improve the cosmetic appearance.

Keratosis Follicularis Spinulosa Decalvans of Siemens

This variant of keratosis pilaris atrophicans has shown X-linked dominant mode of inheritance, hence the most severe manifestations are found in males. It begins in infancy with numerous milia and horny follicular plugs on the nose and cheeks, and later on the eyebrows, scalp, neck and body. Faint erythema may be present. Scarring alopecia of scalp, eyebrows, eyelashes become apparent in childhood and progresses until puberty. It is often restricted to the patches and rarely proceeds to full baldness. Remnant hairs of the eyelashes typically protrude in different directions. Axillary and pubic hair thinning is frequently observed. Patches of eczema, particularly of the scalp, may be seen. After puberty, progression slowly subsides.

Keratosis follicularis spinulosa decalvans is frequently associated with palmoplantar keratoderma and photophobia, which is predominant in children and improves after puberty.

Various exfoliants and keratolytics have been used for the treatment of this disorder but with limited success.

FOLLICULITIS DECALVANS

Folliculitis decalvans is an inflammatory alopecia characterized by erythematous scaling and small rounded or oval patches of scarring surrounded by perifollicular pustules.

The exact etiology is unknown. Bacterial folliculitis caused by Staphylococcus aureus is often associated with this disorder, but whether this is primary or secondary process is unclear. It is also found to be associated with a long history of seborrheic dermatitis and a low grade pustular reaction in the hair follicles, resulting in a peripherally spreading inflammatory disease and alopecia.

Histopathologically, the pustular phase is characterized by polymorphonuclear microabcesses in the upper half of pilosebaceous follicle and a perifollicular plasma cell infiltrate, and the atrophic phase resembles that of lichen planus or lupus erythematosus.

Folliculitis decalvans shows a chronic course and the severe forms may be cosmetically disfiguring especially in males.

The treatment of folliculitis decalvans consists of topical and systemic antibiotics. In severe or protracted cases topical, intralesional or systemic corticosteroids should be combined with long term antibiotics. Systemic retinoids may also be helpful. In many patients, despite the long term and intensive therapy, the disorder persists and results in severe scarring alopecia.

DISSECTING CELLULITIS OF THE SCALP

This disorder, also known as perifolliculitis capitis abscedens et suffodiens of Hoffman, is another inflammatory condition of the scalp leading to scarring alopecia. It occurs commonly in the age group 18 to 40 years and males are more frequently affected than females. It has greater incidence among the Blacks.

It begins with deep inflammatory nodules, primarily over the occiput, that progress to formation of burrowing abscesses over the scalp connected by sinus tracts with seropurulent discharge. As in folliculitis decalvans, Staphylococcus aureus is the most common bacterial isolate. Cicatricial alopecia and keloid formation is frequently seen. This disorder appears to have a slightly greater incidence in patients with acne conglobata and hidradenitis suppurativa where the condition is described as "Follicular occlusion triad of Pillsbury".

Treatment consists of topical and systemic antibiotics with intralesional and systemic steroids. Surgical incision and drainage of abscesses, excision with grafting and X-ray epilation are occasionally used for refractory cases, but the course of this disorder is chronic with remissions and relapses over many years.

ACNE KELOIDALIS

Acne keloidalis (Folliculitis keloidalis) is a chronic destructive scarring folliculitis and perifolliculitis of nape of the neck (occasionally the beard area) which begins as follicular papules and pustules, and progresses to form keloidal papules, nodules and plaques.

It is more common among Blacks, between the ages of 14 and 25 (postpubertal age group). The exact etiology of this disorder is not known but it appears to be related to a persistent infection (most commonly streptococcal or staphylococcal), with a tendency towards granulomatous change followed by eventual destruction of normal structures and their replacement by hypertropic connective tissue and plasma cell infiltrate.

Treatment consists of long term systemic antibiotics and intralesional corticosteroids. Cryosurgery and radiation therapy may be helpful. In long term cases with severe scarring, excision and plastic repair may be beneficial.

PSEUDOPELADE

Pseudopelade of Brocq is a nonspecific scarring form of alopecia of the scalp, of unknown etiology, generally seen in adults. It is characterized by multiple round or oval or irregularly shaped non hairy cicatricial patches of varying sizes which appear shiny, ivory white or slightly pink and are atrophic. Lesions generally appear at the vertex of the scalp and they coalesce to form finger-like projections resembling "footprints in the snow". A few hair containing dilated hair follicles are seen in between the patches.

Histopathologically, the affected areas reveal perifollicular and perivascular infiltrate composed mainly of lymphocytes with few histiocytes. In late stages, dermis shows extensive fibrosis.

Treatment of this disorder includes infiltration of triamcinolone acetonide (2.5 mg/ml) into the alopecia patches at an interval of 6-8 weeks which may be only temporarily beneficial. In unresponsive cases, multiple punch autograft technique of hair transplantation may provide a reasonable cosmetic improvement.

ALOPECIA MUCINOSA

Alopecia mucinosa (follicular mucinosis) is an inflammatory disorder characterized by sharply defined follicular papules or infiltrated plaques, with scaling, loss of hair and accumulation of mucin in the sebaceous glands and the outer root sheaths of affected hair follicles. It is a relatively uncommon condition occurring in both children and adults. Lesions are distributed primarily on the face, scalp, neck and shoulders, and are usually devoid of hairs.

Three different morphologic forms of this disorder have been described:

- Flat rough patches consisting of grouped follicular papules.
- Scaly plaques formed by the coalescence of follicular papules.
- Nodular boggy infiltrated plaques with overlying erythema and scaling.

Etiology of this disorder is unknown. In young patients (of age less than 40 years) it occurs as a benign idiopathic condition. In older patients (above 40 years) it may occur as a first sign of an accompanying reticulosis, usually mycosis fungoides.

Alopecia mucinosa should be differentiated from lichen spinulosus, pityriasis rubra pilaris, tinea infection, pityriasis alba, granulomatous diseases and the papulosquamous group of disorders. The diagnosis of alopecia mucinosa can be established by the histopathologic examination of the cutaneous biopsy from the affected area. The histopathologic features include intracellular edema, loss of cohesion between cells, formation of cystic spaces and accumulation of mucin within the external root sheath and sebaceous glands. Mucin shows metachromatic staining with Geimsa's stain, PAS negativity and stains with Alcian blue and is digested by hyaluronidase.

Generally, especially in children and young adults lesions of alopecia mucinosa resolve spontaneously. In some cases, topical or intralesional corticosteroid and radiation therapy have been beneficial.

HYPERTRICHOSIS

Hypertrichosis is a condition of non-androgen-dependent, diffuse or localized patterns of excessive hair growth in a male or female without evidence of masculinism or menstrual abnormality. It must be distinguished from hirsutism, which is characterized by an androgen-dependent hair pattern with excessive facial and body terminal hair distributed in a male pattern. The abnormal hair growth patterns found in patients with hypertrichosis are not caused by abnormal hair shaft formation, but are probably due to delayed anagen termination. While the underlying mechanism of hypertrichosis is unclear, the cloning of several genes that affect hair growth and the availability of mouse models provide a variety of candidate genes for study. The angora (go) gene has been shown to have a regulatory function in hair growth. The go/go recessive mutation produces abnormally long hair in mice. This gene has been shown to be a mutant allele of fibroblast growth factor 5, a signaling molecule that is localized to the outer root sheath of the lower 1/3rd of the hair follicle. No human homologue for the angora mouse has yet been found.

Hypertrichosis can be present in a diffuse or localized pattern.

DIFFUSE HYPERTRICHOSIS

Primary Hypertrichosis

Primary hypertrichotic condition, whether localized or generalized, are rare in pediatric patients and of unknown origin. Primary generalized hypertrichosis includes various entities.

Hypertrichosis lanuginosa: This is an exceedingly rare inherited disorder characterized by persistence or an acquired excessive production of lanugo hairs. At birth, the child is covered with a coat of profuse, usually fair, silky, fine hair up to 10 cms in length, involving all the usual hair bearing areas of skin and blending with the hair of scalp and eyebrows. Accentuation of hair growth may be seen over the spine and pinnae. Profuse hair growth in the ear canal can lead to infection and hearing deficit and matted hair in the diaper area may be troublesome. At puberty, there may be no conversion to terminal hair in secondary sexual hair areas with long, fine, lanugo hairs persisting in pubic and axillary areas and in the beard.

Two clinical forms of congenital hypertrichosis lanuginosa have been described:

1. The dog face type is an autosomal dominant disorder. In this type, the affected person develops typical lanugo hair growth of several inches in length over the first years of life which persists and is associated with other congenital anomalies.
2. The monkey face type is of uncertain heredity and the affected child bears lanugo hair at birth. It is associated with a high incidence of infant mortality. The surviving patients develop a simian like facies.

In adults, an acquired form of hypertrichosis appears to be strongly associated with internal malignancy.

Ambras syndrome: This is a unique form of diffuse congenital hypertrichosis in which the hair, which may demonstrate pigmentation and medullation, is said to be vellus rather than lanugo hair. The excessive hair growth is seen on face, ears and shoulders persisting throughout the lifetime. The long hair on the face uniformly covers brow, eyelids, nose and cheeks. A number of dysmorphic facial features have occurred in these patients.

X-linked dominant hypertrichosis: This condition has been recently mapped to chromosome X_q24-q27.1 in which the affected individual have a diffuse terminal hair hypertrichosis present at birth, most severe on face, upper chest, back and pubic area, and may show improvement on trunk and limbs after puberty in some cases.

Prepubertal hypertrichosis: It has been reported that some children have diffuse hypertrichosis at birth which progresses during early childhood without any associated abnormalities. Profuse terminal hair growth will be seen on back, proximal limbs and temples spreading across the brows and merging with bushy eyebrows. An inverted fir tree type of hypertrichosis is seen on the back centering the spine. It is not known whether this condition is an abnormality or just the extreme form of normal hair growth as similar pattern of hair growth is seen in some racial groups. However it has been found that serum dihydrotestosterone levels are elevated in several of these patients suggesting that endocrinal abnormality may be the basis of this condition.

Hypertrichosis as Part of Other Genetically Determined Disorders

Hypertrichosis occurs as one of the features of a number of genetically determined syndromes with its onset in the neonatal period or in childhood. Some of these syndromes include Cornelia de Lange's syndrome, Coffin Siris syndrome, hypertrichosis with gingival fibromatosis, hereditary porphyrias like congenital erythropoietic porphyria, familial porphyria cutanea tarda and hepato-erythropoietic porphyria, Cantu syndrome, leprechaunism, Seip-Berardinelli syndrome, mucopolysaccharidoses, Barber-Say syndrome, Rubenstein-Taybi syndrome.

Drug Induced Hypertrichosis

Neonatal hypertrichosis can occasionally occur as a feature of fetal alcohol syndrome and also occur due to maternal use of minoxidil. Drugs like diazoxide, which is used in neonates with hyperinsulinemia leads to a dose-dependent hypertrichosis of the brow, limbs and back. Other drugs which may be responsible for hypertrichosis in infants and children include cyclosporine, penicillamine, diphenylhydantoin, and minoxidil. Each drug may show a unique pattern of excessive hair growth, for example, minoxidil causes hypertrichosis primarily involving the face, shoulders and extremities. In addition, drugs such as oral contraceptives, systemic corticosteroids, and occasionally other drugs such as psoralens and streptomycin sulfate, may increase hair growth, although not to the extent usually seen with earlier mentioned drugs. Discontinuation of drug use will resolve this cosmetic adverse effect. If the drug cannot be discontinued, then other common methods of hair removal such as depilatory agents and shaving may be used.

LOCALIZED HYPERTRICHOSIS

Nevoid Hypertrichosis

This condition refers to single or multiple localized patches of terminal hair growing from skin of normal color and texture or in association with other abnormalities like underlying lipoatrophy. Other abnormalities which have been reported in patients with nevoid hypertrichosis include areas of lipoatrophy and streaky depigmentation away from the areas of hypertrichosis, developmental delay and seizures, congenital lung cyst, congenital malrotation of the gut, multiple skeletal, dental and ocular abnormalities. In a recently reported case, a patient had Blashcko-distributed pattern of depigmented hypertrichosis associated with short stature, scoliosis, developmental delay and seizures, microphthalmia, eyelid coloboma and other structural ocular abnormalities. In another case with multiple patches of congenital nevoid hypertrichosis there was an associated epidermal nevus, hypopigmented hairless streaks and retinal pigmentary abnormality, and the hypertrichosis spontaneously resolved by 2 years of age.

Hypertrichosis Cubiti

Hypertrichosis cubiti or "hairy elbows syndrome" is a condition characterized by presence of profuse vellus hairs, symmetrically at birth or develop during infancy on the extensor surfaces of the elbows, extending from midhumerus to midforearm and spontaneously resolves at puberty. Both dominant and recessive patterns of inheritance have been reported but some cases are apparently sporadic. This uncommon form is usually not associated with any abnormalities and represents only a cosmetic problem. There has been isolated case reports of hypertrichosis cubiti associated with short stature.

Anterior Cervical Hypertrichosis

This condition is characterized by a congenital patch of hypertrichosis at the sternal notch and lower anterior aspect of the neck. The mode of inheritance is most likely autosomal recessive. Although usually an isolated phenomenon, it may be associated with peripheral sensory and motor neuropathy with or without retinal abnormalities.

Posterior Cervical Hypertrichosis

In posterior cervical hypertrichosis, excessive hair growth is seen at birth on the cervical vertebrae associated with underlying kyphoscoliosis. An X-linked recessive or autosomal dominant pattern of inheritance has been observed.

Lumbosacral Hypertrichosis or Faun Tail Deformity

Here a congenital localized patch of hypertrichosis is seen on the sacral midline. It is commonly seen in association with various cutaneous malformations like sacral dimple, lipoma, hyperpigmentation, port-wine stain, dermoid cyst, sinus tract and aplasia cutis. This developmental defect often overlies bone and spinal cord defects, most commonly spina bifida occulta and diastematomyelia. If undetected and uncorrected surgically, complications may ensue with advancing age. As the vertebral column grows disproportionately with respect to the spinal column, fibrous bands that connect the skin to the spinal theca pull on the spinal theca and may result in neurologic abnormalities. The most common defects are foot drop, nocturnal enuresis, and backache, sometimes developing as late as adolescence or adulthood. Computed tomographic and/or MRI myelography are diagnostic.

Hypertrichosis with Cranial Meningoceles, Encephaloceles and Heterotopic Meningeal or Brain Tissue

This is represented by a peripheral collar or hypertropic hair, a tuft of hair near by or overlying hair or sometimes prominent or patulous hair follicle orifices may be seen. Scalp lesions show longer, thicker and darker hair compared to the surrounding normal hair. Presence of such a patch anywhere on the body, away from the scalp, signals about a neural lesion. The membranous form of aplasia cutis with a hair collar is now recognized as a form fruste of a neural tube closure defect. A congenital patch of hypertrichosis has been reported in a patient, over the lumbar area, away from the spine, overlying the meningeal tissue. Displacement of meningeal cells along nerves during embryogenesis may be the possible mechanism in this case.

Hairy Cutaneous Malformations of Palms and Soles

This condition is characterized by familial occurrence of circumscribed patches of hair growth on palms and soles due to presence of ectopic hair follicles. Exaggerated skin markings in a geometric pattern over the involved skin have been reported in one family. It presents at birth and persists throughout lifetime.

Scrotal Hair

There have been reports of several infant boys developing scrotal hair within first 3 months of life without any clinical or biochemical evidence of excessive androgen production. The condition was non progressive and hair usually disappeared by age of 18 months.

Hypertrichosis with Focal Facial Dermal Dysplasia

An unusual variant of focal facial dermal dysplasia has been reported in a patient who had multiple, scar like, circular, atrophic lesions, each surrounded by a fine rim of hair, present on both the temples extending onto the cheeks. These lesions are believed to follow an embryonic fusion line.

Hemihypertrophy with Hypertrichosis

Hemihypertrophy is a rare congenital disorder characterized by enlargement of the whole or a part of one side of the body. The skin is usually normal but cutaneous abnormalities like hyperpigmentation, telangiectasia, abnormal nail growth and hypertrichosis have been reported.

Localized Hypertrichosis in Association with Nevi or Tumors

Congenital melanocytic nevi may be covered at birth with dense, dark terminal hair over part or their entire surface **(Figure 13.10)**. On scalp, hair overlying the nevus will be darker and thicker than the surrounding normal hair. In areas other than scalp, degree of hairiness of the nevus is usually proportional to its degree of elevation. A varying degree of hypertrichosis is seen over congenital smooth muscle hamartoma with a characteristic feature of transient piloerection or elevation of the lesion after it is rubbed [Pseudo-Darier sign]. Becker's nevus usually presents in late childhood or adolescence as a patch of thickened, pigmented, hypertrichotic skin but congenital cases have been reported, although usually lacking hypertrichosis in the neonatal period. Plexiform neurofibroma often shows hyperpigmentation with irregular outlines over the lesions and hypertrichosis of varying degree may also occur. There have been case reports of hypertrichosis over the lesions of sclerosing tufted angioma.

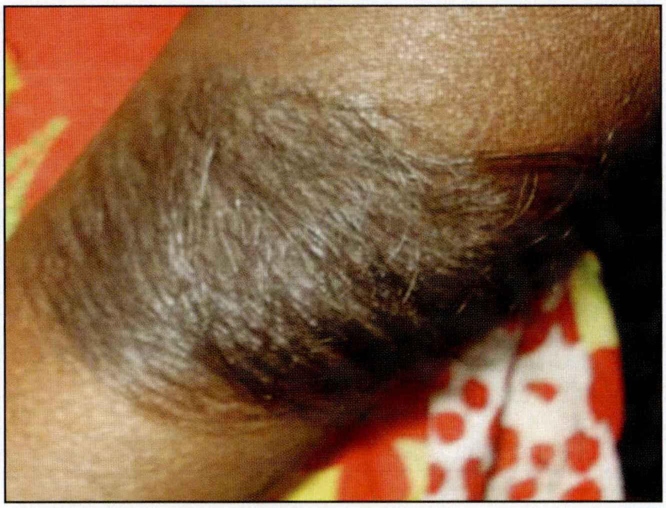

FIGURE 13.10: Localized hypertrichosis (congenital nevomelanocytic nevus)

HYPERTRICHOSIS DUE TO LOCAL HEAT AND CUTANEOUS HYPEREMIA

Hypertrichosis can occur due to local heat and cutaneous hyperemia at the sites of PUVA therapy, chickenpox scars, insect bites, at the edges of burns, areas of chronic excoriation, under a plaster cast, over inflamed joints, thrombophlebitis, stasis dermatitis, chemical irritation or hormonal stimulation.

MANAGEMENT OF HYPERTRICHOSIS

Long term removal of unwanted hair is a challenge. The need for treatment depends on the degree of hypertrichosis and the psychosocial needs of the child. The current available treatment methods for removal of excessive hair include bleaching, trimming, physical and chemical depilatories, electrolysis, intense pulsed light therapy and laser hair removal.

Bleaching is a quick and easy process that removes natural hair pigment partially or totally, lightening the hair to a yellowish hue. The active ingredient is hydrogen peroxide which softens and oxidizes the hair. Occasionally bleaching results in skin irritation.

Trimming of the hair is a recommended option for young children with either localized or diffuse hypertrichosis.

Physical depilation includes tweezing or plucking, shaving and waxing. Tweezing is a slow, tedious painful process suitable only for localized hypertrichosis. Shaving is not usually preferred because the diameter of the cut hair at the surface is greater than that of the uncut tapered hair. Wax epilation is a painful process for the removal of fine vellus hair using cold, warm or hot wax with the effect lasting up to 4-6 weeks. But it is associated with various adverse effects like folliculitis, skin irritation. Another drawback of this procedure is the requirement for the hair to be a minimum length of 2 to 3 mm to be grasped by the wax. Since it is too painful and traumatic, this method may be an option only for older adolescents rather than children.

Chemical depilatories contain sulfides, thioglycolates and enzymatic depilatory agents which breakdown hairs by cleaving their cysteine linkages. Sulfides are more effective but the generated hydrogen sulfide releases an unpleasant odor and can irritate the skin. Thioglycolates are the most commercially available depilatories. They are less odiferous and less irritating but take long time to act. Enzymatic depilatory agents are not very effective. The associated adverse effects are localized irritation and allergic contact dermatitis.

Permanent hair removal methods such as electrolysis and Laser therapy have not been studied in prepubertal children, and their use has been limited in older children and adolescents.

Electrolysis, a permanent hair removal technique, can be accomplished by either galvanic electrolysis or thermolysis or blend of these two methods. It is a tedious procedure and even in the best of the hands, one can expect up to 25% regrowth. Permanent hair removal can occur only if the needle is inserted deep into the follicle, enabling the current to travel to the germinating bulb directly because hair is not an electrical conductor. The adverse effects include pain, postinflammatory erythema and whealing, bruising, swelling and postinflammatory hyperpigmentation.

Laser therapy and intense pulsed light therapy are the newest available permanent hair removal systems. These techniques remove unwanted hairs through selective photothermolysis of melanin-rich structures, thus affecting only the hair with minimal absorption by surrounding tissues. Lasers are capable of hair removal include ruby, diode, Nd: YAG and alexandrite. Occasionally, posttreatment erythema, edema, blisters and hyperpigmentation occur. As with traditional electrolysis, laser electrolysis is uncomfortable for children, which limits its usefulness.

A recent treatment for retarding the excessive hair growth (not removing hair) is **eflornithine hydro-**

chloride cream. It reversibly inhibits the enzyme ornithine decarboxylase present in hair follicle which is essential for the hair growth. Fifteen percent eflornithine hydrochloride cream has to be applied twice daily to the affected area. Local irritation with burning, stinging, and tingling can occur as adverse effects. Safety and effectiveness of this treatment in children have not been established.

HIRSUTISM

Hirsutism implies an excessive growth of terminal body hair in females in an androgen-induced hair pattern or male sexual pattern [upper lip, chin, sideburn areas, neck, anterior chest, breasts, linea alba, abdomen, upper inner thighs and legs]. Hirsutism may be a sign of an endocrine disorder involving the adrenal glands and/or the ovaries, the two organ source for androgens in women, or may even occur in many patients without any clinical evidence of disturbed endocrine or metabolic function which is classified as idiopathic hirsutism **(Table 13.6)**. The cause for idiopathic hirsutism is assumed to be increased stimulation of the hair follicles of genetically predisposed females by normal levels of androgenic hormones.

PATHOGENESIS

The four primary circulating androgenic steroids in females are dehydroepiandrosterone (DHEA) and its sulfate (DHEA-S), androstenedione and testosterone. Approximately 50% of the testosterone is secreted from the ovaries and adrenal glands. The remainder is produced from metabolism of the prehormones in the liver, fat and skin. Testosterone overproduction overwhelms the liver's clearance capabilities and the excessive testosterone appears in the circulation. The hair follicle then becomes a site to metabolize the excess testosterone. Testosterone binds to androgen receptors in the hair follicle. Follicular enzyme 5α reductase transforms the receptor bound testosterone to 5α dihydrotestosterone which is metabolized to androstanediol. The activated hormones stimulate follicular proliferation, resulting in the growth of terminal hair.

The incidence of hirsutism in any population is difficult to assess, since the range of normal is quite wide, subject to individual acceptance, and includes that which is not always socially acceptable in a particular culture. Latin, Jewish and Welsh women in general have more hair than their counterparts of Northern European, Japanese and Indian heritage. In such cases the physician should be aware as to what is normal and acceptable to some individuals, yet unacceptable and a source of anguish to others.

TABLE 13.6: Causes for hirsutism

Idiopathic
Ovarian
Polycystic ovary syndrome
Hyperthecosis
HAIR-AN syndrome [Hyperandrogenism, Insulin Resistance, Acanthosis Nigricans]
Tumors
Adrenal
Congenital adrenal hyperplasia
21-hydroxylase deficiency
11- hydroxylase deficiency
Tumors
ACTH-dependent Cushing's syndrome

A detailed history and thorough physical examination will give a clue to decide whether the endocrinologic evaluation is required. If a post pubertal female develops hirsutism along with other signs of virilization like acne, clitoral hypertrophy, deepening of the voice, decrease in breast size, frontotemporal balding and infrequent or absent menses, then the abnormalities of the pituitary, adrenals or ovaries must be ruled out. In such cases, minimal laboratory investigation for excessive androgen production should include free plasma testosterone, urinary 17-ketosteroids, serum DHEA-S levels, morning and evening cortisol levels, serum LH and FSH ratio and pelvic USG.

TREATMENT

Hirsutism cannot be cured, only suppressed. The problem is cosmetic, and the decision of treatment must be made after consideration of the potential side effects of the medication.

If the ovarian or adrenal disease is diagnosed, it should be dealt with appropriately under the guidance of a gynecologist or endocrinologist. Drugs used in the treatment are oral contraceptives preferably ones containing 35 to 50 mg of estrogen (ethinyl estradiol) to reduce free plasma testosterone levels, low dose prednisolone (5 mg/day) or dexamethasone (0.5 mg/day) to suppress adrenal gland production and lower DHEA-S levels, cyproterone acetate (50 to 100 mg/day) with ethinyl estradiol

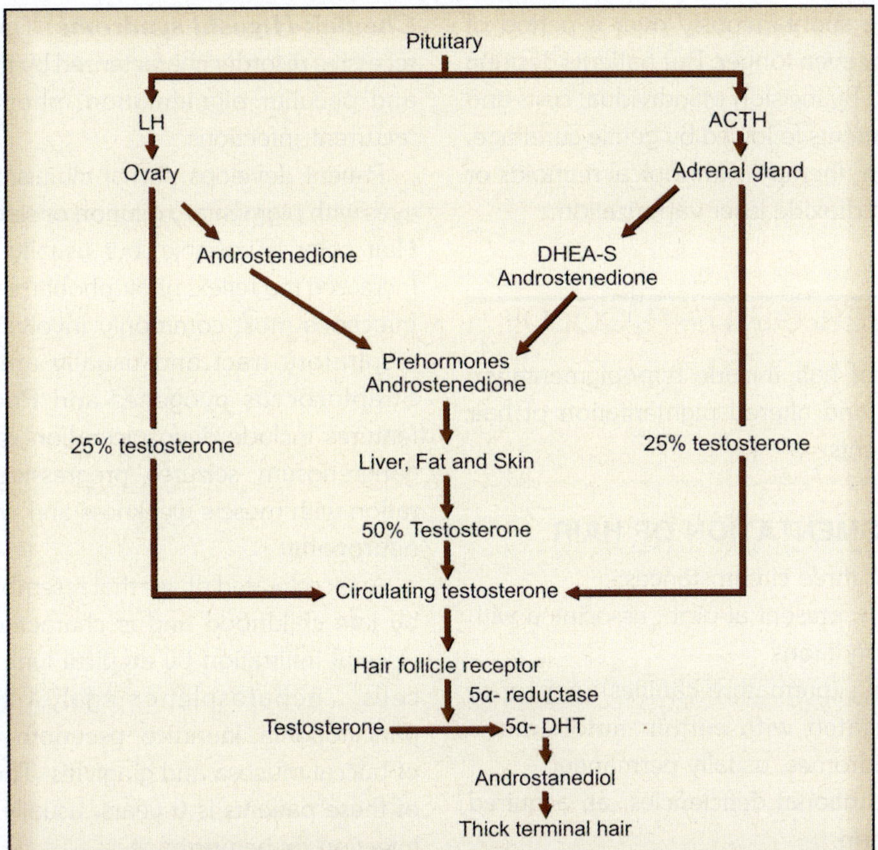

Note: ACTH- Adrenocorticotrophic hormone; DHEAS- Dehydroepiandrosterone sulfate; DHT- Dihydrotestosterone; LH- Lutenizing hormone

Flow Chart 13.2: Pathogenesis of Hirsutism

(0.5 mg/day), spironolactone (50 to 200 mg/day) or cimetidine (300 mg, 5 times a day) which are androgen receptor competitive inhibitors.

The excessive hair can be removed by one of the several methods like bleaching, shaving, plucking, waxing, chemical depilatories, electrolysis, laser and intense pulsed light therapy or eflornithine hydrochloride cream.

ERUPTIVE VELLUS HAIR CYSTS

Eruptive vellus hair cysts are developmental abnormality of the vellus hair follicle with occlusion at the follicular level, presenting as 1 to 2 mm skin colored to variably pigmented follicular papules, most commonly on the anterior chest.

The exact etiology of this condition is not known. An autosomal dominant pattern of inheritance has been suggested. These cysts are commonly seen in children between 4 and 18 years of age but can occur at any age. The lesions are soft and sharply demarcated follicle oriented round or dome shaped papules with a smooth surface but central puncta. Umbilication and hyperkeratotic crusts have been noted. Umbilicated papules with histological evidence of transepithelial elimination may explain the spontaneous disappearance of lesions. These follicle oriented papules show no tendency to grouping. They may be skin colored, yellow, blue, red or hyperpigmented mainly distributed on the anterior chest, also seen on upper and lower extremities, face, neck, abdomen, axillae, posterior trunk and buttocks. There are reports of families in which milia, eruptive vellus hair cyst and steatocystoma multiplex all occurred, with some individuals showing more than one type of lesion. This led to the conclusion that these three types of lesions can be considered as subtypes of multiple pilosebaceous cysts.

The histologic features of eruptive vellus hair cyst include small, mid to upper dermal keratinizing cysts filled with lamellar keratin and small-diameter nonpigmented hair shafts.

These cysts resolve spontaneously over a period of few months to years or even longer. But patients desiring therapy can be treated by incision of individual cysts and expression of their contents followed by gentle curettage, light electrodessication, therapy with topical retinoids or lactic acid and carbon dioxide laser vaporization.

ABNORMALITIES OF HAIR COLOR

Pigmentary changes of hair include hypopigmentation (diffuse or localized) and altered pigmentation of hair due to exogenous agents.

DIFFUSE HYPOPIGMENTATION OF HAIR

This may occur under three circumstances:-

i. Primary condition, present at birth, associated with certain genetic conditions
ii. Premature graying (premature canities), appear at later age, associated with certain autoimmune diseases and syndromes, usually permanent.
iii. As a result of nutritional deficiencies, an acquired reversible condition.

Primary Diffuse Hypopigmentation of Hair

This presents at birth as a part of a wide range of genetic conditions **(Table 13.7)**. The color of the hair may range from simply fairer than expected to silvery color.

TABLE 13.7: Primary diffuse hypopigmentation of hair

Absent hair color
Tyrosinase negative albinism
Diluted hair color (often yellowish)
Tyrosinase positive albinism
Silvery color
Chediak-Higashi
Griscelli syndrome
Elejalde syndrome
Fairer than expected
Isolated pili torti
Uncombable hair
Fairer than expected, sometimes silvery
Menke's syndrome
Alternating light & dark color (flag sign)
Phenylketonuria
Homocystinuria
Very light (almost white)
Oast house disease

Chediak-Higashi syndrome: This is a rare autosomal recessive disorder characterized by incomplete, decreased and peculiar pigmentation, photophobia and severe recurrent infections.

Patient develops partial albinism of the hair, skin or eyes with pigmentary dilution or slate gray pigmentation. Hair color is variable, but usually has a silvery sheen. Increased red reflex, photophobia, strabismus is common. Infections most commonly involve the skin, lungs and respiratory tract and usually are due to S. aureus, Streptococcus pyogenes and Pneumococcus. Other features include deep ulceration resembling pyoderma gangrenosum, seizures, progressive neurologic deterioration with muscle weakness and cranial and peripheral neuropathy.

An accelerated phase that resembles lymphoma occurs by late childhood and is characterized by widespread visceral infiltration by atypical lymphoid and histiocytic cells, hepatosplenomegaly, lymphadenopathy, pancytopenia, jaundice, pseudomembranous sloughing of buccal mucosa and gingivitis. The mean age of death of these patients is 6 years, usually from overwhelming infection or hemorrhage.

The circulating neutrophils, melanocytes, renal tubular cells and neurons show giant granules which are thought to result from markedly delayed discharge of lysosomal and perioxidative enzymes from cells, perhaps because of a defective protein involved in membrane fusion. Hair shafts have finely clumped pigment granules. Diminished chemotaxis of neutrophils and decreased antibody-dependent cellular cytotoxicity and NK cell function are often associated.

The treatment of choice is bone marrow transplantation, which corrects the immunologic status but does not affect pigment dilution. Antibiotics for recurrent infections, acyclovir, high dose intravenous gamma globulin, vincristine, cyclosporine and prednisone have been used to control the accelerated phase. Interferon has been demonstrated by some authors to partially restore NK cell function.

Griscelli syndrome: This is an uncommon autosomal recessive disorder characterized by hypomelanosis of the skin and hair, and immunodeficiency.

Although pigmentary dilution of the skin may be seen, hypomelanosis in Griscelli syndrome may be limited to an abnormal appearance of the hair, described as silvery gray or grayish golden. Histologic and ultrastructural studies show large pigment clumps with in hair shafts and an accumulation of melanosomes in melanocytes with poorly pigmented adjacent keratinocytes.

Frequent pyogenic infections and acute episodes of fever, hepatosplenomegaly, neutropenia, thrombocytopenia, progressive neurologic deterioration and lymphohistiocytosis occurs. Patients with Griscelli syndrome have hypogammaglobulinemia and defective cell-mediated immunity. Neutrophils do not show giant granules.

Griscelli syndrome has been uniformly fatal but now can be reversed by successful bone marrow transplantation.

Elejalde syndrome: Elejalde syndrome (Neuroectodermal melanolysosomal disease) is another silvery hair syndrome with bronze skin after sun exposure **(Figures 13.11A and B)** and severe neurologic dysfunction.

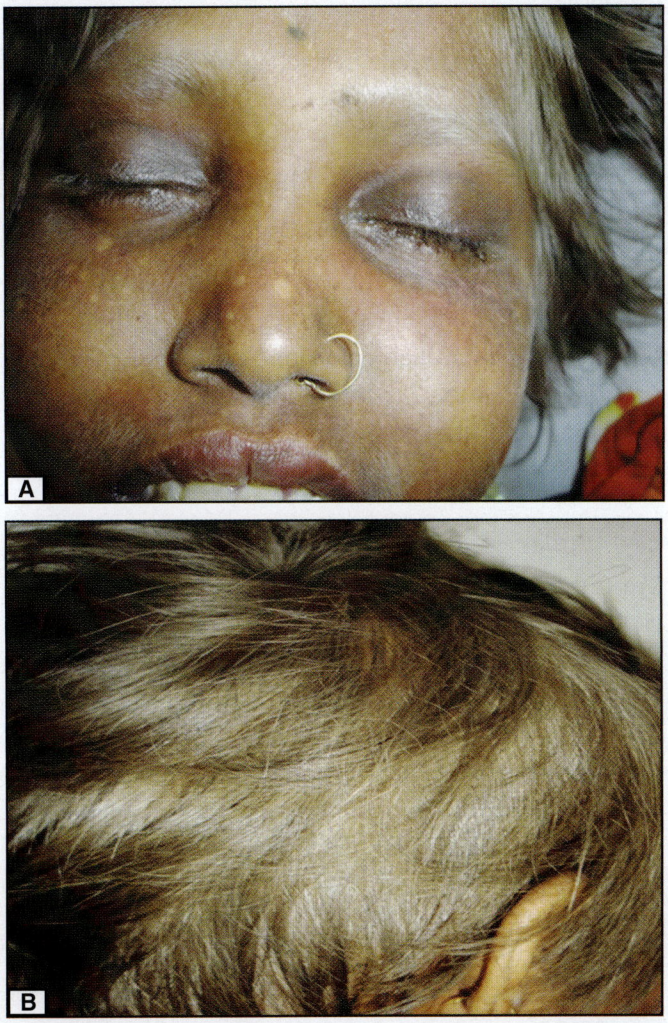

FIGURES 13.11A AND B: Silvery hair in Elejalde disease

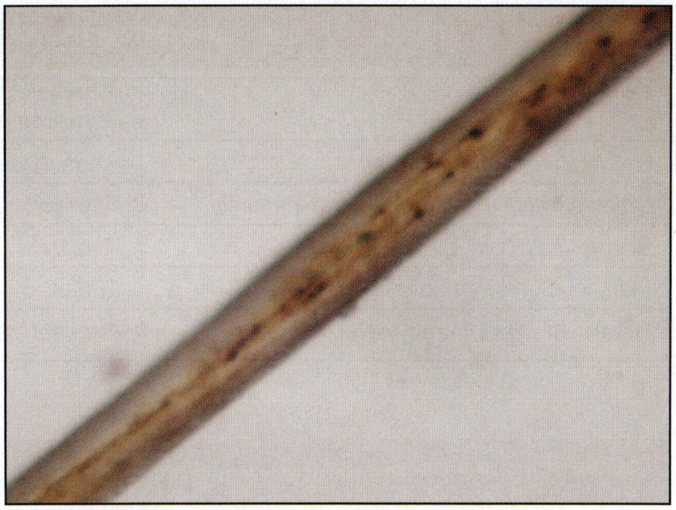

FIGURE 13.11C: Light microscopy of hair showing irregular clumps of melanin in Elejalde disease

Psychomotor impairment is a constant feature and may be observed in the newborn or during infancy. Seizures, severe hypotonia, hemiplegia, quadriplegia, ataxia, ocular abnormalities and mental retardation that is usually of a severe degree are also seen.

While the impairment of the nervous system is more severe in Elejalde syndrome, the defects in cellular or humoral immunity of Chediak-Higashi and Griscelli syndrome are not seen in Elejalde syndrome **(Table 13.8)**. Similar to Griscelli syndrome, no neutrophils with giant intracytoplasmic granules are found, although microscopic examination of hair shafts shows an irregular distribution of abnormally small or large clumps of melanin **(Figure 13.11C)**. It has been postulated that Elejalde syndrome is allelic to Griscelli syndrome.

Therapeutic measures have included the use of steroids, anticonvulsants and antipyretics. They have been unsuccessful in all the patients. Thus, whether any medical therapy can be recommended for these patients is unclear.

Premature Graying (premature canities)

Premature canities refers to diffuse lose of hair color, especially of scalp hair, at an age earlier than that generally accepted as physiologic (before the age of 20 years in whites and 30 years in blacks). This occurs due to reduction in the activity of melanocytes in the hair follicles. It may be seen as an early sign of various conditions mentioned in the **Table 13.9** but occasionally it may occur in the apparent absence of any dermatologic or systemic cause.

TABLE 13.8: Differences between Chediak- Higashi, Griscelli and Elejalde syndrome

Characteristics	Chediak-Higashi syndrome	Griscelli syndrome	Elejalde syndrome
Neurologic dysfunction	Less severe	Less severe	More severe
Defects in cellular and humoral immunity	Present	Present	Absent
Silvery gray hair	Present	Present	Present
Melanin clumps in hair	Small	Large	Irregular, small and large
Neutrophil giant intracytoplasmic granules	Present	Absent	Absent

TABLE 13.9: Premature graying of hair

Endocrine disorders
Addison's disease
Hypothyroidism
Hyperthyroidism
Premature aging syndromes
Progeria
Werner syndrome
Genodermatoses
Rothmund-Thomson syndrome
Dyskeratosis congenita
Others
Generalized vitiligo
Wide spread alopecia areata
Pernicious anemia
Down's syndrome

TABLE 13.10: Localized hypopigmentation of hair

White forelock
Piebaldisim
Waardenburg syndrome
Multiple white patches
Tietz syndrome
Patchy
Vitiligo
Patchy/ vitiligo
Vogt-Koyanagi-Harada syndrome
Alezzandrini syndrome
Regrowing hair, reversible
Alopecia areata
Tuberous sclerosis
Halo nevus
Halo around neurofibroma

Acquired Reversible Diffuse Hypopigmentation

This condition results from various nutritional deficiencies. In protein malnutrition, kwashiorkor, hair appears light colored and may show alternate dark and light bands corresponding to the periods of adequate diet and malnutrition. This is referred to as 'flag sign'. Severe iron deficiency can also occasionally lead to light colored hair.

LOCALIZED HYPOPIGMENTATION OF HAIR (POLIOSIS)

Poliosis refers to a localized patch of white hair due to absence or deficiency of melanin in a group of neighboring hair follicles. Conditions featuring poliosis are listed below **(Table 13.10).**

ALTERED PIGMENTATION OF HAIR DUE TO EXOGENOUS AGENTS

Drugs

Certain drugs can alter the hair color reversibly, restoring back the original color once the drug is discontinued. Few of these drugs are used in children. Chloroquine causes progressive lightening and silvery coloration in blonde individuals. α-interferon causes progressive lightening and etretinate causes lightening of normally dark hair.

Chemicals

Various chemicals, usually encountered in industrial setting, can cause hair discoloration. In children, copper used as an algae retardant in swimming pools and present in excessive amounts in household tap water, can lead to green discoloration of the hair. It can be treated by topical application of a chelating agent containing EDTA or penicillamine containing shampoo or by application of an aqueous solution of 1.5% 1-hydroxyethyl diphosphonic acid.

BIBLIOGRAPHY

1. Alonso L, Fuchs E. The hair cycle. J Cell Scien 2006; 119: 391- 3.

2. Bertolino AP. Alopecia areata. A clinical overview. Postgrad Med 2000; 107: 81- 05, 89- 90.
3. Connolly M, Berker D. Disorders of hair in children. Curr Pediatr 2003; 13(6): 429- 37.
4. de Berker D, Sinclair R. The hair shaft: normality, abnormality and genetics. Clin Dermatol 2001; 19: 129- 34.
5. Drake LA, Dinehart SM, Farmer ER, Goltz RW, Graham GF, Hordinsky MK, et al. Guidelines of care for androgenetic alopecia. American Academy of Dermatology. J Am Acad Dermatol 1996; 35 (3 pt 1): 465- 9.
6. Fleming CJ, Mackie RM. Á- IFN induced hair discoloration. Br J Dermatol 1996; 135: 337- 38.
7. Habif TP. Hair diseases. In: clinical dermatology: a color guide to diagnosis and therapy. 3rd edn. St. Louis: Mosby, 1996; 720- 60.
8. Hamm H, Traupe H. Loose anagen hair of childhood: the phenomenon of easily pluckable hair. J Am Acad Dermatol 1989; 20: 242- 48.
9. Han A, Mirmirani P. Clinical approach to the patient with alopecia. Semin Cut Med surg 2006; 25(1): 11- 23.
10. Jackson EA. Hair disorders. Primary care 2000; 27: 319- 32.
11. Krause K, Foitzik K. Biology of the hair follicle: The basics. Semin Cut Med Surg 2006; 25(1): 2- 10.
12. Madani S, Shapiro J. Alopecia areata update. J Am Acad Dermatol 2000; 42: 549- 66.
13. Messinger ML, Cheng TL. Trichotillomania. Pediatr Rev 1999; 20: 249- 50.
14. Paller AS, Mancini AJ. Disorders of pigmentation. In: Hurwitz Clinical Pediatric Dermatology. 3rd edn. Philadelphia: Elsevier Saunders, 2006; 265- 306.
15. Pierard- Franchimont C, Pierard GE. Teloptosis, a turning point in hair shedding biorhythm. Dermatology 2001; 203: 115- 7 .
16. Sawaya ME, Shapiro J. Androgenetic alopecia. New approved and unapproved treatments. Dermatol Clin 2000; 18: 47- 61.
17. Shapiro J, Wiseman M, Lui H. Practical management of hair loss. Can Fam Physician 2000; 46: 1469- 77.
18. Shapiro J. Alopecia areata update. Dermatol Clin 1993; 11: 35- 45.
19. Shapiro J. Topical immunotherapy in the treatment of chronic severe alopecia areata. Dermatol Clin 1993; 11: 611- 7.
20. Sperling LC, Cowper SE. The histopathology of Primary cicatricial alopecia. Semin Cut Med Surg 2006; 25(1): 41- 50.
21. Sperling LC. Hair disease and systemic disease. Dermatol Clin 2001; 19: 711- 26.
22. Springer K, Brown M, Stulberg Dl. Common hair loss disorders. Am Fam Physician 2003; 68(1): 93- 102.
23. Tosti A, Jorizzo M, Piraccini BM. Androgenetic alopecia in children: report of 20 cases. Br J Deramtol 2005; 152: 556- 9.
24. Tosti A, Misciali C, Piraccini BM. Drug induced hair loss and hair growth: incidence, management and avoidance. Drug Saf 1994; 10: 310- 17.
25. Tosti A, Peluso AM, Misciali C. Loose anagen hair. Arch Dermatol 1997; 133: 1089- 93.
26. Tosti A, Piraccini BM. Diagnosis and treatment of hair disorders: An evidence based atlas. New York: Taylor & Francis group, 2007..
27. Vashi RA, Mancini AJ, Paller AS. Primary generalized and localized hypertrichosis in children. Arch Dermatol 2001; 137: 877- 84.
28. Vesper JL, Fenske NA. Hair darkening and new growth associated with etretinate therapy. J Am Acad Dermatol 1996; 34: 860.
29. Wade MS, Sinclair RD. Disorders of hair in children other than alopecia. Clin Dermatol 2002; 20: 16- 28.
30. Whiting D. Chronic telogen effluvium. Dermatol Clin 1996; 14 (4): 723- 31.
31. Whiting DA, Dy LC. Office diagnosis of hair shaft defects. Semin Cut Med Surg 2006; 25(1): 24- 34 .

14

Disorders of Nail

Rashmi Sarkar
Vijay Kumar Garg

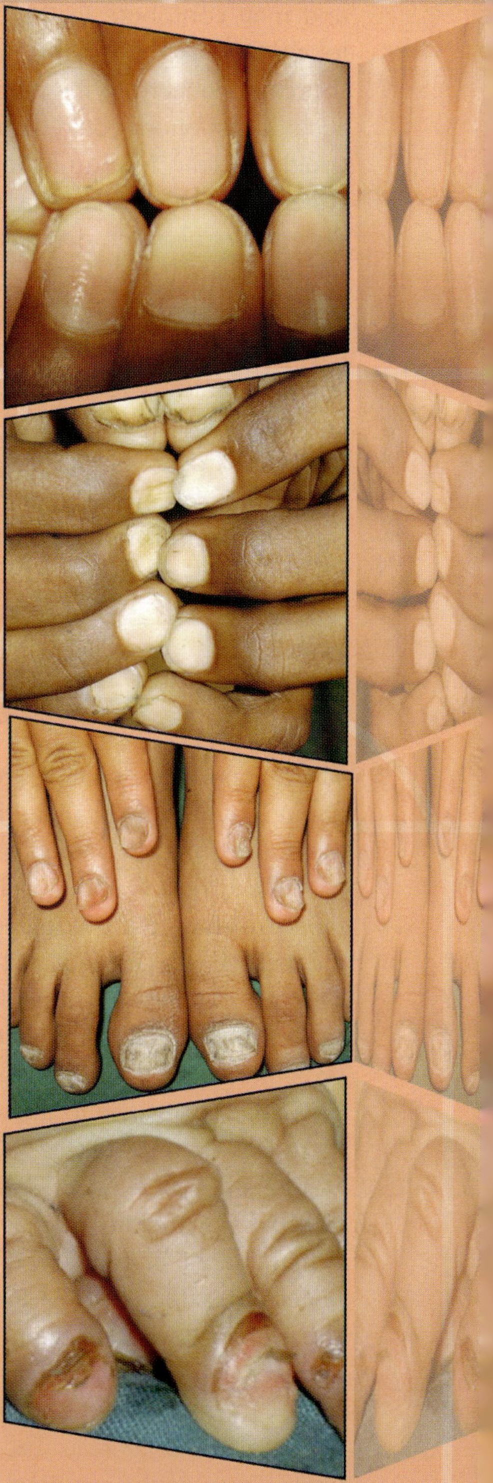

INTRODUCTION

The human nail is a hard plate like structure, which, although seemingly unimportant is more than a cosmetic appendage. It protects the tips of the fingers and toes, maker fine grasping more efficient, is used for scratching and may contribute to the precision and sensation of touch. Different childhood nail presentations may be a source of concern to the parents as they worry whether such presentations could be uncomfortable for the child, could affect any future function or suggest any underlying systemic disorder. Hence, a knowledge of pediatric nail disorders is useful to dermatologists to address parental concerns.

Nail disorders are a rather uncommon cause of consultation in childhood. These disorders may be congenital and hereditary or acquired. There are some conditions which are typically seen in children such as twenty nail dystrophy (TND), whereas diseases such as onychomycosis are uncommon. Common nail disorders due to dermatological disease and traumatic nail abnormalities account for 90 to 95% of all childhood nail disorders.

ANATOMY

The nail first appears as a structure called the matrix, at about 10 weeks of gestational life. It is from the nail matrix, that the nail plate grows out and begins to get keratinized by the 15th week and is well formed at birth. The nail unit consists of four specialized epithelia: The nail matrix, the nail bed, the proximal nail fold and the hyponychium. The nail matrix is a germinative epithelial structure that gives rise to a fully keratinized nail plate. It consists of a proximal and distal region which due to their diagonal orientation gives rise to the upper and lower portion of the nail plate respectively.

The nail plate is a rectangular, translucent and transparent structure which is derived from keratinocytes within the nail matrix, which begins proximal to the nail plate and extends to the lunula, the white half-moon shaped portion often seen through the nail plate. It appears pink due to the vessels of the underlying nail bed. The nail plate is surrounded by the nail folds proximally and laterally. The cuticle is formed from the horny layer of the proximal nail fold and it intimately adheres to the underlying nail plate and prevents the separation from the proximal nail fold. The hyponychium is a distal continuation of the nail bed and marks the separation of the nail plate from the digit. The nail plate grows throughout life. In the fingernails the average nail growth is 3 mm/month and in toenails 1-1.5 mm/ month.

In the newborn, the nails are thin and soft, and may present a certain degree of koilonychia. When the toenails are very short at birth, they may appear to grow into distal digital pulp and resemble ingrowing toenails. Normal nail growth, however, ensues, unless congenital malalignment is present. Nail growth rates in children are similar to adults and the fastest value of nail growth (150 mm/day) is reached during adoleslescence.There are numerous physiologic and pathologic factors which may affect nail growth **(Table 14.1).** Due to the brief arrest of growth, during the first few days of life, there can be transitory arrest in nail growth with the development of Beau's lines at the base of the nails at about 4 weeks of life. These are physiological and can occur in 20-25% of healthy newborns.

TABLE 14.1: Factors that alter normal nail growth rate

Slower	Faster
Physiologic	
Females	Males
Toes	Fingers
First and fifth digits	Third digit
Winter	Summer
Night	Day
Pathologic	
Severe infections	Psoriasis
Chronic illness	Erythroderma
Hypothyroidism	Hyperthyroidism
Malnutrition	Biting
Congestive heart failure	Arteriovenous shunts
Nerve injury	Pregnancy
Ischemia	Typing
Chemotherapy	A V Shunts

PATHOLOGICAL CHANGES OF THE NAIL APPARATUS

ALTERATIONS IN THE NAIL PLATE

Beau's lines are uniform transverse grooves or furrows originating under the proximal nail fold that move distally

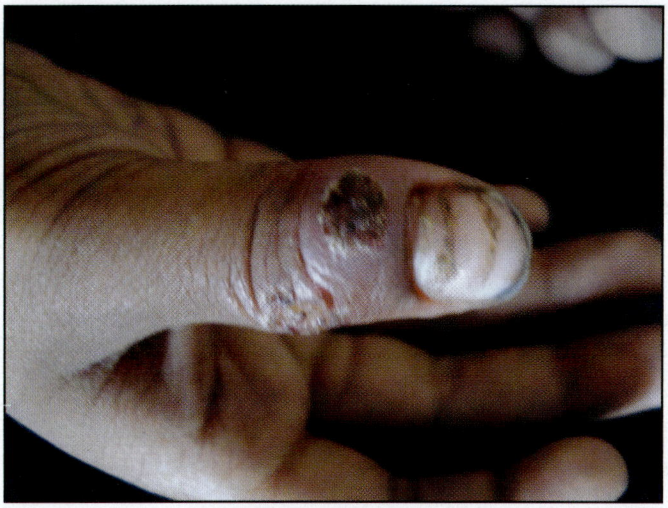

FIGURE 14.1: Beau's lines

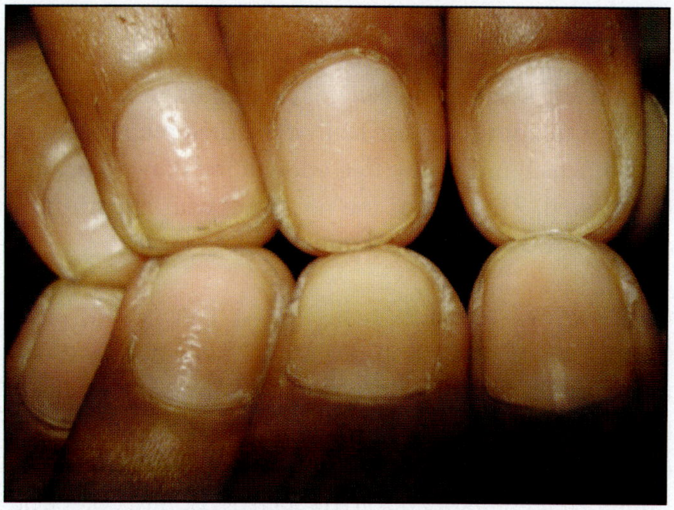

FIGURE 14.2: Nail pittings

with the nail growth **(Figure 14.1)**. These develop due to arrest in nail plate formation due to any stressful condition, systemic illness or toxins. Narrow depressions indicate that the insult was brief whereas a sloping trailing border with wide depressions represents a gradual protracted resolution of the illness. Although all the nails are equally affected, deformities are frequently noted on thumbnails, or toenails due to their slower growth rate. Physiologic Beau's lines may be noted in 4 to 10 weeks old infants as a result of birth trauma. They are similar to the process of telogen effluvium hair loss, which is commonly observed in newborns and their mothers.

Onychomadesis

Onychomadesis is the spontaneous separation and subsequent shedding of the nail plate. Severe illnesses, drug toxicities, severe intrauterine distress, local illnesses such as eczema, paronychia and trauma to the nail matrix can result in this condition. It is a transient phenomenon and new plate usually grows back.

Washboard Nails

Washboard nail is a self induced deformity of the thumbs produce by the habit tic of pushing the proximal nail fold back with the index finger. They consist of close, irregularly placed, transverse grooves and ridges that only extend part way across the breadth of the nail plate. Healing of the nail fold occurs by stopping the behavior.

Pitting

This is a common nail disorder in children.

Etiology: Various theories for the formation of nail pits include pinpoint areas of aberrant keratinization (clusters of dyskeratotic cells or parakeratotic columns), matrix invasion by inflammatory cells (neutrophils microabscesses, as in psoriasis or lymphocytic exocytosis, as in pityriasis rosea), or localized spongiosis (as in eczema). It appears that spaces remain in place of loose cellular or acellular material that has been sloughed once the nail plate becomes exposed from under the proximal nail fold.

Clinical features: Pits are punctate depressions which may be small and shallow or large and deep, involving few or all 20 nails **(Figure 14.2).** Isolated clusters of pits are found in normal persons or those who have suffered localized trauma to the nail matrix. Shallow pits which are randomly distributed are seen in inflammatory dermatoses e.g. psoriasis. Regularly spaced pits arranged in transverse rows resembling Beau's lines are characteristic of alopecia areata.

Multiple Longitudinal Nail Grooves

These are a prominent finding with thin nail plates due to any cause. They may be due to decreased nail matrix volume or of alterations of normal ridged configuration of the matrix and nail bed. These nail findings may be seen in patients with lichen planus, chronic graft versus host disease, psoriasis, Darier's disease, alopecia areata, connective tissue diseases, frostbite or chilblains.

Onychauxis

Thickening or hypertrophy of the nail plate due to any cause is termed onychauxis. It should not be overinterpreted in children under the age of 10 years. Toenail thickening could just represent a reactive change, in the early stages of walking. The immature muscles of the foot can direct the toe so that the digit pulp is plantar flexed, which makes the free edge of the nail tap against the ground. This makes the nail react with hypertrophy and also subungual hyperkeratosis.

Diseases of the Nail Bed

Oncholysis or separation of the nail plate from the nail bed may be caused by numerous diseases in a child. It may be accompanied by accumulation of subungual debris. The various causes of onycholysis in children are: trauma; inflammatory disorders such as psoriasis, alopecia areata, lichen planus, dermatitis, drugs such as tetracyclines, retinoid and antineoplastic agents; chemicals such as alkaline detergents, organic solvents, cosmetics, depilatories and nail polish removers; systemic diseases such as connective tissue diseases; hypo or hyperthyroidism and iron deficiency anemia and infections such as onychomycosis, candidiasis, herpetic whitlow, bacterial paronychia and warts.

ALTERATIONS IN NAIL SIZE

Anonychia/Micronychia

Anonychia refers to total or partial absence of nails at birth and is rare. Congenital anonychia may be an isolated inherited trait or may be associated with other malformations of ectodermal or mesodermal origin. Acquired anonychia may occur due to severe inflammatory involvement of the nail unit as in Stevens-Johnsons Syndrome or may occur after pterygium formation.

Micronychia or nail hypoplasia can occur in children whose mothers have been exposed to anticonvulsant drugs, alcohol or warfarin. The degree of hypoplasia may vary from a minimal decrease in size to complete absence on different digits of the same patient.

Polyonychia

This condition may accompany any of the micronychias. Radiological evaluation should be done of the digits for underlying bone duplications. A history of maternal teratogen exposure should be sought and chromosomal analysis should be beneficial. Polyonychia and polydactyly may be inherited as an isolated autosomal trait, or may be associated with trisomy 13 or Laurence Moon-Biedl syndrome.

DISEASES OF THE NAIL BED

ONYCHOLYSIS

Onycholysis or separation of the nail plate from the nail bed can frequently be accompanied by accumulation of subungual debris. Causes of onycholysis in children include trauma; inflammatory disorders such as psoriasis, alopecia areata, lichen planus and dermatitis: drugs such as organic solvents, depilatories, nail polish removers, cosmetics, systemic diseases such as connective tissue diseases, hypo- or hyperthyroidism, iron deficiency anemia and infections such as onychomycosis, candidiasis, bacterial paronychia, warts and herpetic whitlow.

TRAUMATIC NAIL DISORDERS

Ingrown nails are a frequent disorder in school going children. An important predisposing factor is congenital malalignment of the great toenails. Improper nail trimming, occlusive footwear and traumatic injuries may also contribute to the development of nail ingrowing.

The clinical features of ingrown toenails can be divided into three stages.

Stage 1: Embedding of the nail spicula within the lateral nail fold producing pain, redness, and swelling of the nail fold. Treatment is conservative with extraction of the spicula and introduction of a package of non-absorbent cotton under the lateral corner of the nail every few days.

Stage 2: There is formation of granulation tissue that covers the nail plate. Topical steroids of high potency under occlusion for a few days can be used for treatment followed by conservative treatment as in stage 1.

Stage 3: The epidermis of the lateral nail fold covers the granulation tissue. Surgical treatment with selective destruction of the lateral horn of the nail matrix is required.

NAIL BITING AND ONYCHOTILLOMANIA

It has been estimated that upto 33 percent of 7 to 10 years old bite their nails for short periods of time, with the incidence increasing to 45 percent during adolescence. Nail biting could be familial, can result from poorly manicured nails or from anxiety and stress from sibling rivalry, parental disharmony or boredom.

The complications of nail biting (onychophagia) are ingrown nails, paronychia, or warts. It may be a sign of pathology such as Lesch-Nyhan syndrome or onychotillomania. Nail biting is discontinued by most children as they grow up. Treatment consists of minimizing precipitating stresses and also relaxation imagery techniques. Frequent application of distasteful topical preparations on the nail and peruingual skin can be discouraging for children to bite and chew their fingernails.

PARONYCHIA

Paronychia usually follows minor trauma, ingrown nails or sucking of the thumbs and fingers. Acute paronychia is usually caused by Staphylococcus aureus or herpes simplex virus or candida. Paronychia is characterized by erythema, swelling, pus formation and pain of the proximal or lateral nail folds with wet glistening or dry fissured surfaces. Whenever required, cultures should be taken to identify the responsible organism. Treatment would include application of clotrimazole solution several times daily when candida is suspected, incision and drainage of the abscess, systemic antibiotics or acyclovir depending on the etiology and prevention of finger sucking in children.

LEUKONYCHIA

Leukonychia or white nails, may present with total or partial involvement or striate or punctate configurations. Leukonychia can actually result from opacification of the nail plates by abnormal keratinization, retention of cell nuclei or formation of air pockets from reabsorbed acellular debris. The causes of hereditary or congenital leukonychia are associations with duodenal ulcer, sebaceous cysts and renal calculi, or LEOPARD syndrome. Punctate leukonychia can be caused by minor repeated trauma to the nail matrix or congenital candidiasis. The transverse striate variety is associated with Stevens-Johnson syndrome, febrile illness, metal poisoning or chemotherapy. Total leukonychia can be seen in vitiligo or treatment with sulfonamides. Punctate leukonychia regresses by avoiding traumas.

NAIL CHANGES IN PRIMARY CUTANEOUS DISORDERS

ECZEMA

Childhood eczema affects the periungual tissues and thus causes inflammation of the nail matrix which, in turn, will give rise to nail abnormalities such as transverse ridges, grooves or Beau's lines. Onycholysis may also result due to eczematous involvement of fingertips. In childhood, the eczema may be part of atopic dermatitis or irritant dermatitis for which finger or thumb sucking is a common cause. The complications can be loss of cuticle and paronychia. Treatment would consist of preventing finger and thumb sucking and also treatment with moderate or high potency steroids.

LICHEN PLANUS

Nail lichen planus is considered to be very rare in children and is more common in boys than girls. It may be underestimated in children due to lack of skin or mucosal lesions and the general reluctance to perform nail biopsies. Lichen planus of the nails in children may have three different clinical presentations: Typical nail lichen planus, 20-nail dystrophy **(Figures 14.3A and B)**, and

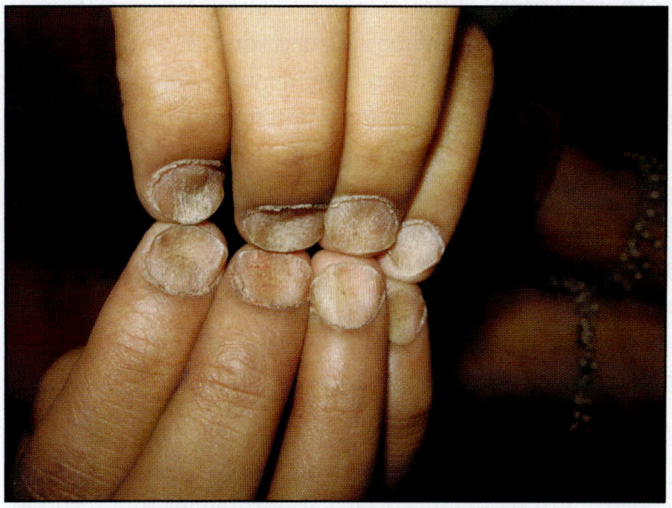

FIGURE 14.3A: Lichen planus of nail

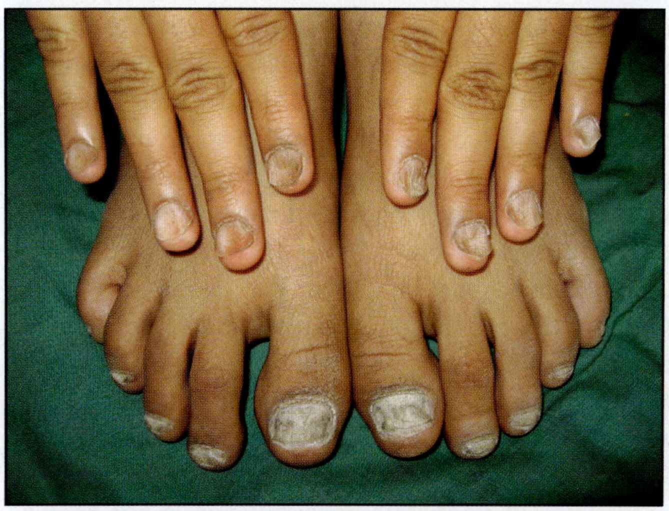

FIGURE 14.3B: Twenty nail dystrophy (lichen planus)

idiopathic atrophy of the nails. In most cases, nail lichen planus in children has the same characteristics as that of adults, i.e. diffuse nail ridging, thinning, splitting and dorsal pterygium. If this variety is not treated, it may produce nail matrix destruction with scarring in both adults and children.

Twenty nail dystrophy will be discussed separately. Idiopathic atrophy of the nails is more common in Indians and has an acute and rapid course that leads to painless nail destruction. Systemic steroids are effective in treating this condition and prevent destruction of the nail matrix. Oral prednisolone 0.5 mg/kg every other day for 2-6 weeks may be helpful.

PSORIASIS

Nail involvement in childhood psoriasis varies from 7 to 39% and the clinical manifestations are nearly the same as that of adults, although nail bed involvement is usually absent or mild. Nail pitting is a common feature of psoriasis in children with large, deep, irregularly scattered pits within the nail plate. The other important feature is onycholysis surrounded by an erythematous border as well as salmon patches. Subungual hyperkeratosis and splinter hemorrhages are rare in children with psoriasis. Nail psoriasis has a chronic unpredictable course and complete remissions are uncommon.

TWENTY NAIL DYSTROPHY

Synonym: Trachyonychia

Twenty nail dystrophy or trachyonychia describes a spectrum of nail plate surface abnormalities that result in roughness of the nails. This condition is caused by several inflammatory disorders which disturb nail matrix keratinization such as LP, psoriasis, alopecia, areata, eczema and pemphigus vulgaris. The definitive diagnosis can only be established by a nail biopsy which would either reveal typical features of lichen planus or psoriasis in trachyonychia, or spongiotic changes in trachyonychia due to alopecia areata.

The patients may be divided into two major groups: One with personal history or clinical evidence of alopecia areata; second with isolated nail involvement (idiopathic trachyonychia). In upto 12% of children with alopecia areata, this nail disorder is observed either preceding or following the onset of hair loss by years. The exact prevalence of idiopathic trachyonychia is not known. Trachyonychia can be opaque or shiny. In the former, the nails show excessive longitudinal striations with loss of nail lustre. The surface of the nail plate is brittle, friable and covered with small scales or keratin. In shiny trachyonychia, nail roughness is less severe and is caused by numerous small pits.

Twenty nail dystrophy is a benign condition and may not involve all 20 nails. It can regress spontaneously over several years. Nail scarring does not usually occur. Nail fragility can be treated with topical emollients and administration of systemic biotin.

WARTS

Warts are common on skin areas bordering the nail plate, especially in habitual biters. The nail plate may be displaced or compressed by the enlarging growth. In young children, surgical procedures should be avoided and treatment should be as conservative as possible. Topical immunotherapy with strong sensitizers such as squaric acid dibutylester (SADBE) or diphencyprone 2% in acetone used for 21 days followed by weekly applications with dilutions selected according to the patient's response may be effective. Complete cure usually requires 3-4 months.

GENODERMATOSES

Epidermolysis Bullosa

Nail changes are common yet not specific to the EB subtypes **(Figures 14.4A and B)**. Permanent nail loss may be caused by extensive and repetitive blistering. In autosomal recessive junctional epidermolysis bullosa, the nails appear thick and short and develop recurrent periungual and subungual hemorrhagic blisters.

PACHYONYCHIA CONGENITA

Synonym: Jadassohn-Lewandowsky Syndrome

Pachyonychia congenita, is an autosomal dominant disorder characterized by hyperkeratosis of the nails beds, and often the palmoplantar skin. Although four different types of pachyonychia congenita have been recognized, nail abnormalities are a constant feature and usually develop in childhood. Progressive nail changes include gross thickening of nails with discoloration from yellow to brown. Subungual hyperkeratosis that is most pronounced distally is severe, resulting in elevation of

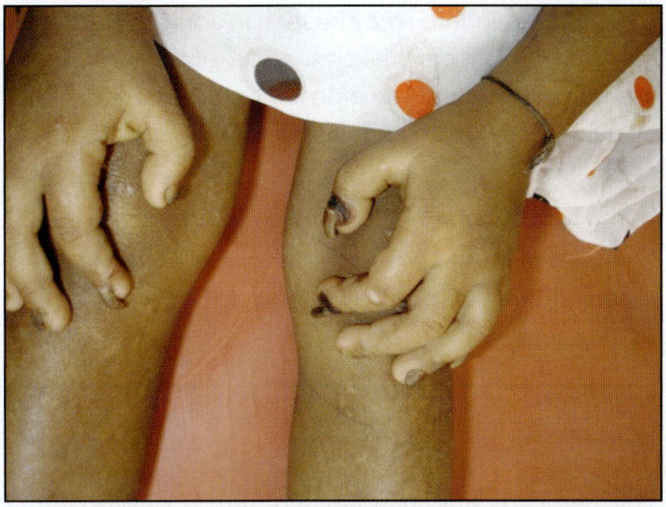

FIGURE 14.4A: Nail changes in recessive dystrophic epidermolysis bullosa

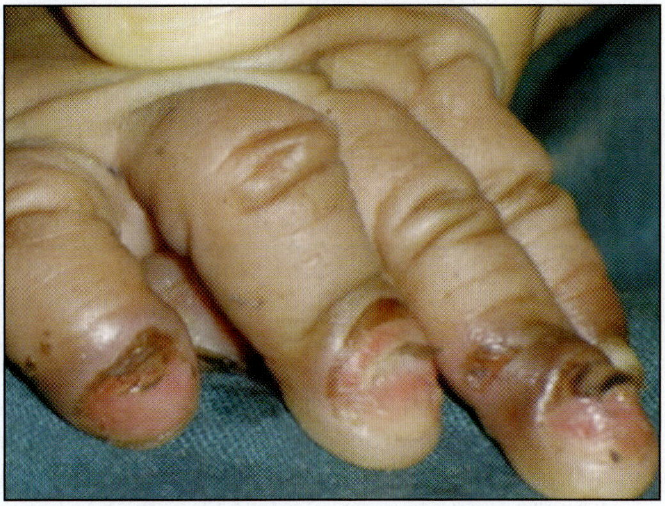

FIGURE 14.4 B: Absence of nail in dystrophic epidermolysis bullosa

the nail plate and separation from the nail bed at the tip of the finger. The condition can be treated surgically or by using a carbon dioxide laser with excision of the hyperkeratotic nail bed.

NAIL PATELLA SYNDROME

This is an autosomal dominant disorder that presents with congenital absence or hypoplasia of the nails and patella associated with other bone and kidney abnormalities. The thumb nails and great toenails are affected most severely. Nail changes consist of the characteristic triangular shaped lunula, as well as ridging, spooning, discoloration and cracking. The characteristic bone abnormalities are absent or present as hypoplastic patella, radial head abnormalities and iliac crest exostosis. A nephropathy may develop in 40% of all cases and 5.5 to 8% of cases may develop renal insufficiency. There is no specific treatment for the affected nails.

ECTODERMAL DYSPLASIAS

The children affected with ectodermal dysplasias present with dystrophic nails, the nails showing variable features depending on the different syndromes. Nail hypoplasia is frequently associated with thickening of the nail plate.

PERIUNGUAL FIBROMAS

Periungual fibromas in children are usually a sign of tuberous sclerosis. They appear as firm, flesh colored, smooth tumors that originate in the periungual groove and usually extend outward over the nail plate. A groove may be produced in the nail plate due to compression of the nail matrix. These are usually asymptomatic and require no treatment. Large lesions may require surgical excision.

NAIL CHANGES IN SYSTEMIC DISORDERS

KOILONYCHIA

Koilonychia refers to spoon-shaped nail plates. There is a central concavity surrounded by upturned lateral and distal margins **(Figure 14.5)**. Koilonychia may be seen in newborns and young infants which spontaneously resolve over a few years. Sometimes, in psoriasis or onychomycosis, distal subungual debris from the hyponychium may alter the direction of the growth of

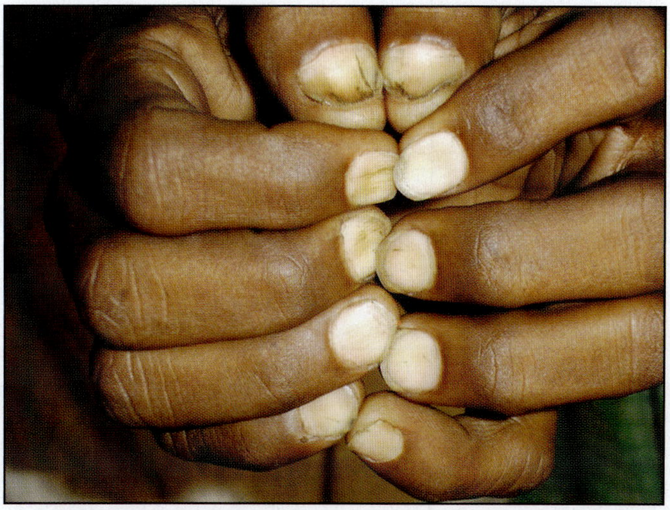

FIGURE 14.5: Koilonychia (iron-deficiency anemia)

the nail. Transitory koilonychia in children is a physiological disorder which recovers when the nail plate thickens with age.

Isolated koilonychias may be inherited as an autosomal dominant trait or may be associated with other syndromes. Koilonychia has been also associated with iron deficiency anemia. Although the mechanism of spooning in this condition remains speculative, it could be coincidental. Other systemic associations with koilonychias may be hemochromatosis, hypothyroidism, lichen planus, and the 20 nail dystrophy seen in children.

CLUBBING

Clubbing is recognized as a reliable sign of internal disease. This deformity results from hypertrophy and hyperplasia of the fibrovascular support stroma of the distal phalanx. An early sign of clubbing is increased flexibility of the proximal nail plate due to softened edematous underlying tissues. When viewed laterally, the angle formed by the proximal nail fold and nail plate exceeds 180 degrees.

Clubbing is seen in children with cyanotic congenital heart disease, cystic fibrosis, inflammatory bowel disease, malignancy such as Hodgkin's or non-Hogdkin's lymphoma, hypertrophic pulmonary osteoarthropathy as well as pachydermoperiostosis.

TABLE 14.2: Causes of clubbing in children

System	Disease
Pulmonary	Cystic fibrosis Bronchiectasis Tuberculosis Aspergillosis Sarcoidosis Pulmonary fibrosis Tumors
Cardiovascular	Cyanotic congenital heart disease Subacute bacterial endocarditis Myxomas
Gastrointestinal	Inflammatory bowel disease Parasitosis Cirrhosis Chronic active hepatitis
Endocrine	Gardner syndrome Hypervitaminosis A Malnutrition
Hereditary	Pachydermoperiostosis Familial, isolated

Localized clubbing may be seen in aortic or subclavian artery aneurysm, brachial plexus injury, trauma, Mafucci's syndrome, gout and sarcoidosis. The causes of clubbing in children are given in **Table 14.2.**

SHELL NAILS

These are very similar to clubbed nails. They have been observed to be associated with bronchiectasis.

SPECIFIC NAIL CHANGES IN CARDIOPULMONARY DISEASES

The nail beds are cyanotic and Terry's onychodermal band is prominent in cyanotic congenital heart disease. A late clinical feature is clubbing. Chronic pulmonary disease, lymphedema and yellow, thickened, slow growing, onycholytic nails constitute the yellow nail syndrome, which is rare in children. The nail changes may precede or follow onset of pulmonary disease.

ENDOCRINE AND RHEUMATOLOGIC DISEASES

Dystrophic nails may be seen in hyperthyroidism or Grave's disease which has its onset in puberty. Brittle nails with horizontal furrows and leukonychia may be seen in hypoparathyroidism. The resistance to infections with candida albicans is diminished. Nailfold capillary loops as well as periodic acid-Schiff positive deposits are observed in some endocrine and rheumatologic diseases. Capillary dilatation can be observed in juvenile diabetes mellitus, whereas capillary dilatation and dropout can be seen in childhood scleroderma and dermatomyositis.

NAIL CHANGES ASSOCIATED WITH CHEMOTHERAPY IN CHILDREN

Nail matrix cells are continuously dividing and are frequently affected by chemotherapy. Chemotherapy induced nail changes may involve the nail matrix (e.g. Beau's line/onychomadesis, melanonychia), nail bed (e.g. onycholysis, subungual hemorrhage/hematoma), and proximal nail fold (e.g. paronychia, periungual pyogenic granuloma). The chemotherapeutic agents commonly inducing nail changes are cyclophosphamide, doxorubicin/

daunorubicin, 5-fluorouracil and vincristine. Transverse leukonychia, Murehrcke's lines (paired, white, transverse lines parallel to the lunula that disappear with pressure and do not grow out with the nail), Beau's lines, Mee's lines and trachyonychia are other changes seen in children receiving chemotherapy.

BIBLIOGRAPHY

1. Chen W, Yu YS, Liu YH, Sheen JM, Hsiao CC. Nail changes associated with chemotherapy in children. J Eur Acad Dermatol Venerol 2007;21:186-90.
2. de Berker D. Childhood nail diseases. Dermatol Clin 2006;24: 355-63.
3. Joste A, Piraccini BM, Cambiaghi S, Joreizzo M. Nail lichen planus in children. Clinical features, response to treatment and long term follow up. Arch Dermatol 2001;137:1027-32.
4. Khemani C, Khubchandani R. Beau's lines. Indian Pediatrics 2007;44:47.
5. Pappert A, Scher RK, Cohen JL. Nail disorders in children. Pediatric Clinics of North America 1991;38(4):921-40.
6. Rogers M. Nail manifestations of some important genetic disorders in children. Dermatologic Therapy 2002;15:111-120.
7. Sarkar R,Jain RK. Pachyonychia congenital type II. Pediatr Dermatol 2004;21(4):517-18.

15

Disorders of Cutaneous Appendages

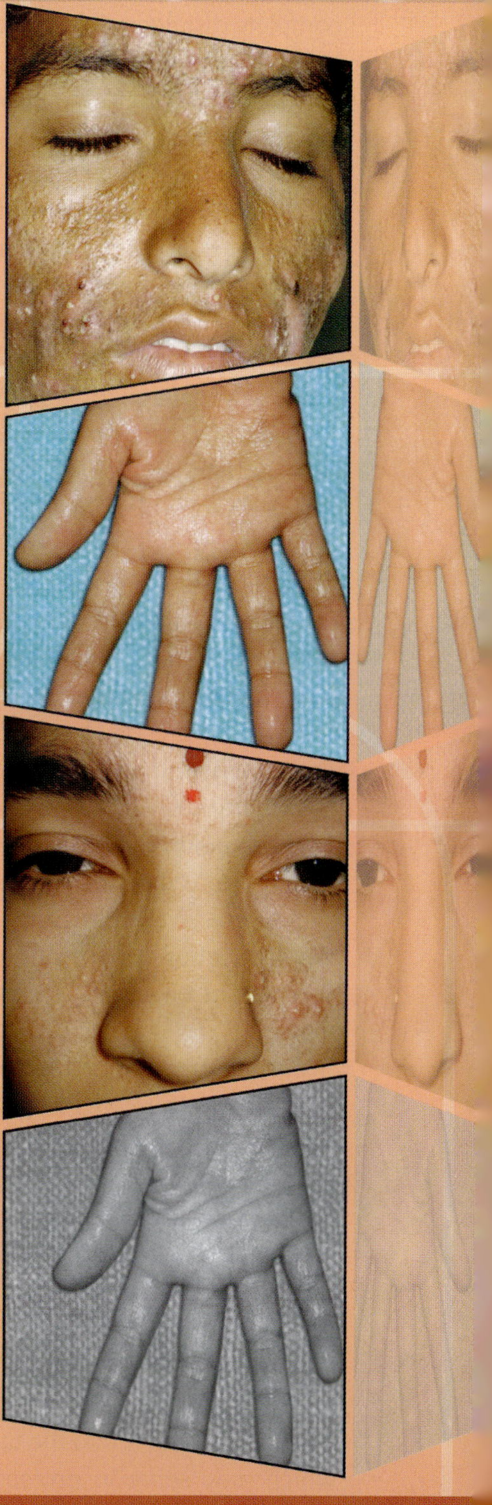

Devinder Mohan Thappa
Sowmya Kaimal

DISORDERS OF SEBACEOUS GLANDS

ANATOMY AND PHYSIOLOGY OF SEBACEOUS GLANDS

Sebaceous glands are holocrine in nature, secreting by complete disintegration of the glandular cells. Each gland consists of a series of lobes, each with a duct lined by keratinized squamous epithelium. Ducts of individual lobules converge towards the main sebaceous duct, which opens into the pilary canal. Acini within each gland vary in differentiation and maturity. The synthesis and discharge of the lipid contained in the sebaceous cells requires more than one week. Sebaceous glands are present everywhere, except on the palms and soles. These are largest and most numerous on the face, scalp, upper trunk, external auditory meatus and anogenital area. Free sebaceous glands open directly onto the surface of the skin, and these include the Meibomian glands of the eyelids, Tyson's glands of the prepuce, and Fordyce's spots on the margin of the upper lip.

Sebaceous glands are functional since its formation, sebum being the first demonstrable glandular product of the human body. The glands reach peak activity in the third trimester, and their secretion forms part of the vernix caseosa in the newborn. They remain active in the neonatal period and then involute and remain quiescent till puberty.

Human skin surface lipid contains glycerides, free fatty acids, wax esters, squalene, cholesterol esters and cholesterol. Wax esters and squalene are produced by the sebaceous glands only. Squalene is an important component of sebum and is virtually unique to human species.

Sebum has several functions in humans. The lipid film controls moisture loss from the epidermis and protects the skin from fungal and bacterial infection. The view that sebum may have a fungistatic property is supported by the fact that fungi preferentially colonize areas that are not rich in sebaceous glands. This is also the reason for rare occurrence of tinea capitis after puberty, when there is increased sebum production.

The colonization of the skin by *P. acnes* may have an immunomodulatory role. The sebaceous gland also secretes vitamin E into the upper layers of the facial skin, which may serve to protect skin surface lipid and the upper stratum corneum from harmful oxidation. Androgens are responsible for the development and maintenance of sebum secretion in both sexes, and are the most important hormones controlling sebaceous gland activity. Administration of testosterone dramatically increases the size of the sebaceous glands and the sebum output of pre-pubertal boys. In adult males, the glands are almost but not maximally stimulated by endogenous androgen. The secretion of sebum by adult women is only a little less than that of normal men. The effect of progesterone on sebaceous glands is controversial, but estrogens undoubtedly depress sebaceous activity. Many pituitary hormones including gonadotrophins, growth hormone, and alpha-melanocyte-stimulating hormone (α-MSH) promote sebum secretion.

ACNE

The term acne encompasses a group of disorders, including acne vulgaris and its variants. Acne vulgaris is a common and easily recognizable dermatological disorder. It is seen in almost all individuals at some stage of life. Small, non-inflamed acne lesions may not be more than a slight nuisance, but, in individuals with more severe inflammatory nodular acne, pain, social embarrassment and both physical and psychological scarring can affect the quality of life immensely. The pediatric dermatologist and the pediatrician have an important role in shaping the future of youngsters prone to acne. Approximately 40% of adolescents below the age of 15 years will develop acne and in 15% of these patients, the acne is sufficiently troublesome to merit a visit to their physician. Pubertal acne may last 3-6 years, but significant clinical lesions may last much longer, often more than 8 years. In a minority of patients, this can persist for more than 20 years.

There are four key factors in the pathogenesis of acne. These include:

- Follicular epithelial hyper-proliferation and resultant follicular plugging
- Excess sebum
- Presence and hyperactivity of *Propionibacterium acnes*,
- Inflammation.

The earliest lesion present in acne vulgaris is the micro-comedone which is the precursor of other acne lesions. This lesion is characterized by follicular plugging. The stimulus for micro-comedone formation is still unknown.

Leading hypotheses implicate androgen hormones, alterations in follicular linoleic acid levels, and the inflammatory cytokine interleukin-1a (IL-1a). Subsequently, the micro-comedones fill up with *P. acnes*, whose cell wall and biological byproducts are chemo-attractant and pro-inflammatory. Later, inflammatory cells infiltrate the follicle, diffuse through the follicular wall, and produce enzymes that disrupt the follicular wall.

The degree of inflammation seen in acne vulgaris may be dependent upon individual immune responsiveness to *P. acnes*. Likewise, there may be individual variability in the response of the sebaceous gland androgen receptor to circulating androgens. Recently, the toll-like receptor 2 (TLR-2) has been implicated in the pathogenesis of acne. TLR-2 is a pattern recognition receptor that is activated by *P. acnes*. When bound, TLR-2 activates a transcription factor that up regulates production and the release of pro inflammatory cytokines like interleukin-12 and interleukin-8 from monocytes. TLR-2 is expressed on the infiltrating inflammatory cells around the pilosebaceous follicle in individuals with acne. Its expression increases as the acne lesion ages and becomes more inflamed.

The role of androgen hormones in the pathogenesis of acne has also been carefully evaluated. Overall, circulating androgen hormone levels are normal in individuals with acne who do not have other signs or symptoms of hyper-androgenism. The enzyme 5α-reductase type 1 has been studied in those with and without acne. It is present in the sebaceous gland and converts testosterone to the more potent androgen receptor ligand, dihydrotestosterone (DHT). It has been hypothesized that those with acne might have more active 5α-reductase type1. However, no statistically significant difference in enzyme activity has been observed to date between those with and without acne.

CLINICAL FEATURES

Acne is a disease of the pilosebaceous follicles and therefore affects the face and upper trunk. Physical signs of acne are seborrhea, non-inflamed lesions (whiteheads, blackheads), superficial inflamed lesions (papules, superficial pustules) and deep inflamed lesions (nodules). Scarring can occur at any age including as early as 9 or 10 years.

Seborrhea is due to excessive production of sebum by acne-prone follicles.

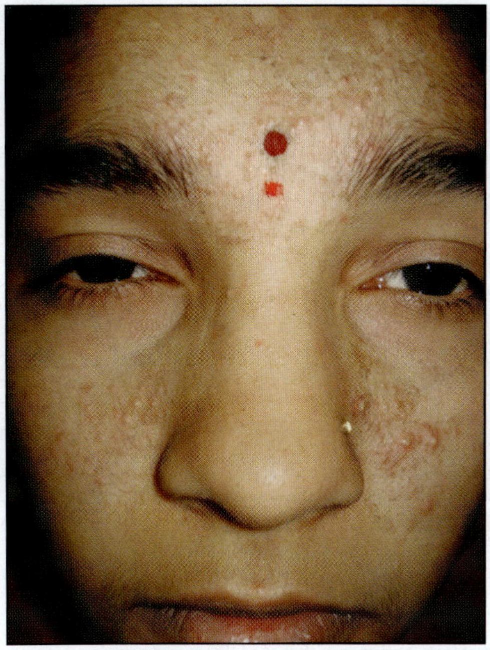

FIGURE 15.1: Acne vulgaris

Blackheads or open comedones vary in size from almost microscopic to 2-3 mm. The black tip of the comedone results from oxidization of melanin. Whiteheads, or closed comedones, outnumber blackheads by as much as 10 or 20 to one. They are very small, usually less than 1 mm, skin-colored, pink or white papules or macules. Non-inflamed lesions precede inflamed lesions **(Figure 15.1)**. They can be seen 2-3 years prior to the onset of significant inflammatory acne and it is perhaps at this early stage that intervention could prevent the development of significant clinical acne.

Papules can vary in size from 0.5 to 9 mm and develop through a phase of natural progression lasting from a few to 14 days. These may be bright red, termed as 'active papules' or dull red termed as 'less active papules'. Similarly, pustules can be divided into active and less active pustules depending on their size and intensity. The duration of the pustule is less than that of the papule because of the patient's natural tendency to squeeze these lesions. Nodules refer to large inflammatory lesions (1 cm/>) and may persist for many weeks to months **(Figure 15.2)**. These usually produce scarring.

Scarring is not infrequent in the pediatric age-group and can either be associated with loss or increase of collagen. Loss of collagen may present as fairly well-defined depressed scars which are irregular, occur particularly on the face and are referred to as 'ice-pick' scars. 'Atrophic macular scars' present as superficial,

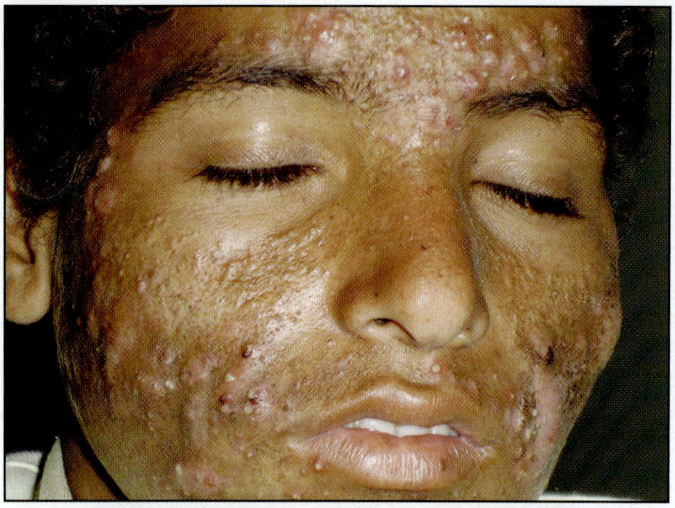

FIGURE 15.2: Nodulocystic acne in adolescent

shallow depressions with wrinkling of the epidermis. Scarring associated with increased collagen, like hypertrophic scars and keloids are less frequent.

The initial site of acne is often the face, particularly the cheeks and forehead, but with time, lesions frequently spread to involve all areas of face, as well as the neck and trunk. Rarely a patient is seen with little or no facial acne but considerable truncal acne. In extreme cases, it may extend to the arms, forearms, as well as to the buttocks and upper thighs.

Acne can precede menarche, but 85% of the patients presenting to the pediatric dermatologist will have established menstruation. Pre-menstrual flare of the acne is evident in about 20% of children compared to 65% of adults. Acne can cause considerable psychological morbidity as evident by increased anxiety, depression, loss of social esteem and inability to mingle with the peers. Significant acne and scarring in adolescence may hamper relationships with opposite sex, as well as difficulties in future employment. Hence, the importance of treating acne early should be emphasized.

DIFFERENTIAL DIAGNOSIS

The commonest misdiagnosis is rosacea (occurs in older individuals, has facial flushing, typically pustules occurring over erythematous background, localization of lesions to mid-face, absence of seborrhea, comedones, nodules, cyst or scarring). Perioral eczema /dermatitis may be mistaken as acne in females, but the lesions are itchy, the skin is dry and there are no comedones. Whiteheads may resemble milia (present predominantly in infraorbital location and are whiter). Acneiform eruptions are sudden onset, follicular monomorphic eruptions characterized by papules and pustules resembling acne, induced by exposure to various drugs or chemicals. Rarely acne vulgaris need to be differentiated from pityrosporum folliculitis, acne agminata, adenoma sebaceum, pseudofolliculitis barbae and plane warts.

TREATMENT

The patho-mechanism of acne suggests that combination therapy should be utilized as early as possible, preferably at the beginning.

In mild comedonal acne with a few inflammatory lesions, topical retinoids are thought to be the treatment of choice. This affects the micro-comedone formation and lead to a decrease in these lesions. Addition of antimicrobial therapy is synergistic to this action. For inflammatory lesions, benzoyl peroxide and/or topical antibiotics, along with the topical retinoid, speed up the clearing of lesions.

For moderate to severe acne, oral antibiotics combined with topical retinoids are appropriate. In severe, refractory cases oral isotretinoin is the treatment of choice. Topical therapy should be used for the entire duration of acne treatment; used alone in mild acne, combined with oral therapy in moderate to severe cases and as maintenance therapy when oral treatment has been discontinued. Oral antibiotics should initially be continued for 6 months but occasionally several courses may be necessary, each for 6 months duration. A subgroup of patients may require treatment for up to 48 months and when required, this is safe in the pediatric age group.

Multiple whiteheads are a major cause of poor response. Multiple macrocomedones rarely respond to topical retinoids. It is usually necessary to treat these lesions with light cautery after applying of a local anesthetic cream. The aim is to produce thermal damage encouraging the patient's own local immune mechanisms to aid resolution of the lesions.

Antibiotic resistance of *Propionibacterium acnes* is another important reason for treatment failure. Patients who fail to respond to adequate antibiotic treatment or relapse while on antibiotic therapy or in those who have been treated with multiple different topical and systemic antibiotics, *P. acnes* resistance should be suspected. It is more likely to develop with erythromycin (65%), clindamycin (65%), tetracyclines (40%) and doxycycline (40%) but less frequent with trimethoprim and rarely encountered with minocycline. Combination of benzoyl peroxide dramatically reduces *P. acnes* count in case of erythromycin resistance. Treatment with isotretinoin may occasionally be necessary.

A further cause of poor response is cystic acne. A recent large nodule should be treated for 5 days with the topical application of a potent steroid such as clobetasol propionate cream applied sparingly twice daily or by intralesional injection of triamcinolone. If a large nodular lesion has been present for over two weeks, then cryotherapy is the preferred treatment. Patients can often tolerate 20s freezing with little discomfort. The aim of this treatment is to encourage polymorphonucleocytes to enter into the nodule, which is developing early fibrosis, and redirect the process from one of fibrosis towards resolution. In addition to the treatment of individual nodular lesions, severe acne requires oral isotretinoin. Severe acne in the absence of nodulocystic lesions and acne variants also respond poorly to conventional therapy.

Oral isotretinoin should be prescribed at the onset in a patient with severe acne. Patients with moderate acne unresponsive to repeated courses of antibiotic therapy, those at risk of scarring and those with significant psychological disturbance related to their acne should also receive this therapy. Isotretinoin is uniquely effective as it acts on all four major etiological factors in acne. The recommended dose is 0.5-1.0 mg/kg per day for an average period of fourth month. The dose of the isotretinoin can be adjusted to optimize response and minimize side-effects. These consist predominantly of mucocutaneous symptoms of cheilitis, conjunctivitis, xeroderma, dermatitis and secondary skin infection with *S. aureus*.

Treatment guidelines for acne vulgaris are summarized in the **Table 15.1.**

All patients with acne expect and deserve a brief explanation of their disease. Diet, dirt, soap and water, topically applied acne gels, and realistic expectations for cures seem to be the most important subjects to emphasize in the written or oral teaching of patients with acne. Poor compliance is undoubtedly the most important reason for the treatment failure. In order to improve compliance, especially in less educated people, the strategy of the treatment has to be very carefully prepared. The following action plan can facilitate patient treatment adherence **(Flow Chart 15.1)**.

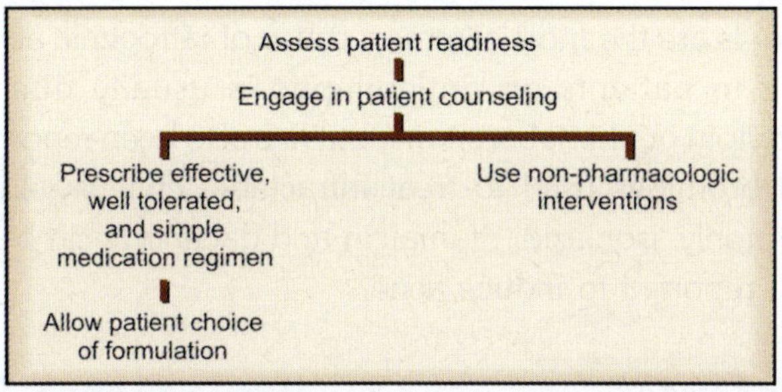

Flow Chart 15.1: Dermatologic plan of action for facilitating treatment adherence

ACNE VARIANTS

Neonatal, Infantile and Juvenile Acne

Acne may rarely occur in neonates or in the first 18 months of life and often persists until the age of 3 or 4 years. Males are more frequently affected and the face is virtually always involved.

TABLE 15.1: Treatment guidelines for acne vulgaris

Grade 1 (Mild)	**Grade II-III (Moderate)**	**Grade IV (Severe)**	**Maintenance**
Topical retinoids Benzoyl peroxide (BPO) or topical antibiotic	Topical retinoids BPO or topical antibiotic Oral antibiotic Hormone therapy (females only)	Isotretinoin or Topical retinoids, oral antibiotics, hormone therapy (females only)	Topical retinoids ± BPO

The sebaceous glands of neonates produce a considerable amount of sebum in the first few weeks of life due to the effect of maternal androgens. Many infants have tiny whitish yellow papules over the nose, forehead and cheeks as a result of the sebaceous hyperplasia. After three months of age the glands atrophy, seborrhea declines and the lesions disappear over a 2-3-month period.

Mild, predominantly inflammatory lesions should be treated with benzoyl peroxide predominant comedones should be treated with a topical retinoid. A combination of both therapies is necessary for mixed pattern. Moderate cases require 6 months of oral erythromycin 125 mg twice daily.

Drug-induced Acne

Steroids are the most common cause of iatrogenic acne. Acne in patients on antiepileptic is usually due to phenytoin or phenobarbitone, but has also been reported with bromides used to treat intractable epilepsy. Less commonly, isoniazid, rifampicin and dactinomycin have been reported to induce acne.

Acne Excoriee

Some anxious patients may pick and scratch their lesions producing the clinical picture of acne excoriee. The importance of not picking their skin must be emphasized to patients. Systemic treatment is often required as they are often reluctant to use topical therapy.

Acne Fulminans

Acne fulminans is a rare ulcerative form of acne which most commonly affects adolescent boys. It has an acute onset and is associated with systemic symptoms such as fever, weight loss, arthralgia, myalgia, erythema nodosum and hepato-splenomegaly.

Etiology is uncertain; presence of microscopic hematuria, erythema nodosum, increased response to *P. acnes* antigen in skin tests and depressed response to intradermal purified protein derivative in some patients are all in favor of an abnormal immunological response.

These patients require urgent dermatological review and admission to hospital is occasionally necessary. Immediate treatment is oral prednisolone, at an initial dose of 0.5-1.0 mg/kg per day, which should be continued for a minimum of 2-3 months to prevent relapse. It should be combined with oral isotretinoin.

Hyperandrogenism

Hyperandrogenism should be considered in a young girl, especially between 18 months and 7 years of age. These children present with acne, precocious puberty, hirsutism, menstrual dysfunction and obesity. The most common cause of hyperandrogenism in a teenage girl is polycystic ovary syndrome. The differential diagnosis includes exaggerated adrenarche, late-onset congenital adrenal hyperplasia, virilizing tumors, Cushing's syndrome, hyperprolactinemia, acromegaly and local abnormalities of androgen action or metabolism. Plasma-free testosterone is a sensitive indicator of hyperandrogenism. The pattern of response of plasma-free testosterone, DHEA and cortisol to dexamethasone suppression testing identifies the source of excess androgen.

Gram-negative Folliculitis

This occurs as a complication of long-term antibiotic therapy. Clinical features usually consist of sudden onset of multiple pustules frequently localized to the perioral and perinasal areas. Occasionally the condition can present with nodular lesions or simply as flare of ordinary acne. The organisms isolated include *Escherichia coli*, *Proteus*, *Pseudomonas* and *Klebsiella*. The existing antibiotic has to be changed to trimethoprim 300 mg twice daily or isotretinoin. As relapse common when trimethoprim is stopped, isotretinoin is often the treatment of choice.

Acne Conglobata

This is a very severe form of acne characterized by deep nodules, interconnecting sinuses and grouped comedones. This rarely occurs in children. Isotretinoin is the preferred mode of therapy but relapse is common and re-treatment with isotretinoin is frequently required.

Steatocystoma Multiplex

This is a nevoid condition that shows a mixture of keratinizing epithelium, and sebaceous lobules, attached to the epidermis by a thin epidermal strand histopathologically. It is an uncommon condition, associated in some patients with type 2 pachyonychia congenita (Jackson-Lawler syndrome). These cases are found to have mutations in the keratin 17 (K17) gene. Clinically, lesions are multiple, smooth, elastic, yellow dermal swellings (few mm to 20 mm) on the trunk and limbs. They tend to appear or enlarge at puberty, with little tendency to spontaneous resolution. When the cysts rupture, inflammation may occur, with lesions mimicking acne conglobata; this is termed steatocystoma multiplex suppurativa. The condition is difficult to treat. Surgical excision can be done for larger cysts. Antibiotics (tetracycline/ minocycline) or oral isotretinoin do not affect the primary disease process, but may be given for short periods of time to tide over episodes of inflammation.

DISEASES OF ECCRINE SWEAT GLANDS

ANATOMY AND PHYSIOLOGY OF HUMAN ECCRINE GLANDS

Eccrine sweat glands are tubular coiled adnexal structures which produce and secrete sweat directly on to the skin-surface. The gland consists of a secretory coil in the lower dermis and subcutaneous tissue and a duct leading through the dermis to the intra-epidermal sweat duct unit.

These are distributed over the entire skin surface, including the glans penis and the foreskin, but absent on lips, external ear canal, clitoris and labia majora. They are most numerous on the palms, soles and axillae. The glands vary in size from person to person and this probably accounts for individual as well as regional variations in sweat secretion (maximal individual rate ranging from 2 to 20 ml/min/gland).

Embryologically, eccrine sweat glands are derived from a specialized down-growth of the epidermis known as the eccrine gland germ. Normally, 2–4 million such glands are present at birth, which may become fully functional only by the age of two years. New eccrine glands are not developed after birth.

The physiological stimuli for sweating include thermal, osmotic, mental and gustatory stimuli. Thermoregulatory sweating occurs especially on the upper trunk and face, but also on the whole body surface, including the palms and soles. Rise of core temperature is nine times more efficient than skin-surface temperature in stimulating sweating. Mental stimuli produce sweating especially on the palms and soles, perhaps to improve the grip at times of activity.

The functioning of eccrine sweat glands is dependent on intact non-myelinated C fibers of sympathetic nerve which are cholinergic.

The major function of sweat is thermoregulatory. Other minor functions include excretion of metabolites as well as absorption of topical medications.

CLASSIFICATION OF ECCRINE SWEAT GLAND DISORDERS

Hyperhidrosis (HH)

1. Generalized or involving large area
   a. Associated with a past history of spinal cord injuries
      i. HH caused by autonomic dysreflexia
      ii. HH with orthostatic hypotension
      iii. HH caused by post-traumatic syringomyelia
   b. Associated with peripheral neuropathies
      i. HH in familial dysautonomia (Riley-Day syndrome)
      ii. HH caused by congenital autonomic dysfunction with universal pain loss
      iii. HH on exposure to cold
   c. Associated with probable brain lesions
      i. Episodic HH with hypothermia (Hines-Bannick syndrome)
      ii. Episodic HH without hypothermia
      iii. Episodic HH with hypertension after brain injury
      iv. Olfactory HH
   d. Associated with intra-thoracic neoplasms or lesions
      Paroxysmal unilateral HH (caused by cervical rib, osteoma, pulmonary adenocarcinoma, bronchial cancer, mesothelioma)
   e. Associated with systemic illnesses
      Pheochromocytoma, Parkinson's disease, thyrotoxicosis, diabetes mellitus, congestive heart failure, menopause, anxiety, poisoning (insecticides, herbicides, mercury)
   f. Night sweats (nocturnal diaphoresis)
      i. Lymphoma (Hodgkin's disease)
      ii. Others (tuberculosis, endocarditis, hyperthyroidism, diabetes mellitus, insulinoma, vasculitis, pheochromocytoma, carcinoid, drug withdrawal, dysautonomic states, acromegaly)
   g. Compensatory
      i. After sympathectomy
      ii. Associated with diffuse anhidrosis
2. Localized or HH of relatively small area (<100 cm^2)
   a. Idiopathic unilateral circumscribed HH (nevus sudoriferous or functional eccrine nevus)
   b. Gustatory sweating associated with

i. Encephalitis, syringomyelia, diabetic neuropathies, herpes zoster parotitis, parotid abscesses, thoracic sympathectomy
ii. Auriculotemporal or Frey syndrome

c. HH reported to be associated with
Blue rubber-bleb nevus, glomus tumor, POEMS syndrome, burning foot syndrome (Gopalan's), causalgia, pachydermoperiostosis, pretibial myxedema

3. Emotional (palms, soles or axillae)

Hypohidrosis or Anhidrosis (AH)

1. Generalized or AH of relatively large area
   a. Caused by poral occlusion
      i. AH in papulosquamous, dermatitic or ichthyosiform lesions
      ii. AH in xerosis (including xerosis of atopic patients)
      iii. Acquired generalized AH (tropical anhidrotic asthenia?)
   b. Caused by absence of the sweat gland
      Anhidrotic ectodermal dysplasia (Christ-Siemens-Touraine syndrome)
   c. Caused by paucity, atrophy or dysfunction of the sweat gland
      i. AH in systemic sclerosis
      ii. AH in Fabry's disease (?)
   d. Caused by neuropathy
      i. Congenital sensory neuropathy
         - Type II (Riley-Day syndrome)
         - Type IV (congenital insensitivity to pain with AH)
      ii. Progressive segmental AH with Adie's atonic pupils (Ross' syndrome)
      iii. Progressive isolated segmental AH without tonic pupils
      iv. Autonomic insufficiency syndrome (postural hypotension and AH)
      v. Chronic idiopathic anhidrosis
      vi. Diabetic neuropathy
      vii. Guillain-Barre syndrome
      viii. Fabry's disease (?)
2. Localized or AH of relatively small area
   a. Caused by damage to the glands by infection, trauma, tumors, morphea, scars or inflammatory infiltrate
   b. Caused by local denervation (?)
      i. Incontinentia pigmenti (?)
      ii. Dermatomal vitiligo (?)
   c. Miscellaneous
      i. Follicular atrophoderma (Bazex syndrome)
      ii. Sjögren's syndrome

Sweat Retention Syndromes

1. Miliarias
   a. Miliaria crystallina
   b. Miliaria rubra (prickly heat)
   c. Miliaria profunda
2. Tropical anhidrotic asthenia
3. Transient acantholytic dermatoses (Grover's disease)
4. Dyshidrosis (pompholyx).

Chemotherapy-associated Eccrine Reactions

1. Neutrophilic eccrine hidradenitis
2. Eccrine squamous syringometaplasia.

HYPERHIDROSIS

Hyperhidrosis is the generalized or localized excessive production of sweat. There may be marked inter-individual physiological variation in thermoregulatory sweating. Generalized hyperhidrosis may be secondary to a variety of causes, important among which are; emotional outbursts, hypoglycemia, shock, pheochromocytoma, thyrotoxicosis, Cushing's syndrome, cocaine abuse, familial dysautonomia (Riley-Day syndrome), brain tumors or defervescence in patients with chronic infections. Hyperhidrosis related to systemic disease may persist during sleep, unlike that related to emotional stimuli.

Localized hyperhidrosis may be classified as
- Gustatory,
- In association with cutaneous disease
- Idiopathic.

Physiologic gustatory hyperhidrosis occurs over the lips, nose and forehead in normal individuals after eating spicy foods. This is postulated to be due to the release of substance P after intra-oral exposure to capsaicin.

Emotional or mental activity may increase sweating in certain areas, commonly, on the palms, soles and axillae. It is useful to keep in mind that mental activity (such as solving arithmetic) devoid of any clear emotional content may also provoke sweating.

Some primary cutaneous disorders are known to be associated with localized hyperhidrosis. Idiopathic circumscribed hyperhidrosis is a condition where the affected area may sweat continuously, or more commonly, with mental activity. Such an area may show normal histology or eccrine gland hypertrophy, and is therefore also called functional eccrine nevus or nevus sudoriferous.

PALMOPLANTAR HYPERHIDROSIS (FIGURE 15.3)

The sweating of palms and soles may be continuous or phasic. When continuous, it is worse in the summer and not so clearly precipitated by mental factors. When phasic, it is usually precipitated by minor emotional or mental activity, and seasonal variation is not marked. Palmoplantar hyperhidrosis, which occurs quite frequently in children, may be so severe that sweat drips from the fingertips on to the floor, or soaks through clothing and shoes. This causes great embarrassment and interferes with daily activities such as writing or playing a musical instrument. It may also be an aggravating factor in certain dermatoses such as juvenile plantar dermatosis, epidermolysis bullosa (Weber- Cockayne type), pompholyx, contact dermatitis (to footwear) and pitted keratolysis.

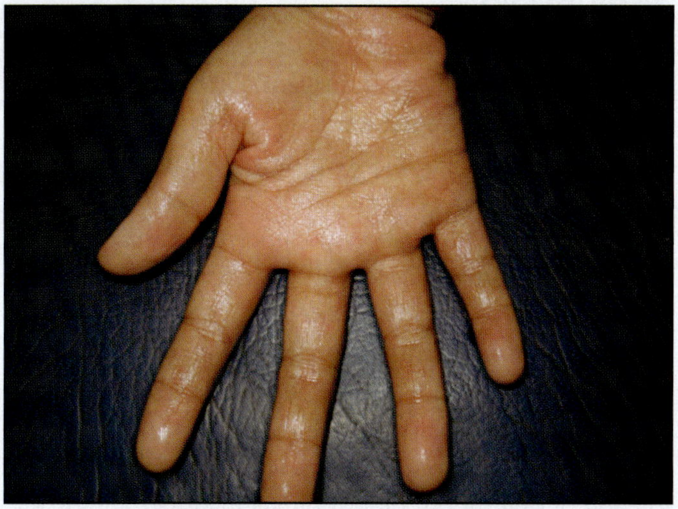

FIGURE 15.3: Palmar hyperhidrosis.

It is important to delineate the area of sweat dysfunction. This is achieved by certain test agents like starch-iodine, bromophenol blue, quinizarin, and the food dye edicol ponceau. In the starch-iodine test, iodine solution is applied to the affected area and surrounding normal skin. Starch powder is then sprinkled over the painted area and blown off. Individual sweat droplets show up as minute black dots at the eccrine pores. Due to significant regional and individual variations in the maximal sweat rate, care should be taken in interpreting the rate of sweating in a given patient. Therefore, it is important to obtain baseline maximal sweat rate (assessed by intradermal injection of 0.01% pilocarpine or methacholine).

TREATMENT OF HYPERHIDROSIS

See **Table 15.2.**

TABLE 15.2: Modalities of treatment for hyperhidrosis

A. *Medical*
1. Topical:
   Antiperspirants -
   - 20% aluminum hexahydrate in alcohol
   - 2 to 5% tannic acid solution
   - 5 to 20% formalin solution
   - 10% glutaraldehyde

   Anticholinergics—0.5% glycopyrronium bromide cream
   Topical 0.5% clonazepam
   Iontophoresis
   Botulinum toxin A injection
2. Systemic:
   - Tranquilizers—diazepam, clonazepam, amitriptyline
   - Anticholinergics—propantheline bromide, glycopyrrolate, oxybutynin, benztropine mesylate
   - NSAIDs—indomethacin
   - Calcium channel blockers—diltiazem
   - Clonidine hydrochloride

B. *Surgical:*
- Sympathectomy
- Excision of axillary sweat glands
- Liposuction
- Excision of hyperhidrotic skin

In general, choice of treatment of hyperhidrosis should be directed by the primary cause. Topical agents include anticholinergics and eccrine duct blocking agents (antiperspirants). Powders such as corn-starch may be temporarily beneficial. Topical anticholinergics are not reliable in general, except for topical 0.5% glycopyrronium bromide cream, which has been found to be effective for gustatory hyperhidrosis in diabetics. If hyperhidrosis involves a relatively small area, a number of topical antiperspirants may be used. Formalin soaks (1%) have been used for hyperhidrosis of the feet, but are unsuitable for the hands and axillae. Glutaraldehyde (10%) in a buffered solution is also suitable only for the feet because of its staining property. In addition, the later may cause allergic sensitization. Aluminium chloride is considered to be the best, but may irritate the skin and damage clothes. Other newer salts, such as aluminium chlorhydrate and hexahydrate may be cosmetically more acceptable. Solutions containing 20% aluminium chloride in absolute ethanol are applied at least two hours after bathing, left on overnight under occlusion, nightly at first, and then once in 1-4 weeks for maintenance. Mild irritation of the skin may be helped by a weak topical steroid.

Topical methenamine is a condensation product of formaldehyde and ammonia, which releases formaldehyde in solution, which in turn precipitates protein plugs in the sweat duct. It has been found that methenamine (10% solution) is superior to iontophoresis and faster acting than glutaraldehyde for palmoplantar hyperhidrosis, with fewer side effects.

Tap water iontophoresis is probably the most effective noninvasive method for controlling localized palmoplantar hyperhidrosis. It is thought that iontophoresis produces strong acidity by the generation of H^+ ions within the sweat duct. This results in leakiness of the sweat duct and sweat recycling that results in occlusion and collapse of the sweat pore lumen. This procedure enhances transdermal drug delivery when added to the water. Anticholinergic agents (e.g. poldine methyl sulfate, glycopyrronium bromide, atropine) may be added to the water, but this may cause mild side effects (dry mouth and eye) due to systemic absorption. Direct current is usually used, with each palm or sole being able to tolerate up to 0.2 mA/cm^2 of galvanic current without burn. Stinging can be avoided by a thin application of petrolatum. Treatment is for 30 minutes, initially 3 times a week, but once euhidrosis is achieved, monthly treatments may be sufficient for maintenance.

Botulinum A toxin has recently been used to treat localized hyperhidrosis, and is found to be very effective. The toxin blocks the release of acetylcholine from presynaptic terminals of the neuromuscular junction, and intradermal injection of small doses irreversibly inhibits sympathetic cholinergic production of sweat. Each axilla usually requires 12 injections, hands 20, and each foot 24-36 injections. The benefit begins within 48 hours after injection and lasts for 6-8 months, after which repeat injections may be necessary. Transient reduction of thenar and hypothenar muscle power is a minor problem after palmar injections. Also, the pain of injection makes the procedure difficult to perform without nerve blocks or general anesthesia, especially in children.

Use of oral anticholinergic agents is limited by side effects such as drowsiness, flushing and tachycardia, as well as their contraindication in asthmatic patients. However, low doses of glycopyrrolate (1-3 mg per oral once a day), or propantheline bromide (15 mg night dosage) may bring relief from symptoms in some individuals. Small doses of clonazepam may also be useful.

Axillary hyperhidrosis may be reduced by surgical curettage of the axillary vaults or tumescent liposuction of the axillae, with long-lasting benefit.

Finally, the most aggressive treatment for palmoplantar hyperhidrosis is transthoracic endoscopic sympathectomy done at the T_2-T_3 level. Results of surgery are gratifying, with a low recurrence rate, and this is an acceptable option in children with severe disability arising from palmar or axillary hyperhidrosis. Significant complications include Horner's syndrome, bradycardia requiring a cardiac pacemaker and rarely, postoperative pneumothorax. However, these are uncommon. Compensatory hyperhidrosis occurs in up to 80% of patients on the trunk, legs and face. This is more common in warm climates and is usually mild.

ANHIDROSIS

Anhidrosis or the absence of sweating may result either from an abnormality of the sweat gland or an insult to the central or peripheral nervous system, such as spinal cord transection, Horner's syndrome, familial sensory neuropathy and leprosy. Certain medications such as antihistamines and tricyclic antidepressants may produce significant anhidrosis due to their anticholinergic effects. Localized areas of anhidrosis are of little clinical importance except that these may help in the diagnosis of neurological lesions and leprosy. Generalized anhidrosis characteristically occurs in anhidrotic ectodermal dysplasia. Otherwise normal premature or full-term infants under the age of one month may show widespread anhidrosis. Severe anhidrosis may impair heat regulation to such an extent that it may result in hyperpyrexia.

Hypohidrosis may be an accompaniment of certain disorders where plugging of the sweat duct is a feature; these include miliaria, psoriasis and atopic dermatitis. Ross' syndrome is a rare condition in which widespread hypohidrosis occurs, with patchy, sometimes very striking, compensatory hyperhidrosis, tonic pupils and loss of deep tendon reflexes. Compensatory hyperhidrosis may be a feature in patients with hypohidrosis.

Whenever extensive anhidrosis is present, measures such as air conditioning or a fan, cool soaks and light clothing should be undertaken to reduce the likelihood of a heat stroke.

MILIARIA

Miliaria is one of the most common disorders of eccrine sweat glands. It denotes retention of eccrine sweat at various levels of the skin. Based on the level of ductal obstruction, there are three types of miliaria:

- miliaria crystallina (sudamina); ductal obstruction in the stratum corneum;
- miliaria rubra (prickly heat); ductal obstruction within the stratum malpighii;
- miliaria profunda (mamillaria); ductal obstruction at or below the dermoepidermal junction.

The characteristic histopathological finding in miliaria crystallina is an intracorneal or subcorneal vesicle arising from the acrosyringium of the sweat duct. In miliaria rubra, there are spongiotic vesicles in the stratum malpighii, which may be in communication with sweat ducts and a chronic inflammatory infiltrate surrounding the ducts. An amorphous, PAS- positive, diastase-resistant material can frequently be identified in the acrosyringium, which in older lesions, is replaced by a parakeratotic plug. In miliaria profounda, rupture of the intradermal duct below the dermoepidermal junction is seen with marked lymphocytic infiltration of the adjacent dermis, as well as spongiosis of the intraepidermal portion of the duct.

The role of bacterial colonization and overgrowth on the skin surface has been extensively studied to explain the pathogenesis of miliaria. A complex PAS-positive extracellular polysaccharide substance (EPS) produced exclusively by *Staphylococcus epidermidis* has finally been confirmed to have a central role in the pathogenesis of miliaria.

Miliaria crystallina is characterized by a diffuse crops of 1 to 2 mm, monomorphic superficial asymptomatic vesicles on a non-inflamed base, typically appearing on the trunk, sometimes resembling "drops of water." The onset occurs after days to weeks of excessive exposure to heat and humidity, especially in tropical areas or during summer months. Miliaria crystallina may also be frequently seen following profuse sweating accompanying persistent febrile illnesses, or in response to drugs that induce sweating, such as bethanechol. The individual vesicles are extremely fragile, rupturing spontaneously or with slight friction, and resolve with a superficial branny desquamation. Therapy is generally not required because the eruption is self-limited. Miliaria crystallina may occur in the neonatal period due to delay in patency of the sweat ducts after birth.

It occurs most commonly on the head, neck and upper trunk and may be confused with other vesicular eruptions in this age group

Miliaria rubra is the clinically most significant manifestation of eccrine sweat retention. The primary lesion is an erythematous non-follicular macule or papule which may be topped by a minute vesicle. Pustule may form in some of the lesions, and if widespread, the term 'miliaria pustulosa' is used. Characteristically, miliaria rubra is accompanied by paroxysmal pruritus or a stinging sensation, which is frequently exacerbated by stimuli that induce sweating. It tends to occur in hot, humid environments but there is a wide individual susceptibility. Episodes of miliaria are typically followed by periods of anhidrosis in affected sites, sometimes lasting up to several weeks. Rarely, extensive miliaria may lead to hyperpyrexia and heat exhaustion.

Miliaria rubra affects up to 4% of neonates, most commonly in the flexural areas, face and scalp, with a peak at 11th to 14th day of life. Secondary infection may supervene either as impetigo or as multiple staphylococcal abscesses, known as 'periporitis staphylogenes', commonly seen in school-going children.

Treatment of miliaria consists of avoidance of excessive clothing, excessive use of soap and contact of the skin with irritants. The condition may persist for 2 to 3 weeks and subsides when poral obstruction is gradually relieved. Oral ascorbic acid and topical application of lanolin may be helpful. Calamine lotion is probably effective in relieving discomfort.

Miliaria profunda is usually seen in tropical environment after repeated episodes of miliaria rubra. The cutaneous findings can be subtle and are characterized by pale or flesh-colored, 1 to 3 mm papules located predominantly on the trunk and extremities, which represents a deep-seated sweat retention vesicle. These lesions are asymptomatic, and individual papules may become more prominent when the patient sweating. Other common findings include compensatory facial hyperhidrosis and inguinal and axillary adenopathy. Because of widespread inactivation of eccrine sweat glands, patients with miliaria profunda are predisposed to the development of tropical anhidrotic asthenia when exposed to prolonged heat stress. These patients have associated malaise, weakness, dyspnea, and tachycardia leading to hyperpyrexia and exhaustion. Isotretinoin has been reported to be helpful in the treatment of miliaria profunda.

ECCRINE BROMHIDROSIS

Eccrine sweat is usually odorless, but under some circumstances, it may attain odor.

Eccrine bromhidrosis is a foul-smelling condition resulting due to presence of volatile metabolic byproducts of cutaneous microbial flora produced from components of stratum corneum softened by sweat. This occurs in many hyperkeratotic conditions such as exfoliative erythroderma of atopic dermatitis, psoriasis, lamellar ichthyosis, hyperkeratosis palmaris et plantaris, and pitted keratolysis. Treatment is by keratolytic agents followed by bacteriostatic washes (chlorhexidine) or topical antibiotics (clindamycin, erythromycin, metronidazole).

Metabolic eccrine bromhidrosis occurs in specific metabolic diseases, such as fish odor syndrome (trimethylaminuria). The foul odor may result in serious psychological and social problems, as well as difficulties in attending school. Dietary restriction rapidly corrects this malodor.

Acquired exogenous eccrine bromhidrosis may be a sign of ingestion of a toxin, but is usually accompanied by additional features of toxicity such as seizures and altered sensorium. Acquired bromhidrosis may sometimes be the sole manifestation of a foreign body in the nose or other orifices.

NEUTROPHILIC ECCRINE HIDRADENITIS

There are several causes of neutrophilic eccrine hidradenitis, of which commoner is chemotherapy-associated.

This is an inflammatory disorder of eccrine sweat glands, seen in children and adults, which develop within weeks of initiating chemotherapy for a malignancy. The initial reports were associated with cytarabine and doxorubicin but other antineoplastic drugs as well as zidovudine may also result in this condition.

The most common associated malignant neoplasm is acute myelogenous leukemia (64%), followed by various other leukemias and solid tumors. The eruption typically consists of erythematous, edematous papules and plaques which may be pruritic and painful. Onset is often associated with fever and neutropenia. The sites affected in decreasing order of frequency are the extremities, trunk, periorbital region, neck, face, ears, and palms. The eruption begins approximately 10.6 days (mean 8 days) after the institution of chemotherapy and usually resolves in 2-3 weeks. Histopathology reveals a dense neutrophilic infiltrate around the eccrine coils, with infiltration and necrosis of the ductal epithelium. Treatment is mainly symptomatic.

There are recent reports of neutrophilic eccrine hidradenitis involving the palms and soles of healthy children and young adults. Healthy children present with a rapid onset of tenderness of the palm and/or feet, with erythematous to purple, deep-seated papules, nodules and plaques, mainly limited to the palmoplantar surfaces. Therapies include topical/ systemic steroids and ibuprofen; the response is rapid with resolution of lesions in 7-10 days.

GRANULOSIS RUBRA NASI

Granulosa rubra nasi (GRN) is a rare disease involving the eccrine glands of the nose. The pathogenesis of GRN remains obscure. Most cases are genetic, transmitted either in autosomal dominant or autosomal recessive pattern.

It begins in early childhood, manifesting as hyperhidrosis of nose, which becomes diffusely erythematous after several years. The tip of the nose is involved initially, but the erythema may spread to the rest of the nose, cheeks, upper lip, and chin. Fine erythematous papules and beads of sweat are commonly seen in the erythematous area. Vesicles and small cysts have also been noted occasionally. The condition may be mildly pruritic. Other associated conditions include volar hyperhidrosis and poor peripheral circulation. Although GRN usually resolves spontaneously at puberty, sometimes it may persist indefinitely, with telangiectasia being the predominant feature. Histopathological examination reveals dilatation of the dermal blood vessels and lymphatics with a mild mononuclear cell infiltrate. These changes are invariably accompanied by cystic dilatation of the eccrine ducts.

DISEASES OF APOCRINE GLANDS

Apocrine sweat glands are so named because of the characteristic shedding of the apical portion of the cell during secretion. These are larger than eccrine glands, situated in the subcutaneous tissue, and have a tubular duct, which opens into the neck of the hair follicle above the sebaceous gland. These glands are located only in certain areas – the axillae, perianal region and areolae of the breasts. These are poorly developed in childhood and begin to enlarge around puberty due to androgen effect. These do not have any thermoregulatory function and secrete small quantities of odorless oily secretion. Bacterial decomposition of this secretion on skin surface is responsible for the odor of sweat. The ducts have an adrenergic sympathetic nerve supply and are stimulated by circulating epinephrine.

APOCRINE BROMHIDROSIS (OSMIDROSIS)

This is a disorder of the apocrine glands manifesting after puberty, where the sweat is malodorous, which is more pronounced in summer. A number of compounds are liberated from the odorless apocrine secretions by axillary bacteria, like trans-3-methyl-2-hexanoic acid, certain short chain fatty acids and ammonia. These compounds lead to body odor. The condition may be controlled by the use of topical antiseptics, deodorants, and antiperspirants.

APOCRINE CHROMHIDROSIS

Apocrine chromhidrosis or pigmented sweat is a disorder where yellow, blue or green discoloration of sweat occurs among 10% population of pigmented races. The sweat contains lipofuscin, which stains skin and clothing. It is most common in the axillae, but has been reported on the face and areola as well. The pigmentation increases with emotional, manual or pharmacologic stimulation and the color is accentuated on Wood's lamp examination.

Pseudochromhidrosis is due to bacterial pigment production in sweat and this can be identified by cultures. Treatment of true axillary apocrine chromhidrosis is unsatisfactory, although topical capsaicin has been reported to be successful in facial and nipple chromhidrosis. Pseudochromhidrosis is treated with topical or systemic antibiotics.

APOCRINE MILIARIA (FOX-FORDYCE DISEASE)

Fox-Fordyce disease is the apocrine counterpart of miliaria. The etiology is unknown. Obliteration of the apocrine duct at the infundibulum is thought to be the cause. Histopathology shows apocrine duct obstruction by keratin debris (with consequent apocrine sweat retention), surrounding spongiosis and a dermal inflammatory infiltrate. The disease starts in adolescence, more frequently in females. A chronic intensely pruritic papular eruption occurs in the axillae, and to a lesser extent in the ano-genital region and around the breasts. Itching may be provoked by emotional stimuli, and the disease runs a chronic persistent course until menopause.

Topical and intralesional steroids provide some relief. Topical clindamycin, UV radiation, and topical and systemic retinoids have all been reported to be useful. Severe cases may require electrocautery, surgical excision of the affected skin, or subcutaneous removal of the apocrine glands.

HIDRADENITIS SUPPURATIVA

Hidradenitis suppurativa is a disease involving apocrine sweat glands, characterized by chronic inflammation and discharge, with sinus tract formation. The exact cause is unknown; plugging of the apocrine sweat duct, subsequent bacterial infection, rupture and inflammation has been postulated as the causative factors. However, it may involve sites without apocrine glands like lateral thighs and infra-mammary area; hence, it is possible that apocrine glands may only be secondarily affected by follicular occlusion.

Histopathology shows deep folliculitis, keratin plugs, follicular rupture and a dense mixed inflammatory infiltrate in the dermis. Frank abscesses are often seen, and dense fibrosis with sinus tract formation occurs in chronic lesions. Pseudocarcinomatous hyperplasia may occur in the overlying epidermis.

Onset of the disease is usually at puberty, and is commoner in females. Lesions begin as tender deep-seated inflammatory papules and nodules in axilla and groin. Lesions then become suppurative, with abscess formation and purulent discharge. Sinus tract and puckered scars are formed later in the course of the disease. Open comedones are often seen. Other components of the follicular occlusion triad/tetrad may be seen, such as conglobate acne, perifolliculitis capitis and pilonidal sinus. The disease runs a chronic relentless course. Long-term complications include fistula formation, anemia, hypoproteinemia, interstitial keratitis, arthropathy, amyloidosis and squamous cell carcinoma.

The disease is difficult to treat. Prophylactic measures include local hygiene, weight reduction, avoidance of

TABLE 15.3: Eccrine and apocrine gland tumors

Tumor	Age	Clinical features	Treatment
Eccrine nevus	Birth/ early childhood	Three clinical presentations: localized area of hyperhidrosis; solitary pore discharging mucinous material; skin-colored plaque in a linear configuration. Association: comedones (nevus comedonicus)	Comedonal variants: topical tretinoin 0.1% cream. Hyperhidrosis: topical aluminium chloride 20% Cryotherapy/ curettage Excision
Eccrine poroma	>40 yrs; reported in children (4 yrs)	Asymptomatic moist, exophytic, pink/ red/skin-coloured nodules (up to 1-2 cm) on palms and soles	Complete surgical excision
Eccrine spiradenoma	Children, young adults	Solitary bluish/skin-colored dome shaped intradermal nodules on trunk or extremities, may be painful/tender	Complete surgical excision with margin control
Syringoma	Adolescence/ early adulthood, females>males (2:1)	Single/ eruptive/ linear presentation; 1-3 mm flat-topped, flesh-colored/ translucent/yellowish papules on lower eyelids and upper cheeks. Other areas – axillae, groin, chest, and abdomen. Proliferate during puberty/ pregnancy/ perimenstrual period/ on OCPs. Association: Down syndrome.	Topical/ systemic retinoids; superficial ablation by electrodesiccation/ cryotherapy/ chemical peels/ CO_2 laser; surgical excision
Apocrine hidrocystoma/ cystadenoma	Adults/ elderly; unique forms in children	Solitary cystic, translucent, skin-colored/ bluish papule or nodule (less than 1.5 cm); periorbital region (near the outer canthus); pigmented forms reported; multiple lesions in Goltz syndrome, ectodermal dyplasia	Surgical excision or punch biopsy (diagnostic and therapeutic); CO_2 laser for multiple lesions
Syringocystadenoma papilliferum	Birth/ adolescence	Small grouped, translucent or slightly pigmented, umbilicated papules on the scalp or face, that grow rapidly and become verrucous at puberty; solitary/ linear/ zosteriform presentations reported; one third arise within a sebaceous naevus	Surgical excision

irritant deodorants/ antiperspirants and occlusive clothing, and regular washing with antiseptics. Antibiotics may be used to tide over acute episodes of bacterial infection. Isotretinoin, dapsone, sulfasalazine, intralesional steroids and cryotherapy have all been tried with varying success rates. Surgery is the only curative mode of therapy; it consists of excision of the involved skin and exteriorization of sinuses, with healing by secondary intention or split thickness skin grafting.

TUMORS

Salient features of eccrine and apocrine gland tumors have been presented in **Table 15.3.**

BIBLIOGRAPHY

1. Coulson IH. Disorders of sweat glands. In: Burns T, Breathnach S, Cox N, Griffiths C, Editors. Rook's Textbook of Dermatology. Massachusetts: Blackwell Science 2004;45.1-45.23
2. Cunliffe WJ. Acne. In: Harper J, Oranje A, Prose N editors. Textbook of pediatric dermatology. First edition. Oxford; Blackwell Publications 2000;639-54.
3. Eady EA, Farmery MR, Ross JI, Cove JH, Cunliffe WJ. Effects of benzoyl peroxide and erythromycin alone and in combination against antibiotic-sensitive and -resistant skin bacteria from acne patients. Br J Dermatol 1994; 131: 331-6.
4. Harper JC. An update on the pathogenesis and management of acne vulgaris. J Am Acad Dermatol 2004; 51: S36-8.
5. Healy E, Simpson N. Acne vulgaris. Br Med J 1994; 308: 831-3.
6. Heckmann M, Ceballos-Baumann AO, Plewig G. Hyperhidrosis Sudy Group. Botulinum toxin A for axillary

hyperhidrosis (excessive sweating). N Engl J Med 2001; 344:488-93.
7. Katsambas AD. Why and when the treatment of acne fails. Dermatology 1998; 196: 158-61.
8. Koo J. How do you foster medication adherence for better acne vulgaris management? SKINmed 2003; 2(4): 229-233.
9. Layton AM, Knaggs H, Taylor J, Cunliffe WJ. Isotretinoin for acne vulgaris—10 years later: a safe and successful treatment. Br J Dermatol 1993; 129: 292-6.
10. Leyden JJ. A review of the use of combination therapies for the treatment of acne vulgaris. J Am Acad Dermatol 2003; 49: S200-10.
11. Phadke VA, Joshi RS, Khopkar US, Wadhwa SL. Comparison of topical methenamine, glutaraldehyde and tap water iontophoresis for palmoplantar hyperhidrosis. Indian J Dermatol Venereol Leprol 1995;61:346-348.
12. Rai R, Srinivas CR. Iontophoresis in dermatology. Indian J Dermatol Venereol Leprol 2005;71:236-41.
13. Sato K, Ohtsuyama M, Samman G. Eccrine sweat gland disorders. J Am Acad Dermatol 1991;24(6):1010-4
14. Shalita AR. Acne revisited. Arch Dermatol 1994; 130: 363-4.
15. Sigurdsson V, De Wit RF, De Groot AC. Infantile acne. Br J Dermatol 1991;125:285.
16. Silverman R, Baran R. Nail and appendageal abnormalities. In: Shachner LA, Hansen RC, Editors. Pediatric Dermatology. Philadelphia: Mosby/ 2003;561-88.
17. Simpson NB, Cunliffe WJ. Disorders of the sebaceous glands. In: Burns T, Breathnach S, Cox N, Griffiths C, editors. Rook's Textbook of Dermatology. Massachusetts: Blackwell Science; 2004;43.1-43.75.
18. Treatment of hyperhidrosis. Dermatologic Clinics. 1998; 16(4):863-9.
19. Viehman GE, Shea CR. Adnexal disorders. In: Harper J, Oranje A, Prose N. Textbook of Pediatric Dermatology. Oxford: Blackwell science; 2000;765-79.
20. Walton S, Cunliffe WJ, Keczkes K, Early AS, McGarrigle HH, Katz M, Reese RA. Clinical, ultrasound and hormonal markers of androgenicity in acne vulgaris. Br J Dermatol 1995; 133: 249-53.
21. Wenzel FG, Horn TD. Nonneoplastic disorders of the eccrine glands. J Am Acad Dermatol 1998;38:1-17
22. Yu CC, Cook MG. Hidradenitis suppurativa: disease of follicular epithelium rather than apocrine glands. Br J Dermatol 1990;122:763-7.

16

Disorders of Keratinization

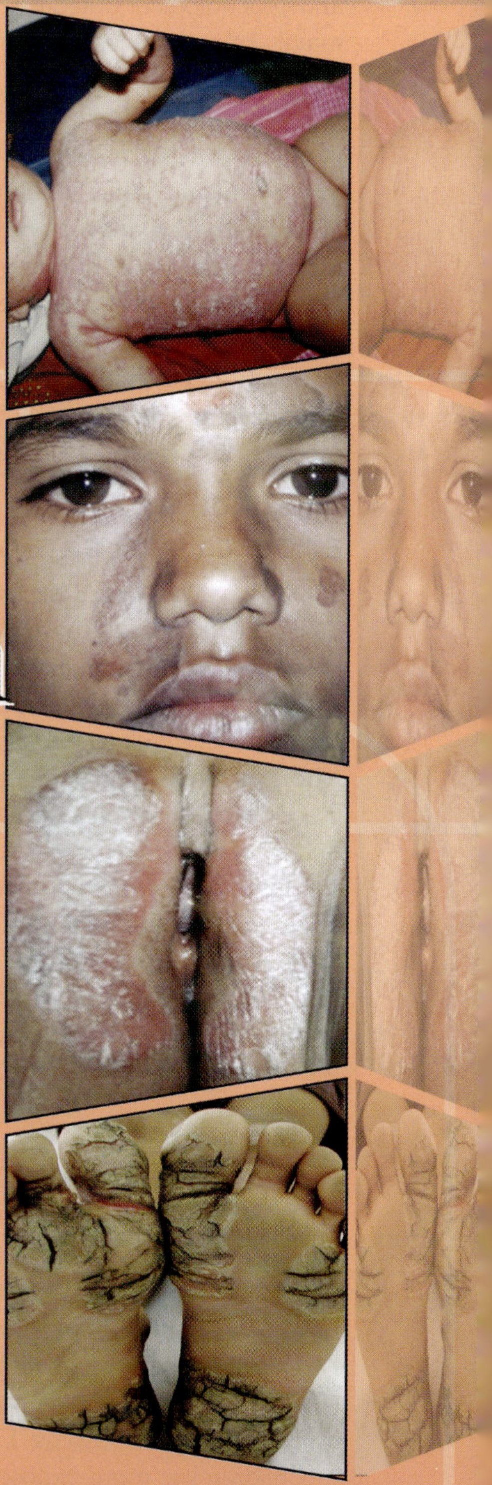

Childhood Psoriasis

Erythroderma in Children

Sunil Dogra, Dipankar De

Lichenoid Eruptions and other Papulosquamous Disorders

Ragunatha S

CHILDHOOD PSORIASIS

It is aptly said that children are not simply small adults and that is true for childhood psoriasis as compared to psoriasis in adults. The childhood psoriasis differs in epidemiology, clinical features, treatment options, and long-term clinical and psychological outcome. Our discussion will remain mainly limited to these differences rather than exhaustive discussion about psoriasis as a whole.

Psoriasis is a chronic, inflammatory, hyperproliferative papulosquamous disorder involving skin, nails and joints. There is altered differentiation of the keratinocytes and other internal organs may be involved rarely. The disease is highly variable in duration, severity and morphology. Non-pustular psoriasis can be classified according to the age of onset. Type 1 has an age of onset less than 40 years, often heritable, and associated with HLA Cw6; whereas type 2 has an age of onset more than 40 years, often sporadic and not associated with HLA Cw6. Childhood psoriasis, thus by definition is type 1 disease.

ETIOLOGY AND PATHOGENESIS

The exact cause of psoriasis is unknown. The accumulating evidence indicates that psoriasis is precipitated by concerted action of multiple disease genes in a particular individual, triggered by environmental factors. Some of these genes regulate inflammation and immunity as a whole, whereas others are unique to psoriasis.

Genetic factors influence the pattern psoriasis, severity and age of onset. The best evidence for genetic basis for psoriasis comes from twin studies. Psoriasis is concordant about three times as often in identical twins as in fraternal twins. The lifetime risk of acquiring psoriasis is 0.04, 0.28, and 0.65 if no parent, one parent and both of the parents are affected by psoriasis; if one sibling is affected then the corresponding figures are 0.24, 0.51, and 0.83 respectively.

Several genetic factors such as HLA Cw6 and HLA DR7, as well as polymorphisms in the apolipoprotein E gene, α_1-antitrypsin inhibitor gene and interleukin 1 receptor antagonist gene contribute to an early onset and more severe course of psoriasis. A number of genetic loci have been identified by genome wide linkage scans, and two loci have been replicated: PSORS1 on chromosome 6 within the major histocompatibility complex, and PSORS2 on chromosome 17q.

Children are more exposed to infections and trauma rather than drugs and alcohol. The most important triggering factor for psoriasis in children is infections. There is strong association (26 to 97%) between streptococcal infection and childhood psoriasis, especially the guttate variety. Some authors emphasize the necessity to screen pediatric patients with guttate psoriasis very thoroughly including swabbing of both the pharynx and perianal area in these patients. The role of precipitating factor is apparently more important in childhood onset psoriasis compared to adult onset psoriasis. In a study, a higher rates of apparent precipitation or exacerbation of disease by pharyngitis (27.9 *vs* 12.2%), stress (50.4 *vs* 42.7%), and trauma (49.6 *vs* 38.9%) was found. A much lower rate of triggering factor has been observed in other studies.

Drugs can induce psoriasis in children like in adults. The most important drugs implicated in childhood are antimalarials and systemic corticosteroids. Pustular flare in psoriasis can be precipitated by sudden withdrawal of oral corticosteroids.

Psoriasis is an inflammatory disorder with T cell abnormalities. Milieu of abnormal expression of cytokines leads to abnormal keratinocyte differentiation and proliferation. Overall, the pathogenesis of psoriasis in different age groups is similar.

HISTOPATHOLOGY

Histopathology of psoriasis in children is essentially similar to that in adults. The picture varies with the stage of the lesion. Immediately below the parakeratotic stratum corneum, there is collection of neutrophils (spongiform pustules of Kogoj). Munro's microabscesses, commonly seen in the early lesions, are located within the parakeratotic stratum corneum. The spongiform pustules of Kogoj and Munro's microabscesses are considered to be pathognomonic of psoriasis. Epidermis is acanthotic and stratum granulosum is absent. There is regular elongation of rete ridges with bulbous thickening at the lower portions. The dermal papillae are elongated and edematous. There is suprapapillary thinning of the epidermis. The capillaries within the edematous papillary dermis are dilated and tortuous. A predominantly mononuclear inflammatory infiltrate is present in the dermis.

CLINICAL FEATURES

General Data/Epidemiological Data

Psoriasis in childhood is a disease of many forms that may change over time. Its true incidence is unknown.

The disease may start at any age. Congenital psoriasis has been described. Epidemiological data suggest that in 37% of psoriasis patients the disease appears before the age of 20 years, in 27%, by the age of 15 years, in 10%, by the age of 10 years, in 6.5%, the disease manifest before the age of 5 years and in 2%, by the age of 2 years. Nyfors and Lemholt, in a review of the literature from Scandinavia, reported that 45% of adult psoriatics from that region had onset of disease before the age 16 years. Incidence estimates have been hampered by a lack of clarity about defining childhood psoriasis. Psoriatic diaper rash with dissemination is the most outstanding example of this and controversy exists over the terminology and validity of its inclusion within the classification of psoriasis.

It is commonly found that girls with psoriasis outnumber boys (even up to the proportion of 2:1), though there are studies to suggest that both sexes may be affected equally as in adults. It may reflect different referral patterns based on gender issues for the various study locations. There is no significant difference of the mean age of onset and duration of psoriasis between male and female patients, though there are studies to suggest that the disease appears early in girls.

Variable familial incidence has been described in childhood psoriasis, ranging from 9.8 to 89% of patients. In a study from northern India, family history was positive in 4.5% of patients, and the low incidence was ascribed to ignorance of family members to the presence of disease, or the disease might have appeared after the point of time when it was enquired.

The frequencies of some types or patterns of psoriasis differ between adults and children, with several adult types rarely described in children. Overall childhood psoriasis differs from adult onset psoriasis in following aspects:

- Greater familial incidence,
- Twice as common in females,
- More frequently pruritic,
- The lesions are relatively thinner, softer, and less scaly,
- Certain clinical variants/features are less common in childhood, like erythroderma, arthropathy, localized and generalized pustular psoriasis, whereas guttate psoriasis is commoner,
- Common precipitating factors are infections, physical and psychological trauma compared to adults,
- Greater tendency for more extensive and severe forms of the disease,
- Frequency of remissions has been found to be greater in pediatric onset psoriasis than adult disease.

In general majority of children have mild disease. In the large series reported from India, most children (93.7%) had a mild form of the disease with a body surface area of involvement of < 20% similar to that reported from Kuwait. An earlier disease onset is believed to be associated with a history of familial occurrence and a poorer prognosis; however, an Indian study did not find any positive correlation between the age of onset, severity of involvement, and family history.

FORMS OF PSORIASIS IN CHILDREN

Morphology

Morphology of lesions is often similar to that seen in adults **(Figure 16.1)**. Classic chronic plaque lesions are well-defined, erythematous with silvery scales. The scalp is the most commonly affected site of involvement (58% of patients) followed by the appearance of lesions on the extensor surface of the extremities, and trunk. In contrast with adult psoriasis, the face and ears are often involved in children. Flexors and diaper regions, which are trauma prone, have been found to be more commonly involved in infants and young children.

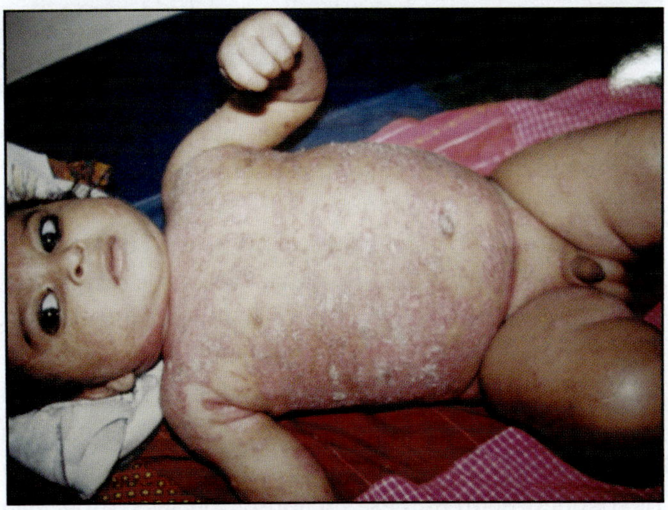

FIGURE 16.1: Psoriasis vulgaris

Plaque psoriasis (Figures 16.2A and B): In children, plaques are often smaller and the scales softer and finer than adults. In dark-skinned children, the scale may be subtle and it presents as hypopigmentation, the scale becoming obvious only when the lesions are scratched. In different studies on childhood psoriasis, plaque psoriasis

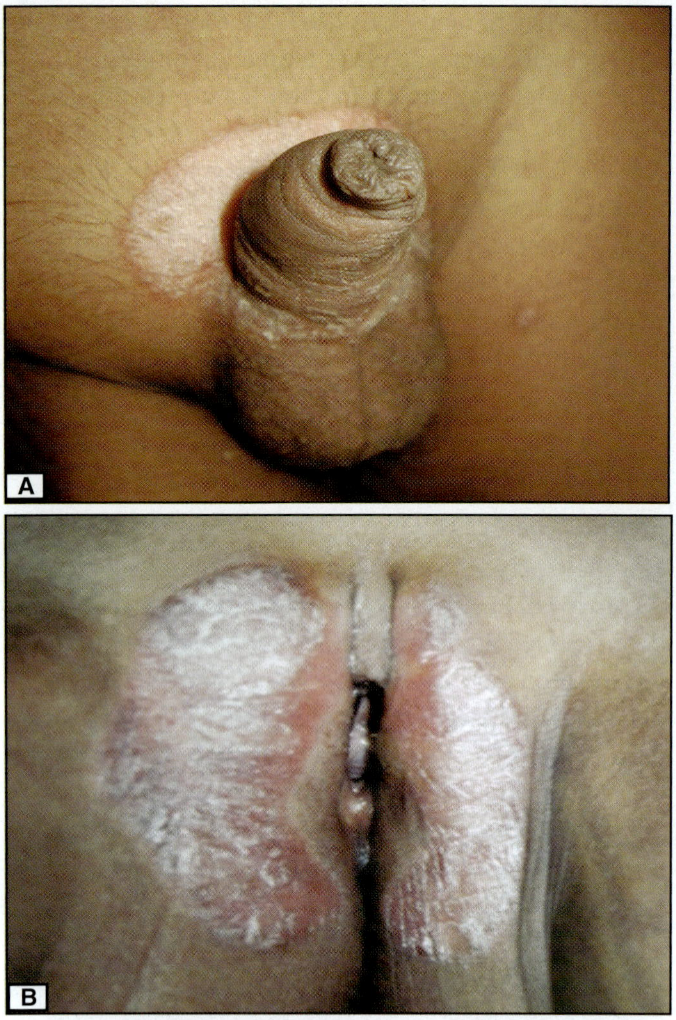

FIGURES 16.2A AND B: Plaque psoriasis

is the most common morphological type reported to vary from 34 to 84%. In a study from northern India, 60% of 419 patients had plaque psoriasis at the time of presentation. Involvement of scalp **(Figure 16.3)**, palms and soles **(Figure 16.4)** by plaque lesions is commoner in children. An incidence of 12.8% for only plantar lesions has been reported in sharp contrast with a previous study in Australia where plantar involvement was reported to be only 4%. This may be due to the habit of walking barefoot or wearing sandals in India, leading to a degree of koebnerization at these friction-prone sites, especially in children who are generally more active.

Facial lesions in childhood psoriasis is common; published incidence being 18- 46%. This high incidence is particularly common in geographic areas with less sunny days. A 4.7% incidence of facial lesions has been reported from India. Children in the tropics are exposed to the ultraviolet rays of the sun throughout the day and hence, involvement of the sun-exposed sites, such as face

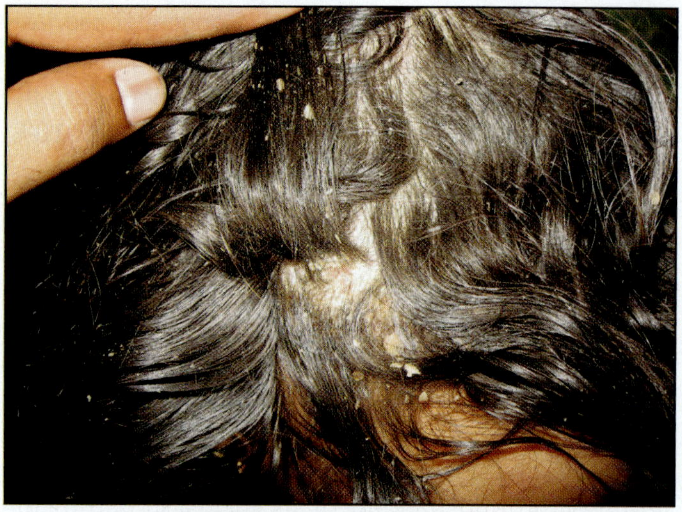

FIGURE 16.3: Scalp psoriasis

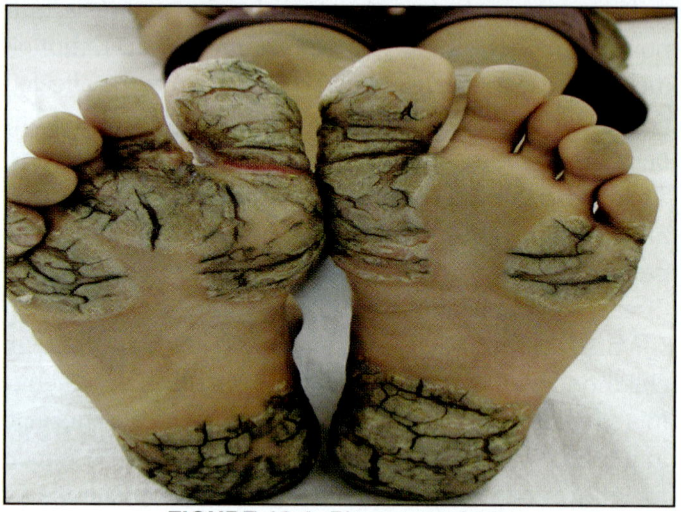

FIGURE 16.4: Plantar psoriasis

may be less frequent. Likewise, facial involvement was less common in the patient series from Australia, and the Middle East, where sun exposure is more. The facial lesions may be subtle or florid. Characteristically, these are more clearly demarcated than eczematous patches, are less itchy, and commonly have an annular configuration. A common site is under the eyes. This may be the only manifestation of psoriasis in less than 5% of children or occur as part of a more generalized rash.

Guttate psoriasis: This form of psoriasis occurs most often in children and young adults. The term is derived from Latin *gutta* (a drop). Guttate psoriasis appears in showers, often a week after streptococcal pharyngitis. An association with perianal streptococcal dermatitis has also been described. The lesions vary from 2 to 3 mm to 1 cm in diameter, and are round or slightly oval. The small papular lesions are characteristically topped with silvery scales. The lesions are particularly common over the trunk and proximal extremities. These appear frequently over the face, ears and scalp, and are unusual over palms and soles. Guttate psoriasis may resolve spontaneously with time, may resolve faster with anti-streptococcal antibiotics, or the lesions may gradually increase in size to become chronic plaque lesions.

In the published reports, frequency of guttate psoriasis varies from 6.4 to 44%. Guttate psoriasis was the most common type of psoriasis observed in Denmark. In a study from India, only 9.7% children had guttate lesions. In a poor/developing set-up, repeated episodes of subclinical infection may not allow building up of critical levels of streptococcal antigens required to trigger guttate psoriasis. Genetic and environmental factors may also play some role in this disparity.

Flexural psoriasis: This inverse variant of psoriasis most frequently affects the napkin area and the axillae in children. Flexural psoriasis of the genital and the peri-umbilical areas is common, and may be the isolated finding. Two clinical variants in the diaper distribution are described, i.e. localized psoriatic diaper rash and psoriatic diaper rash with dissemination. However, validity of their inclusion within the spectrum of psoriasis is a matter of debate. Clinically it may be difficult to differentiate from infantile seborrheic dermatitis. A significant proportion of patients with psoriatic diaper rash are considered to develop classical lesions of psoriasis subsequently. Psoriatic diaper rash is brighter red, better demarcated, often more shiny than seborrheic dermatitis and lacks the greasy yellowish scale that is present in the later.

In the study from India, only 0.4% of patients had diaper area involvement. This rarity can be explained by infrequent use of the western-type of diapers in India. Increased bacterial and fungal growth associated with thick and occlusive diapers may initiate psoriasis lesions in predisposed individuals.

Pustular psoriasis (Figures 16.5 and 16.6): Pustular psoriasis can be divided into generalized and localized (palms and soles). Three forms of generalized pustular psoriasis can be seen in children;

- Acute generalized pustular psoriasis of von- Zumbusch,
- Annular and circinate variety,
- Pustular lesions localized to plaques of psoriasis.

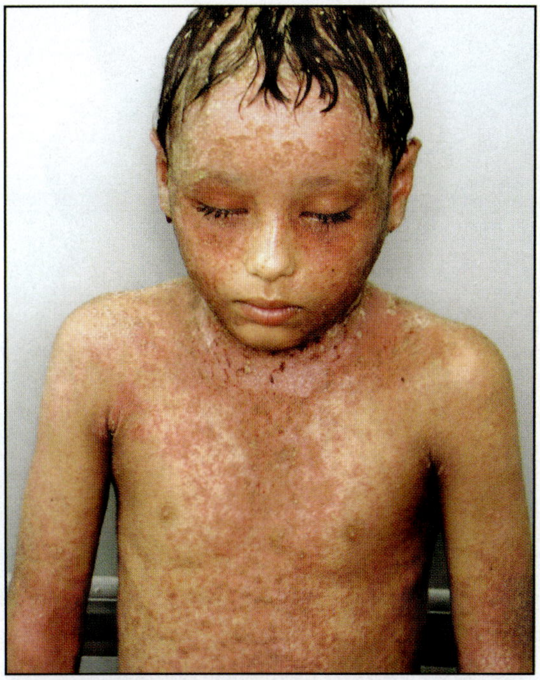

FIGURE 16.5: Unstable psoriasis with pustulation

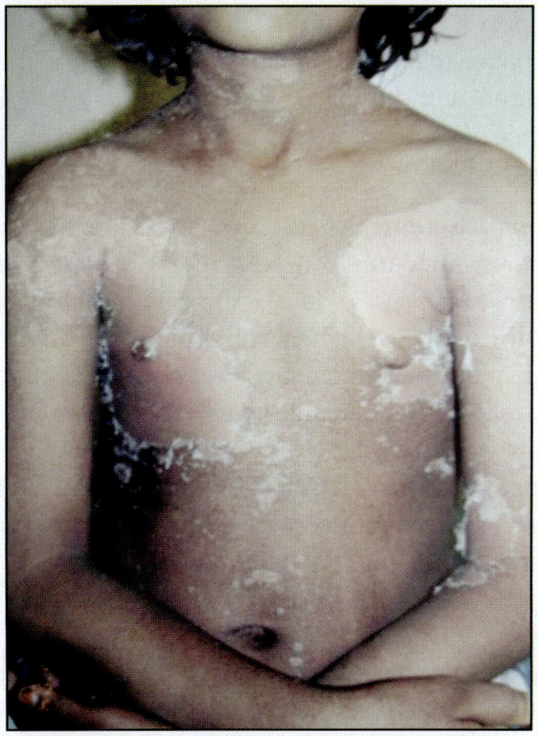

FIGURE 16.6: Subsiding pustular psoriasis

In one study, only 0.4% each had generalized pustular psoriasis and localized pustular psoriasis. Annular pustular psoriasis has been noted to have more benign course than generalized pustular psoriasis.

Erythrodermic psoriasis (Figure 16.7): This variant is also rare in children. It may start *de novo* or may

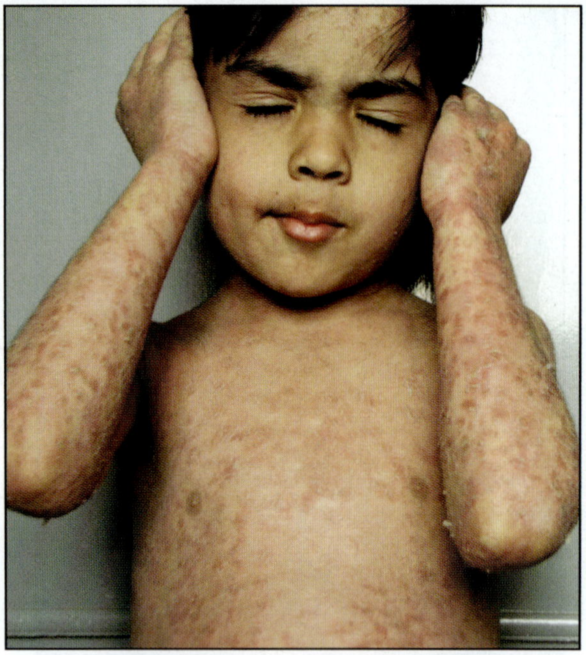

FIGURE 16.7: Psoriatic erythroderma

develop in a patient with plaque type of psoriasis with exacerbation following chronic irritation of topical therapy or sudden withdrawal of systemic therapy. A 0.7% incidence of psoriatic erythroderma in children has been reported.

Nail involvement: Severe nail changes are uncommon in children and are seen particularly in longstanding chronic psoriasis cases. Pitting is the most common feature seen particularly in children with arthropathy. In a study, frequency of isolated nail involvement was 2.3% where as overall nail involvement was noted in 31% of all children with psoriasis.

Joint involvement in psoriasis is uncommon. Children with psoriatic arthropathy alone may not develop psoriatic skin lesions even after long-term follow-up.

Psoriatic Diaper Rashes

Psoriatic diaper rash is bright red, well-demarcated and often very shiny. It lacks the yellow scale that may be present in seborrheic dermatitis. Diagnosis is mostly clinical as confirmation by skin biopsy is difficult in the pediatric age group. However, many patients who initially presented with psoriatic diaper rash with dissemination have subsequently developed other forms of psoriasis. It has been classified as localized psoriatic diaper rash and psoriatic diaper rash with dissemination. The former is well-demarcated, confluent, bright red rash confined to the diaper area, often with a glazed appearance; where as the later (previously referred to as psoriasiform diaper dermatitis or psoriasiform seborrheic dermatitis) starts with a well-demarcated erythematous plaque localized to the diaper area, followed by few scattered lesions on the trunk and thereafter an explosive spread occurs to the face, neck, trunk, and finally the limbs. Frequency-wise, it is perhaps the most significant form of psoriasis in infancy. In a review of 1,262 cases of childhood psoriasis, a history of psoriatic diaper rash in more than 20% of cases was noted; however, it did not appear to be related to the future development of any particular clinical type of the disease. The data on history of psoriatic diaper rash is often incomplete and possibly subject to recall bias.

Eczema/psoriasis Overlap

In this condition, there are scaly erythematous patches with overlapping features of eczema and psoriasis, often with a history of discoid eczema in infancy **(Figure 16.8)**. Most patients have a family history of both atopic disease and psoriasis.

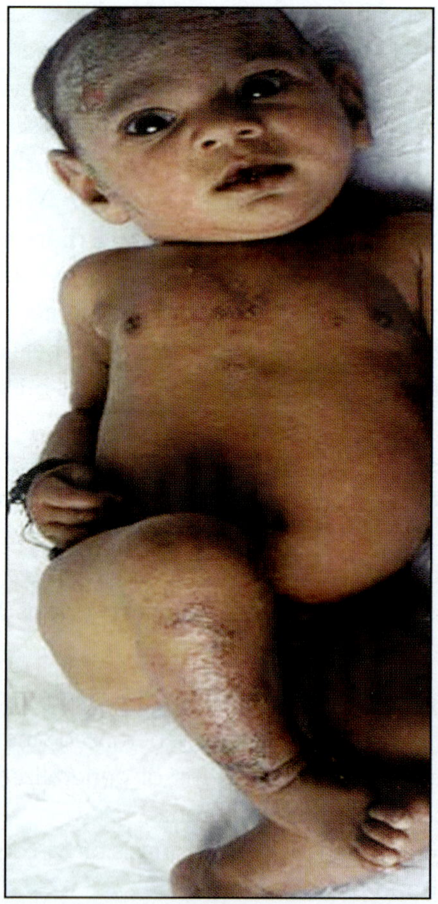

FIGURE 16.8: Eczematous psoriasis

DIFFERENTIAL DIAGNOSIS

In infancy and early childhood, the most important differential diagnoses are seborrheic dermatitis and nummular eczema (atopic eczema). At a later stage, psoriasis can be confused with pityriasis rubra pilaris, tinea corporis and pityriasis rosea.

Atopic dermatitis can be differentiated from psoriasis in majority of the patients. However, patients with initial diagnosis of nummular eczema may develop classical lesions of psoriasis later on or vice versa, the so called spectrum of eczematous psoriasis. Pityriasis lichenoides chronica can closely resemble guttate psoriasis.

Psoriatic nail involvement should be differentiated from onychomycosis, lichen planus, and trachyonychia. Psoriatic scalp involvement should be differentiated from tinea capitis.

TREATMENT

The objective of the treatment of psoriasis in children is to improve the physical and psychological symptoms, minimizing the effect of disease on psychosocial development and limiting the adverse effects of drugs on future health. In young children, compliance to long- term treatment is dependent almost entirely on the parents. Education of the child and parents concerning the nature of psoriasis is especially important to encourage a positive approach to the condition and its treatment. Through the school years and adolescence, considerable support is needed to cope with the reactions of other children. Practical advice should be given about cosmesis, participation in sports, etc. Psoriasis has been shown to have an adverse effect on the quality of life in children; this can be improved considerably by treatment.

Psoriasis can usually be treated effectively in children with topical agents including emollients, coal tar, corticosteroids, dithranol and calcipotriol. In those who do not respond, consideration should be given first to day care or in-patient treatment which may be combined with UVB phototherapy. Systemic therapy should be used only under circumstances such as resistant erythrodermic, generalized pustular or arthropathic psoriasis.

Avoidance/Removal of Triggering Factors

There is a strong association between pharyngitis and the clinical activity of psoriasis, especially in guttate psoriasis, with considerable anecdotal evidence that treating the infection improves psoriasis. This is particularly the case in recurrent guttate psoriasis for which prophylactic antibiotics or tonsillectomy has been advocated. Unfortunately there are no controlled trials.

Topical Therapy

Most children with psoriasis can be managed with topical treatment.

Coal tar is helpful in all age groups and particularly in plaque psoriasis. However, it is an irritant, especially when used on the face and flexures, sites frequently affected in children. In older children, the smell of coal tar limits its suitability.

Dithranol may be applied as short contact therapy under careful parental supervision. In an open study of 58 children aged 5–10 years treated with dithranol at concentrations up to 1%, remission was achieved in 47.

Topical corticosteroids may be used in inflammatory psoriasis or in combination with topical treatments that may produce irritation, such as calcipotriol. They are also widely used on the face, ears, flexures and genitals.

Calcipotriol has been rigorously evaluated in children. In an un-controlled study of 66 children aged 2–14 years, twice daily application of calcipotriol ointment (50 mg/g) up to 45 g/week/m^2 for 8 weeks was found to be effective without alteration of serum calcium. Irritation and facial rashes were not more frequent than in adults. In a subsequent trial in 77 children, treated as above but with the ointment base as control, the Psoriasis Area and Severity Index (PASI) was reduced by 52% in the treated group and by 37% in the control group. In UK, Daivonex cream and ointment (calcipotriol 50 μg/g) are licensed for use in children with a maximum dose of 75 g/week for children aged over 12 years and 50 g/week for those aged over 6 years.

Tazarotene, a topical retinoid, has recently been licensed for use in adults but as yet there are no data on the efficacy and safety in children.

Phototherapy

Topical therapy may be combined with UVB phototherapy in children who are mature enough to comply. In the absence of any clear evidence concerning the long-term safety of UVB, a variety of divergent opinions have been expressed as to the role of UVB phototherapy in children. Parents should be informed that there may be a slight increase in photoaging and risk of skin cancer. UVB may be useful in the treatment of guttate psoriasis. PUVA is contraindicated in young children but may be used in adolescents if necessary.

UV treatment to children must be administered in an appropriate environment with constant supervision by parents and trained professional staff. As compliance with eye protection may be difficult in children, phototherapy with UVB (NBUVB) or UVA is usually preferred to PUVA (photochemotherapy).

Systemic Therapy

There are no controlled trials in this age group but most experiences have been with retinoids which are probably the second-line drugs for children. Methotrexate and cyclosporine appear to be effective in children but more efficacy and safety data are required.

Many of the treatments used in adults have been used in children but are not licensed for use in this age group.

Indications: Systemic therapy should only be considered in extreme circumstances such as resistant erythrodermic, pustular or arthropathic psoriasis. Pustular and erythrodermic psoriasis may settle with bland topical treatment and hospitalized supportive care, unless very severe.

Methotrexate (MTX): MTX is an anti-metabolite, a synthetic analogue of folate. It is a competitive inhibitor of the enzyme dihydro folate reductase responsible for the conversion of folic acid to reduced folate cofactors, i.e. tetrahydrofolate which are required for metabolic transfer of 1- carbon units as in DNA synthesis. Recent investigations have suggested that MTX possesses both immunomodulatory and profound anti-inflammatory properties.

The side-effect profile of MTX is not favorable for its use in children as an antipsoriatic agent except in select situations like generalized pustular psoriasis, psoriatic erythroderma, psoriatic arthropathy or recalcitrant severe plaque type psoriasis. Since late 1950s, MTX is the gold standard of therapy in psoriasis and even in the era of biologicals, it continues to be an agent with which other systemic medications are compared. The advantages of MTX are its efficacy, affordability and convenient weekly oral dose. Meticulous use of MTX may avert the long term or serious side effects. The tolerability and efficacy of MTX in the treatment of childhood psoriasis is not yet established. The available evidence in this age group comes largely from a few studies involving small number of patients. In a previous report from India, MTX is used successfully in 7 children (3 to 16 years of age) having severe disease without any significant side effects or biochemical and hematological alterations. MTX has been used successfully in children as young as 2 years suffering from generalized pustular psoriasis and 3.5 years.

The long- term use of MTX with attendant risk of hepatic fibrosis is the main concern while using it in children with a chronic disease like psoriasis. However, the natural course of psoriasis and the pharmacokinetics of MTX may delay this effect. As psoriasis in general is more severe in winter, MTX can be tapered to complete withdrawal when the disease is controlled with seasonal change and manageable with topical medications. MTX has been detected in liver for up to 116 days after the last dose. Thus intermittent drug free intervals may allow the liver to recover from drug induced toxicities. Advances in the non- invasive assessment of liver fibrosis may eventually further reduce the need for liver biopsy to detect extent of MTX induced liver damage.

In a recent study by Kaur et al (in press), involving 24 children, the authors have concluded that MTX is cheap, easily available, reasonably safe drug to be used in severe childhood psoriasis with success in resource-poor set-up and will continue to be a paradigm in the new era of biologicals. Considering the long-term side effects of systemic agents like MTX, these should be used only by experienced dermatologists with adequate facilities for patient monitoring. However, there are no guidelines or consensus on the use of systemic therapies in childhood psoriasis and it is used mostly empirically. Relatively less data regarding the use of systemic therapies may be attributed to the rarity of severe forms of the disease in the pediatric age group.

Retinoids: The major limitation of the use of oral retinoids (acitretin) in children is the risk of growth retardation due to premature closure of epiphyses on long-term use. Most experience has been reported with retinoids which, on the basis of the published data, appear to be the second line drug for using in children. Premature epiphyseal closure is of particular concern with use of retinoids in children; this risk is minimized by using the lowest possible dose, 0.25–0.6 mg/kg of acitretin, which is often effective, although up to 1 mg/kg may be used. Monitoring the patient with a bone scan every 12–18 months has been recommended for children on retinoids, but in contrast to ichthyosis, continuous treatment over long periods may not be necessary in psoriasis.

Cyclosporin (CYA): The limitation of CYA is its cost and renal toxicity. Although it is not licensed for use in dermatological diseases in children, it has been investigated in childhood atopic dermatitis. The use of CYA in childhood pustular psoriasis has been reported. Though there are reports of favorable response with CYA in childhood psoriasis, Mahe et al have reported total ineffectiveness of this drug in 4 cases. CYA is generally effective in doses of 2.5-5 mg/kg per day in adults. Pharmacokinetics of CYA, including intestinal absorption, distribution in body fluids and tissues, metabolism and elimination is different in children, thus requiring higher doses for similar therapeutic effects with potential risk of dose dependent toxicity.

Hydroxyurea: Experience regarding use of hydroxyurea as systemic agent in treatment of childhood psoriasis is limited. Hematological side effects are of concern at this age group.

Etanercept: It is a TNF-α antagonist, recently introduced in the treatment of psoriasis; however, its use in childhood psoriasis is limited. Guidelines for the use of biological agents in pediatric age group need to be established. The limitation of use of etanercept in childhood psoriasis is its cost and the twice weekly injection schedule may not be liked by children.

Psoriasis should not adversely affect the life-expectancy or development of children. Whether the childhood-onset predicts a milder or more severe form of psoriasis, is controversial. Though there is little data to support, it is well recognized that children who have an episode of guttate psoriasis, may never develop chronic plaque disease.

A chronic disfiguring skin disease, such as psoriasis, in childhood is likely to have profound emotional and psychological effects, and hence requires special attention. It is essential to understand the morphological type, natural history and exogenous and endogenous factors responsible for the increased morbidity of this disease in order to help the young sufferers with psoriasis. The management of psoriasis in children differs from adults in several important aspects including the emphasis on educating the family, dealing with the emotional aspects of the disease and eliminating triggering factors. More evidence is needed about the effectiveness and long-term safety of topical therapy, phototherapy and systemic therapy in children.

ERYTHRODERMA IN CHILDREN

Erythroderma is conventionally defined as erythema, scaling and infiltration involving more than 90% of body surface area. This cut-off mark of 90% is little contentious as a person with the same dermatosis of similar severity with involvement of 85% body surface (non-erythrodermic) area might have similar prognosis as that of an erythrodermic patient. Moreover, assessment of body surface area is subjective; a given patient might be erythrodermic as per the assessment of one physician and non-erythrodermic by another. Thus, it may be preferable to define erythroderma as generalized erythema and scaling with minimal sparing of normal skin.

Previously, erythroderma and exfoliative dermatitis were differentiated by presence of scaling. A patient having scaling and erythema was supposed to have exfoliative dermatitis. The terms are, however, used interchangeably in recent times.

Erythroderma has been studied extensively in adults. There are few case series of erythroderma in neonates and infants as well. But there is a grey area between erythroderma in infancy and adulthood that is erythroderma in childhood, where surprisingly no studies have been done. Childhood erythroderma seems to be a transition zone between erythroderma in other two age groups, where the causes of erythroderma may be overlapping. As discussion of erythroderma in adults is beyond the scope of this chapter, we would limit our discussion in neonatal and infantile erythroderma, and more particularly to those dermatoses which can persist in childhood.

EPIDEMIOLOGY

Neonatal and infantile erythroderma is an uncommon entity. In a study of 19,000 pediatric patients seen over 6 years period, 20 were of neonatal eythroderma, accounting for an incidence of 0.11%. However, the denominator in calculating incidence was total pediatric population. So, exact age wise incidence is not known.

The diagnosis of primary cause of erythroderma in children is difficult, because of poor specificity of clinical signs and histopathological features. In a study, there were 51 patients of erythroderma presenting within first year of life. In these, the cause of erythroderma could be established on an average after 11 months of onset. The underlying causes of erythroderma in their study were immunodeficiency (30%), ichthyosis (24%), Netherton's syndrome (18%), eczematous or paupulosquamous dermatitis (20%), and erythroderma of unknown origin in 10% of patients. They did not include erythroderma with blistering into consideration. In a study, the causes of erythroderma were infections (40%), ichthyosiform erythroderma (25%), atopic dermatitis (15%), infantile seborrheic dermatitis (10%) and unidentified in 10% of the patients.

CAUSES AND CLINICAL FEATURES OF ERYTHRODERMA

Infectious Causes

a. Staphylococcal scalded skin syndrome
b. Toxic shock syndrome
c. Scarlet fever
d. Generalized congenital candidiasis.

Staphylococcal scalded skin syndrome (SSSS): This disorder is caused by 'epidermolytic toxins (ETA) A or B', produced by *Staphylococcus aureus* phage group 2. ETA specifically cleaves desmoglein 1 in human skin leading to disruption of desmosomes in the epidermal granular layer resulting in epidermal splitting as seen in pemphigus foliaceous. Particularly neonates are susceptible to SSSS because of renal immaturity and associated ineffective renal clearance of the toxin as well as lack of specific immunity to the toxin. It can occur in children below 5 years of age, more particularly in those with acquired renal impairment or immunodeficiency. Bullous impetigo is caused by same toxins, thus can be considered as localized variant of SSSS in normal immunocompetent children.

Affected children initially have a faint red generalized erythema associated with cutaneous tenderness, fever and toxic look. Periorificial and flexural accentuation is characteristic. Nikolsky's sign may be elicited in the early stage even without frank blisters. Within a day or two, large flaccid bullae and erosions start appearing in and around the flexures and orifices which may subsequently generalize, sparing the mucous membranes. Healing is usually complete within a week following superficial desquamation. Acantholytic cells may be observed in Tzanck smear. Histopathology is diagnostic and differentiates from toxic epidermal necrolysis.

Toxic shock syndrome: Toxic shock syndrome is a toxin mediated illness affecting multiple organs. It is caused by toxins produced by *S. aureus*, predominantly 'toxic shock syndrome toxin-1 (TSST-1)'. Though commonly seen in menstruating women with poor tampon hygiene, it may occur in children. It is clinically characterized by rash, hypotension, and involvement of at least three organ systems;

- Muscle involvement characterized by myalgia and rhabdomyolysis,
- Renal involvement with azotemia,
- Hepatic involvement as evidenced by elevated liver enzymes and serum bilirubin,
- Thrombocytopenia,
- Toxic encephalopathy.

The rash is characteristic having generalized scarlatiniform erythema. Other mucocutaneous manifestations include strawberry tongue and mucosal congestion involving conjunctiva, oropharynx, and vagina. Desquamation of palms and soles appear after 1 to 2 weeks of rash. Diagnosis is mainly based on constellation of clinical features. Appropriate investigations should be ordered to detect internal organ system involvement.

Scarlet fever: Scarlet fever is a toxin mediated illness caused by pyrogenic exotoxin (erythrogenic toxin) produced by group A beta- hemolytic streptococci usually harbored in a pharyngeal infection. This occurs primarily in children below 10 years of age. Constellation of clinical features includes fever, associated constitutional symptoms, exanthema and enanthem. The rash appears after 1-2 days of the onset of fever and pharyngeal symptoms starting over the head and neck followed by caudal progression involving trunk and extremities. Even in patients with extensive involvement, palms and soles are usually spared. The rash is characterized by blanching erythema with a rough sand-paper feel. The erythema is marked over the flexures and pressure points with Pastia's lines appearing over axillae and antecubital fossae. As the rash fades after 4-5 days, exfoliation starts first over the periauricular areas and then progressing in the order of appearance of the rash. The exfoliation over palms and soles are in the form of thick sheets while in other areas, it is of branny quality.

The pharynx is beefy red with exudative pharyngitis occasionally extending up to the soft palate and uvula. The tongue initially is coated with bright red erythema over the margin and tips. Erythematous hypertrophied papillae projecting through the white coat gives rise to 'white strawberry' appearance. Subsequently, the coating is sloughed off leaving behind bright red tongue with 'red strawberry' appearance.

The condition may mimic rubella, infectious mononucleosis, drug-induced maculo-papular rash and Kawasaki disease. However, the classic constellation of clinical features is diagnostic of this entity which has become rare nowadays.

Congenital candidiasis (generalized): Congenital candidiasis is easy to recognize when it is in its fully expressed form. Immediately after birth, when the maculopapular erythema of the trunk is the only manifestation, it may be difficult to differentiate form other similar entities. Pustules appear over the trunk and rapidly extend to involve the extremities. The involvement of the palms and soles is said to be classical of generalized congenital candidiasis. In some neonates, the umbilicus may be studded with pustules, which is considered to be pathognomonic. KOH mount from the pustule would confirm the diagnosis.

Ichthyosis and Related Syndromes

a. Bullous and non-bullous ichthyosiform erythroderma
b. Lamellar ichthyosis
c. Harlequin ichthyosis
d. Keratitis-ichthyosis- deafness syndrome
e. Sjögren-Larsson syndrome
f. Conradi Hunermann syndrome
g. Neutral lipid storage disease
h. Trichothiodystrophy
i. Netherton's syndrome

Presence of collodion membrane at birth is an important feature in differentiating between different ichthyosis presenting with erythroderma. Almost 90% of neonates with non-bullous ichthyosiform erythroderma and lamellar ichthyosis have collodion membrane at birth. Other erythrodermic ichthyosiform disorders which occasionally present as collodion baby are Conradi Hunermann syndrome, neutral lipid storage disease, and trichothiodystrophy.

Bullous ichthyosiform erythroderma (BIE): It is an autosomal dominant disorder, where defect is in keratin synthesis or degradation involving keratins K_1 and/K_{10}. In the neonatal period, it is characterized by mild generalized erythema. Skin fragility and blisters appear at the sites of minor trauma and localized areas like hands, feet, knees, napkin area, etc. are involved. In childhood, erythroderma fades and is followed by hyperkeratosis over joint flexures. In these areas characteristic yellow, waxy scales (hystrix like) develop. Cobblestone keratosis develops over dorsum of the hands and feet. Palmoplantar hyperkeratosis can be appreciated in two-thirds of patients. In the neonatal period, it may mimic SSSS and epidermolysis bullosa. Though clinical features are characteristic, histopathology may be helpful in difficult cases.

Non-bullous ichthyosiform erythroderma (NBIE) (Figures 16.9 and 16.10): In this autosomal recessive

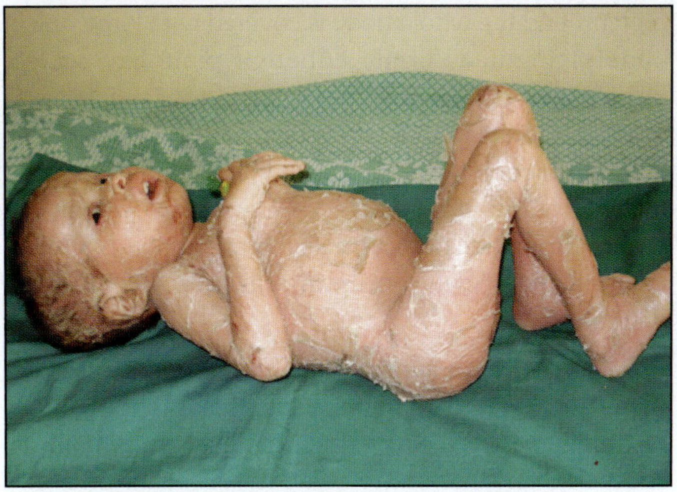

FIGURE 16.9: Infantile erythroderma (NBIE)

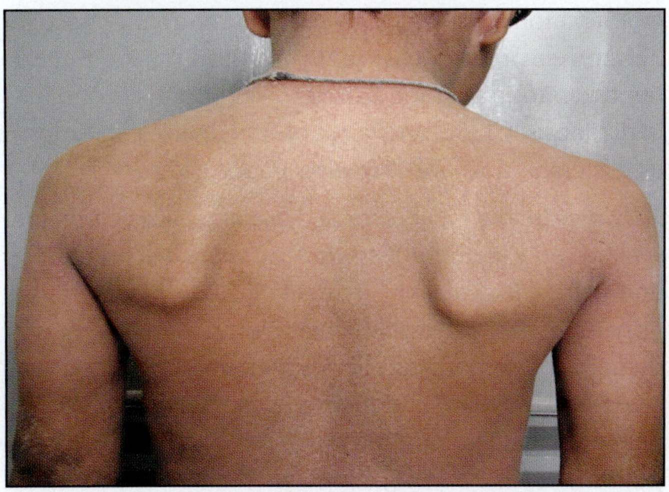

FIGURE 16.10: Childhood erythroderma (NBIE)

condition, almost 90% of neonates present as collodion babies, while the rest are erythrodermic since birth. When the collodion membrane is shed, generalized erythroderma is evident, the intensity of which is decreased as the child grows. Palmoplantar involvement is present and hyperkeratosis is common. The condition mimics congenital psoriasis, trichothiodystrophy and neutral lipid storage disease.

Lamellar ichthyosis (LI): Most neonates with this autosomal recessive ichthyosis presents as collodion baby. After shedding of the membrane, the erythema is evident, which is less intense than NBIE. Scales of LI are large, dark, plate-like and adherent with intervening deep fissures. Palmoplantar keratoderma may be associated. Other features include scarring alopecia, ectropion and hypoplasia of acral and nasal cartilages. Unlike BIE and NBIE, LI does not improve with age.

Harlequin ichthyosis: Infants with this condition are preterm and the whole body is covered with large, thick, hyperpigmented, firmly adherent plate-like scales. Firm adherence of the scales leads to deep fissures running into the dermis simulating Harlequin's costume. Ectropion, conjunctival edema, and eclabium give rise to characteristic grotesque facies. Hands and feet may be encased in mitten like casts. The presentation is striking in itself and should not be mistaken with any other dermatosis.

Sjögren-Larsson syndrome: This autosomal recessive condition due to deficiency of fatty alcohol: NAD oxidoreductase is characterized by congenital ichthyosis, spasticity, and mental retardation. At birth, after the collodion membrane is shed, the skin is dry and minimally erythematous. Scales when present are fine. A peculiar lichenification, occasionally topped by verrucous hyperkeratosis over the flexures is characteristic and aids in diagnosis. Characteristic macular retinal lesions known as glistening dots are seen after infancy.

KID syndrome is characterized by generalized erythema, scaling, and leathery skin. Linear spiny hyperkeratosis and hystrix like scaling occurs. Follicular hyperkeratosis appears over the trunk. Fixed, orange-colored, well demarcated hyperkeratotic plaques over head and face resembling erythrokeratoderma is characteristic. There is palmoplantar keratoderma with pebbly appearance. Most patients have scarring alopecia. There is associated congenital sensorineural deafness. A keratoconjunctivitis that progresses to neovascularization and pannus formation usually begins during infancy.

Neutral lipid storage disease is an autosomal recessive condition, manifesting as collodion membrane or congenital erythroderma which resembles mild to moderate NBIE. Muscle involvement ranges from subclinical myopathy with elevated muscle enzymes to marked proximal muscle weakness. Hepatosplenomegaly and cataract without much visual impairment may be associated.

Netherton's syndrome is an autosomal recessive disorder comprised of erythroderma, hair shaft defects and atopy. Erythroderma of varying severity is an early feature. During childhood, the characteristic lesion of ichthyosis linearis circumflexa becomes apparent in the form of erythematous, annular or polycyclic patch with an incomplete advancing double edge of scale. Hair shaft defects like trichorrhexis invaginata (bamboo hair) leads to brittle, lusterless, and sparse hairs.

Inflammatory Dermatoses

a. Atopic dermatitis
b. Seborrheic dermatitis
c. Psoriasis
d. Diffuse cutaneous mastocytosis
e. Toxic epidermal necrolysis.

Atopic dermatitis (AD): In the neonatal and early infantile period, it is difficult to differentiate between atopic dermatitis (AD) and infantile seborrheic dermatitis (SD). AD is characterized clinically by pruritus, relapsing course, dermatitis in classical distribution depending upon the age, personal or family history of atopy and other features. Itch response is not properly developed before the age of 3 months. However, when the child presents with erythroderma, differentiation from other conditions becomes difficult. Yates et al have suggested that distribution of the skin lesions is the only reliable criteria for differentiation between AD and SD. If the dermatitis involves the axillae or groins, it is more likely to be SD while if it involves the forearms or shins, it is more likely to be AD. In infants with atopic erythroderma using disposable napkins, due to persistent humidity in the local area, the groins are usually spared. Family history of atopy, age of onset and history of associated pruritus does not reliably differentiate between AD and SD. The major points which indicate towards a diagnosis of AD are; the child is well and thriving even when there is erythroderma with occasional irritability, the distribution of rash as has already been described and rapid improvement in the activity of the disease with appropriate treatment.

Seborrheic dermatitis (SD): The rash most commonly appears during second week to second month of life. Most common area of onset is the napkin area. Other areas that can initially be involved are face, scalp and trunk. On the scalp, the vertex and frontal areas are the sites of predilection. On the face, the typical seborrheic areas are most severely involved. The other areas of involvement are the sides of the neck, sides of the face, temples, retroauricular areas and the umbilicus. The rash is characterized by well-defined areas of erythema and scaling. Lichenification which is characteristic of AD is never seen in SD. The scale in SD is rather characteristic which is adherent, yellow-brown in color, large and greasy over the scalp while drier and smaller in other areas. Itching is not a significant component of SD unlike in AD.

Erythrodermic psoriasis (Figure 16.11): This is rare in children. It may start *de novo* or may follow plaque type of psoriasis with exacerbation following irritant reaction due to topical therapy or sudden withdrawal of systemic therapy.

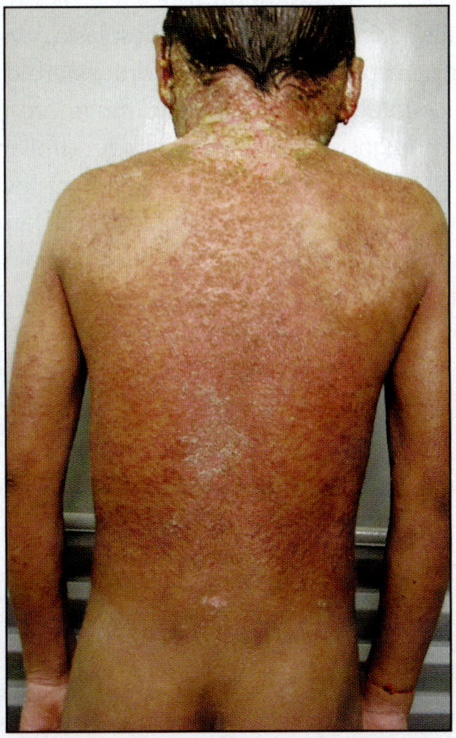

FIGURE 16.11: Childhood erythroderma (Psoriasis)

Diffuse cutaneous mastocytosis: This variant of mastocytosis is rare. Due to diffuse infiltration of the skin by mast cells, it is thickened and often yellowish in appearance. Widespread, firm papular lesions on the background of infiltration give the skin a leathery appearance. Cutaneous folds are often exaggerated, more so in the axillae and groins. Pruritus is usually absent. Mild pressure or trauma to the skin induces mast cell release with development of urticaria which can progress to bullae formation. Episodic flushing which can be associated with headache, dyspnea, wheezing and diarrhea may occur.

Toxic epidermal necrolysis (TEN): It is a disease of adulthood and less common in children. In majority of cases, the diagnosis is straightforward, but in infants it may pose diagnostic difficulty from SSSS. A nonspecific prodrome precedes the onset which is characterized by macular rash appearing first over the face and neck and gradually extending over extremities and trunk. Rapidly spreading atypical target lesions are characterized by irregular pale macules with dusky center. These are flat unlike typical target lesions, tender and Nikolsky's sign can be elicited. In some patients, flaccid hemorrhagic bullae may appear. Subsequently large sheets of necrotic skin may peel off leaving moist erosions. Mucosal involvement is universal which may appear parallel to or preceding the rash. The oral cavity is always affected. The conjunctiva as well as anogenital mucosa may be involved. Initial erythema and burning sensation is followed by extensive dull red erosions coated with grayish white pseudomembrane. Hemorrhagic crust over the lips, more particularly over vermilion borders is characteristic. In a minority of patients with TEN, the so-called TEN without spots, diffuse erythema proportionate to the erythroderma with occasional sparing of the mucosa can occur.

Leiner's Disease

This is a conglomeration of clinical features including acquired erythroderma, diarrhea, and failure to thrive. The diarrhea may be severe and chronic. The dermatitis is often erosive and can be generalized. It has often been described as like that of seborrheic dermatitis. These children are unusually susceptible to infection. Though deficiency of complement component 5 (C_5) was thought to be causative, its role has subsequently been refuted.

Omenn's Syndrome

This disorder of reticuloendothelial system is of significance as it is often misdiagnosed and the earliest manifestation is most commonly cutaneous. It is clinically characterized by erythematous rash appearing during the neonatal period which gradually evolves into erythroderma. Other associated features are hepatosplenomegaly, generalized lymphadenopathy, recurrent infections, chronic diarrhea, and failure to thrive. Thus, apart from the lymphadenopathy, this disorder is almost similar to Leiner's disease. Histopathology of the skin biopsy specimen shows dense perivascular lymphohistiocytic infiltrate, with numerous eosinophils. Basic architecture of the lymph nodes is distorted with dense infiltrate of similar lymphohistiocytic and eosinophilic cells.

Other immunological disorders which may present with erythroderma are hypogammaglobulinemia and DiGeorge syndrome. Though rare in infants, graft versus host disease and cutaneous T cell lymphoma may present with erythroderma in children.

Metabolic and Nutritional Disorders

a. Multiple carboxylase deficiency
b. Essential fatty acid deficiency
c. Acrodermatitis enteropathica
d. Protein malnutrition (branched chain amino acid deficiency)

Multiple carboxylase deficiency: Holocarboxylase synthetase deficiency and biotinidase deficiency are autosomal recessive disorders. In well developed cases, both have similar morphology and skin manifestation is a prominent finding. The presenting manifestation for holocarboxylase synthetase deficiency is lactic acidosis in the neonatal period which may be fatal in the absence of timely diagnosis. Progressive erythroderma with alopecia follows. Severe bacterial and viral infections, as well as neurological abnormalities are other associated features. In biotinidase deficiency, the clinical features are similar, though of lesser severity and appear later than holocarboxylase synthetase deficiency.

Essential fatty acid deficiency: Essential fatty acids are polyunsaturated fatty acids not synthesized in the body and thus deficiency occurs exclusively in the setting of malnutrition. Linoleic acid is biologically the most important essential fatty acid.

This condition arises due to long-term parenteral nutrition and disorders of fat malabsorption. It is clinically characterized by growth retardation, alopecia, eythroderma with occasional weeping intertriginous erosions. Systemic manifestations include anemia, thrombocytopenia, fatty liver, and increased susceptibility to infection.

Protein malnutrition (amino acid disorders): It is presumed that normal concentrations of amino acids are required for normal keratinization. Thus various amino acid deficiencies are associated with dermatological manifestations. Acrodermatitis enteropathica like exfoliative erythema may occur in leucine, and isoleucine deficiency. Other metabolic abnormalities involving amino acids which may present with acrodermatitis enteropathica like clinical presentation may occur in neonatal citrullinemia, methylmalonic acidemia, propionic acidemia, carbamoyl phosphate synthetase deficiency, and arginine deficiency.

APPROACH TO A CHILD WITH ERYTHRODERMA

In fully expressed cases with typical features, diagnosis is straightforward. However, the diagnosis is difficult where the disease is not fully manifested, presents with atypical features, or two or more dermatoses present with overlapping features. According to a study, variables like congenital disease, skin induration, presence of large scaling plaques, alopecia with or without dysplasia, evolution of the lesions, response to topical corticosteroid therapy, presence of infection, or failure to thrive are helpful in reaching a diagnosis. In another study, similar findings were noted; congenital onset, evolution of the disease, family history of atopy, pruritus, presence of large scaling plaques, and sites of predilection after partial clearance are the features important to consider to reach a diagnosis. However, their findings were based on the primary dermatosis in their patient cohort, which may not have been representative and comprehensive encompassing all causes of neonatal erythroderma. We propose that the following features should be considered while dealing a child with erythroderma and individual feature may indicate one or a set of diagnoses **(Table 16.1)**.

MANAGEMENT OF CHILDHOOD ERYTHRODERMA

The management of erythroderma depends on the primary dermatosis, the diagnosis of which is largely clinical

TABLE 16.1: Features and possible diagnosis of erythroderma

Feature	Possible diagnoses
a. Onset at birth or early neonatal period	SSSS, Generalized cutaneous candidiasis
b. Collodion membrane	NBIE, LI, Conradi Hunermann syndrome, Neutral lipid storage disease, Trichothiodystrophy
c. Bullae	SSSS, TEN, BIE, DCM
d. Diarrhea	Leiner's disease, Omenn's syndrome
e. Increased susceptibility to infection	Leiner's disease, Omenn's syndrome, Multiple carboxylase deficiency, Essential fatty acid deficiency
f. Central nervous system symptoms	Sjögren's Larsson syndrome, Multiple carboxylase deficiency
g. Failure to thrive	Leiner's disease, Omenn's syndrome, Essential fatty acid deficiency
h. Hypotension	TSS
i. Hepatosplenomegaly/ lymphadenopathy	Omenn's syndrome
j. Skin tenderness	SSSS, TEN
k. Nikolsky's sign	SSSS, TEN
l. Strawberry tongue	TSS, Scarlet fever
m. Desquamation of palms and soles	TSS, Scarlet fever
n. Palmoplantar keratoderma	BIE, NBIE, LI, KID syndrome
0. Mucosal erosions	TEN
p. Alopecia	Netherton's syndrome, Leiner's disease, Omenn's syndrome, Multiple carboxylase deficiency
q. Systemic abnormality	TSS

SSSS—Staphylococcal scalded skin syndrome, NBIE—Non-bullous ichthyosiform erythroderma, LI—Lamellar ichthyosis, TEN—Toxic epidermal necrolysis, BIE—Bullous ichthyosiform erythroderma, DCM—Diffuse cutaneous mastocytosis, TSS—Toxic shock syndrome

in majority of the cases. Investigations can be undertaken to arrive at a diagnosis or detecting complications arising out of erythroderma. The following investigations may be useful in reaching a diagnosis:

- Demonstration of fungus, bacteria (*Staphylococcus aureus, Streptococcus pyogenes*), or scabies mite in appropriate clinical specimen;
- Complete hemogram,
- Skin biopsy which might have to be done repeatedly or multiple biopsies might have to be taken simultaneously from different sites;
- Hair mount to detect hair shaft disorders,
- Serum zinc and alkaline phosphatase levels to confirm acrodermatitis enteropathica,
- Essential fatty acid estimation,
- Plasma amino acid levels,
- Biotinidase/ holocarboxylase synthetase levels.

The investigations to detect complications are renal function tests, liver function test including total protein and albumin levels, serum electrolytes and urine for routine and microscopic examinations. When sepsis is suspected, repeated blood cultures may be helpful. Erythroderma in children, more particularly in neonates and infants, may be life-threatening if the diagnosis is missed and associated complications are not adequately addressed. Potential complications include anemia, dehydration, hypoalbuminemia, hypernatremic dehydration, hypothermia, hyperpyrexia, and septicemia. Other complications which may be encountered are hypokalemia, edema, and loss of muscle mass. Thus, these issues should be taken care of in addition to the proper management of the underlying dermatosis.

Treatment at hospital is preferable. Protein and electrolyte balance, circulatory status, and body temperature require frequent monitoring. Cooling and overheating should be avoided. Serum electrolytes and renal function should be assessed regularly. Adequate fluid intake should be ensured. Appropriate antibiotics should be considered in every case as staphylococcal superinfection may exacerbate erythroderma.

The prognosis depends on the primary cause of erythroderma. Infective causes and drug-induced erythroderma except TEN is expected to have best prognosis, if detected early and managed properly. So is the case with nutritional deficiency states. However, management of ichthyotic erythroderma is difficult and may be associated with complications of long-term use of retinoids. Immunodeficiency disorders have the worst prognosis. The mortality in the patient cohort of a study was quite high (16%). The causes of mortality were either due to the primary dermatosis or the complications arising thereof. In 67% of the survivors, severe erythroderma persisted at a mean follow-up period of 5.5 years.

LICHENOID ERUPTIONS AND OTHER PAPULOSQUAMOUS DISORDERS

The term "lichenoid" is used to describe both clinical and histopathological changes that occur in certain skin diseases. Clinically, lichenoid means flat topped, shiny, polygonal papules of different sizes resembling tree moss or lichen on the rock. Histopathologically, it refers to band like inflammatory infiltrate in the papillary dermis obscuring the dermo-epidermal junction along with vacuolar degeneration of basal keratinocytes. Certain dermatological conditions present, clinically and/ or histopathologically, as lichenoid lesions. Lichen planus is the prototype of lichenoid eruptions. Other dermatoses that occur commonly in children include lichen nitidus, lichen striatus, lichen sclerosus, pityriasis lichenoides, lichen aureus, pigmented purpuric lichenoid dermatosis of Gougerot and Blum (PPLD), Gianotti-Crosti syndrome (GCS), graft-versus-host disease (GVHD) and frictional lichenoid eruption.

LICHEN PLANUS

Lichen planus (LP) is a papulosquamous disorder of unknown etiology that affects skin, hair, nail and mucous membrane. It was first described by Erasmus Wilson in 1869. The disease is characterized by violaceous to purple flat topped pruritic papules distributed symmetrically over flexor aspects of wrists, legs, and oral and genital mucous membranes.

Epidemiology

Lichen planus is common in adults with equal sex incidence. Childhood LP is rare constituting 1-4% of total cases of LP and 0.13% of total cases seen in pediatric dermatology. LP is extremely rare in infants and the youngest documented case is in a 3-week-old neonate. Familial cases of LP have been reported indicating involvement of genetic factors in the pathogenesis. Familial LP is characterized by early age of onset, generalized involvement including oral mucosa, and prolonged course with relapses.

Etiopathogenesis

The exact etiology of LP is unclear. However, the association of LP with hepatitis C infection and hepatitis B vaccination has been reported. Recently, cell mediated autoimmune response targeting basal keratinocytes has been suggested. The trigger for autoimmune response may be an alteration in the antigenicity of keratinocytes caused by a virus or a drug or an allogenic cell.

Clinical Features

Various clinical types of LP are described based on morphology, configuration and predominant site of involvement. The clinical manifestations and types of LP are similar in both adults and children. However, certain clinical types are common or rare in children compared to adults. Classical LP is the commonest type as in the adults **(Figures 16.12 to 16.15)**. The mucosal and nail involvement is less common in children. Linear LP is more frequently seen in children than adults, whereas actinic LP is less common. A large case series from India, obtained over a long period of time demonstrated occurrence of LP over eyelids and palmo-plantar region which are previously not described in the literature.

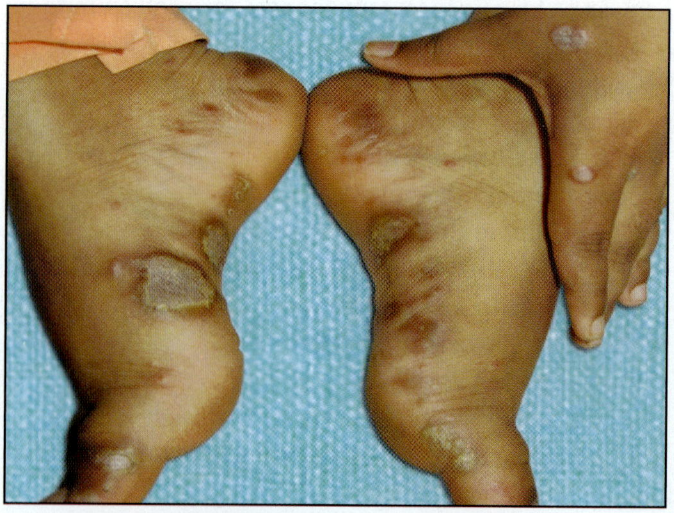

FIGURE 16.12: Lichen planus

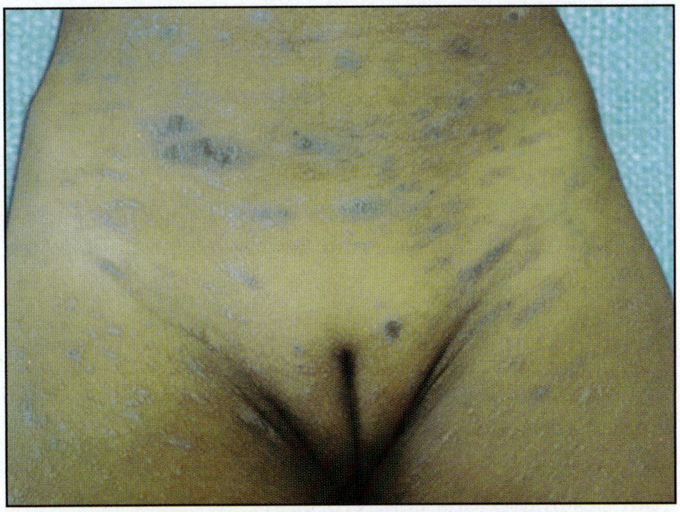

FIGURE 16.13: Generalized lichen planus

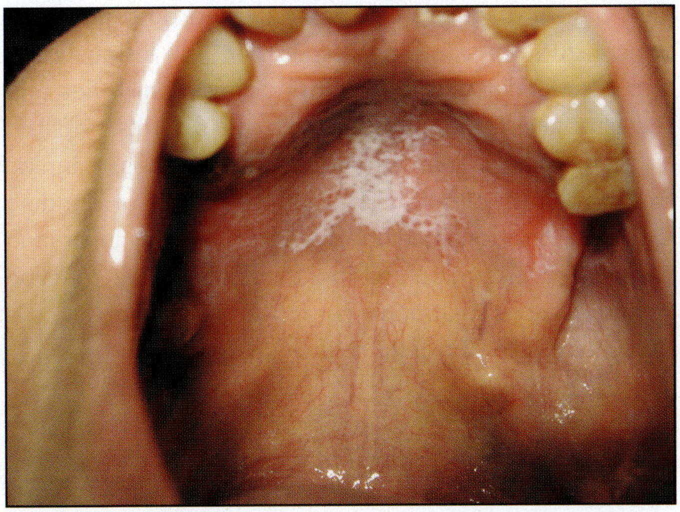

FIGURE 16.14: Oral lichen planus

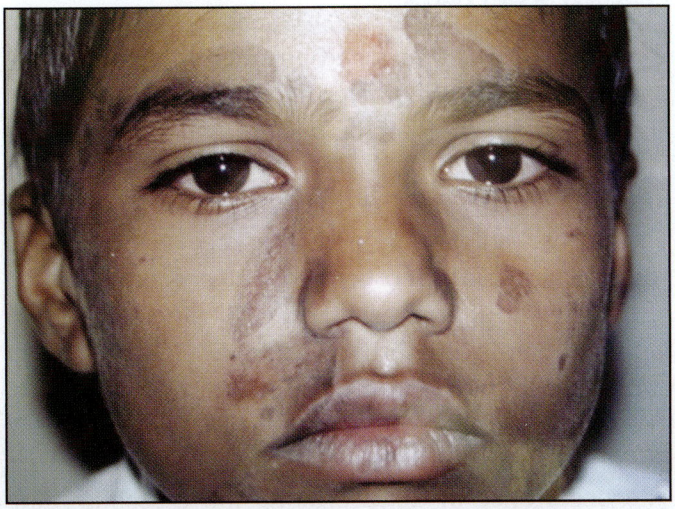

FIGURE 16.15: Actinic lichen planus

Differential Diagnosis

The differential diagnosis of LP includes conditions with lichenoid eruptions such as lichen nitidus, lichenoid drug eruptions, and graft-versus-host disease. LP also needs to be differentiated from psoriasis and pityriasis rosea. Violaceous, flat-topped papules with Wikham's striae, distribution of the lesions, involvement of mucus membrane and histopathological features help in distinguishing LP from other disorders.

Laboratory Investigations

Routine blood investigation-including complete hemogram and blood chemistry are usually normal in LP. In some cases, skin biopsy is required to confirm the diagnosis. The characteristic features are wedge-shaped hypergranulosis, saw tooth acanthosis, basal cell vacuolization, band-like lymphocytic infiltration obscuring dermo-epidermal junction and civette or colloid bodies in the lower epidermis and upper dermis.

Treatment

The response to therapy in children is similar to that in adults. Various treatment modalities have been used. Topical corticosteroids are mainstay of treatment for localized and classical LP. Dapsone has been found to be effective in chronic and recurrent LP. Short course of systemic corticosteroids can be used in the treatment of acute and wide spread disease. Narrow band ultraviolet therapy is a safe and effective therapy for generalized disease.

Course and Prognosis

In approximately 2/3rd of patients acute generalized LP tends to resolve spontaneously in 8 to 15 months leaving behind post inflammatory hyperpigmentation. Malignant transformation of mucosal and hypertrophic LP has not been reported in children. Patients with familial LP are at increased risk of carcinomatous change.

LICHEN NITIDUS

Lichen nitidus is a clinically and pathologically distinct inflammatory disorder commonly occurring in children.

Epidemiology

The disease is common in preschool and school-going children.

Etiopathogenesis

The etiology of LN is unknown. Familial cases of LN have been reported. LN has also been reported in association with atopic dermatitis, Crohn's disease, and Juveline chronic arthritis. In some cases, the lesions may involve photo-exposed areas. This pattern is also noticed in advanced HIV. All these associated diseases suggestature that LN is a result of immune alterations. In some cases, sun exposure may also play a role in the pathogenesis.

Clinical Features

LN is clinically characterized by well demarcated, monomorphic, pinhead sized, flesh colored to violaceous, shiny papules distributed over abdomen, chest, glans penis and upper extremites. The lesions are usually asymptomatic and show Koebner phenomenon in almost 100% of cases **(Figures 16.16A and B)**.

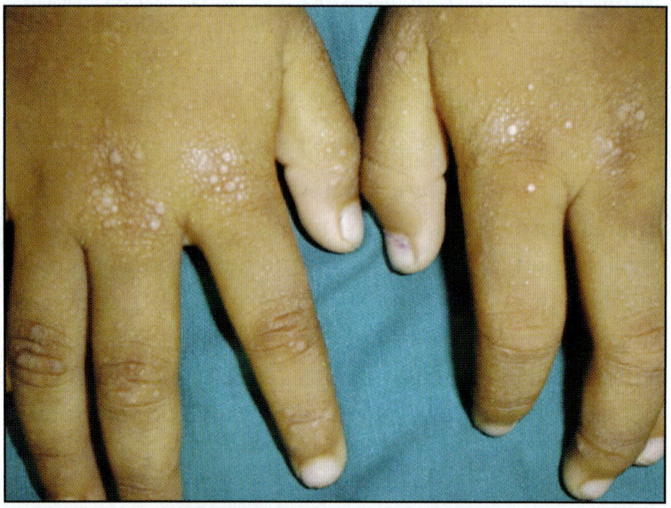

FIGURE 16.16A: Lichen nitidus

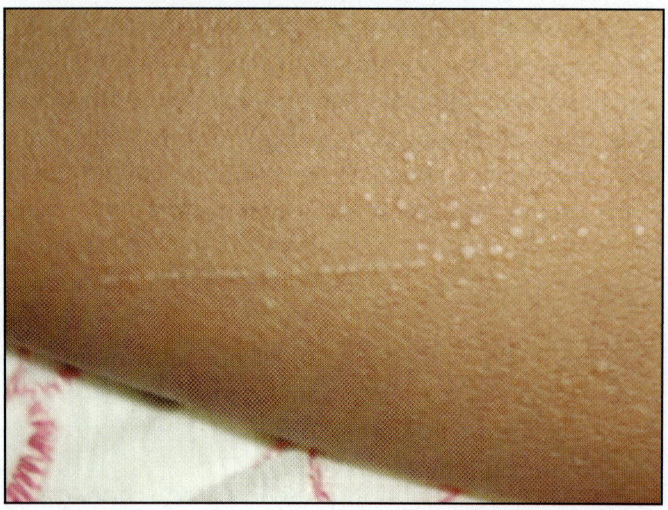

FIGURE 16.16B: Lichen nitidus with Koebnerization

Photodistributed pattern has also been reported. Generalized lesions with the involvement of palms and soles have been described. The lesions over palms and soles are usually keratotic resembling sand paper. Nails and oral mucosa may be affected. The former presents with linear ridges and pits indicating inflammation of nail matrix and the latter with minute grayish flat papules on the buccal mucosa.

Differential Diagnosis

The important differential diagnoses are early lesions of lichen planus, and frictional lichenoid eruptions. LN with lesions on photo-exposed areas needs to be differentiated from polymorphous light eruptions.

Diagnosis

The clinical diagnosis can be confirmed by histopathological study of skin biopsy specimen. LN lesions show circumscribed infiltrate of lymphocytes, histiocytes and few plasma cells spanning the width of 2-3 dermal papillae. The overlying epidermis shows parakeratosis, thinning and basal vacuolization. The rete ridges of surrounding epidermis are elongated and incline towards the infiltration resembling a claw clutching the ball. There may be granulomatous infiltration composed of epithelioid cells and multinucleated giant cells.

Treatment

There is no specific treatment for LN. Most of the cases undergo spontaneous remission. Topical corticosteroids may hasten the resolution of lesions in some children.

LICHEN STRIATUS

Lichen striatus is an acquired uncommon dermatosis of unknown etiology characterized by lichenoid papules arranged along the Blaschko's line.

Epidemiology

The disease is common in children between 5 and 15 years of age. However, younger children may also be affected. Though female preponderance has been reported, there is consensus on equal sex incidence. There are no known racial or hereditary predispositions.

Etiopathogenesis

The occurrence of disease along the Blaschko's line suggests somatic mutation in the early stage of embryogenesis. Lichen striatus is not an inherited disorder as the mutation is postzygotic. The outbreak of disease among non related children living together suggests a role of environmental factor. In addition, family history of atopy has been reported in 85% of cases. Thus, the interaction of factors such as genetic, environmental and atopy at a certain age may be responsible for manifestation of lichen striatus.

Clinical Features

The patients of lichen striatus commonly present with linear hypopigmentation **(Figure 16.17)**. However, the disease initially manifests as asymptomatic, small, erythematous, scaly, flat-topped papules arranged as continuous or interrupted band along the Blaschko's line. The lesions are usually localized to limbs but can involve trunk, neck, face and buttocks. The lesions may be multifocal involving more than one body part, unilateral or bilateral. Post inflammatory hypopigmentation is the usual sequel which takes months to years to resolve.

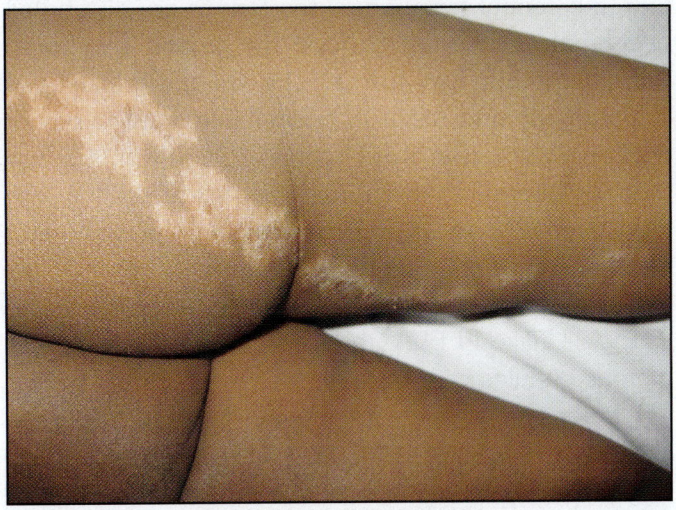

FIGURE 16.17: Lichen striatus

Rarely nail involvement can occur either as sole manifestation or in association with adjacent skin lesions. Unlike LP, the involvement is restricted to single nail and a part of the nail plate is affected.

Differential Diagnosis

Lichen striatus should be differentiated from disorders which follow Blaschko's line such as lichen planus, psoriasis, nevus unius lateris, epidermal verrucous nevus, and nevus depigmentosus (hypopigmentation).

Diagnosis

The diagnosis of lichen striatus is mainly clinical. Histopathological features may help in differentiating lichen striatus from other disorders. The early lesions show epidermal hyperkeratosis with focal parakeratosis and a dense perivascular lymphohistiocytic infiltrate is noticed in the dermis. There may be band-like or periappendageal infiltration.

Treatment

Lichen striatus is benign condition which usually undergoes spontaneous resolution. Reassurance regarding the course and prognosis is all that is required. Topical corticosteroids may be helpful in hastening the resolution.

LICHEN SCLEROSUS

Lichen sclerosus is an inflammatory disorder of skin predominantly involving genitalia resulting in progressive sclerosis or scarring of the affected part.

Epidemiology

Lichen sclerosus affects all age groups with 10-15% of cases occurring in children. There is a female preponderance with female to male ratio of 10:1. The disease shows a bimodal distribution in prepubertal and postmenopausal female patients.

Etiopathogenesis

Exact etiology of lichen sclerosus is not yet clear. However, association of lichen sclerosus with autoimmune disorders, certain human leukocytic antigens (HLA), and *Borrelia burgdorferi* infection has been suggested. The peak incidence of the disease in prepubertal girls and postmenopausal women, both being low-estrogen states, suggests a role of hormones.

Clinical Features

The initial lesions of lichen sclerosus are well demarcated, ivory-white to pink, flat-topped, small papules that slowly coalesce to form thin plaques. There may be koebnerization. As the disease progresses, the atrophy of lesions occurs with prominent follicular openings. Pruritus of variable intensity is usually present. In girls, the labia, and perineal and anal areas are involved resulting in a pattern often described as "figure of 8", Keyhole", "hourglass", and "butterfly" lesions. In boys, glans penis and prepuce are involved resulting in white sclerotic ring at the preputial opening, phimosis, recurrent balanitis, dysuria and eventually difficulty in micturition. The vaginal mucosa is spared because the disease affects only cornified stratified squamous epithelium. Though uncommon, the neck and shoulders are common extragenital sites of involvement. Trunk, arms, and face are less frequently involved. The extragenital lesions are usually asymptomatic.

Diagnosis

The clinical diagnosis, when in doubt, can be confirmed by characteristic histopathological features. The epidermis is atrophic with relative hyperkeratosis. In early stages, liquefactive degeneration of basal keratinocytes, chronic inflammatory infiltrate in the upper dermis abutting the epidermis and homogenization upper dermis are diagnostic of lichen sclerosus. In later stages, the middermis shows inflammatory infiltration.

Treatment

The ultrapotent clobetasol proprionate applied at night with gradual tapering is effective in the treatment of childhood lichen sclerosus. Though the symptoms are alleviated within a few days, the return of normal color and texture of skin takes several months. Topical tacrolimus has been used successfully in the treatment of lichen sclerosus.

About 5% of patients may develop local squamous cell carcinoma. It occurs in patients with chronic hyperkeratosis or erosions.

PITYRIASIS LICHENOIDES

Pityriasis lichenoides is a benign lymphoproliferative disorder grouped under parapsoriasis. Pityriasis lichenoides occurs in two forms, pityriasis lichenoides et varioliformis acuta (PLEVA) or Mucha-Habermann disease and pityriasis lichenoides chronica (PLC).

Epidemiology

Pityriasis lichenoides is a disorder of young adults and children. It is commonly seen in school-going children (5-10 years). Pediatric age group constitutes 19-38% of cases of pityriasis lichenoides. It exhibits a variable male predominance. The onset of the disease at birth and infancy has been reported.

Etiopathogenesis

The presence of clonal T- lymphocytes and occasional progression of PLC to mycosis fungoides suggests that pityriasis lichenoides is a cutaneous lymphoproliferative disorder. Benign nature of the condition is due to vigorous host immune response mediated by CD8+ suppressor T-lymphocytes. Another explanation proposes immunologic response to unidentified infectious agents. The immune response includes both immune complex and cell mediated hypersensitivity reactions.

Clinical Features

PLEVA presents as recurrent crops of erythematous papules which undergo vesicular, pustular, necrotic or hemorrhagic surface changes. The lesions are found at different stages of evolution. The duration of the disease depends on the distribution of lesions. Therefore, PLEVA is classified as peripheral, central and diffuse forms. In the peripheral form the lesions are predominantly distributed over extremities with longer duration of disease than the central form where the lesions are distributed over trunk. In the diffuse form the lesions last shorter than the other two forms. The lesions are usually symptomatic and result in postinflammatory hypo- or hyperpigmentation, and typical varioliformis scars. Mucha-Habermann disease is a variant presenting with high degree of fever, and hemorrhagic necrosis and ulceration of established PLEVA lesions.

The PLC can occur separately or in association with PLEVA. Unlike PLEVA, the lesions in PLC are erythematous papules with mica-like scales **(Figure 16.18)**. The lesions progress to form minimally elevated plaques.

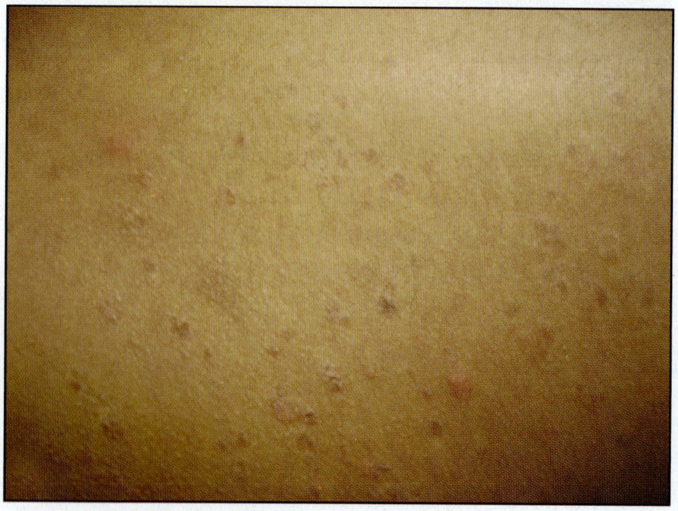

FIGURE 16.18: Pityriasis lichenoides chronica

Differential Diagnosis

PLEVA should be differentiated from lymphomatoid papulosis, varicella, insect bites, impetigo, vasculitis and scabies. PLC should be differentiated from psoriasis, lichen planus, pityriasis rosea, parapsoriasis and secondary syphilis.

Lymphomatoid papulosis is a cutaneous lymphoproliferative disorder clinicallly similar to PLEVA. The lesions are localized to a part of the body. Lymphomatoid papulosis is rare in children. The presence of atypical lymphocytes (CD_4+ T cells/Natural killer cells) and absence of interface dermatitis distinguish lymphomatoid papulosis from PLEVA.

Diagnosis

Recurrent crops of lesions, presence of pleomorphic lesions, distribution of lesions and the duration of disease helps in the clinical diagnosis. When the diagnosis is in doubt, histopathological examination of involved skin will substantiate the diagnosis. PLEVA is characterized by dense perivascular and diffuse lymphocytic infiltration, exocytosis of erythrocytes, vacuolar degeneration of basal cells, epidermal necrosis, parakeratosis and hyperkeratosis. Histopathological features of PLC are similar to PLEVA but changes are less severe. The cellular infiltration is less dense and more superficial than PLEVA.

Treatment

In most of the patients the disease remits spontaneously over months to years depending upon the distribution of lesions. Oral antibiotics are the mainstay of therapy. Erythromycin or tetracycline (>10 years of age) have been found to be effective in PLEVA. Antihistamines and topical corticosteroids may be useful. Acute flares of PLEVA and Mucha-Habermann disease are often controlled by systemic corticosteroids. Phototherapy with ultraviolet (UV) B light provides the best therapeutic response. Photochemotherapy (PUVA) has also shown therapeutic benefit. In refractory cases methotrexate (weekly dose), cyclosporine, or retinoids can be considered.

OTHER SKIN DISEASES WITH LICHENOID ERUPTIONS

Lichen aureus

Lichen aureus (LA) belongs to the group of pigmented purpuric disorders. LA is rare in children accounting for 17% of cases. Slight female preponderance has been reported in one study. The exact etiology of the condition is unclear. However, the presence of extravasated erythrocytes in the dermis suggests either increased vascular pressure as a result of vascular insufficiency or increased permeability of the vessels. Medications such as nonsteroidal anti-inflammatory drugs, diuretics and ampicillin have also been implicated. Clinically, LA presents as characteristic asymptomatic gold, copper or rust colored lichenoid papules or macules on the lower limbs. Pruritus may be present in some cases. The lesions may remain stationary or slowly enlarge and coalesce. The lesions are usually unilateral and may show segmental distribution. Rarely, abdomen, neck, trunk, face, forearm or fingers may be involved. Apart from extravasated erythrocytes; hemosiderin deposition; and perivascular lymphocytic infiltration that are characteristics of pigmented purpura, LA lesions also show a band like lymphohistiocytic infiltrate in the papillary dermis with a Grenz zone. The disease in children is self limiting. Treatment with topical corticosteroid is often ineffective.

Pigmented Purpuric Lichenoid Dermatosis of Gougerot and Blum

PPLD is a type of pigmented purpuric dermatoses. It is extremely rare in children with equal sex incidence. The etiopathogenesis is similar to that of LA. Unlike LA, the PPLD presents as bilaterally symmetrical asymptomatic minute lichenoid papules with erythema and scaling. The predominant sites of involvement are legs, thighs, lower part of abdomen and rarely, the arms. Mild pruritus may be present in some cases. Histopathologically, PPLD lesions show epidermal parakeratosis and spongiosis along with perivascular lymphocytic infiltration and extravasation of erythrocytes in the dermis.

The treatment is usually symptomatic, as the disease is self limiting. Fluorinated topical corticosteroids, systemic steroids, PUVA, vitamin C, and vitamin D have been found to be effective.

Gianotti-Crosti Syndrome

Gianotti-Crosti syndrome (GCS) is a viral exanthematous disorder affecting mainly children aged 2-6 years (see Chapter on viral exanthemas for details). The disease frequently occurs in boys and it is common in spring and early summer. A prodrome of fever, malaise and upper respiratory tract symptoms precedes sudden onset of skin lesions. The eruption usually starts on the thigh and buttocks, and then spreads to involve extensor extremities and face. The lesions are flat, pink to red-brown relatively nonpruritic papules with bilaterally symmetrical distribution. Koebner phenomenon can occur early in the course of the disease. Papulovesicles may be seen especially in children younger than 1 year of age. Purpuric lesions may occur at the site of trauma. Histopathology of papules shows psoriasiform hyperplasia, hyperkeratosis, focal parakeratosis and focal spongiosis. Lichenoid histology has also been reported. The disease resolves spontaneously within a few weeks. Treatment is usually symptomatic with antihistamines.

Graft-versus-Host Disease

Graft-versus-host disease (GVHD) occurs when immunologically competent foreign cells are administered to an immunocompromised patient. GVHD is commonly seen following bone-marrow transplantation. Depending upon the duration between transplantation and the onset of disease, GVHD is divided into acute and chronic forms. Acute GVHD occurs 5 to 40 days after transplantation and chronic GVHD occurs weeks to months after transplantation. Lichenoid eruptions are seen in chronic GVHD. The lesions are morphologically similar to LP. However, the distribution of lichenoid papules tends to be diffuse with a background of diffuse poikiloderma. Over the limbs the lesions are often arranged in a reticular configuration. The oral involvement manifests as ulcerations of lips, buccal mucosa and tongue. Histopathological changes are similar to that of lichen planus except for less intense inflammatory infiltrate. The combination of systemic corticosteroid and cyclosporine or azathioprine is used to treat the condition.

Frictional Lichenoid Eruption

Frictional lichenoid eruption is also known as recurrent papular reaction of childhood, summertime pityriasis of elbows and knees, recurrent papular eruption of childhood, and summertime lichenoid dermatitis of the elbows. It is common in children of 3 to 12 years of age and boys are affected more frequently than girls. The lesions consist of mildly pruritic, skin colored, 1-2 mm lichenoid papules distributed on the back of the hands, fingers, elbows, and knees. A history of contact with abrasive materials like sand, grass, wool, fabric, etc. is usually elicited. An association with atopy has been suggested. The histopathological changes are non specific. The condition is self-limiting and resolution may be hastened by topical corticosteroids.

PITYRIASIS ROSEA

Pityriasis rosea (PR) is self-limiting papulosquamous disorder of unknown etiology commonly occurring in adolescents and children.

Epidemiology

The disease occurs equally in both sexes. Fifty percent of cases occur in patients of less than 20 years of age. The incidence of PR in children less than 4 years is 4%.

Etiopathogenesis

Exact etiology of the disease is not yet clear. Various infections and drugs are implicated in the etiopathogenesis of PR. The clinical features, course of the disease, occurrence of the disease in clusters and absence of recurrences in majority of cases indicate viral etiology. Human herpes viruses (HHV), like HHV-7 and HHV-6 have been implicated in the etiology of PR. However, the evidences in favor of role of HHV-7 and HHV-6 are inconsistent and contradictory.

Clinical Features

The prodromal symptoms are usually absent in most of the cases. However, in severe PR there may be prodrome of pharyngitis, malaise, headache and lymphadenopathy. The characteristic lesion of PR is a single-isolated patch, called herald patch that occurs in 70% of patients. It is a well demarcated, annular, erythematous, oval patch with fine peripheral scale usually found on the trunk or upper arm or neck. After a span of 2 to 21 days, a secondary eruption consisting of small erythematous papules appear in crops with characteristic 'above knee above elbow' distribution sparing face and distal extremities **(Figure 16.19)**. Itching may be present in 25% of cases. The lesions are round to oval with their long-axis along the lines of skin cleavage, resembling a 'Christmas-tree' on the back. The secondary lesions also show a 'Collarette of scale'. In some cases, the lesions occur only on the face or distal extremities or axilla or groin. This clinical variant is called inverse PR which is difficult to diagnose in the absence of herald patch. Other clinical variants, though rare, have been reported **(Table 16.2)**. Oral mucus membrane involvement in the form of erythematous patch has been reported in 16% of patients.

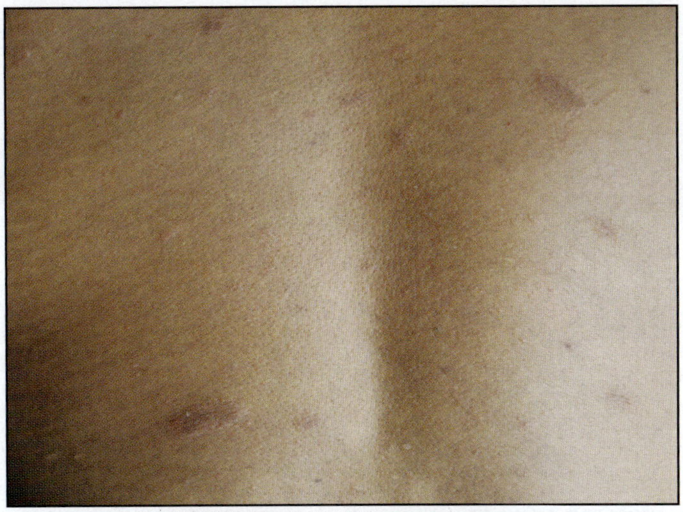

FIGURE 16.19: Pityriasis rosea

TABLE 16.2: Clinical variants of pityriasis rosea
1. Classical—PR with herald patch and secondary eruption
2. Inverse—PR involving distal extremities
3. Papular—PR with only papular lesions
4. Pustular—PR with pustular lesions
5. Vesicular—PR with concomitant vesicles
6. Urticarial—PR with whealing along the border of the patch
7. Purpuric—PR with tiny purpuric spots
8. Erythema—multiforme like- PR with target lesions
9. Gigantic—PR with secondary eruption around the herald patch
10. Localized—Cervicocephalic form (scalp), Girdle (axilla or groin)
11. Pityriasis circinata et marginata of Vidal- PR with circinate and confluent lesions
12. PR with only herald patch (single or multiple)

Differential Diagnosis

There are several differential diagnoses depending upon the stage of the disease. The herald patch should be differentiated from tinea corporis. The well established disease should be differentiated from lichen planus, psoriasis, and pityriasis versicolor. PR-like eruptions are also seen in pediculids and epidermodysplasia verruciformis. Erythema dyschromicans perstans and parapsoriasis which follow skin cleavage lines are other differential diagnoses. In the absence of herald patch, secondary eruption should be differentiated from secondary syphilis especially in sexually active patients. Presence of eosinophilia and absence of herald patch help in distinguishing PR-like drug eruptions from PR.

Treatment

Usually no treatment is required apart from reassurance regarding the course and prognosis of the disease. The lesions clear spontaneously within 6 weeks, but may take as long as 5 months. If pruritus is present, antihistamines, topical calamine lotion and topical corticosteroid can be used. Oral antibiotics (erythromycin) and antivirals (acyclovir) have been tried to shorten the course of the disease.

PITYRIASIS RUBRA PILARIS

Pityriasis rubra pilaris (PRP) is a chronic skin disease characterized by keratotic follicular papules that coalesce to form widespread erythroderma, and palmoplantar keratoderma. PRP is an acquired disorder though familial cases have been described.

Epidemiology

PRP is worldwide in distribution with an estimated prevalence of 1 in 5,00,000. Males and females are equally affected. In children circumscribed type (7-24%) is more common than classical (4-14%) and atypical (4-14%) types.

Etiopathogenesis

The exact etiology of PRP is not yet clear. The histopathological features suggest that it is a disorder of abnormal keratinization. The role of bacterial superantigens has been suggested.

Clinical Features

PRP is divided into six types. These are classic adult (Type I), atypical adult (Type II), classic juvenile (Type III), circumscribed juvenile (Type IV), atypical juvenile (Type V) and HIV infection associated PRP (Type VI). The characteristic presentation is follicular, erythematous keratotic papules with central plugs along with yellow colored keratoderma of palms and soles. These follicular papules over period of several weeks to months coalesce and evolve into erythroderma. During this stage diagnostic 'island of sparing' of skin surface is noticed. In Type III PRP the lesions spread in a cephalo-caudal direction. The scalp and face usually show bran-like diffuse scaling. In Type IV PRP, the lesions are localized to elbows and knees **(Figures 16.20A to C)**. These two juvenile forms manifest in the first decade of life. The familial Type V

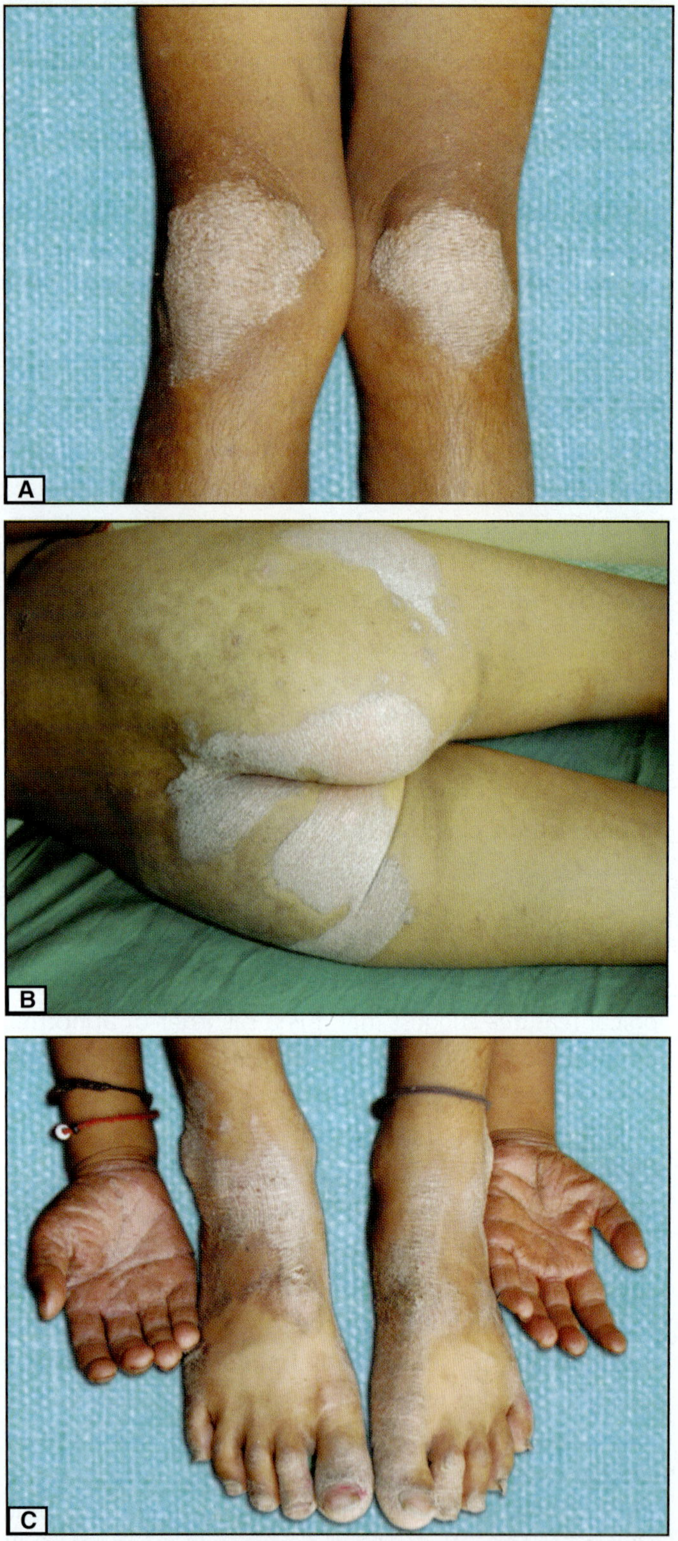

FIGURES 16.20A TO C: Juvenile circumscribed pityriasis rubra pilaris

PRP is rare and occurs at birth or in the first few years of life. It presents as diffuse erythema with prominent follicular papules. Palmoplantar keratoderma referred as 'keratodermic sandal' occurs in most of the cases in

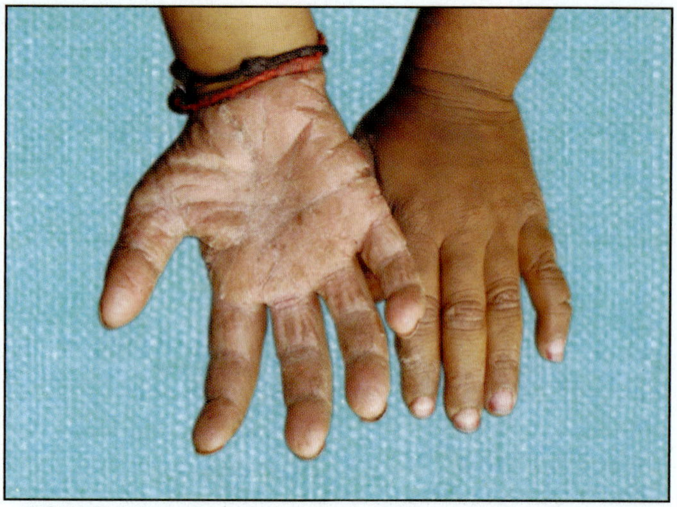

FIGURE 16.21: Palmar involvement in pityriasis rubra pilaris

children **(Figure 16.21)**. It may precede or follow skin lesions. Sometimes the keratoderma may be severe enough to cause contractures. Koebner phenomenon has been noticed in 10% of children with PRP. Nails may be dystrophic with thickening, transverse striations and subungual debris.

Differential Diagnosis

The differential diagnoses of Type III and IV PRP include phrynoderma, lichen spinulosus, and psoriasis. Type V should be differentiated from ichthyosiform erythrodermas and erythrokeratodermas.

Phrynoderma is a discrete follicular keratotic disorder characterized by keratotic perifollicular papules with central plug predominantly distitributed over elbows, knees and buttocks. Rarely there may be generalized and widespread lesions. The deficiency of various nutritional factors such as vitamin (Vit) A, Vit B-Complex, Vit E and essential fatty acids has been implicated in the etiology of the condition. Good response to Vit A, Vit B-Complex and topical keratolytics has beeen reported.

Lichen spinulosus is characterized by skin colored keratotic follicular papules with central filiform spines grouped into patches over neck, trunk, buttocks and extremities.

The ichthyosiform erythrodermas and erythrokeratodermas lack follicular papules. The psoriasis can be distinguished by histopathological features.

Diagnosis

The diagnosis can be established by characteristic clinical features of PRP. However, in some cases histopathological study may be required to distinguish PRP from psoriasis. The involved skin in PRP shows follicular keratosis, alternate orthokeratosis and parakeratosis, and mononuclear infiltration around the follicle.

Treatment

The course of the disease is characterized by exacerbations and remissions. Some children may eventually develop typical psoriasis. Irrespective of extent of involvement and mode of onset, the disease usually clears in 6 months to 1 year of time.

The patients with mild or localized PRP may respond to topical keratolytics, calcipotriol, and emollients. Extensive or severe PRP requires systemic therapy with retinoids, methotrexate, high-dose Vit A (>100000 U/day), UVB, cyclosporine or azathioprine. Oral isotretinoin and acetretin are the most effective therapeutic agents. The therapy is continued for at least 4-6 months with regular monitoring of side effects of retinoids.

PARAPSORIASIS

Parapsoriasis is a group of cutaneous T cell lymphoproliferative disorder with close relationship with malignant lymphoproliferative disease. Clinically it is characterized by persistent, scaly and inflammatory skin lesions. Parapsoriasis is classified into two types namely, small plaque parapsoriasis (SPP) and large plaque parapsoriasis (LPP).

Epidemiology

Parapsoriasis is mainly a disease of adults with male preponderance. Rarely, it can occur in children. In a study, 5% of SPP and 20% of LPP cases were children.

Etiopathogenesis

Parapsoriasis is a cutaneous T cell lymphoproliferative disorder with 1- 10% of dominant T cell clones. However, the percentage of clonal cells is less than what is seen in mycosis fungoides. LPP is considered as a clinically benign end of mycosis fungoides spectrum because of malignant transformation that occurs in some cases over a period of time. The dominant clonality has also been described in follicular mucinosis, pagetoid reticulosis, primary erythroderma and nonspecific chronic spongiotic dermatitis. These disorders have given rise to the concept of clonal dermatitis. Though, cases of clonal dermatitis are benign, progression to mycosis fungoides has been reported. It has been postulated that each of the above mentioned diseases including LPP are potentially at the risk of progression to mycosis fungoides through an intermediate clonal dermatitis.

Clinical Features

SPP presents as asymptomatic well demarcated patches or thin plaques with fine scaling predominantly distributed over trunk and proximal extremities. The lesions measure less than 5 cm. A digitate pattern on the sides of the trunk resembling a finger print is a distinct variant of SPP. LPP presents as asymptomatic or mildly pruritic, irregular or oval, well demarcated or ill-defined patches or thin plaques, measuring more than 5 cm. The surface of the lesions shows fine scaling and wrinkling. There may be telectectasia and mottled pigmentation resulting in poikiloderma. Retiform parapsoriasis is a variant of LPP characterized by wide spread scaly macular and papular eruptions arranging in a zebra-like or net-like pattern.

Differential Diagnosis

SPP should be differentiated from nummular eczema, psoriasis, tinea corporis and mycosis fungoides. The differential diagnoses of LPP include the diseases with poikilodermatous skin lesions such as Rothmund-Thomson syndrome, Bloom's syndrome, dyskeratosis congenital, systemic lupus erythematosus, dermatomyositis, radiodermatitis and mycosis fungoides.

Diagnosis

The diagnosis of parapsoriasis is mainly clinical. The associated clinical findings and relevant investigations differentiate other diseases (see above) from parapsoriasis. Skin biopsy is required to distinguish LPP from mycosis fungoides. The histopathological features of SPP are similar to that of spongiotic dermatitis with mild superficial perivascular lymphocytic infiltrate. The advanced lesions of LPP show epidermal atrophy, marked exocytosis of lymphocytes and a band-like lymphocytic infiltrate in the papillary dermis. Poikilodermatous changes are also seen.

Treatment

SPP usually requires no treatment. Topical corticosteroids and UVB therapy may be used in symptomatic patients. LPP can be treated with topical potent corticosteroids, UVB and PUVA therapy. In case of malignant transformation, local radiotherapy is useful.

Parapsoriasis runs a chronic, slowly progressive course over many years. However, 10-30% of LPP cases will progress to mycosis fungoides. Therefore, long-term follow up with repeated biopsy is essential.

LYMPHOMATOID PAPULOSIS

Lymphomatoid papulosis is a recurring, self healing, papulonodular eruption with the histopathological features of a T-cell lymphoproliferative disorder.

Epidemiology

Lymphomatoid papulosis is rare in children.

Etiopathogenesis

Lymphomatoid papulosis is a T-cell lymphoproliferative disorder with predominant CD4 T-lymphocytes. Cases with predominant CD8 T-lymphocytes or Natural Killer cells have been described. The cause for proliferation is not known. However, virus induced process has been suggested. Similar to parapsoriasis, T-cell clonality has been identified.

Clinical Features

Lymphomatoid papulosis presents as recurrent crops of asymptomatic, erythematous papules and nodules predominantly distributed over trunk and extremities. The varying numbers of lesions develop at the interval of months to years. The lesions may undergo necrosis and ulceration. The lesions spontaneously resolve in weeks to months with varying degrees of pigmentary changes or atrophic scarring. Pustular and vesicular variants have been reported. Only CD30+ large cell anaplastic lymphoma has been reported to develop in pediatric age group. Mycosis fungoides and Hodgkin's lymphoma develop in adults. However, regular follow up is essential in children with lymphomatoid papulosis to detect any malignant transformation.

Differential Diagnosis

The important differential diagnoses include insect bite reaction, pityriasis lichenoides, lymphoma and pseudo-lymphoma.

Diagnosis

The clinical course, absence of lymph node involvement, the type of cellular infiltrate and characteristic histopathological findings of lymphomatoid papulosis help in differential diagnosis. Depending upon the morphology of atypical cells, three histopathological subtypes have been described. Type A is characterized by large cells with vesicular nuclei, prominent nucleolus and abundant cytoplasm. These cells are CD30+. There may be multinucleated cells resembling Reed-Sternberg cells of Hodgkin's lymphoma. Type B is characterized by smaller, cerebriform cells with scanty cytoplasm resembling atypical cells of mycosis fungoides. Type C is characterized by abundant Type A cells resembling CD30+ large cell anaplastic lymphoma.

Treatment

Only severe cases require treatment, though there are no therapeutic guidelines for treatment in children. The treatment modalities include superpotent topical corticosteroids, intralesional or oral corticosteroids, oral antibiotics, UVB and PUVA therapy. Methotrexate may be considered in very severe cases.

BIBLIOGRAPHY

1. Bekkenk MW, Kluin PM, Jansen PM. Lymphomatoid papulosis with a natural killer-cell phenotype. Br J Dermatol 2001;145:318-22.
2. Burden AD. Management of psoriasis in childhood. Clin Exp Dermatol 1999;24:341-5.
3. Chan ES, Cronstein B. Molecular action of methotrexate in inflammatory diseases. Arthritis Res 2002;4:266-73.
4. Chen W, Schramm M, Zouboulis CHC. Generalized lichen nitidus. J Am Acad Dermatol 1997;36:630-1.
5. Chuh AA, Peiris JS. Lack of evidence of active human herpesvirus-7 infection on three cases of pityriasis rosea in children. Pediatr Dermatol 2001;18: 381-83.
6. Connelly EA, Spraker MK. Differential diagnosis of neonatal erythroderma. In: Harper J, Oranje A, Prose NS ,editors. Textbook of pediatric dermatology. Oxford: Wiley Blackwell 2006;105-17.
7. Dadlani C, Orlow SJ. Treatment of children and adolescents with methotrexate, cyclosporine, and etanercept: review of the dermatologic and rheumatologic literature. J Am Acad Dermatol 2005;52:316-40.
8. Dicken CH. Treatment of classic pityriasis rubra pilaris. J Am Acad Dermatol 1994;31:997-9.
9. Dogra S, Kumaran MS, Handa S, Kanwar AJ. Methotrexate for generalized pustular psoriasis in a 2-year-old child. Pediatr Dermatol 2005;22:85-6.
10. Garzon MC, Paller AS. Ultrapotent topical corticosteroids in the treatment of childhood genital lichen sclerosus. Arch Dermatol 1999;135:525-8.
11. Gelmetti C, Cerri D, Grimalt R. Lichen aureus in childhood. Pediatr Dermatol 1991;8:280-3.
12. Glometti C, Rigoni C, Alessi E. Pityriasis lichenoides in children: a long-term follow up of eighty-nine cases. J Am Acad Dermatol 1990;23: 473-78.

13. Grills C, Burge S. Methotrexate: improving safety profile. Australas J Dermatol 2006;47:178-81.
14. Handa S, Sahoo B. Childhood lichen planus: a study of 87 cases. Int J Dermatol 2002;41:423-27.
15. Hawrot AC, Metry DW, Theos AJ, Levy ML. Etanercept for psoriasis in the pediatric population: experience in nine patients. Pediatr Dermatol 2006;23:67-71.
16. Juanqin G, Zhiqiang C, Zijia H. Evaluation of the effectiveness of childhood generalized pustular psoriasis treatment in 30 cases. Pediatr Dermatol 1998;15:144-6.
17. Kennedy D, Rogers M. Lichen striatus. Pediatr Dermatol 1996;13:95-9.
18. Kosuge H, Tanaka-Taya K, Miyoshi H. Epidemiological study of human herpevirus-6 and human herpesvirus-7 in pityriasis rosea. Br J Dermatol 2000;143:795-98 .
19. Kotrulja L, Murat-Susic S, Husar K. Differential diagnosis of neonatal and infantile erythroderma. Acta Dermatovenereol Croat 2007;15:178-90.
20. Kumar B, Dhar S, Handa S, Kaur I. Methotrexate in childhood psoriasis. Pediatr Dermatol 1994;11:271-73.
21. Kumar B, Jain R, Sandhu K, Kaur I, Handa S. Epidemiology of childhood psoriasis: a study of 419 patients from northern India. Int J Dermatol. 2004;43:654-8. .
22. Laeijendecker R, Van Joost T, Tank B, Oranje AP, Neumann HAM. Oral lichen planus in childhood. Pediatr Dermatol 2005;22 (4):299-304.
23. Luis-Montoya P, Dominguez-Soto L. Vega-Memije E. Lichen planus in 24 children with review of literature. Pediatr Dermatol 2005;22 (4):295-98.
24. Mahe E, Bodemer C, Pruszkowski A, Teillac-Hamel D, de Prost Y. Cyclosporine in childhood psoriasis. Arch Dermatol 2001;137:1532-33.
25. Menni S. Parapsoriasis in two children: A clinical, immunophenotypic and, immunogenotypic study. Pediatr Dermatol 1994;11:151.
26. Nanda A, Al-Ajmi HS, Al-Sabah H, Al-Hasawi F, Alsaleh QA. Childhood lichen planus: A report of 23 cases. Pediatr Dermatol 2001;18 (1):1-4.
27. Patrizi A, Neri L, Marini R, Guerrini V. Lichen aureus with uncommon features in a child. Pediatr Dermatol 1996;13:173.
28. Piamphongsant T, Akarapant A. Pityrisis rubra pilaris: a new proposed classification. Clin Ex Dermatol 1994;19:134-38.
29. Powell J, Wojnarowska F. Childhood vulvar lichen sclerosus: an increasingly common problem. J Am Acad dermatol 2001;44:803-6.
30. Pruszkowski A, Bodemer C, Fraitag S, et al. Neonatal and infantile erythrodermas. A retrospective study of 51 patients. Arch Dermatol 2000;136:875-80.
31. Roenigk HH Jr, Auerbach R, Maibach H, Weinstein G, Lebwohl M. Methotrexate in psoriasis: consensus conference. J Am Acad Dermatol 1998;38:478-85.
32. Romani J, Puig L, Fernandez-Figueras MT. Pityriasis lichenoides in children: clinicopathologic review of 22 patients. Pediatr Dermatol 1998;15:11-6.
33. Sanchez-Regana M, Creus L, Umbert P. Pityriasis rubra pilaris: A long-term study of 25 cases. Eu J Dermatol 1994;4:593-97.
34. Sarkar R, Basu S, Sharma RC. Neonatal and infantile eythrodermas. Arch Dermatol 2001;137:822-23.
35. Sarkar R. Neonatal and infantile eryhtroderma: 'The red baby'. Indian J Dermatol 2006;51:178-81.
36. Sehgal VN, Srivastava G. Erythroderma/ generalized exfoliative dermatitis in pediatric practice: an overview. Int J Dermatol 2006;45:831-39.
37. Sharma PK, Yadav TP, Gautam RK. Erythromycin in pityriasis rosea: a double blind placebo-controlled clinical trial. J Am Acad 2000;42:241-44.
38. Sharma R, Maheshwari V. Childhood lichen planus: A report of fifty cases. Pediatr Dermatol 1999;16 (5):345-48.
39. Shieh S, Mikkola DL, Woods GS. Differentiation and clonality of lesional lymphocytes in pityriasis lichenoides chronic. Arch Dermatol 2001;137:305-8.
40. Siddiqui J. Clonal dermatitis: A potential precursor of CTCL with varied clinical manifestations. J Invest dermatol 1997;108:584.
41. Simon M. Large plaque parapsoriasis: Clinical and genotype correlations. J Cutan Pathol 2000;27:57.
42. Tilly JJ, Drolet BA, Esterly NB. Lichenoid eruptions in children. J Am Acad Dermatol 2004;51:606-24.
43. Van Neer FJMA, Toonstra J, Van Voorst PC. Lymphomatoid papulosis in children: a study of 10 children registered by Dutch Cutaneous Lymphoma Working Group. Br J Dermatol 2001;144:351-4.
44. Vanderhooft SL, Francis JS, Holbrook KA. Familial pityriasis rubra pilaris. Arch Dermatol 1995;131:448-53.
45. Yates VM, Kerr RE, MacKie RM. Early diagnosis of infantile seborrhoeic dermatitis and atopic dermatitis—clinical features. Br J Dermatol 1983;108:633-8.
46. Zibrel GM, Gellis SE, Kadin ME. Lymphomatoid papulosis in children. J Am Acad Dermatol 1995;33:741-48

17

Vesiculobullous Disorders

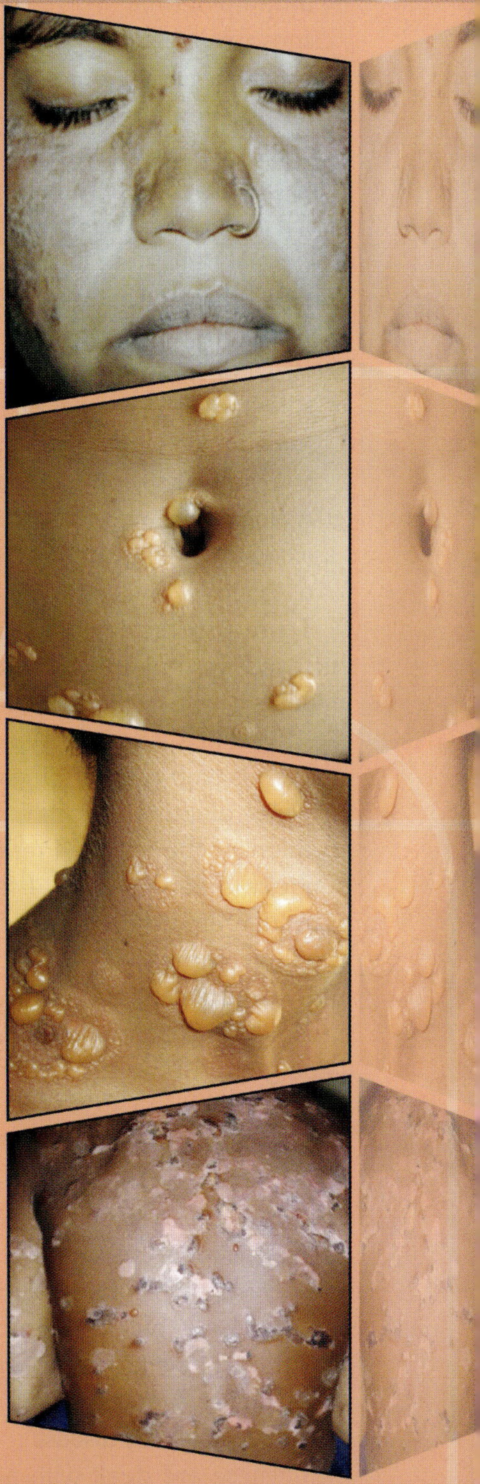

Chitra S Nayak

INTRODUCTION

Vesicle is a fluid-filled lesion on the skin that measures less than a centimeter in diameter. A similar lesion, greater than a centimeter is designated as bulla. Depending upon the level of fluid collection, these can be classified as:

- Intra-epidermal
  sub-corneal
  supra-basal
- Sub-epidermal.

Though the definitive diagnosis is possible by histopathological examination, there are certain clues by which the level of blistering can be assessed clinically. Intra-epidermal bullae are flaccid and rupture easily whereas subepidermal bullae are usually tense.

There are two clinical signs, which help to determine the level of split in the skin:

- Nikolsky's sign is the separation of the skin by shearing force applied to the normal-appearing area adjacent to a bulla/over a bony prominence.
- Asboe-Hansen sign (bulla spread sign) is the peripheral extension of the margin of an intact bulla on application of torsional/tangential pressure over it.

These signs are demonstrable in clinical conditions with intra-epidermal bullae, like pemphigus, erythema multiforme, toxic epidermal necrolysis and staphylococcal scalded skin syndrome. When the split is in the upper epidermis (sub-corneal), it gives rise to scaling, whereas presence of crusts indicate lower epidermal (suprabasal) location of the lesion. Presence of scarring and milia suggests a sub-epidermal location of the bullae, but secondary infection in intra-epidermal lesions may also produce scarring.

In children, blistering disorders can be categorized broadly as hereditary and immune-mediated. There is a large group of hereditary blistering disorders which can be classified as:

I. Mechano-bullous disorders:
   1. Epidermolysis bullosa-
      Epidermolysis bullosa simplex (EBS)
      Junctional epidermolysis bullosa
      Dystrophic epidermolysis bullosa
      Transient bullous dermolysis of newborn
   2. Ectodermal dysplasia with skin fragility
   3. Kindler syndrome
   4. Hailey-Hailey disease

   These are dealt with at length in the chapter on genodermatoses.

II. Immunobullous disorders are as follows:
   1. Pemphigus — Pemphigus vulgaris, Pemphigus foliaceous, Paraneoplastic pemphigus
   2. Bullous pemphigoid
   3. Dermatitis herpetiformis
   4. Chronic bullous disease of childhood
   5. Epidermolysis bullosa acquisita
   6. Bullous systemic lupus erythematosus

Various bacterial, viral and fungal infections may be associated with blistering. Non-infectious localized blistering may be due to phototoxicity or photo-allergy, contact dermatitis due to physical or chemical agents or mastocytosis. All these conditions have been detailed in the respective chapters. In the following section, immunobullous disorders will be discussed.

IMMUNOBULLOUS DISORDERS

The nonhereditary bullous diseases of childhood are essentially autoimmune disorders with autoantibodies directed against structural components of the skin.

PEMPHIGUS

Pemphigus consists of severe, chronic, occasionally fatal blistering disorders with flaccid bullae appearing on normal looking skin and mucous membranes. The blister formation in pemphigus results from acantholysis which is loss of cohesion between epidermal cells owing to disappearance of the intercellular bridges. Pathogenic autoantibodies (IgG) are generated against desmosomal components; cadherins (glycoproteins), desmoglein-1, 3, desmocollins and cytoplasmic plaque proteins, plakoglobin and desmoplakin-I and II. These autoantibodies bind to the cell surface inducing secretion of plasminogen activators which initiates the process of acantholysis.

The clinical variants of pemphigus are:

- Pemphigus vulgaris
- Pemphigus foliaceous
- IgA pemphigus
- Drug induced pemphigus
- Paraneoplastic pemphigus

Pemphigus Vulgaris

Pemphigus vulgaris (PV) is a chronic vesiculo-bullous disorder uncommon in children, but with a better prognosis than in adults. The PV antigen is a desmosomal cadherin known as desmoglein-3 (130-kDa), with more intense expression on lower epidermis and mucous membrane.

Oral mucosal lesions are found in 95% of the affected patients and are usually the initial lesion in the majority. Mucosal lesions rupture readily and patients present with painful erosions that heal slowly. The anogenital area, conjunctiva, vermilion borders of lips, pharynx and larynx may be involved. As skin lesions may follow the oral mucosal lesions after months, children with severe recurrent or chronic erosive mucous membrane disease should be examined carefully and a mucosal biopsy taken if needed.

The primary cutaneous lesions of pemphigus vulgaris are vesicles or bullae (usually 1 centimetre or less, later increasing to several centimetres in diameter) arising on normal looking skin. New lesions may appear with itching, burning or local discomfort. Nikolsky's sign is demonstrable in the active phase of the disease. Vesicles and bullae rupture easily leaving painful erosions that may bleed and heal slowly with crust formation. Childhood PV has been reported with other autoimmune disorder like vitiligo.

Tzanck smear demonstrates acantholytic cells. Histopathological examination of fresh lesions show characteristic features. Early histopathological changes include intercellular edema with loss of cohesion between epidermal cells leading to suprabasal clefts and bullae formation. Eosinophilic spongiosis is present. The basal cells, though separated from each other, remain attached to the basement membrane giving the "row of tombstones" appearance. There are eosinophils and acantholytic cells in the cleft.

Direct immunofluorescence (DIF) of the peri-lesional normal-appearing skin shows IgG and C3 bound to the intercellular spaces throughout the epidermis. Similar findings are demonstrable in the outer root sheath of plucked anagen hairs from scalp and constitute a non-invasive technique of tissue sampling for DIF study in children with suspected pemphigus. Indirect immunofluorescence (IIF) studies from the sera of patients with pemphigus vulgaris show IgG antibody binding to intercellular space. Levels of circulating antibody correlate with disease activity; increases in titres may precede clinical flares and clinical improvement may be reflected in decreased titres.

Pemphigus vegetans, a variant of pemphigus vulgaris is very rare in children. It usually involves the flexural and intertriginous areas. Small pustules are seen at the periphery of ruptured bullae and hypertrophic vegetations are present after healing.

Pemphigus Foliaceous

Pemphigus foliaceous is a superficial form of the disease, which, though rare in children is commoner than pemphigus vulgaris at pre-pubertal age. The targeted antigen is desmoglein-1 (160 kDa), which is homologous to desmoglein-3, but expression is more in the upper epidermis.

The course is milder than pemphigus vulgaris and prognosis in children is better than in adults. Slowly spreading arcuate, crusted plaques develop in the scalp, face, upper chest, abdomen and back. Pruritus, pain and burning may occur but patients are not severely ill. There may be progression to severe generalized exfoliative dermatitis. Mucosal lesions are rare and if present at all, small inconspicuous erosions are seen.

Tzanck smear demonstrates acantholytic cells. Histopathological findings in pemphigus foliaceous are similar to those of pemphigus vulgaris with acantholysis and intra-epidermal bullae formation, which is located in the granular layer or may be subcorneal. Direct and indirect immunofluorescence patterns are similar to pemphigus vulgaris.

Variants of pemphigus foliaceous

In Senear-Usher syndrome or pemphigus erythematosus, lesions are localized to the butterfly area of face, scalp, upper chest and back **(Figure 17.1)**. Antinuclear antibody test may be positive.

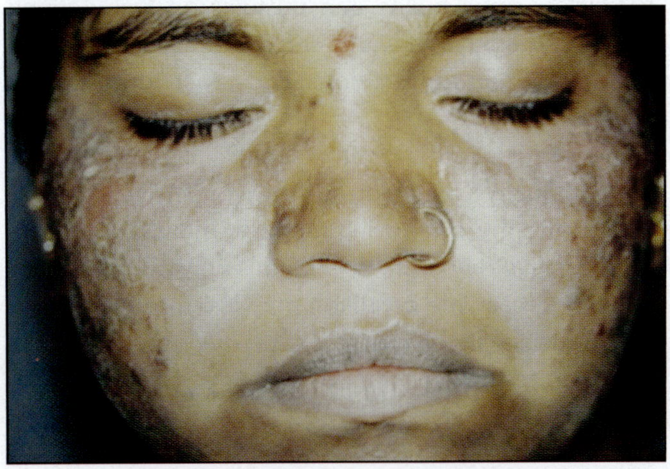

FIGURE17.1: Pemphigus erythematosus

Fogo selvagem (wildfire) is also known as endemic pemphigus or Brazilian pemphigus. It is endemic in Brazil and other South American countries and 15% of the affected patients are children. The name has been derived because of the typical distribution of lesions on sun-exposed skin, burnt appearance and the painful burning sensation of the lesions. Hyperpigmentation, hyperkeratosis and loss of hair over scalp and body are prominent features. The black fly *Simulium nigrimanum* is thought to be the vector for transmission of this endemic disorder.

Drug Induced Pemphigus

Drug induced pemphigus is rare in children. Penicillamine and captopril, the commonly implicated drugs, possess sulfhydryl groups which interact with the sulfhydryl groups in desmoglein 1 and 3, thus modifying the antigenicity of the desmoglein. Several months of exposure to the drug is needed for onset of the disease. The initial rash is morbilliform, urticarial or annular which evolves into blistering. Drug induced pemphigus rarely involves oral mucosa and resembles pemphigus foliaceous more than pemphigus vulgaris. There are reports of isotretinoin, enalapril and certain vaccines inducing pemphigus vulgaris and amoxicillin inducing pemphigus foliaceous.

IgA Pemphigus

IgA pemphigus is characterized by intercellular deposition of IgA rather than IgG. There are two subgroups of this entity,

- Subcorneal pustular dermatosis (SPD)
- Intraepidermal neutrophilic IgA dermatosis (IEN)

Vesicles, small bullae and pustules on well-defined background erythema with a serpiginous outline are the usual presentation. Erosions and crust formation is common.

The pustules resolve with a superficial scale or scale-crust and finally a faint blotchy brown hyperpigmentation without atrophy or scarring remains. Individual lesions last about five days with new lesions appearing as older ones disappear. The condition may last for five to eight years. Mucosal involvement is rare. IgA pemphigus has been reported in an infant as young as one month of age.

The auto-antigen is desmosomal protein desmocollin 1 for the SPD type. There may be no identifiable autoantigen in the IEN type or the patients may have circulating antibodies against desmoglein 1 and 3.

Histopathological examination of intact lesion reveals subcorneal blister filled almost entirely with neutrophils. Immunofluorescence analysis may not show immune deposits.

Paraneoplastic Pemphigus

Paraneoplastic pemphigus is a rare autoimmune disorder occasionally seen in children. Castleman's disease characterized by massive growth of lymphoid tissue in the retroperitoneum or mediastinum is the underlying malignancy in most pediatric patients. Sarcoma, T-cell lymphoblastic lymphoma and myofibroblastic tumor may be the underlying malignancies and sometimes no such tumor is detected. Paraneoplastic pemphigus has been reported in an eleven year old girl with underlying inflammatory myofibroblastic tumor.

There is intractable stomatitis especially of the labial mucosa and resembles Stevens-Johnson syndrome. Two-thirds of the patients show conjunctival involvement, sometimes leading to symblepharon and visual impairment. Skin changes may be bullous or lichenoid or resemble erythema multiforme. The trunk and extremities are more commonly involved. Palmoplantar involvement and paronychia resulting in nail shedding are often seen. Mucosae of the tracheo-bronchial tree are also involved and fatal bronchiolitis obliterans may occur.

Histopathological examination shows intraepithelial acantholysis, keratinocyte dyskeratosis and basal cell vacuolar changes, a combination of the histologic features of pemphigus and Stevens-Johnson syndrome. Direct immunofluorescence is usually negative but immunoblotting shows several circulating autoantibodies directed against desmosomal and hemidesmosomal proteins.

The differential diagnosis of paraneoplastic pemphigus includes Stevens-Johnson syndrome, toxic epidermal necrolysis, pemphigus vulgaris, bullous and cicatricial forms of pemphigoid, lichen planus pemphigoides and mucosal infections from herpes or candida. Any child or adolescent with paraneoplastic pemphigus should be screened for malignancy which includes a complete physical examination of the liver, spleen or lymph nodes, complete blood count, serum protein electrophoresis and computerized tomography of the chest, abdomen and pelvis.

Neonatal Pemphigus (Pemphigus neonatorum)

Pemphigus neonatorum is a clinical entity, where neonates of mothers suffering from pemphigus develop skin lesions due to transplacental transfer of anti-desmoglein antibodies. It is a distinct entity different from primary pemphigus at the neonatal period.

The distribution of desmoglein in neonatal epidermis differs from that of adult. Desmosomes of subcorneal keratinocytes in newborn contains both desmogleins-1 and 3, unlike adults, where only desmoglein-1 expression is observed. The suprabasal layers in neonates have predominantly desmoglein-3 and much less desmoglein-1, which in adults show only desmoglein-3. This may explain the fact that pemphigus vulgaris is the major clinical type in neonatal pemphigus, pemphigus foliaceous occurring only rarely. Even if neonatal desmoglein-1 is destroyed by transplacentally transferred maternal anti desmoglein-1 antibody, this damage is made up by presence of desmoglein-3. Neonates of mothers with pemphigus foliaceous and high titres of anti desmoglein-1 antibody may develop neonatal pemphigus. Neonatal pemphigus is not seen in infants of mothers with active fogo selvagem.

Mothers may or may not have active disease during pregnancy. Occurrence of lesions in the newborn in absence of active maternal disease during pregnancy indicates that neonatal skin is more sensitive to pemphigus antibodies than the maternal skin is. The child is born with flaccid bullae and erosions. Oral mucosal lesions are rare. There are reports of still-birth but its relation with neonatal disease severity or antibody titre is not clear. However, it may be the sequela of severe disease in the mother requiring intensive therapy.

Histopathological features are similar to the classical diseases and DIF study is positive but the antibody titre detected by IIF is usually lower than the mother. Skin lesions heal by subsequent 3 weeks with fall in the titre of maternal antibody in the sera of neonate. Hence aggressive therapy is not required for the neonate. A monitoring of the serum antibody titre for pregnant women with pemphigus, irrespective of disease activity has been suggested.

Differential Diagnosis

Pemphigus vulgaris in childhood may be mistaken as other commoner vesiculo-bullous disorders at this age group. These include staphylococcal scalded skin syndrome, bullous contact dermatitis, erythema multiforme, Stevens-Johnson syndrome, epidermolysis bullosa, chronic bullous disease of childhood, bullous mastocytosis etc. The superficial and serpiginous crusted lesions of pemphigus foliaceous and IgA pemphigus and the intertriginous vegetative lesions of pemphigus vegetans may resemble impetigo. Oral lesions may resemble herpetic gingivostomatitis, aphthous stomatitis or Stevens-Johnson syndrome.

Treatment

The treatment of choice for pemphigus is systemic corticosteroid therapy, given either as high doses orally (1-2 mg/kg/day) or as intravenous pulse. Oral corticosteroids used are prednisolone or methylprednisolone. Adjuvant therapy with immunosuppressive agents like cyclophosphamide, azathioprine, and mycophenolate mofetil provides the advantage of steroid-sparing. Azathioprine is the most commonly used drug in this group.

At many centres in India, intravenous steroid pulse therapy is administered with or without adjuvant therapy with an immunosuppressive agent. Dexamethasone is used for pulse steroid therapy with the dose depending on the weight of the patient. A rough guide for the dosage is:

- If the patient is 30 kg or less, 48 mg dexamethasone.
- If the patient is between 31-49 kg, 72 mg dexamethasone.
- If the patient is 50 kg and over. 96 mg dexamethasone.

Injection dexamethasone is added to 500 ml of 5% dextrose and given on three consecutive days, repeated every four weeks till lesions heal and for nine months thereafter. In children, cyclophosphamide is best avoided as an immunosuppressive agent because of its gonadal toxicity. Azathioprine (1-3 mg/kg/day), mycophenolate mofetil (2-3 g/day), cyclosporine (5 mg/kg/day) or dapsone may be added as a steroid sparing agent with oral steroids. Azathioprine must be given daily when pulse intravenous steroids are used. After this, oral Azathioprine is continued for a further nine months and then stopped.

Intravenous immunoglobulins are reported to be useful as adjunctive therapy in pemphigus. Anti-CD20 monoclonal antibody (rituximab) has been reported to be successful in treatment of refractory pemphigus vulgaris.

BULLOUS PEMPHIGOID

Bullous pemphigoid (BP) is a disorder with tissue-bound and circulating IgG antibodies directed against hemidesmosomal BP 230 and BP 180 antigens, located in the basement membrane zone (BMZ).

Usually a disorder of the elderly, but BP may rarely occur in children. About 70 patients with childhood BP have been reported till now of which 20 are infants. The childhood disease may be associated with other disorders like ulcerative colitis, Crohn's disease, autoimmune membranous glomerulopathy, psoriasis, hyper IgE syndrome and has also been reported following several vaccinations and drugs. Unlike adult-onset BP, association with malignancies has not been found.

It is characterized by large, tense, subepidermal bullae that appear on an erythematous or urticated skin or rarely on normal-looking skin and associated with mild to severe itching. Tense bullae of varying size evolve over weeks to months, some of which may be hemorrhagic. The blisters may occur at the edge of annular or polycyclic plaques. Unlike adults and older children, infants tend to get bullae on the face, palms and soles. Nikolsky sign is absent. The lesions heal with hypo or hyperpigmentation and milia formation. The prognosis is good unless other systemic disorders are associated.

Peripheral blood eosinophilia and increased IgE level are the usual features in childhood BP. Tzanck smear is negative for acantholytic cells but may demonstrate plenty of eosinophils. Skin biopsy is taken from a fresh lesion, which shows subepidermal blister, filled with inflammatory cells like neutrophils and eosinophils. Dermis shows mixed inflammatory infiltrate, particularly in perivascular location and intercellular edema. DIF study from perilesional skin shows deposition of IgG and C3 at the basement membrane. IIF study to demonstrate circulating anti BMZ antibody is positive in 70% cases. In children, blister fluid and urine are the non-invasive alternative samples for IIF study.

Variants

Localized vulvar pemphigoid: It is a very rare clinical variant of BP seen only in childhood. Localized erythema of the vulva followed by tense hemorrhagic bulla formation associated with pain and pruritus is the clinical presentation. Erosions and adhesions complicate the course of the disease but scarring is absent. Other mucosae are not involved.

Mucous membrane pemphigoid (Cicatricial pemphigoid): Mucous membrane pemphigoid is very rare in childhood. The target antigens are located in BMZ but are diverse in nature. It presents as recurrent blistering of one or several mucosal surfaces; oral cavity, conjunctiva, vulvar, penile, anal and mucosae of nasopharynx, esophagus and larynx. Rarely lesions start on the skin, thereafter localizes to mucosae otherwise *de novo* mucosal lesions occur. Intact vesicles on mucosal surfaces are rare but erosions are commonly seen. In patients with oral mucosal involvement, desquamative gingivitis is common. It differs from classical BP by the severe scarring of the involved mucosae.

Erosions and ulcerations give rise to scarring during healing. There may be severe ocular complications like symblepharon, misdirected eyelashes, corneal opacity, xerosis (due to obliteration of lacrimal glands and puncta) and blindness. Genital lesions lead to vaginal or meatal stenosis. Synechia formation between labia majora and minora, which is a hallmark feature of this disorder in adult females, is not seen in children. Anal lesions may result in painful fissures or damage of anal sphincter. Esophageal and laryngeal stenosis may lead to life-threatening situations. The disorder may continue till adulthood.

Histopathological examination of a fresh lesion on mucosa reveals subepidermal bulla formation with dense cellular infiltrate in the dermis, composed predominantly of neutrophils with or without scarring. DIF study reveals linear deposits of IgG, IgA and C3 in the BMZ. IIF study may or may not demonstrate circulating autoantibodies.

Differential Diagnosis

The widespread tense blisters of BP have to be differentiated from other bullous disorders at this age-group, like chronic bullous disease of childhood, epidermolysis bullosa, bullous mastocytosis, bullous SLE, childhood pemphigus and erythema multiforme. Indirect immunofluorescence with salt split skin is required for exact localization of the immune deposits and thereby help in diagnosis.

Localized vulvar pemphigoid has to be differentiated from mucous membrane pemphigoid localized to genital mucosa. Pemphigus vulgaris involving mucosa, Stevens Johnson syndrome, herpetic gingivostomatitis, Behcet's disease include the differential diagnosis of mucous membrane pemphigoid.

Treatment

Localized blisters in BP, localized vulvar pemphigoid or mucous membrane pemphigoid may be treated with potent topical corticosteroids like halobetasol propionate or clobetasol propionate. Widespread BP requires systemic treatment with any of the following agents:

- Prednisolone (1-2 mg/Kg /day)
- Dapsone (1-2 mg/Kg /day),
- Sulphapyridine(10-50 mg/Kg/day)
- Erythromycin (500mg three times /day)
- Tetracyline in older children (500 mg four times/day)

Systemic steroid brings rapid relief to widespread disease, and has to be tapered slowly thereafter. Other agents show variable effectiveness when used in less severe disease. Erythromycin with or without niacinamide (500 mg three times /day) has been beneficial in children.

Pemphigoid Gestationis (herpes gestationis) in Newborn

Pemphigoid gestationis is an autoimmune bullous disorder occurring in pregnancy, similar to bullous pemphigoid. Neonatal cutaneous involvement may occur rarely due to transplacental transfer of maternal anti-BMZ antibodies. The affected newborns present either at birth or within first 3 days of life with a generalized, mild, erythematous rash with or without bullae. The condition is self-healing and the lesions subside completely by one month.

Histopathology reveals a subepidermal bulla with eosinophilic infiltration. DIF study shows linear deposits of IgG and C3 at BMZ. Symptomatic topical treatment is adequate for this condition in neonate.

This condition has to be differentiated from pemphigus neonatorum, which is possible by eliciting the history of maternal illness, histopathological examination and DIF study.

DERMATITIS HERPETIFORMIS (DUHRING'S DISEASE)

Dermatitis herpetiformis (DH) is a disorder of adults and rare in infants and children. Gluten-sensitive enteropathy may be associated with DH. Only 10% individuals may have the onset of disease before 16 years of age. Its occurrence is very rare before 2 years of age, presumably because of absence of exposure to gluten in diet before this age.

It is characterized clinically by an intensely pruritic, grouped papulovesicular or occasionally, bullous lesions with a predilection for extensor surfaces of the body. Urticarial lesions may be present. The lesions are distributed symmetrically on the elbows, knees, sacrum, buttocks and shoulders, and rarely on the face, neck and scalp. The minute, clear, tense vesicles are rarely seen intact as they rupture easily when scratched and excoriated papules are commonly seen. The course is chronic lasting for indefinite period with frequent exacerbations and remissions.

Some children may have chronic diarrhoea, due to associated gluten-sensitive enteropathy. However, frank features of malabsorption may not always be present and intestinal mucosal changes found in endoscopy may be the evidence of this association.

Biopsy from an urticated pre-bullous lesion or a fresh vesicle shows papillary tip microabscesses, subepidermal bulla and neutrophilic infiltration. However, these features are not specific of DH and may be found in BP and chronic bullous disease of childhood. DIF study from the uninvolved skin demonstrates granular deposits of IgA at the tips of the dermal papillae and constitutes the diagnostic hallmark for DH.

In absence of clinical features suggestive of gluten sensitive enteropathy, the child should be investigated for it. Screening for malabsorption include estimation of complete blood count, liver function tests, serum calcium, iron, folate and vitamin B12 levels. If facilities are available, small intestinal biopsy should be undertaken for children with DH to assess the state of the mucosa, depending upon which gluten free diet may be advised. A baseline complete blood count and G6PD levels should be estimated before starting therapy with dapsone.

Insect bites, atopic dermatitis, urticaria, scabies and pityriasis lichenoides *et* varioliformis acuta are differential diagnoses of childhood DH. In presence of bullous lesions, other bullous dermatoses of childhood should be ruled out.

Dapsone (1-2 mg/kg/day) or sulphapyridine (250 mg/day) is the drug of choice for DH. It effectively relieves the symptoms as well as suppresses the eruption of skin lesions. The relief is often dramatic within 24 hours and helps to confirm a diagnosis while histopathological reports are awaited. Once the lesions have healed, the minimum dose required for suppression of the disease may be continued for longer duration. Regular monitoring of blood counts is essential in patients on such long-term therapy.

Institution of gluten-free diet brings remission to both cutaneous and intestinal symptoms. This may also reduce the minimum suppressive dose of sulphonamides. Achieving a gluten-free diet in Indian set-up is difficult where many communities are strictly vegetarian. Hence adherence to such a diet requires high motivation and family support.

Application of iodinated medicaments or intake of drugs containing iodides may precipitate an acute attack of the disease and should be forbidden for children with DH.

CHRONIC BULLOUS DISEASE OF CHILDHOOD (LINEAR IgA DISEASE OF CHILDHOOD)

Chronic bullous disease of childhood (CBDC) is the pediatric counterpart of the adult linear IgA disease (LAD). The location of the targeted antigens is at the BMZ, and a dual expression, both at lamina lucida and lamina densa has been detected.

Adult LAD has been reported to be associated with autoimmune disorders like Crohn's disease, SLE, dermatomyositis, hyper and hypothyroidism, autoimmune hemolytic anemia, vitiligo, diabetes mellitus etc. Different infectious agents have been reported to be associated with the onset of CBDC; these include α-hemolytic streptococci, *S.typhi*, measles virus, hepatitis A virus, Epstein-Barr virus etc.

It is reported to be seen commonly in developing countries, where the pediatric population is higher. However, in a series of patients reported from India, the incidence was stated to be lower compared to other countries. The onset of the disease is during the pre-school years. There is abrupt eruption of tense, clear or hemorrhagic bullae on normal or erythematous skin of the face, scalp, abdomen, anogenital region, buttocks, inner thighs, legs and dorsa of feet. Multiple bullae may be arranged in characteristic annular or rosette-like fashion surrounding a central crust, assuming "cluster of jewels" or "string of pearls" appearance **(Figures 17.2A and B)**. Pruritus is variable ranging from minimal to very severe. Oral and genital mucous membranes are mainly involved in children but any mucosa may be affected and the lesions may heal with scarring and related complications.

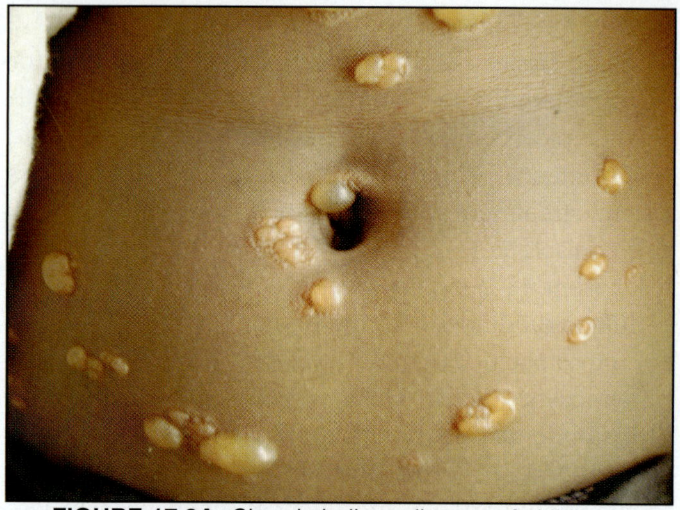

FIGURE 17.2A: Chronic bullous disease of childhood (cluster of jewels pattern)

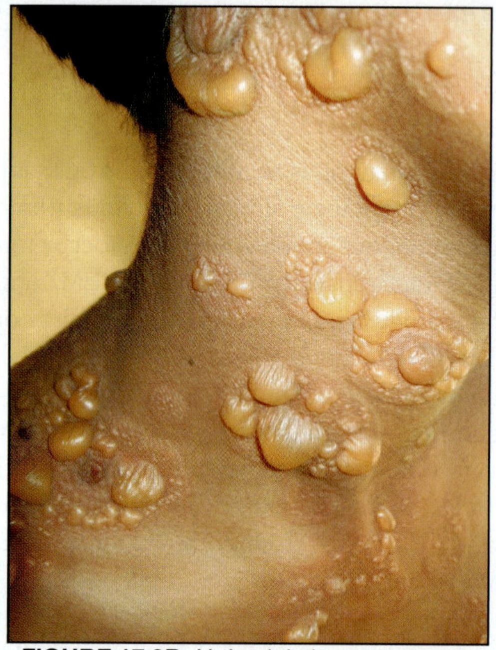

FIGURE 17.2B: Urticarial plaques topped with bulla (CBDC)

Initial episode may be associated with marked systemic features like fever, malaise and anorexia. Spontaneous remission within a few months to years is the rule and the disease does not usually continue till puberty.

Histopathological examination reveals a subepidermal bulla with edema of the adjacent dermal papillae and a dermal infiltrate of neutrophils, eosinophils and mononuclear cells.

These features are not distinctive and do not differentiate CBDC from other disorders like BP and DH. DIF study from perilesional uninvolved skin is mandatory for diagnosis and it shows linear band of IgA deposits along the BMZ, pathognomonic of this condition. Circulating anti IgA antibodies are found in 80% children by IIF study.

CBDC should be differentiated from other bullous disorders of childhood.

Localized skin lesions and mucosal lesions may be treated with potent topical steroid. Dapsone is the drug of choice (1-2 mg/Kg/day) for CBDC. Other effective sulphonamides are sulphamethoxypyridazine and sulphapyridine. Dapsone clears the existing lesions and suppresses the disease activity **(Figures 17.3A and B)**. Once the patient is in remission, the drug has to be tapered off very slowly over months. Some patients may relapse while tapering and needs reinstitution of the same dosage. Maintainance dose to control the disease has to be continued in these patients till remission is achieved.

Cases not responding adequately to dapsone, with frequent relapse, or when these drugs are contraindicated are treated with systemic steroid (prednisolone 1 mg/Kg /day), which shows very good response but cannot be continued for long because of related side effects. Steroids can be used in combination with dapsone or azathioprine.

Other drugs which have been used in patients with CBDC are erythromycin, oxacillin, dicloxacillin and colchicine. Colchicine is a safe and effective alternative to dapsone in G-6-PD deficient patients.

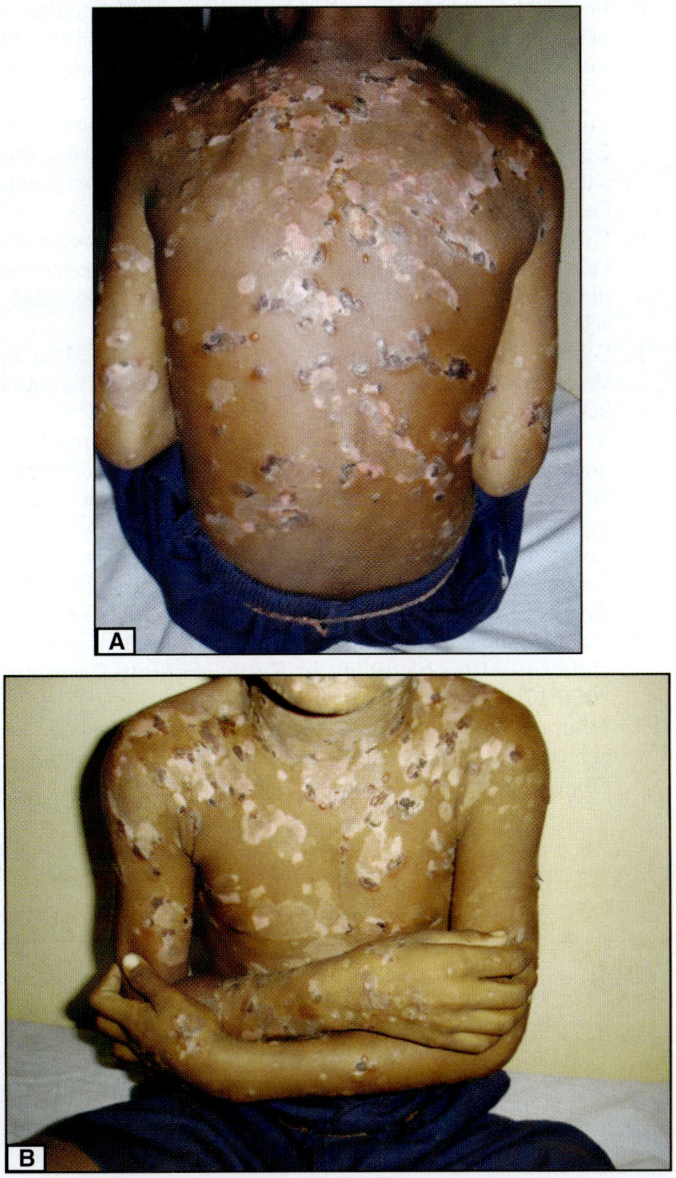

FIGURES 17.3A AND B: Resolving lesions of CBDC following treatment with dapsone

EPIDERMOLYSIS BULLOSA ACQUISITA

Epidermolysis bullosa acquisita (EBA) is an acquired subepidermal immunobullous disorder. Young adults are the common sufferers, but the disorder may affect the pediatric age group.

There is circulating IgG autoantibodies directed against type VII collagen in the sub lamina densa of BMZ.

Lesions tend to involve the trauma-prone areas like hands, elbows, feet and knees (non-inflammatory variant), simulating autosomal dominant dystrophic epidermolysis bullosa.

Nail dystrophy may be present in this type. Children may develop more widespread inflammatory variant of the disease. Individual lesions are tense bullae on erythematous or urticated background, with or without pruritus, simulating BP. Healing may occur with atrophic scarring with or without milia formation. Mucosal involvement with resultant scarring may be present.

Histopathological examination from a fresh vesicle reveals subepidermal bullae and neutrophilic infiltrations at the dermo-epidermal junction. Features are not distinctive and may be mistaken with BP. DIF study from perilesional skin reveals broad, linear, band-like deposit of IgG at the BMZ. Complement, IgM and IgA may also be found. IIF study shows circulating IgG antibodies and staining on the dermal side of the blister is found in salt split skin preparation.

The non inflammatory variant has to be differentiated from dystrophic epidermolysis bullosa, which is a congenital mechanobullous disorder. The inflammatory variant has to be differentiated from other childhood subepidermal bullous disorders.

EBA has a chronic course with remissions and exacerbations but has a better prognosis in children than in adults.

Avoidance of trauma is suggested in presence of acral and oral lesions. Systemic corticosteroid (prednisolone 1-2 mg/Kg/day) is the drug of choice and brings remission usually. In lack of response, dapsone may be added. Topical steroid may be useful for mucosal lesion.

BULLOUS SYSTEMIC LUPUS ERYTHEMATOSUS

It is a clinical variant of SLE where sudden eruption of tense, subepidermal blisters predominate the clinical picture. The antibodies are directed against type VII collagen in BMZ. The clinical features resemble those of bullous pemphigoid or dermatitis herpetiformis. Young women are most often affected with pruritic vesicles and tense bullae with occasional erythematous macules and papules which heal leaving post-inflammatory hypo or hyperpigmentation. Most commonly involved areas are those exposed to sun and also flexor and extensor skin surfaces and oral mucosae.

Immunofluorescence examination shows IgG deposition, sometimes IgM, IgA or C3 at the basement membrane and upper dermis. Granular, linear and mixed patterns have all been described. Prognosis is usually favourable and largely determined by the course of the associated systemic lupus erythematosus. Dapsone is fairly effective in controlling the eruption. Systemic corticosteroids with or without additional immunosuppressive agents have led to variable response.

BIBLIOGRAPHY

1. Chorzelski T, Karczewska Dyduch A, Kasner J, PieniazekW. Epidermolysis bullosa acquisita in a 4-year-old boy. Pediatr Dermatol 2000;17:157-8.
2. Erbagci Z. Childhood bullous pemphigoid in association with hyper immunoglobulin E syndrome. Pediatr Dermatol 2008;25:28-33.
3. Fenniche S, Benmously R, Marrack H, Dhaoui A, Ammar FB, Mokhtar I. Neonatal pemphigus vulgaris in an infant born to a mother with pemphigus vulgaris in remission. Pediatr Dermatol 2006;23:124-27.
4. Jain R, Dogra S, Sandhu K, Handa S, Kumar B. Coexistence of vitiligo and pemphigus vulgaris in an Indian patient. Pediatr Dermatol 2003;20:369-70.
5. Kanwar AJ, Sandhu K, Handa S. Chronic bullous dermatosis of childhood in north India. Pediatr Dermatol 2004;21:610-12.
6. Kong HH, Prose NS, Ware RE, Hall III RP. Successful treatment of refractory childhood pemphigus vulgaris with anti-CD 20 monoclonal antibody (Rituximab). Pediatr Dermatol 2005;22:461-64.
7. Kuenzli S, Grimaitre M, Krischer j, Saurat JH, Calza A-M, Borradori L. Childhood bullous pemphigoid: report of a case with life threatening course during homeopathy treatment. Pediatr Dermatol 2004;21:160-63.
8. Paller AS, Mancini AJ. Bullous disorders of childhood. In: Paller AS, Mancini AJ, (editors). Hurwitz clinical pediatric dermatology, Philadelphia: Elsevier Saunders; 2006;3:345-63.
9. Schoeffler A, Roth B, Causeret A, Knitakis J, Faure M, et al. Vulvar cicatricial pemphigoid of childhood. Pediatr Dermatol 2004;21:51-3.
10. Smitt JHS. Pemphigus, pemphigoid and epidermolysis bullosa acquisita. In:Harper J, Oranje A, Prose N, (editors). Textbook of pediatric dermatology, Oxford: Blackwell Publishing 2006;1(2):855-77.
11. Sousa L, Bajanca R, Cabral J, Fiadeiro T. Dermatitis herpetiformis: should direct immunofluorescence be the only diagnostic criterion? Pediatr Dermatol 2002;19:336-39.
12. Tay Y-K, Ang P. Treatment of linear IgA bullous dermatosis of children with colchicine:In Reply. Pediatr Dermatol 2000;17:157.
13. Tidman MJ, Garzon MC. Vesiculobullous disease. In: Schachner LA, Hansen RC, (editors). Pediatric Dermatology. Edinburgh: Mosby 2003;3:683-712.

18

Disorders of Pigmentation

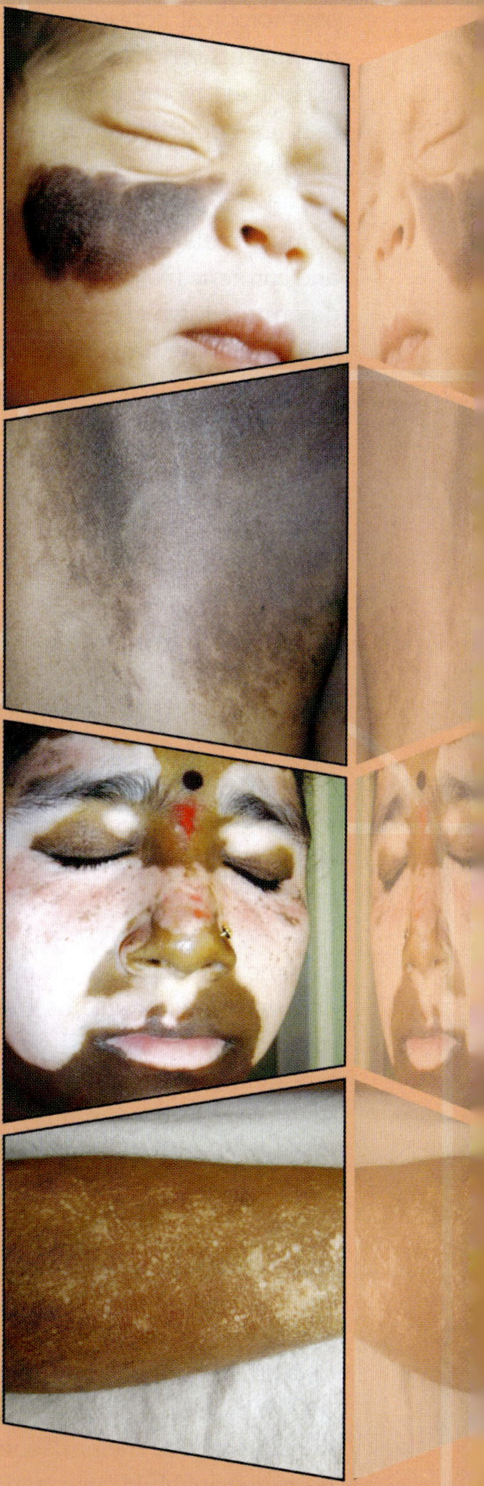

Manjunath Shenoy

INTRODUCTION

Disturbances in melanin pigmentation are among the most conspicuous of all dermatologic disorders especially in the Indians. They are frequently encountered diseases in the infants and childhood, and may lead to devastating psychological consequences to the afflicted individuals or parents. In this chapter the author refers almost exclusively to the melanin related pigmentary disorders that are common amongst the newborn, infant and the childhood.

Normal skin color is an admixture of chromophores namely melanin (brown), hemoglobin (red and blue), and carotene (yellow). Constitutive skin color is genetically determined, which is seen in the habitually sun shielded areas like inner arms. Genetically predetermined capacity of the skin to darken on exposure to solar radiation is responsible for facultative skin color. Melanocytes situated in the epidermis perform the function of synthesizing melanin. Fitzpatrick and Breathnach proposed an epidermal melanin unit, a functional unit composed of one Melanocyte and 36 keratinocytes. Skin color is mainly determined by the type, number and size of melanosomes transferred from melanocytes to the surrounding keratinocytes. This is the base for the Fitzpatrick phototyping; darker skin types (Fitzpatrick phototype 4 to 6) have larger and numerous melanosomes compared to lighter skin types (Fitzpatrick phototype 1 to 3). Melanosomes are packaged mainly with eumelanin, synthesized from the amino acid tyrosine by the action of copper dependent enzyme tyrosinase. Phenylalanine hydroxylase and tyrosine hydroxylase are other two enzymes involved in the melanin synthesis, and along with tyrosinase explains the "three enzyme theory" of melanogenesis. (6R)-L-erythro-5, 6, 7, 8-tetrahydro biopterin ($6BH_4$) is the cofactor that controls the activities of these three enzymes. $6BH_4$ levels correlate with Fitzpatrick phototypes with increased levels in the darker skin types and on UV exposure. Melanocytes and keratinocytes are capable of autocrine de novo synthesis, regulation and recycling of $6BH_4$, and are capable of controlling melanogenesis.

There are several factors that control melanogenesis and thus skin pigmentation. Pro-opiomelanocortin (POMC) derived peptides (Ex. α-MSH and β-MSH) can directly control melanogenesis. Melanocyte stimulating hormone (α-MSH) was earlier considered as a pituitary hormone with exclusive pigmentary functions. Now it is known that several cells including keratinocytes and melanocytes can produce α-MSH. It has a potent anti inflammatory action in addition to stimulation of melanin synthesis. Corticotrophin releasing hormone, which was thought to stimulate production of adrenocorticotrophic hormone (ACTH), is known to have multiplicity of functions including production of POMC and release of α-MSH. Other hormones like ACTH, estrogens, progestogens and possibly testosterone in some pathologic conditions may stimulate melanogenesis either directly or by the release of MSH peptides from the pituitary.

Understanding biology of pigmentation is crucial in understanding pathophysiology of disorders of pigmentation. Pigmentary disorders in the newborn and childhood may be transient or permanent, localized/segmental or diffuse. Abnormalities in the production of melanin and transfer of melanosomes to keratinocytes are the proposed causes of such disorders. Major concern in these lesions is whether they represent cutaneous manifestation of a neurocutaneous disorder, especially when they occur in pediatric patients. Common disorders of adults such as vitiligo and post inflammatory pigmentary alterations are not uncommon in childhood. It is also important to remember that there are a group of inflammatory disorders where the lesions are hypopigmented right from their onset. Certain disorders of pigmentation such as chemical leukoderma and idiopathic guttate hypomelanosis are not common in childhood. There is no standard classification of pigmentary disorders. Following classifications **(Tables 18.1 and 18.2)** can be considered for the purpose of understanding the pathophysiology.

CLASSIFICATION

This classification does not cover all disorders but this gives an insight to the pathogenesis of pigmentary ailments. Diagnosis of these disorders is mainly based on the clinical features. Histopathology with or without special stains is complementary, but is mandatory in certain conditions like melanoma. Wood's lamp can be a useful tool to intensify the pigmentary alterations when dealing with some hypopigmented lesions and melasma. Dermoscopy (also called as dermatoscopy, epiluminescence microscopy, incident light microscopy and surface microscopy) is a noninvasive technique that has been used to increase the accuracy of diagnosing pigmented skin lesions. In spite of better diagnosis, therapy for many

TABLE 18.1: Causes of hyperpigmentation

Genetic	Freckles Lentigines Café au lait macules
Endocrinal	Addison's disease Cushing's syndrome
Metabolic	Haemochromatosis Porphyria
Nutritional	Malabsorption Kwashiorkor
Drugs	Photosensitizing drugs Psoralens Minocycline
Postinflammatory	Lichen planus Eczema Macular amyloidosis
Tumors/paraneoplastic	Acanthosis nigricans Benign Melanocytic tumors Malignant melanoma Mastocytosis

TABLE 18.2: Causes of hypopigmentation

Genetic	Albinism Piebaldism Phenylketonuria Waardenburg's syndrome Chediak–Higashi syndrome: Tuberous sclerosis
Endocrinal	Hypopituitarism
Chemical	Contact with substituted phenols (in rubber industry) Chloroquine and hydroxychloroquine
Post inflammatory	Eczema Pityriasis alba Psoriasis Sarcoidosis Lupus erythematosus Lichen sclerosus et atrophicus Cryotherapy
Infections	Leprosy Pityriasis versicolor Syphilis Yaws
Tumors	Halo naevus Malignant melanoma
Miscellaneous	Vitiligo

diseases is limited and often ineffective. With increasing understanding of biology of pigmentation and pathogenesis of these disorders, it is expected to have better therapeutic options in the future.

It is advised to understand the following terms and their definitions since they are used frequently in this chapter.

Hyperpigmentation: Increase in pigmentation. Excess melanin or other pigments, endogenous or exogenous (iron, tattoos).

Melanosis/hypermelanosis: Increase in pigmentation due to excess melanogenesis. Hyperpigmentation and hypermelanosis are generally used synonymously.

Hypopigmentation/depigmentation: Reduction (hypo-) or total loss (de-) of pigmentation.

Hypomelanosis/amelanosis: Reduction (hypo-) or total absence (a-) of pigmentation because of abnormal melanogenesis since birth.

Leukoderma: Hypo- or depigmentation following an inflammatory skin disease.

Dyschromatosis: Any alterations in color of the skin; often refers to combination of hyper- and hypopigmentation; others use it to refer to pigmentary changes not related to melanin.

Poikiloderma: Combination of atrophy, telangiectases, and hypo- as well as hyperpigmentation.

DISORDERS OF HYPERPIGMENTATION

Hyperpigmented lesions in children may be transient or permanent or localized or diffuse. When they occur at birth or soon after, it may be an expression of mosaicism of pigmentary system. Most of these disorders are not understood at molecular levels. Acquired disorders are also seen frequently and conditions like acanthosis nigricans and hemochromatosis are very significant. Diseases that are common in the newborns and childhood are discussed in the following sections.

FRECKLES (EPHELIDES)

Freckles occur more frequently in the light skinned and probably inherited as an autosomal dominant trait. They are not seen at birth, but gradually appear during infancy or late childhood. They are seen mainly over the sun exposed area, and they darken in summer and fade during winter. They are well circumscribed brown macules occurring on face, back, chest and forearms sparing the mucosa. Appearance of freckles is an early manifestation of xeroderma pigmentosum, and the diagnosis may be delayed until other manifestations like photosensitivity and eye symptoms occur.

Histopathologically freckles show increased melanin without melanocyte proliferation or epidermal elongation.

LENTIGINES

Lentigenes may be present at birth and their number may increase in the later life. A typical lentigene is a small, discrete, brown or black macule occurring at any cutaneous or mucosal area. Lentigenes are benign lesions that do not require any treatment. Long term PUVA photochemotherapy may lead to appearance of small brown macular lesions called as PUVA lentigo.

Presence of multiple lentigines on the cutaneous or mucosal surfaces may have an association with a multisystem disease. **Table 18.3** gives a list of some important syndromes and the features of them. Patients of *LEOPARD syndrome* may also have Café au lait spots, junctional nevi, and abnormal pigmentation of the iris and retina. Lentigines in *Peutz-Jeghers syndrome (PJS)* appear in infancy or childhood usually on the lips **(Figure 18.1)** and buccal mucosa and, less commonly, on the eyelids and dorsa of the fingers. Increased incidence of gastrointestinal and other malignancies has been noticed in PJS. Earlier defined as "NAME" or "LAMB" syndrome, an association of myxomas, pigmentation and endocrine overactivity is currently known as *Carney complex*.

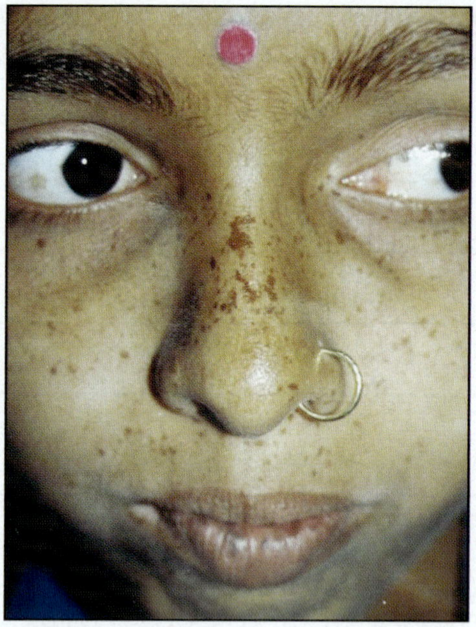

FIGURE18.1: Lentigines (Peutz-Jeghers syndrome)

Characteristically there is relative hypertelorism and centrofacial spotty pigmentation that involves the vermilion border of the lips and the conjunctiva.

Histologically lentigenes are characterized by an increase in the basal epidermal melanocyte activity with melanocyte hyperplasia. Dermoscopy reveals a light brown regularly meshed and narrowly spaced pigment network.

CAFÉ AU LAIT SPOTS

Cafe au lait spots (CALS) are macules with uniform brown pigmentation, distinct margins and variable

TABLE 18.3: Familial lentiginoses: Clinical manifestations and genetics

Syndrome	Genetics	Clinical features
Peutz-Jeghers Syndrome	Autosomal dominant	Gastrointestinal hamartomas and other tumors, polyps of the respiratory and renal collecting systems, thyroid, breast, testicular and ovarian neoplasms.
Multiple Lentigenes (LEOPARD) Syndrome	Autosomal dominant	Electrocardiographic abnormalities, ocular hypertelorism, pulmonary stenosis, abnormalities of the genitalia (hypogonadism), retardation (mental), and deafness (sensorineural)
Carney Complex	Autosomal dominant	Cardiac myxomas, Pigmentation (lentigines, ephelids, Nevi), cutaneous myxomas, testicular tumors, pituitary adenomas,
Cronkhite-Canada Syndrome	Sporadic	Lentigines on the backs of the hands, diffuse pigmentation of the palms and volar aspects of the fingers, gastrointestinal polyposis, alopecia and nail abnormalities
Centrofacial Lentiginosis	Autosomal dominant	Developmental anomalies of skeletal, neural tube
Laugier- Hunziker Disease	Unknown	Lentigines, other pigmented lesions

TABLE 18.4: Disease associations with multiple Café au lait spots	
Syndrome	**Clinical features**
Neurofibromatosis type 1	Cutaneous neurofibromas, CNS tumors, Iris hamartomas, Skeletal defects
McCune-Albright syndrome	Polyostotic fibrous dysplasia, Precocious puberty, thyrotoxicosis, Pituitary gigantism
Watson syndrome	Pulmonary stenosis, low intelligence, facial dysmorphic features, axillary freckling
Multiple lentigenes syndrome (LEOPARD Syndrome)	Lentigenes, Electrocardiographic abnormalities, ocular hypertelorism, pulmonary stenosis
Multiple mucosal neuroma syndrome	Mucosal neuromas, thyroid carcinoma, pheochromocytoma, parathyroid adenama
Fanconi's anemia	Limb abnormalities, renal anomalies, pancytopenia
Russel-silver syndrome	Short stature, asymmetry, limb defects
Bloom's syndrome	Short stature, poikiliderma, photosensitivity

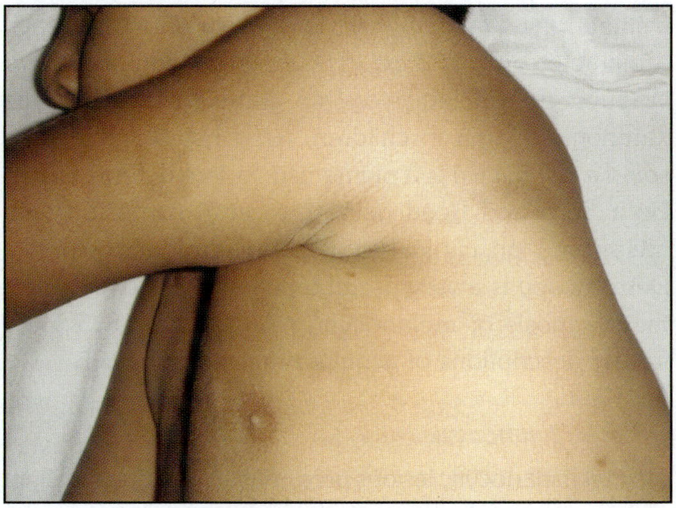

FIGURE 18.2: Café au lait spots

contours **(Figure 18.2)**. They are seen at birth or early infancy and enlarge during childhood proportionate to the body growth, and then remain stable. Most children with CALS have no associated abnormalities. They measure from a few millimeters to several centimeters. If children have multiple large CALS, it may be a sign of one of the few heritable disorders as mentioned in **Table 18.4**.

Histopathologically CALS are characterized by increased epidermal melanin without melanocyte proliferation. Ultrastructural examination reveals giant pigment granules.

MELANOCYTIC NEVI

Melanocytic nevi are one of the common pigmentary lesions in pediatric dermatology. It was found in about 1% of pediatric outpatients attending dermatology department in a South Indian hospital, and most of them (78%) presented in less than one year of age. Melanocytic nevi can be congenital or acquired. Acquired melanocytic nevi are so common that some believe they cannot be considered as a defect. However, despite the high prevalence, melanocytic nevi are pathologic in the sense that they represent an aberrant or neoplastic proliferation of cells. Malignant potential of congenital nevi and certain acquired nevi is well known.

Congenital Melanocytic Nevi

Congenital melanocytic nevi are present at birth (1 to 3% of all newborns) or soon thereafter. They vary considerably in size and are commonly classified as small (<1.5 cm), large (1-20 cm), and giant (>20 cm) nevi. These nevi have a variable malignant potential which is proportional to their size **(Figures 18.3A and B)**. Small and medium sized lesions are pale macular lesions at birth, which grow less rapidly, darken and develop terminal hairs over a period of years. Rare giant lesions (bathing-trunk nevus) are obvious at birth, and the surface becomes warty and nodular as the infant grows. The *Nevus Spilus* is a variety of congenital melanocytic nevus, characterized by a light brown patch stippled with dark macules or papules.

Ultrastructurally congenital nevi have characteristic increased melanocytes in the epidermal basal layer with nevus cells disposed in the deep reticular dermis between the collagen bundles and adenexal structures. Dermoscopic pattern is variable with a reticular or a globular pattern. They are light brown or dark brown in

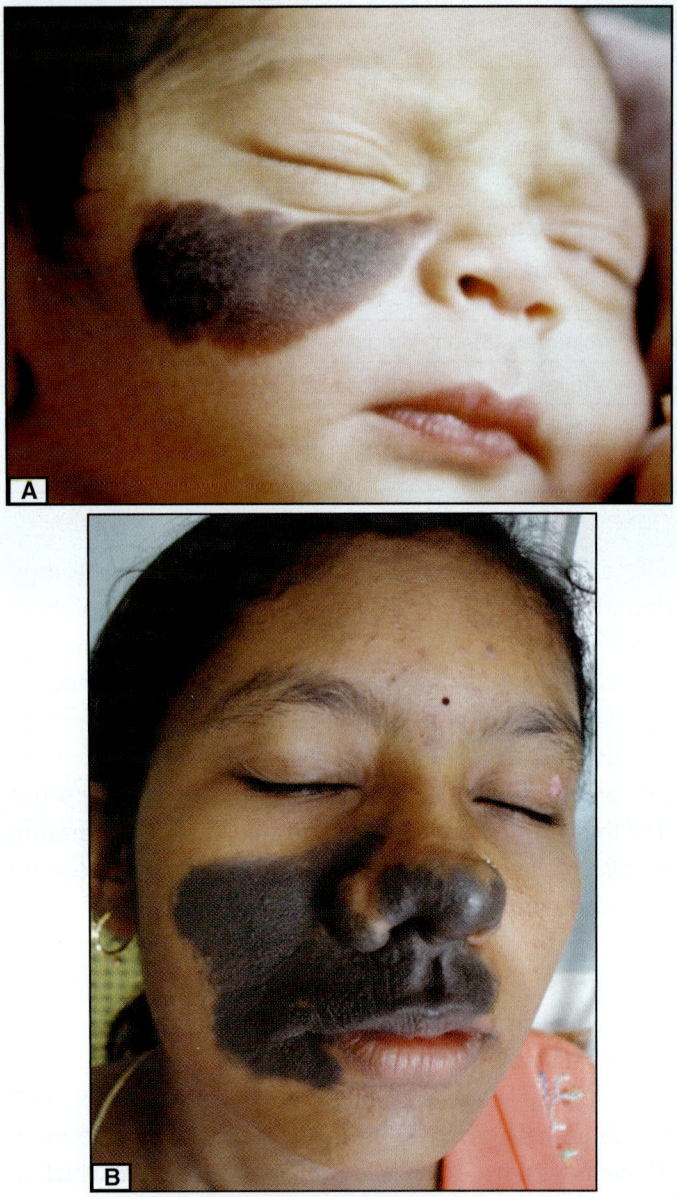

FIGURES 18.3 A AND B: Congenital nevomelanocytic nevus

color with globules of various colors and size placed irregularly in the lesion.

Nevi are often removed for cosmesis by tangential or shave excision. Large lesions may require complete excision with sutured closure, even if they are benign. Excision may not be possible for many giant lesions. A simple conservative excisional biopsy is a reliable means to diagnosis if concern exists regarding the possibility of melanoma.

Acquired Melanocytic Nevi

Acquired melanocytic nevi are almost universal with their frequency gradually increasing during childhood and adolescence. They can be classified in to junctional, compound and intradermal nevi. *Junctional nevus* is a small uniformly brown macule slightly larger than a lentigo. *Compound nevus* is a raised lesion with color ranging from a natural pigmentation to very dark. *Intradermal nevus* is elevated, dome shaped and not pigmented. *Halo Nevus,* which is particularly common in older children and adolescents, is a compound nevus with surrounding depigmented halo. The natural history of the halo nevus is the gradual spontaneous disappearance of the nevus cells accompanied by a centripetal extension of the depigmented zone resulting in a circular white macule. *Meyerson's nevus* is the term that describes a nevus that has developed a surrounding inflammatory reaction. *Spitz nevus* usually appears in childhood and rapidly grows over 3 to 6 months to reach a diameter of 1 to 2 cm. They may be confused for a vascular tumor like pyogenic granuloma or juvenile xanthogranuloma in children. *Reed nevus (pigmented spindle cell nevus)* is a pigmented variant of Spitz nevus. Both Spitz and Reed nevi may cause confusion with melanoma on clinical and histopathologic grounds. Dermoscopy is a very useful tool that helps clinician for the diagnosis of melanocytic nevi. **Table 18.5** gives further descriptions of acquired melanocytic nevi.

Dermal Melanocytic Nevi

Dermal melanocytic lesions presumably arise due to failure of migration of melanocytes from the neural crest to the epidermis during fetal life. These lesions occur at birth or in early childhood, and they have a characteristic slate gray or blue color. Potential for malignancy is very low however incidents of malignant transformation in blue nevi and Ota's nevi are reported. *Mongolian spot* is present at birth, which deepens over a period of life and then diminishes **(Figure 18.4)**. They are seen in all races but the incidence is up to 90% in Mongolic race. *Ota's and Ito's nevi* are more frequently reported in the Asians. Ota's nevi are more common in females. They are not visible at birth, gradually appear and darken in childhood, persist in adulthood. They are generally unilateral but bilateral lesions have been reported. *Blue nevus* usually appears during puberty. **Table 18.6** gives the description of various types of dermal nevi. Treatment of these lesions is mainly for the cosmetic reasons. Q-switched Alexandrite or Nd:YAG laser used in multiple sittings significantly reduces the pigmentation.

TABLE 18.5: Acquired melanocytic nevi: clinical, histopathologic and dermoscopic findings

Type	Clinical features	Histopathology	Dermoscopy
Junctional nevus	Unpalpable uniformly pigmented small brown macule	Cluster of melanocytic proliferation at the dermo-epidermal junction (DEJ)	Regularly meshed, narrowly spaced pigmentary network
Compound Nevus	Round or oval, pigmented, raised lesions	Nests of nevoid melanocytes at the DEJ and dermis.	Network of uniform and regular brown globules
Intradermal Nevus	Raised, nonpigmented and dome shaped lesion	Nevoid cells remaining free in the dermis alone	No characteristic features
Halo Nevus	Appearance of a halo of depigmentation around an existing nevus.	Intense Lymphocytic infiltration around the dermal Melanocytes	Characters of the associated nevus
Meyerson's Nevus	Nevus with scaly and pruritic surrounding zone	Nevus with spongiotic dermatitis	Characters of the associated nevus
Spitz Nevus	Firm and rounded nodule with a red brown color due to high vascularity	Interlacing bundles of spindle shaped nevus cells in the dermis.	No pigmentary network. Homogenous, light brown or red color
Reed Nevus	Densely pigmented dark brown or a black nodule	Junctional melanocytic proliferation with spindle shaped nevus cells in dermis	Diffuse pigmentation with peripheral streaks ("Starburst") in most cases

TABLE 18.6: Types of dermal nevi with clinical features and histopathology

Nevus	Clinical Features	Histopathology
Mongolian spot	A macular blue-gray pigmentation in the sacral area	Widely scattered melanocytes in the collagen and neurovascular bundles
Ota's Nevus	Patchy blue pigmentation of sclera and periorbital area	Increased dermal melanocytes with fibrosis and melanophages.
Ito's Nevus	Patchy blue pigmentation of acromio-clavicular area and upper chest	Increased dermal melanocytes with fibrosis and melanophages.
Blue Nevus	Slightly raised, well demarcated diffuse blue pigmentation seen over the lumbosacral region or extremities.	Dendritic melanocytes distributed singly and in clusters in the deep dermis

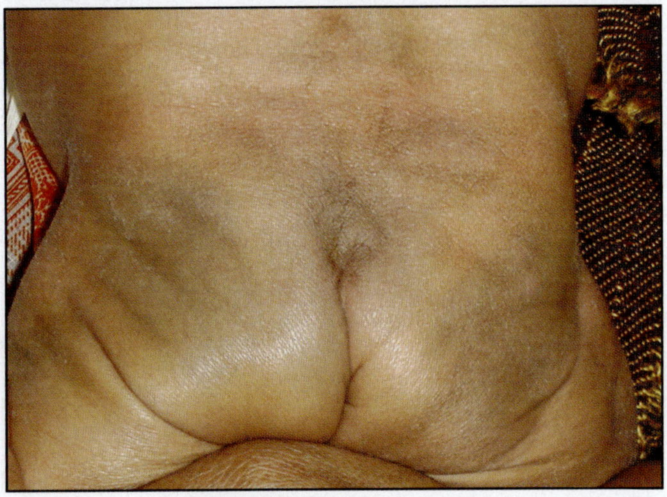

FIGURE 18.4: Mongolian spot

CHILDHOOD MELANOMA

A detailed discussion of melanomas is beyond the scope of this chapter. It is a rare disease in children (1 to 3% of pediatric malignancies), but incidence of childhood melanomas seems to be increasing. Approximately 50% of them arise from a preexisting lesion, most frequently a giant congenital melanocytic nevus. Most of them occur before puberty. There is a higher incidence of nodular melanomas in childhood. Rapid increase in the size of the lesion, bleeding, pruritus, color changes and lymphnode enlargement are the common features that suggest the appearance of melanoma from a nevus.

SEGMENTAL HYPERMELANOSIS

Segmental hypermelanoses are features of cutaneous mosaicism of pigmentary system, and they present at birth or in early childhood. They are sharply unilateral following a dermatome usually without any associated systemic involvement. The term *Linear and whorled nevoid hypermelanosis* is used clinically when there are swirls and streaks of macular hyperpigmentation following the lines of Blaschko. It may have associated serious internal defects that need further evaluation. In an Indian study, 26 children with pigmentary anomalies and CNS manifestations, majority of them presented before the age of 2 years (Anita Pinheiro et al). Surveillance until 2 years is hence recommended. Incontinentia pigmentii that attains pigmentary stage in childhood should also be considered as a cause of such segmental lesions.

BECKER'S NEVUS

Becker's nevus or Becker Melanosis is a sporadic asymptomatic irregular brown patch, most commonly located over the shoulder **(Figure 18.5)**, upper chest, or back. It appears around puberty and is followed several months to years by the appearance of terminal hairs within and in close proximity of the patch. Androgens may play a role as evidenced by its peripubertal development, male preponderance, hypertrichosis and occasional development of acneiform lesions within the patch. Rarely hypoplasia of underlying structures, such as breast or pectoral muscle hypoplasia has been reported. Surgical excision of the lesions with primary closure may not be feasible in many cases who desire it to be removed for cosmetic purposes. Q switched lasers or Erbium YAG lasers have been used with variable success to remove pigmentation and hypertrichosis.

Histopathologically basal layer demonstrates hyperpigmentation resulting from increased melanin. Melanosomes are increased in keratinocytes, and giant melanosomes may be found in both keratinocytes and melanocytes

PUNCTATE OR RETICULATE PIGMENTARY DISORDERS

Dermatopathia pigmentosa reticularis **(Figure 18.6)** is a rare inherited disorder presenting at birth or in early childhood, characterized by reticulate hyperpigmentation of trunk and proximal limbs, mild nonscarring alopecia, and mild onychodystrophy. *Franceschetti-Jadassohn (Naegeli) syndrome* is an autosomal dominant condition with gray-brown reticulate pigmentation of the trunk and neck that fades after adolescence. *Dyskeratosis congenita* is an X-linked condition presenting in male children, characterized by reticulate hyperpigmentation, nail dystrophy, hyperkeratosis and atrophy of the palms and soles, leukokeratosis of mucosal surfaces and blood dyscrasias. *Reticulate acropigmentation of Dohi* is an autosomal dominant condition presenting in the first decade of life with hyperpigmented and hypopigmented macules forming a reticulate pattern on the dorsa of the hands and feet **(Figure 18.7)**, varying in its intensity and the extent of involvement.

Poikiloderma is the term used when there is a triad of reticulate pigmentation, atrophy and telangiectasia. Rothmund–Thomson syndrome, Bloom's syndrome and Cockayne's syndrome are classical examples of

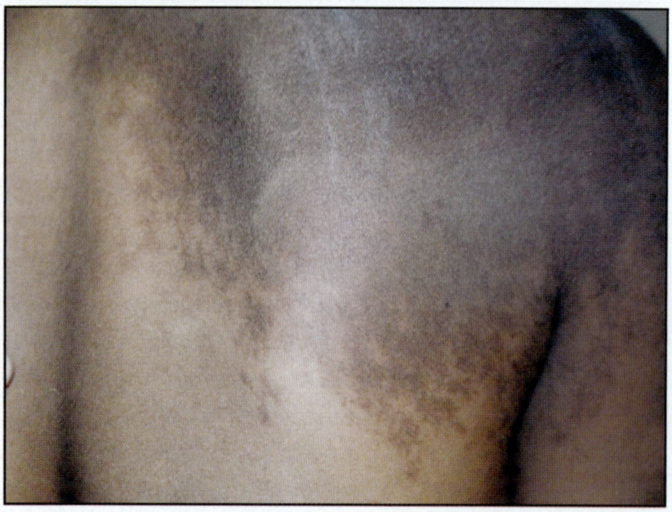

FIGURE 18.5: Becker's nevus

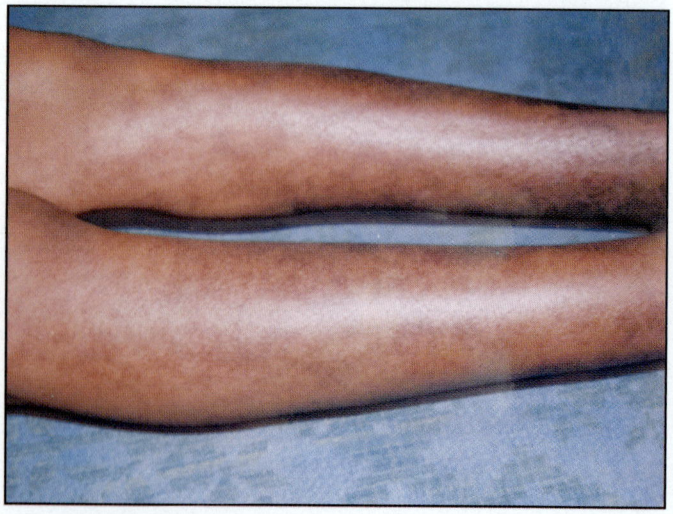

FIGURE 18.6: Dermatopathia pigmentosa reticularis

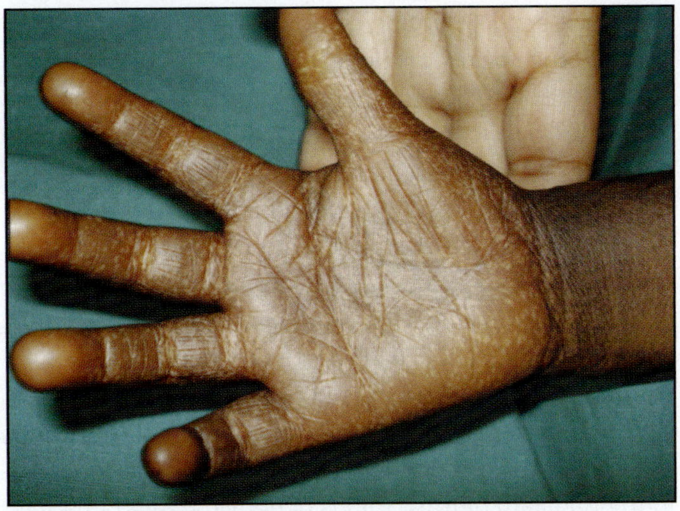

FIGURE 18.7: Acropigmentation of Dohi

poikilodermas. Similar cutaneous changes can also be seen in irradiation, connective tissue diseases and lymphoreticular disorders.

ACQUIRED HYPERPIGMENTATION

Diffuse hyperpigmentation may have systemic causes such as Addison's disease, drugs, Vitamin B12 deficiency or hemochromatosis. Post inflammatory hyperpigmentation is commonest cause of acquired localized or diffuse pigmentation especially in Indians and other darker skin types. **Table 18.7** gives a list of common causes of diffuse pigmentation that are common in pediatric age group.

Addison's disease results due to destruction of adrenal glands by a possible autoimmune mechanism leading to adrenal insufficiency. Common age at presentation of adrenal insufficiency is 30-50 years, but it can present during infancy or childhood in congenital adrenal hyperplasia and polyglandular autoimmune syndromes. Expression of adrenal cortex antibodies represents a significant risk of progression to adrenal insufficiency. Children have a high risk of progression compared to adults. There is an elevated level of ACTH and MSH. Hyperpigmentation is considered as the hallmark of Addison disease, but normal skin does not exclude the disease. It is prominent on the sun-exposed areas, Palmar creases, nail beds, extensor surfaces, knuckles, elbows, knees, nipples, axilla, perineum, scars formed after the onset of disease and the oral cavity (dentogingival margins and buccal mucosa). Patients with Addison's disease should be treated with mineralocorticoid and glucocorticoid replacement to reduce the drive for excess production of ACTH and MSH. Increased ACTH production (*Cushing's syndrome*) may cause a picture like that of Addison's disease. *Hyperthyroidism*, especially in those with darker complexions may also cause hyperpigmentation similar to that in Addison's diseases. Diffuse hyperpigmentation in *chronic renal failure* and in patients on hemodialysis is said to be caused by an increase in levels of pituitary melanotrophic peptides.

Diffuse pigmentation of hands, feet, face and gums has been reported with *Vitamin B12 deficiency*. It was reversible after B12 administration. *Severe wasting diseases* like malabsorption, AIDS, tuberculosis or neoplasms may be accompanied by diffuse hyperpigmentation. *Kwashiorkor* can present with mixed picture of generalized hypopigmentation and patchy

TABLE 18.7: Causes of diffuse hyperpigmentation in the pediatric age group

Diffuse pigmentation	Punctate and reticulate pigmentation
Addison's disease	Dermatopathia pigmentosa reticularis
Cushing's syndrome	Franceschetti-Jadassohn syndrome
Hyperthyroidism	Reticulate acro-pigmentation of Dohi
Vitamin B 12 deficiency	Dyskeratosis congenital
Malabsorption syndrome	Xeroderma pigmentosum
Kwashiorkor	Bloom's syndrome
AIDS	Rothmund-Thomson syndrome
Hemochromatosis	
Bronze baby syndrome	
Porphyria	
Chronic renal failure	
Adrenoleukodystrophy	
Universal acquired hypermelanosis	
Phototoxic reactions	
Post inflammatory hyperpigmentation	

hyperpigmentation. *Hemochromatosis*, a disorder of iron storage and deposition, can cause a slate-gray (Bronze) hyperpigmentation. Bronzing results from increased melanin production and hemosiderin deposition. Porphyrins, the endogenous photosensitizers, are produced in excess in Hepatic *porphyria* and congenital erythropoietic porphyria. Along with skin fragility, blistering, and hypertrichosis, there is hyperpigmentation on exposed areas of the body.

Adrenoleukodystrophy

Adrenoleukodystrophy is an X-linked acquired generalized hyperpigmentary disorder, characterized by slowly progressive disease of the brain and adrenals of affected children due to accumulation of unsaturated fatty acids. There is uniform macular pigmentation sparing the palms and groin area. *Bronze baby syndrome* is a rare acquired generalized pigmentary disorder of neonates, characterized by generalized gray-brown discoloration which occurs in patients with hepatocellular dysfunction undergoing phototherapy. Generalized dark insidious and progressive pigmentation with its onset in early infancy has been reported rarely, and has been termed as *universal acquired hypermelanosis ("Carbon baby")*.

Urticaria Pigmentosa

Urticaria pigmentosa is the commonest variety of mastocytosis seen in India. This disorder is common in the pediatric age group. Clinically presentation may vary from pigmented macules to violaceous plaques.

Hyperpigmentation can be a sequel of *phototoxic reactions* to systemic or topical medications (Fluoroquinolones, Ketoconazole, Thiazide diuretics, Phenothiazines, Psoralens, retinoids), or from contact with certain plants in conjunction with sun exposure (phytophotodermatitis). Initially there is an inflammatory reaction which is later followed by epidermal hyperkeratosis and melanocytic hyperplasia, causing hyperpigmentation. Certain drugs can cause pigmentation even without sun exposure (Clofazimine, Cyclophosphamide, Adriamycin, Minocycline, Antimalarials). Drugs should be considered as a cause of diffuse pigmentation especially in older children on long term medications.

Post-inflammatory Hyperpigmentation

Post-inflammatory hyperpigmentation (PIH) is a frequently encountered problem in pediatric age group. This excess pigmentation can be attributed to preceding disease processes that include infections, allergic reactions, injuries, phototoxic eruptions, trauma and inflammatory diseases (e.g. lichen planus, discoid lupus and atopic dermatitis). The distribution of the hypermelanotic lesions depends on the location of the inflammatory dermatosis. The color of the lesions ranges from light brown to black. Histopathologically there are epidermal and dermal types of PIH. Epidermal PIH involves increased melanin pigment in the basal cell layer of the epidermis, with or without giant melanosomes in the epidermis. In dermal PIH changes are seen in the upper dermis, with pigment incontinence due to increased numbers of melanophages in the papillary dermis. PIH is generally treated in adults with topical agents that inhibit tyrosinase (ex. Hydroquinone, Arbutin, Kojic acid, Azelaic acid, Aloesin) or enhance epidermal turnover (Retinoic acid, Glycolic acid). Safety of many such agents in children below 12 years is not well established; hence they should be used cautiously.

DISORDERS OF HYPOPIGMENTATION

Hypopigmentation or depigmentation can be congenital or acquired. They may occur in a localized or a diffuse pattern. Diagnosis is usually based on detailed clinical examination, and histopathologic examination is not mandatory in most of the conditions. Wood's light examination can accentuate the hypomelanotic lesions since they appear brighter by contrast to surrounding skin.

Pathophysiology of these conditions is the basis for the classification depicted in **Table 18.2**. However an initial clinical categorization of lesions in to an age based scheme is very useful for the diagnosis. There are three major subdivisions namely birth/early infancy and childhood. Further clinical information of localized, segmental or diffuse areas of involvement helps clinical diagnosis. **Table 18.8** gives a classification based on these clinical findings.

Treatment of these diseases in pediatric age groups should be rationally adapted based on the best available scientific evidence. Several other factors such as expectations of the parents, disease activity and co-morbidities should also be considered. This may also include a dedicated work of a team constituting

TABLE 18.8: Clinical classification of disorders of hypo/depigmentation

	Focal	Segmental	Diffuse
Birth/Infancy	Tuberous sclerosis, Piebaldism, Waardenburg Syndrome	Achromic nevus, Hypomelanosis of Ito,	Oculo-cutaneous albinism, Phenylketonuria
Childhood	Vitiligo, Postinflammatory hypopigmentation	Segmental Vitiligo	Generalized Vitiligo, Postinflammatory hypopigmentation

dermatologist, pediatrician, neurologist and geneticist. In this chapter discussions are mainly relevant to the pediatric age group. Vitiligo has been discussed separately.

ACHROMIC NEVUS

It is also called depigmented nevus or hypochromic nevus. It is characterized by presence of circumscribed hypopigmented macules present at birth or evident within few months after. It is a common condition usually seen on the trunk measuring a few centimeters in largest diameter **(Figure 18.8)**. Larger lesions often show a linear configuration with or without swirls.

Clinical diagnostic criteria for achromic nevus are 1. Hypopigmentation present at birth or onset early in life, 2. No alteration in distribution of pigmentary alteration throughout life, 3. No alteration in texture, or change of sensation, in the affected area, and 4. No hyperpigmented border around the achromic area.

There has been a suggestion to classify these lesions in to Depigmented nevi simplex and complex; simplex group differs from complex group that there is no associated systemic pathology. According to this the complex group includes hypopigmented lesions found in conditions such as tuberous sclerosis and hypomelanosis of Ito.

No medical treatment is likely to be beneficial in the treatment of achromic nevus, and achieving repigmentation is possible only by surgical means of autologous graft with melanocytes or a conventional epidermal graft. Treatment with 308-nm excimer laser has been found effective in a report of a solitary case.

Ultrastructurally some have found aggregates of melanosomes in the melanocytes suggesting a transfer block, where as others have found altered melanosome synthesis.

TUBEROUS SCLEROSIS

Hypopigmented macules of tuberous sclerosis ("ash-leaf spots") are usually present at birth. In 80 percent of persons with tuberous sclerosis, lesions appear by first year of life. They are found commonly on the trunk and lower extremities. They are the earliest indicator of this disorder, and appear before the neurological and other cutaneous markers. Clinically lesions are characterized by a flame or lance-ovate shape measuring about 1-3 cm in their largest diameter **(Figure 18.9)**.

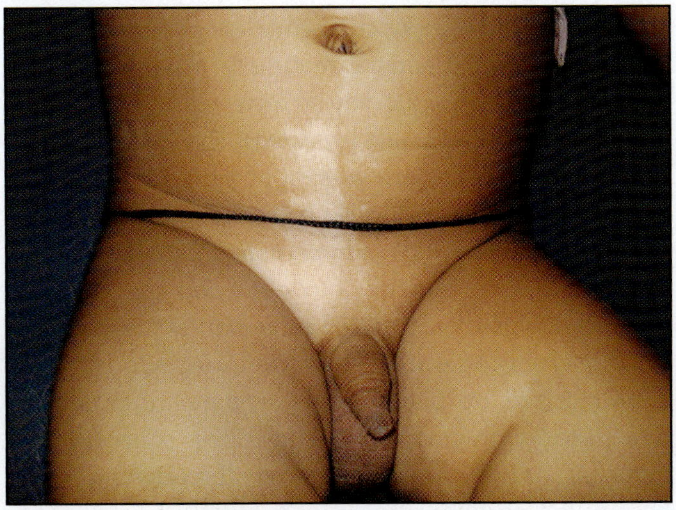

FIGURE 18.8: Achromic nevus

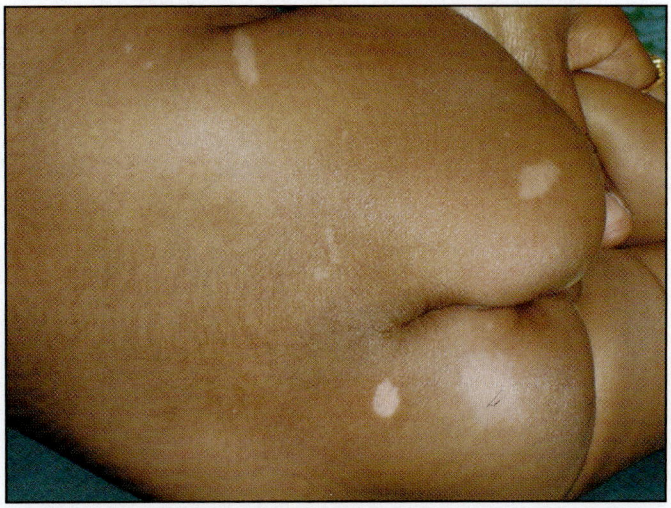

FIGURE 18.9: Ash leaf macules (Tuberous sclerosis)

TABLE 18.9: Disorders exhibiting distribution along Blaschko's lines

Congenital/Nevoid disorders	Acquired disorders
Hypomelanosis of Ito Achromic Nevus Segmental Hypermelanosis Incontinentia pigmenti Verrucous epidermal Nevus Nevus comedonicus Nevus Sebaceous Linear porokeratosis Linear Darier's Disease	Lichen Striatus Linear lichen planus Linear Psoriasis Extragenital lichen sclerosus Segmental vitiligo Linear Morphea and Parry Romberg Syndrome

Although ash-leaf spots are the most characteristic lesions, other hypomelanotic lesions such as polygonal, confetti-like and segmental lesions may also be seen.

HYPOMELANOSIS OF ITO

Hypomelanosis of Ito (HI) is a syndrome characterized by hypopigmented cutaneous lesions along the Blaschko's lines associated with neurologic, skeletal, hair, and dental defects. It is believed to have caused by Chromosomal mosaicism, and it is highly varied in its phenotype. Some believe that Hypomelanosis of Ito results from the somatic mosaicism of the Incontinentia Pigmenti gene. A list of disorders that may follow Blaschko's line is given in **Table 18.9.**

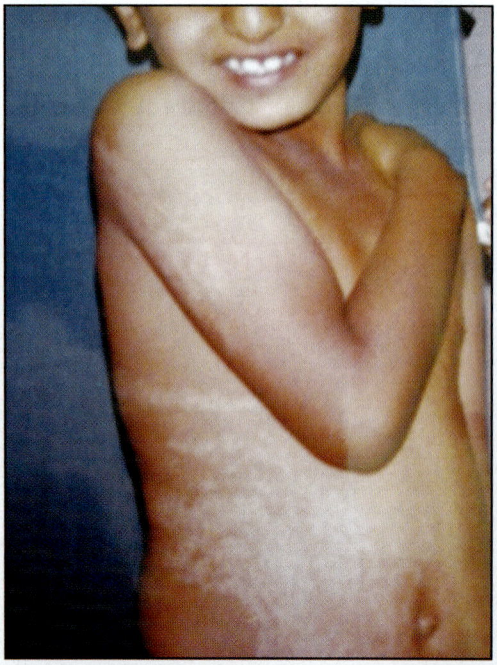

FIGURE 18.10: Hypomelanosis of Ito

HI is present at birth, and patients usually report with in first two years of life. Hypopigmentation is not preceded by vesicular or verrucous lesions; a feature distinguishes it from incontinentia pigmenti. Hypopigmented macules coalesce to form reticulated patches along the Blaschko's lines revealing linear, segmental and whorl like patterns **(Figure 18.10)**. Lesions cover more than 2 dermatomes and are often asymmetrically distributed on both sides of the body. Skin lesions may become pigmented over time and blend well with normally pigmented skin. Associated systemic lesions may cause seizures, mental retardation, developmental delay, deafness and visual problems. Cleft palate, hemi-hypertrophy, nail/ hair/ dental defects, and limb/face/skull anomalies may be evident on examination. Appropriate consultations and imaging studies may be required for the evaluation of the defects. There is no specific treatment for the cutaneous lesions apart from cosmetic coverage.

PIEBALDISM

Piebaldism is a rare autosomal-dominant genetic disorder, characterized amelanotic cutaneous lesions and white hair. The most specific clinical feature is a white forelock (poliosis). Similar lesions may be seen on the ventral chest, abdomen, upper arms and lower legs. These depigmented symmetrical patches are present at birth and are stable throughout life. Occasionally increased pigmentation at the margins and islands of hyperpigmentation within the amelanotic lesions can be noted. The anomaly is caused by defective proliferation and migration of melanoblasts during embryogenesis. *Waardenburg syndrome* is characterized by piebaldism like amelanotic lesions associated with heterochromic irides, sensorineural deafness, and dystopia canthorum (broadening of the base of the nose).

OCULO-CUTANEOUS ALBINISM AND OTHER SYNDROMES WITH DIFFUSE HYPO OR AMELANOSIS

Oculo-cutaneous Albinism

Oculo-cutaneous albinism *(OCA)* constitutes a group of diseases that present with a generalized complete or partial loss of pigmentation of the skin, hair and eye. Mutations in genes that regulate the multistep process of melanin synthesis are responsible for them. OCA type 1 primarily manifests with complete absence of pigment in the skin, hair and the eyes. It presents with generalized amelanosis with photophobia, reduced visual acuity, and nystagmus. OCA type 2 does not present with complete absence of pigment but rather manifests with a minimal or moderate amount of pigmentation persisting in the skin, the hair, and the eyes.

Chediak-Higashi Syndrome

Chediak-Higashi syndrome (CHS) is a rare autosomal recessive disorder characterized by generalized hypomelanosis, slate gray hairs, immune deficiency, bleeding tendencies, recurrent infection, progressive neurologic defects and a lympho-proliferative syndrome. The degree of altered pigmentation can vary from grayish to milky-white depending upon the ethnic background of the patient. Hair color may demonstrate an unusual "metallic" sheen. Ultrastructurally there are characteristic intracellular giant lysosomal granules. Bone marrow transplantation is the only effective treatment.

Characteristic silvery hairs are also a part of *Griscelli and Elejalde syndromes.* Griscelli syndrome (GS) is an autosomal recessive condition characterized by hypomelanosis, silvery hairs, neurological and immune alterations. Elejalde syndrome (ES) is also a recessive disorder characterized by light bronze skin color, silvery hairs and profound neurological deficits without immunological alterations. CHS, GS and ES seem to have some degree of clinical and genetic overlap.

Phenylketonuria

Phenylketonuria *(PKU)* is a rare autosomal recessive condition caused due to deficiency of enzyme phenylalanine hydroxylase. PKU is the commonest genetic disorder leading to mental retardation in the West; however, it is rare in India (0.08%). It is characterized clinically by a fair skin and hair (hypomelanosis), atopic like dermatitis, mental retardation and epilepsy. In suspected children or pregnant women of at-risk families, screening can be done by detection of serum level of phenylalanine or Guthrie test. Prenatal diagnosis of PKU is done ideally after identifying the mutation in the affected child by sequencing the gene, or by linkage analysis. Early treatment constituting of low phenylalanine diet continued throughout life can prevent mental retardation.

Ziprkowski-Margolis Syndrome

Ziprkowski-Margolis syndrome is characterized by amelanosis of skin and hair, heterochromic irides and deaf-mutism. *Cross syndrome* or Oculo-cerebral syndrome with hypopigmentation is characterized by amelanosis of skin, hair and eye with spasticity. Variable amount of depigmentation in the skin, the hair, and the eyes with a bleeding diathesis resulting from a platelet storage pool deficiency are features of *Hermansky – Pudlak syndrome.* Neurological alterations, peculiar facies and Oculo-cutaneous hypomelanosis are seen with *Prader-Willy syndrome.*

ACQUIRED HYPOPIGMENTATION

Pityriasis Alba

Pityriasis alba (PA) is dermatitis of unknown origin characterized by erythematous scaly lesions that resolve leaving round to oval macules of hypopigmentation. Sun exposure, atopic diathesis, infective agents and environmental influences have been regarded as possible factors involved in pathogenesis. It has been regarded as a manifestation of atopic dermatitis; however, it is also known to occur in the non-atopic. Pityriasis alba can affect any race, but it may be more prominent in dark-skinned patients. It is rare in children below 2 years of age and it can be seen in children of all age group and in teenagers. It is a frequent reason for pediatric dermatological consultation because of its chronic course, tendency to relapse, aesthetic impact and its resemblance to more serious disorders like leprosy and vitiligo.

Initial erythematous phase of PA may be conspicuous in individuals with fair complexion. They occur as one or few rounded or oval slightly raised plaques which later subside completely. At this phase there is only persistent fine lamellar or branny scaling and hypopigmentation. It may be conspicuous in dark skinned children and in others it becomes prominent after sun tanning. Individual lesions usually measure 0.5-2 cm in diameter but may be larger. Lesions are often confined to the face especially on the cheeks, but may be seen over the neck, arms, and trunk. Widespread cases overlap with another condition described below termed as progressive macular hypomelanosis. Lesions persist for several months or a year or more and recurrence is common. Initial erythematous phase may be not noticed by many individuals. Important differential diagnosis includes indeterminate leprosy, vitiligo, post inflammatory hypopigmentation and pityriasis versicolor.

Histopathologic changes are nonspecific with acanthosis, mild spongiosis, hyperkeratosis and patchy parakeratosis. Ultrastructural changes are reduced numbers of active melanocytes and a decrease in number and size of melanosomes.

No drug is found consistently effective in treating PA. Reassurance regarding benign nature and self resolution is important. Emollients and mild topical corticosteroid creams like hydrocortisone are used with variable success rates. Tacrolimus was found to be safe and effective in an open-label in the management of PA.

Progressive Macular Hypomelanosis

Progressive macular hypomelanosis (PMH) is a skin disorder characterized by asymptomatic ill-defined hypopigmented spots on the trunk. PMH has a worldwide distribution. It is commonly seen in young females but it is also reported in adolescents. Propionibacterium acne has been implicated in the pathogenesis of PMH.

PMH is stable disease with spontaneous regression. Clinically it is characterized by numerous ill-defined non scaly hypopigmented macules located in the middle and lower back usually in and around the midline. Lesions can also be noticed over the upper back, abdomen, chest and gluteal region. Histologically there is diminished pigment in the epidermis and a normal-looking dermis.

There is no specific treatment for PMH. Application of 1% clindamycin lotion during the daytime, 5% benzoyl peroxide gel at night-time, along with UVA light irradiation was found effective in the management of PMH.

Lichen Sclerosus et Atrophicus (Figure 8.11A)

Lichen sclerosus (LSA) is a chronic inflammatory dermatosis that results in the development of white papules and plaques with epidermal atrophy. LSA has both genital and extragenital presentations, with genital lesions outnumbering extragenital lesions. It is predominantly a disorder of adult population but up to 15% of the cases occur in children.

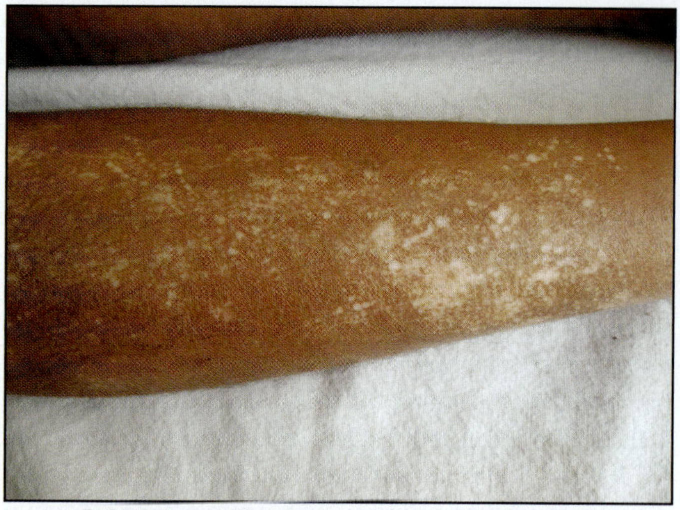

FIGURE 18.11A: Lichen sclerosus *et* atrophicus

Initial lesions are white, polygonal papules measuring few millimeters to centimeters that coalesce into plaques. Regularly placed comedo-like plugs due to obliterated openings of dermal appendages may also be seen. Ensuring atrophy will finally result in to porcelain-white plaque. Vulvar LSA may progress to gradual obliteration of the labia minora and stenosis of the introitus. Male genital lesions are usually noticed over the glans penis and the prepuce. Extragenital lesions may occur anywhere but more so on the back or shoulders.

Hyperkeratosis, epidermal atrophy, lichenoid infiltrate along with homogenization of the dermis is the usual histopathologic features.

Asymptomatic extragenital LSA usually requires no treatment. Vulvar lesions in prepubertal girls may resolve spontaneously. Topical corticosteroids, tacrolimus and a variety of ablative procedures like cryotherapy and lasers are used to control resistant lesions.

Tinea Versicolor

Tinea versicolor (TV) is a common infectious disorder of adolescents and adults, characterized by discrete and confluent scaly hypopigmented macules on the trunk, proximal extremities, face and neck. It is caused by a lipophilic fungus *Malassezia furfur*. Inhibition of tyrosinase by azelaic acid produced by the fungus may be responsible for the hypopigmentation. Variety of topical and systemic antifungal treatment schedules are practiced as therapy to this recurrent dermatosis. Hypopigmentation may persist for very long time in spite of adequate treatment.

Postinflammatory Hypopigmentation

Postinflammatory hypopigmentation is a transient disorder characterized by hypopigmentation of varying shades and sizes resulting after the resolution of a variety of inflammatory dermatosis. In some forms the loss of pigmentation may be complete and permanent due to associated scarring. Common causes in pediatric age group include infections (impetigo, leprosy), inflammatory dermatitis (psoriaisis, lichen striatus, pityriasis lichenoides chronica, DLE, morphea) and due to physical agents (polymorphic light eruptions, burns). In addition, therapies such as use of topical corticosteroids, cryotherapy and laser can also induce hypopigmentation. A number of factors like intensity of preceding inflammation, genetic predisposition and certain poorly understood factors determine the eventual hypopigmentation. It is not certain why some individuals respond with hypopigmentation and others with hyperpigmentation to same trigger. Inherited individual chromatic tendency may be responsible for this.

Morphea and Scleroderma: In *morphea* **(Figure 18.11B)** and *scleroderma*, lesions occur as uneven hypo and depigmented macules or diffuse hypopigmentation with preservation of perifollicular pigmentation. This perifollicular pigmentation is seen as polygonal spots as compared to the oval or round spots seen in vitiligo. In *Discoid lupus erythematosus* (DLE), post inflammatory depigmentation is coupled with atrophy, scarring and follicular plugging.

Lichen striatus : *Lichen striatus* (LS) is a self limiting, linear, inflammatory dermatosis of unknown etiology. It commonly affects children between the ages of 3 and 15 years, but can occur at any age. Initial lesions appear as shiny, flat-topped, erythematous, grouped papules, progress to configure in a linear fashion corresponding to Blaschko's lines. Common site of involvement is leg but can occur on other parts of body. It has a benign, self limiting course with residual postinflammatory hypopigmentation that persists for long time **(Figure 18.12)**.

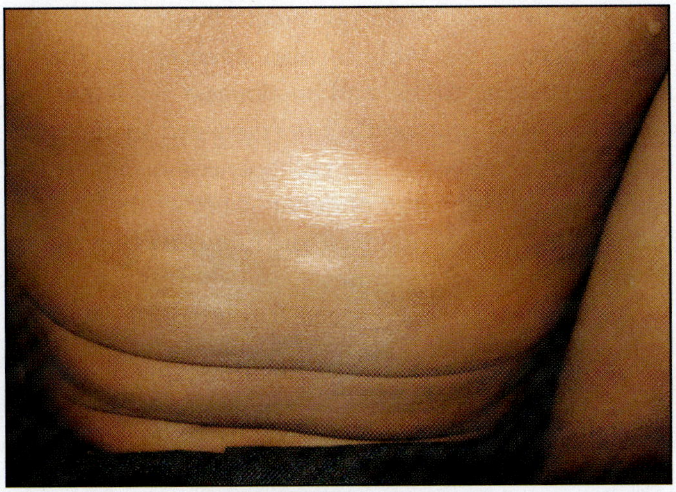

FIGURE 18.11B: Morphea

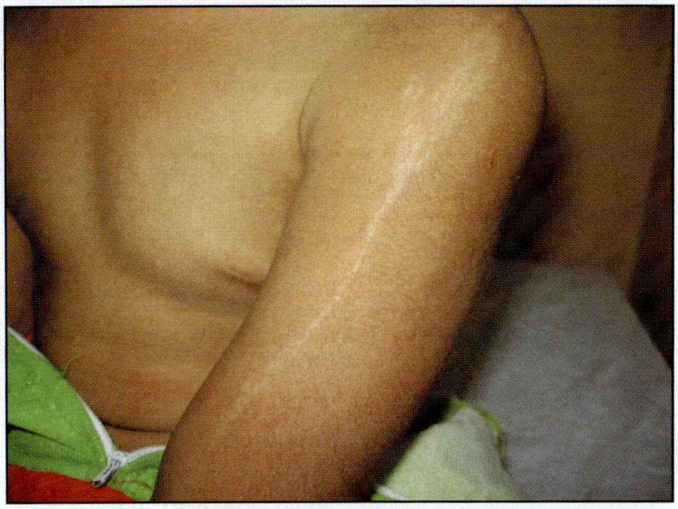

FIGURE 18.12: Lichen striatus

Leprosy: *Leprosy* can present with hypopigmentation especially in indeterminate and tuberculoid varieties. Indeterminate leprosy presents with a single or a few ill-defined macules, with or without sensory impairment. It closely resembles pityriasis alba, but on histopathology infiltration around the cutaneous nerves can be observed. Hypopigmented macules of tuberculoid leprosy (maculo-anesthetic) are characterized by the presence of hypopigmented, hypoesthetic macules with well defined borders. Several factors may be responsible for hypopigmentation in leprosy.

CHILDHOOD VITILIGO

Vitiligo is a common, acquired disorder characterized by depigmentation of the skin marked by the presence of well circumscribed milky white cutaneous macules, with loss of melanocytes on histology. Pathogenesis of vitiligo is complex and not yet fully understood, but it is believed to involve a combination of autoimmune, genetic, and environmental factors. There is a current lack of consensus in definition and methods of assessment of severity of this disorder, which makes it more difficult to compare the efficacy of different treatments.

TABLE 18.10: Salient features of childhood vitiligo as compared to adult vitiligo

Family history	Increased frequency of autoimmune disorders in first and second degree relatives
Autoantibodies	Higher incidence of autoantibodies especially thyroid antibodies
Autoimmune diseases	Higher incidence of autoimmune thyroid disease
Subtypes	Generalized type is the commonest but relatively higher incidence of segmental type
Therapy	Enhanced response to topical steroids, tacrolimus and PUVA

Childhood vitiligo seems to be a distinct subset of vitiligo. Relationship with HLA subtypes has also shown some differences in the pediatric and adult form of diseases. There are certain differences in the clinical features of these two forms of vitiligo, which are summarized in **Table 18.10**. This chapter includes discussion on various aspects of vitiligo with special attention to childhood type.

EPIDEMIOLOGY

Vitiligo occurs worldwide with an overall prevalence of about 1%. The highest of incidence of the condition has been recorded in India. Its incidence ranges from 0.1 to 8.8% in different Indian studies. Nearly all cases of vitiligo are acquired relatively early in life. Almost half the patients present before the age of 20 years. There has been a steady increase in the incidence of childhood vitiligo during the past 2 decades. It is rare in infancy. Few reports of increased incidence of childhood vitiligo in female sex have been reported. Concern about the appearance and its social consequences may lead to early presentation in girls. Family incidence of occurrence in India ranges from 6.25-18% in different regions, however incidence as high as 90.38% among a particular community in Bangalore has been recorded.

In an Indian study on childhood vitiligo, the generalized, non-segmental vitiligo (78%) was the commonest, followed by focal vitiligo (14.4%) and then by segmental vitiligo (4.6%). Grimes et al reported 29% of segmental vitiligo in children as compared to 9% in adults.

ETIOPATHOGENESIS

The pathogenesis of vitiligo has been debated with various hypotheses including, immune, genetic, neural and self destruction. A unifying hypothesis for the etiology has also been proposed, in which final destruction of melanocytes in vitiligo results from a cascade of reactions leading to deregulation of melanogenesis by free radical damage. It is proposed that vitiligo is a psycho-neuro-endocrine-immunologic disease with extra-cutaneous manifestations in genetically predisposed subjects.

An *autoimmune* etiology appears to be the most likely, with melanocytes destroyed by auto-antibodies or specific cell mediated immunity. It has been demonstrated that there is an increased frequency of autoimmune diseases in the first- and second-degree relatives especially in childhood vitiligo. Autoantibodies against thyroid gland and gastric parietal cell, and antinuclear antibodies have been detected in patients. Cytotoxic antibodies against surface and cytoplasmic melanocytic antigens and anti-tyrosinase antibodies have also been detected in the sera. These antibodies may cause destruction of melanocytes or hamper melanocyte function in patients with vitiligo. In children with nonsegmental vitiligo, coexisting autoimmune thyroiditis is also common. Recent work has shown high numbers of cytotoxic T lymphocytes specific for melanocytic antigens, which supports a role of cell mediated immunity in vitiligo. Aberrations in T and NK cell profiles leading to a role for cell-mediated immunity may also be seen in vitiligo. Smyth line chickens (the animal model for vitiligo) also develop blindness, autoimmune thyroiditis, and an alopecia-like feathering defect. A melanocyte specific T-cell mediated autoimmune response is observed in the pathogenesis of Smyth line vitiligo. It is still a matter of debate whether the primary pathogenic role is exerted by humoral or cellular abnormal immune responses.

The earliest evidence suggesting a *genetic* basis for vitiligo comes from the association of other disorders like diabetes mellitus, which have heritable occurrences. Genetic diseases are substantially more prevalent in first degree relatives. Genetic models on basis of family studies include a multifactorial model, a dominant model with incomplete penetration, and a multilocular recessive model. In children and young adults vitiligo inheritance has followed a dominant mode of inheritance with incomplete penetration. Specific HLA haplotypes are strongly but not consistently associated.

Other hypothesis include a *neural* hypothesis, in which it is proposed that neuro-chemical mediator destroys melanocytes or inhibit melanin production; and a *self-destruction* hypothesis, in which it is postulated that intermediate or metabolic product of melanin synthesis causes melanocyte destruction.

Vitiligo is among many diseases in dermatology that can be triggered by psychological stress. As a psycho-cutaneous disorder, it is classified under a disease "sometimes influenced by emotional factors". Onset of the disease is often attributed to a specific life event, crisis or illness. Infections and trauma (Koebner's phenomenon) are other known triggers. A new theory has been proposed based on immunological and ultrastructural evidences that non segmental vitiligo is a melanocytorrhagic disorder, where altered melanocyte responses to friction and other stress induces indolent detachment and subsequent transepidermal loss of melanocytes. Apart from immunologic damage, metabolic deregulations leading to toxic damage of the melanocytes appears also to be relevant.

Segmental vitiligo seems to have some important differences in the etiology, prevalence of associated illnesses and therapy. It has a unilateral and a dermatomal distribution. It is rarely associated with any autoimmune diseases. Neural hypothesis best explains this type of vitiligo. Studies have shown evidence of axonal damage and changes in neuropeptide balance in the nerves of segmental vitiligo lesions. Local injection of physostigmine revealed an associated with a dysfunction of the sympathetic nerves.

A small sub-set of individuals develop *contact/occupational vitiligo* following exposure to particular chemicals (phenolic/catecholic derivatives). This contact/occupational vitiligo and chemical leukoderma present with well-defined, depigmented skin lesions that develop at the site of exposure. Genetic inability of melanocytes to tolerate and/or respond to the oxidative stress may be the cause of these conditions.

CLINICAL MANIFESTATIONS

Clinical features in children are almost same as in adults. Hallmark of vitiligo is appearance of milky white depigmenting macules. Initial lesions are round or oval often with scalloped margins **(Figure 18.13)**. Tendency for confluence and symmetry can be observed in many patients with advancing disease. Lesions are generally well circumscribed with margins being slightly hyperpigmented. Lesions are obviously noted as they have a tendency to appear in exposed parts of the body like face, neck, back of hands, and wrists. Vitiligo often appears after traumatic insults (Kobner's phenomenon) such as a cut or abrasion, thus the knees, elbows, shins and hands are often the sites of initial involvement in children. Clinical relevance of Kobner's phenomenon is not yet established, although it has been postulated that it may indicate active disease. Lesions around the body orifices eyes, nostrils, mouth and genitalia **(Figure 18.14)** are also common. Progression and extension can vary greatly with some patients having a few macules (focal vitiligo) and others having almost whole body involved (universal vitiligo). Mucous membrane involvement as a sole manifestation or as a part of mucocutaneous disease is also common. Loss of color of hairs (leukotrichia) in the lesions may indicate a poor prognosis in regard to repigmentation. Check list for the clinical evaluation is given in the **Table 18.11**.

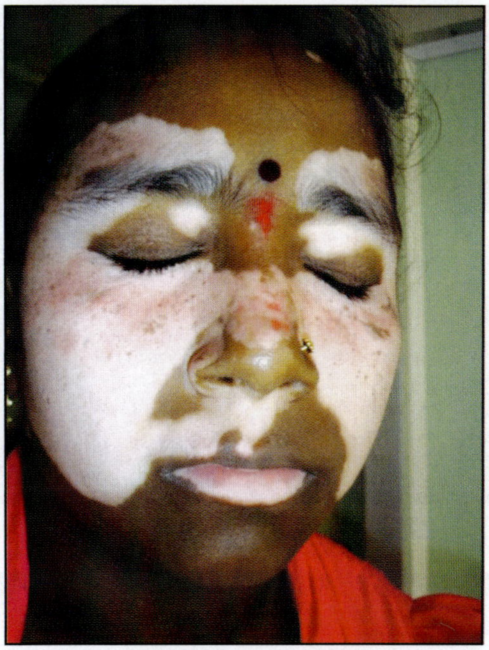

FIGURE 18.13: Vitiligo

Presence of an intermediate color zone between a depigmented macule and normal pigmented surrounding skin gives rise to *Trichrome vitiligo*. During repigmentation a fourth hyperpigmented band may develop which is

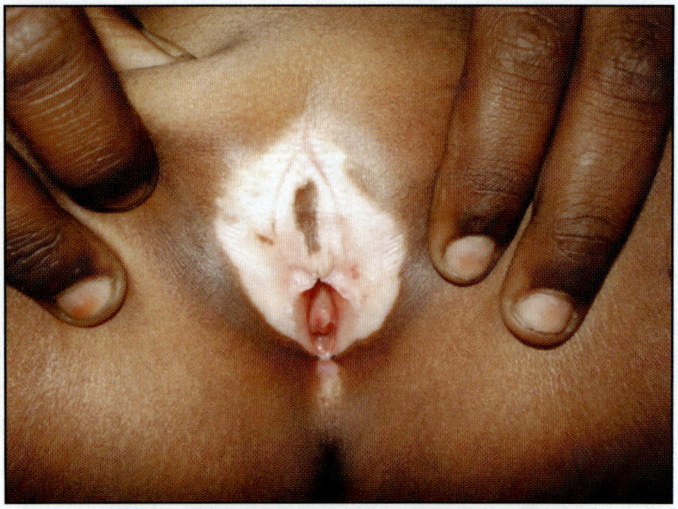

FIGURE 18.14: Genital vitiligo

TABLE 18.11: Checklist for the clinical evaluation of vitiligo

1. Ethnic origin
2. Fitzpatrick Phototype
3. Age of onset
4. Duration
5. Triggering factors
6. Family history of vitiligo and autoimmune disorders
7. Personal history of endocrinal and autoimmune disorders
8. Extent and configuration
9. Disease activity - progressive, stable , repigmenting
10. Koebner's phenomenon
11. Perifollicular pigmentation and trichrome
12. Leukotrichia
13. Mucosal involvement
14. Premature hair graying
15. Halo nevus
16. Ocular lesions

described as *Quadrachrome vitiligo*. A macular perifollicular hyperpigmentation is another feature of repigmenting disease. *Penta-chrome vitiligo* is an infrequent occurrence of sequential display of white, tan, brown, blue-gray hyperpigmentation and the normal skin. Dark skinned patients are more likely to have this variation. *Blue vitiligo* usually describes vitiligo macules occurring at the site of postinflammatory hyperpigmentation. *Confetti vitiligo* describes a condition where a patient develops many small macules (less than or equal to 2 mm) of vitiligo lesions. *Inflammatory vitiligo* exhibits an erythematous, raised border in a vitiligo macule.

Segmental vitiligo is a distinct variety characterized by a sharply unilateral involvement and a segmental or quasi-dermatomal distribution **(Figure 18.15)**. One segment is involved in most patients, but two or more segments even with contralateral distribution may rarely occur. Involvement of several dermatomes in a Blasckoid pattern may also be seen. Lesion involving trigeminal dermatome is the commonest presentation. Segmental vitiligo has an early onset, rapid spread, tendency to stabilize in about 2 years, and remain persistent throughout life if no treatment offered.

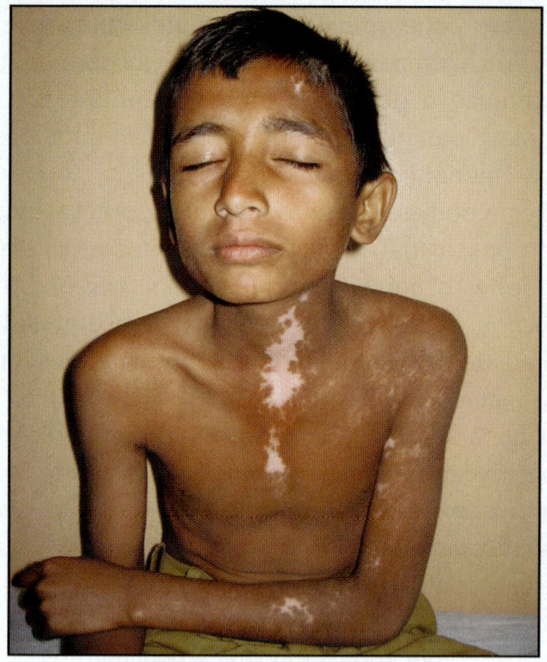

FIGURE 18.15: Segmental vitiligo

CLASSIFICATION

Nordlund established a clinical classification based on extent and distribution, in to localized, generalized and universal vitiligo. Localized variety was classified in to focal and segmental, Generalized variety into acrofacial, vulgaris and mixed (segmental plus vulgaris or acrofacial) types. Collaborating epidemiology, clinical appearance and underlying possible pathogenesis broadly categorizes vitiligo in to nonsegmental (Type A) types and segmental (Type B).

Classification and salient features of the broad categories are described in **Tables 18.12 and 18.13**.

ASSOCIATIONS

Association of dermatological and systemic diseases gives an insight in to the pathogenesis of the disease. Among the various cutaneous disorders associated include alopecia areata, lichen planus, canities, morphea, halo

TABLE 18.12: Classification of vitiligo

Segmental Vitiligo		Depigmented macules distributed in a dermatomal configuration
Nonsegmental Vitiligo	**Focal**	Single or few scattered lesions in a nonsegmental distribution
	Vulgaris	Extensive lesions in a symmetric fashion
	Acrofacial	Distal extremities and face involved in a symmetric fashion
	Universal	Vitiligo involving total or near total body surface
	Mucosal	Lesions limited to mucous membranes

TABLE 18.13: Salient features of non-segmental and segmental vitiligo

	Non-segmental Vitiligo	**Segmental vitiligo**
Possible pathogenesis	Heritable, Autoimmune	Neural
Autoantibodies	Against thyroid gland, gastric parietal cell, ANA	Rare
Onset	Any age	Usually in childhood
Triggering factor	Often present	Absent
Evolution	Variable; Usually progress with appearance of new lesions but can remain stationary or even repigment	A rapid progression followed by stabilization; if untreated persists unaltered there after.
Koebner's phenomenon	May be present	Rare
Halo Nevus	May be present	Absent
Associations	Autoimmune diseases like thyroiditis, Alopecia areata, pernicious anemia, Addison's disease	Rare
Therapy	Variable response to medical treatment; surgical therapy for limited, stable vitiligo.	Variable response to medical treatment; best suited for surgical therapy

Note: ANA=Antinuclear antibody

nevus, melanoma and psoriasis. Systemic associations include hypo and hyperthyroidism, Diabetes mellitus, pernicious anemia, Addison's disease, lymphoma and leukemia. It is important to notice that most of these disorders have possible autoimmune etiology. Autoimmune thyroiditis presented simultaneously or after the onset of vitiligo.

A number of ocular lesions have been described. They include anterior segment (iris) involvement, ring-like peripapillary atrophy around the optic nerve, pigment epithelium atrophy, focal hypopigmented spots and diffuse hypopigmentation. These lesions occur more frequently in patients with periorbital involvement. There are two syndrome associations related to ocular lesions. First among them is *Vogt-Koyanagi-Harada syndrome*; it refers to vitiligo, poliosis and alopecia in association with panuveitis, auditory and neurological defects. Second one is the *Alezzandrini syndrome*, characterized by unilateral retinal degeneration, and ipsilateral vitiligo, poliosis, and, possibly, hearing abnormalities.

A mild degree of subclinical sensorineural hypoacusis was found in many patients with vitiligo.

DIAGNOSIS AND DIFFERENTIALS

Numerous dermatoses may simulate vitiligo, however, the classical lesions in an advanced case is unlikely to be confused with any other dermatoses. However conditions like Pityriasis versicolor, pityriasis alba, postinflammatory hypopigmentation, Tuberculoid and borderline tuberculoid leprosy, nevus depigmentosus, tuberous sclerosis, piebaldism, Waardenberg's syndrome, systemic sclerosis and chemical leukoderma will have to be differentiated by appropriate history and clinical examination. Biopsy may be occasionally needed.

Histopathologically vitiligo is characterized by absence of melanocytes in the lesional skin. Perivascular and perifollicular lymphocytic infiltrate may be observed at the margin of vitiliginous lesions and in early lesions, consistent with cell-mediated immune processes destroying melanocytes.

It is important to evaluate children with vitiligo for the association of systemic involvement, especially the endocrinal and autoimmune diseases. Commonest endocrinal abnormality in childhood vitiligo is a thyroid dysfunction, and estimation of TSH levels is the most cost effective laboratory evaluation. A thorough clinical and laboratory evaluation is required in a child with family history of autoimmune disease.

TREATMENT

Vitiligo is a cosmetic problem in most cases but the social stigma associated with this disease often demands an aggressive approach. Treatment in children may need some alterations; however modalities remain the same as in adults. Major concerns in many established treatments are their safety while using in children. The natural history of vitiligo is unpredictable. Stable non segmental vitiligo may actively progress after a variable time interval. Segmental vitiligo is the better variety since it is the most stable and possibility of systemic disease association is rare.

Primary targets in the management of vitiligo include stabilizing the disease and inducing repigmentation. Most treatment modalities attend both these targets, but response in an individual patient is highly variable. Cure is a distant possibility with the present treatment options, but significant repigmentation can be achieved. Lack of response to one mode of treatment need not be a total failure. It is important to counsel the patient or parents regarding these issues, and to have a long term treatment plan. Various treatments are listed in the **Table 18.14**.

Topical Treatments

Corticosteroids: Topical corticosteroids are considered as the first line treatment of vitiligo. Antiinflammatory effects induced by topical steroids may locally suppress the immunologic changes allowing inactive melanocytes to repopulate affected skin sites and induce repigmentation. Advantages, disadvantages and side effects of topical corticosteroids are explained in the table. Potent topical non-fluorinated corticosteroids mometasone furoate may be used safely in children for a variable period of time. Other preparations like betamethasone valerate and clobetasol propionate have also been used. In general, best results with topical steroids are obtained in limited disease of face and proximal extremities. **Table 14.15** presents the factors to be considered while using topical steroids in children with vitiligo.

Calcineurin Inhibitors: They are primarily used in the treatment of atopic dermatitis. There are evidences to support usefulness of topical *tacrolimus* in vitiligo as a monotherapy or as an adjuvant to other modalities like excimer laser. In a study (Lepe V Et al), 0.1% tacrolimus was almost as effective as 0.05% clobetasol propionate to restore skin color in lesions of vitiligo in children. It

TABLE 18.14: Therapeutic options in vitiligo

Medical	Surgical
Topical	Tattooing
Corticosteroids	Punch grafting
Immunomodulators	Suction blister grafting
Vitamin D analogues	Split thickness grafting
Vegetal catalase and superoxide dismutase	Meshed split skin grafting
Hydroalcoholic extract of human basic fibroblast growth factor	Follicular unit grafting
Cosmetic Camouflage	Cultured epidermal suspension
Phototherapy/Laser	Melanocyte culture transplantation
PUVA – Topical/systemic	Dermabrasion
Broadband UVB	
Narrowband UVB	
Targeted UVB (Micro-phototherapy)	
Excimer laser	
Bleaching	
Systemic	
Corticosteroids	
Nutritional supplements	
Phenylalanine	

does not have a tendency to induce atrophy; hence tacrolimus may be useful for younger patients and for sensitive areas of the skin such as eyelids.

Vitamin D Analogues: *Calcipotriol* has been used topically either alone or in combination with topical steroids or UV radiation in the management of vitiligo. These agents affect the growth and differentiation of both melanocytes as well as keratinocytes, thus they may stimulate melanogenesis. Calcipotriol has given variable results in treatment of vitiligo in different studies.

Other Topical Preparbasic ations

Melagenine, a topical agent derived from placenta, has been used successfully in treating some childhood cases of vitiligo. *Hydroalcoholic extract of human placenta* which promotes melanin synthesis by supplying the amino acid, tyrosine, as well as encouraging copper tyrosinase linkage has shown variable results. *Vegetal catalase and superoxide dismutase* has been used in combination with UVB phototherapy showed some repigmentation of lesions. *Recombinant human basic fibroblast growth factor* has also shown some promises as a safe topical alternate in the treatment of vitiligo. *Pseudocatalase* is another molecule used topically in the treatment.

Cosmetic camouflage is an important tool for limited disease and lesions of face, neck and hands, especially for adolescent girls. Obtaining a color match may be difficult, but they are generally safe.

Bleaching

In adults, bleaching of remaining pigmented skin can be considered using monobenzyl ether of hydroquinone or Q switched ruby laser, for universal vitiligo. This is not recommended for children.

Phototherapy and Lasers

PUVA: Topical or oral 8-methoxypsoralen (or trimethyl psoralen) combined with Ultraviolet A (PUVA) or natural sunlight (PUVASOL) irradiation is effective for treating vitiligo. Oral PUVA is considered for generalized vitiligo where as topical PUVA is considered for vitiligo involving $< 10\%$ body area. Limitations of oral PUVA include gastric intolerance, cataract formation, photo aging and an increased risk of cancer. It is recommended to have photoprotection of skin and eye during treatment and 12 hours following ingestion of psoralens. It is not recommended for children less than 12 years age. Topical PUVA (TUVA) can cause local reactions like erythema and blistering. Total treatments are generally restricted to 100 to 150 Joules given in terms of one to three times a week. With the advent of more effective and less dangerous treatments like narrowband UVB, PUVA may soon be replaced. PUVASOL is still practiced widely in India since it does not require a phototherapy center and its ability to use at home.

UVB phototherapy: Broadband UVB (280 to 320 nm) is used with an initial dose of 20mJ/cm^2 increasing every visit by 20% until minimal erythema develops in the lesional skin. It is said to have success rates equivalent to PUVA.

Latest in the phototherapy advance is the Narrowband Ultraviolet B (NB-UVB) therapy with a wavelength of 311nm, first reported by Westerhof et al. Narrow-band UVB is an effective and well-tolerated treatment option for childhood vitiligo, with definite advantages over PUVA. Some recent studies indicate that it is superior to oral PUVA. It seems to act by local and systemic immunomodulation and by stimulating residual follicular melanocytes. To deliver NB-UVB, wide variety of cabins and panels of TL-01 lights are available. Therapeutic regime includes an initial dose of 150mJ/cm^2 given on three alternate days in a week; 10% increment of dosage until minimal erythema develops. On Type 4 and Indian skin it may range from 150 to 400mj.

Treatment can be continued for up to 12 months in children.

Advantages of NB-UVB Therapy

1. At least as effective or more effective than other treatments like PUVA and broadband-UVB.
2. No prior photosensitization with psoralen needed, hence better patient compliance.
3. Eye and photo protection beyond treatment is not required.
4. Recent guidelines indicate that it is safe in children.
5. Low cumulative dose, hence lesser photodamage.
6. Lesser contrast between normal and repigmented skin.
7. Better efficacy if combined with topical treatments like corticosteroids.

TABLE 18.15: Important considerations while using topical steroids in children with vitiligo

Advantages	1. Home based , unsupervised treatment 2. Can be used in children in almost all age group 3. Cost effective treatment 4. Low incidence of side effects when used judiciously
Disadvantages	1. Useful only in limited disease (< 20% body surface involved) 2. Extra precautions when using on Face, eyelids and body folds
Side effects	Cutaneous atrophy, Striae, Hypertrichosis, acnieform eruptions, Rosacea

Considering all these advantages, NB-UVB may replace PUVA and other forms of phototherapies in future. More controlled studies are required to confirm the safety and efficacy of long-term NB-UVB therapy.

Microphototherapy is a variation of NB-UVB to treat limited segmental and non-segmental vitiligo. The beam of light is focused only on the areas affected by vitiligo. It seems to be the best option for children, as the cumulative dose of radiation is very low and unaffected skin is not irradiated.

Monochromatic Excimer Light (MEL)

Monochromatic excimer light (MEL) has been used to treat adults with either segmental or generalized vitiligo. Its efficacy is not known in children since evidences on its efficacy and safety is lacking in children less than 15 years.

Systemic Steroids

Systemic corticosteroids can control the activity of a rapidly progressive disease, however due to its large number of side effects like weight gain, moon faceies, peptic ulcer, acne, striae etc., its use has been limited to only a few selected cases. Oral mini pulse treatment using betamethasone in a dose of 2.5 – 3.5 mg given on two consecutive days of a week can be considered in children with progressive disease under strict supervision for side effects. This dose should be reduced in a stepwise manner until cessation of new lesions occurs.

Surgical Therapy

Medical therapy can fail if all melanocyte reservoirs are destroyed by a progressive disease. Surgical procedures are usually not recommended for vitiligo in children, however for a highly motivated preadolescent child may be a candidate for surgery. A list of various surgical therapies is given in **Table 18.14**. Epidermal suction blister grafting seems to be the most effective surgical procedure. Grafting is best done for small inactive vitiligo (stable for at least two years) lesions of exposed parts. Absence of new Kobner's phenomenon and a positive minigraft test (repigmentation around 4 to 5 minigrafts placed 3 to 4 mm apart in depigmented skin) are the other factors indicating stability. By definition segmental vitiligo is the most stable form, and the surgical result with this variety is the best. Detailed surgical therapies are not discussed here in this chapter.

CONCLUSION

No single therapy for vitiligo can be regarded as the most effective. Face and neck respond best to all therapies, but distal extremities and lips are least responsive. Topical corticosteroids are the most commonly used drugs for localized vitiligo. Topical immunomodulators like tacrolimus seems to have comparable effectiveness and fewer side effects. For generalized vitiligo, phototherapy with UVB radiation is very effective with fewest side effects. Oral steroids in regular or pulsed therapeutic regimes are efficacious but they should be used cautiously. Surgical therapy can be very successful in stable childhood vitiligo, but requires an expertise. Counseling the afflicted patients or the parents is an integral part of the treatment.

BIBLIOGRAPHY

1. Abagge KT, Marinoni LP, Giraldi S, Carvalho VO, Santini CO, Favret H. Lichen Striatus: Description of 89 Cases in Chiidren. Pediatric Dermatoiogy 2004;21:440-3.
2. Addison Disease. Liotta EA, Elston DM, Brough A, Erickson QL. Last updated 21st February 2007. http://www.emedicine.com /DERM/topic761.htm. Last accessed 10th July 2008.
3. Agrawal D, Shajil EM, Marfatia YS, Begum R. Study on the Antioxidant Status of Vitiligo Patients of Different Age Groups in Baroda. Pigment Cell Research 2004;17:289-94.
4. Albinism. Boissy RE, Nordlund JJ. Last Updated: 29th June 2007. http://www.emedicine.com/derm/topic12.htm. Last accessed 16th July 2008.

5. Aydogan K, Turan OF, Onart S, Karadogan SK, Tunali S Audiological abnormalities in patients with vitiligo. Clinical & Experimental Dermatology 2006;31:110-13.
6. Baba M, Bal N, Efficacy and Safety of Short-Pulse Erbium:YAG Laser in the Treatment of Acquired Melanocytic Nevi. Dermatol Surg 2006;32:256–60.
7. Baharav E, Merimski O, Shoenfeld O, Zigelman R, Gilbrud B, Yecheskel G, Youinou P, Fishman P. Tyrosinase as an autoantigen in patients with vitiligo. Clinical & Experimental Immunology 1996;105:84-8.
8. Banerjee K, Barbhuiya JN, Ghosh AP, Dey SK, Karmakar PR. The efficacy of low-dose oral corticosteroids in the treatment of vitiligo patient. Indian J Dermatol Venereol Leprol 2003;69:135-7.
9. Baskan EB, Baykara M, Ercan I, Tunali S, Yucel A. Vitiligo and ocular findings: a study on possible associations. Journal of the European Academy of Dermatology and Venereology 2006;20:829-33.
10. Becker Melanosis. Rivers JK, Wiseman MC. Last updated 1st October 2007. http://www.emedicine.com/derm/topic48.htm Last accessed 12th July 2008.
11. Bellet JS, Prose NS. Vitiligo in children: a review of classification, hypotheses of pathogenesis and treatment. An Bras Dermatol. 2005;80:633-7.
12. Boissy RE, Manga P. On the Etiology of Contact/Occupational Vitiligo. Pigment Cell Res 2004;17:208–14.
13. Brazzelli V, Prestinari F, Castello M, Bellani E, Roveda E, Barbagallo T, Borroni G Useful Treatment of Vitiligo in 10 Children with UV-B Narrowband (311 nm). Pediatric Dermatology 2005;22:257-61.
14. Briganti S, Camera E, Picardo M. Chemical and Instrumental Approaches to Treat. Hyperpigmentation. Pigment Cell Research 2003;16:101-10.
15. Cario-André MC, Pain CY, Gauthier Y, Taïeb A. The melanocytorrhagic hypothesis of vitiligo tested on pigmented, stressed, reconstructed epidermis. Pigment Cell Research 2007; 20:385-93.
16. Congenital Patterned Leukodermas. Boissy RE, Hoath S. Last Updated: 12th Jan 2007. http://www.emedicine.com/derm/topic325.htm. Last accessed 12th July 2008.
17. Dell'Anna ML, Picardo M A. Review and a new hypothesis for non-immunological pathogenetic mechanisms in vitiligo. Pigment Cell Research 2006;19:406-11.
18. Dogra S, Kanwar AJ. Narrow band UVB phototherapy in dermatology. Indian J Dermatol Venereol Leprol 2004; 70:205-9.
19. Finco O, Cuccia M, Martinetti M, Ruberto G, Orecchia G, Rabbiosi G. Age of onset in vitiligo: relationship with HLA supratypes. Clinical Genetics 1990:39:48-54.
20. Forschner T, Buchholtz S, Stockfleth E. Current state of vitiligo therapy – evidence-based analysis of the literature. Journal der Deutschen Dermatologischen Gesellschaft 2006; **5**:467-75.
21. G Relyveld, H Menke, W Westerhof. Progressive and extensive hypomelanosis and extensive pityriasis alba: same disease, different names? JEADV 2006, 20, 1328–99.
22. Gangopadhyay KA. Bilateral nevus of ota. Indian J Dermatol Venereol Leprol 2000;66:104-5.
23. Gauthier Y, Andre MC, Taieb A. A Critical Appraisal of Vitiligo Etiologic Theories. Is Melanocyte Loss a Melanocytorrhagy? Pigment Cell Research 2003;16:322-2.
24. Giorgi V, Sestini S, Massi D, Lotti T. Melanocyte aggregation in the skin: Diagnostic clues from lentigenes to melanoma. Dermatol Clin 2007;25:303-20.
25. Gupta S, Kumar B. Epidermal Grafting for Vitiligo in Adolescents. Pediatric Dermatology 2002;19:159-62.
26. Handa H, Dogra S. Epidemiology of childhood vitiligo: a study of 625 patients from North India. Ped Dermatol 2003;20:107-10.
27. Handa S, Dogra S. Epidemiology of Childhood Vitiligo: A Study of 625 Patients from North India. Pediatric Dermatology 2003;20:207-10.
28. Hann SK. Vitiligo. Last Updated: 14th april 2005. http://www.emedicine.com/DERM/topic453.htm Last accessed 22nd July 2008.
29. Hartmann A, Brocker EB, Becker JC. Hypopigmentary Skin Disorders Current Treatment Options and Future Directions. Drugs 2004; 64 (1): 89-107.
30. Hemady N, Noble C, An Infant with a Hypopigmented Macule American Family Physician 2007;75:1053-4.
31. Hercogova J, Buggiani G, Prignano F, Lotti T. A rational approach to the treatment of vitiligo and other hypomelanosis. Dermatol Clin 2007;25:383-92.
32. Huggins RH, Janusz CA, Schwartz RA. Vitiligo: A sign of systemic disease. Indian J Dermatol Venereol Leprol 2006;72:68-71.
33. Huggins TH, Schwartz RA, Janniger KC. Vitiligo. Acta Dermato Ven 2005;14:137-45.
34. Inamadar AC, Palit A. Cutaneous mastocytosis: report of six cases. Indian J Dermatol Venereol Leprol 2006;72:50-3.
35. Inamadar AC, Palit A. silvery hair and bronze tan in a child: A case of Elejalde disease. Indian J Dermatol Venereol Leprol 2007;7:417-9.
36. Ingordo V, Iannazzone SS, Cusano F, Naldi L. Dermoscopic Features of Congenital Melanocytic Nevus and Becker Nevus in an Adult Male Population: An Analysis with a 10-Fold Magnification. Dermatology. 2006;212:354–60.
37. Jaisankar TJ, Baruah MC, Garg BR. Vitiligo in children. Internatioal Journal of Dermatology1992;31:621-3.
38. Kanwar AJ, Dogra S, Parsad D, Kumar B. Narrow-band UVB for the treatment of vitiligo: an emerging effective and well-tolerated therapy. International Journal of Dermatology 2005; 44:57-60.
39. Kanwar AJ, Dogra S. Narrow-band UVB for the treatment of generalized vitiligo in children 2005;30:332-6.
40. Kaviarasan PK, Prasad PVS, Joe JM, Nandana N, Viswanathan P. Universal acquired melanosis (Carbon baby). Indian J Dermatol Venereol Leprol 2008;74:38-40.
41. Khandpur S, Sumanth KM. Systematized Nevus Depigmentosus. Indian Pediatrics 2005:42: 1046-7
42. Kim DY, Lee K, Park Y. Use of the 308-nm excimer laser for nevus depigmentosus: A promising treatment for either nevus depigmentosus or vitiligo. Journal of Dermatology 2007; 34: 217–8.
43. Koga M, Tango T. Clinical features and course of type A and type B vitiligo. British Journal of Dermatology 1988;118:223-8.
44. Koga M. Vitiligo; a new classification and therapy. British Journal of Dermatology 1976;97:255-61.
45. Kohli S, Saxena R, Thomas E, Rao P, Verma IC. Prenatal diagnosis of Phenylketonuria. Indian J Med Res 2005; 122:400-03.

46. Kumarasinghe SPW, Tan SH, Thng S, Thamboo TP, Shen Liang S, Lee YS. Progressive macular hypomelanosis in Singapore: a clinico-pathological study. International Journal of Dermatology 2006, 45, 737 –742.
47. Lepe V, Moncada B, Castanedo-Cazares JP, Torres-Alvarez MB, Ortiz CA, Torres-Rubalcava AB. A double-blind randomized trial of 0.1% tacrolimus vs 0.05% clobetasol for the treatment of childhood vitiligo. Arch Dermatol. 2003;139: 651-4.
48. Lernia VD. Linear and Whorled Hypermelanosis. Pediatric Dermatology 2007;24: 205-210.
49. Lichen Sclerosus et Atrophicus. Jeffrey Meffert. Last Updated: Dec 15, 2006. http://www.emedicine.com/derm/topic234.htm. Last accessed 17th July 2008.
50. Masuria BL, Batra A, Kothiwala RK, Khuller R, Sing. Topical mometasone furoate for the treatment of childhood vltiligo. Indian J Dermatol Venereol Leprol 1999;65:219-21.
51. Mukhopadhyay AK. Nevus of Ota associated with nevus of Ito. Indian J Dermatol Venereol Leprol 2004;70:112-3.
52. Njoo MD, Westerhof W, Bos JD, Bossuyt PMM. The Development of Guidelines for the Treatment of Vitiligo. Arch Dermatol 1999;135:1514-1521.
53. Njoo MD,Das PK,Bos JD,Westerhof W. Association of the Köbner Phenomenon With Disease Activity and Therapeutic Responsiveness in Vitiligo Vulgaris. Arch Dermatol 1999; 135:407-413.
54. Nordlund JJ. The melanocyte and the epidermal melanin unit: An expanded concept. Dermatol Clin 2007; 25:271-281.
55. Ongenae K, Geel NV, Naeyaert JM. Evidence for an Autoimmune Pathogenesis of Vitiligo. Pigment Cell Res 2003;16: 90–100.
56. Palermo B, Campanelli R, Garbelli S, Mantovani S, Lantelme E, Brazzelli V et al. Specific Cytotoxic T Lymphocyte responses against Melan-A/MART1, Tyrosinase and Gp100 in Vitiligo by the use of major histocompatibility complex/Peptide tetramers: the role of cellular immunity in the etiopathogenesis of Vitiligo. Journal of Investigative Dermatology 2001;117: 326–332.
57. Panuncio A, Saralegul P, Matteo C, Dorce S, Viganale R. Nevus depigmentosus: Ultrastructural and immunohistochemical study. Med Cut Iber lat Am 2004; 32:36-38.
58. Pasricha JS, Khatian BK, Dash S. Pigmentary disorders in India. Dermatol Clin 2007;25:342-352.
59. Phenylketonuria. Arnold GL. Last Updated: 18th Dec 2007. http://www.emedicine.com/PED/topic1787.htm. Last accessed16th July 2008.
60. Pityriasis alba. Ali M, Zeina B, Mansoor S. Last updated 3rd Apr 2006. http://www.emedicine.com/derm/topic333.htm. Last accessed 12th July 2008.
61. Postinflammatory hyperpigmentation. Schwartz RA, Kihiczak NI, Last updated 28th march 2008. http://www.emedicine.com/DERM/topic876.htm Last accessed 10th July 2008.
62. Rai R, Srinivas CR. Phototherapy: An Indian perceptive. Indian J Dermatol 2007;52:169-75 .
63. Ramaiah A, Mojamdar M, Amarnath VM. Vitiligo in the Ssk Community of Bangalore (a Preliminary Report). Indian J Dermatol Venereol Leprol 1988; 54:251-254.
64. Rao KS, Shetty JN. Acropigmentation of Dohi. Indian J Dermatol Venereol Leprol 1998;64:128-9.
65. Relyveld GN, Menke HE. Westerhof W. Progressive Macular Hypomelanosis: An Overview. Am J Clin Dermatol 2007; 8: 13-19.
66. Retornaz G, Betuel H, Ortonne JP, Thivolet J. HLA antigens and vitiligo. British Journal of Dermatology 1976;95:173-175.
67. Rigopoulos D, Gregoriou S, Charissi C, Kontochristopoulos CG, Kalogeromitros D, Georgala S. Tacrolimus ointment 0.1% in pityriasis alba: an open-label,randomized, placebo controlled study. British Journal of Dermatology 2006;155:152–155.
68. S Handa, R Rai, I Kaur. Segmental vitiligo in northern India. Ind J Dermatol 2000;45:10-13.
69. Schallreuter KU. Advances in melanocyte basic science research. Dermatol Clin 2007;25:283-291.
70. Sehgal VN, Srivastava G. Vitiligo: Compendium of clinico-epidemiological features. Indian J Dermatol Venereol Leprol 2007;73:149-56.
71. Senthilkumar M, Thappa DM. Melanocytic nevi in children: A clinical study. Ind J Dermatol 2006:51(1):26-29.
72. Sharma R, Chandra M. Reticulate Acropigmentation of Dohi-a Report of Two Unrelated Families. Indian J Dermatol Venereol Leprol 2000;66:139-40.
73. Singh N, Thappa DM, Jaisankar TJ, Habeebulla S. A clinical study of vulval lichen sclerosus at a tertiary care hospital in South India. Indian J Sex Transm dis 2007; 28: 87-90.
74. Srinivas CR, Rai R, Kumar PU. Meshed split skin graft for extensive vitiligo. Indian J Dermatol Venereol Leprol 2004;70:165-7.
75. Srinivas CR. Minimal erythema dose (Med) to narrow band ultraviolet-B (NB-UVB) broad band ultraviolet-B (BB-UVB)-A pilot study. Indian J Dermatol Venereol Leprol 2002;68:63-4.
76. Srivastava N, Chand S, Bansal M, Srivastava K, Singh S. Reversible hyperpigmentation as the first manifestation of Vitamin B12 deficiency Indian J Dermatol Venereol Leprol. 2006;72: 389-390.
77. Stratakis CA, Genetics of Carney complex and related familial lentiginoses, and other multiple tumor syndromes. Frontiers in Bioscience 2000; 5:353-366.
78. Stulberg DL, Clark N, Tovey D. Common hyperpigmentation disorders in adults. American family Physician. 2003; 68:1956-68.
79. Tagra S, Talwar AK, Walia RS. Lines of Blaschko. Indian J Dermatol Venereol Leprol 2005;71:57-9.
80. Taieb A, Boralevi F. Hypermelanoses of the newborn and of the infant. Dermatol Clin 2007;25:327-336.
81. Taieb A, Picardo M. The definition and assessment of vitiligo: a consensus report of the Vitiligo European Task Force. Pigment Cell Research 2007;20: 27-35.
82. The Clinical Profile of Children in India with Pigmentary Anomalies along the Lines of Blaschko and Central Nervous System Manifestations. Pinheiro A, Mathew MC, Thomas M, Jacob M, Srivastava VM,Cherian R, Raju R, George R,Pediatric Dermatology 2007:24;11–17.
83. Thoma W, Krämer HJ, Mayser P. Pityriasis versicolor alba. European Academy of Dermatology and Venereology (JEADV) 2005;19:147–152.
84. Travis LB, Silverberg NB. Calcipotriene and Corticosteroid Combination Therapy for Vitiligo. Pediatric Dermatology 2004;21:495-498.
85. Travis LB, Weinberg JM, Silverberg NB.Successful Treatment of Vitiligo With 0.1% Tacrolimus Ointment. Arch Dermatol 2003;139:571-574.
86. Wayte DM, Helwig EB. Halo nevi. Cancer 1968;22:69-90.
87. Yones SS, Palmer RAGaribaldinos TM, Hawk JLM. Randomized Double-blind Trial of Treatment of Vitiligo: Efficacy of Psoralen–UV-A Therapy vs Narrowband–UV-B Therapy. Arch Dermatol 2007;143(5):578-584.
88. Zettinig G, Tanew A, G. Fischer G, Mayr W, Dudczak R, Weissel M. Autoimmune diseases in vitiligo: Do anti-nuclear antibodies decrease thyroid volume? Clin Exp Immunol 2003; 131:347–354.

19

Photosensitivity and Photodermatoses

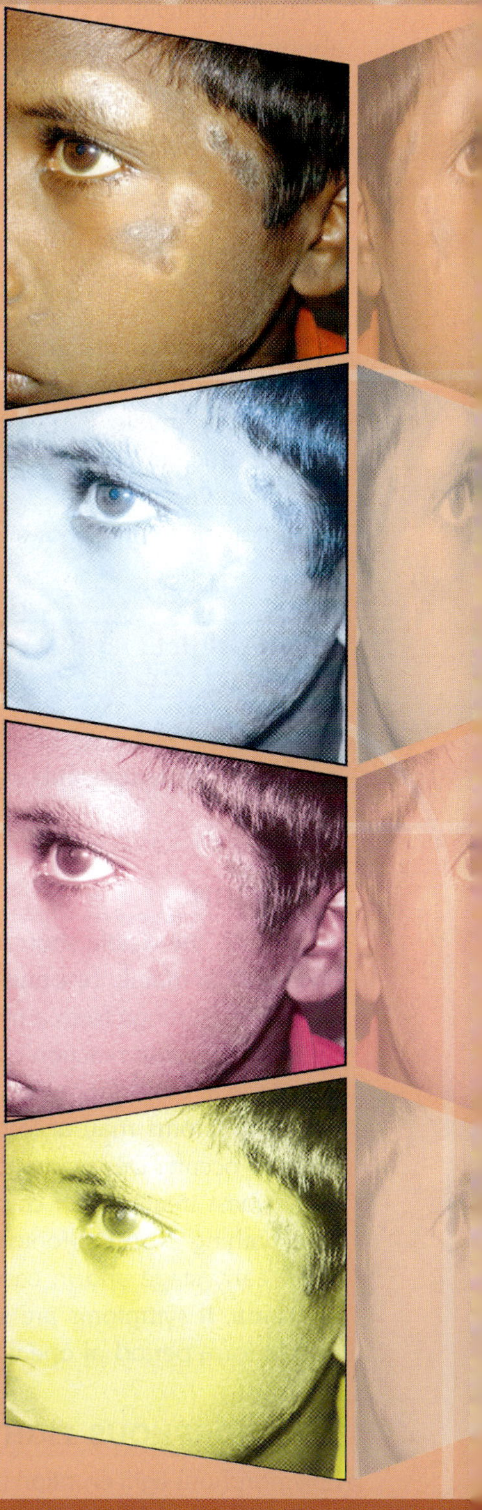

Sacchidanand S

INTRODUCTION

Sunlight emits a wide spectrum of radiation energy. It ranges from radio waves through infrared, visible and ultraviolet (UV) light to X- rays. UVA and UVB are the major rays causing skin reactions.

Photosensitivity is a broad term which describes the abnormal/adverse reactions to sunlight. Disorders of photosensitivity in childhood can be categorized as follows:

GENETIC

- Genodermatoses associated with photosensitivity.

ACQUIRED

- Sunburn
- Polymorphous light eruption
- Juvenile spring eruption
- Hydroa aestivale
- Solar urticaria
- Hydroa vacciniforme
- Phototoxicity and photoallergy

ACQUIRED PHOTOSENSITIVITY DISORDERS

Some of the acquired photosensitivity disorders have genetic predisposition and family history is positive in such cases.

SUNBURN

Sunburn is the visible short-term effect of UV exposure. UVB light is mainly responsible for acute sunburn. The severity may range from a mild asymptomatic erythema to a more intense reaction associated with pain, tenderness edema, vesiculation and bullae formation. Constitutional symptoms may accompany if extensive sunburn reaction occurs. Desquamation occurs within a week.

It is best treated with cold sponging or colloidal oat meal bathing. NSAIDs (topical or systemic) can give relief at an early stage and in cases with mild UVB induced erythema. If symptoms are severe, short course of oral steroid for a period of one week is helpful.

POLYMORPHOUS LIGHT ERUPTION

Polymorphous light eruption (PMLE) is the most common sunlight induced idiopathic disorder. It is an immune mediated, delayed type of hypersensitivity reaction to UV rays (290-400 nm). It is commoner in females in the second and third decade of life. However, it is frequently encountered in the pediatric age group, especially in tropical countries.

There are two forms of PMLE; hereditary and idiopathic acquired PMLE.

Hereditary PMLE

It is an autosomal dominant disorder seen more commonly among native Americans. Onset is in childhood with female preponderance. The majority of these patients are UVA sensitive. Face is the commonly involved site. Chelitis may be an associated symptom with early onset disease.

Idiopathic PMLE

Initial symptoms are burning, itching and erythema after intense sunlight exposure. Clinically lesions consists of a group of polymorphic or pleomorphic lesions, comprised of papules, vesicles, hypopigmented patch or eczematous lesions **(Figure 19.1)**. Interestingly, individual patients tend to develop same type of lesions every year. Nape or 'V' area of the neck, dorsa of the hands and extensor aspects of forearms are common sites of involvement. Grouped papular form is the most common morphology of PMLE. Other less common types of lesions include; plaque, papulo-vesicle, erythema-multiforme like, and rarely hemorrhagic type. Diagnosis is by clinical findings.

Treatment consists of protection from sun exposure, topical steroids, oral steroids. Oral beta carotene and

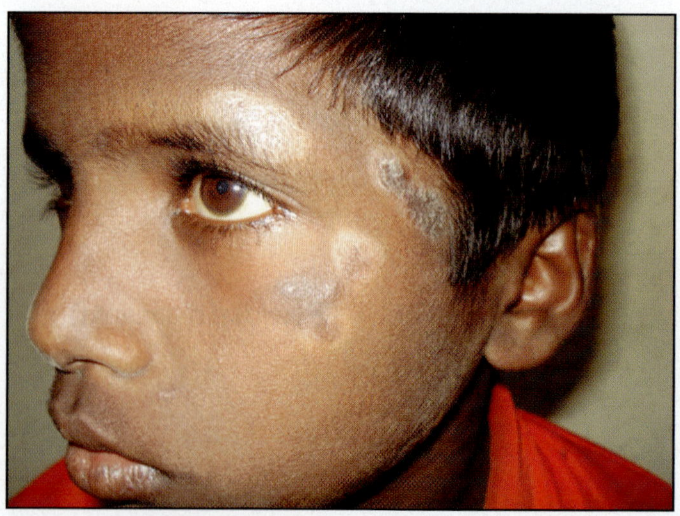

FIGURE 19.1: Polymorphous light eruption

prophylactic phototherapy (PUVA). Full-sleeve clothing, use of sunscreens with maximum SPF and sun avoidance between 11 am and 3 pm are essential for protection. Topical steroids reduce itching and may hasten resolution of the lesions. Short course of systemic steroids may be used for wide spread and very itchy lesions. Controlled exposure to sunlight or artificial UV light induces hardening effect on skin leading to an appreciable tolerance. PUVA is not to be used in children younger than 9 years old. Beta carotene is effective as prophylactic in small percentage of patients. Antimalarials are to be used in older children and adolescents, when sunscreens and UV therapy are not effective.

JUVENILE SPRING ERUPTION

It is a photo-induced spring-time dermatosis seen in children. It is thought to be a subset of PMLE. Usually lesions are seen over the helices of the ears after sun exposure. The eruptions consist of papules and vesicles which heal with crusting. Scarring is not seen. Boys are more commonly affected than girls probably because of lack of the cover of hair and protuberant ears. Topical steroids are helpful to relieve the itching. Interestingly, use of sunscreen does not prevent the recurrence of the disease.

HYDROA AESTIVALE (SUMMER PRURIGO OF HUTCHINSON)

It represents a type of PMLE, seen mainly in children. Intensely itchy papules progress to weeping lesions followed by crusting. Sun unexposed sites like buttocks may also be involved. Lesions do not clear during winter. Evidence of HLA association is also present (HLA DR4). The disorder has a chronic course with persistence till adulthood. Spontaneous remission may be seen in few patients. Sun protection and topical steroids are to be used for relief of symptoms. Thalidomide may be useful to bring complete resolution. Desensitization by UV light is also useful (hardening effect).

SOLAR URTICARIA

It is an uncommon photosensitivity disorder, due to IgE mediated, type I reaction. It is rarely reported in children. It is characterized by erythema, itching and urticarial wheals appearing within 30 minutes of sun-exposure. Location of the lesions may be on both sun-exposed and unexposed area. Antihistamines, antimalarials and corticosteroids are useful in managing these cases. Desensitization can be done with gradual exposure to incremental dosage of natural or artificial light.

HYDROA VACCINIFORME

The disorder starts manifesting by 10 years of age. Clinically, almost similar lesions are found as in hydroa aestivale, except the tense, umbilicated vesicles resembling small pox appearing on sun exposed parts of the face. These heal with scarring. It tends to appear in summer. It follows autosomal recessive inheritance pattern. This is one of the photodermatoses in children which has specific histopathological findings and can be diagnosed from this finding. There is intra-epidermal blister formation, which is filled with acute inflammatory cells and fibrin. It is followed by reticular degeneration and epidermal necrosis. Perivascular neutrophil and mononuclear cell infiltrate is present in the dermis. The disorder usually clears by puberty, like hydroa aestivale. Broad band UVB therapy may be effective therapy. Topical steroids and antimalarials help in controlling symptoms.

PHOTOTOXICITY AND PHOTOALLERGY

Phototoxicity is seen when a photo-sensitizer is absorbed into the skin either topically or systemically in appropriate concentrations and is exposed to sufficient amount of specific wavelength of light (UVA). The reactions are nonallergic skin responses. Certain group of drugs with photosensitive potential are important agents causing this type of reaction.

Phytophotodermatitis is plant-induced photosensitivity. It is the most common phototoxic reaction seen in children. In majority of the cases, the reaction is due to furocoumarin compounds found in plants like, carrot, lemon, lime, wheat, and celery. It may start as mild erythema to severe blistering. Usually healing occurs with hyperpigmentation.

Photoallergy is rarely seen in children. UV light induces a reaction between skin proteins and a chemical or drug to form antigens. A delayed type of hypersensitivity reaction follows with eczematous inflammation. Sunscreens with chemical components, soaps and fragrances in cosmetic products may be the cause of photoallergic reactions in children. Photopatch test confirms the diagnosis. Treatment with anti-inflammatory agents sand avoidance of the offending agent will reduce the reaction.

GENODERMATOSES ASSOCIATED WITH PHOTOSENSITIVITY

Photosensitive genodermatoses are commoner in children. Following is the list of such diseases:

- Xeroderma pigmentosum
- Cockayne syndrome
- Rothmund-Thomson syndrome
- Bloom syndrome
- Hartnup disease
- Smith-Lemli-Opitz syndrome
- Ataxia-telangiectasia
- Kindler syndrome
- Porphyria

All the above diseases are discussed in respective chapters. Correct clinical recognition with supporting investigations will help in the management of such conditions and genetic counselling.

BIBLIOGRAPHY

1. Ferguson J. Polymorphic light eruption and actinic prurigo. Curr Probl Dermatol 1990;2:127-47.
2. Garzon MC, DeLeo VA. Photosensitivity in the pediatric patient. Curr Op Pediatr 1997; 9: 377-87.
3. Gupta G, Man I, Kemmett D. Hydroa vacciniforme: A clinical and follow-up study of 17 cases. J Am Acad Dermatol 2000;42: 208-13.
4. Harris A, Burge SM, George SA. Solar urticaria in an infant. Br J Dermatol 1997;136: 105-7.
5. Horkay I, Emri G, Varga V, Simics E, Remenyik E. Photosensitivity skin disorders in childhood. Photodermatol Photoimmunol Photomed 2008; 24:56-60.
6. Inamadar AC, Palit A. Photosensitivity in children: An approach to diagnosis and management. Ind J Dermatol Venereol Leprol 2005;71:73-9.
7. Jury C, McHenry P, Burden AD, Lever R, Bilsland D. Narrowband ultraviolet B (UVB) phototherapy in children. Clin Exp Dermatol 2006; 31:196-99.
8. Puech-Plottowa I, Michel J. Photodermatosis and photoprotection in children. Arch. Pediatr 2000; 7: 668-79.
9. Stratigos A, Antoniou C, Katsambas AD. Polymorphous light eruption. JEADV 2002; 16: 193-206.
10. Wainwright NJ. Polymorphic light eruption. In: Photodermatology. Ferguson J, Dover JS (Eds) London: Manson Publ Ltd; 2006;29-34.

20

Urticaria, Angioedema and Annular Erythemas

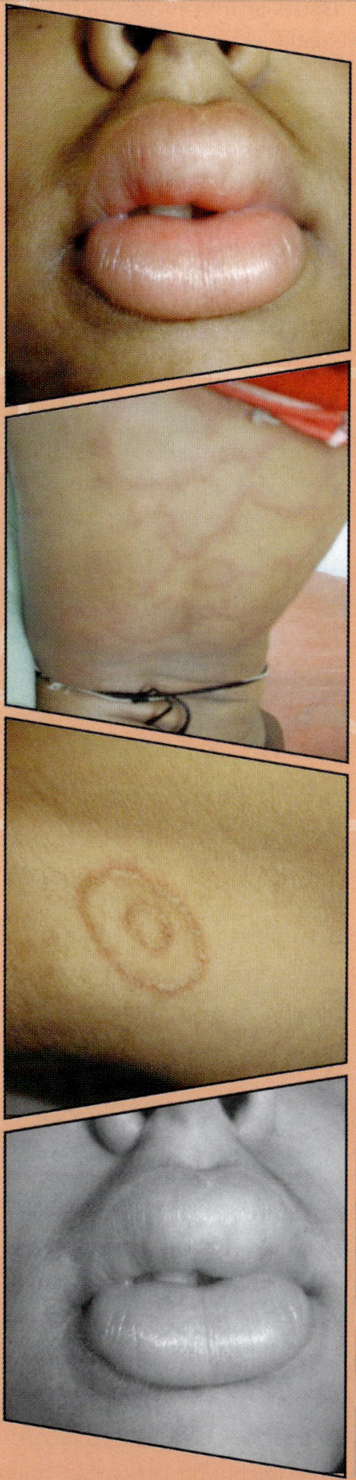

Arun C Inamadar
Ragunatha S

URTICARIA

Urticaria is a Type 1 (immediate) hypersensitivity reaction characterized by evanescent well circumscribed, pruritic, edematous, erythematous plaques (wheals) involving skin or mucous membrane. In angioedema, subcutaneous tissue is involved resulting in diffuse localized painful swellings.

EPIDEMIOLOGY

Urticaria is a common disease occurring at sometime in the life of about 15% of all individuals. In children acute urticaria is common compared to chronic urticaria.

ETIOPATHOGENESIS (FLOW CHART 20.1)

Urticaria represents a Type 1 hypersensitivity reaction where antigens bind to immunoglobulin E (IgE) on the surface of mast cells resulting in activation, degranulation and release of vasoactive mediators such as histamine, prostaglandins and leukotrienes. These substances mediate wheal and flare that are seen in urticaria through vasodilatation and increased permeability of capillaries. The mast cell degranulation can be triggered by both immunological and non-immunological factors.

All the four classic types of Coombs and Gell hypersensitivity reactions can result in urticaria or angioedema. The immediate hypersensitivity is IgE dependent which is commonly triggered by antigens found in foods, drugs (e.g. Penicillin) or latex. The classic example is anaphylactic reaction. Chronic autoimmune urticaria represents Type II hypersensitivity reaction. Immunecomplex mediated urticaria is elicited by activation of complement pathway. Finally, Type IV cell mediated immune response induced urticaria is represented by delayed pressure urticaria.

CLINICAL FEATURES

Clinically, urticaria/ angioedema can be classified as ordinary urticaria, physical urticaria, contact urticaria, and hereditary angioedema. More than one type of urticaria can coexist. Urticaria/ angioedema can also occur as a manifestation of several systemic disorders.

Ordinary Urticaria

Urticaria is considered as ordinary when physical, contact and vasculitic urticarias have been excluded. The child with ordinary urticaria presents with sudden appearance

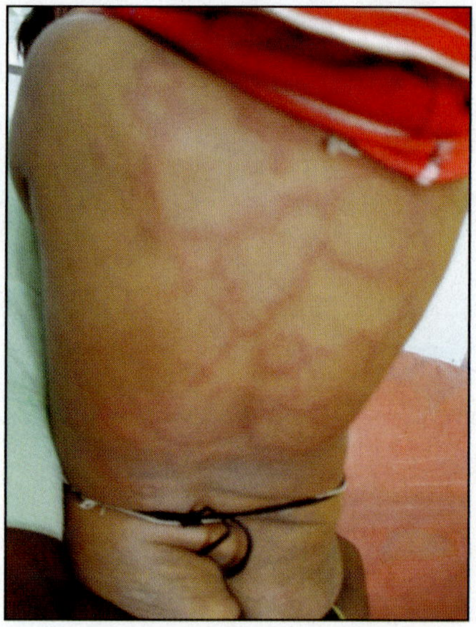

FIGURE 20.1: Acute urticaria

of pruritic erythematous, edematous plaques scattered all over the body. The lesions are evanescent, disappearing within a few hours. If the lesions persist for more than 24 hours, one should suspect other causes of urticarial plaques such as urticarial vasculitis. In most cases plaques may enlarge centrifugally resulting in large polycyclic or annular configuration **(Figure 20.1)**. In 10% of cases of ordinary urticaria, there may be accompanying angioedema. If the urticaria subsides within six weeks it is considered as acute, and if it persists for more than four weeks it is considered as chronic. In chronic urticaria, the causal factors such as infections, foods, food additives, and drugs can be identified only in some of the cases. In others, autoantibodies (IgG_1 and IgG_4) against IgE and FcεR1-α receptor of IgE have been implicated.

When the disease process involves deeper dermal and subcutaneous vessels, angioedema develops. It presents as light red to skin colored, relatively ill-defined deep nodules. There may be burning or stinging or pain instead of pruritus associated with urticaria. The common sites of predilection are lips, eyelids, cheeks, genitalia, tongue, hands, feet and mucous membranes **(Figure 20.2)**. Angioedema can be life-threatening when it occurs as a manifestation of anaphylaxis, serum sickness and hereditary angioedema.

Physical Urticaria

Certain physical factors elicit urticarial lesions when they come in contact with skin. These urticarias are induced by either mechanical or thermal stimuli. The former

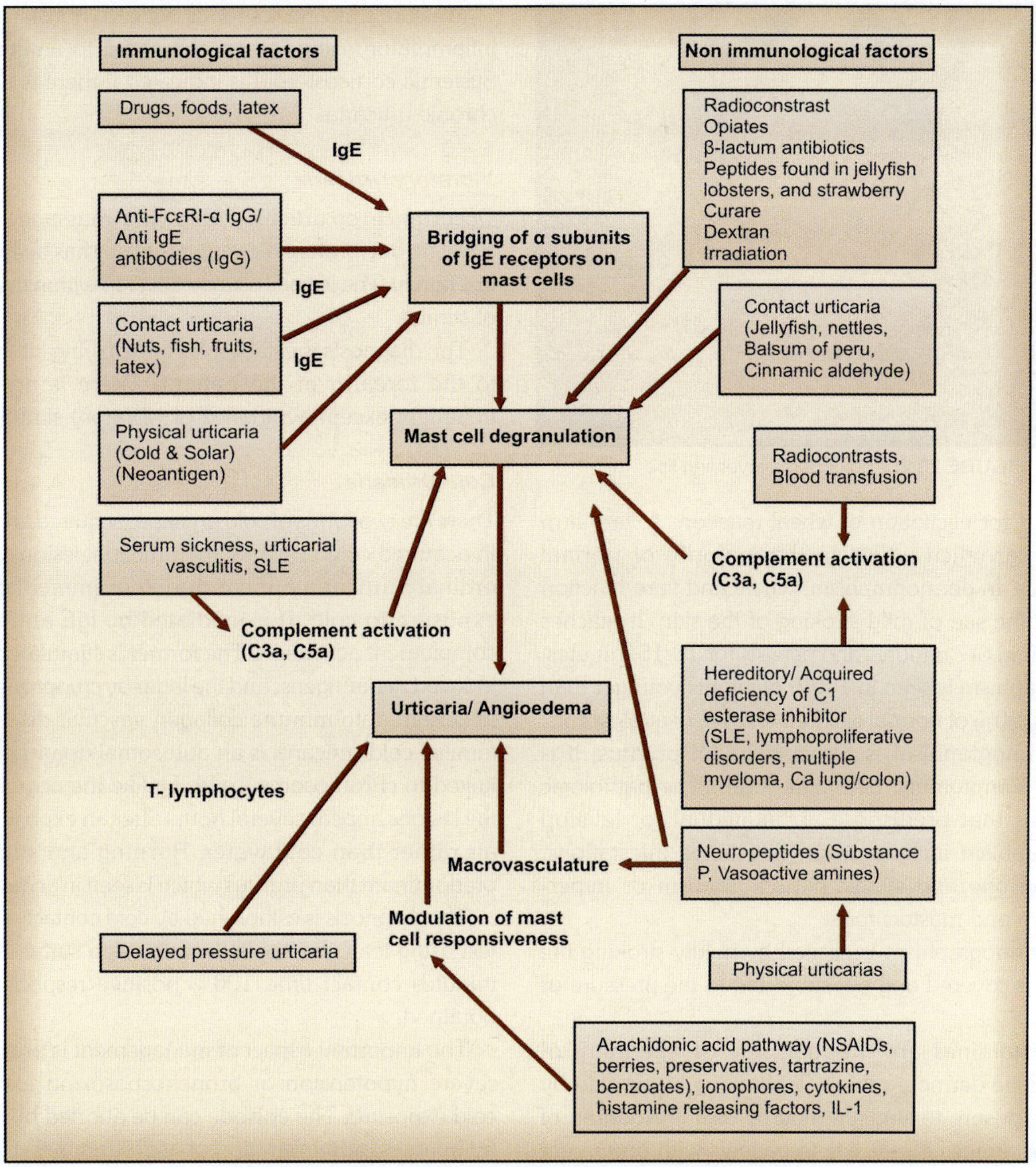

Flow Chart 20.1: Etiopathogenesis of urticaria/angioedema

Note: C—complement; Ig—immunoglobulin; IL—interleukin; NSAIDs—nonsteroidal anti-inflammatory drugs; SLE—systemic lupus erythematosus

includes dermographism, pressure urticaria and vibratory urticaria, and the latter includes cold urticaria, cholinergic urticaria and solar urticaria. The physical factors modify the antigenicity of skin or release chemicals resulting in immunological or nonimmunological degranulation of mast cells respectively. The physical urticarias present with distinct clinical features. These are episodic, localized, and occur following contact with physical stimuli. Young adults and children are commonly affected by physical urticarias. In severe cases there may be hypotention, bronchospasm, respiratory distress and gastrointestinal disturbances. Among physical urticarias, dermographism is the most common followed by cholinergic urticaria. Other types are relatively rare.

Dermographism

An exaggerated triple response of Lewis is referred as dermographism. In triple response of Lewis a firm stroking

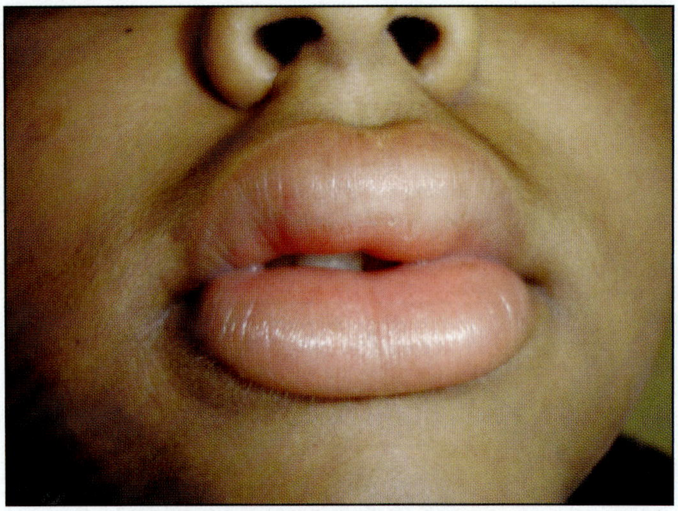

FIGURE 20.2: Angioedema involving lips

is required for elicitation of wheal reaction. A very firm stroking can elicit wheal in the majority of normal individuals. In dermographism, wheal and flare reaction occurs at the site of mild stroking of the skin. It reaches maximum in 6-7 minutes and persists for 10-15 minutes. Dermographism is seen in 100% of infants younger than 6 months, 50% of normal children and 1% of adolescents. If the dermographism is associated with pruritus, it is called as symptomatic dermographism. The pathologic conditions that predispose an individual to develop dermographism include drugs, infections, infestations, arthropod bite and stings, hypothyroidism or hyper-thyroidism and mastocytosis.

The dermographism is elicited by mildly stroking the skin that is covered and not subjected to the pressure or friction.

Antihistamines are the mainstay of treatment of symptomatic dermographism. Hardening of the skin by regular exposure to sunlight may be useful. Addition of H_2 antihistamines is effective in patients with prominent wheal and flare reaction.

Pressure Urticaria

Pressure urticaria is a variant of dermographism usually occurs in association with chronic urticaria. Unlike ordinary urticaria, the lesions are deep, non pruritic and painful. The lesions appear 4-6 hours after the application of pressure. Hence, it is also called as delayed pressure urticaria. The presence of abundant T- helper lymphocytes in the lesion suggests role of Type IV cell mediated immune reaction.

The diagnosis is established by pressure challenge on the shoulder using 15 pounds weight for 15 minutes.

Pressure urticaria responds better to nonsteroidal anti-inflammatory drugs when compared to antihistamines. Systemic corticosteroid is indicated if there is associated chronic urticaria.

Vibratory Urticaria

Occurrence of urticaria following massage, vigorous toweling or vibratory movements of lips has been reported in a family. The lesions usually develop within five minutes of stimuli.

The diagnosis is established by applying kitchen mixer to the forearm of the patient. There is no effective treatment except avoidance of vibratory stimuli.

Cold Urticaria

There are two forms of cold urticaria, acquired and familial. In acquired cold urticaria, the urticarial lesions similar to ordinary urticaria appear during or immediately after exposure to cold. It is mediated by IgE antibodies or complement activation. The former is stimulated by cold-induced neoantigens, and the latter by cryoprotiens found in certain autoimmune collagen vascular diseases. The familial cold urticaria is an autosomal dominant disease linked to chromosome 1q44. Unlike the acquired form, the lesions appear several hours after an exposure to cold air rather than cold water. Burning and stinging are predominant than pruritus which is seen in acquired form.

The diagnosis is established by cold contact stimulation test using ice cube applied on the skin surface. With 20 minutes contact time 100% positive response can be obtained.

The important aspect of management is prevention of severe hypotension or bronchospasm on exposure to cold exposure. The episode can be aborted by prior (30-60 minutes) administration of antihistamines. Cyprohep-tadine is the most effective therapy because of its H_1 and H_2 antihistamine, antiserotonin, and anticholinergic activity. Doxepin can also be used to suppress the cold urticaria.

Cholinergic Urticaria

Cholinergic urticaria is a distinct type of physical urticaria that occurs following heat exposure, exertion or emotional stress. All these stimuli induce sweating followed by appearance of numerous, small, 2-3 mm erythematous lesions with central tiny 1 mm papules. Lesions may be extensive usually sparing palms, soles and axillae. Heating of the skin surface, acetylcholine or sweat is implicated in the pathogenesis of cholinergic urticaria. There is a refractory period of 24 hours during which another episode cannot be induced.

The diagnosis is established by inducing sweating through exercise or hot bath.

Application of cold water to the skin surface before induction of sweating can abort the episode. Another method of prevention of attack is careful induction of refractory period by hot bath. Hydroxyzine is effective in the treatment of cholinergic urticaria when compared to other physical urticarias.

Solar Urticaria

In solar urticaria, the lesions similar to ordinary urticaria appear within five minutes of sunlight exposure. The lesions occur readily on untanned skin. These patients are sensitive to ultraviolet (UV) B, UVA, visible light or entire spectrum of UV radiation. Childhood lupus erythematosus, erythropoietic protoporphyria, and polymorphous light eruption which may occur in association with solar urticaria should be ruled out.

The diagnosis is confirmed by phototesting. By using solar simulator or monochromatic light source the patient is exposed to different spectrum of light. In positive cases, the urticaria is induced within 5-10 minutes.

There is no effective treatment of solar urticaria. Sunscreens are generally ineffective. Systemic agents like chloroquine, β- carotene and antihistamines have been used with some response. Induction of "hardening" by PUVA may be tried.

Contact Urticaria

Certain contactants induce urticarial lesions at the site of contact through immunological or pharmacological mechanisms. In some cases anphylaxis-like systemic reaction may occur.

Aquagenic urticaria is a variant of contact urticaria. It occurs within 30 minutes after exposure to water at any temperature. It is characterized by numerous, small, cholinergic-like erythematous pruritic papules oriented around the follicular openings. Palms and soles are spared. Ingestion of water does not induce the lesions.

The diagnosis is established by application of water (35-36°) compresses to the back of the patient for 30 minutes.

Contact and aquagenic urticaria respond to administration of antihistamines as in ordinary urticaria.

Hereditary Angioedema

Hereditary angioedema is an autosomal dominant disease characterized by repeated attacks of angioedema involving face, extremities and throat associated with abdominal pain. Family history of disease is present in only 25% of patients. Unlike angioedema seen in association with ordinary urticaria, hereditary angioedema is caused by activation of complement due to deficiency of C1 esterase inhibitor. Classical lesions of urticaria do not occur but lesions resembling erythema multiforme may be seen. Acute airway obstruction is a life-threatening complication which occurs in 30% of cases. The episode is usually follows trauma such as surgery, dental manipulations or accidents.

The diagnosis is confirmed by functional assay of C1 esterase inhibitor. The level of C4 is persistently low which may give a clue to the diagnosis.

The hereditary angioedema do not respond to antihistamines, adrenaline or systemic corticosteroids. Acute attacks are managed by fluid replacement, airway maintenance and intravenous infusion of plasma inhibitor concentrate. Prophylactic therapy prior to the surgery can be administered. Danazole 10 mg/kg/day given five days before and for two days after surgery, ε-aminocaproic acid or tranexamic acid are commonly used for prophylaxis prior to minor surgeries. For major surgeries, administration of C1 inhibitor replacement one hour before and during the surgery is recommended. If it is not available, solvent/ detergent- treated fresh frozen plasma along with danazole can be used as an alternative.

DIFFERENTIAL DIAGNOSIS

Important differential diagnoses include urticarial vasculitis, annular erythemas, erythema multiforme, papular urticaria and erythema nodosum leprosum. Rarely urticaria needs to be differentiated from initial urticarial plaques of dermatitis herpetiformis, and bullous pemphigoid.

LABORATORY INVESTIGATION

Urticaria is usually a clinical diagnosis. If in doubt, skin biopsy can be done to differentiate from conditions present as urticarial plaques (see above). Urticaria lasting more than 24 hours, absence of pruritus and lack of expected response inspite of adequate antihistamine therapy are indications for skin biopsy. In children, infection is the predominant cause of urticaria followed by drugs and food-related products. Thorough history and clinical examination helps to identify causes in majority of cases. The laboratory investigation to detect underlying causes should be guided by clinical history and examination.

TREATMENT

The first step in the management of urticaria is identifying and removal of triggering factors. The mainstay of treatment of urticaria is administration of antihistamines. The choice of antihistamine should be based on efficacy, frequency of administration and side-effect profile. First generation sedative antihistamines such as chlorpheniramine, diphenhydramine, deschlorpheneramine, hydroxyzine, cyproheptadine or promethazine, if well tolerated, are preferred over second generation nonsedative antihistamines such as cetirizine, loratidine or levocetirizine. Combining sedative antihistamine at bedtime and nonsedating antihistamine in the morning may be useful. H_2 antihistamines like ranitidine may be added if there is little response after the administration of maximum tolerated dose of H_1 antihistamines. The newborns are at increased risk of developing convulsions as a result of antimuscarinic effect. Older children may show hyperexcitability and irritability. However, the anticholinergic effects are seen only when high dose of H_1 antihistamines are used.

If there is no response to antihistamine therapy, epinephrine and systemic corticosteroids can be considered. Leukotriene antagonists, zafirlukast or montelukast, may be useful when nonsteroidal anti-inflammatory drugs (NSAIDs) are suspected as exacerbating factors.

Anaphylaxis is a medical emergency. Immediate subcutaneous adrenaline (1:1000 dilution) 0.01 ml/kg is life-saving. This can be repeated every 15 minutes if there is no significant response. Airway and intravenous access should be secured to manage laryngeal edema and hypovolemic shock. Supplemental oxygen, corticosteroids and antihistamines can be considered whenever necessary.

ANNULAR ERYTHEMAS

Annular erythemas are vascular reactive patterns categorized into a group of disorders because of their distinctive clinical manifestations. These disorders include two distinct disorders with definite etiology, erythema marginatum and erythema chronicum migrans. Others are grouped under erythema annulare centrifugum and annular erythema of infancy.

CLASSIFICATION

Erythema Annulare Centrifugum (EAC)

EAC is common in young and middle-aged adults but can occur in children. Familial annular erythema which is considered as a subtype of EAC occurs soon after birth.

EAC is idiopathic in most of the cases. However, it has been associated with, infections, drugs, endocrine and hematological diseases, malignancy, hepatic disorders, relapsing polychondritis, sarcoidosis and post-biliary surgery. EAC occurring at the site of pacemaker has also been reported.

Initial lesions of EAC are usually small, pink or red papules which slowly increase in size with central fading resulting in a large annular erythema measuring >10 cm. Two clinical variants of EAC have been described. These are deep variant of Darier and superficial variant of Colcott Fox, also known as erythema gyratum perstans. The latter type shows peripheral collarette of scaling or microvesiculation. There may be associated pruritus. The commonly involved sites are buttocks, thighs, legs, and trunk. The course of the disease is variable. The lesions appear in crops and the individual lesions last for weeks to months and in some cases, for years. The new lesion may occur inside the fading lesion resulting in concentric **(Figure 20.3)**, oval, annular, polycyclic, arciform and semicircular configuration.

Familial annular erythema (FAE) with familial occurrence and eosinophilic annular erythema with predominant eosinophilic infiltration have been described as subtypes of EAC.

Histologically, EAC is characterized by perivascular lymphohistiocytic infiltration. In addition, the superficial variant shows epidermal hyperplasia, spongiosis, parakeratosis and edema of the papillary dermis and the deep variant is characterized by sleeve-like infiltrate, melanophages, mild vacuolization, and necrotic keratinocytes at the dermoepidermal junction.

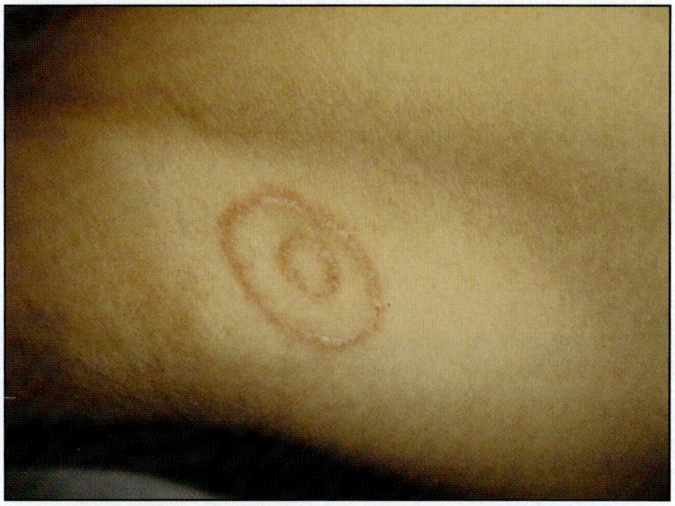

FIGURE 20.3: Erythema annulare centrifugum

Treatment with topical corticosteroids is ineffective. Systemic corticosteroids are usually effective but recurrences are common following therapy. Antihistamines can be used in symptomatic patients.

Erythema Marginatum

Erythema marginatum is usually seen in children in association with acute rheumatic fever. It is one of the major criteria for the diagnosis of rheumatic fever occurring in 10% of children with rheumatic fever. Erythema marginatum can occur following streptococcal infections without rheumatic fever.

The disease presents as asymptomatic, erythematous enlarging annular patches. The border appears as thin red line which evolves into large annular or polycyclic pattern. Each lesion migrates and resolves in an hour or so. The lesions are commonly localized to the trunk and proximal extremities. The cutaneous manifestation resolves within a few days but may recur for many weeks.

Histologically, dermis shows perivascular lymphocytic and neutrophilic infiltrate in the papillary dermis and upper part of reticular dermis. Leukocytoclasia may also be noticed in some cases.

Erythema Chronicum Migrans (ECM)

ECM usually occurs in young and middle-aged adults. It is a cutaneous manifestation of infection caused by *Borrelia burgdorferi sensu lato, B. afzelli* and *B. garinii*. It occurs in association with Lyme disease transmitted by ticks, *Ixodes dommini*. The disease is common in Europe and United States.

Initial lesion is a small erythematous papule with central punctum occurring at the site of tick bite. The initial lesion may be an urticarial or a hemorrhagic papule. Later an erythematous annular ring forms around the papule which enlarges in size up to 30 cm. There may be appearance of small secondary lesions. The child develops fever, malaise, lethargy, arthralgia and arthritis. If untreated neurological or cardiac problems may develop.

Histologically, superficial and deep perivascular infiltration of lymphocytes, histiocytes and a few eosinophils is seen.

The diagnosis is made by clinical features and serology. The organism can be isolated from cutaneous lesions. Once diagnosed prompt treatment with oral penicillin, doxycycline, azithromycin or cefuroxime for 10 days helps in healing of skin lesion, and prevention of systemic complications

Annular Erythema of Infancy (AEI)

As the name itself suggests the disease occurs in infancy including neonatal period. There are no known associations described in the etiology of AEI. However, in some cases, association with Epstein-Barr virus infection and heavy intestinal colonization of *Candida albicans* has been reported.

The clinical features of AEI resemble that of EAC without scaling or vesiculation. The disease is self-limiting over a few months but may be chronic in some cases. Complete resolution of lesions during and recurrence after febrile episodes has been reported in neutrophilic figurate erythema of infancy.

Histologically AEI is characterized by superficial perivascular lymphohistiocytic infiltrate with eosinophils. The epidermis may show spongiosis, mild acanthosis or parakeratosis. AEI with predominantly eosinophilic or neutrophilic infiltration with leukocytoclasia has been described. The latter variant is referred as neutrophilic figurate erythema of infancy.

DIFFERENTIAL DIAGNOSIS OF ANNULAR ERYTHEMAS

The annular erythemas need to be distinguished from each other and from other diseases which present with annular lesions such as neonatal lupus, subcutaneous lupus erythematosus, tinea corporis, pityriasis rosea, urticaria, sarcoidosis, and granuloma annulare. The subtle clinical, pathological and laboratory differences helps in the definite diagnosis.

BIBLIOGRAPHY

1. Annesi G, Signoretti S, Angelo C. Neutrophilic figurate erythema of infancy. Am J Dermatopathol 1997; 19: 403-06.
2. Aoki T, Kojima M, Horiko T. Acute urticaria: history and natural course of 50 cases. J Dermatol 1994; 21(2): 73-75.
3. Baxi S, Dinakar C. Urticaria and angioedema. Immunol Allergy Clin North Am 2005; 25(2): 353-67.
4. Beltrani VS. Urticaria and angioedema. Dermatol Clin 1996; 14(1): 171- 98.
5. Dibbern DA, Dreskin SC. Urticaria and angioedema: an overview. Immunol Allergy Clin North Am 2004; 24(2): 141-62.
6. Dibbern DA. Urticaria: selected highlights and recent advances. Med Clin North Am 2006; 90(1): 187-209.
7. Ghosh S, Kanwar AJ, Kaur S. Urticaria in children. Pediatr Dermatol 1993; 10(2): 107-10.
8. Graham RM, Cox NL. Annular and Figurate reactive erythemas. In: Burns T, Breathnach S, Cox N, Griffith C, edts. Rook's Textbook of Dermatology. 7th edn. Oxford: Blackwell Science, 2004; 59.70- 59.756.
9. Grattan CE. The urticaria spectrum: recognition of clinical patterns can help management. Clin Exp Dermatol 2004; 29(3): 217-21.
10. Hannuksela M. Urticaria in childen. Semin Dermatol 1987; 6: 321- 5.
11. Helm TN, Bass J, Chang LW. Persistent annular erythema of infancy. Pediatr Dermatol 1993; 10: 46- 8.
12. Legrain V, Taieb A, Sage T, Maleville J. Urticaria in infants: a study of forty patients. Pediatr Dermatol 1990; 7: 101- 7.
13. Nopper A, Markus R, Esterly N. When it's not ringworm: Annular lesions of childhood. Pediatr Ann 1998; 27(3): 136-48.
14. Paller AS, Mancini AJ. The hypersensitivity syndromes. In: Hurwitz Clinical pediatric dermatology. 3rd edn. Philadelphia: Elsevier Saunders, 2006; 525-56.
15. Patrizi A, Savoia F, Varotti A, Gaspari V, Passarini B, Neri I. Neutrophilic figurate erythema of infancy. Pediatr Dermatol 2008; 25(2): 255- 82.
16. Sampson HA. Anaphylaxis and emergency treatment. Pediatrics 2003; 111 (6 pt 3): 1601- 08.
17. Steere AC. Lyme disease. N Engl J Med 2001; 345: 115- 25.
18. Troyer C, Grossman ME, Silvers DN. Erythema marginatum in rheumatic fever: early diagnosi by skin biopsy. J Am Acad Dermatol 1983; 8: 724- 8.
19. Volonakis M, Katsarou-Katsari A, Stratigos J. Etiologic factors in childhood chronic urticaria. Ann Allergy 1992; 69(1): 61- 5.
20. Weston WL, Orchard D. Vascular reactions. In: Schachner LA, Hansen RC, edts, Pediatric Dermatology. 3rd edn. Edinburgh: Mosby, 2003; 801- 33.
21. Weyers W, Diaz-Cascojo C, Weyers I. Erythema annulare centrifugum: result of a clinicopathologic study of 73 patients. Am J Dermatopathol 2003; 25: 451- 62.

21

Vascular Malformations, Tumors and Associated Syndromes

Yasmeena Khan
M Naeem Khan

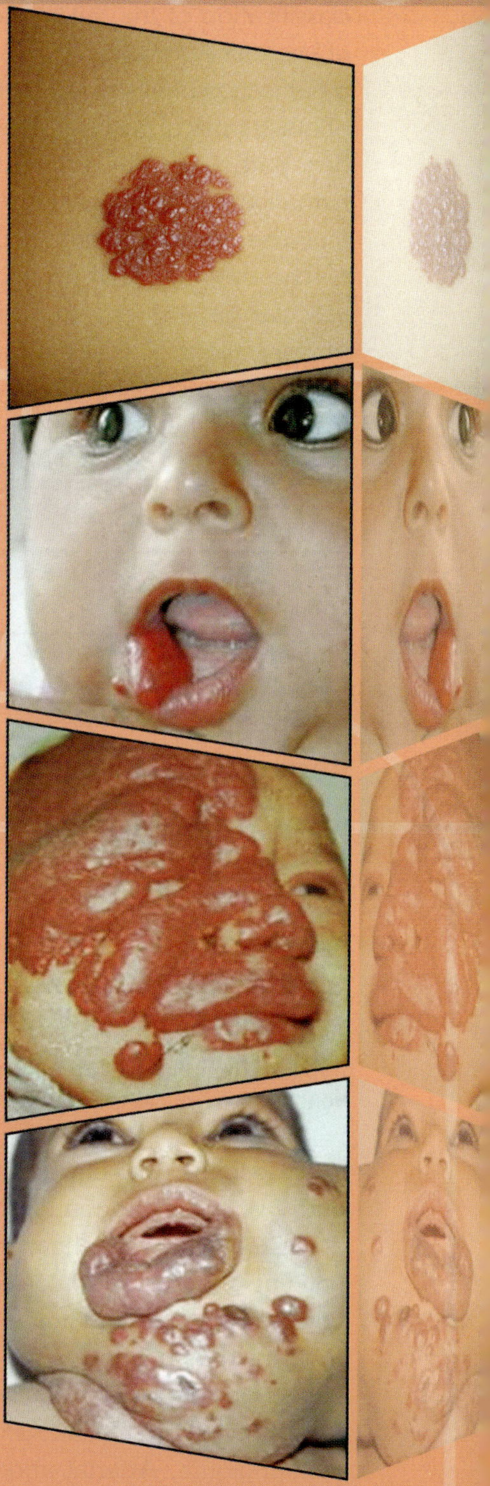

CLASSIFICATION OF VASCULAR ANOMALIES AND TUMORS

Mulliken's biologic classification of vascular anomalies has been widely adopted by the clinicians to differentiate these lesions from vascular birthmarks. This is the accepted classification of the 'International Society for the Study of Vascular Anomalies (ISSVA)'. In 1996, there was slight modification of this classification to reflect the importance of other types of vascular tumors which are clinically and histopathologically different from common infantile hemangioma; these include kaposiform hemangioendothelioma, tufted angioma and others.

The updated ISSVA/biologic classification divides vascular birthmarks into vascular tumors and vascular malformations. This classification **(Table 21.1)** is useful for management of patients and provides a framework for study of these lesions.

TABLE 21.1: Vascular anomalies (ISSVA/Mulliken classification, 1996, modified)

	Vascular malformations	
Vascular tumors	***Simple***	***Combined***
Infantile hemangioma	Capillary	AVF, AVM
Congenital hemangioma	Lymphatic	CVM, CLVM
Miliary hemangiomatosis of infancy		
Tufted angioma	Venous	LVM, CAVM
Kaposiform hemangioendothelioma	Arterial	CLAVM
Hemangiopericytoma		
Glomangioma		
Pyogenic granuloma		
Spindle-cell hemangioendothelioma		

AVF, Arteriovenous fistula; AVM, arteriovenous malformation; CAVM, capillary AVM; CLAVM, capillary-lymphatic AVM; CLVM, capillary-lymphatic venous malformation; CVM, capillary venous malformation; LVM, Lymphatic venous malformation

Despite the clear distinction between vascular tumors and vascular malformations, there are also occasional associations between them. For example, hemangiomas have been observed to coexist with capillary malformations, at the same anatomic site or in close proximity. Pyogenic granulomas, which are vascular tumors, have been noted to arise after laser treatment of capillary malformations. In PHACE (**P**osterior fossa malformation, **H**emangioma, **A**rterial anomalies, **C**oarctation of the aorta, **E**ye abnormalities) syndrome, hemangiomas are associated with structural arterial anomalies. Maffucci syndrome may be associated with spindle-cell hemangiomas (hemangioendotheliomas) and venous malformations.

The recently described entity "multifocal lymphangioendotheliomatosis" is difficult to classify into either category and demonstrates biological and histopathological features of both a vascular malformation and tumor. These associations suggest that there is a common pathologic mechanism shared between two broad categories of vascular anomalies.

INFANTILE HEMANGIOMA

Definition

Infantile hemangiomas are benign developmental vascular tumors which appear during the first month of life, and characteristically have an initial proliferative and a later involutional phase.

Classification

The term hemangioma designates a proliferative blood vessel tumor. The term 'infantile hemangioma' describes the developmental type of hemangioma that arises in early infancy. This type is also termed as 'strawberry nevus' or 'strawberry hemangioma'. The term 'cavernous hemangioma' should be abandoned.

Etiology

Infantile hemangiomas are benign proliferation of vascular elements. Capillary endothelium has the capacity to develop new vessels under certain conditions. This requires the presence of angiogenic factors, and it is possible that infantile hemangioma cells are able to secrete such a factor *in situ*. An imbalance between expression of angiogenic and anti-angiogenic factors within the infantile hemangioma and adjacent normal tissue has been demonstrated.

Recently, it has been recognized that development of infantile hemangioma is a common sequel of chorionic villous sampling. It is anticipated that placental injury leads to increased detachment and release of placental cells into the blood. Infantile hemangioma might therefore result from embolization of fetal placental endothelial cells via the right-to-left cardiac chambers characteristic of the fetal circulation. This hypothesis is supported by the fact that, infantile hemangioma shares immunoreactivity for tissue-specific markers with placental endothelium, in contrast to other vascular tumors and malformations.

Pathology

In the earliest phase of growth of infantile hemangioma, there is a solid mass of proliferating endothelial cells, with few, if any lumina. The nuclei are not pleomorphic, and only occasional mitoses are evident. Later, in the proliferative phase, capillary-sized lumina are apparent, lined by plump endothelial cells. Reticulin staining confirms that each group of endothelial cells is surrounded by a limiting membrane of reticulin fibers. PAS staining shows a thickened basement membrane beneath the endothelial cells lining the lumina. Mast cells are plentiful during the proliferative phase. The onset of involution coincides with an increase in apoptosis. As involution proceeds, the hemangioma becomes progressively more organized, with distinct lobules separated by fibrous septa, containing larger feeding and draining vessels. In children aged two years and older, the number of vascular channels decreases, and the diameter of the lumina increases with flattening of the endothelial lining, resulting in a cavernous appearance. There is a simultaneous progressive increase in intra-lobular connective tissue and fat.

Histopathological features of small, multiple infantile hemangiomas are similar.

Immuno-histochemical Studies

These studies have documented increased expression of basic fibroblast growth factor (BFGF) within the proliferating infantile hemangioma, and its excretion in increased quantities in the urine, which falls as involution progresses.

Immunoreactivity

The endothelial cells comprising infantile hemangioma show intense and persistent immunoreactivity for a number of tissue-specific markers termed Fc gamma RII, Lewis Y antigen (LEY), merosin and GLUTI. This group of markers is highly characteristic of placental microvasculature. However, infantile hemangioma failed to show immunoreactivity for markers of placental trophoblasts.

The location of individual lesions varies. The most superficial lesions are confined to the papillary and subpapillary dermis, while deep lesions may partly extend into the subcutis.

Ultrastructural Studies

Ultrastructural studies show that the proliferative phase lesions comprise of highly active endothelial cells, with multi-laminated basement membrane. Mast cell microvillous projections may be observed alongside the vessel walls, parallel to the basement membrane laminations. During the involution phase, there is evidence of vessel degeneration.

Clinical Features

Infantile hemangiomas are the commonest tumors of infancy, with a prevalence of about 1-3% after the first few days of life, and up to 12%, by the end of the first year. Superficial infantile hemangiomas, sometimes multiple, have also been reported to occur with increased frequency in the fetal alcohol syndrome.

Infantile hemangioma becomes apparent during the first month of life in about 90% of cases, and virtually 100 % by the ninth month. About 65% of infantile hemangiomas are superficial, 15% are deep and 20 % mixed.

In superficial infantile hemangiomas, an initial precursor lesion is often visible on the first day of life. These precursor lesions may appear as a macular area of hyperemia resembling a salmon patch or pale port-wine stain, or a macular area of pallor, resembling a nevus anemicus. A group of small, closely packed angiomas usually develops thereafter within the area, rapidly enlarging and coalescing until the lesion is mature **(Figures 21.1A and B)**. In about 20% of cases, infantile hemangiomas are present at birth without a precursor lesion.

The superficial infantile hemangioma is also known as 'strawberry' nevus or 'strawberry' hemangioma. It is a circumscribed, oval or round, soft, dome-shaped, scarlet-red swelling. The surface may be smooth or lobulated.

About 60% of the infantile hemangiomas occur on head and neck. Next in frequency are the lesions on the trunk, perianal area in both sexes, and the vulva in girls.

In 80% cases, the lesion is single. Apart from the occasional lesion that is fully developed at birth (congenital infantile hemangioma), infantile hemangiomas increase in size over a variable period of 13 to 18 months. However, most of the lesions reach their maximum size within 6-12 months of first appearance.

Mixed Infantile Hemangioma

These are superficial hemangiomas which have a deeper element.

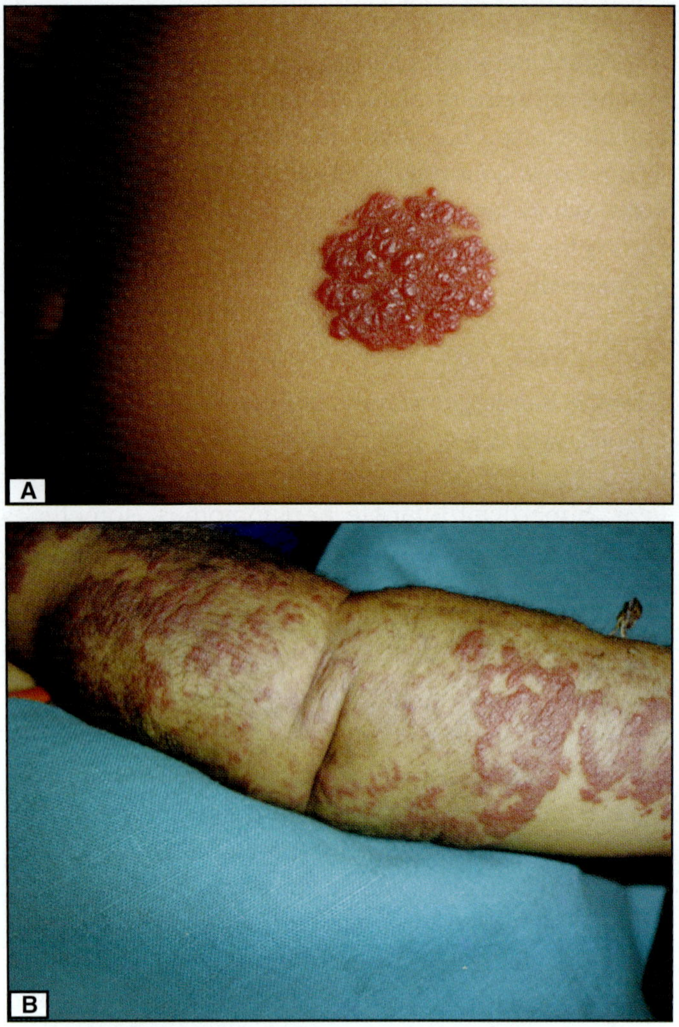

FIGURES 21.1A AND B: Infantile hemangioma

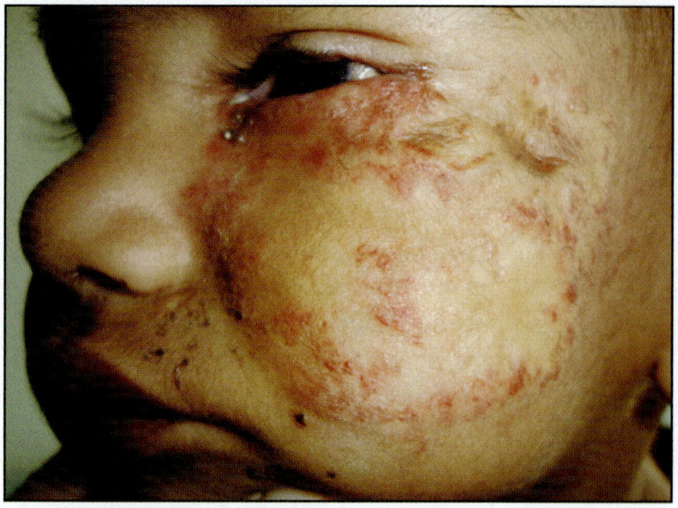

FIGURE 21.2: Spontaneous regression of infantile hemangioma with atrophic scar

Deep Infantile Hemangioma

These are soft, round, warm, bluish masses beneath the normal skin. There may be a few branching telangiectasias or an area of vascular staining on the surface. On palpation, these feel like a 'bag of worms.' A useful feature in distinction from other tumors is that these generally can be compressed to about half of their original size, regaining the original dimensions on release of pressure. These often become larger and darker when the child screams or cries.

Large superficial veins may be present in the peripheral skin of larger infantile hemangiomas.

Virtually 100% of infantile hemangiomas undergo spontaneous regression, which is complete or almost complete in about 95% cases. Resolution of superficial infantile hemangioma is heralded by softening and appearance of focal, grayish surface opacities on the central part of the lesion **(Figure 21.2)**. Infantile hemangiomas on the nose, lips and the parotid area regress slowly and generally incompletely.

Diagnosis

The superficial type of infantile hemangioma is diagnosed easily. The main problem is to distinguish vascular malformations from deep or mixed deep and superficial hemangiomas of infancy. The principal features distinctive of vascular malformations are:

- The history of a lesion present since birth;
- The lack of tendency of spontaneous resolution;
- Frequent co-existence of other elements such as port-wine stain and lymphangioma circumscriptum, in the area of the lesion.

Ultrasound, computed tomography (CT) and MRI are of limited value in making the distinction, as both types of lesions are usually reported as 'hemangioma'. However the distinction is very important, for correct management of the patient.

Differential Diagnosis

Several types of tumor occurring in infancy may present with cutaneous nodules resembling superficial, deep or mixed hemangiomas; these include congenital hemangioma, granuloma telangiectaticum, and fibrous hamartoma of infancy.

Ultrasound scanning can be useful in distinguishing infantile hemangiomas from other soft tumors. CT and MRI scans are useful in delineating the extent of an infantile hemangioma and in evaluating response to therapy.

Complications

1. *Ulceration and hemorrhage* **(Figure 21.3)**.
2. *Infection:* Secondary infection may occur in an ulcerated hemangioma, or following a surgical intervention **(Figure 21.4)**.
3. *Malignant change:* Malignant change may be a complication of hepatic hemangiomas, but it almost certainly never complicates cutaneous infantile hemangiomas.
4. *Heart failure:* Shunting of large volumes of blood through a large infantile hemangioma may lead to high-output heart failure.
5. *Systemic hemangioma:* Visceral hemangiomas may occur with or without coexistent cutaneous infantile hemangioma.

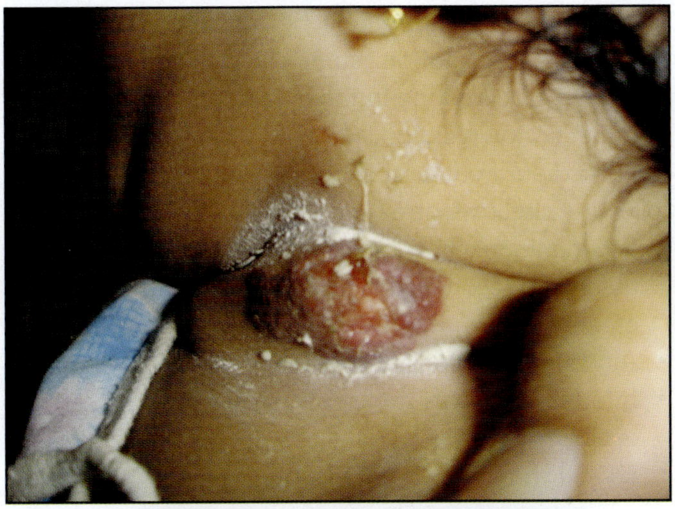

FIGURE 21.3: Ulcerated hemangioma

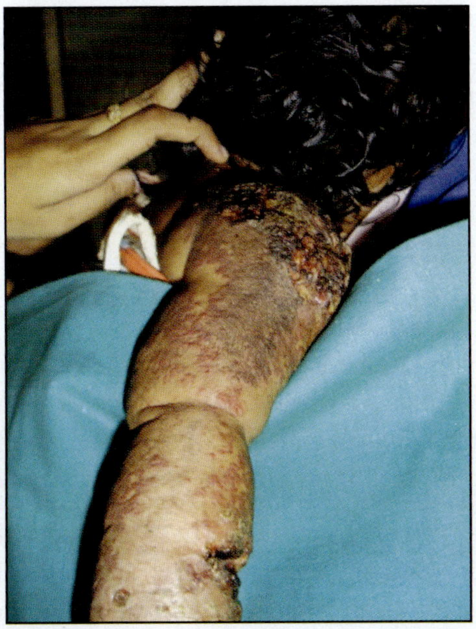

FIGURE 21.4: Hemangioma with superficial infection

6. *Visual impairment:* Infantile hemangioma involving the eyelids and/or the orbit can interfere with vision.
7. *Airway obstruction:* Any infant with a cutaneous infantile hemangioma may have a concurrent subglottic hemangioma. This is most likely if the cutaneous lesion is in the lower part of the face, or the neck.
8. *Obstruction of the external auditory canal:* Infantile hemangiomas that encroach on the ear, particularly those in the parotid area may obstruct the external auditory canal.

Spinal dysraphism and anogenital anomalies: Infantile hemangiomas in the lumbosacral area may be associated with underlying spinal dysraphism, tethered spinal cord, sacral anomalies and genital and renal anomalies. MRI scan is indicated if there is a risk of such an association.

PHACES syndrome (**P**osterior fossa malformation, **H**emangioma, **A**rterial anomalies, **C**oarctation of the aorta, **E**ye abnormalities, **S**ternal cleft and/or **S**upra-umbilical raphe).

An association between posterior fossa brain abnormalities and large facial infantile hemangioma is now well recognized.

Congenital hemangioma: It is now recognized that there is a distinctive type of hemangioma that is already fully developed at birth. These tumors have been detected by ultrasound scan by the 12th week of gestation. Pathologically, these differ from other infantile hemangioma by lack of expression of tissue-specific markers found in placental endothelium.

Clinically, the distinctive feature of these lesions is the lack of proliferative phase, and their tendency to involute very rapidly with the whole process generally being complete within the first year. These tumors have always been single, with an average diameter of 5 cm, enlarging in proportion to the child's growth. The overlying skin often shows telangiectasia. Surgical excision is the best treatment.

Miliary hemangiomatosis of infancy: Occasionally, infants are born with very large numbers, generally many hundreds of small infantile hemangiomas of 'strawberry' type, or develop these within the first few weeks of life. In such cases, the cutaneous lesions are characteristically relatively small, generally between 2 mm to 2 cm in diameter. The lesions may bleed, and quite often at least some are pedunclated. This condition is termed miliary hemangiomatosis of infancy. In cases with multiple infantile hemangiomas, the lesions will rarely exceed 10 in number, in contrast to the miliary hemangiomatosis of infancy, in which lesions will generally number several hundreds, often thousands.

Major complications may supervene, generally due to the presence of associated systemic hemangioma, and these are responsible for a significant mortality. The mean age of death in a large series of patients was around 10 weeks. The most serious of all complications is high-output cardiac failure, which is almost invariably due to shunting through one or more large hepatic angiomas, which may be present at birth.

Apart from the liver, hemangiomas are also commonly present in the gastrointestinal tract, spleen, pancreas, salivary glands, urinary bladder, bone, meninges, brain and eyes.

The Kasabach-Merritt phenomenon has been reported frequently. These cases may demonstrate low-grade thrombocytopenia. In addition, individual hemangioma may result in a wide variety of clinical features due to local pressure.

Investigations

Certain investigations are mandatory in any infant with miliary hemangiomatosis. These include following:

- Complete blood count including a platelet count,
- Urine analysis to exclude bleeding,
- Fecal occult blood testing,
- Chest X-ray to determine the heart size and to rule out lung lesions that might cause arteriovenous shunting,
- Echocardiography to establish cardiac output status,
- Abdominal ultrasound scans to examine the liver.
- Wherever suspected on clinical grounds, lesions in other organs may be sought by appropriate investigations, including technetium-99m scan using red blood cells and MRI.

The small hemangiomas in miliary hemangiomatosis of infancy involute spontaneously, and typically it is more rapid than classical infantile hemangioma, the skin lesions often disappearing by the age of 12 months.

Management of Infantile Hemangiomas

Management is essentially same as for single or multiple infantile hemangiomas. Treatment is not always indicated, and the need for intervention should be guided by careful evaluation of the risk of serious complications. No treatment is indicated where good esthetic outcome is expected and complications appear unlikely. It is helpful to show the parents serial photographs illustrating the spontaneous resolution that has been observed in other cases.

It is important to be aware of the speed with which these lesions can enlarge during their initial phase of growth. The progress of lesions that are still increasing in size should therefore be supervised.

The need for treatment of individual lesions should be carefully and sympathetically considered. Even small lesions may result in major esthetic handicap at certain sites, such as, tip of the nose, lip or forehead. While a good result may ultimately be anticipated following spontaneous resolution, sufficient psychological harm might have been done in the meantime to justify earlier therapeutic intervention.

Immediate treatment should be contemplated in the following circumstances:

- When infantile hemangioma is causing or threatening tissue loss secondary to ulceration (e.g. on the nose or ears),
- Airway obstruction is threatened or feeding is impeded,
- Interference with important structures such as the eyelids,
- Esthetic handicap is significant,

Treatment options include:

1. Systemic corticosteroids;
2. Intralesional corticosteroids;
3. Topical corticosteroids under occlusion
4. Interferon-α-2a
5. Laser therapy
6. Compression bandaging
7. Sclerosant injection
8. Cryotherapy
9. Surgical excision.

An individual case requires careful assessment and observation, knowledge of the advantages and disadvantages of the available therapeutic options, and familiarity with the natural history of this tumor at various sites.

1. *Systemic corticosteroids:* These are the treatment of choice in most situations in which therapy is indicated. Corticosteroids are effective only during the proliferative phase and should therefore be initiated at the first sign

that the patient is developing a significant eyelid lesion, cardiac failure or upper airway obstruction.

Prednisolone should be given at a daily dose of 3-4 mg/kg body weight for 4-8 weeks, followed by gradual reduction of the dose over a period of several weeks. Alternate day dosage regimens tend to be ineffective if used from the start of treatment. If no response is seen after 3-4 weeks, prednisolone therapy should be stopped. A good response is seen in the majority of cases if treatment is started early at a dose no less than 3 mg /kg/ day. Rebound increase in size may occur if treatment is discontinued too soon in rapidly proliferative lesions. Since such lesions continue to proliferate during the first 6 months of life, therapy should be continued until the seventh month. Treatment should also be contemplated when the integrity of the nose, ears, or lips is threatened.

The mechanism by which corticosteroids prevent further growth and reduce the bulk of infantile hemangiomas remains unclear. Corticosteroid molecules bind to the steroid receptors within proliferating hemangiomas, and may thereby inhibit the binding of 17α-estradiol.

Infants tolerate this therapy remarkably well, and it is very unusual for adverse effects to occur that will not reverse within months of discontinuing therapy.

2. *Intralesional corticosteroids:* Intralesional injection of corticosteroids may result in rapid shrinkage of the lesion. This modality has been used successfully to arrest proliferation, to shrink superficial infantile hemangiomas and for lesions on the eyelids.

Combination therapy with systemic and intralesional injection of corticosteroids has also been used.

3. *Topical corticosteroids:* Small hemangiomas of infancy can be treated with potent topical steroids.

4. *Interferon-α-2a:* Experience in complicated cutaneous hemangiomas of infancy has suggested, but not firmly established, the useful effect of both IFN-α-2a and IFN-α-2b. The cost of treatment is substantial.

5. *Laser therapy:* The 585-nm flashlamp-pumped pulsed dye laser can be used to lighten any superficial hemangiomas and to flatten thin lesions (less than 4 nm). The flashlamp-pumped pulsed dye laser has proven valuable for reduction of pain and initiation of healing in ulcerated hemangiomas, where the ulceration has persisted despite good wound care techniques.

Excision using the carbon dioxide laser may be useful for the cosmetic therapy of lesions persisting till adult life, particularly lesions in the mouth, although a degree of scarring is inevitable.

Neodymium:Yttrium Aluminum-Garnet (Nd: YAG) laser, which emits in the near infrared region and can produce photocoagulation up to a depth of 1 cm, has been successful in treating infantile hemangiomas. Treatment of thick hemangiomas with Nd: YAG laser may be improved by using special techniques such as skin surface cooling during irradiation or compression of lesions using cooled glass. Intralesional radiation using light guides has been effective in the shrinkage of large hemangiomas.

The development of the sapphire tip Nd: YAG laser scalpel permits excision with excellent hemostasis, and may prove to be a useful tool in the surgical management of infantile hemangiomas.

6. *Compression:* Compression bandaging can certainly provide temporary reduction of the bulk of the lesion that may allow a child with giant infantile hemangioma on the trunk or a limb to wear normal clothes. Respiratory distress and /or cardiac failure are potential complications of overenthusiastic application of compression to large hemangiomas.

7. *Cryotherapy:* Good results have been claimed for cryotherapy in the treatment of superficial and deep infantile hemangiomas, although there is some risk of scarring.

8. *Sclerosant injection:* Where involution is incomplete and accurate, serial measurements over a period of at least one year show no further involution, the injection of sclerosing solutions may shrink deep infantile hemangiomas. The solutions preferred include sodium citrate 30%, glucose 30% and saturated saline. Using a small needle, 0.5-5.0 ml is injected at fortnightly or monthly intervals. Excellent results have been claimed.

9. *Surgical excision:* Different surgical modalities for the treatment of infantile hemangiomas will be detailed at the end of the chapter.

TUFTED ANGIOMA (SYN. ANGIOBLASTOMA)

This is a rare type of angioma, which is seen most often in pre-pubertal children of either sex. Lesions most commonly are present at birth or appear during early weeks of life. This tumor and the kaposiform hemangioendothelioma together are responsible for the great majority of cases of Kasabach-Merritt syndrome.

Clinical Features

Tufted angioma takes the form of a rather poorly delineated, pinkish macule that evolves into a red or purplish, indurated plaque or nodule, up to 20 cm in diameter. Most lesions are tender or painful, and fine lanugo hair and/or hyperhidrosis are often apparent over the surface of the lesion. These tumors generally appear to behave in a benign fashion, but may progressively worsen in some cases.

Histopathology

There is a lobular proliferation of plump, oval cells surrounding tiny slit-like lumina. These blood vessels are tightly packed and organized in rounded tufts scattered in the dermis, and often described as resembling cannonballs. The tufts may be seen deeper in the dermis, and into the subcutis. Thin-walled lymphatic channels may be seen at the periphery of the cellular masses or throughout the dermis.

Excision is the definitive treatment, although incomplete excision may result in recurrence. Potent topical corticosteroids reduce pain. High-dose systemic corticosteroids may be beneficial, and this treatment should be tried before proceeding to excision.

KAPOSIFORM HEMANGIOENDOTHELIOMA

Kaposiform hemangioendothelioma (KH) is a rare vascular tumor occurring exclusively in childhood. In the majority of the cases, these tumors develop in the retroperitoneum, most often presenting around the age of 1 year. In the skin, KH tends to be a single lesion which initially has the appearance of an innocuous vascular stain. After a variable interval, usually a few months, the lesion starts to grow rapidly to form a mass which is generally complicated by the development of Kasabach-Merritt syndrome.

Histopathology

Kaposiform hemangioendothelioma is composed of lobules or sheets of tightly packed spindle or more rounded endothelial cells and pericytes, with an infiltrative pattern in the dermis, subcutaneous fat and muscles. As in tufted angioma, thin-walled, bloodless vascular channels may be seen at the periphery of the cellular masses or throughout the dermis and subcutis.

Prognosis

Skin lesions appear to have low mortality. Spontaneous regression of skin lesions has been reported.

KASABACH-MERRITT PHENOMENON (SYN.KASABACH-MERRITT SYNDROME, HEMANGIOMA-HEMORRHAGE SYNDROME)

Consumption coagulopathy is an uncommon complication of hemangioma in infancy. It is now clear that this complication almost exclusively occurs in association with tufted angiomas and kaposiform hemangioendothelioma.

Hemorrhage in Kasabach-Merritt syndrome appears to be a consequence of platelet sequestration, with associated consumption of clotting factors within the vascular bed of the angioma.

Cases of Kasabach-Merritt phenomenon presenting to dermatologists will almost always be due to tufted angiomas. These most commonly occur on the trunk, neck and proximal parts of the limbs. The onset of Kasabach-Merritt phenomenon is signaled by a sudden and rapid increase in the volume of the tumor, a change to a deep violet color and by the appearance of ecchymosis. The rapid expansion of the angioma may cause potentially lethal compression of the neighboring vital structures. As a result of the coagulopathy, internal bleeding may occur at different sites and is associated with a significant mortality.

Prognosis

Spontaneous resolution of the coagulopathy can be anticipated within1-6 years (mean 3 years). The coagulopathy resolves but the causative tumor remains. Treatment is indicated only when the patient's life is threatened.

Management

Systemic corticosteroid administration has been reported to have a directly beneficial effect on the disturbed coagulation-fibrinolysis system. Initial dosage of prednisolone should be between 2 and 4 mg/kg per day. When the coagulopathy is severe, prednisolone is ineffective.

Hemostasis can be improved by platelet transfusions. The principal use of this approach is in the preparation of the patient for surgical procedures including embolization. Embolization is an exceedingly valuable treatment, and may result in rapid and permanent reversal of severe acute coagulopathy.

Vincristine has been proven very effective in the Kasabach-Merritt phenomenon. The recommended dose is 1.0-1.5 mg/m^2 per week by slow intravenous infusion for at least 7 weeks, thereafter with decreasing frequency, depending upon the clinical response. This treatment appears to have a rapidly beneficial effect on the coagulopathy and shrinkage of the causative tumor.

Surgical Extirpation

Surgical extirpation of the tumors causing the Kasabach-Merritt phenomenon brings rapid relief of the coagulation defect in many cases, provided adequate intraoperative hemostasis can be achieved.

In general terms, management of patients with Kasabach-Merritt phenomenon should be as conservative as possible. Serial estimation of clotting parameters and platelet counts should be undertaken, and the levels of fibrinogen and fibrin degradation products should be monitored. Oral corticosteroid therapy should be initiated early, and the lesion should be compressed wherever possible. If the situation deteriorates, the relative merits of embolization, surgery, radiotherapy and infusion of vincristine should be weighed up.

Verrucous Hemangioma

Although almost invariably present at birth, verrucous hemangioma may appear later in life. Lesions are single or grouped, occurring mostly on the legs. These tend to start as well-defined, dark-red, macular areas of vascular staining resembling port-wine stains, sometimes progressing to soft, bluish red, vascular swellings. After a variable number of years, lesions start to attain the characteristic bluish black hue and an increasingly verrucous surface. Recurrent bleeding and infection often cause the patient to seek medical advice.

Histopathology

Verrucous hemangiomas are characterized by a hyperplastic epidermis showing orthohyperkeratosis, papillomatosis and irregular acanthosis with elongated rete pegs. The underlying dermis shows vascular spaces of variable size, which are congested with blood filling up the rete pegs. There are lobules of capillaries in the subcutis interposed with fat cells and fibrous tissue. The capillaries are lined by flat endothelium. The endothelium stains strongly with CD34, and the pericytes surrounding these vessels stain strongly with HHf-35.

Differential Diagnosis

These lesions are frequently misdiagnosed as infantile hemangioma or angiokeratoma; sometimes as lymphangioma circumscriptum or verrucous epidermal nevi.

Treatment

Excision is the treatment of choice. Skin grafting is required for larger lesions. There is a tendency for recurrence unless the excision is complete.

DIGITAL VERRUCOUS FIBROANGIOMA

Lesions are generally single and present since birth. They take the form of asymptomatic, soft to firm, dome-shaped nodules on the dorsum of a finger. Initially the lesions are skin-colored, but with time there is a change over to a purplish brown color.

HEMANGIOPERICYTOMA

About 5% of all hemangiopericytomas are congenital. Lesions mostly occur subcutaneously on the head, neck, trunk and limbs, and also internally. The dark red color suggests a vascular origin. The tumors are benign. These may resolve spontaneously or excision may lead to cure. Local complication includes hemorrhage.

GLOMANGIOMAS (SYN. MULTIPLE GLOMUS TUMORS; GLOMANGIOMATOSIS)

Commonest type of glomus tumor is the solitary form, which appears in young adult life. Multiple forms are occasionally seen in children.

Glomus cells are small with eosinophilic cytoplasm and round, centrally placed nuclei. These are considered to be modified smooth muscle cells, lining the endothelial walls of the glomus bodies, found in reticular dermis. Glomus bodies are believed to function as temperature receptors.

The solitary glomus tumor is an encapsulated proliferation of glomus cells lining the lumen of small vessels. In contrast, the childhood types are not encapsulated, and feature larger, more irregular vascular spaces, with fewer glomus cells; this type of lesion is considered hamartomatous and is now called glomangioma. When a substantial proportion of the cells are spindle-shaped resembling smooth muscle, the term glomangiomyoma is used.

Subdivision

Multiple glomus tumors generally have an earlier onset. These are subdivided into three types:

1. **Disseminated multiple glomangiomas:** In this form, compressible red to blue papules or nodules, usually less than 1 cm in diameter, are widely distributed. Total number of lesions is generally less than 10. Pain is less compared to solitary glomus tumors. Familial cases have been reported.
2. **Localized multiple glomangiomas:** The localized type of multiple glomangioma presents as grouped blue nodules. The lesions are usually limited to an area, such as the hand or leg.
3. **Congenital plaque-like glomangioma (Glomangiomatosis):** Plaque-like glomangiomas are extremely rare congenital lesions. These comprise of numerous reddish blue compressible papules, grouped as solitary or multiple plaques, each measuring about 10 to 20 cm across. The papules may be discrete or confluent and the lesions are soft with or without pain. The center of the plaque may be depressed and the affected area may sag. Facial lesions may be very disfiguring. Lesions on the lips present as spherical, soft, bright red nodules.

Natural History

The lesions undergo progressive growth with gradual enlargement of existing lesions and appearance of new lesions at previously unaffected sites.

Differential Diagnosis

Glomangiomas should be differentiated from tufted angioma, congenital plaque-like blue nevi and venous vascular malformations.

Treatment has been disappointing; there is poor response to pharmacological agents and sclerotherapy. Gradual recurrence occurs after surgical resection.

VASCULAR MALFORMATION

Vascular malformations are subdivided into groups based on their vascular components and flow characteristics **(Table 21.2)**. These may be composed of slow-flow capillary, venous, or lymphatic channels, fast-flow arterial channels, or a combination.

TABLE 21.2: Vascular malformations by flow characteristics and vascular components

Slow flow	Fast flow
Capillary malformations	AVMs
Port-wine stains	Combined
Telangiectasia	CAVM
Venous malformation	
Glomuvenous malformations	
Lymphatic malformations	
Macrocystic	
Microcystic	
Combined	
CLM (angiokeratoma)	
CLVM	
CMTC (CVM)	

AVM, Arteriovenous malformation; CAVM, capillary AVM; CLM, capillary-lymphatic malformation; CLVM, capillary-lymphatic venous malformation; CMTC, cutis marmorata telangiectatica congenita; CVM, capillary venous malformation.

PATHOGENESIS

The pathogenesis of vascular malformations is not yet well-understood. It is thought that these arise as a result of abnormalities in the process of normal vascular development. During embryogenesis, the normal vascular system arises via two processes;

- Vasculogenesis: It refers to the process by which vascular channels are formed *de novo* from endothelial cell precursors (angioblasts).
- Angiogenesis: It refers to the development of new vessels from pre-existing vasculature.

Recent studies have provided some insight into the complex processes of normal vasculogenesis and angiogenesis, suggesting that errors result in abnormal vascular channels and vascular malformations.

CAPILLARY MALFORMATIONS OF THE SKIN

Capillary malformations (CM), including telangiectases and port-wine stains **(Figure 21.5)**, are among the most common vascular malformations affecting the skin.

Clinical Features

These slow-flow vascular anomalies are present at birth and have an equal sex distribution. These usually arise sporadically and the incidence is approximately 3 per

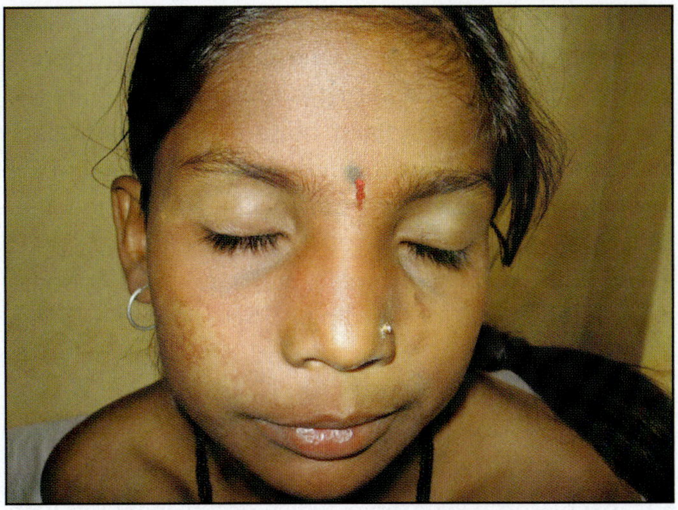

Figure 21.5: Port-wine stain

1000 infants. A CM present at birth may initially be misdiagnosed as bruise or sequel of birth trauma. The lesions may be single or multiple, small patches or involving an entire limb or portion of the face. CMs are frequently present on the head and neck region. In young infants, lesions are usually pale pink macules and patches.

The clinical behavior of port-wine stains is variable according to the anatomic location. The terms 'salmon patch', and 'stork bite' are used to describe a subset of CMs that are very common and located on the central area of the face (glabella, eyelids, nose, and upper lip) **(Figure 21.6)** and the nape of the neck respectively.

The development of blebs and hyperkeratotic areas within the CMs on extremities is virtually always seen in presence of lymphatic or mixed lymphatic-venous malformation. Limb port-wine stains may also be associated with congenital hypertrophy of underlying bone and soft tissues.

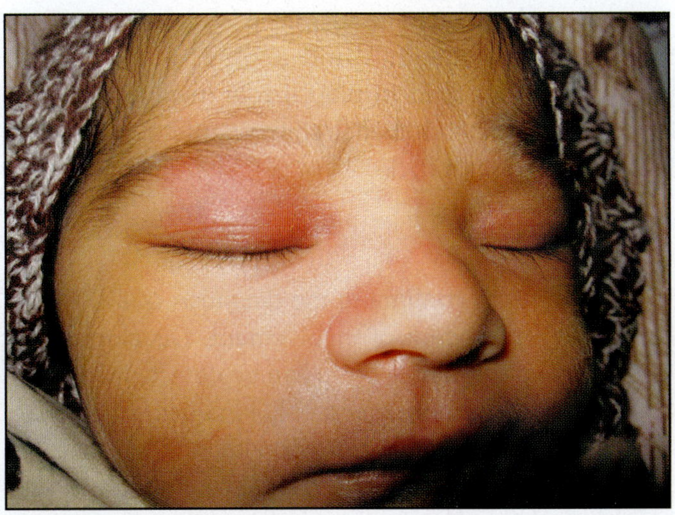

FIGURE 21.6: Salmon patch

CMs of the skin may occur in association with other congenital malformations, including underlying vascular anomalies. Less common anomalies associated with CMs include underlying spinal dysraphism, which classically occur in the lumbar region.

Pathogenesis

CMs are congenital anomalies, believed to represent an error in vascular development occurring during embryogenesis. Histopathology reveals an increased number and ectasia of blood vessels in the dermis. Some studies have suggested that lesions in the V3 dermatome of neck and trunk region tend to be more superficial, whereas lesions in the V2 dermatome and distal extremities have more deep-seated vessels.

Vessel number and depth correlate poorly with age but the mean vessel area and percentage of fullness increase with age. This accounts for the change in color of the lesion from pink to violet with maturity. Immunohistochemical analysis has demonstrated a decreased number of neurons associated with the ectatic vasculature in port-wine stains. It has been hypothesized that an alteration in the neural modulation of vascular flow may be involved in the pathogenesis of these lesions. Alternatively, the reduced density of neuronal cells may be secondary to abnormal vasculature and relative ischemia. There are several reports of autosomal dominant familial cases of CM associated with arteriovenous malformations (AVM), identifying locus CMC1 on chromosome 5q as the genetic region involved. Further genetic mapping has identified RASA1, encoding p120-rasGTPase-activating protein (p120-rasGAP), as the causative defect. p120-rasGAP appears to be integral in signaling for various growth factor receptors that control proliferation, migration, and survival of several cell types, including vascular endothelial cells. Another protein known as developmental endothelial locus-1 (Del-1) may also play a role in some cases of CM. Del-1 is an extracellular matrix protein adhered to by human umbilical vein endothelial cells that have been shown to induce formation of a vascular plexus with a large number of small capillaries. For the majority of patients with CM, however, the molecular pathogenesis has yet to be elucidated.

Diagnosis

CMs are diagnosed on the basis of their clinical appearance. It is important to note that cutaneous erythema overlying a deeper AVM may mimic a CM. Doppler ultrasound evaluation is useful but not always diagnostic. Once the diagnosis of CM is established, the patient should be carefully examined for the presence of underlying vascular malformations and associated congenital anomalies.

Management

Currently, the flashlamp-pumped PDL is the treatment of choice for port-wine stains. The lasers used most commonly employ a wavelength that selectively targets oxyhemoglobin and results in intravascular coagulation, and a pulse duration that limits destruction and heat dissipation to the targeted vasculature without causing damage to the surrounding tissue in the epidermis or dermis. Potassium titanyl phosphate laser has also been shown to produce further lightening of PDL-resitant port-wine stains. However, there may be an increased risk of side effects.

VENOUS MALFORMATIONS

Definition

VMs are slow-flow vascular lesions that are present at birth. These are non-proliferating vascular birthmarks composed of anomalous ectatic venous channels. A variety of terms including 'venous angioma', 'cavernous angioma', cavernous hemangioma', and 'phlebangioma' have been used in the medical literature to describe these anomalies.

Clinical Characteristics

VMs are present at birth but are not always clinically evident. The lesions typically become more prominent as the patient ages. The most pronounced enlargement is usually seen during infancy to puberty, whereas changes are less evident in adulthood. These usually present as soft, compressible blue masses which enlarge when the affected area is in a dependent position or with physical activity. The blue color is pathognomonic and caused by the presence of ectatic anomalous venous channels within the dermis. Head and neck VMs are frequently more extensive than is initially apparent. Facial VMs involve the skin and subcutaneous layers, but often have extension into the muscle and oral mucosa. Lesions on the cheek and temporal area may extend into the infratemporal fossa and parotid gland. As the lesion swells and enlarges, the adjacent or underlying bone may be deformed. Spontaneous, local venous thrombosis may result in the formation of calcifications (phleboliths) within the VM. Localized intravascular coagulation within a VM may result in abnormal coagulation profiles and may lead to episodes of thrombosis and /or bleeding. VM-associated bleeding diathesis usually develops in adolescence or early adulthood.

Differential Diagnosis

Kasabach-Merritt syndrome, which occurs in infants with vascular tumors has to be differentiated.

Pathogenesis

Histopathology of VMs reveals poorly circumscribed lesions composed of irregular, endothelial-lined vascular channels. The lumen walls are thin and deficient in smooth muscle cells. Although the molecular basis of sporadic VMs has yet to be discovered, there have been recent advances in the understanding of familial cases. In 1994-1995, two families were identified to have autosomal dominantly inherited cutaneous and mucosal VMs. Genetic analysis mapped a locus for both these families to the chromosome 9p21. These families shared a mutation resulting in an arginine to tryptophan substitution (R849W), in the gene that encodes for the kinase domain of the endothelial cell receptor Tie2. Earlier studies suggested that Tie2 signaling plays a significant role in the branching and sprouting of the capillary plexus.

Additional research has identified ligands for the Tie2 receptor, angiopoietin-1 and angiopoietin-2. These proteins are believed to play a role in regulating the assembly of nonendothelial components of the vessel including smooth muscle.

Diagnosis

MRI is helpful in confirming the diagnosis of a VM and delineating the extent of involvement. Developmental venous anomalies of the brain can be detected with MRI and may be seen more commonly in patients with head and neck VMs than in general population.

Before any intervention, a coagulation profile should be obtained to rule out an underlying coagulopathy.

Management

The general goals of therapy are to prevent distortion of facial features, limit bony deformities, preserve function, and minimize painful swelling.

Then VMs may be treated with surgical excision, sclerotherapy, or a combination of both. The specific management of these lesions depends on the location of the lesion. It is useful to divide VMs into two broad categories while considering their management:

- Head and neck VMs,
- Trunk and limb VMs.

The most effective management of large head and neck VMs is a combined approach of percutaneous sclerotherapy performed by an interventional radiologist with surgical excision. Postinflammatory hyperpigmentation and infection are potential complications if the overlying skin ulcerates after sclerotherapy.

Patients with extensive limb lesions should be instructed to use compression garments since childhood. Compression helps to decrease the discomfort associated with the lesion, protects the overlying skin, limits swelling, and improves localized intravascular coagulation. Surgery plays a limited role in the management of lesions on extremity, but, if performed, localized coagulopathy must be controlled before surgery.

GLOMUVENOUS MALFORMATIONS

Definition

Glomuvenous malformation (Glomangioma or VMs with glomus cells) is a rare type that exhibits clinical and histopathological features, distinct from typical VMs.

Clinical Features

The lesions become more apparent with maturity, presenting as blue-purple nodules and papules with a 'pebbly' surface. They are often firm and less compressible than typical VMs and may be painful following prolonged compression. They are more frequently confined to the skin and subcutaneous tissues compared to the typical VMs, which may extend into the underlying musculature and joints.

Histopathology

The lesions are characterized by distended venous channels with surrounding glomus cells.

Pathogenesis

Mutations in the gene glomulin, which is located on the chromosome 1p21-22, cause glomuvenous malformations. Studies suggest that glomus cells within the glomuvenous malformations represent abnormally differentiated vascular smooth-muscle cells. Therefore, it has been suggested that the glomulin gene plays a role in the differentiation of vascular smooth muscle cells.

Diagnosis

The clinical features described above help to establish the diagnosis.

Management

It is now recognized that glomuvenous malformations respond differently to treatment than typical VMs. Optimal treatment regimens for this newly recognized entity are lacking. Small, localized lesions can be managed with surgical excision. Sclerotherapy may be less effective and compression garments may increase discomfort.

ARTERIOVENOUS MALFORMATIONS

Definition

AVMs are fast-flow vascular lesions composed of dysmorphic arterial and venous vessels connected directly to one another without an intervening capillary bed.

Clinical Features

Most lesions are visible at birth (40-60 %), and 30% become clinically apparent during childhood. These are more common in the head and neck region. AVMs may progress through four different stages of development. Severity of the lesions can be scored by using the ISSVA-accepted (1990) Schobinger clinical staging.

- Stage I: Lesions are in the quiescent phase, asymptomatic, and usually last since birth until adolescence. During this stage, the AVM may not be apparent or have the appearance of a port-wine stain or involuting hemangioma. Increased warmth, bruit, or thrill suggests presence of high-flow components. Some AVMs remain quiescent throughout the patient's lifetime.
- Stage II: This is the progressive phase, most commonly beginning during adolescence. This stage represents expansion, when the vascular lesions enlarge and darken, deforming the integument and invading

deeper structures. Histopathologically, both arteries and veins undergo progressive dilatation, thinning, and fibrosis. On examination, tortuous draining vessels appear and gradually elongate. Skin changes mimicking Kaposi's sarcoma, known as Stewart-Bluefarb syndrome, may develop in lower extremity AVMs.

- Stage III: This stage grossly mimics Stage II, deep destruction occurs with spontaneous necrosis, chronic ulceration, pain, and hemorrhage. This phase usually develops after years of progressive worsening.
- Stage IV: Cardiac decompensation is the feature of this stage. High-output cardiac failure may result from increased blood flow in the large AVMs.

Pathogenesis

AVMs may arise during early fetal development, due to the failure of regression of arteriovenous channels in the primitive retiform plexus. The embryogenic theory explains the predominance of AVMs in the head and neck region. Although most cases of AVMs are sporadic, there are few inherited syndromes whose molecular genetics have been recently elucidated. A mutation in the gene RASA1, expressing p120-rasGAP, on chromosome 5q, has been identified in families with CMs associated with AVMs, with autosomal dominant inheritance, such as hereditary hemorrhagic telangiectasia. There is speculation that, like hereditary hemorrhagic telangiectasia, sporadic lesions may involve an aberration in the transforming growth factor-β signaling pathway. The fact that transforming growth factor-β is involved in the induction of apoptotic endothelial cell death supports this hypothesis. There is also research to support the idea that a reduced apoptotic process may cause the dysregulation of vascular growth in AVMs.

Although the cause of AVM expansion is unknown, it has been proposed that this may result from dormant arteriovenous communications, dilatation of normal latent arteriovenous shunts by increased pressure and flow, and local ischemia caused by trauma.

Diagnosis

AVMs are diagnosed by clinical findings and radiological features. The differential diagnosis of AVMs includes other vascular malformations and vascular neoplasm. Excessive warmth, unusual pain, and bleeding episodes provide clues but may occur in other conditions. Auscultation of the lesion and bedside Doppler scanners are helpful screening tools. Radiological evaluation is necessary to confirm the diagnosis, delineate the extent of the lesion, and assess the flow characteristics. Angiography is necessary both to assess the extent of the lesion before therapeutic intervention and to guide intra-arterial embolization.

Management

Treatment of AVMs may be difficult. Partial treatment usually results in recurrences that may be more difficult to manage than the initial malformation. Extreme pain, ulceration, bleeding, and gross enlargement of the malformation are indications for treatment. Multimodal treatment, including preoperative embolization and complete surgical resection, is usually necessary for the management of AVMs. Preoperative embolization reduces intraoperative blood loss, allows more complete surgical resection, and therefore, decreases post surgical morbidity and mortality.

Recently, the concept of angiosomes, i.e. the separation of body into compartments of soft tissue and bone defined by vascular supply, has been applied to the head and neck and may guide the treatment strategy for AVMs. Understanding the location and anatomy of head and neck angiosomes may help in more complete embolization by predicting arterial supply. Palliative embolization may be used to treat symptomatic AVMs when combination treatment cannot be performed.

LYMPHATIC MALFORMATIONS

Definition

Lymphatic malformations (LM) are developmental anomalies of the lymphatic system that results in abnormalities in lymphatic flow.

Classification

LM of the skin and subcutaneous tissue represent a diverse group of disorders that may be primary or secondary and localized or diffuse. A diffuse LM is also known as lymphedema.

Acquired or secondary lymphedema is the most commonly recognized disorder of lymphatic tissue. It is most frequently caused by disruption of the normal lymphatic drainage associated with local trauma or infection.

Primary lymphedema is a relatively rare finding. Primary lymphedema can be divided by the age of presentation, into congenital familial Type I (Nonne-Milroy disease), Type II lymphedema praecox (late-onset hereditary lymphedema, or Meig disease), and lymphedema tarda. Milroy disease usually shows autosomal dominant inheritance and often presents at birth with lymphedema of the lower extremities. Lymphedema praecox, representing 80% of patients with primary lymphedema, typically presents within adolescence to 35 years of age with lymphedema of one or both legs. Lymphedema tarda is defined as primary lymphedema presenting after 35 years of age. There are other causes of lymphedema, such as Turner's syndrome and Noonan's syndrome, which are characterized by other congenital anomalies. Most of these conditions are believed to be caused by hypoplasia of the normal lymphatic system.

Localized Congenital Lymphatic Malformations

These LMs are frequently referred to as 'lymphangiomas' and can be divided into following groups:

- Macrocystic (deep)
- Microcystic (superficial, lymphangioma cicumscriptum).

The distinction between macrocystic and microcystic LMs is important because of its relevance in the treatment and prognosis. These two types may also be combined or associated with other vascular malformations.

Clinical Features

Approximately 70% of LMs are present at birth, remainder presenting by 2 years of age. Macrocystic LMs are usually visible at birth and can be diagnosed by prenatal ultrasound. Fifty-five percent to 90% of these lesions are located on the neck or axilla, where they are referred to as cystic hygroma.

These may present as isolated, poorly circumscribed subcutaneous masses that expand over time, as the anomalous channels become ectatic. Although many are asymptomatic, some of these lesions are associated with local pain or tenderness.

Complications depend on the size and location of the lesion. Large LMs are more common in the cervical region of the baby and may impede normal vaginal delivery.

Cervicofacial LMs may also cause airway obstruction, difficulty with feeding and impaired speech development. These may be complicated by recurrent, potentially life-threatening infections following minor trauma, upper respiratory tract infection or poor dental hygiene.

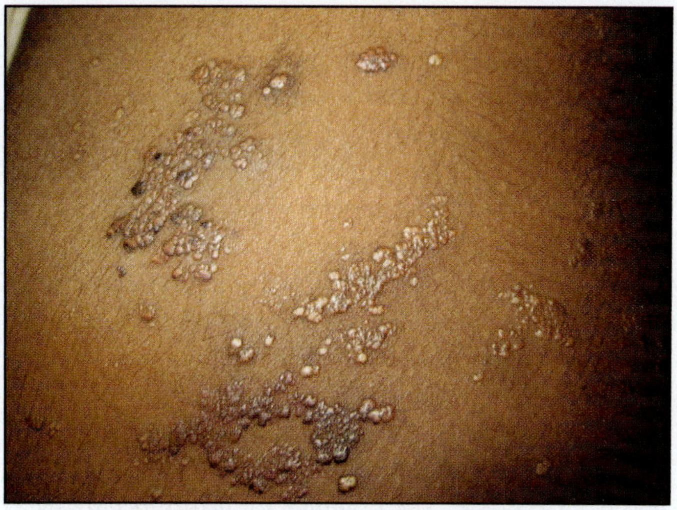

FIGURE 21.7: Lymphangioma circumscriptum

Microcystic LMs are present at birth, like other vascular malformations, but may not be evident until complications such as infection or bleeding make them more obvious. These lesions are frequently located over the proximal limbs, upper arms, axillae and chest. These have been termed 'lymphangioma circumscriptum' because of their common presentation as persistent crops of thin-walled vesicles or hyperkeratotic papules arranged irregularly in groups, usually localized to one region **(Figure 21.7)**. The most common symptom is recurrent oozing of clear fluid. Squamous cell carcinoma may arise within a long-standing congenital lymphangioma circumscriptum. LMs may present in association with CMs.

Pathogenesis

LMs result from an error in the normal development of the lymphatic system and are true malformations rather than neoplasm with inherent growth potential.

Diagnosis

LMs are frequently diagnosed clinically. Radiographic studies are important in confirming and determining the extent of the disease. Macrocystic LMs, such as cystic hygroma, may be detected with prenatal ultrasonography, by visualization of the mass or other signs such as polyhydramnios. By using Doppler flow studies, ultrasonography can also distinguish LM from vascular malformations. MRI is the 'gold standard' for delineating the extent of the lesion and may also be useful in assessing involvement of the deeper structures in cases of 'lymphangioma circumscriptum'.

Management

Important complications of LMs requiring aggressive management is bacterial super infection. These cases should be treated promptly with appropriate antibiotics to cover gram-positive organisms. Symptomatic LMs are most commonly managed with surgical excision.

Sclerotherapy is an alternative to surgical resection. A variety of agents have been used, ethanol, acetic acid, bleomycin and OK-432. For unresectable cases, all these sclerosing agents have been shown to be more effective in treating macrocystic than microcystic LMs.

Variable degrees of success have been reported with continuous-wave and ultra-pulse carbon dioxide lasers, and Nd:YAG laser. The potential for recurrence exists as in other destructive surgical modalities.

ANGIOKERATOMAS

The term angiokeratoma is applied to a number of distinct conditions that share a clinical presentation with asymptomatic hyperkeratotic vascular skin lesions and a histological combination of superficial dermal vascular ectasia and hyperkeratosis. The following variants are recognized:

1. Angiokeratoma circumscriptum
2. Agiokeratoma of Mibelli
3. Solitary papular angiokeratoma
4. Angiokeratoma of the scrotum and vulva
5. Angiokeratoma corporis diffusum.

The angiokeratomas are capillary vascular malformations rather than hemangioma.

SYNDROMES ASSOCIATED WITH VASCULAR MALFORMATIONS

STURGE-WEBER SYNDROME (SYN. ENCEPHALOFACIAL ANGIOMATOSIS)

This term is applied where a facial port-wine stain is associated with an ipsilateral leptomeningeal vascular malformation. Ocular involvement is not a *sine qua non* for this diagnosis.

The syndrome is a developmental malformation of the vasculature of the leptomeninges and facial skin, often also of the eye. There are reports of its occurrence in monozygotic twins, and of facial port-wine stains in first degree relatives.

The cutaneous lesion shows histopathological changes similar to those seen in other port-wine stains.

Control of seizures is essential to minimize brain damage. Anticonvulsants are the first line of treatment, but neurosurgical intervention should be considered early when medical treatment does not secure adequate control.

NEVUS ANEMICUS

Definition

Nevus anemicus is a congenital anomaly of the skin, characterized by macular areas of pallor resulting from reduced blood flow, but having a normal texture and normal melanin pigmentation.

Etiology and Pathology

This lesion is a pharmacological anomaly rather than anatomical. It is considered that nevus anemicus may reflect locally increased vascular reactivity to catecholamines. This is supported by autograft exchange transplantation studies, and by the finding that the pallor can be overcome by local injection of the alpha-adrenergic blocker phentolamine.

Areas of nevus anemicus are often seen in close association with port-wine stain. It has been suggested that this phenomenon may be explained by somatic recombination.

Diagnosis

Diascopy provides the most reliable method to distinguish nevus anemicus from other causes of circumscribed pallor such as hypochromic nevi and vitiligo. Woods's lamp examination does not accentuate the lesion.

Treatment

Treatment is generally not required. Where there is cosmetic disability, the use of camouflage make-up should be considered.

MIXED VASCULAR MALFORMATIONS

CUTIS MARMORATA TELANGIECTATICA CONGENITA (SYN. RETICULATE VASCULAR NEVUS)

Etiology and Pathology

This disorder is a combined capillary and venous malformation. The histopathology remains ill-defined.

Clinical Features

There is a reticulate erythema of variable extent, producing a marble-like effect. Telangiectasia is often visible within the hyperemic areas. The skin in these areas may be atrophic, or may be ulcerated at birth, resulting in linear or reticulate erosions.

Almost any area of the skin may be affected, but involvement of the limbs is more common. The distribution is generally asymmetrical. Fairly sharp midline demarcation is common.

The natural history is gradual spontaneous improvement, although there may be some extension of the lesions during the first few days of life. Generally the reticulate erythema fades more rapidly during the first year and slower thereafter.

Diagnosis

Cutis marmorata, a physiological cutaneous response to cold found in the neonate, usually disappears with warming.

Congenital reticulate erythema with atrophy and telangiectasia may be a feature of neonatal lupus erythematosus. Neonatal lupus erythematosus should be suspected when the head is affected and skin changes are bilaterally symmetrical.

Treatment

Because of the natural tendency of these lesions to fade spontaneously with time, active treatment should not be envisaged during the early years. Tunable dye laser therapy may help in persistent lesions, but often not much effective.

KLIPPEL-TRENAUNAY SYNDROME

Etiology

The association of port-wine stain on a limb with soft-tissue swelling, with or without bony overgrowth, is generally termed Klippel-Trenaunay syndrome. The etiology of the Klippel-Trenaunay syndrome is unknown, but it has been suggested that it reflects defective remodelling of the fetal vascular tree during embryogenesis.

Clinical Features

The most characteristic cutaneous lesion, both clinically and histopathologically, is a port-wine stain. The vascular staining is confined to the hypertrophic limb in about 75% of cases. Occasionally, other types of vascular malformations may be present. The legs are more often affected than arms. The affected part may be larger at birth or undergo more rapid growth or may become apparent gradually. Radiological examination of the hypertrophic bone may show cortical thickening and osteoporosis may appear later.

Venous varicosities of the affected limb are a frequent finding. Pain is a very common symptom. There is a high rate of spontaneous deep-vein thrombosis and pulmonary embolism. Recurrent episodes of septicemia have complicated the course of lower limb Klippel-Trenaunay syndrome. The development of basal and squamous cell carcinoma has been reported.

Differential Diagnosis

The principal differential diagnoses are Parks Weber syndrome and Proteus syndrome.

In rarer Parks Weber syndrome, limb hypertrophy is caused by multiple arteriovenous fistulae **(Figures 21.8A and B)**. Vascular stains of port-wine-stain type may occasionally occur but these are paler. The affected limb is larger, warm, with conspicuous, pulsatile, superficial veins. The enlarged limb is not liable to be deformed, as is frequent in Klippel-Trenaunay syndrome.

In Proteus syndrome, limb hypertrophy and port-wine stains are associated with a variety of distinct structural abnormalities, which distinguish it clearly.

Patients with Maffucci's syndrome may have complex, deep venous and lymphatic malformations in addition to the typical protuberant vascular swellings that may occur on the hands and feet. In such cases, the clinical picture may resemble Klippel-Trenaunay syndrome.

Investigations

MRI scans and contrast venography should be undertaken before undertaking any procedure on the superficial veins.

Management

The majority of patients do well without treatment, or with elastic support alone. Elastic support reduces symptoms of chronic venous insufficiency, decreases swelling caused by lymphatic stasis and protects the limb from minor external trauma.

Pain can be relieved by stripping of superficial venous varicosities.

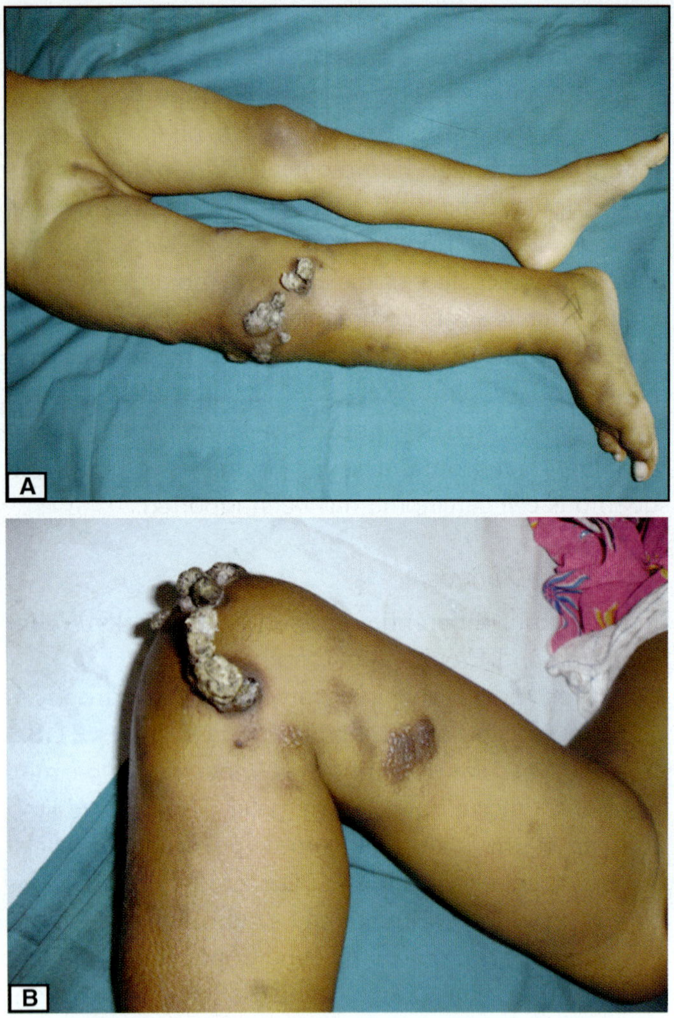

FIGURES 21.8A AND B: Parks Weber syndrome

Patients with Klippel-Trenaunay syndrome should probably be given prophylactic treatment for thrombosis prior to any surgery because of high risk of thrombotic complications.

It is important to recognize any leg length discrepancy as this is likely to lead to scoliosis and early osteoarthrosis of knee and hip.

VENOUS MALFORMATIONS

Blue Rubber Bleb Nevus Syndrome

This is rare disorder comprising of multiple venous malformations of the skin, gastrointestinal tract and, frequently, involvement of other sites.

Clinical features: The lesions may be present at birth, but more often appear progressively during early childhood. The characteristic cutaneous lesions are compressible, blue or purple, soft, rubbery nodules with a wrinkled surface, which have often been simulated to nipples. These are generally small, present in limited numbers and may occur anywhere on the body surface or mucosae of the lips, mouth or glans penis. The lesions may be fairly deep in location, so that only bluish discoloration is visible on the surface. Characteristically, the lesions become painful spontaneously, particularly at night. Once developed, the vascular malformations of the blue rubber bleb nevus syndrome remain unchanged for life, with no tendency to spontaneous regression.

Histopathology: The skin lesions comprise large, blood-filled, vascular lumina in the dermis and subcutaneous fat. The superficially located vascular lumina are often lined only by endothelial cells, whereas the deeper ones have a well-developed vessel wall with smooth muscle. The vascular channels are separated from one another by strands of connective tissue.

Differential diagnosis: Blue rubber bleb nevi need to be distinguished from multiple infantile hemangiomas, Maffucci's syndrome and angiokeratoma corporis diffusum.

Treatment: Patients with blue rubber bleb nevus syndrome mostly require symptomatic treatment of complications. If anemia cannot be controlled by iron supplements or intermittent transfusion, resection of heavily involved lengths of bowel may be indicated. Endoscopic cauterization may also be effective. Successful treatment of the skin lesions with carbon dioxide laser has been reported.

Maffucci's Syndrome (Syn. Dyschondroplasia with hemangioma)

Maffucci's syndrome comprises the association of cutaneous venous malformations with dyschondroplasia.

The skin lesions comprise thick-and thin-walled dermal and subcutaneous vascular spaces, with a single endothelial lining. These lesions are complex venous malformations.

Affected individuals generally have normal appearance at birth, but multiple cutaneous vascular swellings start appearing in infancy. The lesions take the form of soft, bluish, occasionally tender, subcutaneous protrusions. The skin lesions show no tendency to resolve, and grow proportionately with the child. Cavernous lymphangiomas are frequently seen, and may be the sole cutaneous manifestation.

Simultaneously with the cutaneous lesions, the patient develops hard nodules arising from the bones, especially those of the fingers and toes. Pathologically, these are enchondromas, which are radio-lucent. The growth of the affected bones is delayed and distorted due to interference with the epiphyseal cartilage. Pathological fractures are common, which are slow to unite.

A variety of other benign and malignant mesodermal tumors have been reported in Maffucci's syndrome, and the disease has a very high malignant potential.

These patients require careful follow-up. Surgical excision of skin lesions may be justified to improve the patient's appearance.

Gorham's Disease (Syn. Hemangioma with osteolysis)

In this condition, bone is replaced by vascular malformations comprising of ectatic thin-walled sinusoidal blood vessels, and there may be associated cutaneous and soft-tissue vascular or lymphatic malformations. Radiologically, there are lytic bone lesions with little or no sclerosis.

The condition appears to be self-limiting in many cases, but in some patients the disease may be aggressive and ultimately lethal.

SURGICAL ASPECTS OF MANAGEMENT OF PEDIATRIC HEMANGIOMATOUS MALFORMATIONS

Major problem which still prevails is the attempt to bring different forms of vascular lesions under the one heading of hemangiomas. This is termed as International Classification.

There are wide varieties of vascular lesions of different etiology. Hence, no single form of medical or surgical treatment can be applied uniformly to all the vascular lesions (hemangiomas). The most important aspect to remember about hemangiomas is that, these lesions are rarely seen in adults, as most involutes during early childhood and thereafter regress spontaneously. This fact should always be taken into consideration prior to planning invasive management.

Accurate differential diagnosis is essential to avoid mistakes in therapy of other lesions resembling hemangiomas. It is not unusual to have hemangiomatous elements within the lesions of lymphangioma. This is more common in cervical cystic lesions, where lymphangiomatous and vascular elements co-exist. In such lesions, provided there is no respiratory compromise, one can wait for quite sometime for vascular component to regress before the lymphangiomatous part is treated. In majority of the cases of hemangiomas there is no urgency to undertake surgical procedures. However, there are certain indications where surgery may be considered necessary; some of these include an atypical growth, cardiopulmonary de-compensation, large hemangiomas with thrombocytopenia, obstruction to vision, luminal obstruction and rarely, uncontrollable hemorrhage.

Salient features of different forms of hemangioma have been shown in the following figures and specific management suggested.

Large capillary hemangioma of the face has also been termed as 'field fire hemangioma'. Initially these lesions show sudden increase in size for about 6 to 8 months, followed by an arrest in growth and thereafter, regression and involution sets in, which is completed by 3 to 5 years of age. The new born child in **Figure 21.9A** shows remarkable resolution of the lesion at the age of one and half years **(Figure 21.9B)**. Eventually minor surgical procedure may be required to remove the redundant skin and scaring.

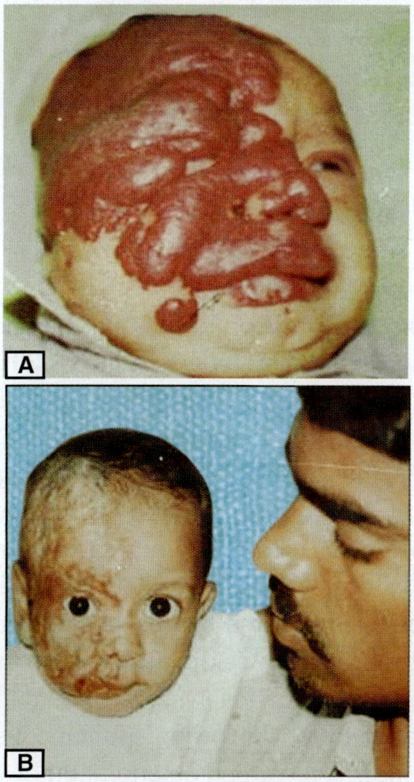

FIGURES 21.9A AND B

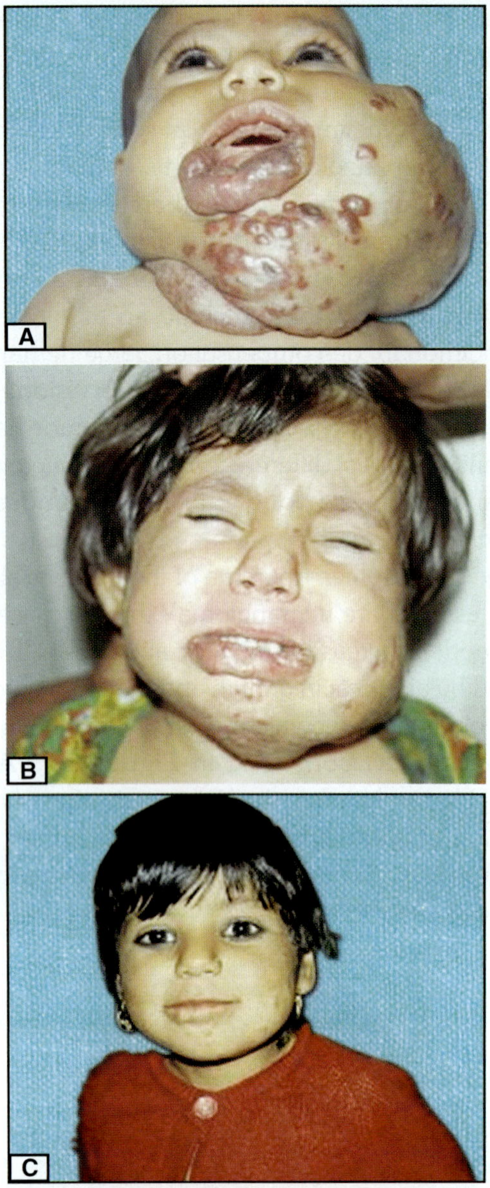

FIGURES 21.10A TO C

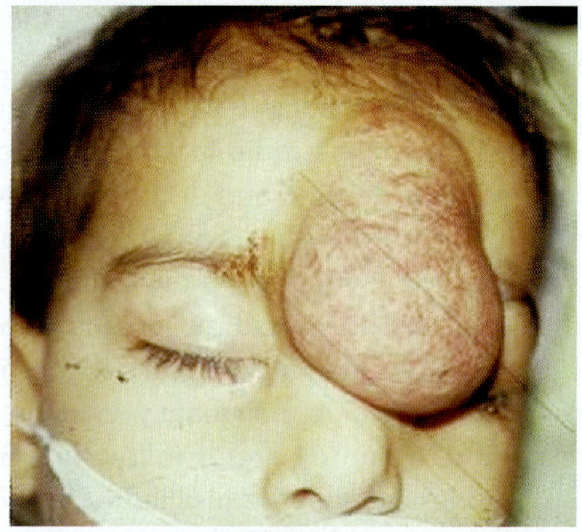

FIGURE 21.11

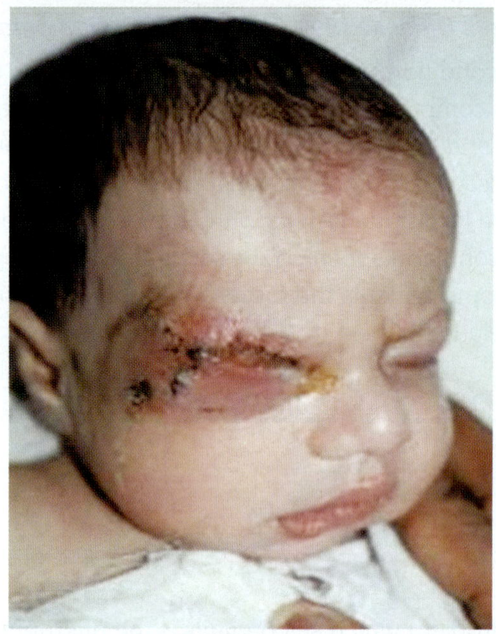

FIGURE 21.12

Remarkable regression of capillary hemangioma has been shown in another patient **(Figures 21.10A to C)** by three years of age. Only lower lip was surgically refashioned with good cosmetic appearance.

Although the capillary hemangioma in **Figure 21.11** is likely to involute spontaneously, because of the obstruction to the vision it is advisable to remove this type of malformations surgically. The child in **Figure 21.12** had hemangioma completely covering the right eye, thus obscuring vision and had to be excised. Cosmetic appearance following such surgery is usually much inferior to that following spontaneous involution but the concerns regarding deterioration of vision is the determinant of surgical excision in such situation.

Occasionally, in the process of regression, hemangiomas may ulcerate because of lack of blood supply. Hemorrhage from such a lesion can be controlled by compression dressings and intra-lesional injection of saline **(Figure 21.13)**.

A small disk-ike lesion of capillary hemangioma **(Figures 21.14 to 21.17)**, although easily amenable to surgical excision, will mostly regress spontaneously with a better cosmetic appearance. About 85% of these lesions regress spontaneously and only few, which have failed to involute completely, should be subjected to surgical removal.

Hemangiomas of lip **(Figures 21.18 and 21.19)** should be allowed to involute, and later surgical reconstruction of the lip may be performed. One such

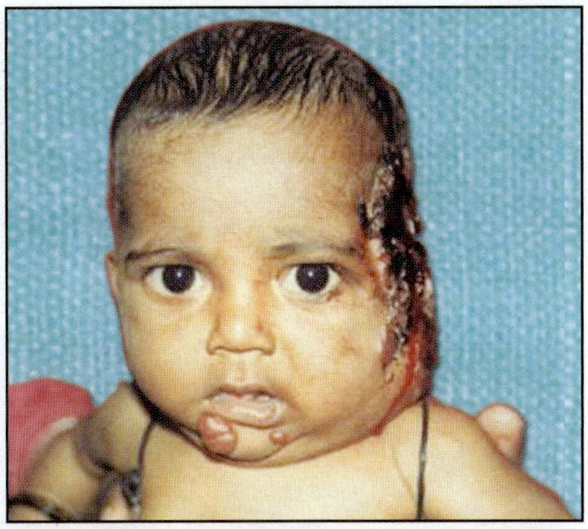

FIGURE 21.13

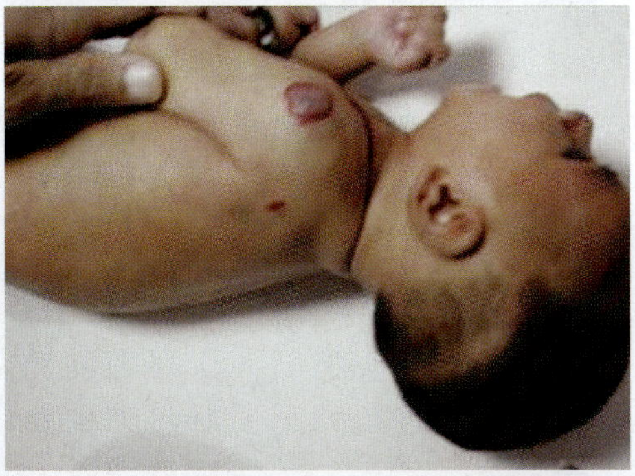

FIGURE 21.14

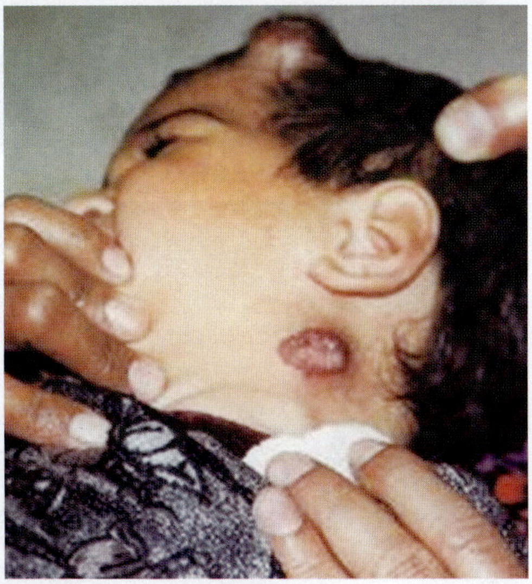

FIGURE 21.15

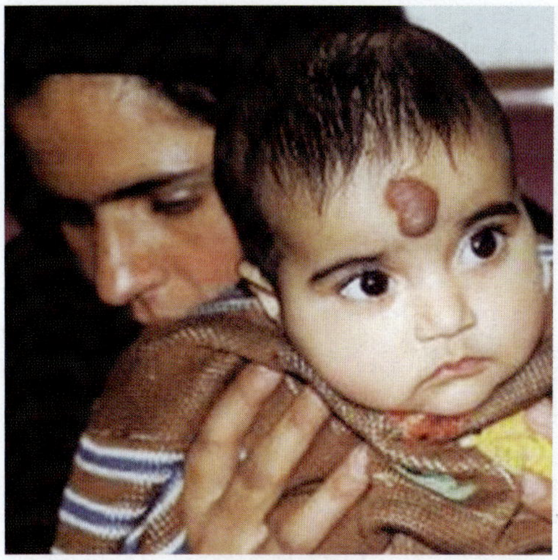

FIGURE 21.16

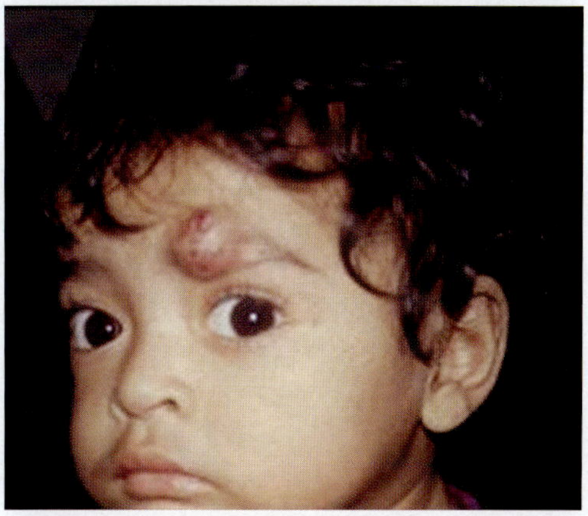

FIGURE 21.17

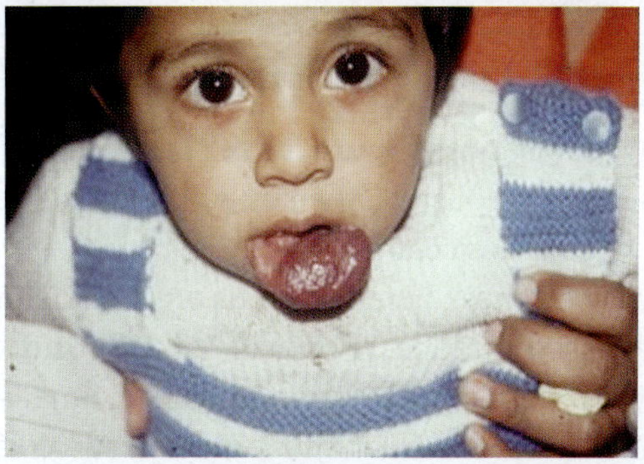

FIGURE 21.18

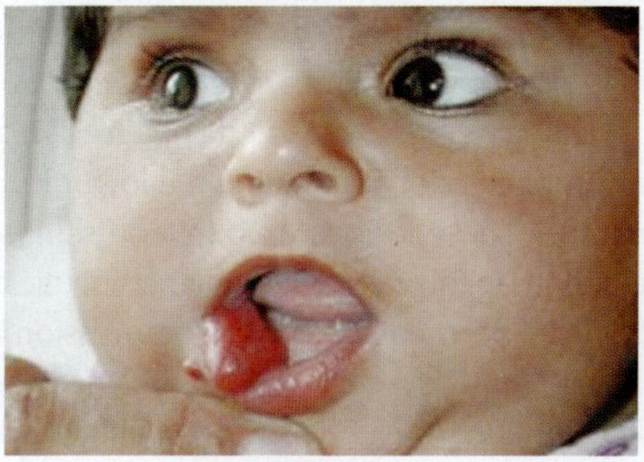

FIGURE 21.19

lesion in a boy **(Figure 21.20)** failed to involute by 8 years of age and at surgery, proved to be neurofibroma.

Regression of capillary cavernous hemangioma **(Figure 21.21)** is slow and the child required systemic therapy with prednisolone for 6 months.

Spider telangiectasias or stellate hemangioma is rare. The lesions have a central feeding vessel with multiple

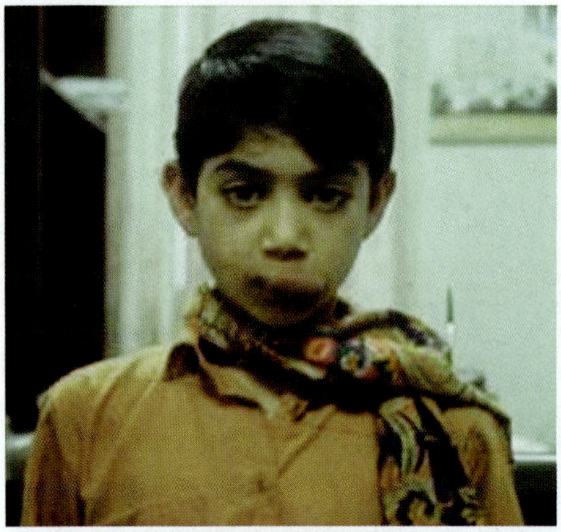

FIGURE 21.20

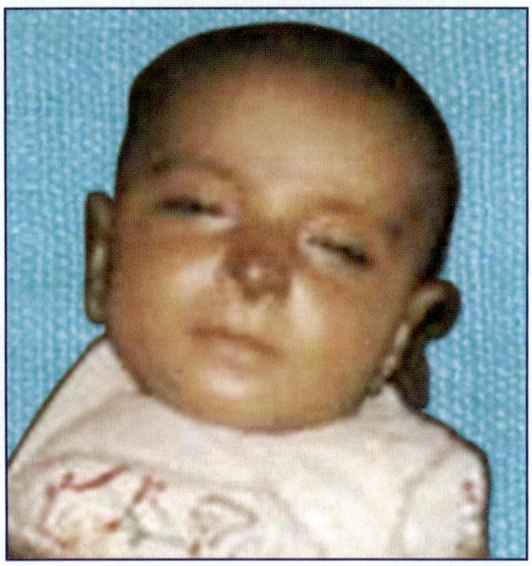

FIGURE 21.21

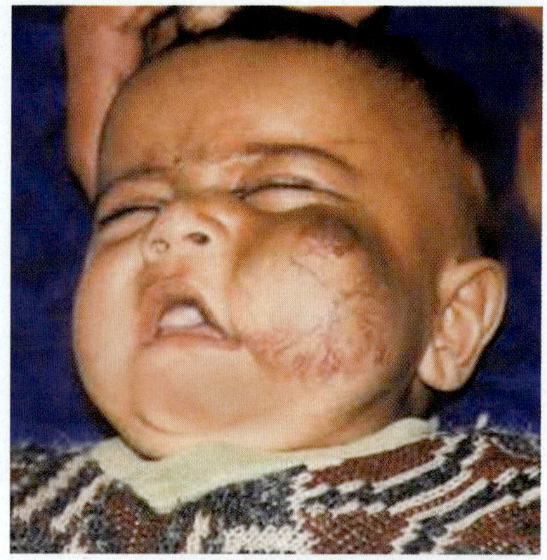

FIGURE 21.22

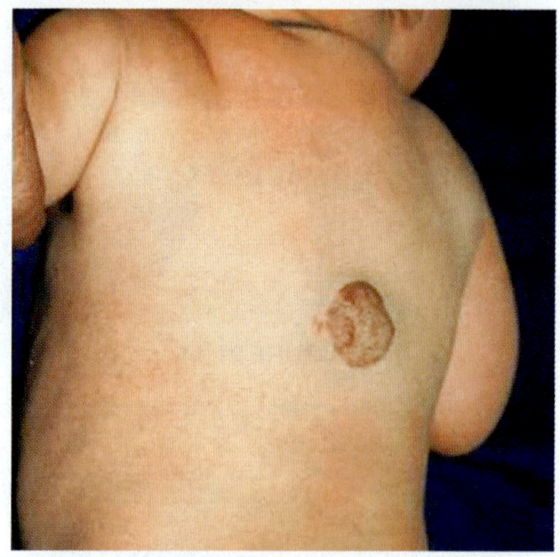

FIGURE 21.23

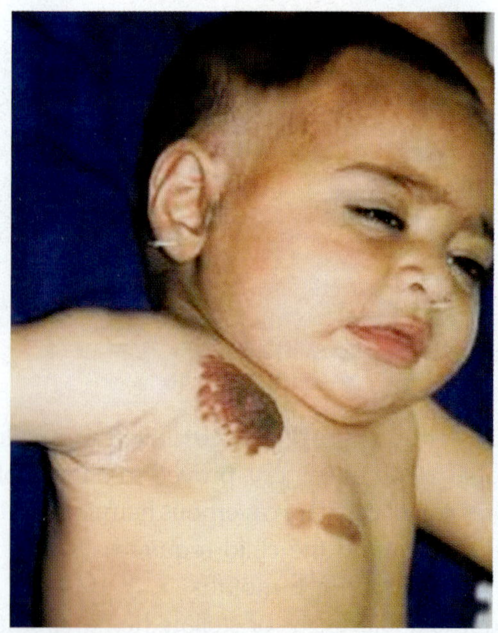

FIGURE 21.24

radiating capillaries **(Figure 21.22)**. About half of these regress spontaneously. Others may be treated with laser or fine needle desiccation.

Strawberry mark hemangiomas are well defined, with slightly raised surface **(Figures 21.23 and 21.24)**. Majority of these involute spontaneously. Smaller lesions on trunk may occasionally be excised to expedite treatment.

Large complex capillary cavernous hemangiomas, especially involving the limbs, are great challenge, as far as the management is concerned. **Figure 21.25** shows a large complex lesion occupying the lower trunk as well as the limbs. These lesions may invade skin, soft tissue and muscles as in this case. Different therapeutic modalities may have to be tried including compression, steroids, embolization and surgery. Many such lesions can be partially managed by use of firm stockings which may even encourage intra-lesional thrombosis and thus may

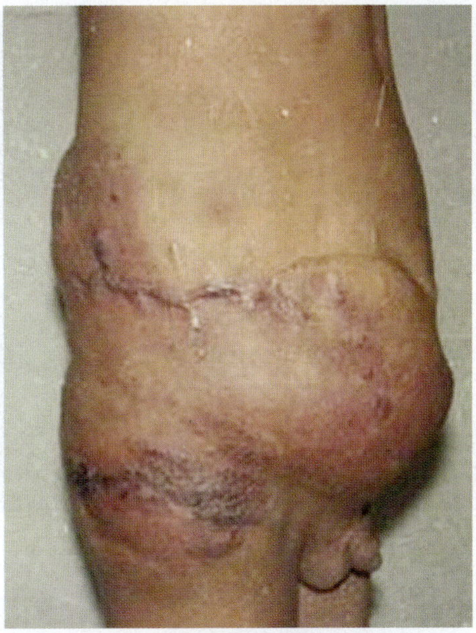

FIGURE 21.25

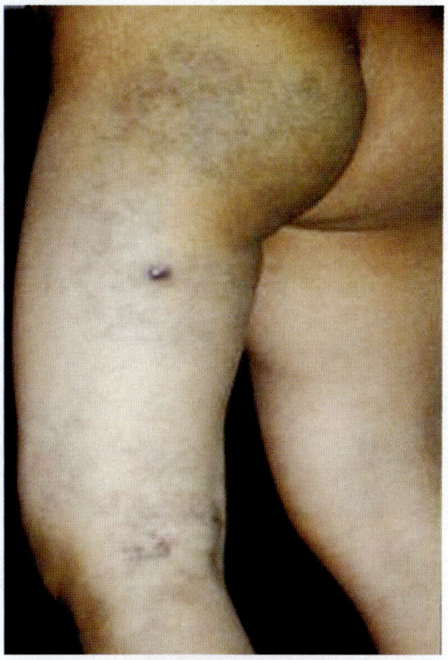

FIGURE 21.27

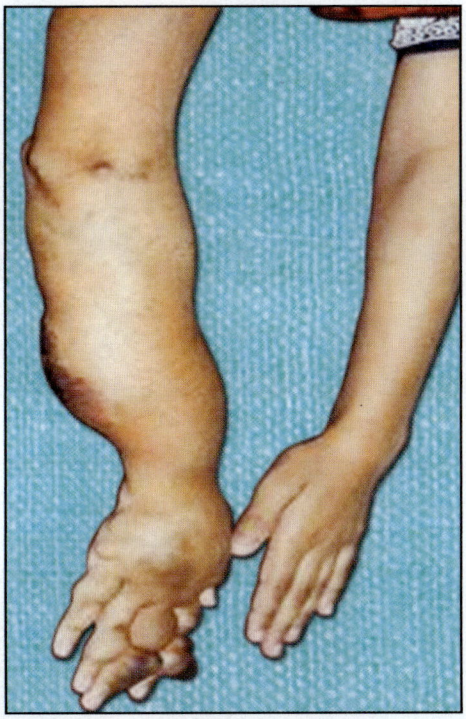

FIGURE 21.26

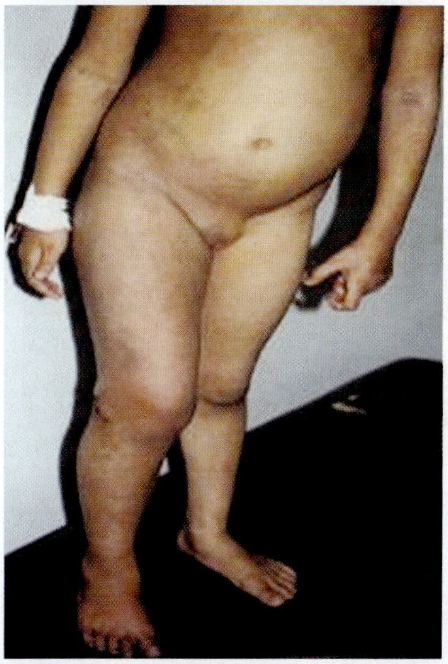

FIGURE 21.28

reduce the size of the hemangioma. Often these diffuse lesions produce enlargement of the affected limb, termed as local gigantism **(Figures 21.26 to 21.28)**. These children often have thrombocytopenia due to platelet trapping.

Ulcerated lesions **(Figures 21.29 to 21.31)** may bleed profusely and may have to be managed by compression dressings, platelet transfusions and large doses of prednisolone therapy. Occasionally, embolization may prove beneficial. Laser treatment is helpful but does not affect the deeper component of hemangiomas.

Cirsoid angioma (racemose aneurysm) and other venous malformations are uncommon entities. These lesions may extend deeply into adjacent tissue and because of proximity to cutaneous nerves, become painful. Arterial embolization seems to offer some benefit. This can be followed by surgical excision. Argon laser therapy has also been found to be helpful **(Figure 21.32)**.

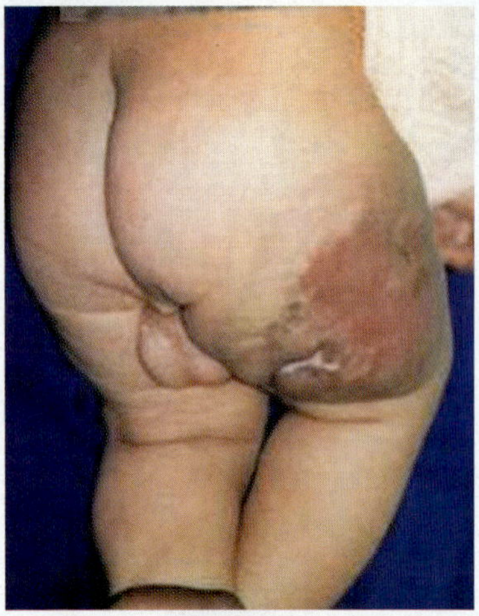

FIGURE 21.29

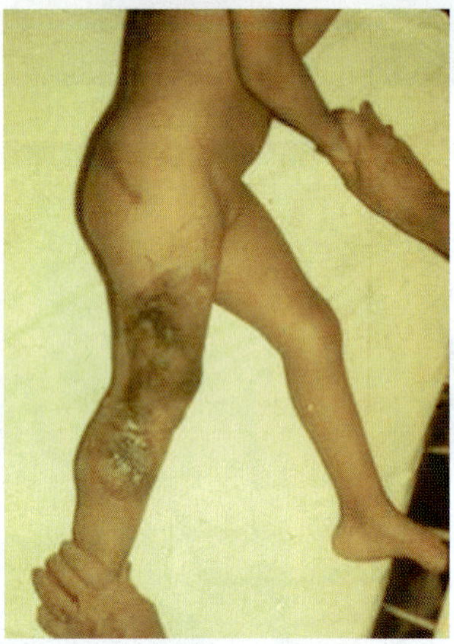

FIGURE 21.30

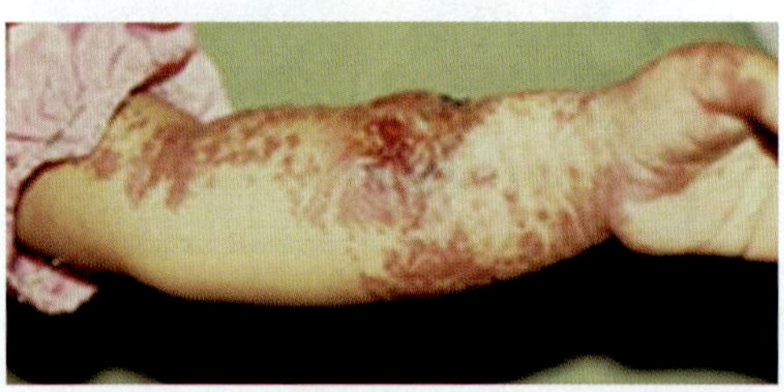

FIGURE 21.31

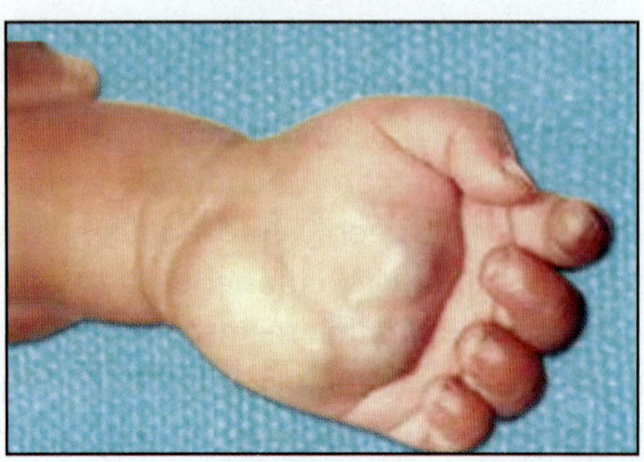

FIGURE 21.32

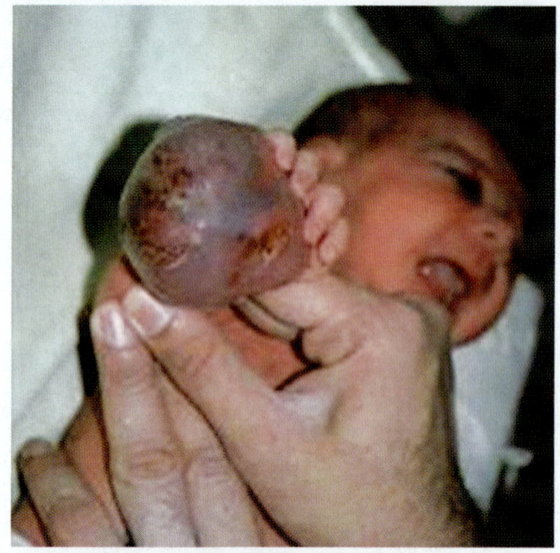

FIGURE 21.33

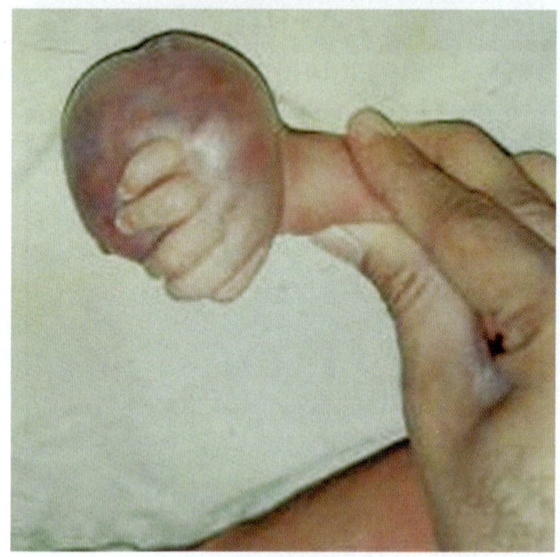

FIGURE 21.34

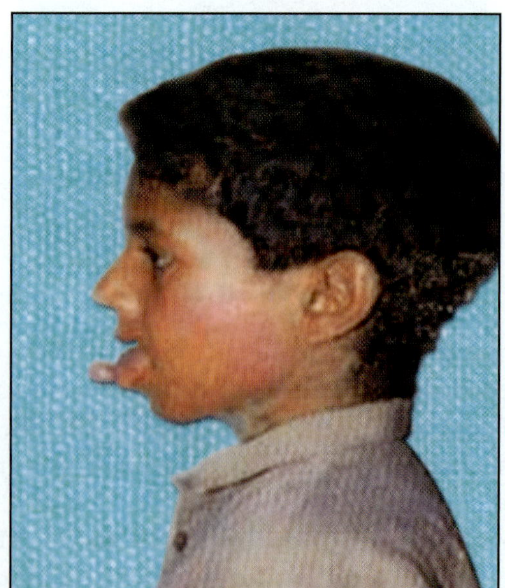

FIGURE 21.35

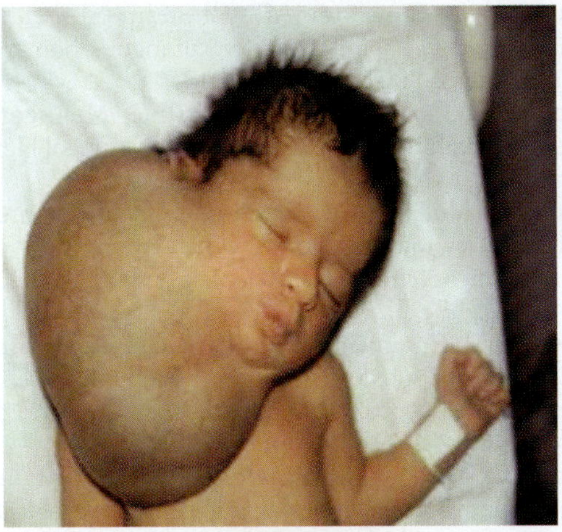

FIGURE 21.36

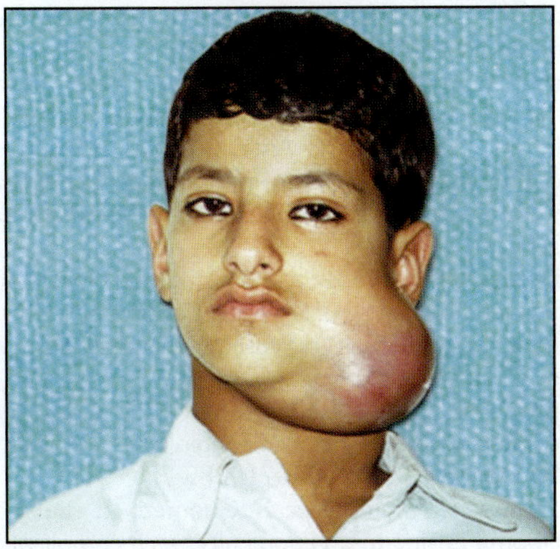

FIGURE 21.37

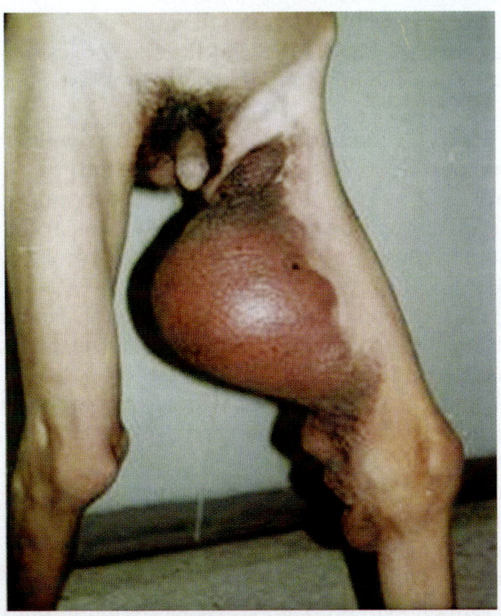

FIGURE 21.38

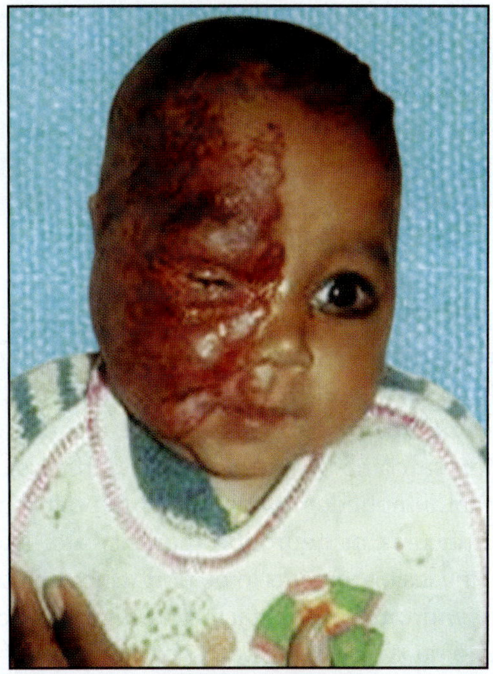

FIGURE 21.39

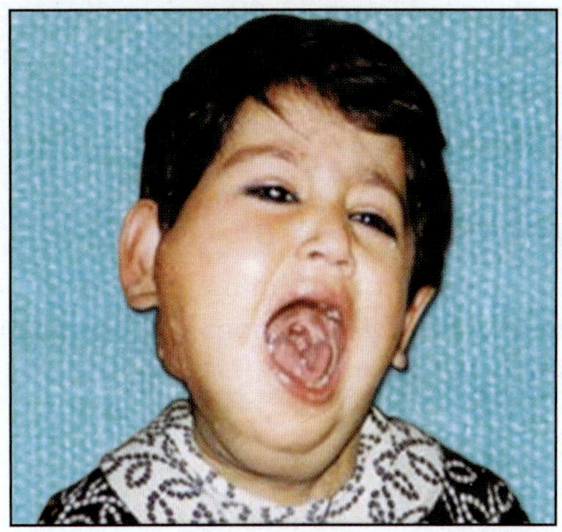

FIGURE 21.40

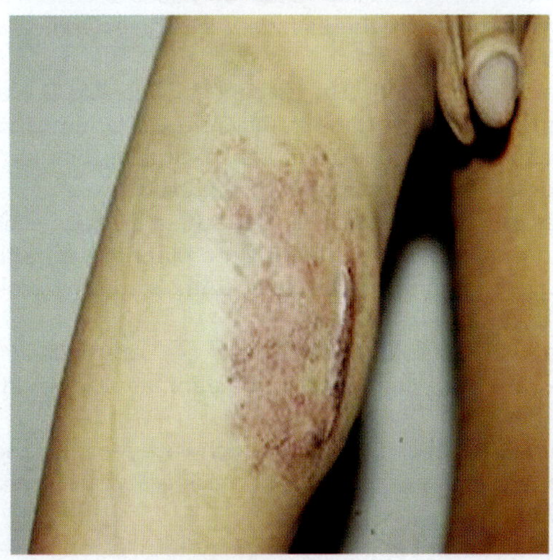

FIGURE 21.41

Rarer lesions like hemangiopericytoma and pyogenic granuloma have also been categorized under the group of hemangioma. Hemangiopericytoma of congenital variety has striking resemblance to congenital fibromatosis. Treatment of these lesions **(Figures 21.33 to 21.35)** is surgical excision. Pyogenic granuloma, which appears to be acquired capillary proliferation, is a fast growing lesion. Removal of this lesion by electrocautery is sufficient.

Hemangiomatous malformations should be differentiated from several other lesions such as lymphangioma **(Figure 21.36)**, rhabdomyosarcoma **(Figure 21.37)**, neurofibrosarcoma **(Figure 21.38)**, abscess, lipoma, congenital lymphedema, idiopathic hypertrophy, *café-au-lait* macules of neurofibromatosis, etc. In **Figure 21.39**, the lesion appears to be port-wine stain of Sturge Weber syndrome but in fact, it is a case of capillary hemangioma which regressed spontaneously.

Figures 21.40 and 21.41 are examples of surgical misadventure. In **Figure 21.40**, facial palsy has occurred after surgical excision of facial hemangioma. In **Figure 21.41** a hemangioma was incised with a misdiagnosis of abscess.

ACKNOWLEDGEMENTS

Surgical Aspects of the management of pediatric hemangiomatous malformations has been contributed by Professor M Naeem Khan.

BIBLIOGRAPHY

1. Auyeung J, Mohanty K, Tayton K. Maffucci's lymphangioma syndrome: an unusual variant of Ollier's disease, a case report and a review of the literature. J Pediatr Opthop 2003; 12: 147-50.
2. Baraldini V, Coletti U M, Cigognetti F, Vercellio G. Haemostatic squeezing and purse-string sutures: optimising surgical techniques for early excision of critical infantile haemangiomas. J Pediatr Surg 2007;42:381-5.
3. Bastarrika G, Redondo P, Sierra A, et al. New techniques for the evaluation and therapeutic planning of patients with Klippel-Trenaunay syndrome. J Am Acad Dermatol 2007;56: 242-49.
4. Batta K, Moss C, Waters R, et al. Early Pulsed dye laser treatment of childhood hemangiomas. Lancet 2003; 361: 348.
5. Ben-AAmitai D, Davidson S, Schwartz M, et al. Sacral nevus flammues simplex: the role of imaging. Padiatr Dermatol 2000; 17: 469-71.
6. Bénateau H, Labbé D, Dompmartin A, Boon L. Sequelae of haemangiomas: surgical treatment. Ann Chir Plast Esthet 2006;51:330-8.
7. Bennett ML, Fleischer AB, Chamlin SL, et al. Oral corticosteroid use is effective for cutaneous hemangiomas. Arch Dermatol 2001; 137: 1208-13.
8. Bloom DC, Perkins JA, Manning SC. Management of lymphatic malformations. Curr Opin Otolaryngol Head Neck Surg 2004; 131: 784-6.
9. Boon LM, Mulliken JB, Enjolras O, et al. Glomuvenous malformation (glomangioma) and venous malformation. Distinct clinicopathologic and genetic entities. Arch Dermatol 2004; 140: 971-6.
10. Bourgeois M, CrimmUins DW, de Oliveira RS, Arzimanoglou A, Garnett M, Roujeau T, Di Rocco F, Sainte-Rose C. Surgical treatment of epilepsy in Sturge-Weber syndrome in children. J Neurosurg 2007;106 (Suppl. 1):20-8.
11. Bree AF, Siegfried E, Sotelo-Avila C, et al. Infantile hemangiomas: speculation on placental trophoblastic origin. Arch Dermatol 2001; 137: 573-7.
12. Bruch-Gerharz D, Gerharz CD, Stege H, et al. Cutaneous vascular malformations in disappearing bone (Gorham-Stout) disease. JAMA 2003; 289: 1479-80.
13. Bucher S, Guerra M, Corrias F, Ribuffo D. Basal cell carcinoma of the nose requiring amputation arising after irradiation for childhood hemangioma. Anticancer Res 2006;26:4767-70.
14. Carvalho VO, Taniguchi K, Giraldi S, et al. Congenital plaque like glomus tumor in a child. Pediatr Dermatol 2001; 18: 223-6.
15. Chiummariello S, Mezzana P, Fioramonti P, Onesti MG, Alfano C, Scuderi N. The use of laser and Varioscope in the management of hemangiomas and vascular malformations. Acta Chir Plast 2006;48:20-5.
16. Clinton TS, Cooke LM, Graham BS. Cobb syndrome associated with a verrucous (angiokeratoma-like) vascular malformation. Cutis 2003; 71: 283-7.
17. De Simone C, Giampetuzzi R, Guerriero C, et al. Squamous carcinoma arising in a venous ulcer as a complication of the Klippel-Trenaunay syndrome. Clin Exp Dermatol 2002; 27: 209-11.
18. Dégardin-Capon N, Martinot-Duquennoy V, Patenotre P, Brevière GM, Piette F, Pellerin P. Early surgical treatment of cutaneous hemangiomas. Ann Chir Plast Esthet 2006; 51:321-9.
19. Di Rocco C, Tamburrini G. Sturge-Weber syndrome. Childs Nerv Syst 2006;22(8):909-21. Epub 2006.
20. Eerola I, Boon LM, Mulliken JB, et al. Capillary malformation-arteriovenous malformation, a new clinical and genetic disorder caused by RASA1 mutations. Am J Hum Genet 2003; 73: 1240-9.
21. Enjolras O, Mulliken JB, Boon LM, et al. Non-involution congenital hemangioma: a rare cutaneous vascular anomaly. Plast Reconstr Surg 2001; 107: 1647-54.
22. Eubanks LE, McBurrney EI. Videomicroscopy of port-wine stains: Correlation of location and depth of lesion. J Am Acad Dermatol 2001; 44: 948-51.
23. Garzon MC, Enjolaras MC, Freiden IJ. Vascular tumors and vascular malformations: evidence for an association. J Am Acad Dermatol 2000; 42: 275-9.
24. Garzon MC, Huang JT, Enjolras O, et al Vascular malformations Part 1 J Am Acad Dermatol 2007;56:353-570.
25. Geh JL, Geh VS, Jemec B, Liasis A, Harper J, Nischal KK, Dunaway D. Surgical treatment of periocular hemangiomas:

a single-center experience. Plast Reconstr Surg 2007;119:1553-62.
26. George M, Singhal V, Sharma V, Nopper AJ. Successful Surgical extirpation of a complex vascular lesion in an infant with Kasabach-Merritt syndrome. Pediatr Dermatol 2002; 19: 340-4.
27. Greene AK, Burrows PE, Smith L, et al: Periorbital lymphatic malformation: clinical course and management in 42 patients. Plast Reconstr Surg 2005; 115: 22-30.
28. Kim HJ, Colombo M, Frieden IJ. Ulcerated hemangiomas: clinical characteristics and response to therapy. J Am Acad Dermatol 2001; 44: 962-72.
29. Kim HJ, Colombo M, Frieden IJ. Ulcerated hemangiomas: clinical characteristics and response to therapy. J Am Acad Dermatol 2001; 44: 962-72.
30. Krebs LT, Shutter JR, Tanigaki K, et al. Haploinsufficient lethality and formation of arteriovenous malformations in Notch Pathway mutants. Genes Dev 2004; 18: 2469-73. Epub 2004 Oct 1.
31. Lahiri A, Kok K, Sharp I, Nishikawa H. Acute exacerbation of macroglossia leading to necrosis of the anterior third of the tongue. J Plast Reconstr Aesthet Surge 2006:59:871-3.
32. Lanigan SW. Taibjee SM. Recent advances in laser treatment of port-wine stains. Br J Dermatol 2004;151:572-33.
33. Lowenstein EJ, Kim KH, Glick SA. Turner's syndrome in dermatology. J Am Acad Dermatol 2004; 50: 767-76.
34. Mallory SB, Rogers E, Berk DR, et al. Congenital plaque-type glomuvenous malformation presenting in childhood. Arch Dermatol 2006; 142: 892-6.
35. Marwah N, Agnihotri A, Dutta S. Central hemangioma: an overview and case report. Pediatr Dent 2006;28:460-6.
36. Metry DW, Hebert AA. Benign cutaneous vascular tumors of infancy. Arch Dermatol 2000; 136: 905-14.
37. Morris PN, Dunmore BJ, Tadros A, et al. Functional analysis of a mutant form of the receptor tyrosine kinase Tie2 causing venous malformations. J Mol Med 2005; 83: 58-63. Epub 2004 Oct 29.
38. Mounayer C, Wassef M, Enjolras O, et al. Facial glomangiomas: large facial venous malformations with glomus cells. J Am Acad Dermatol 2001; 45: 239-45.
39. Naidich HH, Rofsky NM, Rosen R, Karp N. Arteriovenous malformation in a patient with Bannayan-Zonna syndrome. Clin Imaging 2001; 25: 130-2.
40. North P, Waner M, Mizeracki A, et al. A unique microvascular phenotype shared by juvenile hemangiomas and human placenta. Arch Dermatol 2001; 137: 559-70.
41. Poetke M, Philipp C, Berlien HP. Flashlamp-pumped pulsed dye laser for hemangiomas in infancy. Arch Dermatol 2000; 136: 628-32.
42. Puig S, Aref H, Chigot V, et al. Classification of venous malformations in children and implications for sclerotherapy. Pediatr Radiol 2003; 33: 99-103.
43. Rogers M, Lam A, Fisher G. Sonographic findings in a series of rapidly involuting congenital hemangiomas. Pediatr Dermatol 2002; 19: 5-11.
44. Selim MM, Kelly KM, Nelson JS, et al. Confocal microscopy study of nerves and blood vessels in untreated and treated port-wine stains: preliminary observations. Dermatol Surg 2004; 30: 892-7.
45. Senthilkumar M, Thappa DM. Vascular nevi in children. Indian J Dermatol Venereol Leprol 2006; 72: 19-23.
46. Van Lindert Ej, Tan TC, Grotenhuis JA, Wesseling P. Giant cavernous hemangiomas: report of three cases. Neurosurg Rev 2007;30:83-92.
47. Watabe H, Kashima M, Baba T, Mizoguchi M. A case of unilateral dermatomal cavernous haemangiomatosis. Br J Dermatol 2000; 143: 888-9.
48. Wentscher U, Happle R. Linear verrucous hemangioma. J Am Acad Dermatol 2000; 42: 516-8.
49. Werner JA, Eivazi B, Folz BJ, Dünne AA. State of the art of classification, diagnostics and therapy for cervicofacial hemangiomas and vascular malformations Laryngorhinootologie 2006;85:883-91.
50. Won JH, Kim BM, Kim CH, et al. Percutaneous sclerotherapy of lymphangiomas with acetic acid. J Vasc interv Radiol 2004; 15: 595-600.
51. Woo WK, Jasim ZF, Handley JM. Evaluating the efficacy of treatment of resistant port-wine stains with variable-pulse 595-nm pulsed dye and 532-nm Nd:YAG lasers. Dermatol Surg 2004; 30: 158-62.

22

Disorders of Dermis and Subcutaneous Tissue

- Granuloma annulare
- Necrobiosis lipoidica
- Granuloma faciale
- Sweet's syndrome
- Pyoderma gangrenosum
- Scleromyx edema

Sangeeta Amladi, Shankar Savant

- Lipoid proteinosis
- Primary cutaneous amyloidosis
- Foreign body reactions
- Fibrous lesions of the dermis and soft tissue
- Halogenodermas
- Panniculitis
- Lipodystrophy and Lipoatrophy

V K Somani

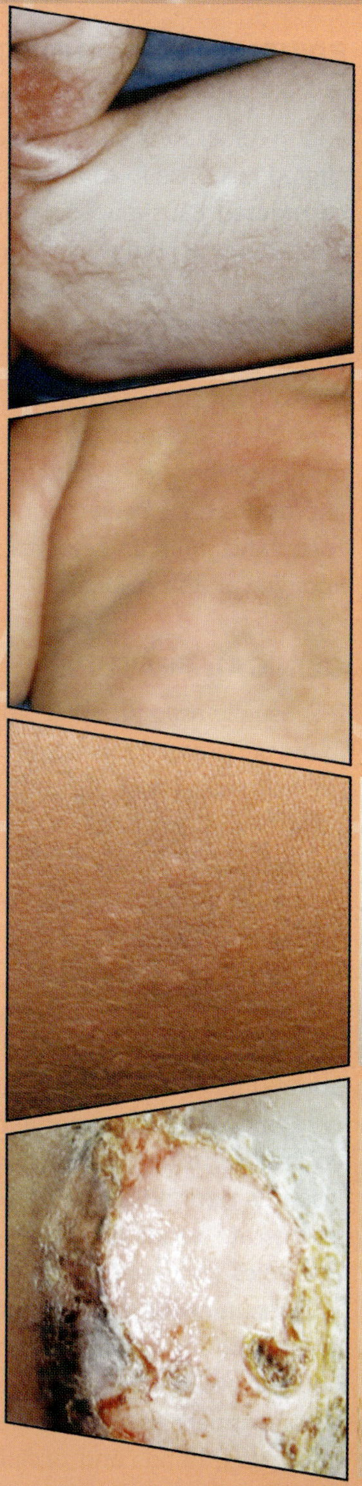

GRANULOMA ANNULARE

INTRODUCTION

It is a benign, inflammatory disorder of dermis and/or subcutis characterized by degeneration of connective tissue and formation of palisaded granulomas.

EPIDEMIOLOGY AND ETIOLOGY

It is a rare disorder predominantly seen in children and young adults. It is perhaps a constitutionally determined altered response to a variety of factors. Trauma has been considered causative or at least a precipitating factor. Occurrence at common sites of injury like dorsa of hands and feet favor this hypothesis but lesions may also appear on sites normally protected from trauma. Sunlight may be the precipitating factor in some patients with lesions on exposed parts. Occurrence of granuloma annulare at sites of insect bite has been documented. Familial incidence has also been described. Granuloma annulare-like lesions have been reported at sites of resolved herpes zoster and rarely in association with tattoos, necrobiosis lipoidica and sarcoidosis.

CLINICAL FEATURES

It is usually asymptomatic. Mild pruritus may be present in the generalized form. Lesions can be painful especially on hands and feet. Four types of granuloma annulare have been described;

- Localized
- Subcutaneous
- Generalized
- Perforating.

The localized type is the most common form found in children. Lesions are single or few in number and approximately 2-5 cm in size. The most common pattern is a ring-shaped or annular lesion composed of skin colored, firm, and smooth papules. The center of the lesion is normal skin **(Figure 22.1)**. Common sites of lesions are hands and feet. Mucous membranes, palms and soles are generally spared.

Subcutaneous granuloma annulare is also known as pseudo-rheumatoid nodule. It commonly occurs in younger children and is rare beyond second decade. The lesions appear as subcutaneous nodules, mostly on pretibial area, hands and occipital area of scalp. They are usually asymptomatic. Diagnosis is difficult in the absence of other typical lesions or histopathology.

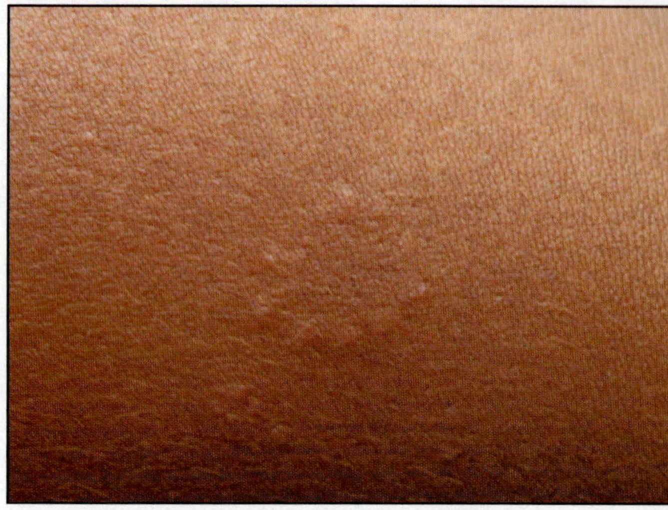

FIGURE 22.1: Granuloma annulare

The generalized form is uncommon. In this type, numerous skin colored papules are distributed symmetrically. Sometimes it clears rapidly. Though in adults generalized granuloma annulare is associated with diabetes mellitus and HIV/AIDS, such association has not yet been observed in the pediatric age group.

Perforating granuloma annulare is rare in children as well as in adults. Clinically it presents as umbilicated papules mostly on the back of hands and sides of fingers.

HISTOPATHOLOGY

Histopathologically granuloma annulare shows palisading granulomas. Histiocytes are arranged either in palisaded or interstitial pattern with sparse lymphocytes. In the center, small quantity of degenerated collagen or fibrin may be present but increased collagen is hallmark of granuloma annulare.

DIFFERENTIAL DIAGNOSIS

The classical clinical picture is not difficult to recognize but may be confused with several other conditions. Tinea corporis shows active border and scaling. Scraping in 10% KOH mount shows fungal hyphae. In tuberculoid leprosy, there is loss of sensation and thickened nerves. Lupus vulgaris presents with surface scaling or crusting and central atrophy. The subcutaneous form mimics subcutaneous nodules but fever, murmur and arthritis are seen in rheumatic fever. Generalized granuloma annulare has to be distinguished from tuberculides, sarcoidosis and lymphoma cutis.

PROGNOSIS AND TREATMENT

It is a self-limiting condition and heals without sequelae. Localized lesions may last from few months to as long as 20 years, although 50% of the cases clear spontaneously within 2 years. Recurrence occurs in about 40% children, but these resolve more quickly than primary lesions.

Since most of the cases of granuloma annulare are asymptomatic, counseling regarding harmless nature of the disease and spontaneous resolution without scarring is most important. Treatment is justified for painful or persistent lesions. Topical or intra-lesional corticosteroids are treatment of choice for localized type of granuloma annulare. Other therapies with variable response are oral chloroquine, dapsone, etretinate, isotretinoin and PUVA therapy.

NECROBIOSIS LIPOIDICA DIABETICORUM

INTRODUCTION

Necrobiosis lipoidica is an idiopathic disorder characterized by indurated plaques located typically on the shins. It usually follows but may precede the diagnosis of diabetes mellitus in children. It is strongly associated with type 1 diabetes mellitus, but has occasionally been reported with type 2 diseases. It is more common in females than in males. Lesions are characteristically located over pre-tibial areas but may also be found elsewhere such as trunk, limbs, face, and scalp.

CLINICAL FEATURES

Necrobiosis lipoidica begins as a painless papule which enlarges to form a plaque with raised rim and a depressed center. The central depressed area becomes waxy, atrophic and reddish brown in color. Telangiectasia may be present. The central atrophic area occasionally ulcerates and may be slow to heal. The size of the lesion is variable, which may be few centimeters or may involve the entire pre-tibial region. Progression of the lesion is slow and persistent over several years.

Lesions located in areas other than the leg may be papular, nodular or plaque-like without central atrophy. Clinically these lesions may resemble granuloma annulare. In rare instances, transfollicular elimination of necrotic material may occur, producing hyperkeratotic plugs. The lesions may coexist with sarcoidosis or granuloma annulare. Rarely, squamous cell carcinoma arising in lesions of necrobiosis lipoidica has been reported.

HISTOPATHOLOGY

The entire thickness of the dermis or its lower two thirds is affected by a process that exhibits variable degree of granulomatous inflammation, degeneration of collagen and sclerosis. Early lesions show superficial and deep perivascular and interstitial mixed inflammatory infiltrate in the dermis. Similar changes are present in septa of adipose tissue. A necrotizing vasculitis with adjacent areas of necrobiosis and necrosis of adnexal structures is also seen.

DIFFERENTIAL DIAGNOSIS

It includes granuloma annulare, sarcoidosis, xanthoma and morphea. In granuloma annulare, waxy yellowish appearance with central atrophy is lacking and association with diabetes mellitus is absent. Annular sarcoidosis presents as erythematous nodules and plaques and can be differentiated histopathologically.

TREATMENT

It is required if the lesion is active and expanding or develops surface ulceration. Topical and intralesional steroids are used for active lesions but may aggravate atrophy; hence the cosmetic result may not be satisfactory. Excision and grafting has been advocated for the chronic ulcerative plaque. Pentoxyphylline and hyperbaric oxygen have been used in few patients.

GRANULOMA FACIALE

INTRODUCTION

Granuloma faciale is an idiopathic cutaneous disorder characterized by red brown plaques on face.

EPIDEMIOLOGY AND ETIOLOGY

It occurs predominantly in middle-aged persons and is less common in children. It is commoner among males. The exact etiology is not clear but is considered a variant of leukocytoclastic vasculitis with prominent eosinophilic infiltrate. Deposition of IgG, IgM and C3 in and around the dermal vasculature has been demonstrated.

CLINICAL FEATURES

Granuloma faciale presents as a solitary asymptomatic reddish brown plaque or nodule with prominent follicular orifices, telangiectasia or scaling on the surface. Lesions never ulcerate. Face is the typical site but rarely extra facial lesions on trunk, extremities and scalp may be accompanied.

HISTOPATHOLOGY

It shows dense polymorphonuclear inflammatory infiltrate in upper half of the dermis which may extend to the lower dermis and subcutis and often around the pilosebaceous follicles. There is a narrow uninvolved Grenz zone beneath epidermis. The infiltrate consists of eosinophils, neutrophils, lymphocytes, histiocytes and few mast cells and plasma cells. Neutrophils are localized around blood vessels. Blood vessels in upper dermis are dilated and eosinophilic fibrinoid material is deposited around some vessel walls. Vascular damage is often very limited.

DIFFERENTIAL DIAGNOSIS

Polymorphous light eruption, granulomatous diseases like rosacea, leprosy, tumid lesions of lupus erythematosus, lymphoma and pseudolymphoma may need to be differentiated.

TREATMENT

It is often quite resistant to therapy; however, since lesions are located on the face, treatment is often desired. Topical or intralesional corticosteroids are recommended as first line therapy. Systemic therapy is reserved for patients who do not respond to above modalities. Dapsone, clofazimine, dermabrasion, CO_2 laser and cryosurgery have been tried.

SWEET SYNDROME (ACUTE FEBRILE NEUTROPHILIC DERMATOSIS)

The term acute febrile neutrophilic dermatosis (AFND) was initially introduced by Sweet in 1964 to describe an uncommon skin condition characterized by painful plaques associated with fever, arthralgia, myalgia and leukocytosis.

EPIDEMIOLOGY

It typically occurs among middle-aged persons. Approximately 5% of the reported cases are in the pediatric age group, between 3 months and 12 years.

ETIOLOGY AND PATHOGENESIS

An upper respiratory tract illness may precede the cutaneous lesions. This has led to the speculation that AFND is a hypersensitivity reaction to a bacterial, viral or alternatively, a tumoral antigen. It has also been proposed that the condition may be a response to inappropriate secretion of cytokines and/or G-CSF (Granulocyte-Colony stimulating factor).

CLINICAL FEATURES

The clinical presentation of Sweet's syndrome is usually distinctive. The patient typically appears ill with persistent high fever, neutrophilia and elevated ESR. Cutaneous lesions occur in few days or weeks. Skin lesions are characterized by abrupt onset of well demarcated, tender, erythematous papules and plaques mostly located on face and upper body. Papules and plaques can coalesce to form large plaques up to 20 cm in diameter. Severe dermal edema may lead to the formation of vesicles and bullae. Plaques may develop yellowish discoloration producing targetoid appearance. Healing usually occurs without scarring. Oral lesions are uncommon.

Widespread lesions occur in hematological disorders. Extracutaneous manifestations of Sweet syndrome are rare but have been described in literature. Ophthalmological manifestations include iritis and conjunctivitis. Arthralgia and myalgia are common. In children, tibial pain with or without related osteomyelitis has been reported. Renal and cardiac manifestations are rare. Proteinuria is most common manifestation of renal involvement.

Criteria for diagnosis of Sweet syndrome:

Major criteria -

1. Acute onset of typical skin lesions
2. Histopathological findings consistent with Sweet's syndrome.

Minor criteria -

1. Fever > 38°C
2. Association with malignancy, inflammatory disorder or antecedent to upper respiratory tract or gastro-intestinal infection

3. Excellent response to corticosteroids.
4. Abnormal laboratory tests at presentation; ESR >20 mm, leukocytosis >8000/cmm, neutrophilia >70%, positive C - reactive protein.

ASSOCIATIONS

In pediatric cases, common associations are osteomyelitis, Fanconi's anemia, leukemia and other hematological malignancies. Inflammatory conditions include inflammatory bowel disease and connective tissue disorders. Infection-related conditions include upper respiratory tract infections, urinary tract infections, viral, fungal and bacterial sepsis. Implicated drugs include minocycline, retinoids, trimethoprim, sulfamethoxazole, diazepam and furosemide. It has also been seen with vaccinations, pregnancy and primary and secondary immunodeficiencies.

HISTOPATHOLOGY

There is dense perivascular infiltrate in upper half of the dermis which may extend throughout the dermis and subcutis. Epidermis is usually spared. In addition, infiltrate may contain scattered lymphocytes, histiocytes and eosinophils. Some neutrophils show nuclear fragmentation (leukocytoclasia). There is no true vasculitis or fibrinoid extravasation; however, vessels often show endothelial swelling.

DIFFERENTIAL DIAGNOSIS

It includes erythema multiforme, vasculitis, Behcet's disease, granuloma faciale, erythema nodosum, bowel-associated dermatitis/arthritis syndrome and bullous pyoderma gangrenosum. Lesions of erythema multiforme are symmetrical, target-like. There is mucosal involvement, absence of lesional pain and constitutional symptoms are mild. Absence of peri-vascular inflammation on histopathological examination can rule out vasculitis. Behcet's disease is characterized by oral and genital aphthosis, arthritis and ocular involvement. The cutaneous lesions are pustular. Histopathological features are either fully developed leukocytoclastic vasculitis or neutrophilic vascular reaction. Nodules of granuloma faciale are typically reddish brown, located mostly on face and not associated with fever.

TREATMENT AND PROGNOSIS

Systemic corticosteroids are the drug of choice, to which excellent clinical response is seen. The recommended pediatric dose is 1-2 mg/kg/day of oral prednisolone. The majority of patients respond within few days but some patients require a maintenance dose for 2-3 months. Recurrences are common (50%) and often occur during tapering of steroids. Oral antibiotics are not effective. There are reports of improvement with colchicine, cyclosporine, dapsone, indomethacin but further studies are required to determine safety and efficacy of these medications in children.

PYODERMA GANGRENOSUM

INTRODUCTION

Pyoderma gangrenosum is a rare, ulcerative, non-infectious neutrophilic dermatosis. It is commonly associated with underlying systemic diseases such as inflammatory bowel disease, arthritis or leukemia. In 1916, Brocq first described pyoderma gangrenosum and later in 1930, Brunsting detailed the morphological features and pathogenesis of the disease.

ETIOLOGY AND EPIDEMIOLOGY

It is more common in adults. Approximately 4% of patients have an onset before 15 years of age. Pyoderma gangrenosum has been reported in infants (4%), aged 1 to 9 months. Although etiology of pyoderma gangrenosum is unknown and very little has been understood about its pathogenesis, an immune mediated process is thought to have an important role. The most common associated defect is a monoclonal or polyclonal gammopathy, but this is not uniformly seen in all patients. There are a few reports suggestive of impaired neutrophil and monocyte chemotaxis and phagocytosis. Histopathological studies have suggested an immune mediated vasculitis. Recent reports indicate a possible autosomal recessive mode of inheritance in some patients.

Common diseases associated with pyoderma gangrenosum are arthritis, inflammatory bowel disease, hepatitis, monoclonal gammopathy, myeloma, SLE, lymphoma, HIV-infection and internal malignancies. Although this disorder can occur without associated conditions but it usually develops in the pediatric age group with a variety of systemic disorders.

CLINICAL FEATURES

Most commonly pyoderma gangrenosum begins as folliculocentric pustules or fluctuant, tender nodules evolving to ulcers with the characteristic violaceous, undermined edge. The base of the ulcer shows granulation tissue, necrosis or purulent exudates **(Figure 22.2)**. Lesions may be single or multiple. In adults, lesions occur on lower extremities and trunk, but in children, these are seen on buttocks, perineal region, head and neck. Pathergy (development of lesion at the site of trauma) has been reported in 20% cases. Koebnerization is evident at sites of trauma including intravenous puncture sites, even at the site of biopsy. Lesions often heal with cribriform scars.

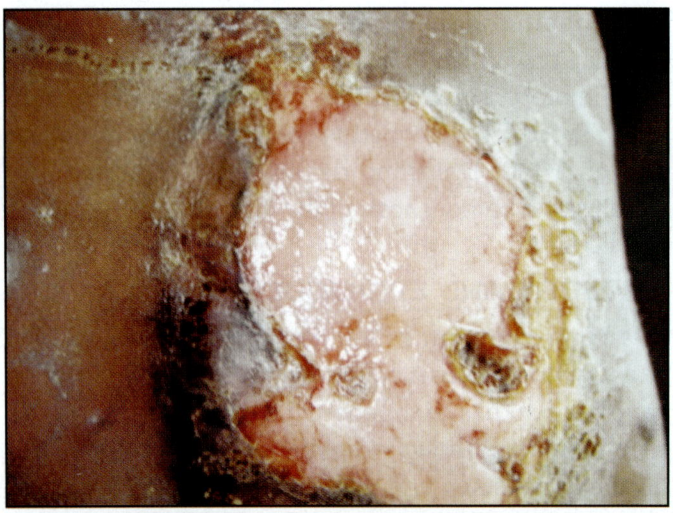

FIGURE 22.2: Pyoderma gangrenosum

The evolution of pyoderma gangrenosum follows one of the two courses; acute rapidly progressive or a chronic indolent course. Other rare forms are bullous, atypical, vegetative or superficial granulomatous pyoderma. Bullous pyoderma gangrenosum is acute and presents with hemorrhagic bullae, mostly on arms and heals with scarring. Vegetative or superficial granulomatous pyoderma presents with painless superficial ulcers with non-purulent base and lacks undermined violaceous border.

HISTOPATHOLOGY

Typical findings include central necrosis and ulceration of the epidermis and dermis surrounded by an acute inflammatory cellular infiltrate mainly composed of neutrophils. Peripheral lymphocytic vascular reaction comprising perivascular and intramural lymphocytic infiltrate without fibrin deposition or mural necrosis is noted.

DIFFERENTIAL DIAGNOSIS

1. Pustules and inflammatory papulonodules are seen in early pyoderma gangrenosum and may mimic folliculitis, furunculosis, insect-bites and vasculitis.
2. The ulcerative stage may simulate deep fungal infection such as cryptococcosis, histoplasmosis or sporotrichosis, atypical mycobacterial infection and ulcerative necrobiosis lipiodica.
3. Other neutrophilic dermatoses such as Sweet's syndrome and subcorneal pustular dermatosis can often be considered in differential diagnosis.

TREATMENT

Though many treatment modalities are available, choice of treatment generally depends on the disease severity as well as the associated systemic disease.

Early or mild lesions are treated with topical therapy, which includes wet compresses, hydrophilic occlusion dressings, topical antibiotics and topical potent corticosteroids. Topical tacrolimus shows good results, but tolerance may be a problem.

If patient is getting multiple lesions or not responding to topical therapy, the drug of choice is oral corticosteroids. Oral prednisolone is started at a dose of 1-1.5 mg/kg and tapered very slowly. Dexamethosone-cyclophosphamide intravenous pulse therapy at half of adult dosage remains the therapeutic choice in case of major side effects of oral corticosteroids or relapse following stoppage of treatment. If case of female children, cyclophosphamide should be replaced with azathioprine. Methotrexate is useful in presence of associated arthritis.

Aggressive surgical debridement and skin grafting and are avoided because of pathergic response. If the patient does not respond to high dose of oral corticosteroids or immunosuppressive drugs, underlying systemic disorders should be ruled out.

PROGNOSIS

The course of the ulcers is quite variable. These may extend rapidly or slowly and may heal at one site while expanding at the other. Spontaneous healing may occur without significant scarring. The course of skin lesions often follows the course of the associated underlying disease.

SCLEROMYXOEDEMA

INTRODUCTION

It is also called 'papular mucinosis' or 'lichen myxoedematosus'. It is a chronic idiopathic disorder characterized by numerous lichenoid papules and nodules due to dermal mucin deposition. The lesions coalesce to form generalized plaques causing extensive thickening and hardening of the skin.

The first description of scleromyxoedema was attributed to Dubreuilh in 1906 and Reitman in 1908. However, it was not until the review of Montgomery and Underwood in 1953, that the disease was distinguished from scleroderma and myxoedema and clinical patterns were described.

EPIDEMIOLOGY AND ETIOPATHOGENESIS

It usually affects middle-aged adults of both sexes. The pathogenesis of scleromyxoedema is unknown. The role of monoclonal gammopathy in patients is still debated. Paraprotein levels do not correlate with either the extent or the progression of the disease.

CLINICAL FEATURES

Confluent papular and sclerotic skin lesions are seen. There is diffuse thickening of the underlying skin. There may be exaggeration of facial ridges and limitation of flexion of the fingers. The involvement of hands may simulate the sclerodactyly of scleroderma. However, the clinical appearance of numerous papules of more or less uniform size, in linear pattern, on erythematous, thickened skin is very distinctive.

DIAGNOSTIC CRITERIA FOR SCLEROMYXOEDEMA

- Generalized papular and sclerodermoid eruptions.
- Microscopic triad of mucin deposition, fibroblast proliferation and fibrosis
- Monoclonal gammopathy
- Absence of thyroid disorder.

HISTOPATHOLOGY

It is characterized by triad of microscopic features;

- Diffuse deposition of mucin in upper and mid dermis
- Increase in collagen deposition
- Marked proliferation of fibroblasts.

The epidermis may be normal or thinned-out by pressure of underlying mucin and fibrosis. The hair follicles may be atrophic and a slight perivascular, superficial lymphohistiocytic infiltrate is often present. The elastic fibers are fragmented and decreased in number. In the localized form, the changes are less characteristic. Mucin accumulates in upper and mid-reticular dermis, fibroblast proliferation is variable and fibrosis is not marked or may be absent.

DIFFERENTIAL DIAGNOSIS

Histopathological examination of skin helps to distinguish localized lichen myxedematosus from papular eruptions that have a similar appearance, such as granuloma annulare, lichen amyloidosis, lichen planus and other lichenoid eruptions. It should be distinguished from systemic sclerosis and scleredema. The presence of papular eruptions especially in linear arrays is a very helpful clinical sign.

TREATMENT

In general treatment is disappointing. Melphalan is the drug of choice; long-term low dose therapy has resulted in gradual resolution of skin lesions, with softening of sclerosis within three months. Plasmapheresis may be beneficial if combined with pulsed corticosteroid or immunosuppressive therapy.

Other therapies reported to be effective are topical betamethasone and dimethylsulfoxide, extracorporeal photochemotherapy and intravenous immunoglobulin.

PROGNOSIS

It is poor despite the introduction of treatment with cyclophosphamide and melphalan. Death may result from complications like bronchopneumonia, coronary occlusion and hematological malignancies.

LIPOID PROTEINOSIS

Syn : Hyalinosis cutis et mucosae. Urbach-Wiethe disease

Salient features

1. Deposition of hyaline-like material into skin, mucosae and viscera.

2. Hoarseness from infancy because of laryngeal infiltration.
3. Skin lesions such as pock-like scarring, waxy infiltration, warty growths.
4. Extracutaneous manifestations like intracranial calcification and upper airway disease.

It was first described in 1929, by Urbach, a dermatologist and Wiethe, an otolaryngologist. Lipoid proteinosis is a rare autosomal recessive disorder, characterized by deposition of hyaline-like material into skin, oral cavity, larynx and internal organs. More than 250 cases have been described. There have been reports of lipoid proteinosis from India, both as isolated cases and in siblings.

ETIOLOGY

Hamada et al, in 2002 mapped the disorder to chromosome 1q21 and identified loss of function mutations in extracellular matrix protein 1 (ECM 1) gene. Later in 2003 they sequenced the ECM1 gene in 10 unrelated patients and concluded that exons 6 and 7 are the most common sites for ECM1 mutations in lipoid proteinosis.

PATHOGENESIS

ECM1 gene encodes a glycoprotein which is involved in skin physiology and homeostasis. It has key roles to play in epidermal differentiation and basement membrane integrity. ECM1 acts as a form of "biological glue" maintaining dermal homeostasis, including regulation of basement membrane and interstitial collagen fibril macro assembly as well as growth factor binding . ECM1 proteins are also expressed in multiple internal organs. Loss of normal function of ECM1 leads to infiltration of various tissues with hyaline-like material, besides the skin and mucosa, and explains the protean manifestations of the disease.

CLINICAL FEATURES

The earliest clinical sign is a hoarse cry, which is either, present at birth or appears in early infancy. It persists for life.

Skin: Skin lesions usually occur during the first 2 years of life and appear in 3 overlapping stages.

1. Initially vesicles, blisters, hemorrhagic or crusted lesions appear mainly over the face and distal extremities. These self-limited lesions heal with varioliform atrophic scarring.
2. Increasing deposits of amorphous hyaline material in the dermis results in generalized skin thickening with waxy, yellow papules and nodules, especially over the face, axillae and scrotum.
3. Verrucous plaques may develop as a result of frictional trauma, over hands, elbows, and knees.

A very classic and pathognomonic feature is a string of bead-like papules along eyelid margins, known as moniliform blapharosis. It is seen in about 50% of individuals. Scalp involvement may lead to patchy or diffuse hair loss.

Oral cavity: The lips, gingiva and tongue may be infiltrated and show pebbling. Tongue may become woody hard with restricted range of movement, impaired gustation and speech impediments. Dental anomalies like hypoplasia or aplasia of lateral incisors, premolars and molars have been reported. Infiltration of the Stensen's duct can lead to recurrent parotitis.

Upper respiratory tract: Involvement of larynx, vocal cords and adjacent structures may cause hoarseness, dysphagia and even airway obstruction in some cases.

Central nervous system: A unique and pathognomonic finding is bilateral, intracranial, sickle or bean-shaped calcifications in the temporal lobe. It is seen in children older than 10 years of age and in at least 70% of cases. Neurologic manifestations include seizures, memory loss and rage attacks.

HISTOLOGY

Hematoxylin-and-eosin staining of early lesions reveals pale pink, hyaline-like thickening of the papillary dermal capillaries. Later lesions reveal hyperkeratosis, occasionally papillomatosis, and a thickened dermis in which diffuse thick bundles of pink hyaline deposits are seen oriented perpendicular to the dermoepidermal junction in diffuse pattern. Lipoid proteinosis is characterized by periodic acid-Schiff (PAS)—positive, but diastase-resistant basement membrane thickening at dermal epidermal junction, surrounding blood vessels and adnexal epithelia, as well as deposition of hyaline material in the dermis. Ultrastructural examination reveals concentric rings of excess basement membrane surrounding blood vessels, and irregular reduplication of lamina densa at dermoepidermal junction resulting in onion-skin appearance.

DIAGNOSIS

Diagnosis is by characteristic clinical features, histopathological and X-ray findings **(Table 22.1)**.

TABLE 22.1: Diagnostic markers

Clinical:
1. Hoarseness of voice
2. Moniliform blepharosis
3. Inability to protrude the tongue beyond the lip margins
Investigatory:
4. Histopathology : PAS positive hyaline-like material
5. Bilateral intracranial calcification

Polymerase chain amplification and direct nucleotide sequencing of ECM1 gene can demonstrate pathogenic mutations and provide definitive evidence for the diagnosis. Recently, rapid diagnosis by skin immonohistochemistry using an anti-ECM1 antibody has been reported.

DIFFERENTIAL DIAGNOSIS

Erythropoietic protoporphyria closely mimics lipoid proteinosis. Presence of scarring mainly in the exposed area, in addition to solar sensitivity distinguishes this from lipoid proteinosis. Histologically hyaline deposition is milder and is absent around sweat coils. The other clinical differential diagnosis includes xanthomatosis, extracellular cholesterolosis, amyloidosis, colloid millium, papular mucinosis, and myxedema.

Prognosis

Disease runs a stable or a slowly progressive course. Life expectancy is normal, but for the risk of respiratory obstruction.

Treatment

No treatment is uniformly successful. Anecdotal reports of successful treatment with various agents—like penicillamine, etretinate, oral dimethyl sulfoxide and potent topical steroids are described. Surgical modalities like dermabrasion and CO_2 laser therapy may be helpful.

PRIMARY CUTANEOUS AMYLOIDOSIS

DEFINITION

Amyloidosis refers to an abnormal extracellular deposition of one of an insoluble fibrillar protein in various tissues associated with changes in the tissue architecture and resultant tissue dysfunction.

Cutaneous amyloidosis is a rare disease in childhood. Most frequent forms seen are macular or lichen amyloidosis. Systemic amyloidosis is observed in children with epidermolysis bullosa, cystic fibrosis and juvenile rheumatoid arthritis. Primary systemic amyloidosis is extremely rare in children.

STRUCTURE AND PATHOGENESIS

Irrespective of the clinicopathologic type or the organ involved, amyloid deposits are composed of paired, linear, nonbranching fibrils that are 7.5-10 nm thick, of indefinite length and are arranged in a loose meshwork. The beta pleated form is abnormal in human tissue and is believed to be responsible for the congophilia and for the protection of amyloid deposits from degradation and phagocytosis, contributing to the progressive and irreversible course of amyloidosis. Primary and myeloma-associated systemic amyloidosis have immunoglobulin light chains as precursors to the amyloid fibril protein, termed amyloid L (AL) whereas in secondary systemic amyloidosis, the deposits are composed of non immunoglobulin amyloid A (AA) protein.

STAINING CHARACTERISTICS

Several stains are employed to demonstrate amyloid in the skin **(Table 22.2)**. Usually a battery of stains is indicated.

TABLE 22.2: Special stains for amyloid

1. Triphenylmethane dyes – methyl violet , cresyl violet
2. Periodic acid-Schiff (PAS)
3. Cotton dyes – congo red, pagoda red, Sirius red, etc. with fluorescence /polarized light microscopy
4. Fluorescent dyes—thioflavin-T and Phorwhite BBU
5. Immunohistochemical staining with anti-SAP
6. Immunohistochemical staining with antikeratin antibody EAB 903 in primary localized cutaneous amyloidosis.

PRIMARY LOCALIZED CUTANEOUS AMYLOIDOSIS (PLCA)

PLCA refers to the deposition of amyloid in normal skin without any visceral involvement. Of the 3 subtypes are described lichenoid and nodular are often not seen in children.

1. Macular amyloidosis (MA)

2. Lichen amyloidosis (LA)
3. Nodular amyloidosis (NA).

ETIOLOGY

In NA, plasma cells produce immunoglobulin light chains that are precursors to the amyloid fibril protein termed amyloid L. Genetic predisposition, as evidenced by familial grouping and racial susceptibility is of importance in both MA and LA.Chronic friction and pruritus are frequently implicated in localization of the lesions of amyloidosis. Amyloid deposits in MA and LA bind to antikeratin antibodies. Two theories have been proposed to explain the origin of amyloid deposits in skin. Hashimoto's theory suggests that there is focal epidermal damage and filamentous degeneration of keratinocytes followed by apoptosis and conversion of these colloid bodies into amyloid in papillary dermis.The secretory theory of Yamagihara et al proposes that the amyloid in MA is secreted by disrupted basal cells and is assembled at the dermoepidermal junction (DEJ).

Histopathology

In nodular cutaneous amyloidosis, an atrophic epidermis overlies large, amorphous, clefted masses of amyloid, extending from the papillary and reticular dermis into the subcutaneous fat. Deposits can also be seen around adnexa, blood vessels, and fat cells. In contrast the amyloid deposits in MA and LA are confined to papillary dermis. The amyloid deposits are usually small and globular, resembling colloid bodies in MA and may escape detection. Epidermis is normal but pigmentary incontinence and melanophages are seen. On the other hand, hyperkeratosis, acanthosis and larger deposits of amyloid characterize LA. The deposits are often large enough to displace the rete ridges laterally.

CLINICAL FEATURES

LA is the commonest and the best known of the three types of PLCA. It presents as a persistent pruritic eruption of discrete hyperkeratotic, hyperpigmented papules distributed mainly on the shins. Other areas like calves, ankle, feet and trunk may also be involved occasionally. The papules may coalesce to form plaques.

MA presents as an eruption consisting of small, dusky-brown or grayish-pigmented macules over the upper back, chest and arms. These macules coalesce to produce a characteristic reticulate or rippled pattern of pigmentation. Associated pruritus may be of variable intensity.

Treatment

Treatment of PLCA, in general, is not satisfactory. Most of the reports are anecdotal. Lichen amyloidosis may respond to dermabrasion, topical DMSO, and etretinate, cyclophosphamide and ciclosporine are reported to be of some benefit in LA.

FOREIGN BODY REACTIONS

Foreign body reaction is generally regarded to be a distinctive type of granulomatous reaction induced by introduction of some extraneous or foreign material into skin or deeper tissues. Other types of reactions like inflammatory, infective and allergic reactions to foreign body may also occur.

Foreign body reaction may develop as a result of

1. Trauma—metal, wood splinters, glass, thorn, etc.
2. Occupational—beryllium, silica, hair, fiberglass
3. Cosmetic—tattoos, silicone, collagen, paraffins, vegetable oils, new fillers
4. Post surgical—suture material, talc, starch
5. Injections—immunization, insulin, calcium salts, vitamin K, oily depot preparations.

PATHOLOGY

After a phase of initial inflammation, the foreign material attracts monocytes which evolve into tissue macrophages. These cells along with epitheloid histiocytes, and foreign body type of giant cells form a granuloma around the foreign body.

DIAGNOSIS

If clinical examination is inconclusive, imaging techniques like plain X-ray, ultrasound, CT scan or even MRI may be considered. Histopathological procedures for, e.g. H&E staining, PAS stain, dark field examination, polarizing microscopy, etc. can also be helpful in some cases.

CLINICAL FEATURES

Clinical features differ and depend upon the mode of injury, type of foreign body, route of entry and presence of infection, toxin, etc. There are certain distinctive forms of foreign body reaction, which can present in children and are described here.

Tattoos

Introduction of insoluble pigments into the skin by trauma, or for cosmetic or medicinal purpose produces tattoos. Tattoos associated dermopathies may be allergic, granulomatous, photosensitive or infective leading to transmission of syphilis, tuberculosis and hepatitis or viral infections like molluscum contagiosum and viral warts. It may show Koebner's response in lichen planus and psoriasis. Allergic reactions are most commonly due to cinnabar (mercuric sulphide) but are also seen with cobalt, chrome and manganese.

Immunization Granulomas

The aluminium hydroxide component of vaccines and toxoids is fairly commonly implicated in causation of immunization granulomas. This type of foreign body reaction has been reported after the use of DPT, influenza and hepatitis B vaccines. Children prone to such reactions should receive non-adsorbed vaccines and toxoids. Recently a foreign body reaction has been reported to the monosodium glutamate component of BCG vaccine in a 7-month-old infant.

Mercury

Prolonged exposure to mercury can cause acrodynia (pink disease), a distinct syndrome restricted to infants and young children. It could be because of an idiosyncratic hypersensitivity reaction.

Calomel containing teething and diaper powders, fungicides in paints, anthelmintics, termite protected wood, laxatives and ammoniated mercury ointments all were the source of mercury. Clinical features may resemble Kawasaki disease. Mercury induced foreign body are relatively rare The granuloma presents as flesh colored to erythematous or hyper pigmented mass, months after the introduction of mercury. Diagnosis can be confirmed by histopathology and scanning electron microscopy.

Carbon

Fire cracker injuries or puncture wound by a pencil can produce discoloration of the skin from the embedded carbon. The deposited carbon can evoke a connective tissue reaction and even keloids.

Silica

Road traffic accidents or sports injuries may produce tattooing of dirt (silicon dioxides) into the skin, leading to silica granulomas. They manifest as black or blue papules or macules generally arranged in a linear fashion. Excision and systemic steroid may help but recurrences are common.

FIBROUS LESIONS OF THE DERMIS AND SOFT TISSUE

Fibromatoses is a group of diseases, characterized by benign proliferation of fibrous or myofibrous tissue. These may be locally progressive but do not metastasize. Many of the childhood lesions tend to resolve spontaneously.

Benign fibromatoses of childhood can be broadly divided into two groups :

I. Those with a generally indolent course
   a. Myofibroma/myofibromatosis
   b. Fibromatosis colli
   c. Fibrous hamartoma of infancy
   d. Nodular fasciitis
   e. Knuckle pads.

II. Those with a potential for a locally aggressive course
   a. Infantile fibromatosis
   b. Plantar palmar fibromatosis
   c. Gingival fibromatosis
   d. Digital fibromatosis
   e. Calcifying aponeurotic fibroma.

KNUCKLE PADS

Definition

Knuckle pads are well defined hyperkeratotic firm thickenings over the extensor aspect of any digital joint. The term is a misnomer, as majority of the lesions occur over the proximal interphalangeal joints.

Etiology

Knuckle pads are usually idiopathic in children. Familial form with onset in childhood also has been reported, where it is transmitted as an autosomal dominant trait. Another category of knuckle pads, associated with other fibrosing conditions usually arises in adulthood. Often repeated trauma is widely believed to be one of the major causes of knuckle pads.

Pathology

Epidermis shows regular acanthosis and compact hyperkeratosis.The dermal connective tissue is hyperplastic.

Clinical Features

Familial forms usually have their onset in childhood, whereas idiopathic variety tends to begin in adolescence. Lesions most commonly occur over the proximal interphalangeal joints, but may occur on any other joints. The onset is insidious and they evolve slowly into the typical smooth, firm, circumscribed, flat or convex plaques over the skin. They are usually asymptomatic. Multiple lesions are part of Bart-Pumphrey syndrome.

Prognosis

Persistence for several years is the rule. Spontaneous resolution has been reported.

Treatment

Topical keratolytics and intralesional corticosteroids have been tried with little result.

PLANTAR PALMAR FIBROMATOSIS

Syn: Palmar fibromatosis – Dupuytren's contracture
Plantar fibromatosis – Ledderhose's disease

Definition

Plantar palmar fibromatosis is a form of fibromatous hyperplasia, involving the plantar or palmar fascia, which may be associated with flexion contractures of one or more digits.

Etiology

Local ischemia and consequently, a build up of free radicals is thought to evoke the fibromatous reaction. Palmar fibromatosis may be inherited as an autosomal dominant trait.

Clinical Features

Palmar fibromatosis generally starts as dimpling of the palmar skin over the head of the fourth metacarpal, or as a nodule. The puckered skin slowly advances until eventually a flexion deformity of the ring and little finger develops.

Plantar fibromatosis usually starts as a nodule over the medial aspect of mid foot.

Treatment

Surgical treatment like complete removal of palmar aponeurosis provides relief. Therapy directed against free radicals, for example, allopurinol and vitamin C have been tried with variable results. Recently collagenase injections have also been tried with good results.

OTHER FIBROMATOSES

Myofibromatosis, fibrous hamartoma of infancy, nodular fasciitis, etc. do not have a distinct clinical picture. They all present as painless subcutaneous or dermal nodules appearing at birth or in the first 2 years of life. Histopathology can help distinguish these benign conditions from one another.

HALOGENODERMAS

Halogenodermas are skin eruptions that result from ingestion of, or exposure to halogen-containing drugs. Neonates can acquire from mother's taking bromides during breastfeeding. The terms iododerma, bromoderma and fluoroderma are used to describe the skin lesions caused by consumption of iodide, bromide or fluoride containing preparations.

PATHOPHYSIOLOGY

Halogenodermas may be regarded as a delayed hypersensitivity reaction. Lymphocyte transformation tests with iodinated human serum albumin have been positive, suggesting that iodine acts as a hapten. Iodides can act as a chemoattractant for polymorphonuclear leukocytes, which release inflammatory mediators. These mediators may be responsible for the hyperproliferative and vegetative lesions seen in halogenodermas. Histopathologic changes of vasculitis in some cases can be attributed to these mediators.

IODODERMA

Iododerma was reported more frequently earlier when iodine was used as an expectorant, sedative, anti-inflammatory and anti-thyroid agent. Nowadays it is a rare clinical entity.

CAUSES

Administration of radiopaque contrast medium for cholecystography, urography and CT scan has led to iododerma. ^{131}I therapy for hyperthyroidism has been reported to induce iododerma of the ankles and feet in 2% of the treated patients. Drugs such as potassium iodide, expectorants and lithium have all been shown to cause iododerma.

CLINICAL FEATURES

Iododerma from radiopaque material generally presents as an acute eruption, whereas it has an insidious onset with oral iodine containing preparations. The lesions may be acneiform, papulonodular, pustular, hemorrhagic or ulcerative and typically involve the seborrheic areas, like face, neck, and upper trunk. Vegetating type of lesions have also been reported. Underlying diseases including multiple myeloma, polyarteritis nodosa, rheumatoid arthritis, lymphoma and glomerulonephritis are thought to predispose patients to iododermas.

BROMODERMA

It is a rare cutaneous reaction that develops after consumption of products containing bromides. It has been reported after administration of syrup containing sodium bromide. Prolonged therapy with drugs containing potassium bromide, for example, anticonvulsants, may also cause bromoderma.

Typically bromoderma presents as pustules, vegetating plaques, or plaques with peripheral pustules. Multiple vegetative or pustular lesions may appear over the legs or other hair bearing areas.

FLUORODERMA

Fluoride gel preparations applied to the teeth for the prophylaxis of post-irradiation dental caries may cause fluorodermas. Numerous, papulonodular skin lesions scattered all over the body may be seen.

Histology

Cutaneous halogenodermas have three main features:

1. Papillomatosis or pseudoepitheliomatous hyperplasia
2. Intraepidermal abscesses with neutrophils, eosinophils and occasionally necrotic keratinocytes
3. A dense, mixed, inflammatory infiltrate in the dermis, composed of neutrophils, eosinophils and histiocytes.

Diagnosis

The diagnosis of halogenodermas generally rests on clinical evaluation and history. Serum and urine bromide or iodide levels are raised. Raised ESR, TLC and eosinophilia are the hematological changes seen.

Treatment

Generally no specific treatment is required. Skin lesions resolve in 4-6 weeks after the causative factor is eliminated. Diuretics may hasten bromide ion clearance from the body. Skin lesions may be treated with systemic steroids.

PANNICULITIS

An inflammatory disorder that is primarily localized in the subcutaneous and/or perivisceral fat is termed panniculitis. The clinical spectrum of panniculitis in children resembles that in adults. Panniculitis can be classified histopathologically as follows:

CLASSIFICATION

I. Septal panniculitis: Erythema nodosum

II. Lobular panniculitis:
   Nodular panniculitis
   a. Idiopathic
   b. Secondary—Pancreatic panniculitis, α1 antitrypsin deficiency panniculitis, lipoatrophic panniculitis, panniculitis associated with crystal deposition–sclerema neonatorum, subcutaneous necrosis of newborn, poststeroid panniculitis, Fat necrosis–cold injury, lymphomatous, cytophagic histiocytic.

III. Mixed panniculitis: LE profundus, scleroderma, subcutaneous sarcoidosis, subcutaneous granuloma annulare, necrobiosis lipoidica, infective panniculitis

IV. Panniculitis with vasculitis
   - Small vessel—leukocytoclastic vasculitis
   - Large vessel—polyarteritis nodosa, erythema induratum.

ERYTHEMA NODOSUM (EN)

This is the most common form of panniculitis and is the prototype of septal panniculitis.

Definition

It is characterised by a sudden onset of symmetric, tender, erythematous, warm nodules or plaques, chiefly affecting shins and less commonly, thighs and forearms.

Incidence

In children the exact incidence is unknown, but the incidence of erythema nodosum in children under 15 years of age was reported to be less than 8% of the total cases of erythema nodosum seen in a series. It is rare before 2 years of age. It occurs 3 times more commonly in females. Sex incidence before puberty is equal.

Pathogenesis

Erythema nodosum is regarded as a hypersensitivity response to a variety of stimuli including drugs, benign and malignant systemic diseases and bacterial, viral and fungal infections.

There is immune complex formation and deposition in the venules of deep dermis and capillary bed of subcutaneous fat, which leads to activation of complement and damage of the vessel walls.

Etiology

Streptococcal infections and tuberculosis are the most frequent etiologic agents of erythema nodosum in children. Other causes are as follows.

Causes

Infection

- Bacteria—*Streptococcus*, GIT pathogens *(Yersinia enterocolitica, Yersinia pseudotuberculosis, Salmonella gastroenteritis, Campylobacter colitis)*, tuberculosis, Tularemia, *Mycoplasma pneumoniae*
- *Chlamydia* viruses
- Cat scratch disease, ornithosis, hepatitis B virus, Epstein-Barr virus
- Mycosis
  - o Superficial infection—T. verrucosus, T. mentagrophytes
  - o Deep infection—Coccidiomycosis, blastomycosis, histoplasmosis
- Inflammatory conditions: Ulcerative colitis, Crohn's disease, sarcoidosis
- Drugs: Bromides, sulphonamides, oral contraceptive pills
- Malignancy: Leukemia, lymphoma

Histopathology

Erythema nodosum is a septal panniculitis with no vasculitis. The septa of subcutaneous fat are thickened and infiltrated by neutrophils in the early stages, and lymphocytes and multinucleated giant cells in late stages. Overlying dermis shows perivascular lymphocytic infiltrate. A histopathological hallmark is the presence of Miescher's radial granulomas consisting of small, well defined, nodular aggregates of histiocytes around a central stellate or banana-shaped cleft.

Clinical Features

Erythematous nodules appear over the shin, knees and ankles bilaterally and may be accompanied by fever, malaise and bodyache. EN lesions are rarely found over areas other than lower legs. Lesions appear in crops and each lesion undergoes changes in color. Eventually the lesions fade over 3-6 weeks, without ulceration, atrophy or scarring.

Investigations

Throat culture, ESR and ASO titres must be done to rule out streptococcal infections. Tuberculosis can be excluded by Mantoux test and a chest radiograph. Other investigations need to be performed as per the etiological agent suspected.

Treatment

Erythema nodosum as a general rule resolves without any treatment. Rest and NSAIDS usually suffice. NSAIDS like indomethacin or naproxen may hasten resolution. Potassium iodide, 360-900 mg/day has been reported to be useful in persistent cases. Potassium iodide is best avoided in children.

IDIOPATHIC NODULAR PANNICULITIS

This is an idiopathic condition characterized by recurrent crops of nodular panniculitis. In some cases panniculits is associated with systemic features like fever, malaise, abdominal pain and arthritis.

Etiology

Generally the condition is idiopathic. However in children, certain precipitating factors have been reported. These include immunization like DPT, oral polio and measles vaccine, infections such as streptococci, *Klebsiella*, *Toxoplasma* and varicella zoster virus and drugs, for example potassium bromide.

Pathology

Panniculitis is typically lobular. Fat lobules are infiltrated by neutrophils and other acute inflammatory cells in the early stages. These are replaced by lymphocytes and macrophages which ingest the fat from damaged lipocytes. Eventually fibrosis supervenes.

Clinical Features

Nodular panniculitis mainly affects adult females. Crops of erythematous, tender, subcutaneous nodules develop over the lower limbs, occasionally involving the trunk and face.

Fever, arthralgia, GIT disturbances, like abdominal pain, melaena, hepatomegaly and splenomegaly have all been reported in association with nodular panniculitis.

Prognosis

Idiopathic nodular panniculitis can be fatal. About 25% died in a series of 27 children.

Treatment

It is mainly symptomatic. Systemic steroids, chloroquine, azathioprine, cyclophosphamide, dapsone and ciclosporin have all been used with variable success.

SECONDARY NODULAR PANNICULITIS

Pancreatic Panniculitis

Subcutaneous fat necrosis and painful nodular panniculitis may result from pancreatic disease. Several pancreatic diseases known to occur in association with pancreatic panniculitis, include acute or chronic pancreatitis, pancreatic pseudocyst, pancreatic islet cell tumors, ductal adenocarcinoma and acinar- cell carcinoma. Circulating lipase and amylase released from the diseased pancreas cause the lesions in subcutaneous tissue via enzymatic destruction of fat. The histopathology is pathognomonic, with necrotic fat containing 'ghost' cells having thick shadowy walls and no nuclei. The reddish, subcutaneous nodules tend to appear over the lower limbs, especially the periarticular region. Ulceration with discharge of a thick, oily material representing liquefaction degeneration of fat is commonly seen.

Pancreatic panniculitis may be associated with arthritis, pleural effusion, ascites and eosinophilia. In such cases prognosis is usually bad. Treatment is generally supportive and hinges around correction of the cause.

α1 Antitrypsin Deficiency Panniculitis

α1 antitrypsin deficiency is caused by decreased hepatic production of a proteinase inhibitor that inhibits both trypsin and other serine proteinases such as elastase. Homozygous deficiency with ZZ phenotype is most commonly associated with panniculitis, although phenotype MZ and MS have also been implicated.

Pathology: A suppurative panniculitis with neutrophils involving both, septal and lobular areas with fat necrosis is often seen.

Clinical features: Certain clinical features are helpful in distinguishing α1 antitrypsin deficiency panniculitis from other panniculitides. The subcutaneous nodules which initially resemble cellulitis are generally located over the trunk and proximal limbs. The nodules tend to ulcerate and discharge oily material that represents necrotic adipocytes. They heal with atrophic scars. Another important feature is the history of antecedent trauma or excessive activity, precipitating the lesions.

α1 antitrypsin deficiency panniculits may be associated with emphysema, hepatitis, cirrhosis, vasculitis, urticaria, etc.

Treatment: Dapsone and doxycycline are effective. For patients with systemic involvement, replacement with α1 antitrypsin is recommended.

Cold Nodular Panniculitis (Figures 22.3A and B)

This variant of panniculitis results from cold injury to fat tissue. Infants and young children are particularly predisposed to develop cold panniculitis.The higher saturated fat content of neonates and infants render them more vulnerable to cold injury. Even a small decrease in an infant's temperature may lead to crystallization of the infants' fat.

Cases of cold panniculitis have been described in the cheeks of children sucking ice cubes, ice packs, or ice lollies (popsicle) or when exposed to cold air. Swimming in cold water may induce cold panniculitis of the scrotum in children. Cold panniculitis involving thighs and buttocks has been described in women riding horses during cold weather.

Cold panniculitis appears as erythematous, indurated plaques occurring 2-3 days after cold exposure. Histopathology shows a lobular panniculitis with an inflammatory infiltrate of lymphocytes and histiocytes. Dermis shows pronounced edema and superficial and deep perivascular lymphocytic infiltrate. Cold panniculitis resolves if further exposure to cold is avoided.

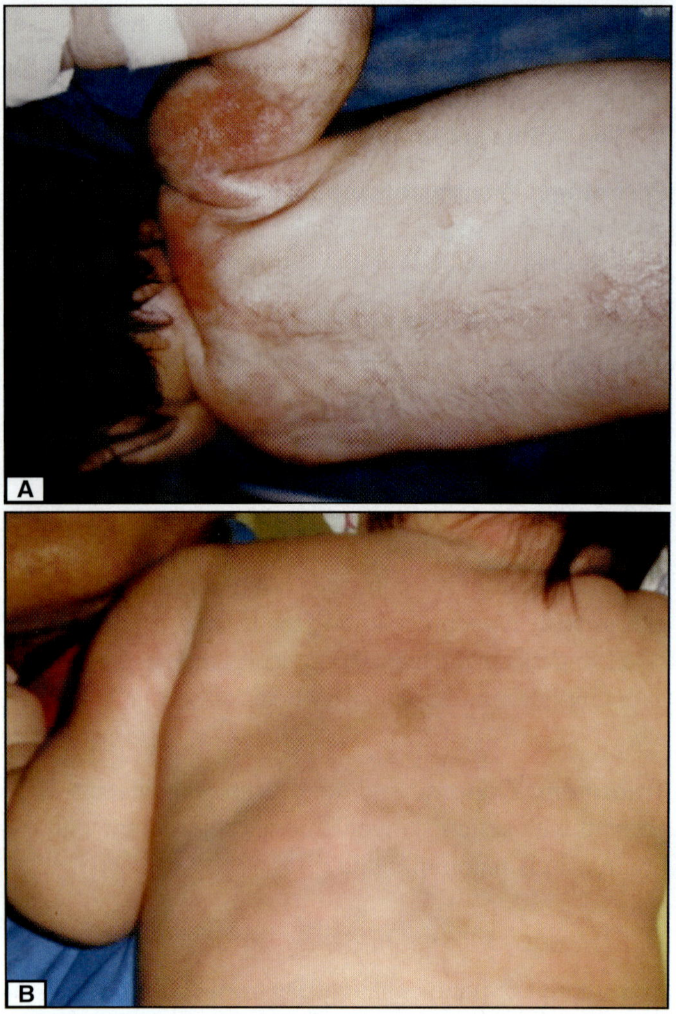

FIGURES 22.3A AND B: Cold nodular panniculitis

Post Steroid Nodular Panniculitis

This type of panniculitis though extremely rare occurs almost exclusively in children who were receiving high doses of systemic corticosteroids and in whom steroids were either rapidly tapered or abruptly stopped. The reasons to receive high dose steroid therapy include rheumatic fever, leukemia, nephrotic syndrome and cerebral edema.

It manifests as subcutaneous nodules or plaques on the cheeks, arms and trunk, areas where there is greatest steroid-induced fat deposition. Panniculitis appears 1-13 days after steroid withdrawal. Nodules vary in size from 0.5 to 4.0 cm and may be painful or itchy.

There is no specific treatment and panniculitis resolves gradually over a period of weeks to months without scarring. If the disease is severe, reintroduction of high dose steroids and gradual reduction is recommended.

LIPOATROPHY (LIPODYSTROPHY)

Lipodystrophies are conditions characterized by a marked reduction or loss of subcutaneous fat. They can be generalized (total), partial or localized and may be congenital or acquired.

LOCALIZED LIPOATROPHIES

Insulin Lipoatrophy

It is more commonly seen in women and children, who require high doses of insulin. It was more common when bovine or porcine insulins were used. The lipoatrophy is considered to be an immunological reaction to impurities in the insulin preparations. Recent studies suggest that insulin lipohypertrophy is more common than lipoatrophy. Atrophy can be noticed 6 months to 2 yrs after the beginning of insulin administration. Lesions may vary from a small dimple to a large area of loss of fat.

Change of insulin to a purified form, especially human insulin results in improvement. Injection sites should be carefully rotated.

Centrifugal Lipoatrophy

It is rare and is characterized by localized loss of fat involving the abdomen usually but occasionally other areas. It generally starts before the age of 3 years. A central large bluish depressed area with a red scaly border develops over the abdomen or groin area and spreads centrifugally. This condition has been mainly reported in Japan, but is reported in caucasians too. The lesion progresses for 3-8 years and then spontaneously resolves to a great extent.

Other

Other forms of local atrophy such as annular lipoatrophy involving an upper limb or semicircular lipoatrophy occurring over anterolateral thighs have been described.

PARTIAL LIPOATROPHY

Familial Partial Lipodystrophy (FPLD) or Kobberling-Dunnigan Syndrome

Familial partial lipodystrophy (FPLD) or Kobberling–Dunnigan syndrome is an autosomal dominant condition with two distinct phenotypes. In Type I FPLD there is complete loss of subcutaneous fat on the limbs, whereas in Type II (Dunnigan) type the involved areas include the limbs and trunk. There is sparing of the face and neck in both the variants. Associated metabolic abnormalities include, acanthosis nigricans, insulin resistant diabetes and hyperlipoproteinemia.

Progressive Partial Lipodystrophy (PPL) or Barraquer-Simons Disease

Progressive partial lipodystrophy occurs predominantly in females, the female to male ratio being 4:1. It presents in the 1st and 2nd decades. It is characterized by a diffuse and progressive loss of subcutaneous fat beginning from the face and scalp and extending down up to iliac crests. There is an apparent and sometimes real deposition of excess fat in the pelvic girdle and lower limbs. Other features are low C3 levels, presence of a circulating polyclonal IgG called "C3 nephritic factor" and progressive membranous mesangiocapillary glomerulonephritis. Insulin dependent diabetes mellitus can occur in about 1/3rd cases of PPL.

Lipodystrophy in HIV Infected Children

Peripheral lipoatrophy is seen in HIV infected children on highly active antiretroviral therapy (HAART) containing protease inhibitors. There is loss of fat in the face, buttocks and limbs with excess fat deposition in the neck, upper back and abdomen.

TOTAL LIPOATROPHY

Congenital generalized lipodystrophy or Berardinelli-Seip syndrome is a rare autosomal recessive condition. There is complete loss of subcutaneous fat appearing at birth or within the first 2 years of life. The mechanical fat of the palms, soles, joints, orbit and scalp is well preserved. Children have increased height and muscular hypertrophy. Scalp hair is abundant and there is generalized hypertrichosis. There is hepatosplenomegaly resulting in protuberant abdomen. Other features are acanthosis nigricans, hyperinsulinemia and insulin resistant diabetes occurring around puberty. The genetic defect is either mutation of the AGPAT2 gene or in the Seipin gene.

Acquired generalized lipoatrophy or Lawrence's syndrome is essentially similar to congenital generalized variety, but develops later in life.

BIBLIOGRAPHY

1. Agrawal SN. Lipoid proteinosis in siblings. Indian J Dermatol Venereol Leprol 2003;69:28-29.
2. Alani RM, Busam K. Acupuncture granulomas. J am Acad Dermatol 2001;45:225.
3. Aronson IK, Zeitz HJ, Variakojis D. Panniculitis in childhood. Pediatr Dermatol 1988;5:216-30.
4. Badalamente MA, Hurst LC, Hentz VR. Collagen as a clinical target. Non operative treatment of Dupuytren's disease. J Hand Surg [Am] 2002;27:788-98.
5. Behr FD, Levine N, Bangert J. Lichen amyloidosis associated with atopic dermatitis: clinical resolution with cyclosporine. Arch Dermatol 2001;137:553-5.
6. Bel S, Bartralot R, Garcia D, et al: Vegetant bromoderma in an Infant. Pediatr Dermatol 2001;18(4):336-8.
7. Bhat Ramesh M. Management of pyoderma gangrenosum – An update. Ind J Dermatol Venereol Leprol 2004;70:329-35.
8. Chan I, Oyama N, South AP et al. Rapid diagnosis of lipoid proteinosis using an anti- extracellular matrix protein 1 (ECM 1) antibody;J Dermatol Sci 2004;35:151-3.
9. Chang WA, Henderson CA. Suppurative panniculitis associated with α1-antitrypsin deficiency (PiSZ phenotype) treated with doxycycline. Br J Dermatol 2001;144:1282-3.
10. Chiu Y, Huang C, Jeng J et al. Foreign body granuloma caused by monosodium glutamate after BCG vaccination. J Am Acad Dermatol 2006;55:s1-5.
11. Cordoro K, Osleber M, Shaffer J et al. Lipoid Proteinosis. www.emedicine.com ;July 2006.
12. D Kemmett, JA Hunter :Sweet's syndrome: a clinicopathologic review of twenty-nine cases. J Am Acad Dermatol 1990;23:503-7.
13. FC Powell, WP Su, HO Perry. Pyoderma gangrenosum: classification and management: J Am Acad Dermatol 1996;34:395-409.
14. Garcia-Porrua C, Gonzales-Gay MA,Vazquez-Caruncho M, et al. Erythema nodosum: aetiologic and predictive factors in a defined population. Arthritis Rheum 2000;43:584-92.
15. Gebauer K, Connor B. Cutaneous mercury granuloma. Australas J Dermatol. 1991;32:129-32.
16. Hamada T, Lipoid proteinosis. Clin Exp Dermatol 2002;27:624-9.
17. Joshi Ketuman, Patel Sarika, Shah Priti P, Parikh Deepak J, Bilimoria FE. Case report: Granuloma faciale. Ind J Dermatol Venereol Leprol 1998;64:291-2.
18. Kaya TI, Kokturk A, Tursen U et al. D-penicillamine treatment for lipoid proteinosis. J Eur Acad Dermatol Venereol 2002;16;286-8.
19. Kennedy CTC. Granuloma Annulare. In: Textbook of Pediatric Dermatology, Harper J, Oranje A, Prose N, editors. 2nd ed. Oxford:Blackwell Publishing 2006;889-900.
20. KN Shivaswamy, Devinder M Thappa. Chandrashekar Laxmisha, S Jayanthi Lipoid proteinosis in two siblings: A report from south India Dermatology Online Journal 2003;9(5):12.
21. Kurizky P, Estrella R, Oliveira J. Vegetating iododerma: A case report. J Am Acad Dermatol. 2007;56:AB135.
22. Lowe NJ, Maxwell CA, Lowe P, et al. Hyaluronic acid skin fillers: Adverse reactions and skin testing. J Am Acad Dermatol 2001;45:930-3.
23. Mancini G, Oranje A, Hollander J, Levy M. Fibromatoses, hyalinoses and stiff skin. In Textbook of pediatric dermatology. Harper J, Oranje A, Prose N, editors. Blackwell Science 2006;1:935-56

24. Nicolas Ortonne, Janine Wechsler, Martine Bagot, Edouard Grosshans, Bernard Cribier. Granuloma faciale: A clinicopathologic study of 66 patients. J Am Acad Dermatol 2005;53:1002-09.
25. Nischal KC, Khopkar Uday. Review article: An approach to the diagnosis of neutrophilic dermatoses: A histopathological perspective Ind J Dermatol, Venereol Leprol 2007;73:222-30.
26. Paller AS, Herbert AA. Knuckle pads in children. Am J Dis Child 1986;140:915-7.
27. Pasricha JS, Seetharam KA. Low dose cyclophosphamide therapy in lichen amyloidosis. Indian J Dermatol Venereol Leprol 1987;53:273-4.
28. Paul AK, Al-Nahhas A, Ansari SM, Islam N: Skin eruptions following treatment with Iodine-131 for hyperthyroidism: a rare and un-reported early/intermediate side effect. Nucl Med Rev Cent East Eur 2005;8(2):125-7.
29. Pedram Geraminejad, James R. DeBloom, Hobart W. Walling. Alpha-1-antitrypsin associated panniculitis: The MS variant;J Am Acad Dermatol 2004:51:645-55.
30. Prendiville JS, Krol Al. Diseases of the dermis and sub-cutaneous tissue. In: Pediatric Dermatology, Schachner L.A, Hansen R, editors. 3rd ed. Edinburgh: Mosby 2003;734-6.
31. Raile K, Noelle V, Landgraf R et al. Insulin antibodies are associated with lipoatrophy but also with lipohypertrophy in children and adolescents with type 1 diabetes. Exp Clin Endocrinol Diabetes 2001;109:393-6.
32. Saxena AK, Nigam PK.Panniculitis following steroid therapy. Cutis 1988;42:341-2.
33. Sumitra S, Yesudian D. Friction amyloidosis—a variant or an etiologic factor in amyloidosis cutis? Int J Dermatol 1993;32:422-3.
34. Tay YK. Erythema nodosum in Singapore. Clin Exp Dermatol 2000;25:377-80.
35. Ter Poorten JC, Hebert AA, Ilkiw R. Cold panniculitis in a neonate. J Am Acad Dermatol 1995;33:383-5.
36. Verroti A, Chiarelli F, Arnerio P, et al. Necrobiosis lipoidica diabeticorum in children and adolescents: a clue for underlying renal and retinal disease. Pediatr Dermatol 1995:12;220-3.
37. Weedon D. The granulomatous reaction pattern. In: Skin Pathology, David Weedon, editor. 2nd Ed. Philadelphia: Elsevier 2002;193-220
38. Wong CK, Breathnach SM, eds. Cutaneous amyloidosis. Clin Dermatol 1990;8(2).

23

Neoplastic Disorders of Skin

- Benign epithelial tumors
- Tumors of the cutaneous appendages
- Benign neoplasias and hyperplasias of melanocytes
- Smooth muscle tumors and skeletal muscle tumors
- Benign neural tumors
- Precancerous lesions

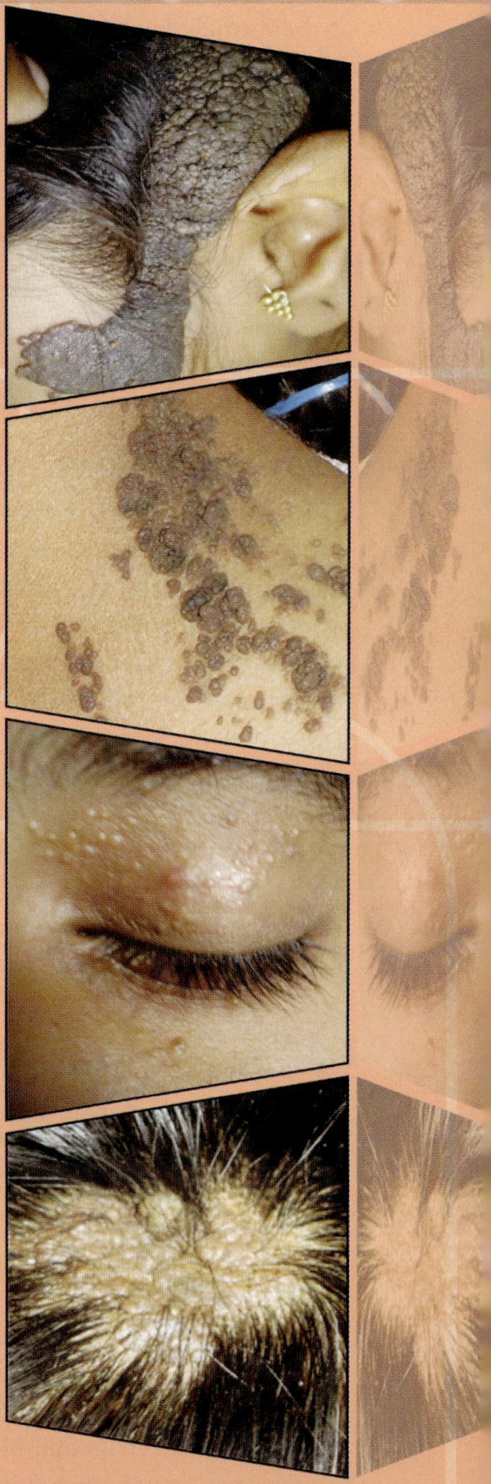

Prabhakar Sangolli

BENIGN EPITHELIAL TUMORS

Benign epithelial tumors are very common. Satisfactory classification is not available.

CLASSIFICATION

- Seborrheic keratosis
- Epidermal nevi
- Verrucous epidermal nevus (VEN)
- Inflammatory linear verrucous epidermal nevus (ILVEN)
- Nevus sebaceus of Jadassohn
- Nevus comedonicus
- Eccrine nevus
- Apocrine nevus
- Becker's nevus
- Epidermal nevus syndrome.

EPIDERMAL NEVUS

Epidermal nevi are hamartomatous proliferation developing from embryonic ectoderm, which gives rise to epidermal related structures including keratinocytes, apocrine glands, eccrine glands, hair follicle and sebaceous glands. Hence, it may be classified into variants based on morphology, extent of involvement and predominant epidermal structures, but they exhibit considerable overlap.

Epidemiology

Incidence of epidermal nevi is about 1 per 1000 live births. Though sporadic in occurrence, familial cases are reported. There is no sex predilection. Most of the VEN especially those on head, appear at birth.

Clinical Features

VEN are characterized by dark verrucous papules and or plaques, mostly appearing along skin tension lines or Blaschko's lines **(Figures 23.1A and B)**. Distribution may be linear/generalized or bilateral. Inflammatory linear verrucous epidermal nevus (ILVEN) is an inflammatory variant of epidermal nevus with itching, erythema and scaling.

VEN enlarge slowly and become stable in adolescence. If extensive, VEN may be associated with abnormalities in other systems. Rarely VEN can develop into basal or squamous cell carcinoma. Mosaicism may result in rare appearance of generalized epidermolytic hyperkeratosis among offsprings.

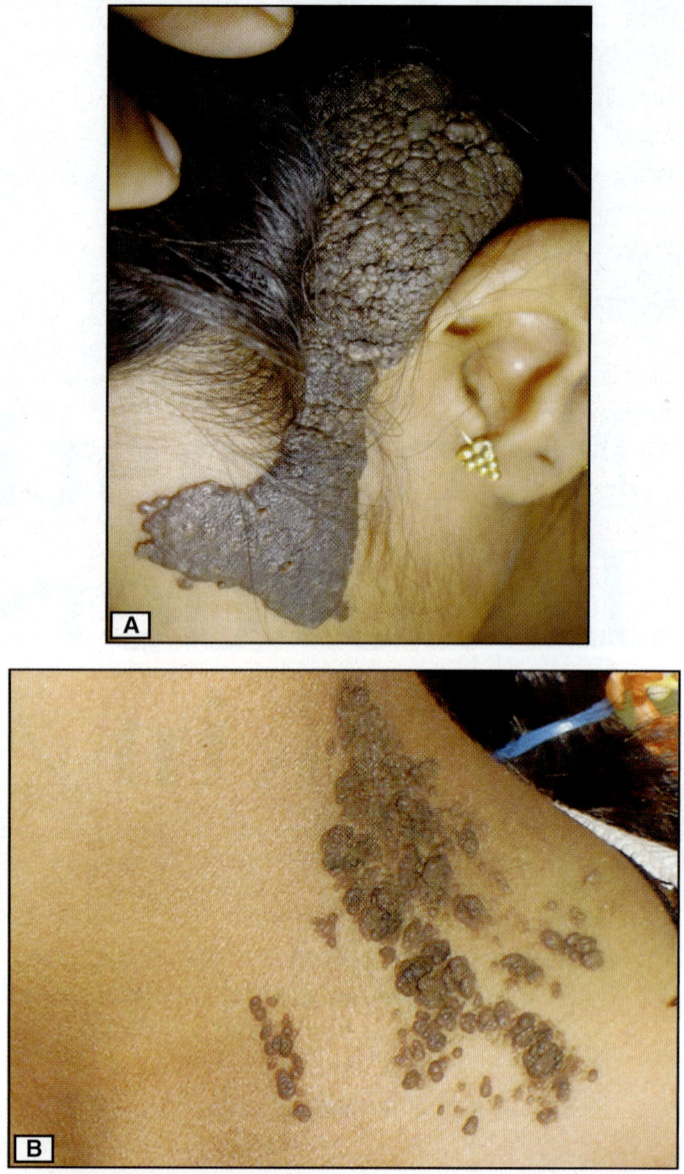

FIGURES 23.1A AND B: Verrucous epidermal nevus

Pathology

Hyperkeratosis, acanthosis and papillomatosis with elongated rete ridges is seen in VEN lesions. Epidermolytic hyperkeratosis display hyperkeratinization, vacuolization of cells in prickle cell layer with large granules in stratum granulosum. ILVEN displays dermal chronic inflammatory cells along with above findings. Alternating hyperkeratosis with parakeratosis is another hallmark of ILVEN.

Differential Diagnosis

Lichen striatus, incontinentia pigmenti (verrucous stage), linear lichen planus and linear psoriasis. The later two could be variants of ILVEN.

Treatment

Though complete deep excision is the ideal treatment, less invasive options include electrofulguration, cryotherapy, CO_2 laser, dermabrasion and TCA peels, which are partially effective but have high recurrence rates.

COMEDO NEVUS

Comedo nevus is a hamartomatous proliferation of pilosebaceous follicle. It may be present at birth or appear at childhood. Lesions resemble comedones occurring over face, arms, chest, often in linear configuration **(Figure 23.2)**.

Histopathology shows dilated pilosebaceous follicles filled with keratinous plugs.

Inflammation in the form of pustules, cysts, scarring and association of systemic defects (nevus comedonicus syndrome) are the well-known complications.

Topical tretinoin, 12% ammonium lactate may be helpful. Oral isotretinoin helps in severe cases.

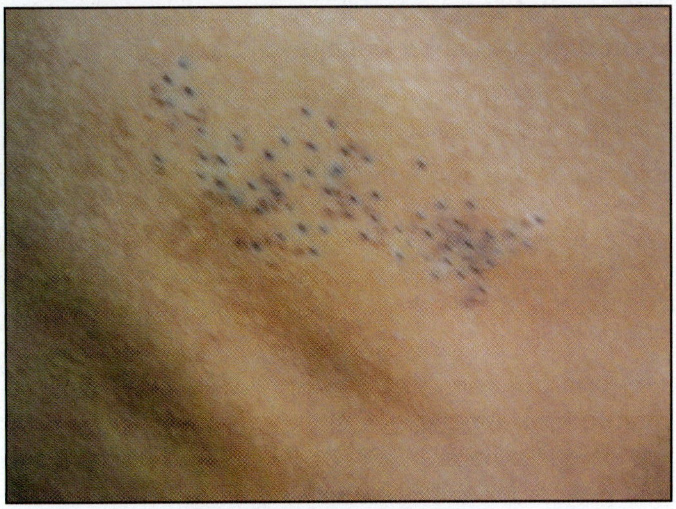

FIGURE 23.2: Comedo nevus

NEVUS SEBACEOUS (ORGANOID NEVUS)

Nevus sebaceous presents as a solitary lesion at birth or early childhood, usually over scalp, in the form of a yellowish plaque with alopecia **(Figure 23.3)**. The lesion becomes conspicuous at puberty.

Histopathologically, increased sebaceous glands, apocrine glands and small hair follicles are seen in the deep dermis with papillomatous epidermal hyperplasia.

Nevus sebaceous may be associated with systemic abnormalities (Nevus sebaceous syndrome), and the tumor has a malignant potential. Different tumors may

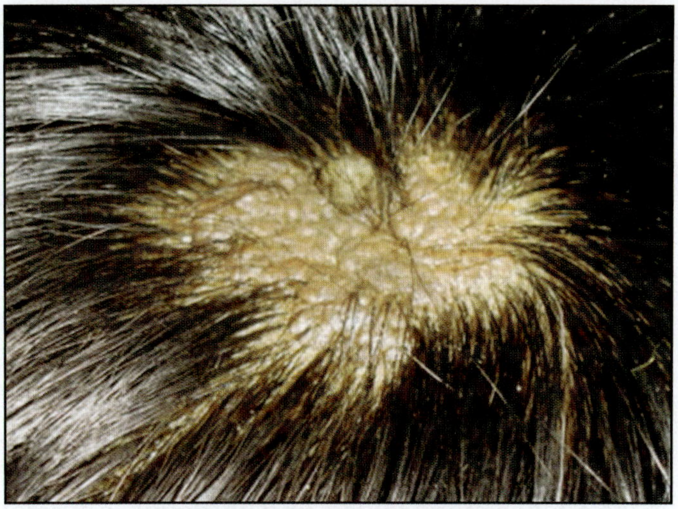

FIGURE 23.3: Nevus sebaceous

arise from existing nevus sebaceous, e.g. trichoblastoma, syringocystadenoma papilliferum and basal cell carcinoma. Surgical excision is the treatment of choice for nevus sebaceous because of risk of malignancy.

ECCRINE NEVUS

Eccrine nevus presents as solitary area of hyperhidrosis or as linear papules/plaques. Eccrine angiomatous hamartoma is commonly seen as a solitary, flesh colored, hyperhidrotic, painful papule or plaque at birth or during childhood. Porokeratotic eccrine ostial and dermal duct nevus presents as congenital, keratotic papules and plaques on distal extremities.

Histopathological examination reveals increased eccrine ducts and coils in dermis. Small blood vessel proliferation (angiomatous hamartoma) or comedo like dilatation or hyperplasia of acrosyringium is the salient feature in porokeratotic eccrine ostial and dermal duct nevus.

In eccrine angiomatous hamartoma surgical excision is the treatment of choice. CO_2 laser therapy is the treatment option for porokeratotic eccrine ostial and dermal duct nevus.

APOCRINE NEVUS

It is a very rare condition seen over the scalp, axillae, or chest, in the form of solitary nodule or as soft masses. Histopathology reveals basaloid proliferation of the epidermis and multiple mature apocrine glands in the reticular dermis. Excision is curative.

EPIDERMAL NEVUS SYNDROME

It is a disease complex of co-occurrence of epidermal, sebaceous, comedo nevi with eye, CNS, skeletal, CVS and urogenital abnormalities. Happle has proposed six types which include Schimmelplening syndrome, nevus comedonicus syndrome, pigmented hairy epidermal nevus syndrome, Proteus syndrome, CHILD syndrome and phakomatosis pigmentokeratotica. Skin lesions are vascular and pigmentary anomalies. Bone cysts, hypertrophy, scoliosis, syndactyly or polydactyly are the bony abnormalities. CNS defects include seizures, mental retardation, hydrocephalus, cortical atrophy, spinal stenosis, etc.

Detailed history taking and thorough physical examination are compulsory for all patients to detect the extent of involvement. Investigations include skin biopsy, CT scan, MRI, electro-encephalography, intravenous pyelography and skeletal radiography. Affected patients need regular monitoring.

LICHEN STRIATUS (BLASCHKO LINEAR ACQUIRED INFLAMMATORY SKIN ERUPTION/ BLAISE)

It affects children between 5 and 15 years of age. Genetic, infective and environmental factors are involved in the pathogenesis. Linear lichenoid eruptions following Blaschko's lines with nail involvement are the characteristic clinical features.

Histopathology reveals hyperkeratosis, focal parakeratosis, spongiosis and lichenoid infiltrate at dermoepidermal junction, around blood vessels and appendages.

Appearance at birth, associated pruritus and lack of spontaneous resolution differentiates ILVEN from this condition. Topical steroid is advised, in case patient complains of itching.

CYSTS OF EPIDERMAL ORIGIN

Epidermal Cyst (Sebaceous cyst)

It is a keratin containing cyst lined by surface epidermis.

Etiopathogenesis: It is the result of inclusion and proliferation of surface cells within the dermis. Production of keratin within a circumscribed space results in cyst formation. Epidermoid cysts arise from occlusion of pilosebaceous follicles, from implantation of epidermal cells into the dermis following penetration injury or following trapping of epidermal cells along embryonal fusion lines. Lining of epidermal cysts is from follicular infundibulum. Palmoplantar cysts may contain HPV 57 and 60.

Epidemiology: Though rare in children, patients with Gardner's syndrome and Gorlin syndrome may have many lesions.

Pathology: Cyst is lined by true epidermis. Within the cyst, keratinous material is arranged in laminated layers. Spillage of contents into the dermis evokes foreign body reaction.

Clinical features: An epidermoid cyst presents as 1-5 cm intradermal or subcutaneous dome-shaped protuberance which is freely mobile over underlying structures. A central punctum which represents plugged orifice of pilosebaceous structure is characteristically present. Face, neck, chest, upper body are the common sites.

Secondary infection is a common complication.

Differential diagnosis: Pilar cyst (mainly seen on scalp), steatocystoma simplex (contains oily fluid), lipoma (soft).

Treatment: Incision and drainage is the treatment modality for infected cyst with antibiotic coverage. Incision and removal of cyst is the definitive treatment.

Dermoid Cyst

It is a rare cyst lined by an epidermis containing various appendages.

Histopathology: Cyst is lined by epidermis and contains mature skin appendages, namely, hair follicles, sweat glands and sebaceous glands. Hairs are present within and project into the cyst cavity.

Clinical features: Lesions are found along embryonal fusion planes. Lateral 1/3rd of the eyebrows, nose and scalp are the common sites. Neck, sternum, scrotum, perineal raphe and sacrum are other sites. These are subcutaneous, mobile, but may be fixed to underlying periosteum. These measure 1-4 cm in diameter.

Complications: Inflammation and infection are common complications. Intracranial communication may exist, especially in frontal, temporal, parietal and occipital regions, and may lead to serious complication.

Differential diagnosis: Other epithelial cysts, glioma, encephalocele.

Treatment: Excision is the treatment of choice after ruling out intracranial extension.

Preauricular Cysts (ear pits)

Pre-auricular cysts arise from incomplete fusion of six tubercles from first two bronchial arches (formation of tragus and pinna). These are present in 1% of the population. Mostly these are asymptomatic, bilateral and appear as cysts or sinuses in front of ears. Secondary infection is a common complication. These are lined by stratified squamous epithelium. Antibiotics in presence of infection and excision are the treatment modalities.

TUMORS OF THE CUTANEOUS APPENDAGEAL

Appendageal tumors of the skin show differentiation toward epithelial components of normal (embryonal or mature) adnexae (eccrine, apocrine, hair follicle and sebaceous units). Lesions may be solitary or multiple. Regional distribution of solitary lesion gives clue to the diagnosis. Multiple lesions exhibit characteristic distribution. Autosomal dominance is the mode of inheritance with or without other organ involvement. Immunohistology helps to unravel the source of the tumors with overlap of visceral malignancies. Cytogenetic and molecular studies throw light on genesis of these tumors.

Histopathology often helps in arriving at correct diagnosis in many patients. These are classified as cysts, hamartomas, hyperplasias, and benign and malignant neoplasms. Cysts are epithelium lined round or oval sac-like lesions. Embryonic malformation with abnormal arrangement of normal skin components is known as hamartoma.

Increase in number of cells with normal arrangement is referred to as cutaneous hyperplasia. Malignant neoplasms exhibit local/distant tissue destructive metastasis.

Complete excision is curative treatment of benign lesions. Superficial ablative therapy, excision, Moh's microsurgery, improvised radio therapy are the modalities used to treat malignancies.

APOCRINE TUMORS

Common sites are head, neck, axillae, genital or perianal skin.

Moll's gland cyst is solitary cyst seen near eyelid.

Hidrocystomas showing eccrine/apocrine differentiation present over eyelids may be seen in ectodermal dysplasia.

HAMARTOMA

Apocrine nevus can be either pure nevus or part of nevus sebaceous.

Supernumerary nipples are seen along the embryonal milk line. These resemble dermatofibroma or melanocytic nevi.

HYPERPLASIA

Juvenile fibroadenoma of breast is seen in teenage females.

Nosology of syringocystadenoma papilliferum is uncertain. Uncommonly it is seen in children at unusual sites like chest, upper arms, and thighs. Epidermal invagination and papilliferous projections with perilesional lymphocyte and plasma cell infiltrate are seen on biopsy. Syringocystadenoma papilliferum co-exists with trichoblastoma in nevus sebaceous. Treatment options include excision and CO_2 laser ablation (in case of lesions at inaccessible sites).

APPENDAGE TUMORS WITH ECCRINE DIFFERENTIATION

Due to broader distribution of eccrine glands, tumor distribution also exhibits similar topography. Histopathologically, these arise from acrosyringium, dermal duct and secretory portion. These exhibit overlap with apocrine tumors.

Cyst: Eccrine hidrocystoma overlaps with apocrine hidrocystoma.

Hamartoma: These are eccrine nevus, eccrine angiomatous hamartoma, porokeratotic eccrine ostial and dermal duct nevus (described earlier).

Benign Neoplasms: Brooke-Spiegler syndrome, also known as familial cylindromatosis manifests with multiple cylindromas, trichoepitheliomas and basal cell carcinomas, arachnoid nevi and spiradenomas.

Syringoma: It is a benign eccrine acrosyringium neoplasm. Familial cases and patients with Down syndrome present with numerous smooth, skin colored or slightly yellowish papules situated on upper half of the face **(Figure 23.4)**.

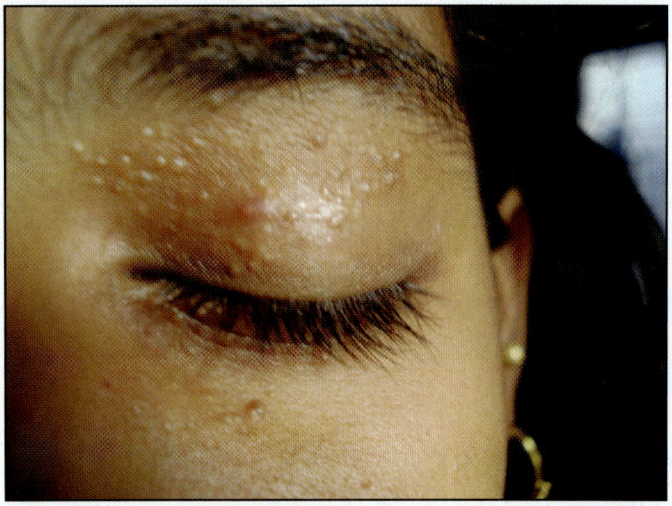

FIGURE 23.4: Syringoma

Histopathology reveals numerous epithelial aggregations of small, solid nests, cords and tubular structures with tadpole shape in the upper dermis. Dermabrasion, electrodesiccation with curettage, Erb:YAG laser resurfacing are usual modalities of treatment.

APPENDAGEAL TUMORS WITH FOLLICULAR DIFFERENTIATION

Cysts

Epidermal cyst: Multiple epidermoid cysts are feature of Gardner's syndrome. Gardner's syndrome, caused by mutation in APC (Adenomatous Polyposis Coli) gene. It is characterized by multiple epidermoid cysts, pilomatricoma, soft tissue tumors, osteomas, retinal epithelial hypertrophy and colorectal polyps. If untreated, patients invariably develop colonic carcinoma.

Hybrid cyst: It is seen as a nodular lesion in head and neck region. It exhibits epidermal and trichilemmal keratinization.

Trichilemmal cyst (pilar cyst): It is a keratin containing cyst on scalp, arising from lower portion of hair follicle. Familial condition with multiple lesions over the scalp is also reported.

Vellus Hair Cyst: Multiple vellus hair cysts are seen at birth or in infancy with presence of multiple pigmented reddish papules on face, trunk, and axillae. Eruptive vellus hair cysts are seen in association with steatocystoma multiplex and hypohidrotic ectodermal dysplasia. Biopsy reveals cystic structures with trichilemmal keratinization.

Hamartoma

Basaloid follicular hamartoma: Familial multiple basaloid follicular hamartomas manifest as numerous flesh colored, micropapules over central face, scalp and neck. These may be associated with myasthenia gravis, alopecia, hypohidrosis or cystic fibrosis.

Histopathology reveals strands of basaloid cells with numerous epidermal connections. Features of follicular differentiation are seen as horn cysts/papillae and rudimentary germs.

Hair Follicle Nevus: These are reported in all age groups. These appear as dome-shaped, skin colored papules and nodules on hair bearing skin especially on face. Variants are faun tail nevus, hairs on palms and soles and Becker's nevus. Hair follicle nevus could be a variant of trichofolliculoma. Histopathology reveals vellus follicles in dermis with surrounding perifollicular connective tissue. Excision is curative.

Linear unilateral basal cell nevus: It presents at birth as numerous cutaneous papules or nodules distributed unilaterally. Unilateral anodontia, diffuse osteoma cutis are the other reported features. Histopathology simulates basal cell carcinoma. Nevus comedonicus resembles basal cell nevus.

Benign Neoplasm

Desmoplastic trichoepithelioma: Rare tumor seen on the face as firm, oblong or annular papule especially around angle of the lip. Histopathology reveals basaloid aggregations in columns and cords surrounded by dense desmoplastic stroma. Sebaceous cells, shadow cells, foreign body granuloma, dermal melanocytic nevus are also seen.

Fibrous papule: Appears as dome-shaped skin colored or pigmented lesion around nose. Multiple fibrous papules are seen in Birt-Hogg-Dube syndrome. On histopathological examination, upper dermis shows poorly formed hair follicles surrounded by fibrous tissue with proliferation of small vessels.

Trichodiscoma: Multiple trichodiscomata may be seen in Birt-Hogg-Dube syndrome. It is also known as "mantleoma".

Trichoepithelioma: This shows a spectrum of histopathological features reflecting mainly differentiation towards hair and hair follicles, particularly follicular germs. Solitary, multiple and desmoplastic are the three types. Multiple trichoepitheliomas present as small papules on the face especially around nasolabial folds, forehead and chin. These may be seen in Brook-Spiegler syndrome, Rombo's syndrome, SLE and myasthenia gravis.

Basaloid cells arranged in cribriform or lace-like pattern surrounded by abundant fibrous stroma with intrastromal clefts; horn cysts are the hallmark histopathological findings.

Cryotherapy, electrodesiccation and CO_2 laser are the treatment modalities.

Trichilemmoma: It is a tumor of the outer root sheath of hair follicle. Multiple facial trichilemmomas represent cutaneous marker for Cowden's syndrome.

APPENDAGE TUMORS WITH SEBACEOUS DIFFERENTIATION

Cysts

Steatocystoma multiplex has been discussed earlier.

Hamartomas

Fordyce's spots and Montgomery's tubercles; these represent occurrence of sebaceous glands on the lips, buccal mucosa and breast areola respectively. Fordyce's spots appear as white or yellowish micropapules on the genital mucosa. Single sebaceous gland or lobule in dermis or submucosa is seen on biopsy, sometimes without sebaceous duct.

BENIGN NEOPLASIAS AND HYPERPLASIAS OF MELANOCYTES

Benign melanocytic proliferative lesions form a spectrum of disorders ranging from a simple increase in epidermal melanocyte numbers to widespread cutaneous infiltration of variously differentiated melanocytes. Melanocytic hyperplasia refers to increased melanocytes in basal layer of the epidermis. Melanocytic neoplasias contain melanocyte nests in epidermis, dermis and other tissues. Cells increase in hyperplasias due to intrinsic cell defect or due to change of local hemostasis. Nevomelanocytes arise from abnormally differentiated melanocytes in neoplasias. Cell nests are hallmark of melanocytic neoplasias.

Hyperplasias are lentigo simplex, agminated lentigines, solar lentigines. Neoplasias include acquired melanocytic nevi (including halo nevi), spitz nevi and blue nevi, congenital nevomelanocytic nevus.

HYPERPLASIAS

Lentigo Simplex

It is a common pigmented lesion among black race. It is due to developmental or intrinsic defect in melanocyte hemostasis and melanogenesis pathway abnormalities.

Multiple lentigines are seen in Peutz-Jeghers syndrome, LEOPARD syndrome, LAMB/MYXOMA syndrome. Clinically present as sharply circumscribed light to dark brown macules. Appearance has no relation to sun exposure.

Combined Lesions of Lentigo Simplex: Two patterns of multiple lentigines are seen. These are agminated lentigines and nevus spilus.

Agminated lentigines consist of group of lentigines arranged in linear distribution. It is a rare disorder with chromosomal mosaicism of neural crest melanoblasts.

These appear at birth or early childhood and may be associated with cerebromacular hypertrophy, epidermal nevus, ocular involvement, etc. Increased numbers of melanocytes are seen in elongated epidermal ridges as in lentigo simplex. Wood's lamp examination helps to differentiate from nevus spilus. Reassurance and periodic assessment is all that is necessary.

Nevus Spilus

Nevus spilus (spilus meaning "spot") is characterized by circumscribed macule/patch of tan pigmentation including scattered, more darkly pigmented melanocytic or nevomelanocytic macules and or papules **(Figure 23.5)**. It represents a localized defect in neural crest melanoblasts with primary genetic defect and followed by intrinsic (growth factor) or UV radiated event. Newborns (0.2%) and school children (1.2%) develop this condition characterized by tan macule with dark flat or raised background. Nevus spilus can be giant in morphology or segmental in distribution. Vascular, CNS or connective tissue anomalies may be associated. Pathology reveals lentiginous melanocytic hyperplasia. Raised lesions contain nevomelanocyte collection in epidermis and or dermis.

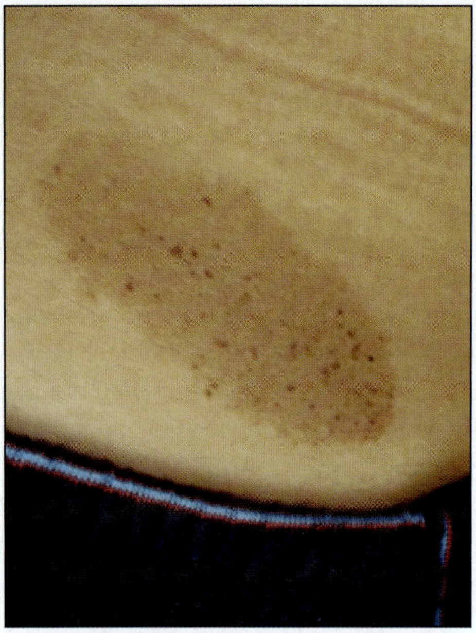

FIGURE 23.5: Nevus spilus

Differential diagnoses include congenital nevomelanocytic nevus, and Becker's melanosis.

Treatment is guided by clinical course and histopathological findings.

NEOPLASIAS

In these lesions, nevomelanocytes are seen in the nests in epidermis and other sites. Nevomelanocytes do not exhibit normal differentiation.

COMMON ACQUIRED MELANOCYTIC NEVUS (AMN)

AMNs are mostly present after birth, slowly enlarge, stabilize, and persist or regress later. These vary from 1 to 43 in numbers in males to 1 to 27 in females, which gradually decrease in number as age advances. It is commoner in Type I and II skin types and triggered by UV radiation. Genetics also play a role. Cells arise from epidermal melanocyte and from Schwann cells in dermis or it could be multiple tissue hamartoma. Biopsy reveals nests of nevomelanocytes in junctional /dermal regions. Epithelioid-like cells are seen in papillary dermis and cells in deeper dermis resemble lymphoid cells, Schwann cells or fibroblasts.

Differential Diagnoses

Differential diagnoses include, blue nevus, dermatofibroma.

Regression of nevi take by neuroid, fibrous (mucous) or fatty degeneration. Though no treatment is necessary, suspicious looking lesion should be completely excised.

EPITHELIOID CELL AND/ OR SPINDLE CELL MELANOCYTIC NEVUS (SPITZ NEVUS)

This tumor constitutes 1-8% of cases.

1. It can present as pink or tan papules with smooth surface that flattens easily with external pressure.
2. A slightly pigmented blue papule often with telangiectasia on the surface resembling fibrous histiocytoma.
3. Dark smooth papule.
4. Agminated brown papule.
5. Large 'congenital nevomelanocytic nevus' like lesions.

Histopathology

Epidermis is hyperplastic with nested epidermal melanocytes with lymphohistiocytic infiltration at DE junction. Cells are giant with mono or multiple nuclei. Kamino bodies and colloid bodies have been seen in 60% patients.

Differential diagnosis include juvenile xanthogranuloma, hemangioma, B-K mole, fibrous histiocytoma.

Treatment

Complete excision with clear margin.

Blue Nevus

It is uncommon in Indian population.

Congenital Nevomelanocytic Nevus (CNN)

These are nevomelanocytic nevi appearing at birth. About 1% of newborns have CNN. Genetic and developmental mechanism play some role in the development of CNN.

CNN have been divided according to largest diameter into small (< 1.5 cm), medium (1.5-19.9 cm) and large (> 20 cm). These have coarse hairs with smooth/pebbly/verrucous/rugose surface **(Figure 23.6).** Giant CNNs can exist in multiple numbers. CNN have been associated with neurofibroma, leptomeningeal melanocytosis which may result in hydrocephalus, seizures, mental retardation or melanoma with poor prognosis. Relative risk of melanoma arising from CNN ranges from 2.3 to 5.7%.

Pathology: CNNs are characterized by nevomelanocytes in the epidermis as well- ordered nests and in the dermis

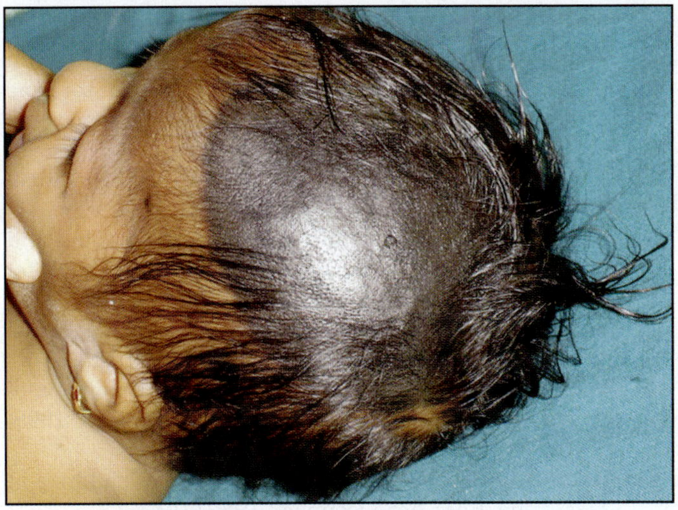

FIGURE 23.6: Congenital nevomelanocytic nevus

as sheets, nests, cords and/or single cells. Other type is known as neuroid type of CNN with Meissner corpuscles, Verocay body and neuroid tubes. Nests of spindle and or epithelioid cells are seen in spindle and/or epithelioid cell type of CNN. Dermal melanocytic type of giant CNN may resemble blue nevus.

Differential diagnosis includes Mongolian spot, lentigo, nevus spilus, VEN, congenital Becker's nevus.

Treatment is planned based on perceived threat of melanoma, cosmetic appearance and functional consideration. Staged excision with or without tissue expanders is the preferred treatment.

BENIGN NEURAL TUMORS

Most of benign neural tumors are markers of genodermatoses. Local excision is curative.

Neurofibroma (NF)

Solitary NF in childhood should alert clinician to look for NF-1. Linear NF are seen due to somatic mosaicism. A 5% of plexiform neurofibroma undergoes malignant degeneration. Diffuse neurofibroma is another variant, presents with plaque over head and neck.

Neurilemmoma

Also known as Schwannoma, neurilemmomas occur as small painful solitary nodules on head in children. It is seen in NF-2. In Gorlin-Knowles syndrome, patients present with multiple neurolemmomas, vaginal leomyoma, multiple CNNs.

Pathology: Neurilemmoma is an encapsulated tumor with biphasic (Antoni's-A and Antoni's-B) pattern.

Neuroma

Neuromas result from disorganized overgrowth of a nerve, usually, seen at the base of supernumerary digit. Multiple neuromas are a feature of MEN 2B syndrome with medullary carcinoma of thyroid and pheochromocytomas. Gorlin sign is conjunctival neuroma in MEN 2B, resulting in a permanently everted eyelid.

Granular Cell Tumor

Multiple granular cell tumors are seen in NF1 patients. Histopathologically, round cells with granular cytoplasm with overlying epithelium exhibit pseudoepitheliomatous hyperplasia. Cells of origin are yet to be elucidated.

Neurothekoma

Neurothekoma or nerve sheath myxomas are rare tumors seen in patients aged 10 to 30 years.

SMOOTH MUSCLE TUMORS

Benign Tumors

Congenital smooth muscle hamartoma (CSMH): This lesion is present at birth or in early infancy. It is seen as pigmented plaque with vellus or terminal hairs, becomes firmer or shows goose bumps when the environment is cold or the lesion is rubbed ("Pseudo Darier's sign"). Trunk, buttocks, or proximal extremities are the commonest sites. Histopathology reveals bundles of smooth muscles throughout dermis. Becker's nevus may overlap with this condition. Michelin tire babies may have CSMH. Excision is not necessary.

Leiomyoma: These mainly arise from arrector pili muscles of hair follicles and also from Dartos'muscle of scrotum. These are painful when palpated. Multiple leiomyoma are seen in Cowden syndrome.

Malignant Tumors

Leiomyosarcomas are seen in children with HIV/AIDS, could be caused due to smooth muscle infection by EBV.

SKELETAL MUSCLE TUMORS

Benign Tumors

Striated muscle hamartoma (rhabdomyomatous hamartoma) are seen on chin. These can be excised easily.

Rhabdomyoma appears before the age of 4 years. It may be associated with basal cell carcinoma syndrome. Excision biopsy with histopathological examination is necessary to rule out rhabdomyosarcoma.

Malignant Tumors

Rhabdomyosarcoma is the commonest childhood sarcoma. Four histopathologic types are described; embryonal, alveolar, botryoid and pleomorphic. Alveolar type may present as blueberry muffin type lesion. Prognosis is bad as by the time diagnosis is established, tumor would have grown rapidly.

Premalignant Lesions

Premalignant lesion is one that has strong likelihood of transforming into a malignancy. Clinically, these demonstrate potential to turn invasive and histopathologically there is cellular atypia.

Actinic keratoses (AK): These can be seen at an early age in patients having skin phototypes I and II and in children with xeroderma pigmentosum, Bloom's syndrome and Rothmund-Thomson syndrome, who may develop AK at very young age.

Bowen's Disease: It is a form of *in situ* squamous cell carcinoma of skin. It is mainly seen after the age of 6 years.

Keloids in Ehlers-Danlos syndrome may undergo malignant change

Epidermodysplasia verruciformis: 30% of the skin lesions undergo neoplastic transformation, in the form of SCC.

Dystrophic epidermolysis bullosa scars develop SCC at early age.

Hence, above mentioned precancerous conditions need close monitoring.

BIBLIOGRAPHY

1. Biggs PJ, et al. The cylindromatosis gene (cyld1) on chromosome 16q may be the only tumour-suppressor gene involved in the development of cylindromas. Oncogene 1996;12:1375.
2. CestaryTF, et al. Nevus comedonicus. Case report and brief review of literature. Pediatr Dermatol 1991;8:300.
3. Chun K, et al. Nevus sebaceous. Clinical outcome and consideration for prophylactic excision. Int J Dermatol 1995;34:538.
4. Dupre A, Christo L.Inflammatory linear verrucous epidermal nevus. A pathologic study. Arch Dermatol 1977;113:767.
5. Gerdsen R, et al. Congenital smooth muscle hamartoma of the skin: Clinical classification. Acta Derm Venereol 1999; 79:408.
6. Green A, et al. Melanocytic nevi in schoolchildren in Queensland J Am Acad Dermatol 1989;20:1054.
7. Happle R. Epidermal nevus syndromes. Semin Dermatol 1995; 14:111.
8. Imai S, Nitto H. Eccrine nevus with epidermal changes. Dermatologica 1983;166:84.
9. Kennedy D, Rogers M: lichen striatus. Pediatr Dermatol 1996;13:95.
10. Kraemer KH, Lee MM, Scot J. Xeroderma pigmentosum: cutaneous, ocular and neurological abnormalities in 830 published cases. Arch Dermatol 1987;123:241.
11. Leung CS, et al. Porokeratotic eccrine ostial and dermal duct nevus with dermatomal trunk involvement: Literature review and report on the efficacy of Laser treatment. Br J Dermatol 1998; 138:684.
12. Maize JC, et al. Adnexal tumours in Cutaneous Pathology. In: Maize JC (editor). Philadelphia:Churchill-Livingstone 1998; 483.
13. Morrell DS, et al. Eccrine angiomatus hamartoma: A report of symmetric and painful lesions of the wrists. Pediatr Dermatol 2001; 18:117.
14. Rogers M, et al. Epidermal nevi and epidermal nevus syndrome. A review of 131 cases. J Am Acad Dermatol 1989;20:476.
15. Swerdlow AJ, et al. Benign melanocytic nevi as a risk factor for malignant melanoma Br Med J 1986;292:1535.
16. Tsuji T, et al. Milia induced by corticosteroids. Arch Dermatol 1986;122:139.
17. Weedon D. Tumors of cutaneous appendages, in Skin Pathology. New York, Churchill-Livingstone, 1997;713.

24

Histiocytoses and Cutaneous Mastocytosis

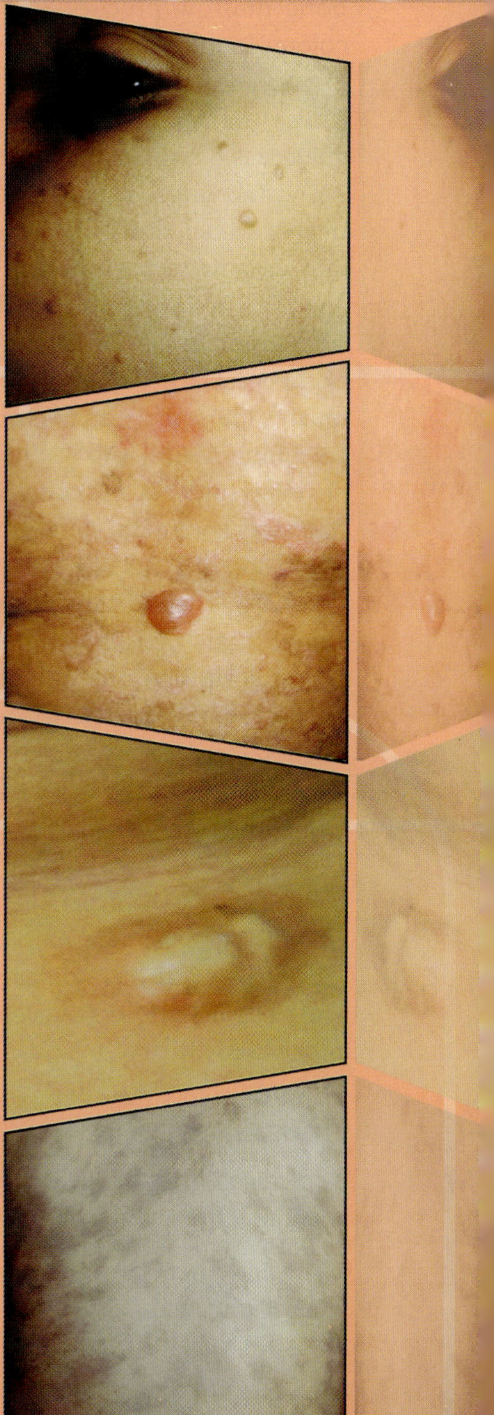

Aparna Palit
Arun C Inamadar

INTRODUCTION

Histiocytoses comprise a group of disorders resulting from proliferation of the bone marrow derived histiocytes and immune related dendritic cells.

Histiocytes are derived from common granulocyte bone marrow precursors, 'granulocyte-macrophage colony forming unit'. Langerhans cells are cutaneous histiocytes, involved in the immune function of the skin. These are located in the suprabasal region of the epidermis of skin as well as mucosa. The cells are large, mononucleated with dendritic processes insinuated between epithelial cells. The nuclei are kidney-shaped and eccentrically located. Electron microcopy reveals specific membrane-bound, tennis racket-shaped, cytoplasmic organelle, Birbeck granules. Langerhans cells possess surface Fc receptors (for binding immunoglobulins), lysosomal enzymes and express major histocompatibility class II (MHC II) molecules. Immunohistochemical study reveals consistent CD1a antigen positivity. Main functions of these cells are antigen presentation and mediation of T cell response.

There are subtle differences between normal Langerhans cells and those seen in patients with histiocytosis. The later cells are larger with a more round configuration because of less number of dendrites, possess vacuolated cytoplasm and clearer, more convoluted nuclei. Cytoplasmic organelles and mitotic figures are commoner in these cells.

Histiocytes other than Langerhans cells (non-Langerhans cell histiocytes) do not possess Birbeck granules and surface markers like CD1a and S-100. However, these have different sets of surface antigens and electron microscopy reveals other types of cytoplasmic organelles.

CLASSIFICATION

According to the classification by Histiocyte society (1987), there are three major classes of histiocytosis, as follows:

Class I: There is massive proliferation of histiocytes due to antigenic stimulation; e.g. Langerhans cell histiocytosis.

Class II: Infection associated and familial hemophagocytic syndromes; e.g. Dorfman's disease (sinus histiocytosis with massive lymphadenopathy), benign cutaneous histiocytosis (juvenile xanthogranuloma).

Class III: Malignant proliferation; acute monocytic leukemia.

CLASS I HISTIOCYTOSIS

The disorders included in this group are broadly known as Langerhans cell histiocytosis (LCH). It is a rare disorder frequent in young children. There are three subgroups under this entity;

- Hand-Schüller-Christian syndrome
- Letterer-Siwe disease
- Eosinophilic granuloma

PATHOGENESIS

There is abnormal proliferation of Langerhans cells, the stimulus for which may be endogenous or exogenous. In patients with LCH, there is raised serum level of granulocyte-macrophage colony stimulating factor (GM-CSF), which induces differentiation and proliferation of Langerhans cells from the bone marrow precursors as well as their local accumulation. Multiple exogenous factors may play a role by acting as the source of antigenic stimulus for proliferation of Langerhans cells. Infectious agents may be involved in the pathogenesis; these include human herpes virus-6, cytomegalovirus and scabies mite.

CLINICAL FEATURES

The disease may be localized (eosinophilic granuloma) or generalized (Hand-Schüller-Christian syndrome and Letterer-Siwe disease). In generalized disease, the commonly involved organs are skin, bone, bone marrow, lymph node, liver, spleen and lungs. There may be clinical overlap of the variants in a given patient. Moreover, progression from one variant to the other may occur.

Eosinophilic Granuloma

This chronic form of the disorder affects mainly adolescent boys and young adults. The lesion may be solitary or multiple, localized bony swelling involving flat bones like skull, ribs, sternum, scapula, pelvis and rarely long bones of the extremities. The lesions may be painful or asymptomatic.

Hand-Schüller-Christian Syndrome

Preschool children (2-6 years) are commonly affected with this subacute variant of the disease. There are lytic bone lesions involving skull and secondarily affecting the pituitary gland and eyes. The children present with exophthalmos and develop diabetes insipidus. Skin involvement may occur.

Letterer-Siwe Disease

This acute, generalized form of the disorder affects infants and young children and is lethal occasionally. Various system involvement occurs which has been described below.

Skin: Cutaneous lesions are common (40%) and usually the initial manifestation. The lesions do not have specific morphology or clinical pattern but resemble other dermatoses like atopic or seborrheic dermatitis. Scalp, face, retroauricular area, chest, mid-back and the diaper area are commonly involved. The lesions start as reddish papules, followed by crusting. Lesions may coalesce to give rise to large sheets of affected areas. Nodules and purpuric or xanthomatous lesions may be present. The nodules may ulcerate. Intertriginous areas show fissuring, maceration and eroded lesions. Pruritus may be associated. Lesions may bleed easily, the feature helpful in considering LCH as a differential diagnosis.

Scalp lesions may give rise to areas of alopecia. Nails may be discolored with longitudinal grooves; brittleness, total dystrophy and paronychia may be present.

Mucosa: Oral and female genital mucosae are involved. Gum bleeding or large oral aphthae may be the presenting features. Premature eruption or loosening of teeth may be present due to involvement of mandible.

Skeletal system: This is the most frequent organ involved (80%) in LCH. Often, especially in older children and young adults, bony involvement may be the sole feature of the disease. Lesions may be single/multiple, asymptomatic/painful. Involvement of skull bones is commonest and the clinical presentation may be varied, simulating chronic otitis media, deafness, proptosis and jaw-lump. Vertebral compression fracture and lytic lesions in long bones may be seen.

Lungs: Pulmonary involvement is commoner in older patients. Symptoms are non-specific and include fever, cough, chest pain, tachypnea and weight loss. Investigations reveal pathology like cysts and bullae in lung parenchyma, resulting in emphysema, nodular or diffuse lung opacities and diffuse interstitial fibrosis.

Other visceral involvements: Hepatosplenomegaly and abnormalities in liver function tests may be seen in up to 50% cases. Abdominal pain, vomiting, bloody diarrhea may result from mucosal infiltration.

Endocrine glands: Involvement of skull bones may result in pituitary dysfunction resulting in diabetes insipidus and growth retardation in children. Other glandular structures like thymus, pancreas, gonads and thyroid may also be infiltrated by Langerhans cells.

Lymph nodes: Cervical lymphadenopathy is commonly seen.

Bone marrow: Late in the course of the disease, bone marrow involvement may occur resulting in pancytopenia.

Central nervous system: Cerebral involvement is rare and usually occurs in patients with advanced skull bone involvement. In addition to the features of pituitary involvement, there may be features of focal cerebral or cerebellar deficits, palsy and seizure due to presence of space-occupying lesions.

Hashimoto-Pritzker Syndrome (Congenital self-healing histiocytosis)

This is a variant of Letterer-Siwe disease, occurring during infancy, where cutaneous involvement is the sole feature of the disease. Multiple papules, nodules or vesicular lesions appear in crops, which may undergo central necrosis resulting in umbilicated or ulcerated surface, simulating viral infections. Distribution is less widespread than Letterer-Siwe disease. Visceral involvement occurs rarely. Skin lesions undergo spontaneous resolution by few weeks to months. Long term follow up of these patients are necessary as some may progress to develop Letterer-Siwe disease.

INVESTIGATIONS

Routine hematological investigations are required to rule out systemic involvement. Skin biopsy is taken whenever there is cutaneous lesion and endoscopic biopsy is undertaken for visceral involvement. Tissue sample is subjected to histopathological examination by light microscopy, electron microscopy and immunocytochemical study.

H&E stained histopathological section is not much informatory and does not help in diagnostic confirmation. Many Langerhans cells are found which are identified as large, vacuolated cells with kidney-shaped, eccentric nuclei with coarse, granular chromatin pattern. Sometimes these cells form granuloma with central necrosis.

Demonstration of Birbeck granules by electron microscopy is confirmatory of the presence of Langerhans cells. However, these are demonstrable in 20-80% of the infiltrating cells in skin specimens and further lower in visceral specimens. Immunocytochemical stains for CD1a antigen, which is consistently found in cells of LCH, may be used as an alternative to electron microscopy for confirmation of diagnosis.

Immunocytochemical studies also help in differentiating the proliferating cells of LCH from normal histiocytes by demonstrating certain surface markers in the former. HLA-DR antigen is expressed more often and there is expression of interferon-α in these proliferating cells, but not in normal cells.

Radiological screening is required to detect bony and visceral involvement. X-ray of involved skull, pelvis and long bones reveal solitary or multiple punched-out osteolytic lesions. Vertebra may show compression fractures. Demonstration of these bony pathologies by X-ray is adequate and MRI is not actually required. However, bone scintigraphy (somatostatin receptor scintigraphy) is a useful tool in detecting multiple active foci of proliferation as well as help in monitoring treatment response.

In presence of pulmonary lesions, chest X-ray and CT scan are helpful. Miliary, interstitial reticulonodular pattern, nodular opacities, cysts or emphysematous changes are seen. Langerhans cells may be normal component of bronchoalveolar lavage fluid (1%), which is increased (5%) in LCH. CT and MRI scan are helpful in detecting other visceral as well as central nervous system involvement.

Patients with suspected diabetes insipidus are evaluated by water deprivation test and estimation of urinary arginine and vasopressin.

COURSE AND PROGNOSIS

Letterer-Siwe disease runs an aggressive course. Prognosis of Hashimoto-Pritzker syndrome and localized solitary eosinophilic granuloma are good, as self-resolution is frequent. However, these two entities may rarely undergo conversion to aggressive Letterer-Siwe disease; hence careful follow-up is necessary in all such cases. Multi-organ involvement has bad prognosis. Patients with restrictive pulmonary disease, cytopenia and liver dysfunction show poor outcome. There may be associated leukemias and lymphomas in patients with LCH, adding to the morbidity and mortality.

DIFFERENTIAL DIAGNOSIS

The skin lesions of Letterer-Siwe disease are to be differentiated from seborrheic dermatitis and atopic dermatitis, which are commonly more severely pruritic. Intertriginous involvement may be confused with candidiasis and scalp involvement in children as tinea capitis. Crusted vesicular eruptions in Hashimoto-Pritzker syndrome may simulate viral exanthema.

TREATMENT

Isolated cutaneous involvement in infants may be treated with topical steroid. Other topical therapeutic modalities are PUVA therapy, topical nitrogen mustard and irradiation which are not suitable for use in young children.

Isolated bone lesion may be treated by curettage or intralesional steroid injection. Surgical decompression may be required in vertebral involvement.

Systemic chemotherapy is indicated when more than three sites are involved. Monotherapy or combination therapy with vincristine, vinblastine, systemic steroid, methotrexate, chlorambucil, cyclophosphamide is administered. Other drugs, which has been used are daunorubicine, cytarabine, etoposide, ciclosporin and interferon.

Bone marrow transplantation and other involved organ transplantation (e.g. liver) may be effective.

CLASS II HISTIOCYTOSIS

This group of disorders involves non-Langerhans cell histiocytes. These have a foamy appearance under light microscope and may express different surface antigens like vimentin, CD68, factor XIIa, anticathepsin B, etc (juvenile xanthogranuloma). Some cells are OKM and Leu3 positive and electron microscopy reveals comma/ 'S'-shaped intracytoplasmic organelles and desmosome like structures (benign cephalic histiocytosis).

The disorders included in this group are categorized into systemic and cutaneous disorders. Systemic disorders may also have cutaneous manifestations as part of the disease. **Table 24.1** represents the clinical features of various systemic class II histiocytoses.

TABLE 24.1: Systemic class II histiocytosis

Type	Age group	Clinical features	Skin lesions	Pathogenic factors	Treatment
Acquired hemophagocytic syndrome	Early infancy	High fever, Hepatosplenomegaly, generalized lymphadenopathy, hemorrhagic episodes. Failure to thrive. Fatal outcome.	Purpuric macules and papules, erythroderma	Infections; EBV, CMV, Tuberculosis, brucellosis Inflammatory disorders; SLE, JRA, Primary immunodeficiency disorders, lymphoma, leukemia	Treatment of infection. High dose steroid , IVIg
Familial hemophagocytic syndrome	Infancy and childhood	High fever, bleeding diathesis, neurological involvement. Fatal outcome.	Purpura	Autosomal recessive, familial. Intrinsic T cell defect and unregulated cytokine secretion.	Systemic steroid, etoposide, intrathecal methotrexate, bone-marrow transplant.
Rosai-Dorfman disease (sinusal histiocytosis with massive lymphadenopathy)	Any age	Low grade fever, massive cervical lymphadenopathy, arthritis, weight loss. Usually self-limited, rare evolution to malignant lymphoma.	Well circumscribed, reddish brown to yellow papules, nodule/plaque.	Probably stimulated by EBV.	Systemic steroid. Chemotherapy/ radiotherapy for progressive disease.
Multicentric reticulohistio-cytosis	Adult	Arthritis involving all joints prior to or following skin lesions. May regress spontaneously	Erythematous papules/ nodules, evoluting to sclerosing lesions.	Reactive proliferation of histiocytes	Systemic steroid, methotrexate, alkylating agents

Most of these represent reactive hyperproliferation of histiocytes due to some infective or inflammatory stimulus. Most of these disorders are better managed by oncologists.

Cutaneous class II histiocytoses are benign, self-healing disorders of unknown etiology. Types of cutaneous class II histiocytosis are as follows:

- Juvenile xanthogranuloma
- Benign cephalic histiocytosis
- Generalized eruptive histiocytoma
- Papular xanthoma
- Xanthema disseminatum

JUVENILE XANTHOGRANULOMA

Juvenile xanthogranuloma (JXG) is a benign, self-healing histiocytosis found in young children.

Skin lesions are present at birth or appear during infancy. Firm, red, smooth, dome-shaped, asymptomatic papules or nodules are the typical initial skin lesions, distributed over head and neck **(Figure 24.1)**, or occasionally disseminated on trunk and extensor extremities. Three clinical patterns are present: the 'small nodular type' (commonest), 'large nodular type', and the 'solitary, giant, congenital' form. The solitary giant lesions are purple-red lesions with central ulcer/crusting and peripheral telangiectasia. These lesions heal with atrophy.

Oral mucosa may be involved with nodules on gingiva, buccal mucosa or tongue and may be confused with other oral tumors. Ocular lesions may give rise to features of chronic uveitis. Some patients may develop visceral nodules, which may or may not be associated with skin

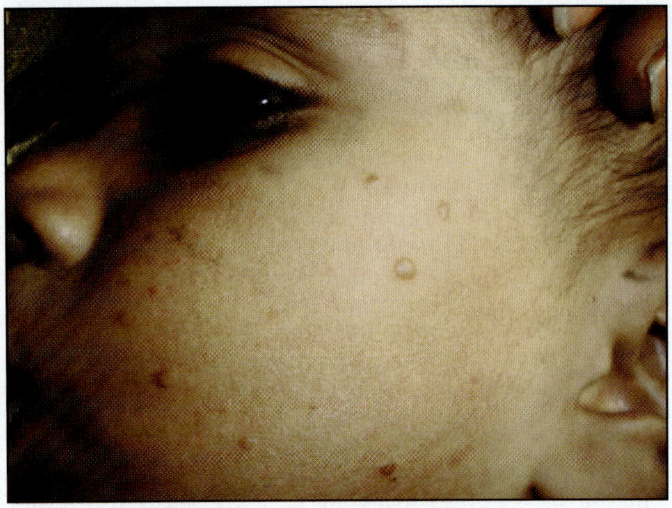

FIGURE 24.1: Juvenile xanthogranuloma

lesions. Tracheal lesions may result in acute respiratory distress.

The lesions gradually attain a yellowish-brown hue, flattened and heal with mild scarring over a period of 3-6 years. Visceral lesions may also undergo spontaneous regression. However, sometimes such lesions may have a progressive course, especially in central nervous system and may result in complications like hydrocephalos.

JXG may occur in association with neurofibromatosis I. In such patients, lesions of JXG develop later than usual and these children are at higher risk of developing myelomonocytic leukemia.

Histopathology reveals granuloma with predominantly histiocytes and other inflammatory cells. The histiocytes have foamy cytoplasm and Touton giant cells are often present.

Older lesions show dermal fibrosis. These histiocytes lack Birbeck granules and surface CD1a antigen.

Self-resolution is common. Hence aggressive treatment is not necessary. Visceral involvement with life threatening complications may necessitate combination chemotherapy.

BENIGN CEPHALIC HISTIOCYTOSIS

Skin lesions start during infancy and male children are more commonly affected. Lesions are yellow-brown, asymptomatic papules (2-4 mm), distributed on face, neck and upper chest. Mucosal or visceral involvements are not found. Lesions slowly regress over years leaving behind atrophic macules.

Histopathologically, there is dense dermal infiltrate with histiocytes along with lymphocytes and eosinophils. The skin lesions may simulate JXG but histopathologically foamy histiocytes and Touton giant cells are absent.

Treatment is not required.

Generalized eruptive histiocytoma is uncommon in children. Crops of small, yellowish brown, smooth papules appear on face, upper trunk and extremities. Spontaneous resolution occurs over many years.

Papular xanthoma also has similar morphology and lesions involute over many years. Xanthoma disseminatum is a rare benign disorder, where both cutaneous and systemic features are present. Skin lesions include numerous yellowish brown papules on face, trunk and flexures, which may coalesce to form plaques. Such reddish yellow plaques are particularly observed on eyelids, conjunctiva and lips. Diabetes insipidus may be present in 50% cases. The disease may resolve over several years or may be persistent and disfiguring .

CLASS III HISTIOCYTOSIS

In this class of disorders there is malignant proliferation of histiocytes and these are very rarely encountered in children. There is clonal proliferation of cells of lymphoid origin and these malignancies are to be differentiated from acute monocytic and myelomonocytic leukemias.

CUTANEOUS MASTOCYTOSIS

Mastocytoses is a group of disorder characterized by localized or generalized infiltration of different tissues by functionally normal mast cells. Any organ may be involved, commonest being skin, designated as 'cutaneous mastocytosis'.

Mast cells are derived from pleuripotent bone marrow stem cells. The mononuclear precursor cells enter the circulation to lodge in different tissues where these undergo differentiation and maturation to form functional mast cells. In skin, these cells are located just below the dermoepidermal junction and also around the blood vessels, nerves and cutaneous appendages. Mast cells are distinct by the property of metachromasia, i.e ability to get stained by basic aniline dyes due to highly acidic intracellular contents.

Mast cells are ovoid/spindle-shaped, mononuclear (occasionally binuclear) and slightly larger than eosinophils. There are numerous metachromatic granules in the cytoplasm. Electron microscopy reveals ridges on cytoplasmic membrane and membrane-bound cytoplasmic granules and lamellae (whorls or scrolls).

Mast cells are store house for different chemical mediators, the principal among which is histamine. The granules contain tryptase and chymase. Few other mast cell products are heparin, chondroitin sulfate, leukotrienes, prostaglandin (PGD_2), interleukins and tumor necrosis factor-α. Surface of mast cells contain high affinity IgE receptors, receptors for C3a, C5a and some other chemokine receptors. c-kit stem cell factor receptors are also present on mast cell surface which play important role in pathogenesis of mastocytosis.

Mast cells contribute to the inflammatory response by degranulation and release of chemical mediators and synthesize interleukins and GM-CSF. However, mast cells are functionally heterogenous and secreted materials as well as the range of action differs depending upon the organ of localization.

PATHOGENESIS

The cause for accumulation of mast cells in different tissues is unknown. Activating mutation of the *c-kit* receptors on mast cell surface may lead to ligand-independent autophosphorylation of the receptors and oncogenic transformation and proliferation of mast cells. Typical childhood disease is linked to Glu-839-Lyc c-kit mutation. The mutation usual in adults is Asp-816-Val is very rare in children and is found only in extensive or progressive cases. This mutation is not seen in familial cases of cutaneous mastocytosis.

Chromosomal anomalies like breaks and trisomy are increased in patients with cutaneous mastocytosis, especially among those with associated hematological disorders.

The mechanisms for systemic symptoms are twofold; massive release of mast cell mediators and organ dysfunction resulting from mast cell infiltration.

CLASSIFICATION

Cutaneous mastocytosis is included under 'indolent mastocytosis' (class IA), in the classification system by Metcalfe *et al*. It includes the following types:

- Urticaria pigmentosa
- Mastocytoma
- Telangiectatic macularis eruptiva perstans
- Diffuse cutaneous mastocytosis

EPIDEMIOLOGY

Cutaneous mastocytosis is a rare disorder. Though occurrence is worldwide, it is commoner among Caucasians. Skin lesions may be present at birth or may appear any time during infancy and childhood. It is mostly sporadic, but familial cases with dominant pattern of inheritance may occur and there are reports of occurrence among monozygotic twins. There is no sex preference.

CLINICAL FEATURES

Clinical pictures of individual variants are described below. Patients may be totally asymptomatic or symptomatic because of only pruritus or severe systemic manifestations.

Darier's sign, i.e., wheal and flare of lesional or non-lesional skin on stroking or rubbing, may be positive is some cases. The disease is congenital in 5% cases, and has been detected *in utero*. Majority (30%) of the patients present during infancy (< 6 months), others by 2 years of age (10%) and the rest (10%) by 15 years. Episodic flushing and pruritus may be associated. Extracutaneous manifestations are seen among 11-33% children. These include gastrointestinal disturbances, pulmonary and neurological symptoms.

Urticaria Pigmentosa

Urticaria pigmentosa (UP) is the commonest clinical variant (70-90%) of cutaneous mastocytosis. In two series of patients with cutaneous mastocytosis from India, the commonest clinical pattern was urticaria pigmentosa.

The skin lesions may be present at birth or appear during infancy. These are in the form of yellowish brown macules or papules in a generalized distribution, more numerous on the trunk **(Figures 24.2A and B).** Face, head, palms and soles are usually spared. In dark-skinned children the skin lesions may be slate-colored. Sometimes plaque or nodular lesions may be present. In acute stage of the disease, few lesions may develop vesicles/bullae. The lesions may be associated with pruritus and/or episodes of flushing on rubbing or towelling the child. Darier's sign may be positive. Mucosal lesions may occur. In older children (>5 years) systemic manifestations like abdominal colic and diarrhea may be associated; otherwise systemic involvement is commoner in adult-onset UP.

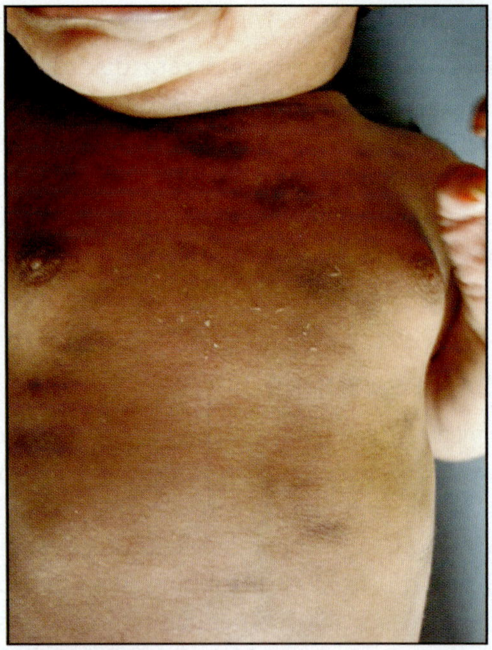

FIGURE 24.2A: Urticaria pigmentosa in infancy

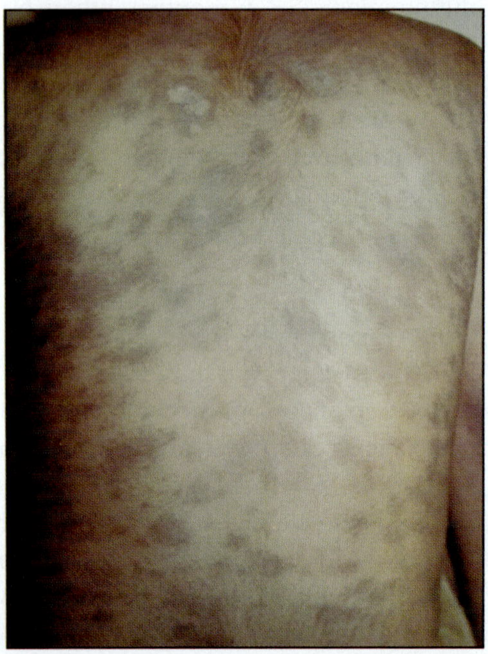

FIGURE 24.2B: Childhood urticaria pigmentosa

Mastocytoma

Mastocytoma may be solitary **(Figure 24.3)** or multiple in children, present soon after birth or usually develop by 3 months of age. This is the most frequent variant observed in childhood.The skin lesions are well-circumscribed, round/oval, yellowish plaque with a *peau d' orange* appearance and may be topped with a vesicle **(Figure 24.4)**. Darier's sign may be positive **(Figure 24.5)**. Systemic manifestations are rarely associated.

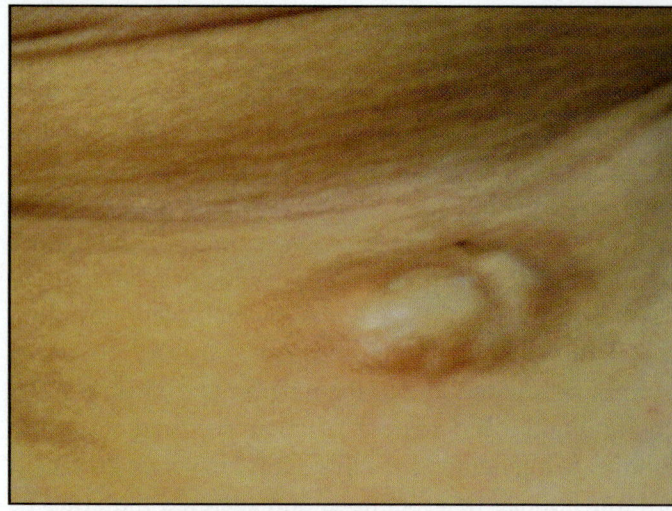

FIGURE 24.3: Solitary mastocytoma.

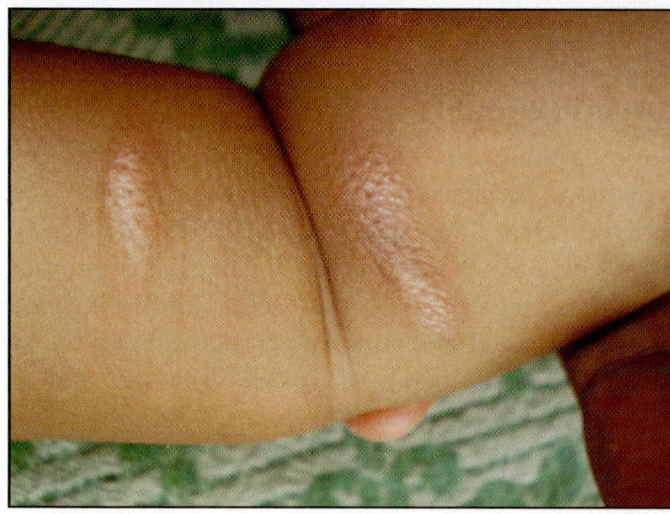

FIGURE 24.4: Multiple mastocytomas (*peau d'orange* appearance)

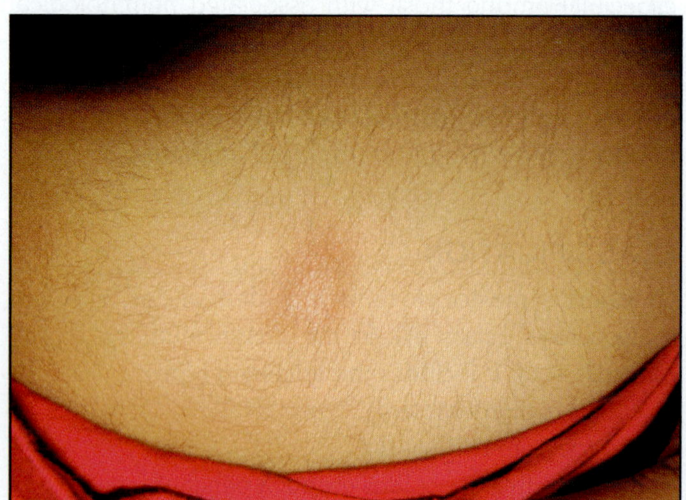

FIGURE 24.5: Positive Darier's sign on a lesion of mastocytoma

Telangiectatic Macularis Eruptiva Perstans

Telangiectatic macularis eruptiva perstans (TMEP) is the rarest variant of cutaneous mastocytosis, which is uncommon in children and usual among adolescents and adults. The skin lesions are in the form of reddish brown, telangiectatic macules occurring mostly on trunk. Darier's sign is usually negative. Familial occurrence with autosomal dominant inheritance pattern has been reported.

Diffuse Cutaneous Mastocytosis

Diffuse cutaneous mastocytosis (DCM) usually starts during infancy, but may persist thereafter as a chronic relapsing disorder. The infant presents with diffuse skin infiltration appreciated as a smooth, leathery appearance, exaggerated skin folds and doughy consistency **(Figures 24.6A and B)**. There may be numerous ill-defined, yellowish papules, known as the xanthelasmoid variant of DCM. Few vesicles or bullae are frequent but sometimes the clinical picture is dominated by large, flaccid bullae, which rupture easily to form erosions, with intervening areas of infiltrated skin. This is known as bullous mastocytosis **(Figure 24.7)**. Sometimes patients may present with erythroderma (erythrodermic DCM).

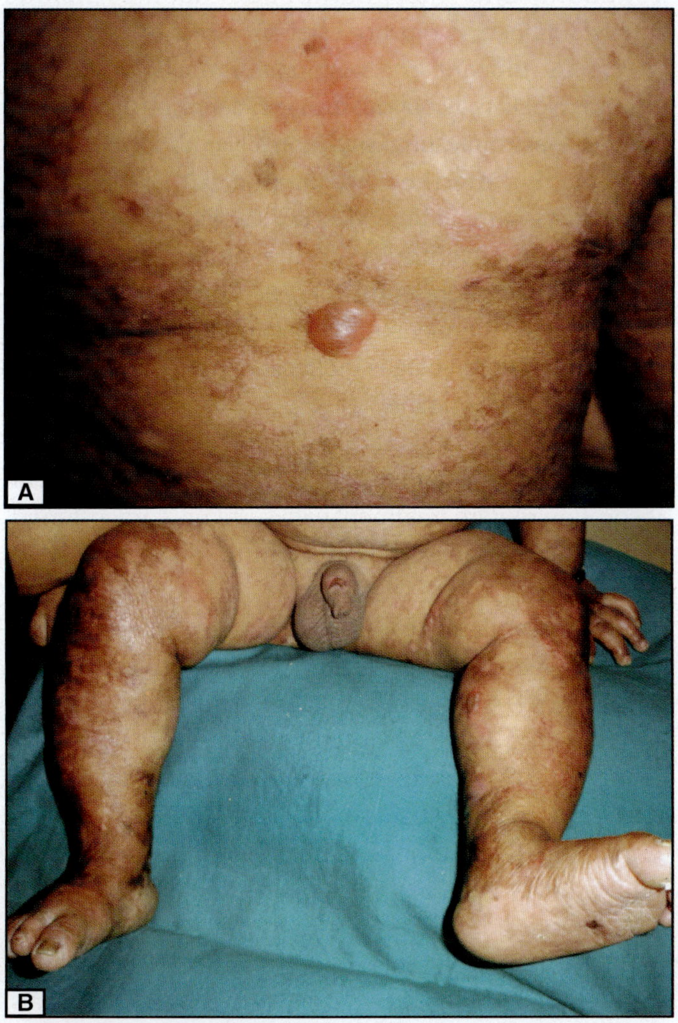

FIGURES 24.6A AND B: Diffuse cutaneous mastocytosis

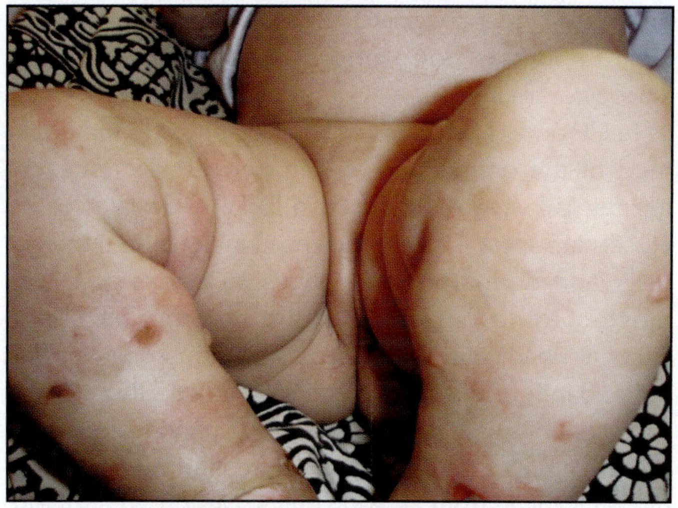

FIGURE 24.7: Bullous mastocytosis

DCM is always symptomatic, associated with intense pruritus and episodes of generalized erythema, flushing and urticaria. Systemic symptoms like vomiting, diarrhea, abdominal colic, restlessness, palpitation, fainting attacks and shock may occur. Neurological symptoms include irritability or depression in infants and poor attention span or impaired short-term memory in older children.

DIAGNOSIS

Diagnosis of cutaneous mastocytosis is mostly clinical, confirmed by histopathology.

Definitive diagnosis depends on demonstration of infiltration of mast cells in histopathological section of biopsied skin specimen. Skin biopsy should be undertaken with due care not to degranulate the mast cells; the precautions are infiltrating the skin with local anaesthetic (without adrenaline) at a distance from the actual site of biopsy; avoidance of rubbing the site and excess handling of the tissue specimen.

In all the clinical variants there is infiltration of mast cells in the dermis. This is demonstrable by H&E stain, but specific mast cell morphology can not be appreciated. Special stains like toluidine blue and Giemsa stain helps in demonstrating the metachromatic granules in the cytoplasm of mast cells. Toluidine blue stain at a lower pH has a higher specificity in demonstrating mast cells. Giemsa stain is not a preferred method as it stains leucocytes also.

In UP and TMEP, mast cells are confined to the upper third of the dermis and also in perivascular location. Infiltrate is sparse and scattered in TMEP and dilated blood vessels are seen. There is increased melanin in the basal layer and dermal melanophages in lesions of UP. In mastocytoma, mast cells are aggregated as a circumscribed, tumor-like mass, which may occupy the entire depth of the dermis and may invade through the subcutaneous tissue. In DCM, a dense band-like infiltrate is seen in upper dermis. Subepidermal bullae are seen if biopsy is taken from an early bullous lesion. In addition, eosinophilic infiltration is seen in all the variants except TMEP.

In absence of definitive histopathological features, biochemical parameters may be assessed to know disease activity. Estimation of levels of mast cell mediators and their degradation products may be helpful, though not specific of mastocytosis. Plasma histamine level is raised. Currently used methods include measurement of serum tryptase and urinary level of histamine metabolites like N-methylhistamine. Serum tryptase level correlates with the course of the disease. N-methylhistamine is an indicator of bone marrow involvement in patients with mastocytosis.

In patients with extensive UP or DCM, systemic involvement should be ruled out. The series of investigations include complete blood count, peripheral blood smear, ultrasonographic scan of liver and spleen, skeletal survey, bone marrow study by aspiration and bone scan. Immunophenotyping of bone marrow cells may help in detecting *c-kit* mutation.

DIFFERENTIAL DIAGNOSIS

Diagnostic confusion may arise in some cases. UP may be mistaken for other dermatoses like histiocytosis, incontinentia pigmenti (in young children) and lentiginosis or generalized lichen planus (older children). Bullous mastocytosis may be mistaken as staphylococcal scalded skin syndrome or any other immunobullous disorders occurring at this age. Erythrodermic DCM has to be differentiated from other causes of infantile erythroderma. Mastocytoma may be confused with juvenile xanthogranuloma or histiocytoma

TREATMENT AND FOLLOW UP

Treatment is mostly symptomatic. Parents should be instructed specifically to avoid known precipitants of mast cell degranulation. These include physical factors like cuddling and toweling, undue exertion or excessive exposure to heat (sunbathing, hot water-bath) and cold. Emotional upset may be a common cause in children. Certain drugs, used in children are known to cause mast cell degranulation and must be avoided. These include; acetyl salicylic acid, atropine, procaine, opioids, skeletal muscle relaxants, iodinated radio-contrast media, intravenous dextran etc. In older children foods like fish, lobster and crabs should be avoided.

Parents of children with asymptomatic UP are reassured and explained avoidance of the above factors. Mastocytoma can be treated by topical potent corticosteroid under occlusion, topical PUVA or excision of individual lesions. Symptomatic UP and DCM require treatment and the therapeutic agents include antihistamines and mast cell stabilizers.

Pruritus, urticaria and flushing are managed with H_1-receptor blockers like hydroxyzine or cetirizine at optimum dosage. Gastrointestinal symptoms like abdominal pain, hyperacidity, diarrhea are treated with H_2-receptor antagonist like ranitidine. Mast cell stabilizers like ketotifen and sodium chromoglycate are helpful in relieving cutaneous symptoms and may be combined with H_2-blockers in the management of gastrointestinal symptoms. Sodium chromoglycate is ineffective in the management of flushing and urticaria.

Children with uncontrollable DCM (bullous/erythrodermic) or significant systemic complications like malabsorption require treatment with systemic corticosteroid. PUVA can be used for treatment resistant UP in adolescents.

Patients with repeated episodes of anaphylactoid reactions, require prophylactic therapy with a combination of H_1 and H_2-blockers. Parents of such patients should be instructed to carry emergency kits with injectable antihistamines, steroids and adrenaline. In children with cutaneous mastocytosis surgical procedures should be carried out with utmost care following prophylactic medication with H_1 and H_2-blockers and adrenaline and systemic steroid in hand.

Follow up in patients with systemic involvement is mandatory. This should be done at 6 monthly intervals, when patient is evaluated by complete blood count, peripheral blood smear and serum (tryptase) and urinary level (N-methylhistamine) of mast cell products. Abdominal ultrasonography is advised at 1 year and bone marrow biopsy and/or bone densitometry are advised at 5th year.

COURSE AND PROGNOSIS

UP and mastocytoma may undergo self-resolution by puberty. These are the types which respond better to available treatment modalities. Bullous and erythrodermic DCM run a relatively chronic course with frequent relapses. Presence of systemic manifestations may be life-threatening at times. Malignant transformation is unlikely in childhood cutaneous mastocytosis. However, if childhood disease continues till adulthood, the course and prognosis simulate adult disease.

BIBLIOGRAPHY

1. Cambazard F, Stephan L-S. The histiocytoses, Langerhans cell and non-Langerhans cell histiocytosis. In:Harper J, Oranje A, Prose N, (editors).Textbook of pediatric dermatology. Oxford: Blackwell Publishing 2006;1(2):1699-1721.
2. Favara BE. Langerhans cell histiocytosis pathobiology and pathogenesis. Semin Oncol 1991;18:3-7.
3. Feger F, Ribadeau Dumas A, Leriche L, et al. Kit and c-kit mutations in mastocytosis: a short overview with special reference to novel molecular and diagnostic concepts. Int Arch Allergy Immunol 2002;127:110-14.
4. Hartman K, Henz BM. Mastocytosis: Recent advances in defining the disease. Br J Dermatol 2001;144:682-95.
5. Huang CY, Chao SC, Ho SF, et al. Congenital self-healing reticulohistiocytosis mimicking diffuse neonatal hemangiomatosis. Dermatology 2004;208:138-41.
6. Imiela A, Carpentier O, Segard-Drouard M, et al. Juvenile xanthogranuloma: A congenital giant form leading to a wide atrophic sequela. Pediatr Dermatol 2004;21:121-3.
7. Inamadar AC, Palit A. Cutaneous mastocytosis: report of six cases. Indian J Dermatol Venereol Leprol 2005;72:50-3.
8. Jain R, Dogra S, Verma S, Mohanty SK, Handa S. Diffuse cutaneous mastocytosis: pseudoxanthomatous variant. J Dermatol 2002;29:354-6.
9. Jih DM, Salcedo SL, Jaworsky C. Benign cephalic histiocytosis: A case report and review. J Am Acad dermatol 2002;47:908-13.
10. Kanwar AJ, Sandhu K. Cutaneous mastocytosis in children: an Indian experience. Pediatr Dermatol 2005;22:85-7.
11. Orange AP, Mulder PGH, Heide R, et al. Urinary N-methylhistamine as an indicator of bone marrow involvement in mastocytosis. Clin Exp Dermatol 2002;27:502-6.
12. Orange AP, Widowati S, Sukardi A, et al. Diffuse cutaneous mastocytosis mimicking staphylococcal scalded skin syndrome: report of three cases. Pediatr Dermatol 1991; 8:147-51.
13. Raveenthiran V, Dhanalakshmi M, Hayavadana Rao PV, et al. Rosai-Dorfman disease: Report of a 3-year old girl and critical review of treatment options. Eur J Pediatr Surg 2003;13:350-4.
14. Sethuraman G, Handa S, Radotra B, Kumar B. Diffuse cutaneous mastocytosis with bullae/bullous mastocytosis: a question of semantics. Pediatr Dermatol 1999;16:409-11.
15. Snow JL, Su WP. Histiocytic diseases. J Am Acad Dermatol 1995;33:1116.
16. Van Gysel D, Oranje AP, Vermeijden I, et al. Evaluation of urinary N-methylhistamine measurement in patients with mastocytosis. J Am Acad Dermatol 1996;35:556-8.

25

Collagen Vascular Disorders and Systemic Vasculitides

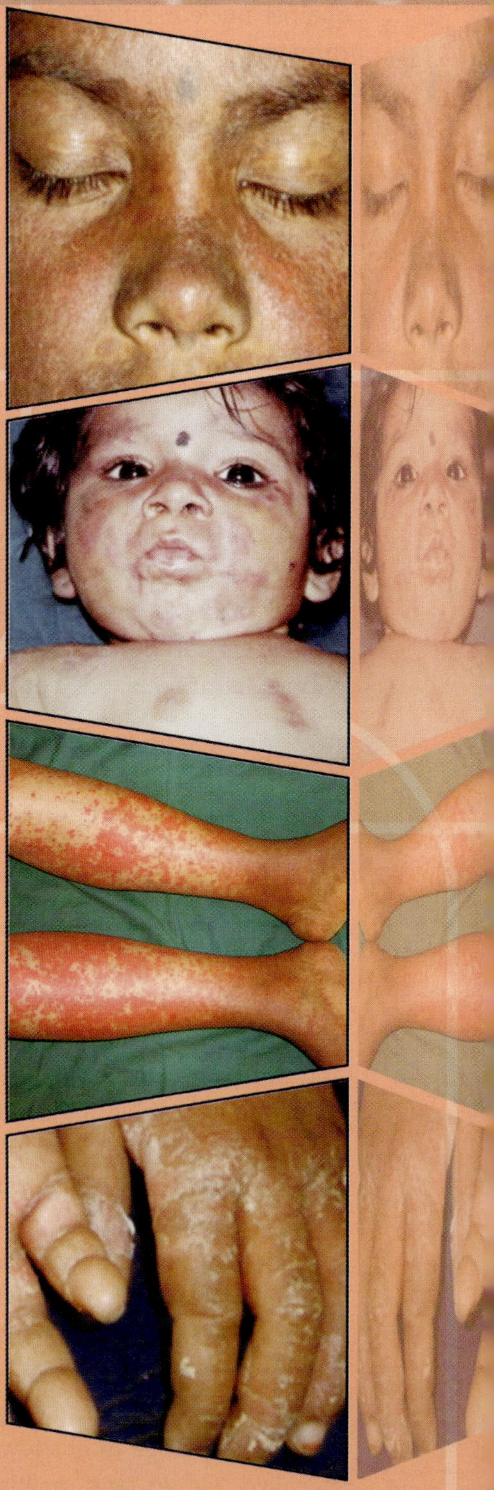

- Lupus erythematosus
- Dermatomyositis
- Systemic sclerosis
- Juvenile idiopathic arthritis
- Mixed connective tissue disorders
- Sjögren's syndrome
- Relapsing polychondritis
- Systemic vasculitides
- Cryoglobulinemia and cryofibrinogenemia

Debabrata Bandyopadhyay

LUPUS ERYTHEMATOSUS

Lupus erythematosus (LE) is a group of autoimmune inflammatory disorders which share, in varying degrees, clinical features, histopathology, and laboratory findings particularly in the form of autoantibodies directed mainly against nuclear antigenic targets. The spectrum of LE ranges from discoid lupus erythematosus (DLE), a chronic, benign, essentially skin-limited form, to systemic lupus erythematosus (SLE), a multisystem disorder with significant morbidity and mortality. Subacute cutaneous lupus erythematosus (SCLE) is an intermediate variant with cutaneous lesions and less prominent systemic affection. Neonatal lupus erythematosus is a distinct pediatric subset of the disease.

From a dermatologic perspective, the lesions of LE are classified as: *chronic cutaneous LE* (DLE, verrucous or hypertrophic LE, tumid LE, chilblain lupus, lichenoid LE or LE-LP overlap, and lupus panniculitis), *subacute cutaneous LE* (annular and psoriasiform), and *acute cutaneous LE* (the lesions generally associated with SLE). Although lesional morphology can often predict the clinical course, it should be recognized that much overlap exists and the typical chronic cutaneous lesions of DLE or lupus panniculitis may actually occur as a part of SLE.

DISCOID LUPUS ERYTHEMATOSUS

The commonest of chronic cutaneous lesions of LE, discoid lupus erythematosus occurs rarely in children. Although DLE may occur in any age, less than 2% of all cases of the disease begin during childhood. In contrast to adult disease, where a female preponderance is seen, the sex ratio is equal in childhood DLE. Genetic factors, as evidenced by histocompatibility antigen associations and familial occurrence, may play an important role in the causation of the disease. DLE has been described in identical twin children. Environmental factors in the form of ultraviolet radiation and traumas have been implicated in the precipitation or aggravation of the lesions.

The lesions of DLE are clinically characterized by well-defined, indurated, and reddish to purplish plaques covered with adherent scales. There may be fine telangiectasia on the surface. The thick scales fill the dilated pilosebaceous follicles and upon removal of the scales, their undersurface may show horny follicular plugs: the so-called 'carpet tack' or 'tin- tack' sign. Untreated or healed lesions may develop persistent hypopigmentation and hyperpigmentation with atrophy. The lesions are usually round or oval, but linear lesions along the lines of Blaschko may occur in childhood DLE. Atrophic lesions of DLE on scalp may eventually develop patches of cicatricial alopecia. Well-circumscribed hyperkeratotic or erosive lesion surrounded by a narrow zone of inflammation may occur on the lip. Mucosal lesions may occur in approximately one fourth of the cases and involve the oral mucosa, nose, eye, or vulva.

Based on patterns of distribution of the lesions, DLE may be classified into localized and disseminated or generalized forms. In *localized DLE*, by far the commoner form, the disease is localized above the neck, typically involving the face, scalp, and ears. In *generalized DLE*, in addition to the head and neck regions, the trunk, upper limbs and other body sites are involved. These lesions tend to be persistent and resistant to therapy. Disseminated disease is more often likely to be associated with laboratory abnormalities in the form of raised ESR, positive antinuclear antibodies, and leucopenia. However, in a study of 27 cases of childhood DLE, no correlation was found between localized and disseminated lesions and evolution to SLE.In contrast to adult cases in which about 5% of cases may progress to SLE, childhood DLE more often occur as a part of systemic disease.

Clinically, DLE may need to be differentiated from conditions like lupus vulgaris, sarcoidosis, polymorphous light eruption, cutaneous lymphoma, and cutaneous lymphoid hyperplasia. DLE is diagnosed by characteristic clinical findings aided by histological evaluation of lesions. Typical histologic findings include hyperkeratosis with follicular plugging, atrophic epidermis, vacuolar degeneration of basal cells, thickening of basement membrane, perivascular and periappendageal dense mononuclear infiltrate often extending to the deep dermis and subcutis, and variable mucin deposition in the dermis. 'Lupus band test', the finding of continuous linear or granular band of immunoglobulin and complement deposition along the dermo-epidermal junction may be positive in 90% of lesional skin on the head and neck region, with much less frequency on lesions on other areas.

Tumid lupus erythematosus is an extremely rare subtype of chronic cutaneous LE in childhood.The lesions are characterized by reddish, edematous, urticaria-like but relatively fixed plaques that occur on the face and other sun-exposed body sites. The lesions are nonscarring and there is no epidermal involvement. Histopathology of lesions shows superficial and deep perivascular and periappendageal mononuclear infiltrate and dermal mucin deposit.

Chilblain lupus is rare variety of chronic LE which preferentially involves the acral areas like tips of toes and fingers, nose and ears but also on the heels, calves, elbows, and knees. The lesions are chilblain-like, painful erythematous or purplish papules and nodules that may be associated with DLE but are more persistent. Histological and immunohistological features are similar to DLE. A monogenic, autosomal dominant form of chilblain lupus that begins in childhood has been described and was mapped to chromosome 3p.

Lupus panniculitis (lupus erythematosus profundus) is a subtype of LE which involves the subcutaneous tissue. Well-circumscribed, non-tender, firm, dermal and subcutaneous nodules often with a rubbery consistency, predominantly involve the cheeks, upper arms, breast, scalp, forehead, thighs, and buttocks. The skin over the surface is usually normal but may ulcerate. A DLE lesion may also overlie a nodule; some prefer to use the designation LE profundus for this type of lesions only. Lesions of lupus panniculitis tend to be very persistent. Atrophy frequently leads to unsightly depressions over the surface of the lesions. Histopathology of the lesions demonstrates infiltration of lymphoid cells in the deep dermis and subcutis often with dermal mucin deposit and hyalinization of collagen. There is usually immunoglobulin and complement deposit along the dermoepidermal junction. A significant proportion of patients may have associated lesions of DLE and some patients may develop systemic features of SLE. Lupus panniculitis has also been described in a child in association with antiphospholipid syndrome.

SUBACUTE CUTANEOUS LUPUS ERYTHEMATOSUS

Subacute cutaneous lupus erythematosus has been rarely described in childhood. The lesions usually begin acutely as erythematous macules and papules that evolve into hyperkeratotic psoriasis-like papulosquamous lesions or annular/polycyclic plaques. The surface of the lesions may be covered with thin, easily removable scales. The margin of the plaques may develop vesicopustules followed by crusting. Lesions of SCLE usually occur over sun-exposed areas (upper back, V area of the neck, shoulder, and face). Unlike lesions of DLE, SCLE lesions are not indurated and heal without scarring. The lesions may however leave prominent post-inflammatory hypo-pigmentation.

SCLE in childhood is characteristically associated with antibody to Ro/SSA nuclear antigen. Homozygous C2 deficiency may also be associated.Histology of both the forms of SCLE may show interface dermatitis with vacuolar damage to basal cells, upper dermal edema, mucin deposits, and an upper dermal perivascular and periappendageal mononuclear infiltrate. Direct immunofluorescent study (lupus band test) usually reveals a linear deposit of immunoglobulins and complement components. The small number of reported SCLE cases in childhood has not been associated with any significant systemic associations.

SYSTEMIC LUPUS ERYTHEMATOSUS

SLE is an episodic multisystem disorder characterized by persistent antinuclear antibody (ANA) seropositivity, widespread inflammation, and immune-complex deposition in key target organs.The clinical manifestation of the disease varies widely in its severity and extent of organ system involvement. The skin is involved in most cases.

Etiology

The pathogenesis of SLE is complex and not fully understood. Familial occurrence of the disease, increased concordance in monozygotic twins, association with certain HLA types, and linkage with certain genes strongly suggest genetic component in the causation of the disease. On the background of this polygenic susceptibility, environmental factors like ultraviolet exposure and exposure to drugs precipitate immune dysregulation resulting in self-reactivity to nuclear and cytoplasmic antigens leading to auto-antibody generation and immune-complex disease. Defect in immune-complex clearance, abnormal antigen presentation, and apoptotic cell death are also implicated.

Epidemiology

About 15 to 20% of all cases of SLE occur during the first two decades of life. The overall incidence during childhood has been estimated at 6 per 100,000 children and the disease is said to be more prevalent in Asian,

African-American, and Hispanic children. Most cases in children occur between the ages of 11 and 15; the disease being rare before the age of three except for neonatal lupus. The sex ratio is approximately 4:1 in favor of females in childhood disease while it becomes 9:1 in adult disease.

Clinical Features

Wide variability in the clinical manifestations is the hallmark of this multisystem illness whose severity may range from a chronic, remitting and relapsing insidious disability to acute, severe, life-threatening illness. Most patients have constitutional symptoms in the form of fever, fatigue, malaise, and weight loss. Joint symptoms and skin lesions are very common manifestations of the disease. Renal and central nervous system manifestations are the most important predictors of long-term survival of children with SLE. Lymphadenopathy and hepatosplenomegaly occur with increased frequency in childhood SLE in comparison to the adult disease. The initial manifestations of childhood-onset SLE are diverse, severe, and often atypical as compared to the adult disease.

Mucocutaneous Manifestations

A wide variety of mucocutaneous lesions may occur in SLE **(Table 25.1)**. About 80% of children have mucocutaneous manifestations at sometime of the illness and about one fourth may have skin changes as their presenting complaint. In a study of 57 children with SLE, cutaneous manifestations were the second most common finding, next to renal involvement.

About half of the patients may have photosensitivity, often manifesting as an erythematous eruption on sun-exposed skin. A characteristic finding is the malar or butterfly rash which takes the form of an erythematous, mildly scaly rash on the cheeks and the nasal bridge **(Figure 25.1)**. There may be associated facial edema. A more widespread erythema involving the ears and chest may also occur **(Figure 25.2)**. The lesions resolve without scarring.

Other Manifestations

Diffuse alopecia may occur as a result of chronic telogen effluvium and increased fragility of hair **(Figure 25.3)**.

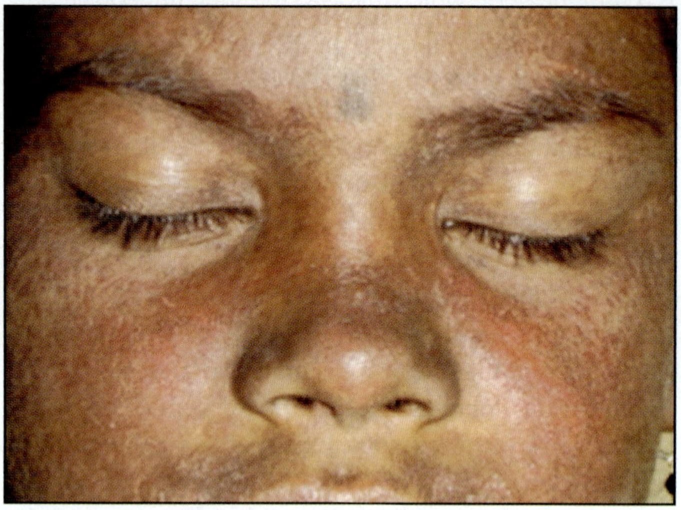

FIGURE 25.1: Malar erythema in SLE

TABLE 25.1: Mucocutaneous manifestations of SLE

Photosensitivity	*Alopecia*
Malar rash	Telogen effluvium
Vascular lesions	'Lupus hair'
Livedo reticularis	Scarring alopecia
Periungual erythema	Alopecia areata
Raynaud's phenomenon	*Mucosal lesions*
Palpable purpura	Oral, nasal, genital erosions/ulcers
Urticarial vasculitis	*DLE*
Digital Gangrene	*SCLE*
Leg ulcer	*Lupus panniculitis*
Chilblain lupus	*Calcinosis cutis*
Atrophie blanche	*Papulonodular mucinosis*
Bullous lesions	Urticaria
Bullae associated with LE-specific lesions	*Erythema multiforme*
'Bullous SLE'	*Ichthyosis*
	Pigmentary changes

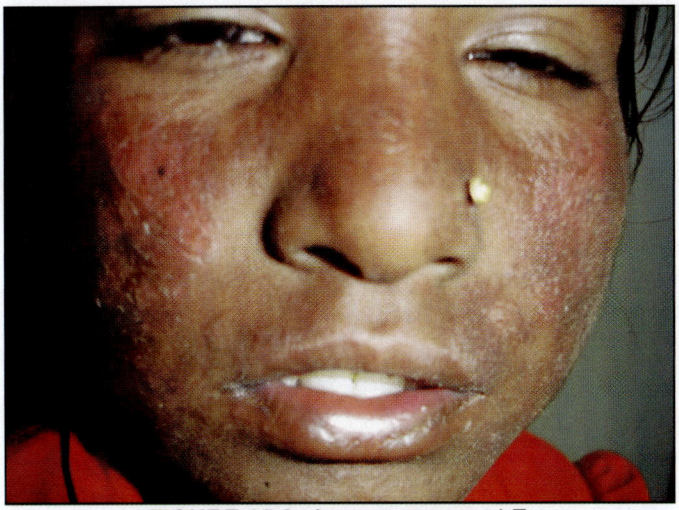

FIGURE 25.2: Acute cutaneous LE

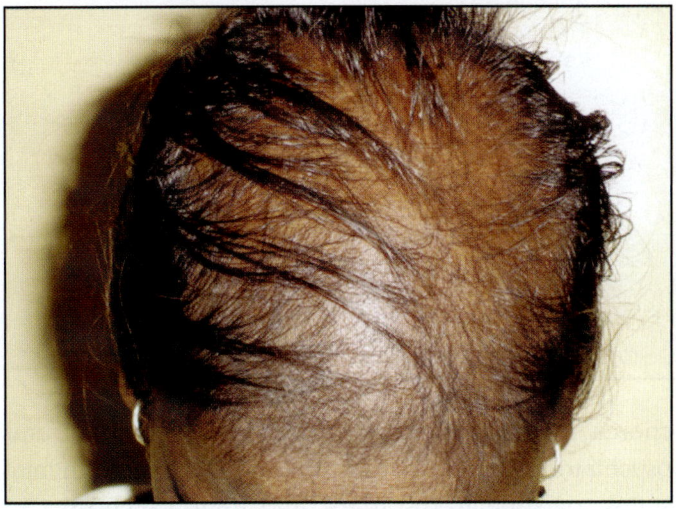

FIGURE 25.3: Diffuse alopecia in SLE

Short, broken, unruly hairs in the fronto-temporal region are termed 'lupus hairs'. Permanent scarring alopecia as in DLE may also be a feature of SLE.

A variety of vascular lesions may occur in a large proportion of cases in the form of vasculitis, periungual erythema, telangiectasia, and nail-fold infarcts. Raynaud's phenomenon, an episodic, reversible vasospasm of acral areas induced by cold exposure may occur in many children and may precede the onset of systemic disease for weeks or months. Livedo reticularis is a persistent, bluish red, reticulated discoloration of the skin, more marked on the lower extremities. Cutaneous small vessel vasculitis in association with SLE may take the forms palpable purpura, cutaneous infarcts, and urticarial vasculitis. Large vessel occlusion from thrombosis or vasculitis may result in digital gangrene. Persistent leg ulcers may result from breakdown of vasculitic lesions.

Bullous lesions in SLE may result from severe liquefaction degeneration of basal cells and dermal edema. A distinct subset of bullous disease in SLE is called bullous SLE. This vesiculobullous eruption usually occurs on an erythematous base in association with pruritus mainly on the sun-exposed skin. Lesions mimic dermatitis herpetiformis or bullous pemphigoid. Localized linear bullous LE along the lines of Blaschko has been described in a child. Subepidermal neutrophilic microabscess, linear deposits of immunoglobulins and C3 along the dermoepidermal junctions, a split at the sub-lamina densa demonstrable on electron microscopy, and presence of antibody to type VII collagen are characteristic features of this disease.

Mucosal lesions, mainly in the form of oral ulcers **(Figure 25.4)**, may occur in about half of the children. Shallow ulcer with a dirty base and surrounding erythema occur mainly on the palate as well as on the buccal mucosa and gingiva. Chelitis, nasal and genital mucosal involvement may occur. Mucosal lesions usually occur during the active phase of the disease.

Other rare cutaneous lesions that may occur in SLE include papulo-nodular lesions from mucin deposits, pigmentary anomalies, widespread ichthyosis, calcinosis cutis, and eruptive dermatofibroma. Herpes zoster may be more frequent and scabies may be severe and of the crusted variety. In addition, it should always be borne in mind that chronic or subacute cutaneous lesions of LE like DLE, SCLE, or panniculitis may occur as part of the mucocutaneous manifestations of the systemic disease.

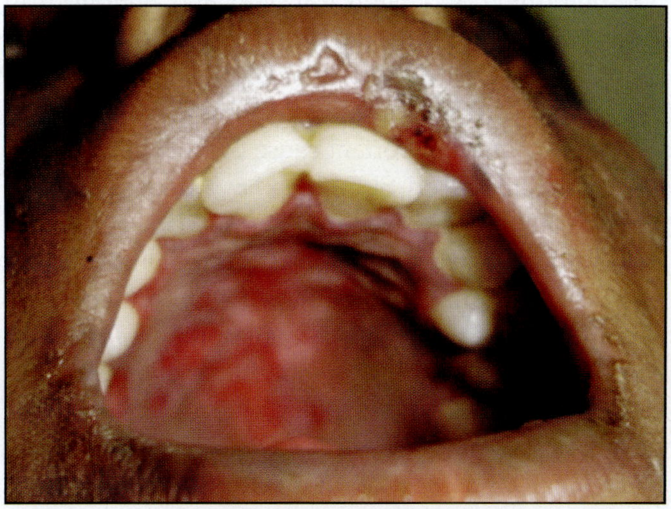

FIGURE 25.4: Oral ulcer in SLE

TABLE 25.2: Systemic manifestations of SLE

Renal Nephritic and nephrotic syndrome Hypertension Renal failure *Musculoskeletal* Arthritis and arthralgia Myositis Avascular necrosis of bones *Neuropsychiatric* Headache Seizure Cerebrovascular disease Peripheral and cranial neuropathy Chorea Personality disorders Psychosis *Cardiac* Pericarditis Endocarditis Conduction defects Valvular insufficiency Ischemia *Hepatosplenomegaly* *Lymphadenopathy*	*Pulmonary* Impaired pulmonary diffusion Acute Pneumonitis Pleuritis Pulmonary hemorrhage Pulmonary hypertension Pneumothorax Infective pneumonia *Gastrointestinal* Abdominal pain Ascites Pancreatitis Mesenteric thrombosis *Hematological* Anemia Thrombocytopenia Leucopenia *Eye* Conjunctivitis Scleritis Episcleritis Uveitis Retinal hemorrhage

Systemic Manifestations (Table 25.2)

Arthritis is among the most common manifestations of childhood SLE. It is present in about 90% of children and in association with fever and fatigue, constitutes the most common presenting feature of the disease. Both small and large joint are involved symmetrically. The arthritis is non-deforming and often transient and migratory in nature. In children, the associated pain is often out of proportion to the degree of clinical inflammation.

Renal involvement is more frequent in children than in adults and is an important cause of mortality. Overall, 60-80% of childhood SLE cases have urinary or renal function abnormalities early in the disease course and in 90% of patients, renal disease occurs within two years from disease onset. Evidence of immune-complex disease, such as anti-dsDNA antibodies or reduced complement level , correlates with active nephritis in most children.

Neuropsychiatric SLE is a frequent cause of morbidity in children and may occur in about one fourth of childhood cases. Seizures, cerebrovascular disease, chorea, recurrent headache, peripheral neuropathy, and psychiatric manifestations in the form of altered mental status, personality disorders, and frank psychosis can occur. Pulmonary manifestations may be an initial or life-threatening complication of SLE in children. Abnormalities of pulmonary functions, pleuritis, pneumonitis, pulmonary hemorrhage, and infectious pneumonia can occur. Cardiac involvement most commonly manifests with pericarditis and pericardial effusion; endocarditis and valvular insufficiency may also occur. Gastrointestinal involvement may occur in about 20% children with SLE, abdominal pain being the most frequent symptom.

Laboratory Findings

SLE is associated with a plethora of laboratory abnormalities reflecting the underlying pathologic and immunologic changes in this multisystem disorder. Routine hematological testing may reveal anemia, leucopenia, and thrombocytopenia. Most children have leukopenia at the onset of the disease and often, leukocytosis does not develop to an appropriate degree even with septicemia. Coomb's test may be positive. A raised ESR may indicate active inflammatory process. Proteins, red blood cells, and casts in the urine and elevated serum creatinine and blood urea nitrogen may indicate the presence and severity of renal involvement. Serum globulin level may be high and there may be reversal of albumin: globulin ratio. However, SLE is mainly characterized by the presence of a host of immunological abnormalities reflecting the presence of autoimmunity. These are more frequently observed in childhood cases than in the adult disease.

Presence of antinuclear antibodies (ANAs) is the hallmark of immunologic abnormalities and this can be documented in nearly all children with SLE particularly when a human cell line (e.g., Hep-2) is used as a substrate in the indirect immunofluorescence test. Owing to its high sensitivity, ANA is a valuable screening test in suspected cases of SLE, but this may be positive in several other connective tissue disorders as well as in 5-10% of normal individuals. Several patterns of immunofluorescence have been described; the peripheral and homogenous patterns being characteristics of SLE. Antibody to double-stranded or native DNA (anti-dsDNA) and anti-Smith (anti-Sm) antibodies are specific for SLE but are less sensitive, found in 50% and 25% of children respectively. Both are associated with an increased risk of renal involvement. Antibody to single-stranded DNA (ssDNA) is non-specific and anti-histone antibodies may be present in drug-induced LE. Antibodies to the ribonucleoprotein antigens Ro/SSA and La/SSB are found with less frequency than in adults except in neonatal lupus. Antiphospholipid antibodies, present in up to 65% of children with SLE, may lead to recurrent thromboses and are associated with increased incidence of neuropsychiatric lupus and chorea. Antibodies to ribosomal P proteins are also found in childhood SLE with CNS involvement and psychosis. Rheumatoid factors, cryoglobulins, and cold agglutinins may also be present.

The immune-complex vasculitis of SLE may activate both the classic and alternate pathways of complement leading to hypocomplementemia. A decreased complement level, indicated by reduced total hemolytic complement (CH50) or reduced individual components (particularly C3 and C4) signify disease activity, particularly renal disease. Hereditary deficiency of early complement components (C1, C2, C3, and C4) is a risk factor for developing childhood onset SLE.

Diagnosis

SLE in childhood may have varied presentations and a high index of clinical suspicion in necessary for diagnosis the disease particularly for children with febrile polyarthralgia or unexplained multisystem disorder with or without a skin rash. Clinical suspicion is substantiated by appropriate laboratory investigations, particularly serological tests for ANA. A skin biopsy is sometimes helpful in diagnosis. Direct immunofluorescence test on non-lesional skin of covered areas (lupus band test) is characteristic of SLE. Detailed clinical examination and laboratory work-up should also focus on detecting the severity and extent of systemic affection. The American College of Rheumatology (ARC) criteria[24] for classification of SLE for the purpose of clinical studies on uniform populations of patients is widely used as diagnostic criteria as well and are applicable to children. For a diagnosis of SLE four of the following 11 criteria should be present concomitantly or sequentially: (1) malar rash, (2) discoid rash, (3) photosensitivity, (4) oral ulcer, (5), arthritis (non-erosive, involving 2 or more peripheral joints), (6) serositis (pleuritis/pericarditis), (7) renal disease (persistent proteinuria more than 0.5 g/day or cellular casts), (8) neurologic disease (seizure/psychosis), (9) hematologic disease (leukopenia, hemolytic anemia, or thrombocytopenia), (10) immunologic disorder (anti-dsDNA/anti-Sm/antiphospholipid antibodies), and (11) antinuclear antibody.

A number of conditions need to be considered in the differential diagnosis of childhood SLE. These include juvenile idiopathic arthritides, dermatomyositis, acute rheumatic fever, acute post-streptococcal glomerulonephritis, drug eruptions, Sjögren's syndrome, infectious mononucleosis, idiopathic seizure disorders, septicemia, and systemic vasculitides.

Treatment

Treatment of lupus erythematosus depends on the severity and extent of local or systemic disease. Some general measures are necessary in all cases with LE. Photoprotection should be adopted by avoidance of direct sun-exposure and use of protective clothing and sunscreens with high SPF. Exposure to excessive cold, heat, or trauma, and unnecessary medications should be avoided. For children requiring long-term treatment for systemic disease, maintenance of adequate nutrition and psychosocial support are necessary.

Cutaneous lesions of DLE or SCLE are best treated with topical corticosteroids. For control of inflammation, relatively potent formulations are often required. For recalcitrant lesions, intralesional triamcinolone acetonide (2.5 to 10 mg/ml) infiltrations may be an option. Topical calcineurin inhibitors like tacrolimus may also be beneficial. Long-term suppression of lesions may be achieved by systemic antimalarial therapy. To avoid the rare complication of retinopathy, ophthalmologic examination before initiation of treatment and six monthly thereafter is indicated. Hydroxychloroquine in the dosage of 5-10 mg/kg/day with a maximum daily dose of 400 mg/day may have to be given for several months for adequate control of disease. Alternative regimens include thalidomide, clofazimine, or systemic and topical retinoids. Lupus profundus in children may also be successfully treated with hydroxychloroquine. Bullous LE respond well to dapsone therapy.

Mild forms of SLE with joint symptoms and myalgia may respond to non-steroidal anti-inflammatory agents like ibuprofen. Antimalarials are also used to manage cutaneous disease or to reduce the required dosage of corticosteroids. Systemic corticosteroids are the mainstay of treatment of all but the mild forms of childhood SLE. For oral therapy prednisolone is generally preferred, which is used in divided dosage initially. For persistent fever, dermatitis, arthritis, serositis, or mild renal disease, low-dose therapy (0.5 mg/kg) is used. Higher dosage of steroids (1-2 mg/kg/day) is indicated for severe renal disease, CNS involvement, or acute hemolytic anemia. Intravenous pulse methylprednisolone therapy (10-30 mg/kg) is also used in severe acute exacerbation of disease. Disease activity is monitored by clinical assessment and decrease in anti-dsDNA and complement levels. After control is achieved, steroid dosage should be tapered to the lowest level that maintains remission. Single morning, or preferably, alternate day therapy is instituted to minimize chances of growth reduction. Children are more prone to infections while on long-term steroids and tuberculosis must be ruled out before starting therapy. Live vaccines should be avoided while on steroids. Children are more likely than adults to develop aseptic necrosis of bones. Osteopenia is a recognized complication and is correlated with the cumulative steroid dosage.High dietary calcium intake and vitamin D and calcium supplementation should be done from the beginning of therapy.

Immunosuppressive agents may be combined with steroid regimens for better response and for their steroid-sparing effects in severe disease. Monthly cyclophosphamide pulse therapy (500 to 750 mg/m^2) for six months is followed by oral maintenance therapy. Azathioprine and methotrexate are useful alternatives. A number of other drugs like mycophenolate mofetil, chlorambucil, tumor necrosis factor inhibitors, cyclosporine A, and rituximab have also been used with variable success.

SLE is characterized by a chronic course with repeated exacerbations and remission and the prognosis is unpredictable in an individual child. Poor outcome is correlated with severe renal and CNS disease. The prognosis however has improved dramatically over the last decades with effective immunosuppressive therapy and a recent study has documented 94% survival at 11 years.In an Indian study, the commonest primary determinant of mortality was found to be uncontrolled disease activity due to delayed diagnosis and treatment.

NEONATAL LUPUS ERYTHEMATOSUS

Neonatal lupus erythematosus (NLE) is a distinct subset of lupus erythematosus occurring in neonates born to mothers who are prone to develop SLE and other connective tissue disorders like SLE, rheumatoid arthritis, Sjögren's syndrome, mixed connective tissue disease, and undifferentiated connective tissue disease.Most of these mothers are HLA DR3 positive. Transplacental transfer of maternal autoantibodies is responsible for the disease. In most cases the antibodies are anti-Ro/SSA autoantibodies, often in association with anti-La/SSB antibodies. A subset of cases are associated with anti- U_1RNP antibodies. Cutaneous manifestations and cardiac involvement, mainly in the form of congenital heart block, are distinct features of this syndrome. About 50% of infants with NLE will demonstrate cardiac conduction defects and about 50% will show skin findings; only 10% have both abnormalities.

The skin rash in NLE is characterized by erythematous scaly lesions particularly on the sun-exposed skin. Facial lesions, particularly around the eyes ('raccoon eyes'), are characteristic. Annular erythematous lesions also occur **(Figures 25.5A and B)**. Besides the head and neck region, the extremities and the palms and soles may also be affected. Discoid lesions, cutaneous atrophy, and telangiectasia can rarely occur. A child may be born with a skin rash or the lesions develop within the first few weeks of life. New lesions rarely occur after three months.

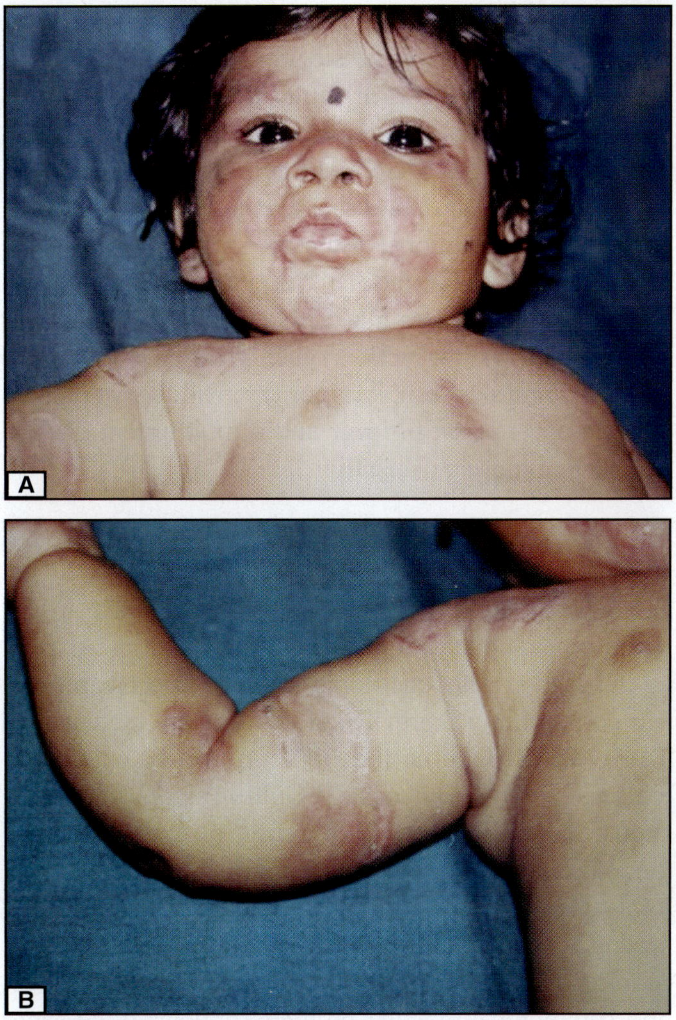

FIGURES 25.5A AND B: Periorbital and annular lesions of neonatal LE

NLE is the commonest cause of congenital heart block. Autoantibody- mediated damage to the conduction tissues of the heart results in fibrosis and calcifications. Complete congenital heart block may occur in isolation or in association with other cardiac defects like myocarditis, septal and endocardial cushion defects, and endomyocardial fibroelastosis. Fetal echocardiography can detect congenital heart block. Cardiac involvement may lead to high neonatal death. Other systemic involvements may also occur. These include hepatic disease with hepatomegaly and abnormal liver function tests and occasional hepatic failure, hematologic abnormalities (anemia, leukopenia, and thrombocytopenia), lymphadenopathy, and splenomegaly. Hydrocephalus and microcephaly have recently been described as important complications in a group of infants.

The characteristic clinical features of cutaneous and systemic involvements help in the diagnosis of NLE. A periorbital erythematous rash in an infant should always raise the suspicion of the disease.The diagnosis can be confirmed by serologic tests (for anti-Ro, anti-La, and anti-U_1RNP antibodies) of both the infant and the mother. A skin biopsy may occasionally be required to demonstrate the vacuolar interface dermatitis characteristic of lupus erythematosus. Echocardiography, ECG, complete hemogram, and liver function tests should be done routinely in suspected cases.

The cutaneous manifestations of NLE are usually transient, remitting with the disappearance of maternal autoantibody from the infants' body following metabolic decay. This usually takes about 6 to 12 months. Topical low to mid-potency steroid or calcineurin inhibitors may be used in conjunction with photoprotective measures. Skin lesions may however leave residual changes in the form of atrophy, scarring, and dyspigmentation.Systemic involvements are treated with systemic corticosteroids. Most children with heart block will need pace-makers. Mothers of affected infants run the risk of having a second affected child. Dexamethasone, given to at-risk mothers from 16th weeks of gestation, may prevent development of congenital heart block, but once established, cardiac lesion cannot be reverted by this mode of treatment.

JUVENILE DERMATOMYOSITIS

Juvenile dermatomyositis (JDM) is a multisystem disease characterized by an inflammatory myopathy and prominent dermatologic manifestations. Apart from striated muscles and skin, other internal organs are often involved. JDM is the most common of the idiopathic inflammatory myopathies in children, accounting for 85% of the pediatric inflammatory myopathies.It is an occlusive small-vessel vasculopathy, involving arterioles and capillaries. Inflammatory myositis without skin changes is termed polymyositis, an uncommon presentation in children. The amyopathic subtype, characterized by pathognomonic skin manifestations of the disease without any clinical evidence of muscle weakness may be present in 3 to 5% of children with JDM.

ETIOLOGY

JDM is believed to be autoimmune in origin, although the precise pathomechanism remains obscure. Some epidemiological studies have documented an antecedent illness a few months before the onset of symptoms of JDM and suggest that disease pathophysiology is mediated by microbial antigens through molecular mimicry. Infectious organisms that have been implicated in the pathogenesis of JDM include viruses like influenza, parainfluenza, hepatitis B, coxsackie B, parvovirus, as well as parasites, such as *Toxoplasma gondii*, and bacterial pathogens such as *Borrelia burgdorferi* and Group A β-hemolytic streptococci. Sun exposure, vaccinations, and drugs such as penicillamine and growth hormones have also been implicated. Genetic data suggest that II major histocompatibility complex allele HLA-DQA1*0501 is a risk factor for development of the disease. The presence of the tumor necrosis factor alpha (TNFα)-308A allele is another common genetic feature and this is associated with increased production of TNF alpha, chronicity of the disease, and pathologic calcifications. Complement activation and enhanced adhesion molecule expression of reactive lymphocytes and blood vessels are thought to be important factors in the pathogenetic pathway for vascular injury. Thus, environmental exposures, specifically infection, in the genetically susceptible child can lead to antigen-driven autoimmune responses that result in the evolution of disease.

EPIDEMIOLOGY

JDM is a relatively uncommon rheumatic disease, accounting for approximately 6% of children with a major connective tissue disease in pediatric rheumatology clinics. The disease affects 2 to 3 children per million children per year. The gender ratio varies in different parts of the world. In most regions, girls are more frequently affected than boys. Indian data suggest that in north India, gender ratio favors the boys, while in south India, girls with JDM are found to outnumber boys. Data on mean age at disease onset also demonstrate worldwide variation. In the United States, the mean age at disease onset is 6.9 years, while in a study from north India, the median age at diagnosis was 12 years, with a range of 2.5 to 16 years and a median duration of disease prior to diagnosis was 12 months.

CLINICAL FEATURES

The clinical features of JDM are dominated by musculoskeletal and dermatological manifestations both of which may be present in about 90 to 100% of the cases. While about one fifth of adult cases of dermatomyositis may be associated with internal malignancies, JDM is not associated with this feature. Pediatric disease, in contrast to the adult variety of dermatomyositis, is characterized by more severe muscle disease, increased incidence of pathologic calcifications, and more small vessel vasculopathy. The disease commonly has an insidious onset with constitutional features like fever, fatigue, malaise and anorexia, together with slowly progressive muscle weakness and skin rash. A minority may however present with an acute onset of fever and a multisystem disease with severe muscle weakness.

Cutaneous Manifestations

The skin changes in dermatomyositis are similar in the pediatric and adult variety of the disease. The lesions may be classified as pathognomonic, characteristic, compatible, less common, and rare. These changes are tabulated in **Table 25.3**. One of the pathognomonic cutaneous features of dermatomyositis is Gottron's papule, a violaceous, flat-topped papule occurring over the interphalangeal or metacarpophalangeal joints, elbow or knee joints and occur in about 70% of children. There may be scaling over the surface of the lesions. Another pathognomonic sign is the Gottron's sign, a confluent, violaceous, and symmetrical macular erythema involving the same regions as the papules. In contrast to SLE, this erythema spares the interphalangeal spaces.

A striking violaceous erythema may involve the face, particularly the eyelids in a symmetrical fashion. This so-called 'heliotrope erythema' (so named because of its similarity to the color of the flower of the heliotrope plant) may be associated with facial edema **(Figure 25.6)**. A confluent violaceous erythema involving the shoulder, upper back, and anterior chest is called the 'shawl sign'. Similar erythematous eruption on the V area of chest is named the 'V-sign'. These erythematous eruptions often spare the photoprotected sites suggesting the role of ultraviolet exposure as a precipitating factor. Periungual telangiectasia and erythema may be associated with thickened, irregular, hyperkeratotic cuticles. Thickened, hyperkeratotic, fissured skin of the palms and fingers may occur. This sign is designated as 'mechanic's hand'. Sometimes, a generalized pityriasis rubra pilaris-like condition may ensue.

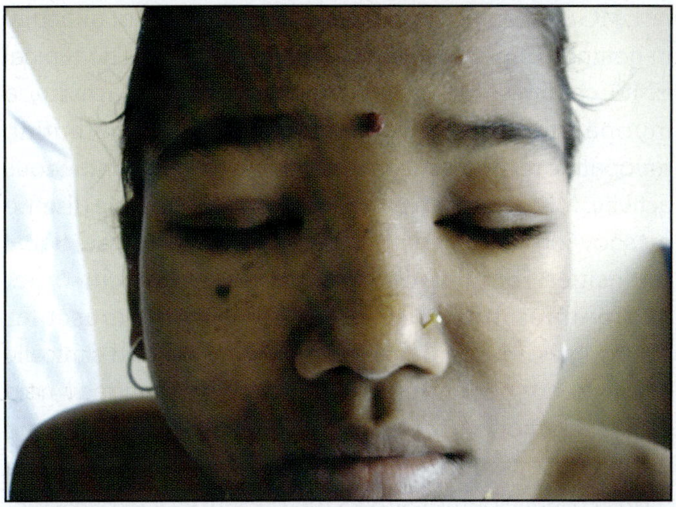

FIGURE 25.6: Periorbital edema in juvenile dermatomyositis

Poikilodermatous skin changes, characterized by mottled hypo- and hyperpigmentation associated with atrophy and telangiectasia may develop in many cases with long-standing disease. These changes are most commonly found over the V-shaped area on anterior chest and neck, upper back, shoulders, and buttock. Partial or complete lipodystrophy may occur particularly in long-standing cases. Slowly-progressive, symmetric loss of subcutaneous tissue occurs often in association with increased triglyceride levels and insulin resistance. Presentation with a generalized anasarca-like condition has been described to occur rarely. Scalp involvement may occur in the form of a diffuse erythema, pruritus, scaling, and a non-cicatricial alopecia. Oral lesions in juvenile DM have rarely been reported. Mucous membrane involvement associated with JDM may include gingival telangiectases, edema, erosions, ulcers, and leukoplakia-like lesions.

TABLE 25.3: Cutaneous manifestations of dermatomyositis

Pathognomonic	*Less common*
Gottron's papules	Erythroderma
Gottron's sign	Facial edema
	Cutaneous vasculitis
	Panniculitis
Characteristic	Lipodystrophy
Heliotrope erythema	
Shawl sign	*Rare*
V-sign	Acanthosis nigricans
Mechanic's hand	Hypertrichosis
Periungual telangiectasia	Follicular hyperkeratosis
	PRP-like generalized rash
	Papular mucinosis
Compatible	Flagellate erythema
Calcinosis cutis	Urticaria
Poikiloderma	Urticarial vasculitis
	Malignant atrophic papulosis

Inflammatory changes of long duration in the skin and muscles frequently lead to calcinosis cutis, a feature characteristically more common in JDM in contrast to adult disease. Incidence of calcinosis cutis is correlated with late diagnosis and less aggressive therapy. Usually occurring a few years after the onset of the disease, some children may have calcinosis from the onset of JDM.Firm to hard, yellowish or skin-colored papules and nodules develop over bony prominences and sites prone to trauma like the knuckle, elbows, knees, buttocks, and around the shoulders. The surface of the lesions may erode, draining a whitish chalky material. The lesions are sometimes painful. Widespread calcification of muscles and fascia may occur in a minority of children. Early diagnosis and aggressive management has resulted in decrease in the incidence of calcinosis to 20 to 35% of children from a previous rate of about 70%.

Musculoskeletal Manifestations

The myopathy commonly involves the proximal limb girdle muscles in a symmetrical fashion. The lower limb muscles are affected initially, followed by the shoulder girdle and proximal arm muscles. Affected children may develop great fatigue of their muscles and have weakness when climbing stairs, walking, rising from a sitting position, combing their hair, or reaching for objects above their shoulders. There may be a nasal intonation to their speech owing to affection of nasopharyngeal muscles and dysphagia may develop. Nasal regurgitation of liquids and palatal speech are early warning signs of impending danger of respiratory failure. Severe weakness of thoracic and respiratory muscles may occur. Involvement of facial or extraocular muscles are rare. The affected muscles may be swollen and tender. Deep tendon reflexes remain intact despite severe muscle weakness. Contractures may later develop in chronic cases. Generalized acute inflammation of the entire striated musculature may occur rarely, particularly in disease with infantile onset. A nondeforming, nondestructive arthropathy may occur in half of the children at some time during the disorder. The small joints of the hands may be affected.

Other Systemic Changes

Pulmonary impairment is one of the most dreaded complications of muscle weakness in dermatomyositis that may lead to mortality. Lung function may be compromised as a result of decreased ventilatory capacity owing to muscle weakness, aspiration pneumonia as a result of esophageal muscle weakness and gastrointestinal reflux, or rarely due to interstitial pneumonitis. Gastrointestinal manifestations are more common in the juvenile disease compared to adult dermatomyositis. Dysphagia may result from impaired functions of the musculature for deglutition. Esophageal reflux may occur. Vasculopathy of the gastrointestinal tract may cause pain abdomen, ulceration, perforation, and bleeding. Malabsorption of nutrients may occur. Cardiac involvement, rarely seen in childhood disease, may manifest as conduction defects or arrythmias. Other than tortuosity of conjunctival vessels, eye disease is limited to premature cataracts from administration of systemic steroids.

A proportion of patients with dermatomyositis have overlapping features of one of the other connective tissue disorders. For making the diagnosis of a true overlap syndrome, the patients must meet the diagnostic criteria for each of the separate disorders. These disorders include SLE, scleroderma, rheumatoid arthritis, mixed connective tissue disease, and polyarteritis nodosa. These patients may have features of dermatomyositis in association with polyarthritis, sclerodactyly, Raynaud's phenomenon, and sicca syndrome.

LABORATORY ABNORMALITIES

Serum levels of muscle enzymes (serum creatine phosphokinase, aldolase, aspartate aminotransferase, lactic dehydrogenase) are elevated in all cases of dermatomyositis in varying degrees. Serial measurements of these enzymes are important in the diagnosis and monitoring response to therapy. Although elevation of serum creatine kinase (CK) is a sensitive and specific indicator of activity of muscle disease activity in JDM, its level may remain normal despite ongoing myopathy, hence levels of all enzymes should ideally be measured. Elevated CPK levels may also be found in other causes of myopathy and after strenuous physical activities. Spurious elevation of serum CK level may occur after trauma of needle insertion for injection of medicines or electromyography (EMG). CK level usually remains low in cases of steroid-induced myopathy. CK elevation is mainly due to the CK-MM isoenzymes, but may also be due to the CK-MB isoenzyme. A CK-MB band signifies regeneration of striated muscles and not cardiac damage.

EMG is often not done in children because of difficulty in getting cooperation during the procedure. The typical EMG changes include increased insertional activity, a myopathic pattern of motor unit action potential, myopathic recruitment pattern, or increased spontaneous activity. MRI scans can provide evidence of muscle disease by showing atrophy, fatty infiltration, or increased signal intensities. Similar changes can be found in other myopathies but MRI can differentiate muscular dystrophies. Muscle biopsy should be taken from clinically involved but not atrophied muscles. MRI scan may help in the selection of the appropriate site. The deltoid and the quadriceps muscles are generally the best sites. Muscle biopsy usually demonstrates the presence of perivascular and perifascicular infiltrate of lymphocytes as well as histiocytes and occasional plasma cells and eosinophils. There may be evidence of atrophy and necrosis and fibrosis in late cases. The vasculopathy of dermatomyositis shows features ranging from endothelial swelling to obliteration and necrosis. Muscle biopsy may be false negative in 10% of cases. Skin biopsy reveals features of interface dermatitis with vacuolar degeneration of basal keratinocytes together with upper dermal perivascular infiltrate. Dermal edema and mucin deposition may also be present. The features are non-specific and indistinguishable from those of SLE and a skin biopsy is generally unhelpful in the diagnosis of dermatomyositis.

A number of autoantibodies **(Table 25.4)** may be found in association with dermatomyositis. Myositis-specific autoantibodies may have varying molecular specificities. The most frequently encountered autoantibodies target different amino acetyl transfer-RNA synthetases. While half of the adult cases may be positive for these antibodies, less than 10% of children are so and routine testing for these antibodies are not recommended in JDM. Antinuclear antibodies (ANA) may be positive in 60-70% of children. Rheumatoid factor may be elevated, particularly in those with overlap syndromes. Neopterin, an aromatic pteridine derived from intracellular guanosine triphosphate, is released primarily by human macrophages and monocytes on stimulation by T-lymphocyte-derived interferon-γ. Serum levels of neopterin is elevated in JDM and as an indicator of muscle strength and function, may be used to monitor disease activity. Quinolinic acid is generated through the metabolism of L-tryptophan in the kynurenine pathway and is produced by macrophages and brain tissue.

TABLE 25.4: Autoantibodies in JDM

Autoantibodies	Specificities	Clinical significance
Jo-1	Histidyl t-RNA synthetase	Myositis-specific antibody Antisynthetase syndrome (interstitial lung disease, polyarthritis, Raynaud's phenomenon, incomplete response to treatment)
Mi-2	Nuclear protein complex	Myositis-specific antibody Shawl sign, cuticular changes, treatment responsive
SRP	Signal recognition particle	Myositis-specific antibody Acute, severe, treatment-resistant form, cardiac disease
PM-Scl	Ribosomal RNA-processing enzyme	Overlap with scleroderma
U_1RNP	Nuclear ribonucleoprotein	Overlap syndrome
Ku	DNA repair protein complex	Overlap with scleroderma
ANA	Nuclear antigens	Amyopathic DM

Elevated urinary excretion of quinolinic acid and neopterin was also correlated with activity of muscle disease in JDM and measurement of these markers in first morning void urine specimens appeared to be as good as, or possibly better than, measurements of their concentrations in plasma. von Willebrand factor antigen, an indicator of endothelial damage, may be elevated; it is often correlated with disease flares.The erythrocyte sedimentation rate (ESR) may be elevated in about half of the cases, but there is little correlation with disease activity.

DIAGNOSIS

Dermatomyositis is clinically diagnosed by the pathognomonic or characteristic skin signs together with evidence of symmetric proximal muscle weakness. Clinical diagnosis is corroborated by laboratory findings of elevated muscle enzymes, EMG studies, and muscle biopsy. The diagnostic criteria require assessment of five components: (1) typical skin rash, (2) symmetric proximal muscle weakness, (3) abnormal muscle biopsy findings, (4) elevated muscle-derived enzymes and (5) abnormal EMG. A definite diagnosis of dermatomyositis can be made if the skin rash and three of the four other criteria are met. A probable diagnosis is suggested by skin rash with two other criteria; and a possible diagnosis is indicated by presence of skin rash plus any one of the other criteria. A thorough systemic review with appropriate investigations should be done to delineate the extent of organ involvement in this multisystem disease. A routine hemogram, urinalysis, stool guaiac, chest X-ray, ECG, and echocardiogram should preferably be done for assessment of every child with JDM.

Cutaneous manifestations of dermatomyositis may need to be differentiated, particularly in its early stages, from conditions like lichen planus, seborrheic dermatitis, contact dermatitis, atopic dermatitis, and polymorphic light eruptions. In its late stages, systemic lupus erythematosus and scleroderma are important differential diagnoses. Proximal muscle weakness of JDM may be mimicked by myopathies and neurological disorders like muscular dystrophies, infectious myopathies, myasthenia gravis, Guillain-Barre syndrome, drug-induced myo–pathies, and myopathies in endocrine disorders like hyper- and hypothyroidism, and Cushing's syndrome.

TREATMENT

The goal of therapy is to improve muscular function, prevent further muscle damage, and prevent disability. The treatment regimen must be initiated promptly and children with JDM should be managed by a multispeciality approach mainly involving rheumatologist, dermatologist, and physical therapist. Stepwise, aggressive treatment directed at achieving rapid and complete control of muscle inflammation is highly successful in minimizing the long-range sequelae of the disease. Hospitalization may be required for children with severe muscle weakness particularly for those with potential for respiratory muscle weakness. General measures include a period of bed rest, particularly in children with severe muscle disease and a program of physical therapy is useful for preventing contracture and deformity, and restoration of muscle strength. For children with dysphagia, elevation of head end of their bed, frequent small meals and not eating before bedtime may be useful. Nasogarstic or intravenous feeding may occasionally be needed.

Systemic steroid therapy is the mainstay of treatment for muscle disease. Early aggressive therapy is associated with better control and improved outcome. Most authorities recommend initiation of therapy with prednisolone in a dose of 2 mg/kg per day in divided dosage tapering to lower dosage and resorting to once daily therapy after clinical improvement and normalization of muscle enzyme values. Intravenous pulse methylprednisolone therapy (30 mg/kg daily or alternate days) is increasingly being favored for acute exacerbations as well as for initial phase of steroid therapy in JDM to minimize adverse effects of high-dose systemic steroid therapy. Overall dosage required may be less than that with oral steroids. This is followed by maintenance oral prednisolone. Most patients will require maintenance treatment for 12 to 24 months to prevent recurrence. Alternate day therapy may be used late in the recovery phase.

For children who do not respond adequately to initial high dosage of systemic steroid or in whom this is associated with unacceptable side effects, the most preferred second-line therapy is with methotrexate. Methotrexate is used orally or as intramuscular injections at a dosage of 1mg/kg per week with a maximum dose of 40 mg/week. Baseline hemogram, liver enzymes and creatinine values must be obtained and repeated periodically for monitoring side effects. Methotrexate may be used from the beginning along with systemic steroids; early intravenous pulse steroid therapy along with methotrexate may be associated with better outcome than either agent alone.Besides methotrexate, adjuvant immunosuppressive therapy may be instituted with other agents like azathioprine (1 to 3 mg/kg/day), cyclosporine (5mg/kg/day), or mycophenolate mofetil in cases not responding to systemic steroid adequately. High dose intravenous immunoglobulin is also used as a steroid-sparing agent in these settings. Rituximab, an anti-CD 20 monoclonal antibody, has also been used with some success. However, there is a lack of high quality randomised controlled trials that assess the efficacy and toxicity of immunosuppressants in inflammatory myositis.

Treatment of cutaneous disease in dermatomyositis is problematic. In many cases there is little correlation of improvement of myopathy with that of skin rash and skin lesions may persist for quite a long time after muscle disease becomes quiescent. Recognition of photosensitivity is important and institution of photoprotective measures with sun avoidance and use of broad-spectrum sunscreens is imperative. Hydroxychloroquine (5 mg/kd/day) and chloroquin have been effective in small open-label clinical trials and their use may have steroid-sparing effect in controlling the systemic disease. Topical corticosteroids and calcineurin inhibitors are sometimes helpful. Methotrexate, mycophenolate mofetil, and sirolimus may also be used to control cutaneous disease. Antihistamines may be used to control pruritus associated with skin lesions. Treatment of calcinosis has been tried with many agents with generally disappointing results. Anecdotal records suggest use of aluminium hydroxide, colchicine, warfarin, the calcium channel antagonist diltiazem, and bisphosphonates. Surgical removal of lesions may sometimes be of help. Early aggressive therapy of myositis is believed to be helpful in preventing calcinosis.

The early and aggressive treatment with systemic corticosteroids has reduced the mortality rate of JDM to less than 10%. Calcinosis has remained an important cause or morbidity. Poor prognostic indicators of childhood dermatomyositis are late initiation of treatment, initial treatment with too low a dose of steroid, recalcitrant disease, and pharyngeal involvement.

SYSTEMIC SCLEROSIS

Systemic sclerosis (scleroderma) is a multisystem autoimmune disorder of uncertain etiology characterized by cutaneous and visceral fibrosis, occlusive microvascular disease, and presence of specific autoantibodies. The term 'progressive systemic sclerosis' is no longer favored as in many instances the disease is not 'progressive'. Scleroderma (literally meaning hard skin) is categorized into two major subtypes, the localized, essentially cutaneous form (morphea and linear scleroderma including the 'en coup de sabre' variety) and the multisystem disorder, systemic sclerosis. The hallmark of systemic sclerosis is diffuse cutaneous fibrosis leading to hidebound skin with associated systemic disease mainly involving the lungs, gastrointestinal tract, heart, kidney, and musculoskeletal system. Systemic sclerosis in children may occur as a part of overlap syndromes, particularly in association with dermatomyositis or systemic lupus erythematosus. No specific treatment of systemic sclerosis exists and the disease is associated with considerable morbidity and mortality.

ETIOLOGY

The etiology of systemic sclerosis remains obscure. The characteristic features of systemic sclerosis are extensive fibrosis, vasculopathy, and activation of immune system. Endothelial alterations may stimulate a cascade of changes involving many cellular elements including T-lymphocytes, fibroblasts, macrophages, and mast cells. Activated cells then secrete several substances that include cytokines and their soluble receptors. These factors cause changes in collagens and extracellular matrix compounds leading to excessive collagen deposition in affected tissues by increased production or defective degradation. Fibrosis is induced by profibrotic cytokines, including transforming growth factor-beta (TGF-beta), interleukin-4 (IL-4), platelet-derived growth factor (PDGF), and connective-tissue growth factor. Serum levels of connective tissue growth factor are elevated in patients of systemic sclerosis and correlated with the extent of cutaneous sclerosis and pulmonary fibrosis. The vasculopathy may be caused by TGF-beta and PDGF, while the paucity of lesional blood vessels in the skin can be attributed to antiendothelial cell autoantibodies.

The cellular immune system may be activated early in the course of the disease and activated T-cells produce the profibrotic cytokine IL-4 and may stimulate B-cells to produce autoantibodies. Autoantibodies to nuclear autoantigens are also believed to be of pathogenic significance as suggested by their high specificity, clustering with specific disease subsets, presence from the very early stage of the disease, and correlation of their titer with disease severity. Genetic factors are also implicated, although familial occurrence of the disease is rare. Scleroderma has been reported in identical twins. Environmental precipitants may include exposure to pentazocine, bleomycin, and vinyl chloride. Ingestion of contaminated rapeseed oil has been responsible for an epidemic of scleroderma-like disease in Spain.

EPIDEMIOLOGY

Systemic sclerosis is a very rare disease in childhood and only 3% of all cases of the disease occur in childhood. The disease may occur at any age and disease onset has been reported to occur at as early as six months of age. The sex incidence is equal in very young children, but beyond eight years of age, girls are three times more likely than boys to be affected with the disease. There is no peak age of onset, the median age of onset in an Indian series was found to be 12 years. Cases have been reported from all over the world and there is no particular racial predilection.

CLINICAL FEATURES

Clinically, there is a broad spectrum of disease ranging from widespread severe skin thickening (diffuse cutaneous systemic sclerosis) to sclerosis limited to the skin distal to the elbows or knees and/or facial involvement (limited cutaneous systemic sclerosis). These two groups of patients have different clinical courses, from rapid progression of skin thickening and early systemic disease in diffuse cutaneous disease to much slower evolution that may take years or decades in limited cutaneous disease. Systemic sclerosis is subtle and insidious in onset and the diagnosis is often delayed for months or years. Analysis of data on 153 children with juvenile systemic sclerosis collected from across the world has shown than Raynaud's phenomenon was the most common symptom, followed by cutaneous induration in approximately 75% of patients, musculoskeletal complaints in one-third of patients, and the most frequently involved internal organs were respiratory and gastrointestinal.Involvement of renal, cerebral, and cardiovascular systems was found to be very rare. Although cutaneous changes occur early in the course of the disease before systemic involvements become clinically apparent, the reverse may rarely occur. Systemic involvement in scleroderma without skin changes is referred to as 'systemic sclerosis sine scleroderma'.

Cutaneous Features

Cutaneous manifestations of juvenile systemic sclerosis are similar to the adult disease. Raynaud's phenomenon is most frequently the presenting symptom. This episodic vascular phenomenon is precipitated by exposure to cold and manifests with the characteristic sequence of color changes of pallor, cyanosis, and erythema involving fingers and toes. Raynaud's phenomenon may also involve the other acral parts like the nose, ear, or lips. The children may have associated pain, numbness, burning and tingling sensations of the affected parts. In tropical climates, Raynaud's phenomenon may be noticeable during the winter months only. Digital ulcers or even gangrene may be the presenting symptom.

The fibrotic process most commonly involves the face and hands and later on progress to affect the proximal areas of upper limbs and the trunk. Initially, the fingers are swollen and shiny with a feeling of tightness. Later on the skin becomes hidebound and the fingers are held in flexion. The pulp of the fingers become atrophic and small painful ulcerations occur which leave pitted scars. Gangrene of the fingers may occur. The fingers eventually become tapered, and with atrophy of the distal phalanx, they are shortened, with the nails curving over the distal part. Similar changes also occur on the feet but with less severity. Dilated nail-fold capillaries could be visible and the nail cuticles may become ragged. Pterygium inversum unguis-like changes may also develop.

In a well-developed case, the facial features are characteristic. The forehead is tight and shiny with loss of furrows, the facial skin is hidebound with smoothening of lines of expression, and the nose becomes pinched and beak-shaped. The oral aperture becomes small with radial furrows round the mouth. The lower eyelid cannot be depressed by the fingers to demonstrate the conjunctiva.

Telangiectasia develops in a large number of cases. Most commonly occurring on the hands, face, lips, mouth and upper trunk, the telangiectatic mats are usually sharply defined in oval, rectangular, of multiangular configurations.

Calcification occurs in scleroderma and most commonly affect the fingers, usually in their palmar aspects. Calcinosis may also occur over other sites like the elbows, knees, and dorsal aspect of feet. The lesions may breakdown discharging a chalky material.

Pigmentary changes frequently occur in systemic sclerosis, mainly in the form of diffuse darkening, or there may be a mottled 'salt and pepper' dyspigmentation owing to areas of hypopigmentation with perifollicular retention of pigmentation.

Systemic Manifestations

Gastrointestinal disease occurs frequently in children with systemic sclerosis. Although any part of the gastrointestinal tract may be involved, esophageal affection is commonest, found in about three-fourth of the cases. Esophageal reflux is the most common disorder. The incidence of reflux disease in children and possible development of esophagitis is more frequent than clinical symptoms suggest. Abnormal esophageal peristalsis occurs resulting in dysphagia; the typical radiological feature being an atonic dilated esophagus containing air in the resting state. Hiatus hernia and lower esophageal stricture can occur. Small and large intestinal involvement may lead to symptoms of colicky abdominal pain, constipation, diarrhea, bloating, and features of malabsorption like steatorrhea.

Pulmonary disease is a major cause of morbidity and mortality in children with systemic sclerosis. Dyspnea on exertion may be attributed to tightness of skin, muscle weakness, or pulmonary interstitial fibrosis. Pulmonary function testing may reveal restrictive lung disease. High resolution computed tomographic scanning (HRCT) is a sensitive indicator of lung disease and may show abnormality in clinically silent pulmonary involvement. Abnormal HRCT results were detected in 91% of a series of juvenile scleroderma.

Musculoskeletal involvement may occur in up to three-fourth of cases. Arthralgia, limited mobility, and contracture of joints may occur. A crepitant tenosynovitis may develop in some. Resorption of bones of terminal phalanges may cause shortening of digits. Myositis with proximal muscle weakness may occur. Diminished cardiac perfusion, myocarditis, arrythmias, cardiomyopathy, and cardiac failure may be manifestations of primary cardiac involvement. Pericarditis may occur leading to pericardial effusion. Pulmonary hypertension may also contribute to cardiac failure. Children with associated myositis may have increased incidence of cardiomyopathy. Renal involvement may occur in about half of the cases. Renal failure may develop acutely with malignant hypertension, but there may be slowly progressive disease in some patients. Regular blood pressure monitoring should be done for timely detection of renal involvement.

CREST syndrome (acronym of *C*alcinosis, *R*aynaud's phenomenon, *E*sophageal dysmotility, *S*clerosis, and *T*elangiectasia) is a subset of limited cutaneous systemic sclerosis which occurs very rarely in children. The telangiectasias occur commonly on the face, upper trunk, and hands. The lips, buccal mucosa, and gastrointestinal mucosa may also be involved, sometimes with GI bleeding.

This subset of the disease has a generally benign, slowly progressive course with favorable prognosis, but pulmonary hypertension and biliary cirrhosis may occur occasionally.

INVESTIGATIONS

Most children with systemic sclerosis have high-titre antinuclear antibodies (ANAs) with speckled patterns. Presence of autoantibodies with a specificity for Scl 70 (topoisomerase 1) correlates with diffuse cutaneous disease and a poor prognosis. Anti-centromere antibodies are rarely found in children, their presence is associated with limited cutaneous disease. Muscle-derived enzymes like creatine kinase, aldolase, or lactate dehydrogenase may be elevated in the serum in children with myositis.

Chest radiography, pulmonary function tests, and HRCT may show abnormal results in children with pulmonary disease. Upper gastrointestinal films and esophageal manometry may indicate functional abnormality of esophagus. X-ray study of hands may document features of digital osteolysis with soft tissue calcifications. Echocardiography and ECG may show abnormalities indicative of heart disease in scleroderma. Abnormal vascular responses in hands with features of occlusive vascular disease may be documented by plethysmographic studies.

Cutaneous histopathologic picture is dominated by collagen abnormalities in the form of swollen, pale, broad collagen bundles that lie parallel to each other with diminution of interbundle spaces in the dermis. Replacement of subcutaneous fat with hyalinized connective tissue may occur. In late states, there is absence of pilosebaceous units and eccrine units. Vascular occlusive changes may be documented. Histologic changes in systemic sclerosis are generally indistinguishable from those of localized scleroderma, but there may be involvement of the papillary dermis and presence of more inflammatory infiltrate in the later.

DIAGNOSIS

Systemic sclerosis can generally be diagnosed clinically by the characteristic features of symmetrical sclerosis of hands and face in association with Raynaud's phenomenon and visceral involvement. Appropriate investigations must be undertaken to delineate the presence and extent of systemic disease. The differential diagnoses of systemic sclerosis are given in **Table 25.5.** The American College of Rheumatology (ACR) criteria for classification of systemic sclerosis has not been validated in children and the classification of juvenile disease is currently under evolution. The provisional classification criteria that appear to be most promising are the presence of proximal sclerosis (proximal to the metacarpophalangeal joints)/induration plus two minor criteria out of nine organ system categories (cutaneous, vascular, gastrointestinal, respiratory, renal, cardiac, neurologic, musculoskeletal, and serologic).

TABLE 25.5: Differential diagnoses of systemic sclerosis

SLE	Phenylketonuria
Juvenile dermatomyositis	Graft-versus-host disease
Mixed connective tissue disease	Generalized morphea
Overlap syndromes	Vinyl chloride disease
Eosinophilic fasciitis	Toxic oil syndrome
Stiff-skin syndrome	POEMS syndrome

TREATMENT

One of the most important general measures in the management of systemic sclerosis is to prevent cold-induced vasospasm by avoidance of cold weather and cool liquids, and by appropriate clothing. Efforts must be made to minimize trauma to the hands. Active exercise and physiotherapy should be undertaken to avoid contractures. Raynaud's phenomenon is treated with vasodilators such as calcium channel blockers like nifedipine or diltiazem as well as angiotensin receptor blockers and pentoxifylline. Application of nitroglycerine patches to the affected areas may also help. Critical ischemic digits in children that are resistant to conventional therapy has been successfully treated with intravenous iloprost.

Treatment of organ-specific manifestations must be undertaken early to minimize morbidity and mortality. Reflux esophagitis is treated with omeprazole and general measures in the form of small-sized bland meals, staying upright after meals, and raising the head-end of the bed. Intestinal bacterial overgrowth is treated with courses of broad-spectrum antibiotics. Subcutaneous injections of octreotide have been successfully used in the treatment of gastrointestinal motility disorders of the disease in the adults. Musculoskeletal symptoms are treated with NSAIDs and aspirin. Renal disease may be treated with administration of captopril for malignant hypertension. Pulmonary arterial hypertension is treated with intravenous administration of prostacyclin analogues like epoprostenol or bosentan, an endothelin receptor blocker. Pulmonary fibrosis in adults has been treated successfully with cyclophosphamide. Systemic steroids is generally avoided in juvenile scleroderma for fear of precipitating renal failure but its use may be appropriate for the management of specific inflammatory disease like myocarditis, myositis, alveolitis, or severe arthritis.

No treatment has given consistent benefit for the cutaneous fibrosis. Penicillamine, which interferes with intermolecular cross-linking of collagen fibrils, has been used with some success in anecdotal reports. Ultraviolet A1 (340-400 nm) phototherapy was also found to be effective in treating cutaneous sclerosis.

The prognosis of systemic sclerosis in children is generally more favorable with significantly better survival than that in the adult disease. In a multinational survey of 135 children, eight children had died at the end of 5-year follow-up, mainly from cardiac failure; the one-year survival was 99%, two-year 97%, and the four-year rate was 95%.

JUVENILE IDIOPATHIC ARTHRITIS

Idiopathic chronic arthritis in children used to be defined and classified in diverse ways. The American College of Rheumatology classification of this group of disorders as 'juvenile rheumatoid arthritis' and the European League Against Rheumatism designation 'juvenile chronic arthritis' were subject to confusion and could not be used interchangeably. In order to facilitate research and treatment, the International League against Rheumatism has devised a unifying set of criteria that reconciled the former classifications by using the term 'juvenile idiopathic arthritis (JIA)'. JIA encompasses juvenile rheumatoid arthritis as well as other arthritic disorders.

JIA is defined as persistent arthritis for more than 6 weeks with an onset at less than 16 years of age, after excluding other causes. The most common rheumatic disease of childhood, JIA is a syndrome consisting of several subtypes **(see Table 25.6)**. Besides involving the joints, it may also produce extra-articular signs and symptoms affecting such organs as the skin, heart, lungs, eyes, liver, and spleen. The systemic onset disease is the only variety with prominent cutaneous involvement.

TABLE 25.6: Classification of juvenile idiopathic arthritis

Types	Proportion (%) of cases	Definition
Oligoarthritis	40-60	Affects one to four joints during the first six months of disease. No systemic onset; rheumatoid factor and HLA-B27 negative; no family history of psoriasis or HLA-B27 positive disease.
2 subtypes:		
a) **Persistent**		Never affects more than four joints
b) **Extended**		Five or more joints affected after first six months of disease.
Polyarthritis		Affection of five or more joints during first six months of disease. Systemic onset to be excluded.
2 subtypes		
a) **Rheumatoid factor positive**	5-10	Rheumatoid factor positivity on at least 2 occasions at least 3 months apart
b) **Rheumatoid factor negative**	20-25	Rheumatoid factor negativity on at least 2 occasions at least 3 months apart
Systemic onset arthritis	10-20	Arthritis with or preceded by daily fever of at least two weeks' duration plus at least one of the following: typical rash, generalized lymphadenopathy, hepatosplenomegaly, serositis
Psoriatic arthritis	5	Arthritis plus psoriasis or at least two of the following: dactylitis; nail pitting; family history of psoriasis in one or more first degree relative.
Enthesitis related arthritis	Undetermined	Arthritis and/or enthesitis, plus at least two of : onset of arthritis in a boy older than 8, sacroiliitis, anterior uveitis, family history of HLA-B27 positive disease.

Rheumatoid factors, which are IgM antibodies against IgG, occur rarely in children and are associated with poor prognosis. In many children, the disease may persist well into adulthood causing lasting disabilities and impairment of physical and psychological growth. Thus, it is important to recognize the disease and institute early treatment to minimize the individual, familial, and societal burden associated with the disease.

ETIOLOGY

The etiopathogenesis of JIA is uncertain, but genetic factors, immune dysfunction, and microbial infections are implicated in the pathogenesis of this diverse group of arthropathies in children. High concordance among identical twins has been recorded and there are associations with certain HLA subtypes pointing towards inherited susceptibility to the disease. Rubella and parvovirus B19 have been implicated as potential cause of JIA. Abnormalities in both the humoral and cellular immune system with production of various proinflammatory cytokines are thought to be responsible for the pathogenesis of the disease.

EPIDEMIOLOGY

JIA occurs in all races with varying prevalence. The incidence is approximately 10-20 cases per 100,000 children. The age incidence varies with the type of disease. Although the disease can occur throughout childhood and adolescence, the peak onset is usually between the ages one and three years and between eight and twelve years. Girls usually outnumber boys in a ratio of 2:1 in the early ages, in the systemic onset disease, however, the sex ratio is equal. Relative frequency of different types may vary according to geographical locations. In an Indian series of 361 children, the relative frequencies of polyarticular, pauciarticular, and systemic onset disease were 46%, 30%, and 24% respectively.

CLINICAL FEATURES

There are three major types of disease onset that correlates with clinical features and future course of the disease. Oligoarthritis involves one to four joints and polyarthritis 5 or more joints during the first 6 months of onset; systemic-onset disease is characterized by prominent systemic features at onset. Fatigue, anorexia, and weight loss may be a feature in many children with severe disease. Young children may not complain of joint pain. Refusal to walk, limping, and assumption of postures guarding the affected joints may be important indications of arthritis.

Oligoarthritis

Oligoarthritis is the commonest variety of JIA and typically involves knee, ankle, and elbows. Monoarticular onset is common and small joints are usually spared. Many children, particularly girls who are ANA-positive, are likely to develop ocular involvement in the form of chronic iridocyclitis. This is often asymptomatic, but may produce symptoms of photophobia, pain, and redness. Permanent visual damage may result if untreated and regular ophthalmic screening is required. Uveitis and ANA-positivity, however, is very rarely documented in Indian children. Severe knee involvement may result in unequal linear growth of legs resulting in limping.

Polyarthritis

Polyarthritis in JIA generally involves the large joints like knees, ankles, wrists, and elbows, but small joints of the hands and feet may also be involved from onset or later. Patterns of small joint involvement are generally similar to the adult rheumatoid disease. Systemic features like low-grade fever, hepatosplenomegaly, and lymphadenopathy may sometimes be present. Involvement of apophyseal joints of spine and the temporomandibular joint is common, subcutaneous nodules are found rarely and are usually found in rheumatoid factor-positive polyarthritis. They occur as firm, non-tender nodules predominantly over the elbows, knees, dorsum of fingers, heels, buttocks and scapular regions. Periungual telangiectasia may be found in some children.

Systemic Onset JIA

Systemic onset JIA, previously known as Still's disease, is characterized by high, spiking fever with daily or twice-daily rise of temperature particularly during the afternoon or evening with rapid defervescence to baseline. Joint symptoms may occur concurrently or there may be a delay of weeks or months. The rash in systemic onset disease is quite characteristic. The lesions are usually discrete, small, erythematous macules often with a surrounding pallor; larger lesions may show central clearing. They are distributed principally over the trunk and proximal limbs sometimes also involving the palms, soles, face, and axillae. The rash is migratory and transient, most often coinciding with the fever and may be more prominent over sites of rubbing with the clothing. Prominent systemic affection may occur in the form of lymphadenopathy, hepatosplenomegaly, and serositis. Pericarditis, myocarditis, pleuritis, pulmonary fibrosis, non-specific abdominal pain, and central nervous system involvement may also occur. The joint affection in half of the cases is oligoarticular with relatively favorable prognosis; in the remaining half the disease takes on a polyarticular, progressive course. Macrophage activation syndrome is a life threatening complication of systemic onset JIA that may occur after viral infections and is characterized by an acute febrile illness with multiorgan dysfunction.

Enthesitis-related Arthritis

Enthesitis-related arthritis in children is characterized by enthesitis (inflammation of tendons and ligaments at their bony attachments) together with variable joint affection. Boys are predominantly affected. Spondyloarthropathy and anterior uveitis are characteristic features.

Psoriatic Arthritis

Psoriatic arthritis in children may present with oligoarthritis, polyarthritis, of enthesitis-related arthritis. In addition there may be typical lesions of psoriasis with characteristic nail involvement.

DIAGNOSIS

As JIA is a diagnosis of exclusion, before assigning a diagnosis of JIA, all other possible causes of juvenile arthritides must be excluded. These should include disorders like rheumatic fever, SLE, infective arthritis, serum sickness, Henoch-Schonlein purpura and hematologic disease like hemophilia or leukemia. There is no specific diagnostic laboratory test for JIA. Non-specific changes include anemia, neutrophilic leukocytosis, and raised ESR and C-reactive proteins. Antinuclear antibodies are present in 40% of patients particularly in girls with oligoarticular disease. They usually show homogenous or speckled patterns of fluorescence using human cell substrates. The rate of ANA-positivity has been reported to be quite low in Indian children. Rheumatoid factor is rarely positive and generally associated with polyarticular disease with rheumatoid nodules and late age of onset. Antibody to cyclic citrullinated peptide (anti-CCP), an autoantibody specific for rheumatoid arthritis, is rarely found in children.

TREATMENT

Recent recognition of the fact that JIA in a significant proportion of cases progresses into adulthood with active disease and considerable disabilities, has tilted the management strategies to a more aggressive mode rather than the conventional conservative approach. The goal of therapy is symptom control and prevention of disabilities while maintaining activities. Treatment modalities that are utilized include a variety of drugs together with a program of physical therapies. Drugs used in the treatment of JIA include non-steroidal anti-inflammatory agents (NSAIDs), systemic and intraarticular steroids, methotrexate and other disease-modifying antirheumatic drugs and immunosuppressants, and biologic-modifying medications. A number of children who reach adulthood with considerable disability may later need orthopedic surgery including joint replacement surgery. In general, the most consistent predictors of a poor outcome in JIA are female gender, polyarticular and symmetrical joint involvement, elevated inflammatory markers and rheumatoid factor positivity.

Oligoarthritis in about one third of cases respond to NSAIDs (like aspirin, ibuprofen, naproxen etc). Intra-articular steroid injections are used for non-responsive cases. Patients who do not respond to intra-articular steroids or with extended disease or small joint affection are treated as polyarticular disease.

For rheumatoid factor negative polyarthritis, NSAIDs may be used for symptom control. Methotrexate should be started early, starting with 10mg/m^2 per week, increased to 15mg/m^2 if the lower dose is ineffective. Sulfasalazine and leflunomide are alternatives. If not effective, anti-TNF drugs like etanercept are used. Systemic steroids may be used for disease flares. Rheumatoid factor positive polyarthritis has a poor outcome and is treated aggressively like adult rheumatoid arthritis, including methotrexate and addition of anti-TNF drugs if methotrexate is ineffective.

Systemic onset JIA may be treated with NSAIDs and systemic steroids are often needed for systemic features like high fever and serositis. Macrophage activation syndrome is treated with high-dose intravenous pulse steroids.

Promising results have been shown in uncontrolled studies using anakinra, an anti-IL6 receptor antibody, thalidomide, or early treatment with a combined therapy with methotrexate, cyclophosphamide, and intravenous pulse steroids. For severe, unresponsive polyarticular or systemic onset JIA, autologous stem cell transplant has been used as a last resort.

MIXED CONNECTIVE TISSUE DISEASE

Mixed connective tissue disease (MCTD) is a systemic autoimmune disorder characterized by a constellation of signs and symptoms referring to a variety of organ systems and a specific antibody profile of high titres of autoantibody to anti-U1 ribonucleoprotein (U1RNP). Although there is a controversy regarding whether MCTD represents a phase in the evolution towards a definitive major connective tissue disease like SLE or scleroderma, it is generally regarded to be a distinct syndrome. The etiology remains uncertain, but genetic, hormonal, and environmental factors have been implicated in the causation of this autoimmune syndrome. Autoantibodies to nuclear ribonucleoproteins may have an inciting role in the pathogenesis.

MCTD is a rare disease in childhood, representing 0.3% of all pediatric rheumatologic diseases. Pediatric onset disease accounts for an estimated one fourth of all cases of MCTD. There is no racial predilection, and the gender ratio is 6:1 in favor of girls. The median age of onset in children is 12 years.

Clinically, MCTD may show a combination of features of connective tissue diseases like SLE, systemic sclerosis, and dermatomyositis. A few patients may eventually progress into classic SLE or systemic sclerosis. The commonest presenting features in childhood are Raynaud's phenomenon and joint symptoms. The arthritis is usually like that of SLE, and characterized by a non-erosive, non-deforming symmetric polyarthritis. Hand edema and stiffness, which constitute some of the core clinical features of adult disease, is less common in childhood MCTD. Mucocutaneous manifestations may occur in the form of malar rash, photosensitivity, heliotrope erythema, periungual telangiectasia, alopecia, and dyspigmentation.

Cardiac disease occurs more frequently in children than in adults and manifestations may include pericarditis, myocarditis, congestive cardiac failure and aortic insufficiency. Nephritis is also more frequent and more severe as compared to adult MCTD. Abnormal esophageal motility and reflux disease may occur. Neurological involvement may occur in the form of seizure, strokes, trigeminal neuralgia, and peripheral polyneuropathy. Myositis may manifest as proximal muscle weakness. Hematologic manifestations are also more frequent than in adult and thrombocytopenia appears to be limited to the childhood disease. Pulmonary involvement, in the form of pulmonary fibrosis and abnormal pulmonary functions tests are less common than in adults.

There are four different sets of diagnostic criteria for MCTD with varying sensitivities and specificities. All require the presence of antibody to U1RNP in association with sets of clinical features, mainly including Raynaud's phenomenon, hand edema and sclerosis, arthritis, myositis, or other visceral changes. Most patients with MCTD have high titres of antinuclear antibodies with a speckled pattern on immunofluorescence as well as rheumatoid factor. Work-ups for patients with MCTD should include tests to detect various systemic affections.

The goal of therapy in MCTD is to control disease manifestations and prevent serious organ damage. Children will require periodic clinical reviews and laboratory evaluations to detect new disease manifestations. Drug treatment generally depends on the severity and extent of systemic affections. Photoprotective measures and antimalarials may be required for cutaneous changes. Non-steroidal anti-inflammatory drugs are used for joint symptoms. Systemic steroids (prednisolone 1mg/kg/day) are used for control of manifestations like myositis or nephritis. Immunosuppressive therapy (with cyclophosphamide or azathioprine), usually with systemic steroids, may be required for nephritis, pulmonary fibrosis, and CNS disease. In unresponsive patients, other agents like cyclosporine and mycophenolate mofetil may be used.

SJÖGREN SYNDROME

Sjögren's syndrome is a systemic autoimmune disease mainly affecting the exocrine glands and usually presents as persistent dryness of the mouth and eyes due to involvement of the salivary and lachrymal glands. Sjögren syndrome may occur alone (primary Sjögren Syndrome), or more commonly, may be associated with virtually any systemic autoimmune diseases (secondary Sjögren Syndrome), especially juvenile rheumatoid arthritis.

Overall, Sjögren Syndrome is a very rare disease in children as compared to adults. The histological hallmark is a focal lymphocytic infiltration of the exocrine glands, and the spectrum of the disease extends from an organ-specific autoimmune disease (autoimmune exocrinopathy) to a systemic process with diverse extraglandular manifestations.

ETIOLOGY

Although the exact mechanisms involved in the etiopathogenic process are not well known, the autoimmune origin of the disease (autoimmune epithelitis) is the hypothesis most commonly postulated in primary Sjögren syndrome. The abnormal responses of both T and B cells against autoantigens contribute to the characteristic histopathological lesions and to alterations in the synthesis of numerous intermediate molecules (cytokines and chemokines), thereby helping to perpetuate the autoimmune process. Later activation of mechanisms of tissue damage (such as apoptosis) leads to chronic inflammation of the exocrine glands, with fibrosis and loss of physiological function. Genetic factors, viral agents like Epstein Barr virus or hepatitis C virus, hormonal influence, and autonomic dysfunctions are also implicated.

CLINICAL FEATURES

The average age of onset is about ten years and girls are predominantly involved. The predominant presenting feature in childhood Sjögren syndrome is recurrent parotitis, parotid swelling, and fatigue. The characteristic functional abnormalities of exocrine glands like the salivary and lachrymal glands results in xerostomia and keratoconjunctivitis sicca. Decreased salivary secretion results in dry mouth, difficulty in chewing and swallowing, and a frothy, ropey saliva. A dry tongue, fissured and cracked lip, and early and severe dental caries are common. Reduced lachrymal secretion leads to dry eyes with a gritty sensation, red eyes, photosensitivity, and reduced production of tears in response to emotion or irritation. Nasal and vaginal dryness may occur. About half of the children with Sjögren syndrome may develop a variety of extraglandular manifestations in the course of the disease **(Table 25.7)**.

DIAGNOSIS

Characteristic clinical features of the disease are slow to develop and the diagnosis is often delayed. Recurrent parotitis and parotid swelling in a child should raise the suspicion of the condition. Rose Bengal staining may detect damaged corneal epithelium and a positive

TABLE 25.7: Extraglandular manifestations of Sjögren syndrome

Musculoskeletal	*Hematologic*
Arthralgia	Leukopenia
Non-erosive arthritis	Autoimmune hemolytic anemia
Myalgia	
	Neurologic
Cutaneous	Cranial and peripheral neuropathy
Hyperglobulinemic purpura	Sensorineural hearing loss
Erythema nodosum	
Annular erythema	*Endocrine*
Raynaud's phenomenon	Autoimmune thyroiditis
Dryness	
Alopecia	*Renal*
Lipodystrophy	Nephritis
	Renal tubular acidosis
Gastrointestinal	
Dysphagia	*Pulmonary*
Achalasia	Alveolitis
Primary biliary cirrhosis	Impaired pulmonary functions tests
Hepatic	*Lymphoreticular*
Autoimmune hepatitis	Lymphadenopathy
	Splenomegaly

Schirmer's tear test (less than 5 mm of wetting of a filter paper inserted beneath the lower lid and kept for 5 minutes) may document decreased tear production.

Parotid gland involvement may be detected by sialography, sonogram and computed tomography. Histopathology of labial minor salivary gland biopsy showing periacinar and periductal lymphocytic infiltrates is diagnostic.

About 80% of cases have at least one positive autoantibody test result (antinuclear antibodies, rheumatoid factor, Ro/SSA, La/SSB); 63% have autoantibodies to SSA or SSB. Antibody against a newly described autoantigen alpha-fodrin was detected in a group of children with primary Sjögren syndrome before anti-SSA or SSB antibody became positive and could be a useful marker for the early diagnosis of SS.

TREATMENT

Reduced salivary flow and its consequences, particularly dental caries needs special attention in the management of Sjögren syndrome. Adequate oral hygiene should be maintained with twice daily brushing, chlorhexidine mouth washes, restriction of refined sugar in the diet, and early treatment of infections like candidiasis. Salivary secretion may be increased by non-specific gustatory stimulants like citric acid and chewing gums. Pharmacologic stimulants like pilocarpine or anethole trithione may be tried. Artificial saliva substitutes containing carboxymethylcellulose or mucin are also used with success. Artificial tears are recommended for ocular affection.

Systemic treatment of Sjögren syndrome is based on treatment of related autoimmune diseases like juvenile idiopathic arthritis or SLE. Primary Sjögren syndrome usually follows a benign course. NSAIDs are used to treat musculoskeletal symptoms. Hydroxychloroquine appears to be beneficial for other manifestations of the disease. Systemic steroids and other immunosuppressants are reserved for severe disease.

RELAPSING POLYCHONDRITIS

Relapsing polychondritis (RP) is a systemic, episodic and progressive inflammatory disorder that affects cartilaginous structures throughout the body. Inflammatory destruction of cartilages followed by fibrosis typically involves the ears, nose, tracheobroncheal tree, eyes, and joints. Respiratory involvement may be a cause of mortality. The cause of RP is unknown, but an autoimmune pathogenesis is suggested by the presence of antibody to type II collagen, a constituent of cartilages. Autoimmunity is also suggested by the association of RP with a number of disorders like SLE, rheumatoid arthritis, MCTD, systemic vasculitides, and autoimmune thyroiditis.

Relapsing polychondritis is a rare disease in children. Fewer than 10% of all reported cases have occurred in children. The auricular cartilage is the commonest site to be involved. The ears become acutely swollen, painful, and red often suggesting an infective cause. The ear lobe is characteristically spared. With progressive disease or repeated affection, the cartilage may eventually be destroyed producing scarring and a cauliflower-like deformity. Audiovestibular damage may occur concomitantly, producing hearing loss. Involvement of the nasal cartilage may cause obstruction and a saddle-like deformity.

Cartilages of the respiratory system may be involved producing one of the most serious manifestations of the disease. There may be cough, dyspnea, airway obstruction or recurrent pulmonary infections. Children may require tracheostomy to maintain respiration. A non-erosive arthritis often involves the small joints of the hands as well as costochondral and sternal joints. Ocular involvement may take the forms of scleritis, episcleritis, iritis, lid edema, and retinopathy. Skin lesions of varying types may occur; these include erythema and edema of skin overlying the cartilages, aphthous ulcers, sterile pustules, livedo reticularis, and cutaneous vasculitis. Cardiovascular system may be involved in the forms of aortitis, aortic aneurysms and regurgitation, pericarditis, and heart block.

There is no specific laboratory test for the diagnosis of RP. Diagnosis of RP is suggested by the characteristic inflammatory involvement of cartilaginous structures. Diagnostic criteria require the presence of any three of more of the following six features: bilateral auricular chondritis, nonerosive polyarthritis, nasal chondritis, respiratory tract chondritis, ocular inflammation, and audiovestibular damage. Histopathology of affected cartilage in its early stage shows a mixed inflammatory infiltrate in the perichondrium, later on there is infiltration of mononuclear cells and macrophages, degeneration of cartilage fibrosis. Differential diagnosis should include other causes of auricular chondritis like infection or trauma, various causes of inflammatory arthritis, and other systemic disorders mimicked by RP. One of the important differential diagnoses in children is 'red ear syndrome', characterized by acute erythema, swelling, and burning pain of a whole ear unilaterally, without sparing the lobes. This condition is short-lived and episodic in nature. RP is treated by systemic steroids (prednisolone 1mg/kg/day) which are tapered to lower dosage after control of inflammation. A low maintenance dose may be required to prevent relapse. Other drugs that have been found to be effective for symptom control and perhaps retarding the disease progress mainly in the adult disease include methotrexate, dapsone, cyclophosphamide, and cyclosporine.

SYSTEMIC VASCULITIDES

Systemic vasculitides constitute a group of heterogenous clinicopathologic entities associated with inflammation of blood vessels. Blood vessels of any caliber in any organ may be involved and inflammatory destruction and obliteration of blood vessels may lead to tissue ischemia and its consequent organ damage and dysfunction. The patterns of vascular involvement vary widely, leading to protean clinical manifestations. There is wide overlap in clinical manifestations and the patients often have non-specific constitutional features initially. Characteristic patterns of organ involvement may develop later requiring revision of initial diagnosis. Delay in diagnosis and misdiagnosis is common, particularly in pediatric cases. Cutaneous involvement is frequent and may provide important visible clues to the diagnosis of vasculitic syndromes. Clinical features that may suggest a diagnosis of vasculitic syndromes in children include prolonged fever of unknown origin; unexplained musculoskeletal symptoms or neuropathy, particularly mononeuritis multiplex; obscure pulmonary, renal, or cardiovascular diseases, particularly in the setting of a multisystem disorder; palpable purpura or gangrene; and laboratory parameters indicative of chronic inflammation. Henoch-Schonlein purpura and Kawasaki disease are the two most common types of systemic vasculitides seen in children.

CLASSIFICATION

Vasculitis may be associated with a number of underlying disorders like infections, malignancies, connective tissue disorders, or drug reactions; these cases are often referred to as the 'secondary' forms of vasculitis as opposed to the 'primary' forms, where no such background are present and vessel damage is believed to be the primary event in causation of the disease. Since the etiopathogenesis of the primary systemic vasculitic syndromes remains largely obscure, this diverse group of diseases is generally classified according to the caliber and size of the blood vessels predominantly involved, the factor most consistently correlated with the clinical manifestations **(Table 25.8)**. It must however be borne in mind that there may be much overlap among the syndromes with respect to the nature of vessels involved.

TABLE 25.8: Classification of systemic vasculitis

- **I. Large-vessel vasculitis** (aorta and its branching arteries)
  1. Takayasu arteritis
  2. Giant-cell arteritis
- **II. Medium-sized-vessel vasculitis** (medium-sized and small arteries and veins)
  1. Polyarteritis nodosa
  2. Kawasaki disease
- **III. Small-vessel vasculitis** (post-capillary venules, arterioles, and rarely capillaries)
  1. Wegener's granulomatosis
  2. Churg-Strauss disease
  3. Microscopic polyangiitis
  4. Henoch-Schonlein purpura
  5. Cryoglobulinemic vasculitis

PATHOPHYSIOLOGY

Vasculitic syndromes are mediated at least in part by immunopathogenic mechanisms triggered by some antigens the nature of which however, may remain obscure in most cases. The final common pathway of vasculitis cannot be explained by a single pathogenic mechanism. Inflammatory damage to vessel wall may be mediated by hypersensitivity reactions in the form of immune complex, autoantibodies, and cellular immune responses. The final effector mechanisms involve a complex interplay of inflammatory cells, cytokines, complements, adhesion molecules, growth factors, and fibrinolytic systems. The ultimate expression of the vasculitic syndrome and its localization may depend on genetic factors, environmental exposures, and local blood flow characteristics.

In immune complex diseases, as in Henoch-Schonlein purpura, circulating immune complexes are deposited in the vessel wall and initiate a sequence of changes involving complement activation, neutrophil chemotaxis, and liberation of tissue-damaging proteolytic enzymes and oxygen free radicals from neutrophils. Pro-inflammatory cytokines are synthesized by damaged endothelium and contribute to the inflammatory process.

Antineutrophil cytoplasmic antibodies are antibodies directed against specific cytoplasmic proteins of neutrophils and are present mainly in the sera of patients with systemic vasculitides like Wegener's granulomatosis, microscopic polyangiitis, and Churg-Strauss syndrome as well as certain other systemic disorders like connective tissue disorders, inflammatory bowel diseases, and autoimmune liver diseases. By indirect immunofluorescence test, two main fluorescence patterns may be seen; a diffuse staining pattern of the cytoplasm (cytoplasmic ANCA, cANCA); and a staining around the nucleus (perinuclear ANCA, pANCA). The proposed mechanisms for pathogenicity of ANCAs include inducing neutrophils to express target antigens on their surface, making them accessible for ANCA; degranulation and oxidative burst of neutrophils; activation of monocytes; induction of expression of adhesion molecules and enhancement of adhesion of neutrophils and monocytes to endothelial cells.

Antiendothelial cell antibodies (AECA) may have roles in diseases like Takayasu's arteritis, Kawasaki disease and may cause endothelial damage by antibody-mediated cellular cytotoxicity with or without participation of complements. AECA may activate endothelial cells and cause increased expression of adhesion molecules thereby promoting migration of inflammatory cells. Cellular immune response and delayed hypersensitivity are important in the granuloma formation in large-vessel vasculitides like Takayasu's arteritis and giant cell arteritis.

Takayasu Arteritis

Takayasu arteritis (TA) is a chronic inflammatory disease of uncertain etiology affecting large vessels like the aorta and its branches. Vascular inflammation leads to occlusion, stenosis, and aneurysmal dilatations. Granuloma with giant cells constitutes the early phase of vascular pathology, which in later states shows sclerosis with little infiltrate. The characteristic obliteration of radial arteries has led to the synonym 'pulseless disease'. The pathogenesis is uncertain, but genetic factors, hypersensitivity to *Mycobacterium tuberculosis*, and autoantibodies like antiendothelial antibodies and anticardiolipin antibodies have been implicated. TA is particularly common in the Asians, Africans, and the Hispanics. TA is generally a disease of young females. It is rarely seen in early childhood. In an Indian series of children and young adults, the female to male ratio was 5:1 and the mean age of onset was 14.

Constitutional features in the forms of fever, fatigue, night sweats, weight loss, arthralgia and myalgia are common in the early pre-pulseless phase of the disease. This is followed by the pulseless phase characterized by audible bruits over the arteries, difference of blood pressure between the arms, loss of pulses and features of ischemia. Hypertension due to renal vascular affection is the commonest presentation; headaches, seizures, angina, and retinopathy may occur. Cutaneous involvement may be present in up to one-fifth of the patients in the form of erythema nodosum-like subcutaneous nodules, pyoderma gangrenosum-like ulcers, cutaneous small-vessel vasculitis, alopecia, xerosis, and atrophy of skin.

Diagnosis of TA may be suggested by the characteristic clinical features. Raised ESR and anemia are common. Plain radiography may detect arterial calcification; Doppler study and MRI scan may help in the assessment of vessel involvement, but angiography remains the gold standard of diagnosis. TA is an eminently treatable condition and five-year survival rate upward of 90% can now be commonly achieved with medical therapy, interventional radiology in the form of balloon dilatation of vessels with or without stents, and vascular surgery. Prednisolone (1-2 mg/kg/day) should be instituted early, tapered to a low maintenance dose which is continued indefinitely. Antitubercular drugs are used concomitantly in appropriate cases. The role of other immunosuppressants like azathioprine and cyclophosphamide are not well-established.

Polyarteritis Nodosa

Polyarteritis nodosa (PAN) is a multisystem disease characterized by segmental necrotizing vasculitis predominantly affecting medium-sized muscular arteries particularly at their branching points leading to nodose swellings, rupture and thrombosis, and eventual ischemic damage to tissues. Although PAN has been described in infants and children, this is an extremely rare disease during childhood. The cause is unknown but streptococcal, and hepatitis B and C virus infections have been implicated in the pathogenesis.

In children, the sex ratio is equal and the peak age of onset is about ten years. The onset of PAN is commonly insidious with constitutional features like fever, fatigue and weight loss. Renovascular hypertension and neurological involvement are common presenting features in children. A multitude of signs and symptoms have been described in PAN, commensurate with the multisystem vascular damage. Renal, cardiovascular, gastrointestinal, and neurologic involvements are commonly encountered. Typically, there is no pulmonary affection. Seizures, psychosis, cardiac failure, abdominal pain, arthralgia and myalgia, sensorimotor peripheral neuropathy (mononeuritis multiplex), and testicular pain may occur. Cutaneous manifestation may occur in the form of subcutaneous nodules along the path of arteries, particularly in the legs, livedo reticularis with or without ulcerations, digital gangrenes, and punched-out ulcers, and purpura. Maculopapular rashes have occurred in six out of eight children in an Indian series.

Infantile PAN is a severe acute illness with high mortality occurring in children below two years of age and characterized by prominent cardiac, renal and CNS involvement. Coronary arteritis with aneurysm, myocardial infarction, congestive cardiac failure, hypertension, neuritis, paralysis and seizures are common features. Benign cutaneous polyarteritis nodosa is the commonest variant of PAN in children and presents with cutaneous features without visceral affection. Painful subcutaneous nodules over lower extremities, livedo reticularis, deep ulcers, and gangrene may occur.

There is no specific laboratory marker for the disease. There may be raised ESR, anemia, hyperglobulinemia, hematuria, proteinuria, and urinary casts as well as ECG changes. Hepatitis B antigens may be found in a small number of children. Sural nerve or muscle biopsy findings or an angiogram that demonstrates aneurysmal dilatations of celiac or renal vasculature may help in establishing the diagnosis. The mainstay of treatment of PAN is systemic steroid given orally (prednisolone 1-2 mg/kg/day) in divided doses or in intravenous pulses. In severe systemic involvement, cyclophosphamide is used together with systemic steroids. PAN-associated Hepatitis B viral infection may be treated with interferon alpha 2b and plasma exchange. PAN in children is associated with a prolonged relapsing course lasting for many years with the possibility of eventual remission in some children.Thus, close follow-up of patients is mandatory. Mortality in PAN is most commonly related to renal failure, hypertensive encephalopathy, and myocardial infarction.

Kawasaki Disease

Kawasaki disease (KS) is an acute, self-limiting, multisystem vasculitis primarily affecting infants and young children. KS typically presents with an acute febrile illness with prominent mucocutaneous manifestations. Prognostically, the most important feature of the disease however, is the cardiological complication of coronary arterial aneurysm that carries significant morbidity and often mortality. KS is now the leading cause of acquired heart disease in the USA and the Western Europe. The etiology of the disease is ill-understood but immune activation and cytokine-mediated endothelial damage initiated by bacterial toxins (e.g. staphylococcal or streptococcal) acting as superantigens is the favored hypothesis for causation of the syndrome.

Epidemiology: The disease occurs worldwide involving all racial and ethnic groups. KS is most prevalent in Japan and in children of Japanese ancestry. In India, the prevalence may be more than the small number of reported cases suggest. The factors suggested to be responsible for this include misdiagnosis, lack or awareness, self-limited nature of the disease, and absence of specific clinical and laboratory features. In Japanese children, the most frequent age of affection is between six and twelve months of age, but in Indian children, most cases occur between one and five years of age. Boys outnumber girls in a ratio of 1.5 to 1. In Indian cases, the ratio has been 5:1.

Clinical features: The most prominent feature in the acute phase is the high fever often spiking to 104° F associated with a toxic appearance. The fever is continuous and usually lasts for about one to two weeks. The skin rash of KS occurs almost universally and develops during the first few days of fever. The rash commonly affects the upper trunk and proximal limbs but may be generalized. The rash is polymorphous, consisting of macules, papules, morbilliform, and sometimes urticarial, and erythema multiforme-like lesions. Vesicles, bullae, and purpura almost never occur. The rash accompanies the fever during the acute phase and desquamates about two weeks later **(Figure 25.7A)**. Psoriatic lesions have been described to appear acutely. A perineal eruption is characteristic and consists of tender erythema and edema

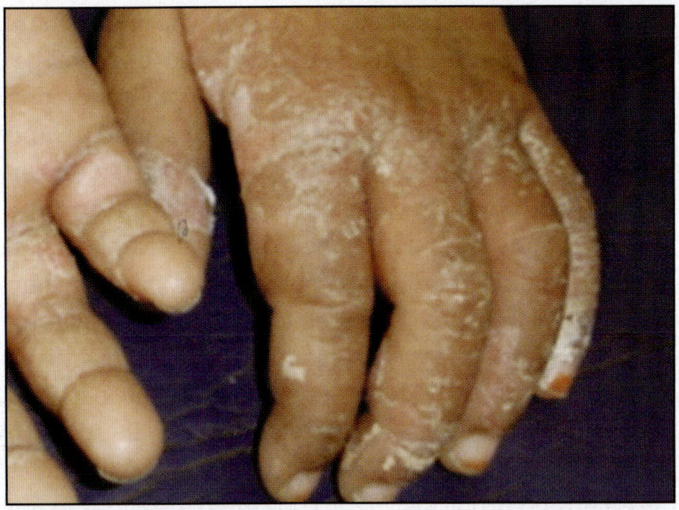

FIGURE 25.7A: Exfoliation of hands in Kawasaki disease

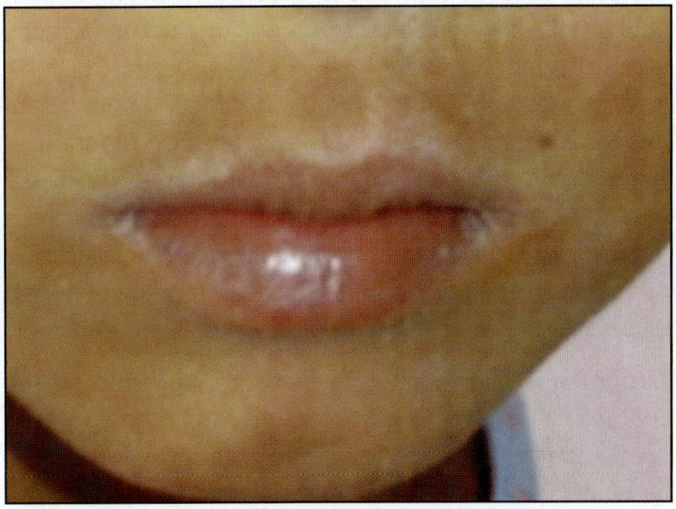

FIGURE 25.7B: Fissuring of lips in Kawasaki disease

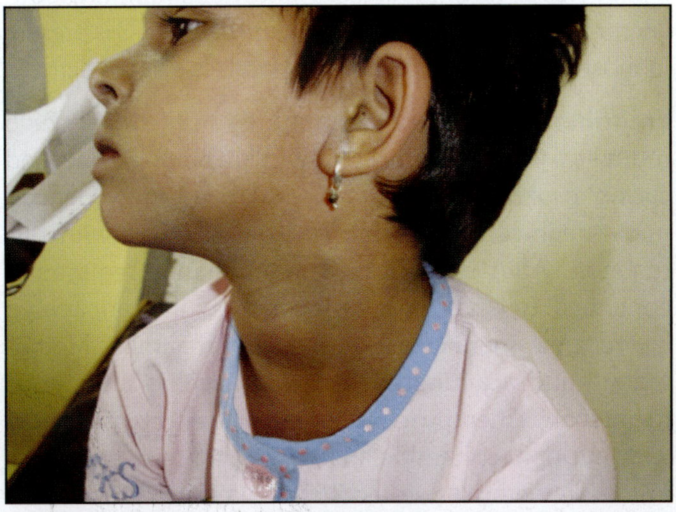

FIGURE 25.7C: Cervical lymphadenopathy in Kawasaki disease

which desquamates after 48 hours. The hands and feet may become edematous and red with swollen fingers. This desquamates after about two weeks in fine peels starting from underneath the tips of the nails, or sometimes as thick casts of palms and soles. Telogen effluvium and Beau's lines and shedding of nails may be late cutaneous features KS.

Oral mucosal lesions are very frequent and tend to affect the lips which are red, dry, and fissured **(Figure 25.7B)** often with bleeding. Pharyngeal hyperemia and red tongue with hypertrophied papillae ('strawberry tongue') are other features. A non-exudative conjunctival injection, more affecting the bulbar conjunctiva in the perilimbal location is a frequent feature. Lymphadenopathy develops in about 75% of children, usually as a non-suppurative, unilateral disease often affecting a single node **(Figure 25.7C)**.

Cardiovascular involvement is the hallmark of systemic affection of KS. Myocarditis and congestive cardiac failure, pericarditis with pericardial effusion, arrhythmia, and valvular heart disease may occur. The most important cardiac complications are aneurysm and ectasia of coronary arteries,, detectable as early as 7 days after the onset of fever by echocardiography and may lead to ischemia and myocardial infarction. Cardiac complication occurs in one-fourth of untreated cases and affects boys more frequently than the girls. Other systemic affections may occur in the form of arthralgia and arthritis, urethritis with sterile pyuria, aseptic meningitis, diarrhea, vomiting and acute abdominal pain, and sensorineural hearing loss.

Diagnosis: Since there is no specific clinical and laboratory features of the disease, it is diagnosed on the basis of diagnostic criteria **(Table 25.9)**. The ESR is raised, there may be presence of pus cells in the urine, and serum transaminase levels may be elevated. Echocardiography is the most sensitive test for early diagnosis of cardiac involvement and should be performed immediately when the diagnosis is suspected and should be repeated in the course of the disease. In a limited number of children, angiography may also be required. A large number of conditions may have to be considered in the differential diagnosis of a child with febrile rash and red eyes. These should include viral exanthems like measles, drug rash (including toxic epidermal necrolysis and Stevens-Johnson syndrome), scarlet fever, toxic shock syndrome, staphylococcal scalded skin syndrome, and connective tissue disorders.

TABLE 25.9: Diagnostic criteria of Kawasaki disease

Fever for at least five days
Plus
4 of the following 5 in the absence of other explanation for the symptoms

1. Bilateral conjunctival injection
2. Mucosal involvement (pharyngeal congestion, fissured lip, strawberry tongue)
3. Polymorphous rash
4. Erythema and edema of peripheral extremities and periungual desquamation
5. Cervical lymphadenopathy

Treatment: Treatment should be initiated early; the best results in the context of cardiovascular complications are obtained if it is initiated within ten days of onset of the disease. The mainstays of treatment are intravenous immunoglobulin (IVIG) and aspirin. A single infusion of IVIG (2 g/kg) is given along with aspirin in the dose of 80-100 mg/kg/day initially for anti-inflammatory effect, followed by a low dose regimen (3-5 mg/kg/day) for its antiplatelet effect continued for months or years for children with risk of coronary artery disease. Death and disabilities in Kawasaki disease is almost always related to cardiac involvement. Long-term follow-up of children should include monitoring of cardiac status, clinically and by regular echocardiography.

Wegener's Granulomatosis

Wegener's granulomatosis (WG) is a systemic vasculitis characterized by necrotizing granulomatous inflammation of small as well as medium-sized vessels involving multiple organs, notably the upper and lower respiratory tracts, and the kidney. The pathogenesis of the disorder is unknown. Aberrant cell-mediated immune response to exogenous or endogenous antigens such as an infection and antineutrophil cytoplasmic antibodies (ANCA) are probably of pathogenic significance.

Clinical features: WG is an uncommon disease involving all age groups and is rarely encountered in childhood. The sex ratio is approximately equal. Constitutional feature like fever, malaise, joint pain, weight loss, and anorexia are common. The characteristic triad of upper respiratory, lung, and kidney involvement may not be evident in all cases. Respiratory tract involvement occurs in more than 90% of patients. Upper airway involvement may lead to sinusitis, purulent or bloody nasal discharge, ulceration and crusting of nasal mucosa, septal perforation leading to saddle-nose deformity, otitis media, and sometimes subglottic stenosis which may lead to airway obstruction. Lung involvement may be silent or there may be symptoms of cough, hemoptysis, breathlessness, or chest pain. Renal disease may be seen in more than 80% of children and is the chief cause of mortality in WG. Mild glomerulonephritis to rapidly progressive renal failure may occur. Ocular involvement may occur in about half of the cases, and manifests with scleritis, episcleritis, conjunctivitis, dacryocystitis, and retrobulbar mass causing proptosis. Neurologic manifestations in the form of cranial neuritis, mononeuritis multiplex and cerebral vasculitis may occur; cardiac involvement with pericarditis, coronary artery disease or cardiomyopathy is less common.

Cutaneous disease has been recorded in about half of the cases. Palpable purpura is the commonest manifestations; these lesions show features of leukocytoclastic vasculitis on histology. Papules, vesicles, petechiae, necrotic papules, pyoderma gangrenosum-like ulcers, and subcutaneous nodules may occur. A strawberry gingival hyperplasia and oral ulcers may occur as mucosal manifestations.

Diagnosis: The diagnosis of WG is suggested by the characteristic symptom complex and confirmed by biopsy of affected tissue which shows necrotizing granulomatous vasculitis. Extravascular granulomas are also seen. Nonspecific findings may include elevated ESR, mild anemia, leukocytosis, thrombocytosis, and hypergammaglobulinemia. ANCA with specificities for proteinase-3 is present in most of the cases and its level parallels disease activity.

Treatment: Untreated cases are associated with high mortality. Combination therapy with prednisolone and cyclophosphamide has greatly improved the prognosis and a high remission rate can be achieved with this regimen. After remission, a maintenance regimen is continued. Relapses are not uncommon; they are treated in the same manner as the induction regimen. Methotrexate and azathioprine are also used as alternative maintenance therapy to reduce adverse effects associated with cyclophosphamide therapy. Long-term trimethoprim-sulfamethoxazole therapy is often used to prevent relapse, this may act presumably by suppressing respiratory infections.

Churg-Strauss Syndrome

Churg-Strauss syndrome (CSS), also known as allergic granulomatosis, is a multisystem disease characterized by asthma, blood and tissue eosinophilia, multisystem vasculitis, and extravascular granulomas. CSS is an uncommon disease which is extremely rare during childhood.

The exact etiology is unknown but aberrant immune reactions are thought to be responsible for the causation. Disease process is characterized by granulomatous reaction in multiple organs with marked tissue eosinophilia and a necrotizing vasculitis involving small and medium vessels.

Three clinical stages have been described in the clinical evolution of CSS. The prodromal phase involves allergic rhinitis and asthma that can last for many years. The second phase manifests with peripheral eosinophilia and eosinophilic tissue infiltration. The hallmark of the final phase is a systemic vasculitis, which, if left untreated, can be fatal. Early in the course of the disease there may be constitutional features such as fever, malaise, anorexia, and weight loss. Pulmonary manifestations often dominate the clinical picture with severe asthma and pulmonary infiltrates. Mononeuritis multiplex is common. Clinical heart disease is seen in 15% and important cause of mortality. In addition to clinical features seen in adults, reported symptoms in children included testicular pain, hypertension, chorea, and seizures. Skin lesions may be seen in about half of the patients and presents with palpable purpura and subcutaneous nodules. Livedo reticularis, pustules and vesicle, and infiltrated papules have also been described. Renal disease is less common and less severe than in WG.

Striking eosinophilia with count more than 1000/ microliter occurs in majority of patients. Raised acute phase reactants are common. In contrast to adult cases, about half of whom are p-ANCA positive, children rarely demonstrate ANCA positivity. Confirmation of diagnosis may be done with tissue biopsy findings, but pathognomonic features are not often detected. Without treatment, CSS carries significant mortality, often due to cardiac disease. Systemic steroid is the cornerstone of therapy and can significantly improve the prognosis. Patients may require low-dose steroids for asthma after the vasculitic symptoms are relieved with initial high-dose therapy. In patients with severe or unremitting disease, combination therapy with cyclophosphamide, azathioprine, infliximab, or methotrexate may be required.

Henoch-Schonlein Purpura

Henoch-Schonlein purpura (HSP) is a multisystem IgA-mediated vasculitic disorder that commonly affects children and adolescents. HSP most frequently affects the skin, joints, kidneys, and gastrointestinal tracts, rarely affecting other organs. HSP is an immune-complex vasculitis which may occur in response to a variety of causes. Infective agents like group A streptococci, mycoplasma, Epstein-Barr and varicella virus, parvovirus B19, *Bartonella henselae* and campylobacter have been implicated, as well as vaccinations for typhoid, measles, cholera and yellow fever. Familial occurrence has been reported and HSP may occur in children with C2 complement component deficiency.

Clinical features: Most cases of HSP occur between the ages 2 and 11, with a peak age of onset at 5 years, the mean age of onset of Indian children is however higher than in the West. There is often a history of upper respiratory tract infection before the acute onset of the disease. The classic tetrad of clinical features of HSP involves the skin, GI tract, kidneys, and joints. Manifestations often occur sequentially, the first sign is often the purpura in majority of children. The palpable purpuric rash comes in crops and most frequently involve the legs **(Figure 25.8A)** and buttocks, lesions on trunk, face, and upper extremities are rare. Lesions above the waist have been associated with increased chance of renal involvement. In some children, petechial lesions may predominate over palpable purpuric lesions. Sometimes, vesiculobullous lesions, erosions and ulcers, necrosis, gangrene, and erythema multiforme-like lesions may

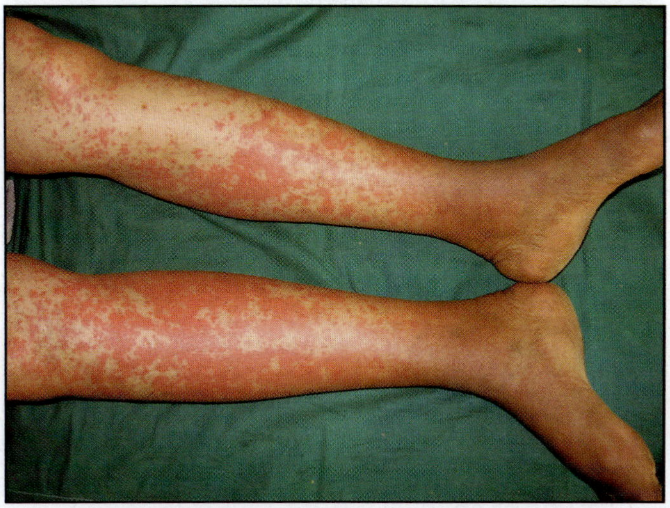

FIGURE 25.8A: Henoch-Schönlein purpura

occur. Subcutaneous edema of scalp, face, extremities, and penoscrotal area may occur and has been described in about half of the children in and Indian series. Oral, nasal, and genital petechiae may occur. Acute, painful scrotal swelling may occur due to vasculitis of scrotal vessels and this may mimic testicular torsion.

More than 85% of affected children may have gastrointestinal signs and symptoms in the forms of colicky abdominal pain, nausea and vomiting, hematemesis and melena, and ileus. Hemorrhage and perforation, pancreatitis, cholecystitis, and intussuception may occur rarely. Clinical evidence of renal involvement may be seen in about half of the cases. Renal affection may range from transient hematuria to rapidly progressive glomerulonephritis. Renal involvement may not be apparent for weeks after the onset of rash, necessitating long-term follow-up of children to detect this prognostically important complication. Arthritis in HSP may be seen in 75% of children and mainly affects the larger joints like knees, ankles **(Figure 25.8B)**, and elbow. Other joints like those of hands and feet may also be involved in a symmetric or asymmetric fashion. There is redness, swelling, and warmth around the joints, but effusions are unusual. The transient, non-migratory arthropathy usually resolves within days without any sequelae.

Apart from the classic tetrad of involvement, other systems are occasionally involved. Neurological involvement may manifest as headache, seizures, intracerebral hemorrhage, or paresis. Guillain-Barre syndrome has been described to occur in Indian children. Pulmonary infiltrates and pulmonary hemorrhage may occur.

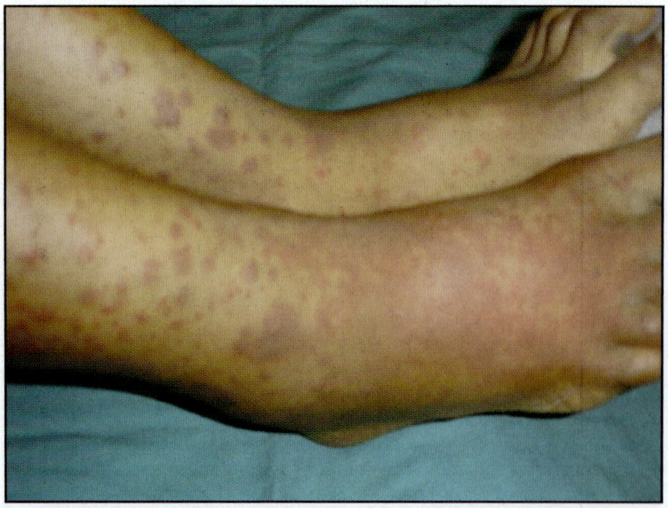

FIGURE 25.8B: Right ankle joint arthritis in Henoch-Schönlein purpura

Diagnosis: The diagnosis of HSP is readily suggested when the classical tetrad is seen, but incomplete forms are common and need to be differentiated from a wide variety of conditions. The differential diagnoses of HSP should include other forms of cutaneous small-vessel vasculitides, bleeding and coagulation disorders, post-streptococcal glomerulonephritis, rheumatic fever, SLE, sepsis, and disseminated intravascular coagulation. Other causes of acute abdomen and GI bleeding should be excluded. In doubtful cases, a skin biopsy may be helpful by demonstrating features of leukocytoclastic vasculitis and deposition of IgA and C3 on direct immunofluorescence test.

Treatment: General supportive care is all that may be needed for most of the children. Non-steroidal anti-inflammatory agents are used for joints symptoms. Systemic steroids are used for gastrointestinal hemorrhage or severe symptomatic disease. Prednisolone (1-2mg/kg/day in divided dosage) is used for at least a week and then rapidly tapered based on clinical improvement. There is no evidence that systemic steroids can otherwise modify the course and duration of the disease or the frequency or severity of renal manifestations. In children with progressive renal disease, various regimens have been used including oral prednisolone, cyclophosphamide, azathioprine, and plasma exchange.

HSP is generally a self-limiting disease with a single episode of manifestations. The course of the disease usually last for 4 to 6 weeks, but in some children there may be one or two recurrences. In younger children the disease tends to be milder and of shorter duration with few complications and recurrences. Morbidity and mortality is principally determined by the extent and severity of systemic involvement, mainly renal and gastrointestinal affection. Long-term follow-up is necessary for children with kidney involvement and in about 5% of children end-stage renal disease may occur.

CRYOGLOBULINEMIA AND CRYOFIBRINOGENEMIA

CRYOGLOBULINEMIA

Cryoglobulins are circulating immunoglobulins complexed with other immunoglobulins or proteins that precipitate in the cold and dissolve on re-warming. Based on their immunoglobulin constituents, cryoglobulins are classified in three groups, types I, II, and III. Type I cryoglobulins are single monoclonal immunoglobulins usually associated with an underlying hematologic malignancy like multiple myeloma or B-cell lymphoma. Type II and type III cryoglobulins are called mixed cryoglobulins as they consist of a mixture of immunoglobulins in the form of immune complexes. Type II cryoglobulins are single monoclonal immunoglobulins, usually IgM rheumatoid factors, complexed with polyclonal IgG. Type III cryoglobulins are polyclonal immunoglobulins complexed with polyclonal IgG or other proteins. Mixed cryoglobulins may be present in association with a number of disorders like connective tissue disorders, malignancies, and infections such as hepatitis C viral infection. Mixed cryoglobulinemia without a detectable primary cause is called essential mixed cryoglobulinemia.

Clinically, type I cryoglobulinemia are typically associated with Raynaud's syndrome, acrocyanosis, and arterial thrombosis. The most common clinical manifestations of mixed cryoglobulinemia are cutaneous vasculitis, arthritis, peripheral neuropathy, and glomerulonephritis. Cryoglobulinemic vasculitis may present with a variety of cutaneous manifestations like purpura, papules, nodules, urticaria, skin necrosis, livedo reticularis, and bullous and ulcerated lesions.

Renal disease may develop in up to 30% of patients. Hypertension, edema, and life threatening rapidly progressive renal disease may occur. Neurological manifestation occurs usually in the form of peripheral neuropathy. Arthralgia and arthritis, hepatosplenomegaly and vasculitic affections of GI tract and eyes may occur.

Evaluation of the patients should include a search for an underlying rheumatologic disease such as SLE, rheumatoid arthritis, Sjogren's syndrome, Hepatitis C and HIV infections, and lymphoproliferative disease. Rheumatoid factors are almost always positive, and hypocomplementemia occurs in 90% of patients. Raised ESR and anemia occur commonly. Treatment of cryoglobulinemia is based on identification and management of any underlying condition. Cutaneous and joint symptoms may be managed by non-steroidal anti-inflammatory agents. Severe systemic affection like renal disease may be treated with systemic steroids with cytotoxic agents. Treatment with interferon-alpha and ribavirin may be beneficial in Hepatitis C-associated cases. Plasmapheresis has also been used with success. Mortality is uncommon in Cryoglobulinemic vasculitis, long-term prognosis depends primarily on severity of renal disease.

CRYOFIBRINOGENEMIA

Cryofibrinogens are plasma proteins that reversibly precipitate in plasma with added anticoagulants but not in serum. In contrast, cryoglobulins precipitate in both serum and plasma. The precipitate is composed of fibrinogen, fibrin, fibrin degradation products and other plasma proteins. Cryofibrinogenemias are classified as primary, when no underlying disorder could be detected, and secondary, when the condition is associated with connective tissue disorders, infections, and malignancies.

Clinical features of cryofibrinogenemia commonly include cutaneous affection, mainly in the form of purpura, ecchymoses, necrosis, livedo reticularis, gangrene, and painful ulcerations induced by cold. Arterial and venous thrombosis may occur. Treatment of secondary cryofibrinogenemia is that of the underlying disease. Protection from cold is essential. Fibrinolytic therapy such as stanozolol has been used with success.

BIBLIOGRAPHY

1. Wimmershoff MB, Hohenleutner U, Landhaler M. Discoid lupus erythematosus and lupus profundus in childhood: report of two cases. Pediatr Dermatol 2003; 20: 140-45
2. Cherif F, Mebazza A, Mokni M, El Euch D, Azaiz MI, Dhahri AB. Childhood discoid lupus erythematosus: a Tunisian retrospective study of 16 cases. Pediatr Dermatol 2003; 20: 295-98.
3. Requena C, Torrelo A, de Prade I, Zambrano A. Linear childhood cutaneous lupus erythematosus following Blaschko line. J Eur Acad Dermatol Venereol 2002; 16:618-20.
4. Moises-Alfaro C, Berron-Perez R, Carrasco-Daza D, Gutierrez-Castrellon P, Ruiz-Maldonado R. Discoid lupus erythematosus in children: clinical, histopathologic, and follow-up features in 27 cases. Pediatr Dermatol 2003; 20: 103-7.
5. Sonntag M, Lehmann P, Megahed M, Ruzicka T, Kuhn A. Lupus erythematosus tumidus in childhood. Report of 3 patients. Dermatology 2003; 207:188-92.
6. Lee-Kirsch MA, Schulz MG, Rüschendorf H, Pfeiffer AS Ballarini A, Gahr M et al. Familial chilblain lupus, a monogenic form of cutaneous lupus erythematosus, maps to chromosome 3p. Am J Hum Genet 2006; 79:731-37.
7. Amato L, Coronella G, Berti S, Moretti S, Fabbri P. Subacute cutaneous lupus erythematosus in childhood. Pediatr Dermatol 2003; 20: 31-4.
8. Ciconte A, Mills AE, Shipley A, Marks R. Subacute cutaneous lupus erythematosus presenting in a child. Australas J Dermatol 2002; 43: 62-4.
9. Ravi VM, Balachandran C. Subacute cutaneous lupus erythematosus (SCLE) presenting in childhood. Dermatol Online J 2005; Aug 1; 11(2) : 27.
10. Cassidy JT. Systemic lupus erythematosus, Juvenile dermatomyositis, Scleroderma, and Vasculitis. In: Harris ED, Budd RC, Genovesic MC, Firestein GS, Sargent JS, Sledge CB. eds. Kelly's Textbook of Rheumatology. Philadelphia: Elsevier Saunders. 2005; 1579-96.

11. Bader-Meunier B, Armengaud JB, Haddad E, Salomon R, Deschenes G, Kone-paut I, et al. Initial presentation of childhood-onset systemic lupus erythematosus: a French multicenter study. J Pediatr 2005; 146:648-53.
12. Wananukul S, Watana D, Pongprasit P. Cutaneous manifestations of childhood systemic lupus erythematosus. Pediatr Dermatol 1998; 15: 342-6.
13. Roholt NS, Lapiere JC, Wang JI, Bernstein L LJ, Woodley DT, Eramo LR. Localized linear bullous eruption of systemic lupus erythematosus in a child. Pediatr Dermatol 1995; 12: 138-44.
14. Benseler SM, Silverman ED. Neuropsychiatric involvement in pediatric systemic lupus erythematosus. Lupus 2007; 16: 564-71.
15. Richer O, Ulinski R, Lemelle I, Ranchin B, Loirat C, Piette JC et al. Abdominal manifestations in childhood-onset systemic lupus erythematosus. Ann Rheum Dis 2007; 66: 174-78.
16. Tan EM, Cohen AS, Fries JF, Masi AT, McShane DJ, Rothfield NF. The 1982 revised criteria for the classification of systemic lupus erythematosus. Arthritis Rheum 1982; 25:1271-77.
17. Willems m, Haddad E, Niaudet P, Kone-Paut I, Bensman A, Cochat P, et al. Rituximab therapy for childhood-onset systemic lupus erythematosus. J Pediatr 2006; 148: 623-27.
18. Singh S, Devidayal , Kumar L, Joshi K. Mortality patterns in childhood lupus-10 years' experience in developing country. Clin Rheumatol 2002; 21:462-5.
19. Sawant S, Amladi ST, Wadhawa SL, Nayak CS, Nikam BP. Cutaneous neonatal lupus erythematosus with unusual features. Indian J Dermatol Venereol Leprol. 2007; 73:250-2.
20. Boros CA, Spence D, Blaser S, Silverman ED. Hydrocephalus and macrocephaly: new manifestations of neonatal lupus erythematosus. Arthritis Rheum. 2007;57:261-6.
21. Cooper RM, Butler DF, Ghali F, Grimwood RE. Periorbital cutaneous neonatal lupus. Skinmed 2007; 6:145-6.
22. High WA, Costner MI. Persistent scarring, atrophy, and dyspigmentation in a preteen girl with neonatal lupus erythematosus. J Am Acad Dermatol 2003; 48:626-28.
23. Wargula JC. Update on Juvenile Dermatomyositis: New advances in understanding its etiopathogenesis Curr Opin Rheumatol 2003;15: 595-601.
24. Ramanan AV, Feldman BM: Clinical outcomes in juvenile dermatomyositis. Curr Opin Rheumatol 2002; 14:658-662.
25. Chowdhary V, Wakhlu A, Agarwal A, et al.: Outcome in juvenile dermatomyositis. Indian Pediatr 2002, 39:931-5.
26. Mahesh A, Panchapakesa Rajendran C, Rukmangatharajan S, Rajeswari S, Vasanthy N Parthiban M. Juvenile dermatomyositis-clinical and laboratory profile. J Indian Rheumatol Assoc 2005: 13 :4-7
27. Peloro TM, Miller OF, Hahn TF, Newman ED. Juvenile dermatomyositis: a retrospective review of a 30-year experience. J Am Acad Dermatol 2001; 45:28-34.
28. Rider LG, Schiffenbauer AS, Zito M, Lim KL, Ahmed A, Zemel LS et al. Neopterin and quinolinic acid are surrogate measures of disease activity in the juvenile idiopathic inflammatory myopathies. Clinical Chemistry. 2002;48:1681-88.
29. Singh S, Bansal A. twelve years experience of juvenile dermatomyositis in North India. Rheumatol Int 2006; 26: 510-15.
30. Al-Mayouf S, Al-Mazyed A Bahabri S. Efficacy of early treatment of severe juvenile dermatomyositis with intravenous methylprednisolone and methotrexate. Clin Rheumatol 2000; 19: 138-41.
31. Majithia V, Harisdangkul V. Mycophenolate mofetil (CellCept): an alternative therapy for autoimmune inflammatory myopathy. Rheumatology (Oxford) 2005; 44: 386-9.
32. Levine TD. Rituximab in the treatment of dermatomyositis: an open label pilot study. Arthritis Rheum 2005; 52: 601-7.
33. Sakkas LI. New developments in the pathogenesis of systemic sclerosis. Autoimmunity 2005; 38:113-6.
34. Senecal J, Henault J. The pathogenic role of autoantibodies to nuclear autoantigens in systemic sclerosis. J Rheumatol 2005; 32:1642-49.
35. Misra R, Singh G, Aggarwal P, Aggarwal A. Juvenile onset systemic sclerosis: a single center experience of 23 cases from Asia. Clin Rheumatol 2007; 26:1259-62.
36. Martini G, Foeldvari I, Russo R, Cuttica R, Eberhard A, Ravelli A et al. Systemic sclerosis in childhood: clinical and immunologic features of 153 patients in an international database. Arthritis Rheum 2006; 54:3971-8.
37. Zulian F, Woo P, Athreya BH, Laxer RM, Medsger TA Jr, Lehman RJ, et al. The Pediatric Rheumatology European Society/American College of Rheumatology/European League against Rheumatism provisional classification criteria for juvenile systemic sclerosis. Arthritis Rheum 2007; 57:203-12.
38. Foeldvari I, Zhavania M, Birdi N, Cuttica RJ, de Oliveira SH, Dent PB, et al. Favourable outcome in 135 children with juvenile systemic sclerosis: results of multi-national survey. Rheumatology (Oxford) 2000; 39:556-9.
39. Singh S, Salaria M, Kumar L, Minz R, Datta U, Sehgal S. Clinico-epidemiological profile of juvenile rheumatoid arthritis at Chandigarh. Indian Pediatr 1999; 36:449-54.
40. Adib N. Silman A. Thomson W. Outcome following onset of juvenile idiopathic inflammatory arthritis: II. Predictors of outcome in juvenile arthritis. Rheumatology 2005; 44:1002-07.
41. Kotajima L, Aotsuka S, Sumiya M, Yokohari R, Tojo T, Kasukawa R. Clinical features of patients with juvenile onset mixed connective tissue disease: analysis of data collected in a nationwide collaborative study in Japan. J Rheumatol 1996; 23:1088-94.
42. Ramos-Casals M, Tzioufs AG, Font J. Primary Sjögren's syndrome: new clinical and therapeutic concepts. Ann Rheum Dis 2005; 64:347-54.
43. Houghton K, Malleson P, Cabral D, Petty R, Tucker L. Primary Sjögren syndrome in children and adolescents: are proposed diagnostic criteria applicable? J Rheumatol 2005; 32:2225-32.
44. Kobayashi I, Kawamura N, Okano M, Shikano T, Mizumoto M, Hayashi Y, et al. Anti-alpha-fodrin autoantibody is an early diagnostic marker for childhood primary Sjögren syndrome. J Rheumatol 2001; 28:363-5.
45. Singh S, Dass R. Clinical approach to vasculitides. Indian J Pediatr 2002; 69:881-8.
46. Bandyopadhyay D. The spectrum of leukocytoclastic vasculitis: etiology, classification and approach to management. in Recent Advances in Dermatology. Ghosh S. ed. New Delhi: Jaypee Brothers. 2004; 31-55.
47. Sridhar MR, Goel H, Anirudh D, Lodha R, Kabra SK. Kawasaki disease:are we missing the diagnosis? Indian J Pediatr 2005; 72:873-75.
48. Khubchandani R, D'Souza S. Kawasaki disease in India. Pediatr Rheumatol Online J 2004; 2:2
49. Boyer D, Vargas SO, Slattery D, Rivera-Sanchez YM, Colin AA. Churg-Strauss syndrome in children: a clinical and pathologic review. Pediatrics 2006; 118:e914-16
50. Kumar L, Singh S, Goraya JS, Uppal B, Kakkar S, Walker R et al. Henoch-Schonlein purpura: the Chandigarh experience. Indian Pediatr 1998; 35:19-25.
51. Florentino DF. Cutaneous vasculitis. J Am Acad Dermatol 2003; 48:311-40.

26

Skin in Systemic Diseases and Multisystem Disorders

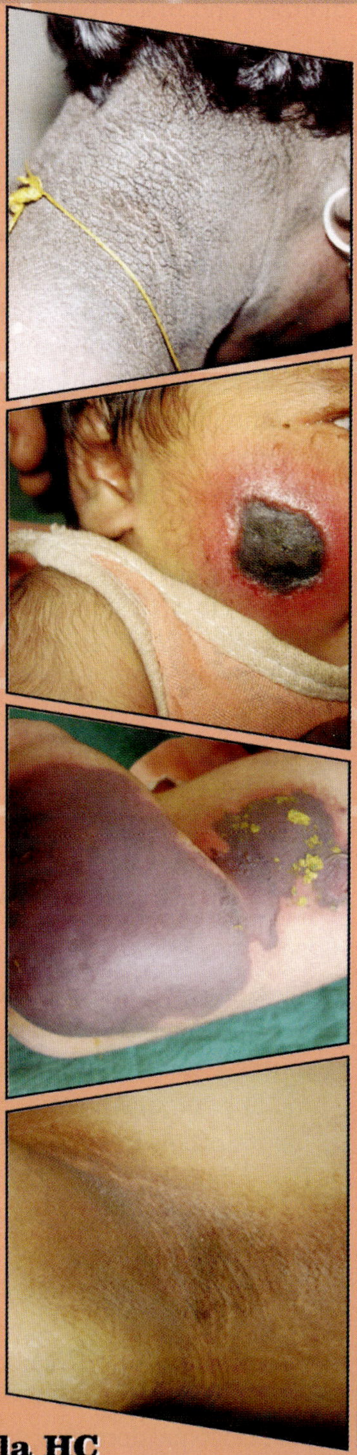

- Cutaneous manifestations of GIT disorders
- Cutaneous manifestations of Hepatobiliary disorders
- Cutaneous manifestations of Renal disorders
- Cutaneous manifestations of Cardiovascular and pulmonary disorders
- Graft versus host disease

Sanjeev Grover

- Cutaneous manifestations of Endocrinal disorders and carcinoid syndrome
- Neurocutaneous disorders
- Psychocutaneous disorders
- Cutaneous manifestations of internal malignancy
- Purpura fulminans
- Systemic amyloidosis
- Sarcoidosis
- Behcet's disease
- Pruritus

R Rajagopal, T Rajkamal, Sudhanshu Shukla, Mangala HC

CUTANEOUS MANIFESTATIONS OF GASTROINTESTINAL TRACT

Disorders of the pharynx, esophagus, stomach, pancreas and intestines that may lead to skin changes include dysphagia, gastrointestinal bleeding, abdominal pain, diarrhea and malabsorption.

DYSPHAGIA

Skin abnormalities that occur with dysphagia:

1. Infections: Oral candidiasis may extend to the pharynx and esophagus and cause dysphagia.
2. Blistering diseases: Extensive esophageal involvement with blisters, erosions, and strictures can occur in hereditary epidermolysis bullosa, particularly in recessive dystrophic and junctional forms. Acquired immunobullous disorders, such as pemphigus and dermatitis herpetiformis can affect mucosa.
3. Oro-oculo-genito-cutaneous syndromes: The mucosae may be involved in Stevens-Johnson syndrome, toxic epidermal necrolysis and Behcet's syndrome. Oral ulceration, occurring at least three times in a 12-month period, is usually seen on the nonkeratinized epithelium and may be difficult to distinguish from ulceration of Crohn's disease.
4. Collagen vascular diseases: Dysphagia occurs in dermatomyositis and systemic sclerosis. Ulcers in the mouth and pharynx may occur in systemic lupus erythematosus.

GASTROINTESTINAL BLEEDING

Vascular Abnormalities

- Hereditary hemorrhagic telangiectasia presents as a familial pattern of epistaxis with telangiectasia on the mucosal surfaces and arterivenous malformations in multiple organs. Hemorrhage from gastrointestinal lesions occurs in 10 to 40% of patients.
- Blue rubber bleb nevi: The venous malformations look and feel as their name suggests and project into the gut lumen. In contrast to the cutaneous lesions, they bleed easily, causing anemia and less commonly, acute hemorrhage.

Inherited Defects of Connective Tissue

In the autosomal dominant vascular type of Ehlers-Danlos syndrome, Type IV, rupture of the bowel, often involving the sigmoid colon, account for one-quarter of all complications and 8 % of all deaths. Thirteen percent of patients with pseudoxanthoma elasticum experience gastrointestinal bleeding.

Kaposi's Sarcoma

The gut is a common site for Kaposi's sarcoma. Involvement is commonly asymptomatic, but severe bleeding may occur.

ABDOMINAL PAIN

Abdominal pain in association with skin abnormalities may occur in following conditions:

- Herpes zoster
- Urticaria and angioedema
- Porphyria
- Anderson-Fabry disease
- Vasculitis
  - o Henoch-Schönlein disease
  - o Collagen vascular disease
  - o Malignant atrophic papulosis
- Polyposis
  - o Gardner's syndrome
  - o Peutz-Jeghers syndrome
  - o Canada-Cronkhite syndrome
  - o Neurofibromatosis
  - o Ulcerative colitis
- Inflammatory bowel disease
- Pancreatitis.

Angioedema

Acute attacks of urticaria or angioedema may be associated with abdominal pain. Edema of the bowel wall, mucosal thickening and free fluid is evident in ultrasonography. This is especially true in the autosomal dominant hereditary angioedema. Treatment is with administration of purified C1 esterase inhibitor concentrate.

Porphyria

In the rare variegate porphyria; skin involvement and attacks of acute abdominal pain coexist. The skin shows changes identical to those of porphyria cutanea tarda. Drugs such as griseofulvin and estrogen can precipitate this attack.

Anderson-Fabry Disease (Angiokeratoma corporis diffusum)

It is a rare X-linked recessive multisystem lysosomal storage disorder caused by deficiency of alpha-galactosidase. Clinical symptoms include painful neuropathy, progressive renal, cardiovascular, cerbrovascular and gastro-intestinal dysfunction.

Vasculitis

Henoch-Schönlein purpura is palpable, especially on the legs and buttocks, and may occur in conjunction with joint swelling. Up to 76% of patients have gastrointestinal involvement ranging from colicky abdominal pain, nausea, and vomiting to bloody diarrhea.

Malignant atrophic papulosis is an idiopathic systemic obliterative vasculopathy. Recurrent crops of porcelain-white atrophic papules with an elevated erythematous border are the characteristic skin lesions. Gut vessels are involved in half of the cases, which manifest itself clinically as bleeding, abdominal pain, malabsorption and bowel perforation.

Polyposis

Among the polyposis, Peutz-Jeghers syndrome is common in children. It is an autosomal dominant condition. Polyps occur mainly in the small intestine, but can also occur in the stomach and colon. The usual presentation is melena or intussusceptions. The cutaneous feature is lentiginosis, predominantly in perioral, periorbital, and intraoral areas. Perianal and acral lentiginosis occurs. The pigmented macules appear early in childhood and may fade with increasing age, although the mucosal lesions persist.

Inflammatory Bowel Disease

Skin lesions in ulcerative colitis and Crohn's disease are:

- Contiguous skin involvement—Oral/perianal granulomatous lesions, perianal skin tag (75-80%), fissures and sinus tracts
- Metastatic cutaneous Crohn's disease—Granulomatous lesions in other body parts
- Reactive cutaneous lesions—Pyoderma gangrenosum, Erythema nodosum, aphthous ulcers
- Rashes at ileostomy and colostomy sites
- Cutaneous manifestations of nutritional deficiency.

Both ulcerative colitis and Crohn's disease may present with abdominal pain, gastrointestinal bleeding, or diarrhea. The skin complications of the two diseases are similar, although some occur with different frequencies; in particular, granulomatous lesions are much more common in Crohn's disease.

Pyoderma gangrenosum: Up to one half of patients with pyoderma gangrenosum may have inflammatory bowel disease, and 5% of pediatric patients with ulcerative colitis and 1% of children with Crohn's disease will develop the condition. The severity and extent of the ulceration in pyoderma gangrenosum may be linked to the activity of the underlying disease, and it may heal with effective treatment of the underlying disease.

Granulomas: Oral granulomatous nodules are common in Crohn's disease, where these may coalesce to give a "cobblestone" appearance. Granulomas may also occur in the perineum, at colostomy and ileostomy sites, and in association with scars, sinuses, and fistulas. Very rarely, granulomas occur at sites not contiguous with the bowel, such as the trunk and limbs: the so-called 'metastatic cutaneous Crohn's disease'.

Erythema nodosum: Pediatric patients with ulcerative colitis and Crohn's disease may have erythema nodosum in 15% cases.

***Aphthous ulcers*:** In inflammatory bowel disease or celiac disease, aphthous ulcers may be the presenting feature. More than 50% children with Crohn's disease present with oral aphthae.Patients with both dermatitis herpetiformis and celiac disease are more likely to have aphthous ulcers than those with dermatitis herpetiformis alone.

Malnutrition: Cutaneous signs of nutritional deficiencies may occur in both the cases.

Pancreatitis

Bruising of the skin around the umbilicus (Cullen's sign) or in the flanks (Grey Turner's sign) are well-known features of acute pancreatitis.

DIARRHEA AND MALABSORPTION

Skin changes due to malabsorption include:

Non-specific signs:

1. Acquired ichthyosis and pruritus: Patients generally have pallid, dry, rough, scaly skin that is usually itchy. Eczema (asteatotic eczema or eczema craquele) may develop.
2. Hair: Hair growth is slow, falls out easily and becomes grey. The root diameter and proportion of anagen hairs decrease. Lanugo hair may develop.

Kwashiorkor causes hair to become hypo pigmented, varying from red-yellow to white, and curly. There may be alternating pale and dark bands on hair. Type 2 vitamin D dependent rickets have alopecia totalis.

3. Nails: Nails grow more slowly, become brittle and may develop fissures. Multiple pigmented bands may appear. Koilonychia occurs in iron deficiency.
4. Skin color: Malabsorption can lead to hyperpigmentation, which is most pronounced on the face. Vitamin B12 deficiency causes pigmentation of the distal extremities in a glove and stocking pattern.

Specific signs:

1. Vitamin A deficiency: Xerosis, wrinkled skin covered with fine scales, occasionally accompanied by deep erosions (dermomalacia).
2. Vitamin B 3 deficiency: Causes pellagra with its triad of diarrhea, dermatitis and dementia.
3. Vitamin C deficiency: Follicular keratoses, hemorrhage and corkscrew hairs.
4. Vitamin K deficiency: Impaired coagulation leads to purpura.
5. Vitamin B12 deficiency: Symmetric glove and stocking hyper pigmentation, with a lemon pallor of skin elsewhere.
6. Iron deficiency: Angular stomatitis, smooth painful tongue and fragile nails with longitudinal ridging and koilonychia. Hair changes include diffuse scalp alopecia with fragile hair.
7. Zinc deficiency: Hereditary cause is acrodermatitis enteropathica; clinical features start at weaning with eczematous or vesiculobullous lesions on hands and feet and periorificial area. Other features are progressive alopecia and failure to thrive.
8. Linoleic acid deficiency: Epidermis becomes hyperkeratotic(phrynoderma), resulting in diffuse xerosis, scale and erythema with brittle nails and capillary fragility.

Other Malabsorption Syndromes

Celiac disease: This disorder is associated with dermatitis herpetiformis which is an intensely pruritic, chronic, recurrent papulovesicular disease. Improvement of psoriasis in a small number of patients who were treated with gluten free diet suggested the possibility that celiac disease and psoriasis may be associated. Patients with psoriasis have a high frequency of positive IgA anti-gliadin antibodies but do not have an increased incidence of celiac disease.

Whipple's disease: This disorder is another cause of malabsorption and diarrhea accompanied by skin manifestations. Diffuse pigmentation is common but buccal mucosa is not involved. Subcutaneous nodules may occur. The disorder usually presents with arthralgia and abdominal features like pain, diarrhea and malabsorption, leading to weight loss.

CUTANEOUS MANIFESTATIONS OF HEPATOBILIARY DISORDERS

When skin lesions occur in association with liver disease, they are usually not specific to a particular hepatic pathology. The most florid lesions generally appear in patients with chronic active hepatitis and cirrhosis, but such changes may also occur in the absence of hepatic diseases.

Main cutaneous changes in liver disease are:

1. Pruritus
2. Icterus
3. Telangiectasis
4. Xanthelasma
5. Parotid swelling
6. Rhagades
7. Spider angiomas
8. Dollar paper markings
9. Acne vulgaris
10. Loss of secondary male hair growth
11. Gynecomastia
12. Collateral veins
13. Purpura
14. Striae
15. Palmar erythema
16. Gonadal atrophy
17. Dupuytren's contracture
18. Nails; white nails, opaque nails, white banded nails, watch glass deformity and patchy whiteness.
19. Edema.

ITCHING

Pruritus often complicates hepatic disorders associated with cholestasis or biliary tract obstruction and sclerosing cholangitis but it is less common in hemochromatosis and autoimmune chronic active hepatitis. In viral hepatitis, itching is usually missed as an early sign of the disease, but it is florid in the later icteric phase. The symptoms are generally most severe at acral sites and areas of tight clothing and are more prominent nocturnally. Disappearance of pruritus may accompany severe deterioration of hepatic function. Some drugs like erythromycin, phenothiazines, and nitrofurantoin may also induce cholestasis and cause pruritus.

The precise mechanism of itch in obstructive liver disease remains unclear. It was believed to be due to the presence of bile salts in the skin, but the intensity of itch does not correlate with bilirubin or bile acids levels in chronic liver failure. However, the partial relief of itching by bile salt chelators and the disappearance of pruritus when liver cells fail suggest hepatic synthesis of at least one of the agents contributing to pruritus. Although patients with cholestasis may have elevated levels of plasma histamine, the therapeutic response to antihistamines is limited, and it is unlikely that release of histamine play an important role in the pathogenesis of hepatobiliary itch. Improvement in hepatic itch after administration of drugs that block the action of opiates suggests that endogenous opioids may be important in the pathogenesis.

Treatment of the underlying cause is the primary mode of management. Less specific options include ursodeoxycholic acid, cholestyramine, phenobarbital, anabolic steroids like stanozolol, rifampicin, antihistamines and dietary intervention to supplement polyunsaturated fatty acids. Phototherapy of various types, sunlight, UVA, UVB, photoirradiation of plasma and extracorporeal photophoresis may be effective, but ongoing treatment is generally required. Oral nalmefene may be useful in the long-term control of pruritus of cholestasis. Other treatments include hemoperfusion or plasma perfusion through charcoal coated beads, plasmapheresis, infusion of albumin and slow intravenous lidocaine. On the basis that endogenous opiates may play a role in this symptom, and that these have a circadian rhythm regulated by light, bright light therapy to the eyes was studied and found to reduce cholestatic itch in a short-term study.

NAIL CHANGES IN LIVER DISEASE

The nails of many patients with liver disease are normal and nail abnormalities are less constant. Nail color changes include diffuse white discoloration with an invisible lunula, proximal white and distal pink color (Terry nails) and white bands (Muehrke's bands). Altered digital blood flow, soft tissue overgrowth and hypo-albuminemia may all contribute. Lunula may be red in patients with hepatic cirrhosis. Patients with cirrhosis also show clubbing, curved nails, thickened nails, longitudinally ridged nails, watch glass deformity, striations and brittleness.

Azure blue nails are seen in Wilson's disease. Azure nails are also seen in patients with argyria or following treatment with busulfan or antimalarials. In hemochromatosis, koilonychia is probably the most common nail abnormalities, but it is not related to anemia.

SKIN AND OTHER PIGMENTARY CHANGES

Jaundice is first visible as a yellowish hue of the sclerae and soft palate before it becomes generalized. It is due to hyperbilirubinemia. Carotenemia may have a similar appearance but does not affect the sclera; skin discoloration following mepacrine and busulphan therapy may simulate jaundice, but these usually also cause subungual pigmented bands. A muddy grey colored hyperpigmentation occurs in chronic liver disease of any cause. It is due to hypermelanosis with normal numbers of melanocytes, but the precise mechanism is uncertain. Guttate hypomelanosis, a condition in which small white macules, sometimes with a central spider, appear on the skin of the buttocks, back, thighs, and forearms, may occur in cirrhosis. In hemochromatosis, there is a striking metallic grey or bronze-brown discoloration of the skin with accentuation over sun exposed areas. Associated dietary deficiency may cause the pigmentary changes of pellagra.

VASCULAR CHANGES

Patients with chronic liver disease often have telangiectatic changes, mainly on the light exposed skin. Numerous tiny telangiectases sometimes give the impression of a diffuse almost exanthematous redness. This change is known as 'dollar paper markings'. These fade on pressure and rarely pulsate.

Spider Nevus/angioma

It is the most representative and classic vascular lesion of chronic liver disease. They are commonly found over hands and fingers in children, unlike in adults where it is more commonly found on the face, neck, forearms, and upper part of the chest. It may regress with improvement of the underlying conditions.

Palmar Erythema

There are two clinical forms of 'liver palm'. In the first, there is an exaggeration of normal mottling; the hands are warm and bright red, especially over the palm, the dorsa of hands, the fingers, and the nail bases. In the second, there is well-demarcated redness of the hypothenar eminence spreading on to the fingertips. The mottling blanches on pressure and it flushes synchronously with the pulse rate.

Portal-systemic collateral vessels may develop as caput medusae, and may be an important clue to the existence of portal hypertension.

Purpuric lesions occur mainly on the lower limbs. These are secondary both to acquired clotting defects such as thrombocytopenia and to vascular fragility.

Hepatitis and the skin: Cutaneous striae may appear in patients with chronic active hepatitis. In the pre-icteric phase, patients may present with a discrete, transient, maculopapular, urticarial, or petechial rash. Other features include pyoderma gangrenosum, urticaria, vasculitis, scleroderma, and splinter nail hemorrhages, depending on the underlying cause of hepatitis.

DISORDERS INVOLVING BOTH SKIN AND LIVER

1. Arginosuccinic aciduria
2. Dermatomyositis
3. Drug hypersensitivity syndrome
4. Eruptive neonatal angiomatosis
5. Graft-versus-host disease
6. Hereditary hemorrhagic telangiectasia
7. Histiocytosis
8. Immunodeficiency states
9. Mastocytosis
10. Mucocutaneous lymph node syndrome
11. Porphyrias: Porphyria cutanea tarda, variegate porphyria, erythropoietic protoporhyria, hereditary coproporphyria
12. Sarcoidosis
13. Syphilis
14. Systemic lupus erythematosus
15. Tuberous sclerosis.

CUTANEOUS CHANGES IN RENAL DISORDERS IN CHILDREN

CUTANEOUS FINDINGS

The sequelae of renal failure are complex and involve multiple systems. In uremia the skin tends to be dry, often associated with perifollicular keratosis and fine scaling. This may be due to the reduction in the eccrine sweat glands and may be due to high diuretic regimens. Usually the body hair is sparse. The various other cutaneous findings are:

Pigmentation

Anemia presenting as pallor is an early and common sign in renal failure resulting from reduced erythropoiesis and increased hemolysis. In many cases a diffuse brown hyperpigmentation is seen which is accentuated in sun exposed areas. It is attributed to increased melanogenesis as a result of increased tissue levels of beta-MSH, which is poorly dialyzable and not excreted normally in uremia. The yellow hue observed in uremic patients is attributed to the retention of carotene, urochromes and other yellow pigments.

Increased nail pigmentation confined to the distal nail occurs. This distal brown or normal red color, combined with a proximal white appearance is a distinctive pattern known as the 'half-and-half nails.'

Purpura, scattered ecchymoses and petechiae are common and due to increased vascular fragility, mild thrombocytopenia or more marked platelet dysfunction.

Wound healing is delayed and patients may be more susceptible to pressure sores.

Pruritus

Generalized pruritus is the most important dermatological symptom of renal insufficiency. It is graded as moderate and severe and correlates strongly with severity of renal failure. Hemodialysis can initiate pruritus as well as improve it. The cause of pruritus in renal failure is obscure. Possible causes are increased urea, slowly accumulated pruritogens, and increased phosphorous and magnesium in the skin. It may also occur due to drug reactions since uremic patients are frequently on numerous medications. UVB radiation is an effective therapy in such cases as it may cause reduction in skin phosphorus levels. UVA, oral cholestyramine and activated charcoal are alternatives. Erythropoietin can alleviate pruritus.

Calcification and Calciphylaxis

Calcifying panniculitis, a rare clinical feature in uremia, is caused by a mechanism known as calciphylaxis. It is invariably associated with a high serum and calcium levels. Metastatic skin calcification is a rare finding, and usually presents as papular or nodular cutaneous lesions around large joints or flexural sites. Cutaneous necrosis or gangrene may develop due to thrombosis of blood vessels as a result of metastatic calcification in blood vessel walls associated with hyperparathyroidism and renal failure.

Perforating Disorders

Perforating collagenosis, Kyrle's disease or perforating folliculitis occurs in renal failure.The conditions are rare in chilgren. Hyperpigmented papules with central keratinous plug, more commonly affecting the extensor surface of the limbs and face are involved.

Nevi

Immune suppressed Caucasian children, such as patients on chemotherapy acquire more nevi than their siblings. Increased total number of nevi is a risk factor for melanoma development.

Tables 26.1 and 26.2 represent cutaneous features of patients with renal impairment.

MULTISYSTEM DISORDERS

Sarcoidosis is a multisystem granulomatous disease with unknown cause and widespread manifestations. Skin lesions are found especially about the eyes, nose, nasolabial folds and mouth. Patients may have renal manifestations like nephrocalcinosis and nephrolithiasis resulting from secondary effects of hypercalcemia.

RENOCUTANEOUS SYNDROME

Skin involvement in renal disease may be due to affection of the systems by the same basic process, and secondary to the non-specific pathologic and clinical changes that accompany renal insufficiency regardless of its etiology.

TABLE 26.1: Uremia related cutaneous findings in children (Silverberg et al)

Finding	Transplant	Dialysis	Medical management
Xerosis(%)	100	100	0
Pruritus(%)	50	69	25
Half-and-half nails(%)	40	19	0
Melanocytic nevi(%)	40	31	25
Average number of nevi(%)	5.5	3.6	1.1

TABLE 26.2: Drug related findings in patients with uremia (Silverberg et al)

Finding	Transplant	Dialysis	Medical management
Moon facies(%)	80	44	25
Striae(%)	50	25	50
Hypertrichosis(%)	60	69	50
Gingival hypertrophy(%)	50	69	25
Onychoschizia(%)	53	63	25
Infectious disease findings			
Tinea versicolor(%)	0	6	50
Warts(%)	60	19	25
Acral warts(% of all warts)	67	83	100
Herpes zoster(%)	10	25	0
Folliculitis(%)	0	12	0
Onychomycosis(%)	10	12	0

Fabry's Disease

In Fabry's disease, in addition to diffuse angiokeratomas there is renal deposition of glycosphingolipids. There is associated proteinuria, microscopic hematuria and lipiduria. Early death occurs in this condition due to the renal failure. Renal transplantation restores the deficient enzyme, alfa-galactosidase A, and results in the improvement of the condition.

Neurofibromatoses (von Recklinghausen's disease)

The neurofibromatosis Type 1, in addition to the cutaneous neurofibromas and *café-au-lait* macules, there may be obstruction to the urinary outflow secondary to impinging neurofibroma. Nephroblastoma is a recognized association of neurofibromatosis and renal polycystic disease.

Tuberous Sclerosis Complex

It is a genetic disorder with multi-organ hamartomatosis. The classical renal lesion is angiomyolipoma, renal cysts may occur in association or as an isolated finding.

Nail-Patella Syndrome (Fong's syndrome; Hereditary onychodysplasia)

Renal lesions are usually asymptomatic. The patient shows protienuria, hematuria and reduced creatinine clearance and presents as chronic glomerulonephritis.

Oral-facial-digital Syndrome

Polycystic disease of the kidneys and liver occurs commonly in this condition.

von Hippel-Lindau Syndrome (VHL)

VHL represents one of the hereditary kidney cancer syndromes. Renal lesions are either simple cysts or adenocarcinomas.

CARDIAC DISEASES AND SKIN

Many cutaneous abnormalities are associated with cardiac disease. General symptoms include cyanosis, erythema, flushing and digital clubbing. Multi-system disorders and inherited diseases are also associated with cutaneous and cardiac abnormalities.

The various congenital/inherited conditions affecting the heart and skin are:

1. Ehlers-Danlos syndrome
2. Cutis laxa
3. Marfan's syndrome
4. Psuedoxanthoma elasticum
5. Werner's disease
6. Progeria
7. Cockayne's syndrome
8. Fabry's disease
9. Noonan's syndrome
10. LEOPARD syndrome
11. Tuberous sclerosis
12. Neurofibromatosis
13. Incontinentia pigmenti.

GENERAL CUTANEOUS SIGNS OF CARDIAC DISEASES

Cyanosis

Bluish discoloration of the skin and mucous membranes due to increased amounts of reduced circulating hemoglobin. Cyanosis is apparent when reduced hemoglobin exceeds 5 mg/dl. It also results when non functional hemoglobin-like methemoglobin is present in the blood. The lips, nail-beds, ears and malar prominences are recognized sites of cyanosis.

Most common congenital cardiac lesion associated with cyanosis is tetralogy of Fallot.

Differential cyanosis involving the lower extremities, but sparing the upper extremities occurs in patients with patent ductus arteriosus and pulmonary hypertension. Mild cyanosis of the lips and cheeks without clubbing of the fingers may suggest mitral stenosis.

Flushing

Flushing of the face, neck, chest may occur from carcinoid tumors. Pheochromocytoma may cause periodic facial flushing associated with sweating and hypertension. A combination of flushing and cyanosis may be seen in patients with ductus arteriosus, patent foramen ovale and left sided cardiac lesions.

Flushing seen with systemic mastocytosis is a result of histamine release from mast cells.

Erythema

Dilated skin capillaries and increase in the amount of saturated oxygenated hemoglobin lead to redness of the skin. Massive capillary dilatation in erythroderma and exfoliative dermatitis may result in high output cardiac failure.

A distinct discoloration of the skin, termed "erythremia" (combination of cyanosis and redness) affecting the tongue, lips, nose, ear lobes, conjunctiva and finger tips with nail clubbing may be seen in polycythemia.

Palmar erythema, primarily involving the hypothenar eminence, the thenar eminence and the finger tips may be associated with high output cardiac failure.

Clubbing

Clubbing is characterized by the proliferation of the connective tissue between the nail matrix and the distal phalanx. Cardio-pulmonary causes of clubbing include cyanotic congenital heart disease, subacute bacterial endocarditis, congestive heart failure and suppurative lung disease.

CONGENITAL AND INHERITED DISORDERS

The various congenital and inherited cardiac disorders associated with cutaneous manifestations are:

Marfan's Syndrome

Marfan's syndrome, an inherited disorder of connective tissue, is caused by a mutation in the fibrillin gene, a major component of extracellular fibers. Mitral valve prolapse and aortic aneurysm occur and 90% of early deaths results from cardiovascular complications. Aortic root involvement and valvular heart disease can be diagnosed by echocardiography in these patients.

Ehlers-Danlos Syndrome

It is a heterogeneous group of inherited disorder of connective tissue, characterized by fragility of the skin and blood vessels.

Cardiac disease is limited to Types 1, 3 and 4 and can include herniation of the mitral valve leaflets.

Pseudoxanthoma Elasticum

Pseudoxanthoma elasticum (PXE) is an inherited connective tissue disorder affecting the organs with predominant elastic tissue. Patients develop angina, congenital heart failure and mitral valve prolapse. Mitral valve prolapse may be a direct expression of damage to the valve cusp by disease itself, or secondary to other cardiovascular defects causing valve dysfunction. The collagen is also abnormal. Atheromatous changes develop at an early age and aneurysm of the aorta and myocardial infraction may develop.

Fabry's Disease (Angiokeratoma corporis diffusum)

The cardiac changes in Fabry's disease include mitral valve prolapse, congestive cardiac failure, conduction defects, cardiomyopathy, myocardial infarction and cardiovascular accidents. Mitral valve prolapse has been documented in affected males and heterozygote females.

Noonan's Syndrome

This is an autosomal dominant disease with variable phenotypic expression that affects 1:1000 to 1:2500 live births. The clinical features include hypertelorism, epicanthal folds, depressed nasal root, low-set ears, a low posterior hair line, webbed neck and short stature. Ninety percent of the patients have pectus excavatum or pectus carinatum. Approximately 50% of patients have congenital cardiac abnormalities. Pulmonary valve stenosis, hypertrophic cardiomyopathy, septal defects and patent ductus arteriosus are features. Cutaneous findings include lymphedema, dystrophic nails, keloid formation and keratosis pilaris atrophicans.

LEOPARD syndrome

It is inherited as an autosomal dominant disorder. It consists of multiple lentigines, ECG abnormalities, ocular hypertelorism, pulmonary stenosis, abnormalities of genitalia, retardation of growth and sensorineural deafness. The cardiac involvement includes conduction disturbances and anatomic malformations such as hypertrophic cardiomyopathy and subaortic stenosis.

Progeria

This is a rare disorder with markedly accelerated aging. The cardiovascular changes include severe generalized atherosclerosis and fatal coronary thrombosis can occur in the childhood.

Tuberous Sclerosis

There may be cardiac hypertrophy and rhabdomyomas.

MULTISYSEM DISEASES

The various common multi-system disorders associated with cardiocutaneous manifestations are:

Behcet's Disease

Various cardiac abnormalities have been described but are rare. Pericarditis, myocarditis, coronary artery aneurysm or occlusion, conduction abnormality and aortic insufficiency have been reported. Coronary artery aneurysm and thrombotic coronary occlusion have been associated with vasculitis.

Kawasaki Disease

Kawasaki disease is an acute self-limited vasculitis of childhood that is characterized by fever, bilateral non exudative conjunctivitis, erythema of the lips and oral mucosa, changes in the extremities, rash, and cervical lymphadenopathy. Coronary artery aneurysms or ectasia develop in 15 to 25% of untreated children and may lead to ischemic heart disease or sudden death. Patients may die of myocardial infarction.

Rheumatic Fever

Erythema marginatum and subcutaneous nodules constitute the major cutaneous criteria for diagnosis of rheumatic fever.

Erythema marginatum is a transient gyrate erythema situated mainly on the trunks and proximal parts of the limbs. It may occur at any time during the course of the disease. Within hours it expands to form figurate lesions with dull red borders, which fade in 1-2 days. The lesion is not specific for rheumatic fever.

Subcutanous nodules occur around the elbow and knee joints, almost exclusively in patients with rheumatic carditis.

Subacute Bacterial Endocarditis

Petechiae are the most common mucocutaneous manifestations.

Osler's nodes, Janeway lesions, subungual splinter hemorrhage are the cutaneous manifestations of subacute bacterial endocarditis.

Osler's nodes are small exquisitely tender, red papules present on the digital tufts. Janeway lesions are faint red, macular, non-tender lesions present on the palms and soles. Both the lesions are due to immune complex deposition, but the initial event may be a micro-embolus.

Sarcoidosis

Though highest incidence occurs in the third and fourth decades, childhood sarcoidosis may also occur. Extensive pulmonary fibrosis leads to cor pulmonale while direct myocardial involvement may result in dysrhythmias, conduction disorders, heart failure or sudden death. Involvement of hilar lymph nodes, bronchi, alveoli results in obstructive or restrictive lung dysfunction.

SKIN IN THE DISEASES OF RESPIRATORY SYSTEM

Some common diseases of respiratory system and their cutaneous manifestation are enumerated below:

YELLOW NAIL SYNDROME

Yellow nail syndrome consists of a triad of yellow nails, primary lymphedema and pleural effusion. The respiratory findings in addition to pleural effusion (unilateral or bilateral) include sinusitis and bronchiectasis.

PULMONARY ARTERIOVENOUS FISTULA

This is a congenital abnormality of capillary development that may not become clinically apparent until late adolescence. Osler-Rendu-Weber disease (hereditary hemorrhagic telangiectasia), may be present in one-third to half of such patients.

CYSTIC FIBROSIS

Cystic fibrosis is an autosomal recessive disorder of the exocrine glands that subsequently involves the tracheo-bronchial tree, pancreas and gastrointestinal tract and increased amount of electrolytes in the sweat.

ATOPIC DIATHESIS

The association of atopic eczema, with asthma and hay fever form the components of atopic diathesis.

CARCINOID SYNDROME

Flushing of the skin may be associated with wheezing and dyspnea during the acute episodes.

LÖFFLER'S SYNDROME

The skin lesions of Löffler's syndrome are non-specific and highly pruritic initially, progressing to erythematous, serpiginous, tunnel-like tracts; older lesions are frequently excoriated and crusted. Patchy urticaria or erythematous papular eruptions may be present in visceral larva migrans. There will be significant peripheral esonophilia.

SARCOIDOSIS

Pulmonary involvement is the major feature in chronic sarcoidosis, about 30% of such patients also having skin lesions. Involvement of hilar lymph nodes, bronchi, alveoli results in obstructive or restrictive dysfunction.

DERMATOLOGICAL MANIFESTATIONS OF ENDOCRINE DISORDERS

INTRODUCTION

Examination of the skin can often provide valuable clues to various underlying endocrine disorders. However, some findings, such as changes in texture of skin and hair, vitiligo, hyperpigmentation, acanthosis nigricans (AN), and alopecia areata, are not uniquely related to specific hormonal abnormalities. Cutaneous features associated with hyper- or hypo-function of some of the major endocrine glands in children has been discussed in the following section. Cutaneous features of androgen excess and syndromes resulting from dysfunctions of multiple endocrine glands will be discussed separately.

DISORDERS OF THYROID GLAND

Hyperthyroidism

The causes and clinical features of hyperthyroidism in children are similar to those of adulthood.

The affected children have emotional lability, a nervous psyche, palpitation, tremor, heat intolerance, sleep disturbance and fatigue with or without exophthalmos.

Cutaneous manifestations include a warm, moist, smooth, velvety skin, with occasional hyperpigmentation of shin, feet and nails. There is marked palmo-plantar hyperhidrosis, palmar erythema and facial flushing may be present. Nail growth is rapid and several changes observed are onycholysis, Plummer's nail (distal upward curvature), koilonychia and hapalonychia (softening of nail plate).

Specific cutaneous features of hyperthyroidism include:

- Pretibial myxedema (thyroid dermopathy): Well-defined, reddish-brown, waxy and translucent papule and plaques occur classically on shin, but other body areas may also be involved. The lesions have a tumid appearance with "peau d' orange" on the surface and occasionally hypertrichosis may be present. Ophthalmopathy may be associated. The lesion occurs due to localized accumulation of acid mucopolysaccharides. Histopathologically, there is perivascular and periadnexal hyaluronic acid deposits, revealed by alcian blue/toluidine blue stain.
- Thyroid acropachy: This is rare in children. This is characterized by bony thickening involving the distal parts of the long bones of extremities along with proliferation of the overlying soft tissues. These changes are manifested clinically as widening of wrists and ankles and radiologically as subperiosteal new bone formation (fluffy/homogeneous). There is grade IV clubbing of the fingers and thyroid dermopathy and ophthalmopathy may be present.

Hyperthyroidism may be associated with generalized pruritus and autoimmune disorders like urticaria, alopecia areata and vitiligo.

Hypothyroidism

Hypothyroidism during childhood can be categorized in to two types:

- Congenital, the features of which are evident at birth. This may occur due to agenesis of the thyroid gland, enzymatic defect leading to faulty synthesis of thyroxin or due to maternal causes like presence of anti-thyroid antibody, ingestion of anti-thyroid drugs or an iodine-deficient state during pregnancy.
- Acquired, which is evident by 5-6 years of age and may result due to several causes like inborn error of thyroxin synthesis, surgical/radiotherapy induced ablation of the gland, intake of antithyroid drugs and Hashimoto's disease in older children.

In both the cases, the child is lethargic with poor food intake, constipation and a hoarse cry. The typical appearance includes a short stature, broad hands with stubby fingers, protuberant abdomen with occasional umbilical hernia, thick lips and macroglossia. Overall, the face is dull and expressionless. There is gross psychomotor delay and cold intolerance in the affected children.

Cutaneous features include dry, coarse, cool skin with a sallow complexion and puffiness of face, hands and feet due to myxedematous state. The hair is coarse and brittle with a low frontal hair line in neonates with congenital hypothyroidism. Older children may have hypertrichosis of back and shoulders and loss of hair on lateral third of eyebrows.

There may be persistent cutis marmorata in the neonatal period. Other features in such children include carotinemia, easy bruising and purpura, eruptive/tuberous xanthomas, ridged, brittle nails with markedly slow growth, delayed dentition, hypothermia and delayed tendon reflexes.

DISORDERS OF PARATHYROID GLAND

Primary parathyroid disorders are very rare in infancy and childhood. If encountered, these are usually in association with familial multiple endocrine neoplasia syndromes or chronic renal failure.

Commonest cutaneous manifestation of hyperparathyroidism is calcinosis cutis, resulting from metastatic calcification. In presence of renal insufficiency, cutaneous changes of uremia may be associated.

Cutaneous changes of congenital (idiopathic) hypoparathyroidism include altered skin texture, which is rough, thick, dry, and scaly. Scalp and eyebrow hair is thin, sparse and nails are short, thin and crumbled due to brittleness. Very rarely extensive calcification of skin and subcutaneous tissue may occur. Acquired (post-surgical) hypoparathyroidism may be associated with complete loss of hair and nails following episodes of tetany. A grayish black pigmentation may occur on face and distal extremities.

DISORDERS OF ADRENAL GLAND

Cushing's Syndrome

Cushing's syndrome may result from different causes of glucocorticoid excess including Cushing's disease and iatrogenic corticosteroid therapy.

Most notable clinical feature is the Cushingoid habitus which include alteration in body fat distribution to the central regions (truncal obesity), including the cheeks (moon facies), upper back (buffalo-hump), and supraclavicular fossae. Common cutaneous findings include facial plethora, atrophy and telangiectasia of the skin, easy bruisability and broad purplish striae occurring on the flanks, lower abdomen, upper thighs, breast, hips, and buttocks. Hirsutism and acneiform eruptions may be present. There is increased susceptibility to superficial fungal and bacterial infections and impaired wound healing.

Addison's Disease

Addison's disease is associated with adrenocortical insufficiency. The hallmark sign of Addison's disease is diffuse blue-black hyperpigmentation caused by increased melanin deposition in the skin. Hyperpigmentation is most noted in sun-exposed areas and also on the palms and soles (especially palmar creases), in the axilla and perineum, and on the nipples. Darkening of existing nevi, all mucous membranes, scars, and hair can also occur, as well as longitudinal pigmented bands on the nails. Pigmentation in the oral cavity involves gingiva, tongue, hard palate and buccal mucosa, and it is streaky. Intensity of the color in buccal mucosa and tongue may wax and wane with treatment and constitutes a sensitive indicator of the need for replacement steroids. Vitiligo occurs in 10-20% of patients with autoimmune adrenal insufficiency.

DISORDERS OF PITUITARY GLAND

Hyperpituitarism

Hypersecretion of the pituitary gland results in gigantism in children (before the epiphyseal closure) and acromegaly in adults (following epiphyseal closure). Hence, clinical features of acromegaly are not seen among children; however, children with gigantism may develop features of acromegaly during adolescence.

Growth hormone excess results in various cutaneous changes; skin is increased in area, and appears as folds on scalp and excess skin on nose and extremities, termed in general as dermatomegaly. In addition, there is increase in thickness of skin, giving a doughy consistency.

There is a gradually progressive facial coarsening with furrowing of the scalp (cutis verticis gyrata), prominent supra-orbital ridges, droopy eyelids, bulbous nose, prominent nasolabial folds, thick lips, lantern jaw and large chin. Excessive sebaceous and sweat glad activity gives rise to an oily facial skin and palmo-plantar hyperhidrosis. Occasional features include hypertrichosis and hyperpigmentation. Skin tags and acanthosis nigricans may be associated.

Hands and feet become spade-shaped with stout, square fingers and heel pad thickness increases.

Hypopituitarism

Pituitary insufficiency (Simmond's disease/Sheehan's syndrome) produce subtle cutaneous changes which include generalized pallor (combined effect of anemia, decreased cutaneous blood flow and absence of melanocyte secreting hormone) and hypotrichosis. The skin texture may be thin and smooth or coarse and dry depending upon the predominant deficiency of growth hormone or thyroid stimulating hormone (TSH) respectively. The nail growth is slow and hair shaft is thin. In adolescents, there is sparse or absent axillary/pubic hairs and micropenis in boys due to deficiency of gonadotropins.

DISORDERS ASSOCIATED WITH ANDROGEN EXCESS

Congenital Adrenal Hyperplasia (Adrenogenital syndrome)

Clinical features of congenital adrenal hyperplasia (CAH) vary with the sex of the child.

Female children are born with ambiguous genitalia (clitoromegaly, fused labia majora, common urogenital tract). Male children are born with subtle features like enlargement and hyperpigmentation of the external genitalia. There is precocious puberty in both the sexes. In childhood, accelerated bone age and rapid linear growth occurs, but there is short stature in adolescence and adulthood due to premature closure of the epiphyses. Females may develop hirsutism, acne and menstrual irregularities. In adult life disturbed reproductive function is present much more commonly among females.

The pathogenesis involves impaired peripheral synthesis of cortisol in the adrenal cortex due to congenital deficiency of enzymes like 21-hydroxylase (commonest), 11-β-hydroxylase, and 3- β-hydroxysteroid dehydrogenase. Classic 21-hydroxylase deficiency results from mutation of *CYP21* gene (6p). The pituitary stimulation of the adrenal gland remains intact with overproduction of precursor molecules which are converted to androgens. In patients with 21-hydroxylase deficiency, there is deficiency of aldosterone and features like salt-wasting (hyponatremia, hyperkalemia), hypovolemia, dehydration and failure to thrive may be associated.

Diagnosis is possible by high serum level of 17-hydroxy-progesterone, a substrate of 21-hydroxylase. Prenatal diagnosis is possible by DNA analysis of cells obtained by chorionic villus sampling or amniocentesis. Treatment includes replacement therapy with glucocorticoids and mineralocorticoid and supplementation of minerals. Reconstructive surgery for the ambiguous genitalia should be undertaken during infancy.

Polycystic Ovary Syndrome (Stein-Leventhal syndrome)

The clinical manifestations of polycystic ovary syndrome (PCOS) start during adolescence. It includes a combination of symptoms and signs like hirsutism, acne vulgris, menstrual irregularities (oligomenorrhea/amenorrhea) and obesity. Acanthosis nigricans is often found in these patients and may be present as a part of HAIR-AN syndrome. PCOS constitutes one of the most common endocrine disorders among females.

Insulin resistance is common in affected patients and they run the risk of developing Type 2 diabetes mellitus in adulthood. Diagnosis is established by ultrasonographic demonstration of enlarged, cystic ovary in combination with hormonal assays to estimate excess circulating androgen and deranged gonadotrophin secretion. Treatment of acne and hirsutism in adolescent girls is mandatory to minimize the psychological impact. However, it should always be combined with anti-androgen or other specific therapies.

CUTANEOUS MANIFESTATIONS OF DIABETES MELLITUS

Cutaneous changes are common in patients with diabetes mellitus (DM). Some of these have distinct association with DM while in some other conditions such relation is not established. Majority of these disorders occur in adulthood and associated with DM of long duration.

Necrobiosis Lipoidica Diabeticorum (NLD)

NLD is a distinctive cutaneous marker of DM, though not absolutely specific. It occurs classically on the shin of adult diabetic patients who have already developed micro-angiopathy and neuropathy. The lesion begins as asymptomatic, small, erythematous papule enlarging into an annular plaque, which then extends centrifugally and exhibits an erythematous raised border with a brown to yellow depressed atrophic center, surface telangiectasia with or without mild scaling. Lesions are usually multiple and bilateral and occur three times more commonly in females. Histopathologically, NLD is characterized by granulomatous inflammation and degenerative changes in collagen and elastic fibers associated with altered extracellular matrix deposition. Lesions are most commonly treated with potent topical steroids or intralesional corticosteroid injection.

Diabetic Dermopathy

Diabetic dermopathy (shin spots) are multiple, 0.5-1.0 cm, round or oval, dusky red to brown, indurated papules with scaling. It is found most commonly on bilateral pretibial areas. Lesions are persistent and may regress spontaneously.

Diabetic Bullae

Asymptomatic, large bullae may occur spontaneously the lower legs, feet, and hands of patients with DM. The bullae are sub-epidermal and usually heal within several weeks without significant scarring

Various other manifestations that may be associated with diabetes in children are erysipelas like erythema on legs and feet, pyoderma, generalized pruritus, skin tags, stiff joints and scleredema diabeticorum, finger pebbles on dorsal aspect of knuckles and distal finger and localized lipodystrophy in children getting insulin injections.

Acanthosis Nigricans

Acanthosis nigricans (AN) is an indicator of high risk for development of Type II diabetes mellitus **(Figures 26.1A and B).** Obesity, hyperinsulinemia and a state of insulin resistance are predisposing factors for the development of AN and obese children have more severe involvement. HAIR-AN syndrome is a combination of *H*yper*A*ndrogenism, *I*nsulin *R*esistance and *A*canthosis *N*igricans.

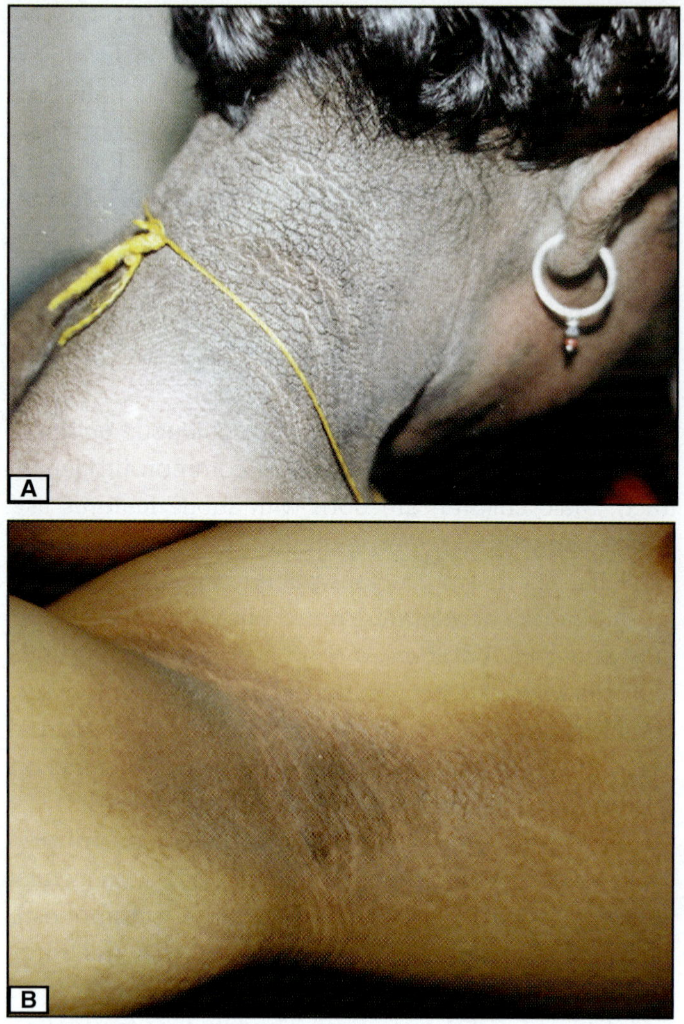

FIGURES 26.1A AND B: Childhood acanthosis nigricans

SYNDROMES ASSOCIATED WITH MULTIPLE ENDOCRINE GLAND DYSFUNCTIONS

Multiple Endocrine Neoplasia Syndromes

This is a group of autosomal dominant familial syndrome where benign or malignant neoplasia involves multiple endocrine glands (MEN syndromes). Some of these disorders are associated with cutaneous manifestations.

MEN I (Werner's syndrome): The endocrine glands involved in this disorder are adrenal, anterior pituitary, thyroid, parathyroid and endocrine pancreas. Clinical features of hyperparathyroidism and prolactinoma may be present. There may be associated carcinoid tumors (bronchial/foregut) or malignancies of parathyroid or thymus glands. The affected gene is *MEN I* located at 11q13.

Cutaneous lipomas and hamartomas-like collagenoma and facial angiofibromas are common in these patients. Facial angiofibromas appear in adulthood and may even involve the vermillion border and upper lip; otherwise, it is indistinguishable from adenoma sebaceoum of tuberous sclerosis. Collagenoma found in this disorder are discrete, small and papular. Pigmentary changes include few *café au lait* macules and multiple confetti-like hypopigmented macules.

MEN II (MEN II A/Sipple syndrome): The endocrine glands involved in this disorder are thyroid, parathyroid and adrenal glands. There is medullary thyroid carcinoma, pheochromocytoma and parathyroid hyperplasia. Lichen amyloidosis may be an associated feature in this disorder.

MEN III (MEN IIB/mucosal neuroma syndrome): Multiple mucosal neuromas are the prominent feature in this disorder, which may be present at birth or appear during childhood. The lesions occur as pinkish white translucent papules and nodules involving anterior one third of tongue, gingiva, lip (usually upper lip), nose, conjunctiva and eyelids. The lip is diffusely enlarged with a bubbled appearance. Eye lesions occur at the conjunctiva, limbus and eyelids, the later resulting in altered appearance like thickening of the eyelid margin and displacement of eyelashes. Viscera-like larynx and intestine are frequently involved and symptomatic, giving rise to diarrhea, intermittent intestinal obstruction and failure to thrive. Patients have a Marfanoid habitus.

Endocrine involvements include medullary thyroid carcinoma, pheochromocytoma and parathyroid hyperplasia. This disorder is associated with activation mutation of *RET* proto-oncogene.

Autoimmune Polyglandular Syndromes

Autoimmune polyglandular syndrome (APS) comprises of various combinations of endocrinological and non-endocrinological disorders. The most distinct clinical entity in this group is APECED syndrome (APS1), comprised of Autoimmune Polyendocrinopathy, Candidiasis, Ectodermal Dystrophy, which undergoes AR transmission.

Clinical manifestations start during childhood. The principal clinical features consist of adrenocortical failure, hypoparathyroidism and mucocutaneous candidiasis, presence of two of which is required for the diagnosis. Any of the clinical variants of oral candidiasis is present in all patients by 2 years of age and may extend to pharynx and esophagus and other areas like perineum, nail and periungual tissue may also be involved. Other associated cutaneous and systemic disorders are: alopecia areata, insulin-dependent diabetes mellitus, autoimmune thyroiditis, chronic active hepatitis and gonadal failure.

APS2 is the symptom complex resulting from adrenocortical failure, thyroiditis and diabetes mellitus and APS3 is a combination of vitiligo, alopecia areata, pernicious anemia and diabetes mellitus.

NEUROCUTANEOUS DISEASES

INTRODUCTION

The neurocutaneous diseases are genetically determined disorders having both cutaneous and neurological involvement. Since the skin and nervous system share a common embryological origin, it is not surprising that there are a large number of neurological conditions associated with cutaneous manifestations.

Advance in molecular genetics has allowed the neurocutaneous diseases to be classified according to inheritance pattern:

- Autosomal disorders **(Tables 26.3 to 26.5)**
- X-linked disorder
- Chromosomal disorders
- Lethal mutations surviving by mosaicism.

TABLE 26.3: Autosomal dominant neurocutaneous disorders
• Neurofibromatosis 1
• Neurofibromatosis 2
• Tuberous sclerosis complex
• Mucosal neuroma syndrome
• Nevoid basal cell carcinoma syndrome
• LEOPARD syndrome
• Piebald trait with neurological defects
• Waardenburg syndrome
• Noonan's syndrome (cardiofaciocutaneous syndrome)
• Osler-Weber-Rendu syndrome
• Vareigate porphyria
• KID syndrome
• Verbov Sharland syndrome
• Preaxial anonychia with neurologic defects

X-LINKED DISORDERS

Affected females with X-linked disorders have mild clinical manifestations. Some X-linked neurocutaneous diseases occur almost exclusively in girls because the underlying genes exert a lethal effect on male embryos. Rarely the male patients with gonotype XXY may show the manifestations of these disorders. **Tables 26.6 and 26.7** presents the clinical pictures of some of the disorders in this group.

LETHAL AUTOSOMAL MUTATIONS SURVIVING BY MOSAICISM

Few autosomal mutations result in early death of the embryo. However, in a mosaic state, the affected embryo can survive. Clinical features of some of these disorders are presented in **Table 26.8.**

CHROMOSOMAL DISORDERS

Common disorders in this group are Ullrich Turner syndrome, Klinefelter's syndrome and Trisomy 21, which have been detailed in 'genodermatoses section.

TABLE 26.4: Clinical features of some disorders following autosomal dominant inheritance pattern

Disorder	Cutaneous anomalies	Neurologic anomalies	Other anomalies
Nevoid basal cell carcinoma syndrome	Multiple basal cell carcinoma Plantar and palmar pits Milia Epidermoid cysts	Intracerebral calcification Hydrocephalus Agenesis of corpous callosum Medulloblastoma Mild mental deficiency	Jaw cysts Hypertelorism Bone anomalies (spine,ribs,fingers) Ovarian fibromas
LEOPARD Syndrome (Lentiginosis, ECG abnormalities, Ocular hypertelorism, Pulmonic stenosis, Abnormal genitalia, Retardation of growth, sesorineural Deafness)	Generalized lentigenes	Disturbed EEG wave activity Diffuse encephalopathy Deafness Mild mental retardation	Genital hypoplasis Cardiac defects Ocular hypertelorism Pulmonic stenosis Retardation of growth
Piebald trait with neurologic defects	Patchy leukoderma White forelock	Defective motor coordination Cerebellar ataxia Mental retardation Hearing loss	
Waardenburg syndrome	Patchy leukoderma White forelock Synophrys	Neurosensory hearing loss	
Noonan syndrome (Cardiofaciocutaneous syndrome)	Curly or woolly hair Multiple melanocytic naevi Keratosis pilaris Lymphedema	Mild mental retardation	
Osler-Weber-Rendu syndrome	Multiple vascular dilatations	Vascular lesions of the brain or the spinal cord Cerebral abscess	

PSYCHOCUTANEOUS DISORDERS IN CHILDREN

INTRODUCTION

The relation between the skin, the nervous system and the psyche is intimate. The nervous tissue and a considerable part of the skin share a common embryonic origin; the ectoderm. Psychological problems related to a child's medical condition can have long-term implications in the form of social development, stress management, treatment of these problems may even be more important for children than it is for adults.

Dermatological disorders in relation with psychological, psychosocial and sometimes psychiatric factors are as follows:

1. Multifactorial dermatological disorders that can be substantially influenced by psychological factors, e.g. psoriasis, vitiligo, etc.
2. Dermatologic disorders resulting from psychiatric illness, e.g. factitious dermatoses, body dysmorphic disorder.
3. Psychiatric illness developing as a result of skin disease, e.g. reactive depression, adjustment disorders.
4. Comorbidity with other psychiatric disorders, e.g. alcoholism.

In this section the disorders relevant to pediatric age group will be discussed. The first three groups are important in respect to pediatric population.

It has been estimated that the effective management of at least one third of patients attending skin department

TABLE 26.5: Clinical features of some disorders with autosomal recessive inheritance pattern

Condition	Cutaneous anomaly	Neurological anomaly
Neutral storage disease	Congenital ichthyotic erythroderma Mild ichthyosis with fine scaling	Muscular weakness Ataxia Neurosensory hearing loss Nystagmus
Refsum's disease	Mild ichthyosis Accentuated palmar creases Yellowish hue of melanocytic nevi	Neurologic anomalies Anosmia Neurosensory hearing loss Peripheral neuropathy Cerebellar ataxia intention tremor
Sjogren-Larsson syndrome	Ichthyosis with areas of lichenification	Pathologic reflexes Muscular hypertonia Spastic paraplegia Mental retardation
Multiple sulfatase deficiency	Mild ichthyosis	Severe psychomotor retardation Metachromatic leukodystrophy
Tay syndrome (IBIDS syndrome)	Congenital ichthyosis Sulfur deficient brittle hair Dysplastic nails Hypoplasia of subcutaneous tissue	Mental retardation Microcephaly Intracerebral calcifications Mild hearing loss Spasticity Ataxia Hemiparesis
Brittle hair syndrome (BIDS syndrome)	Hair trichothiodystrophy	Mental retardation Ataxia Intention tremors
Bjornstad syndrome	Pili torti	Neurosensory deafness
Shapira syndrome	Sparse, brittle, light colored hair	Developmental delay Short stature Ataxia Unsteady gait
Elejalde syndrome	Silvery hair showing irregular distribution of melanin clumps Peculiar bronze-colored skin	Hypotonia Hemiplegia Ataxia Severe mental retardation Nystagmus Blindness
Cross syndrome	Silvery hair Generalized hypopigmentation	Microcephaly Mental retardation Spasticity Ataxia Cerebellar hypoplasia
Xeroderma pigmentosum	Photosensitivity Diffuse freckled hyper and hypopigmentation Multiple skin cancers	Mental retardation Microcephaly Cortical atrophy Ventricular dilatation
Hartnup disease	Increased photosensitivity Pellagroid skin changes	Progressive cerebellar ataxia

TABLE 26.6: Clinical features of some disorders following X-linked inheritance pattern (male lethal)

Disorder	Cutaneous anomalies	Neurologic anomalies
Focal dermal hypoplasia	Linear and patchy lesions of dermal hypoplasia Herniation of fatty tissue Poikiloderma Periorificial papillomas	Mild mental retardation Meningomyelocele Hydrocephalus Defects of optic nerve
Incontinentia pigmenti It is caused by NEMO gene mutations	Linear lesions of inflammation resulting in pigmentary disturbance	Psychomotor retardation Microcephaly Seizures Spasticity Cerebellar ataxia
CHILD syndrome (congenital hemidysplasia with ichthyosiform naevus with limb defects)	CHILD nevus	Hypoplasia of ipsilateral hemisphere Hypoplasia of cranial nerves Defects of spinal cord Reduced sensation to touch and heat
MIDAS syndrome (microphthalmia, dermal aplasia, and sclerocornea)	Linear lesions of dermal aplasia involving mainly the face and neck	Microcephaly Focal dysplasia of brain Agenesis of corpus callosum
OFD 1 syndrome	Linear or patchy areas of hairlessness Multiple facial milia	Porencephaly Partial agenesis of corpous callosum Hydrocephalus Mental retardation

TABLE 26.7: Clinical features of some disorders following X-linked inheritance pattern (non-lethal variants)

Disorders	Cutaneous anomalies	Neurologic anomalies
Parington 2 syndrome	Generalized reticular hypopigmentation in men Linear skin lesions in women	Seizures Hemiplegia
Menkes disease	Brittle hair showing characteristic kinking Light skin complexion	Mental retardation Seizures Hypothermia
Bullous dystrophy of Mendes de Costa type	Generalized macular hyper- and hypo-pigmentation Total hair loss	Microcephaly Mental retardation
Albinism-Deafness syndrome	Pigmentary disorders of the piebald type	Neurosensory deafness
Lesch-Nyhan syndrome	Severe lesions of self mutilation mainly on the lips and the fingers	Delayed motor development Choreoathetosis
Adenoleukodystrophy	Cutaneous anomalies Bronze-discoloration of skin Diminished hair growth	Spastic paresis Sensory disturbances Urinary incontinence

TABLE 26.8: Clinical features of some disorders where lethal autosomal mutations occur (surviving by mosaicism)

Disorder	Cutaneous anomalies	Neurologic anomalies
Sturge-Weber-Klippel-Trenaunay syndrome The syndrome is characterized by a rather too often bilateral involvement.	Telangiectatic nevi showing lateralization	Leptomeningeal angiomatosis Spinal angiomatosis Seizures Hemiplegia
Encephalocraniocutaneous lipomatosis	Hairless fatty tissue nevus of the scalp	Multiple intracranial lipomas Porencephaly Vascular dysplasia Mental retardation Seizures
Speckled lentiginous nevus syndrome	Speckled lentiginous nevus of a papular type	Segmental dysesthesia Hyperhidrosis Muscular weakness
Nevus comedonicus syndrome This syndrome is characterized by nevus comedonicus in combination with ipsilateral cataract and skeletal defects.	Nevus comedonicus	EEG abnormalities
Neurocutaneous melanosis	Giant melanocytic nevus	Leptomeningeal melanocytosis

depends upon the recognition and treatment of emotional factors. While in disorders like dermatitis artefacta the influence is primary and pathogenic, the relationship between mind and skin are more complex, e.g. the intractability of atopic dermatitis may be a response to an impaired parent-child relationship. There are evidence based studies showing that stressed patients with psoriasis have longer disease duration and counseling can be effective in reducing disease severity in these patients. Disfiguring skin lesions (e.g. intractable atopic eczema, psoriatic lesions on face and port-wine stains) may profoundly influence the emotional development of a child which is also affected by the attitude of the parents and later of teachers. With the approach of puberty, a disfiguring skin disease (acne vulgaris) becomes a cause for increasing anxiety in many teenagers and may hinder them in developing easy relationships with the opposite sex.

There are chemical mediators which translate an emotion to a cutaneous lesion. These are neurotransmitters and hormones that can be produced directly in skin by nerve fibers or other cells such as keratinocytes, Langerhans cells and perhaps Merkel cells. These include neuropeptides, substance P, substance Y, vasoactive intestinal peptide (VIP), calcitonin gene-related peptide, MSH and these entire bind to cell surface receptors.

PSYCHOLOGICAL IMPORTANCE OF SKIN

Newborn babies require the stimulus of stroking and caressing which favors emotional development. Massaged babies gain weight as much as 50% faster than unmassaged babies. Swaddling clothes provide an environment of warmth, touch and decreased stress as demonstrated by reduced heart rate, better feeding and longer sleep patterns in neonates. Children who live in emotionally destructive homes may show growth arrest as a response to the withdrawal of love and touch. Many of the alternative medical therapies such as aromatherapy and kinesthesiology show clinical effects related to the measurable effects of touch. Furthermore, patients who are regularly touched by their carers show quicker improvement than those who do not and these effects are measurable at all ages.

A classification of psycho-cutaneous disorders with an emphasis on usefulness for dermatologists has been presented in **Table 26.9.**

DERMATOLOGICAL DELUSIONAL SYMPTOMS

A delusion is a disorder of the content of thinking. Delusions are beliefs that are not true to fact and cannot be corrected to by an appeal to reason of the individual.

TABLE 26.9: Classification of psycho-cutaneous disorders

Category	Specific disorder
Delusional beliefs of skin	Parasitosis Smell Impregnation and contamination
Disorders of body image	Body dysmorphic disorder (dysmorphophobia) Atypical pain disorders such as glossodynia and essential vulvodynia. Dermatological hypochondriasis Anorexia nervosa.
Phobic states	Venereophobia and AIDS phobia Mole phobia Wart phobia Erythrophobia
Obsessive compulsive disorder	Hand washing
Group and mass population reactions	Sick building syndrome Epidemic hysteria
Dermatoses primarily factitious in origin	Dermatitis artefacta Artefact by proxy Witchcraft syndrome Dermatological pathomimicry Dermatitis simulate Malingering Compensation neurosis Münchausen's syndrome Münchausen's syndrome by proxy Deliberate self-cutting Self-mutilation Religious stigmata and psychogenic purpura
Dermatoses aggravated by harmful habits and compulsions	Lichen simplex Neurotic excoriation Prurigo nodularis Acne excoriee Hair plucking Trichotillomania Trichophagia Nail destruction Onychotillomania Lip-lick cheilitis Knuckle biting Disorder of neglect of self-care (syn. Diogenes syndrome)
Dermatoses caused by accentuated physiological responses	Hyperhidrosis Blushing
Dermatoses in which emotional precipitating or perpetuating factors may be important	Vesicular eczema of the palms and soles Atopic dermatitis in the adult Seborrheic dermatitis Psoriasis Some cases of localized or generalized pruritus Alopecia areata Aphthosis Rosacea Chronic urticaria

DELUSIONS OF PARASITOSIS

The patient with delusions of parasitosis has an unshakable conviction that his or her skin is infested by parasites which must be differentiated from parasitophobia—the fear of becoming infested. Delusions of parasitosis in adolescents should be regarded with utmost concern as it may be a feature of drug abuse (amphetamine or cocaine) or may be a part of delusion shared with another member of a family (folie a deux).

Delusions of perception may follow diseases in the non-dominant hemisphere and so delusions of parasitosis is sometimes seen in patients after a cerebrovascular accident involving that side of the brain.

BODY DYSMORPHIC DISORDER (DYSMORPHOPHOBIA, DERMATOLOGICAL NON-DISEASE)

This term is used to describe patients rich in symptoms but poor in signs of organic skin disease. The dermatological non-disease was originally thought to be uncommon, but screening over the last decade has revealed a prevalence of 12%.

Some children may be examples of monosymptomatic hypochondriacal psychosis in that they have an isolated delusion. They socialize poorly and do not like contact with other people. The disorder most often comorbid with dysmorphophobia is major depression (60-80%). An obsessional premorbid personality can be found in few patients and comorbidity with obsessional compulsive disorder may be seen in up to 30%. Dysmorphophobic symptoms in a teenager or adult may be the presentation of schizophrenia. Comorbid psychiatric conditions include social phobia, trichotillomania, substance abuse, avoidant personality disorder and anorexia.

Uncommonly, the delusional type of body dysmorphic disorder (BDD) runs in a family where the parents imposes a delusional idea upon the child who in turn develops the idea that his/her child has a bodily defect (BDD by proxy). There is a definite risk of suicide in patients with BDD. Most patients with dysmorphophobia perceive the solution to their problems in dermatological or plastic-surgical terms.

ANOREXIA NERVOSA AND BULIMIA

Anorexia nervosa is a phobia about body weight. It may be associated with other psychodermatoses, BDD and self-injurious behaviors. Skin manifestations includes xerosis, hair effluvium, brittle nails, cheilitis, diffuse hypertrichosis, poor wound healing, etc. These are common in restrictive type of anorexia nervosa as opposed to bulimic type where hair and nail changes are prominent.

EPIDEMIC HYSTERIA SYNDROME

Common closed community, like school-children may show epidemic complaints of itchy dry skin and transient rash. In some studies these outbreaks involved 50-100 children aged 7-12 years with symptoms lasting two weeks where no cause could be found. Girls outnumbered boys (3:1). It has been suggested that the precipitating factors may be illness of a favorite teacher or student, rigid teaching regimens and parental pressure for academic success.

SELF-INFLICTED AND SIMULATED SKIN DISEASE

Lichen Simplex

This is very rarely an isolated disorder in children. It results from constant rubbing or scratching. Aggression and hostility related to anxiety caused by emotional disturbance may lead to scratching. This can be treated successfully with behavior therapy to break the itch-scratch cycle.

Acne Excoriée

Brocq in 1891 described acne excoriee in adolescent girls under emotional stress, who picked and squeezed acne lesions. Excoriations can be found predominantly around the hair line, forehead, pre-auricular cheek and chin. Chronic lesions show white atrophic scarring with surrounding hyper pigmentation. Patients sometimes respond to simple topical acne therapy, most require systemic antibiotics and isotretinoin. These patients tend to be psychologically dependent, and the benefits of simple supportive consultation and psychotherapy should not be underestimated.

Trichotillomania

Trichotillomania is defined as the irresistible urge to pull out hair, accompanied by a sense of relief after it has been plucked.

There are two distinct age groups; the majority present during childhood and the fewer chronic cases are probably the continuation of childhood or adolescence-onset disease. It occurs more frequently in females but below the age of 6 years boys outnumber girls. It is more severe in females.

The early onset group (2-10 years), show a benign self-limiting course and probably most of them suffer from a habit disorder. The association with nail biting, thumb sucking, skin picking, nose picking, lip biting and cheek chewing is well documented. In children there are associations with anxiety and dysthymia, learning disability and iron deficiency.

Clinical features*:* The revised DSM-IV-R diagnostic criteria for trichotillomania are:

- Recurrent pulling out of one's own hair resulting in hair loss.
- An increasing sense of tension immediately before pulling out the hair or when attempting to resist the behavior.
- Pleasure, gratification or relief following pulling out of the hair.
- The disturbance is not better accounted for by another mental disorder. The disturbance provokes clinically marked distress and/or impairment in occupational, social or other areas of functioning.

The hair pulling is usually not a response to any skin symptoms but is either a conscious deliberate act, or more often, a subconscious act in some children being part of hypnogogic state. Some patients may have incomplete awareness until the pattern is established. Most patients pull hair from the vertex, but temporal, occipital and frontal hair loss in children may be more obvious on the side of manual dominance. The hair loss may be minimal, commonly a solitary patch but visible hair thinning may progress to virtual total depilation, significantly so in adult women. Typically the hairs are short, irregular, broken and distorted. The hair feels like stubble because of fractured hair shafts, in contrast to alopecia areata which is much smoother. The eyelashes, eyebrows, facial and pubic hair may also be affected.

Trichotillomania may be associated with hair licking, chewing and eating (trichophagia). Patients may swallow long strands of hair with a small percentage developing gastro-intestinal bezoars. There should be high index of suspicion in children with trichotillomania who present with abdominal pain, weight loss, nausea, vomiting, anorexia and foul breath. Gastric trichobezoars may cause intestinal bleeding, pancreatitis, obstructive jaundice and life-threatening intestinal obstruction (Rapunzel syndrome) necessitating a laparotomy.

Trichotillomania can be easily differentiated from alopecia areata and tinea capitis clinically. In tinea capitis the texture of the infected hairs is abnormal and the scalp surface may be scaly.

Treatment*:* Usually support from the treating dermatologist is sufficient; behavior therapy and habit reversal are also helpful. The diagnosis is often unacceptable to the parents who have not observed the child pulling the hair and find it difficult to believe that the problem is self-inflicted. Drug treatments include tricyclic antidepressants and SSRIs like fluoxetine. Other drugs include citalopram and pimozide.

Onychotillomania and Onychophagia

Compulsive habits of nail picking and nail biting are common in children and adolescents. Etiological factors include stress, imitation of family members and exchange of thumb sucking habit. Nail biting is usually confined to the finger nails but nail picking, especially in adults, may involve all digits. Damage to cuticles and nails causes paronychia nail dystrophy and longitudinal melanonychia. In chronic cases trichotillomania may be associated.

Onychotillomania is often denied by the patient but some admit the habit. Most commonly it is a compulsive action at the time of stress. Successful response to treatment has been shown with clomipramine and pimozide.

Factitious Skin Disease

Factitious behavior cannot be defined easily as the level of intention is variable. The DSM-IV-TR criteria for factitious disorder include:

- Intentional feigning of physical or psychological signs or symptoms.
- The motivation is to assume the sick role.
- External incentives for the behavior are absent (e.g. economic gain, avoiding legal responsibility or improving physical well-being, as in malingering).

Dermatitis Artefacta

It is an artefactual skin disease caused entirely by the actions of the fully aware patient on the skin, hair, nails or mucosae. These patients conceal the responsibility of their actions from the doctors. Children beyond the age of 8 years may be affected. The ratio of female to male varies from 4:1 to 20:1. In half of the subjects, the lesions are on the face, particularly in children. In many cases, the psycho-social stress of a major life event may be apparent. Children and adolescents commonly show anxiety and immaturity of coping styles in response to a dysfunctional parent-child relationship, bullying, physical body changes or sexual and substance abuse.

The characteristic of dermatitis artefacta is the vague history. The patient describes the sudden appearance of lesions with little or no prodrome. Lesions appear at the same stage of development in crops or groups, either symmetrically or scattered apparently at random. There is lack of history of significant progression of lesions from an initial lesion to its fully developed state. The most common site of involvement is the face, dorsa of the hands, forearms and most frequently the non-dominant hand. Crude destructive processes are the result of thermal, chemical or instrumental injury. Excoriations, punched out necrotic areas, blisters can be seen. Children produce purpura on the chin by sucking on cups and limbs by direct mouth suction. There may be unexpected complications to the artefactual damage leading to severe infections such as cerebral abscess which may be life threatening.

Factitious Cheilitis

There is persistent and often gross crusting and scaling of the lips, which follows continued biting, picking or licking in emotionally immature or disturbed patients of both sexes.

Nail Artefact

Chronic paronychia caused by the insertion of nails, pins or splinters has been recorded in children. The characteristic lesions show purpura and hemorrhage around the nail fold but subungual hemorrhage and pustules may also be seen.

TREATMENT

First treat the cutaneous damage by topical/systemic antibiotics and anti-inflammatories.

Later there is a need to identify the nature and extent of the psychological problem. Direct confrontation with the patients should be avoided, but usually it is possible to infer that his or her activities are known but are regarded with understanding and sympathy. However, chronic persistent self damage is predictive of long term emotional illness and referral to a child psychiatrist is imperative.

Münchausen's Syndrome by Proxy

Here the illness in a child is fabricated by the parents (usually the mother), or someone in the loco parentis which may include health professionals. The victims have a persistent or recurrent illness that cannot be readily explained. The diagnosis remains descriptive. Symptoms do not respond to treatment and laboratory tests are incongruous. Rarely, the parents exhibits the syndrome themselves and produce proxy lesions on the child.

The victims are usually infants or toddlers with a mean age of 40 months at diagnosis. The most common presentation in one series was bleeding, CNS depressions, apnea, diarrhea, vomiting, fever, and skin rash. The long-term consequences of childhood victimization might contribute to the development of factitious disease in adult life.

Hyperhidrosis

States of fear, rage and tension can induce an increase of sweat secretion. Perspiration in the human has two distinct forms: thermal and emotional.Under conditions of prolonged emotional stress, excessive sweating or hyperhidrosis may lead to secondary skin changes, rashes, blisters, and infections; therefore, it may underlie a number of other dermatological conditions that are not primarily related to emotions.

Psychogenic Pruritus

The affected patients present with intractable or persistent itch for which no pruritic physical illness or dermatological illness can be found. In some individuals intense scratching can induce an ultimate feeling of pleasure which may be related to release of opioids in the CNS.

Most dermatological disorders have a psychosomatic or somatopsychic component. A combination of sympathetic approach to the patient and family, psychotropic drugs, hypnosis, bio-feed techniques, behavioral therapy, group therapy can be used in clinical practice.

CUTANEOUS MANIFESTATIONS OF INTERNAL MALIGNANCIES

INTRODUCTION

Cutaneous manifestations of internal malignancies can be grouped into the following categories:

1. Direct tumor spread
2. Genetically determined syndromes with cutaneous manifestations, where there is increased predisposition to develop internal malignancy
3. Cutaneous markers of exposure to carcinogens
4. Paraneoplastic syndromes
5. Non-specific lesions.

DIRECT TUMOR INVOLVEMENT OF THE SKIN

In the pediatric age group, skin involvement from visceral tumors is uncommon.

However, cutaneous involvement from lymphoma and leukemia may be seen, the lesions presenting as solitary or multiple nodules.

GENETICALLY DETERMINED SYNDROMES WITH INCREASED PREDISPOSITION TO MALIGNANCY

a. Muir-Torre syndrome: The essential features are sebaceous tumors of the skin, with or without keratoacanthomas, in association with more than one visceral nedoplasm.
b. Gardner's syndrome: Intestinal polyposis, with a high rate of malignant transformation, epidermoid cysts of the face, scalp and trunk, osteomas of the maxilla, mandible, and cranial bones, fibromas, desmoids and other tumors of the skin and subcutaneous tissue are the clinical features
c. Cowden syndrome: The distinctive cutaneous lesions are multiple trichilemmomas grouped around the mouth, nose and ears. Other cutaneous lesions are lipoma, hemangioma, neuroma, vitiligo and xanthoma. Juvenile xanthogranuloma can be associated with café-au-lait macules and acromelanosis. There is a great risk of patients developing breast and thyroid carcinomas.
d. Basal cell nevus syndrome: It comprises of multiple basal cell carcinomas, jaw cysts, palmo-plantar pits, skeletal abnormalities and a tendency of malignant disease. The most common malignant tumor is medulloblastoma.
e. Mucosal neuroma syndrome: A probable variant of MEN-2A, Sipple's syndrome, whose features are oral, nasal, upper gastrointestinal tract and conjunctival neuromas associated with medullary carcinoma of thyroid and pheochromocytoma. The neuromas are typically soft to firm intradermal nodules.

CUTANEOUS MARKERS OF EXPOSURE TO CARCINOGENS

Chronic arsenic toxicity can be manifested by arsenical melanosis, plantar and palmar keratosis, and Bowen's disease. There is also an increased risk of internal neoplasia including tumors of the urogenital region, mouth, esophagus and lung.

NON-SPECIFIC LESIONS

The manifestations can be grouped according to the characteristics of the manifestations in the following groups.

Lesions Secondary to the Deposition of Substances in the Skin

a. Icterus: A late manifestation of internal malignancy occurring secondary to obstruction of the bile duct or gross intrahepatic obstruction.
b. Melanosis: Caused by abnormal deposition of melanin pigments in skin. A mild darkening of the skin may be seen with ACTH producing tumors and diffuse melanosis can be secondary to malignant melanoma.
c. Xanthoma: Plane xanthoma may be the predominant feature of juvenile chronic myeloid leukemia.

Vascular and Hematological Abnormalities

a. Flushing: Pronounced flushing with wheezing and abdominal pain may be a manifestation of carcinoid tumors.
b. Palmar erythema: It is an associated feature with hepatic failure which may be secondary to either a primary or a metastatic tumor.
c. Telangiectasia: Telangiectatic vessels may be the first evidence of skin metastases of many cancers. Genaralized telangiectasia can be a presenting factor of malignant angioendotheliomatosis and progressive telangiectasia have been associated with carcinoid tumors.

d. Purpura: Lymphoma is the most common cause of purpura associated with malignant disease.
e. Vasculitis: Leukocytoclastic vasculitis can be associated with malignant neoplasms as renal carcinoma, leukemia and lymphoma.
f. Cutaneous ischemia: Peripheral ischemia has been associated with many malignant neoplasms, including carcinoma of stomach, small bowel and kidney as well as lymphoma and leukemia.

Bullous Disorders

a. Pemphigus: There is a well-defined association of pemphigus vulgaris with thymoma. Paraneoplastic pemphigus described in association with lymphoma, thymoma, Waldenstrom's macroglobulinemia, sarcoma which has a very poor prognosis.
b. Cicatrical pemphigoid: Antiepiligrin cicatrical pemphgoid has an increased risk of occurrence in solid tumors.
c. Linear IgA dermatosis: Reported in association with lymphoma, myeloma, chronic lymphocytic leukemia, carcinoma of the bladder and esophagus.

Infections and Infestations

a. Herpes zoster: Patients with leukemia and lymphoma have an increased risk of herpes zoster, but occurs late in the course of the disease. Segmental herpes zoster also can occur after radiation therapy. Disseminated herpes zoster is commonly associated with underlying malignant disease.
b. Demodex folliculitis: A particular association has been identified with Demodex folliculitis in children with acute lymphoblastic leukemia on maintenance chemotherapy.
c. Other infections and infestations: Bacterial, fungal, yeast and severe scabies are common in immuno-compromised conditions as in advanced malignancies.
d. Pruritus: When it occurs with malignant disease, pruritus is most commonly associated with lymphoma and leukemia.
e. Clubbing: Is usually associated with neoplasms of the chest, especially, bronchogenic carcinoma. It may also be seen in diffuse intestinal lymphoma.

Collagen Vascular Disease

a. Dermatomyositis: Though adults with dermatomyositis need to be examined thoroughly for evidence of an associated malignancy, in children dermatomyositis is not significantly linked to malignancy.
b. Lupus erythematosus: Only rarely associated with lymphoma or thymoma.
c. Scleroderma: Systemic sclerosis is rarely associated with internal malignancy.

CUTANEOUS PARANEOPLASTIC SYNDROMES

Changes of the skin can be a marker for an internal malignancy, however, the relationship of the marker with the malignancy is variable. These markers can be grouped according to the major clinical manifestation. These are specific when rare and the tumor is also very uncommon but the problem arises when the marker is a common dermatosis as seborrheic keratosis in Leser-Trelat sign.

Some cutaneous manifestations of the cancers are paraneoplastic syndromes, i.e. dermatoses secondary to the cancer. To qualify as a true paraneoplastic syndrome two essential criteria are to be fulfilled:

- The dermatosis must only develop after the development of the malignant tumor
- Both the dermatosis and the malignant tumor follow a parallel course; complete removal of the cancer results in clearing of the dermatosis and recurrence of the cancer causes relapse of the dermatosis.

Some of the paraneoplastic markers are as follows:

a. Acanthosis nigricans: The malignant variant which is of sudden onset and has a rapid progression is usually secondary to adenocarcinoma, ususlly intra-abdominal, commonly gastric.
b. Acquired ichthyosis: Though it is a late manifestation of lymphoma, it may precede the diagnosis by several years.
c. Palmar hyperkeratosis: There are two groups of patients with palmar hyperkeratosis and associated malignant tumors:
   - Diffuse palmar hyperkeratosis
   - Punctuate palmar hyperkeratosis.

   Diffuse variety is also known as tylosis and is a manifestation of esophageal carcinoma but needs to be differentiated from the childhood variant which has uniform thickness associated with benign conditions. Punctate variety is associated with increased risk for cancer of the breast and uterus.

d. Tripe palms: A rugose thickening of the palms that is strongly associated with visceral cancer.
e. Multiple eruptive seborrheic keratosis- Also known as the sign of Leser-Trelat. It is a regular feature in association with multiple internal malignancies
f. Erythema gyratum repens: It is a cutaneous eruption consisting of concentric raised erythematous bands moving in waves over the body surface in a wood-grain pattern. Found in association with tumors of the lung, bladder, cervix, stomach and esophagus.
g. Sweet syndrome: Most commonly seen with acute myelocytic leukemia, myelo dysplastic syndrome, multiple myeloma and lymphoma.
h. Conditions related to release of hormone: Skin conditions resulting from the hormones released by the metastatic tumors into the systemic circulation. Hirsutism may result from excessive androgen release by gonadal or adrenal tumors. Hypertrichosis lanuginose acquisita may occur secondary to internal malignancy. Gynecomastia in the males can be produced by excess of androgens secreted by tumors of the testis.

PURPURA FULMINANS

DEFINITION

Purpura fulminans (PF) is a acute onset, rapidly fatal severe reaction characterized by large ecchymotic patches mainly involving extremities occurring commonly in children usually following an infectious disease. It is a life-threatening disorder characterized by cutaneous hemorrhage and necrosis, hypotension, fever and disseminated intravascular coagulation

ETIOLOGY

It is characteristically associated with meningococcal septicemia and may occur as a sequel to a number of other infections, such as streptococcal infections, varicella, and measles. Asplenic patients and patients with meningococcal meningitis are at special risk for developing PF. In the neonate, its occurrence is suggestive of protein C deficiency.

PATHOPHYSIOLOGY

Associated with Infections

The Gram-negative diplococcus *Neisseria meningitidis* is a major infective cause for precipitating PF. In meningococcemia, a severe bleeding tendency often simultaneously exists with severe thrombosis in the microvasculature of the skin, often in a glove-and-stocking distribution that may necessitate amputation of digits or limbs. Meningococcal infection affects the following three main pathways of coagulation:

- Endothelial injury results in platelet-release reactions. Along with stagnant circulation due to local vasoconstriction, platelet plugs form to start the process of intravascular thrombosis. In the plasma, soluble coagulation factors are consumed, and the natural inhibitors of coagulation (e.g. tissue factor pathway inhibitor antithrombin III) are down-regulated; this process further encourages thrombosis .
- The protein C pathway is thought to be crucial in the development of purpura fulminans. A similar rash is seen in neonates with congenital protein C deficiency and in older children who develop antibodies to protein S after varicella infection. Protein C and S levels are low in children with meningococcal disease, but similar levels exist in patients with septic shock, whether or not a severe rash develops. The inability to activate protein C in the microvasculature because of endothelial down-regulation of thrombomodulin or associated cell-surface proteins appears to play a role.
- The fibrinolytic system is also down-regulated in meningococcal disease, reducing plasmin generation and removing an aspect of endogenous negative feedback to clot formation. In addition, plasminogen activator inhibitor levels are dramatically increased, further reducing the efficacy of endogenous tissue plasminogen activator.

Protein C Deficiency

In the rare inherited homozygous or compound heterozygous state, protein C deficiency is associated with severe life-threatening neonatal purpura fulminans or massive venous thrombosis.

Protein C is a 62-kD glycoprotein, synthesized in the liver as a zymogen, which circulates in the blood at a concentration of 4 mcg/ml. Activation of protein C requires conversion of the single-chain zymogen into a 2-chain serine-protease–like enzyme required for catalytic activity. Physiologically, this activation occurs on phospholipid cell surfaces by the action of thrombin when bound to the endothelial cell proteoglycan, thrombomodulin. Once activated, activated protein C (APC) binds to the cell-

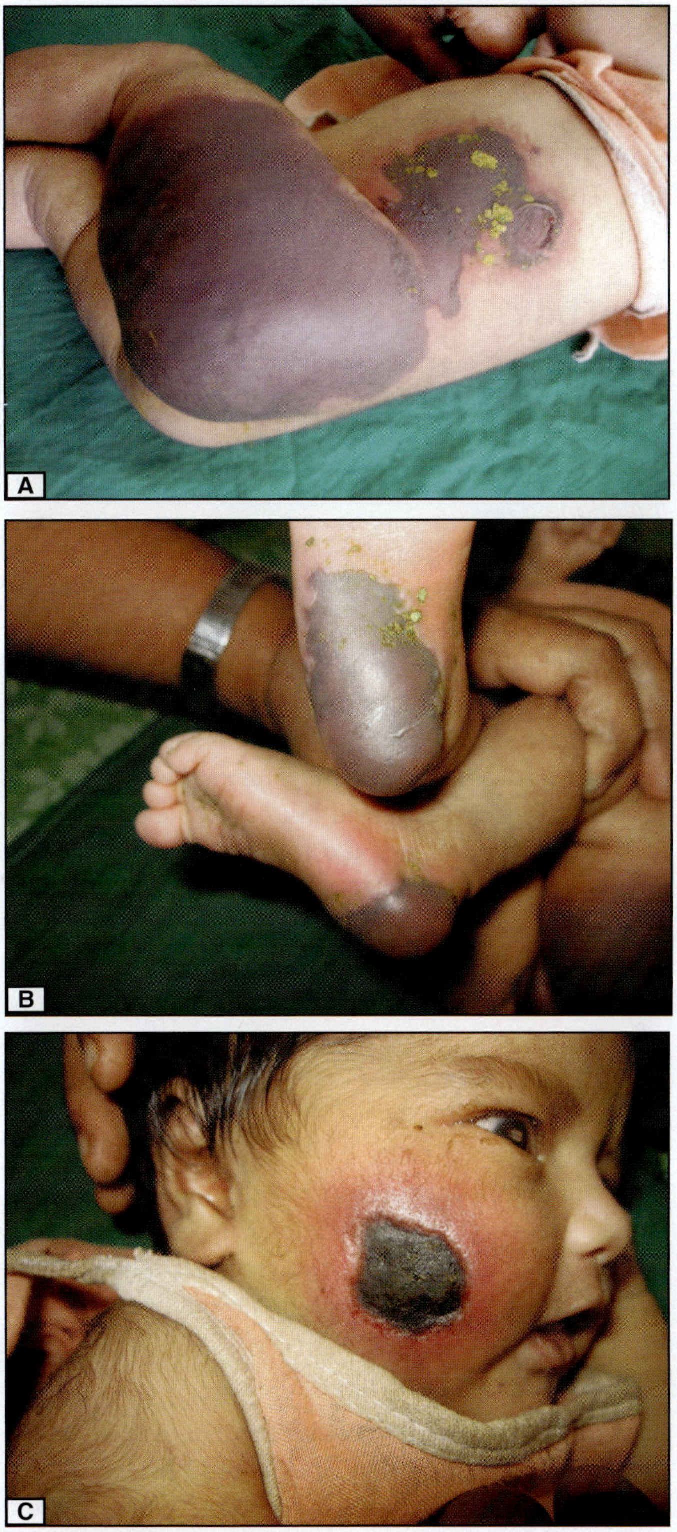

FIGURES 26.2A TO C: Purpura fulminans

surface–bound anticoagulant cofactor, protein S. The APC/protein S complex then proteolyses activated procoagulant cofactors factor VIII and factor V, thereby retarding fibrin formation by preventing activation of procoagulant proteins, factor X and prothrombin. Histopathology shows platelet thrombi occluding blood vessels, with non-inflammatory necrosis.

CLINICAL FEATURES

Lesions are characterized by the development of more or less symmetrical and well-defined lakes of confluent ecchymosis without petechiae, mainly on limbs, trunk and face.

The onset is sudden, and the lesions enlarge rapidly, with coalescence and often with the development of hemorrhagic bullae with central necrosis. There is a surrounding erythema and the lesions are tender **(Figures 26.2A to C)**. Acral cyanosis may be noted in the presence of large arterial pulses. The patient is frequently febrile. Vascular thrombosis is a particular feature of this disorder. There is a substantial danger of internal hemorrhage, shock and death.

TREATMENT

Heparin 50 to 100 mg/kg as bolus dose followed by 10 to 15 mg/kg/hour was the treatment of choice earlier. The dose has to be titrated in such way that clotting time remains between 25 to 30 minutes and the treatment may be continued up to 5 weeks. Currently, the treatment of choice is rapid transfusion of fresh frozen plasma. Hyperbaric oxygen may be used to save the gangrenous part.

COURSE AND PROGNOSIS

The lesions are rapidly progressive with severe systemic toxicities. Even with excellent care mortality is high.

SYSTEMIC AMYLOIDOSIS

INTRODUCTION

Amyloidosis is the term used for a group of diseases where one or more body organs accumulate various insoluble proteins (amyloid) in amounts to cause dysfunction of the organ system. Organs often affected include the heart, kidney, gastrointestinal tract, nervous system and skin. Amyloidosis of the skin is called cutaneous amyloidosis. In this condition, amyloid-like proteins are deposited in the dermis layer of skin which are characterized by the extracellular deposition of several unrelated proteins that exhibit similar histological, immunofluorescence, and ultrastructural features.

Amyloid deposits contain (in addition to the fibrillar component) a nonfibrillar protein referred to as amyloid-P (Am-P). This protein is identical to normal plasma globulin, known as serum amyloid-P (SAP). Am-P constitutes 14% of the dry weight of amyloid. This protein is also found in the microfibrillar sheath of elastic fibers. SAP is closely related to the acute phase reactant C-reactive protein (CRP) and has been shown to be an elastase inhibitor. SAP and the beta-pleated sheet configurations are thought to protect amyloid deposits from degradation and phagocytosis, leading to persistence of the deposits.

Systemic amyloidosis is rare in children. Primary, secondary and heredo-familial forms may occur.

PRIMARY SYSTEMIC AMYLOIDOSIS

This variant is exceedingly rare in children. Amyloid deposition occurs in various organs like kidney, liver, heart and spleen. Mucocutaneous lesions may occur in 30-40% patients and include macroglossia, periorbital waxy papules and plaques with ecchymosis and pinch purpura. Rarely bullous lesions may be seen. Rectal biopsy is diagnostic.

SECONDARY SYSTEMIC AMYLOIDOSIS

This occurs as a complication of many chronic inflammatory diseases such as rheumatoid arthritis, osteomyelitis, cystic fibrosis and cutaneous diseases like epidermolysis bullosa. It is also known as amyloid A (AA) amyloidosis and is the commoner form of systemic amyloidosis. In developed countries, juvenile rheumatoid arthritis (JRA) is the commonest cause of secondary systemic amyloidosis in children and 50% of the patients with JRA die as a result of renal amyloidosis. The kidney, liver and spleen are the organs affected. Cutaneous involvement is rare and clinical features are similar to the primary form of the disease. Muckle-Wells syndrome is an autosomal dominant disorder where chronic, recurrent episodes of urticaria start during adolescence, followed by progressive deafness and amyloid nephropathy in adult life.

HEREDO-FAMILIAL SYSTEMIC AMYLOIDOSIS

In this rare form of systemic amyloidosis, neuropathy starts during adolescence and patients present with painless ulcers, atrophic scars and sclerodermatous skin changes.

SARCOIDOSIS

Sarcoidosis is a granulomatous disorder involving viscera or skin. In children two different forms of sarcoidosis are seen. The first is early-onset starting before the age of 4yrs. The other form occurs in late childhood and more closely resembles adult-onset sarcoidosis.

ETIOLOGY

Sarcoidosis is a disease of unknown etiology. Two main postulations regarding pathogenesis are infections and genetic and familial factors

Infections

Many infectious agents have been implicated in the pathogenesis of sarcoidosis but culture and response to antimicrobial agents has always been negative. It may be possible that disease may represent an unusual host response to one or more infectious agents. Serological studies have shown that patients with sarcoidosis have raised levels of antibodies to *M. paratuberculosis*. A recent study has reported that acid fast cell wall deficient form of *M. tuberculosis* was grown from blood of patients with active sarcoidosis.

Genetic and Familial Factors

Familial sarcoidosis is well recognized. In ethnic groups known to have a high prevalence of sarcoidosis, the probability that an index case will have a sibling with sarcoidosis is about 10%. Family aggregates of the disorder occur either on genetic basis or require a common environmental exposure during childhood. In certain populations sarcoidosis is commoner in persons with HLA BW-15 and HLA DRB1. HLA type can influence the pattern of the disease rather than occurrence.

EPIDEMIOLOGY

Sarcoidosis has a world-wide distribution and affects all races and ethnic groups. It primarily affects adults between 20-40 years of age, but may also affect children. Childhood sarcoidosis is a rare disease with an estimated incidence of 0.22-0.27/100 000 in one study. Most children manifest during early second decade of life, commonest age being between 13-15 years. However, an apparently distinct form of sarcoidosis affects children under the age of 4 years. In the United States, the disease is 2-10 times more common in Hispanic and black children than it is in white children. However, affected children under the age of 4 years are more commonly white.

Skin involvement is seen in about 77% of younger children (<4 yrs) and 24-40% of older children. There are a few reports of isolated cutaneous sarcoidosis in children. Some patients have isolated musculo-cutaneous involvement.

IMMUNOLOGY

The factors which trigger the granulomatous immune response in patients with sarcoidosis is not clear. These granulomas often undergo spontaneous resolution over months to years, but may also lead to scarring and functional impairment of vital organs.

Patients with sarcoidosis display a combination of depressed cell-mediated immunity and increased humoral immune response. The circulating T lymphocytes are usually decreased and B-lymphocytes may be normal or increased. The granulomas are T-lymphocyte related. Patients are usually anergic to skin test antigens. This deficiency of delayed hypersensitivity is persistent and often does not change when patients improve clinically. Serum immunoglobulin levels may be normal but IgG is elevated in about half of the patients. Serum complement, reflecting an acute phase reaction, may be increased.

HISTOPATHOLOGY

All affected organs have the similar histopathological features i.e, aggregates of epithelioid cells with pale staining nuclei forming discrete sarcoid granulomas.

Granulomas are surrounded by an inconstant and variable rim of lymphocytes (naked granuloma). Caseation is typically absent but fibrinoid necrosis may be seen at the center. In cutaneous sarcoidosis the granulomas are present in the deeper dermis and are less well defined in the erythrodermic disease. Epidermal changes include hyperkeratosis, parakeratosis, acanthosis, atrophy and spongiosis. Lichenoid reaction may also be seen at times. Two types of inclusion bodies are found in giant cells of sarcoid granulomas. These are Schaumann bodies and asteroid bodies and are not specific for the disorder but can be correlated with the chronicity of the disease.

CLINICAL FEATURES

Table 26.10 presents the predominant clinical features of both the categories of childhood sarcoidosis.

TABLE 26.10: Comparative features of sarcoidosis in children

Feature	< 4 years (%)	>4 years (%)
Skin involvement	80	40
Eye involvement	60	45
Arthritis	55	5
Bone lesions	50	20
Lymphadenopathy	40	45
Fever	35	24
Weight loss	32	18
Lung involvement	22	17

Cutaneous lesions occur in 10 to 100% of cases and are of two types: specific and non-specific. Specific lesions include angio-lupoid lesions, nodule, plaque, lupus pernio, nail deformities and psoriasiform lesions. Nonspecific lesions are rare in children.

SPECIFIC LESIONS

Maculopapular Form

It is uncommon and usually observed in prodromal stage of the disease as transient, ill-defined, yellowish maculo-papular rashes. Slight scaling is occasionally present.

Nodular Form

Usually single or countable lesions are present. Nodules are soft/firm, round, well circumscribed red or yellowish initially and later become violaceous or purplish brown. In the process of healing the lesions develop central depression and later replaced by telangiectatic marks or yellowish fibrotic and atrophic patches.

Papular Form

The lesions are painless, well defined papules measuring 1 to 5 mm occurring mainly over the face and extensor extremities. Lesions are orange to yellow initially and later change to brownish red and heal with a pale, yellowish white telangiectatic scar. Occasionally the lesions become confluent evolving into an erythematous plaque. This form of sarcoidosis has a better prognosis.

Angio-lupoid Form

This is a rare but characteristic form. Generally one or two soft hemispherical lesions with livid hue are seen, most often on the side of nasal bridge. Other less common sites include cheek and inner edge of eyebrow. Spontaneous resolution occurs less frequently.

Annular Form

This is mainly found in chronic stage and shows central clearing. Lesions are found usually on forehead, face and neck. Central area may be depigmented and scarred.

Erythema Nodosum

Erythema Nodosum may be present in 16 to 30% of patients with sarcoidosis. Lesions are tender nodules on extremities.

Lupus Pernio

This appears as a relatively common skin manifestation. It generally affects older patients. Lesions are large bluish red to dusky or violaceous, infiltrated soft doughy nodules and plaques, distributed symmetrically over nose, cheeks, ears, fingers, hands and toes. The skin over the lesion is stretched with enlargement of pilosebaceous follicles. Ulceration occurs rarely. Turkey ears (enlargement of involved ear lobe) are seldom seen. Nasal involvement is associated with swelling, ulceration and crusting of nasal vestibule and patient may present with breathing problems. Lupus pernio may be associated with chronic visceral sarcoidosis.

UNUSUAL AND ATYPICAL FORMS

Unusual and atypical forms of cutaneous lesions include the following:

- Alopecia of skin and shin
- Atrophic form (localized to legs or generalized)
- Erythrodermic form
- Hyper or hypopigmentation around central indurated lesion
- Ichthyosiform
- Lichenoid form
- Psoriasiform
- Verrucous form
- Cutaneous calcinosis.

Nail Changes

Nail changes are rare and not seen in children. These include pitting, cracking, longitudinal ridging, thickening, fragility, opacity and loss of nail plate. These may be associated with sarcoid dactylitis, cystic bone changes of phalanges and lupus pernio.

Mucosal Involvement

Oral mucosa is not commonly involved but nasal mucosal involvement is often seen in lupus pernio. Diffuse pale yellow plaques, nodules or ulceration of palate, buccal mucosa and pharynx are seen.

Eyes

Ocular involvement is extremely common in children (50%). Uveitis is the commonest manifestation and develops with acute pain in the eyes with misty vision in one third of patients while others develop the chronic form. Anterior uveitis is common in self limiting sarcoidosis whereas posterior uveitis is more often associated with chronic disease. Other ophthalmic manifestations include iridocyclitis, retinochoroiditis, iris nodules, phlyctenular conjunctivitis and keratoconjunctivitis sicca. Marked visual impairment occurs in few children.

Uveo-parotid Fever

This is characterized by febrile illness and triad of uveitis, parotid enlargement and facial palsy. This is quite rare in children.

Skeletal System

Osseous involvement is also rare in children. When present however, the metacarpals, metatarsals, and phalanges are the bones most frequently affected. Joints show symmetrical boggy synovitis without much pain and limitation of movements. Radiological findings are usually negative. Joint involvement may lead to contractures.

Pulmonary Involvement

Pulmonary involvement is the earliest and most frequently observed manifestation in adults but also occurs in most children with this disorder. Symptoms referable to the lungs are usually mild and often consist of a dry hacking cough, with or without mild to moderate dyspnoea. The X-ray Chest shows enlarged lymph nodes and small round opacities. "Staging" or identifying the degree of lung involvement can help to determine the progress of the sarcoidosis. A scale of 0-3 is commonly used with Stage 3 having the highest amount of lung involvement. In a few cases, only the X-ray Chest is needed to make the diagnosis.

Systemic Sarcoidosis is Classified in to Four Stages

Stage 0—Normal chest X-ray (5-10%)
Stage 1—B/L hilar lymphadenpathy (35-45%)
Stage 2—Stage 1 with parenchymal lung involvement of fluffy or coarse type
Stage 3—Chronic stage with fibrosis and pulmonary insufficiency

DIAGNOSIS

Only after the common causes of granulomas are ruled out, the diagnosis of sarcoidosis is made. An evaluation to detect sarcoidosis should include the following:

Histopathological examination of the skin lesions is confirmatory. Sometimes the diagnosis is made by obtaining tissue samples from the lung, liver, or enlarged lymph nodes.

Thorough clinical examination of all patients is to be carried out to screen for other organ involvement. Other investigations include estimation of serum angiotensin converting enzyme (ACE) level and serum and urinary calcium level. Imaging techniques like CT scan and gallium scan reduces the need of invasive visceral biopsy.

TREATMENT

Fifty to 75% of the patients diagnosed with sarcoidosis improve without treatment. Those with persistent disease should be treated with anti-inflammatory drugs, to which some may respond.

Topical Therapy

For isolated cutaneous lesions like lupus pernio and plaque sarcoidosis, high potency topical steroids or intralesional steroids may be used. Tacrolimus, which inhibits hapten induced production of Th1 cytokines and TNFα by T cells, has been recently reported to be beneficial when used topically in cutaneous sarcoidosis.

Systemic Therapy

In presence of widespread organ involvement, systemic therapy is indicated. Different systemic treatment modalities include corticosteroids, antimalarials, methotrexate, cyclophosphamide and azathioprine. When required, corticosteroids and antimalarials are the mainstay of systemic therapy in children.

Other drugs under study for use in treating sarcoidosis are etanercept, infliximab, pentoxyphylline and thalidomide.

COURSE

The natural course of sarcoidosis in childhood is insidious and often regresses completely after many years. Mortality is reported to be 5 percent and tuberculosis has been estimated to occur in 10 percent of children with sarcoidosis.

BEHCET'S DISEASE

Behcet's disease is a complex multisystem inflammatory disorder of unknown etiology. It is predominantly characterized by recurrent oral and genital aphthae associated with relapsing uveitis or iritis, cutaneous lesions, arthritis and rarely genital and neurological manifestations.

First description of this disorder was probably given by Hippocrates. The disease is named after the Turkish dermatologist Hulusi Behcet, who in 1937 described patients with recurrent oro-genital ulcerations and uveitis.

EPIDEMIOLOGY

Behcet's disease occurs predominantly in young adults and is uncommon in children, who account for 5% of all cases. There is no sex predilection at this age group. There appears to be significant familial aggregation. A survey among Israeli children revealed the mean age of diagnosis to be 10.7 years and the initial symptom of all patients was recurrent ulcerative stomatitis.

ETIOLOGY AND PATHOGENESIS

The exact cause of Behcet's disease still remains unknown. An association with HLA- B5 and HLA-B51 has been established. Three hypotheses have been proposed regarding pathogenesis; viral, autoimmune and defective fibrinolytic activity. The possibility of antibody mediated immune response in the pathogenesis had surfaced after a few cases of transient neonatal Behcet's disease in offsprings of mothers with Behcet's disease have been described, suggesting that an antibody –mediated immune process may have a role in this disorder. The basic pathology underlying the disease is a vasculitis of small and medium sized arteries with cellular infiltrations leading to fibrinoid necrosis and narrowing and obliteration of the vascular lumens.

CLINICAL FEATURES

Oral and genital aphthae are the most common (60%) presenting features and are essential for the diagnosis of Behcet's disease.

The oral ulcerations begin as vesicles or pustules, may occur anywhere on the oral mucosa, and present as superficial erosions indistinguishable from apthous stomatitis or it may present as deeply punched out necrotic ulcers. These tend to appear in crops and are characterized by superficial grayish erosions that vary in size from a few millimeters to a centimeter in diameter. The ulcer base is covered with a yellowish grey exudates and the margin is surrounded by a red halo. The aphthous lesions whether in the mouth or genitalia, persist for 7-14 days and usually heal without scarring. They recur at irregular intervals varying from weeks to months. Deep crateriform necrotic ulcerations with raised margins called 'periadenitis mucosa necrotica recurrens (Sutton's disease)', are distinctive, usually very painful, and frequently heal with scarring.

Cutaneous lesions are variable. Seen in approximately 70% of patients, these consist of lesions simulating erythema nodosum, sweet's syndrome and pyoderma gangrenosum. Other lesions include pseudofolliculitis, acneiform lesions, pustular vasculitic lesions (including pathergy lesions) and palpable purpura. Cutaneous pathergy occurs as erythematous sterile pustule after 24-48 hours at a needle prick site.

Ocular manifestations including anterior or posterior uveitis and retinal vasculitis are less common in children but more severe than adults and may progress to blindness. Intense periorbital pain and photophobia are associated.

Musculoskeletal involvement includes acute onset, migratory, asymmetrical, non erosive oligo- arthritis. Large joints are mainly involved.

Neurological manifestations are present in fewer than 25% of patients. Though there are wide array of neurological manifestations as cerebral venous sinus thrombosis, benign intracranial hypertension, cranial nerve palsies, brain stem lesions, pyramidal or extra pyramidal lesions and psychosis, only meningo-encephalitis is considered to be a diagnostic criteria. These occur later in the course of the disease (generally an average of two to five years after the disease-onset) and indicate a poor prognosis.

Behcet's disease affects the systemic blood vessels, leading to aneurysms, arterial occlusions, venous occlusions and varices that can be fatal. The principal features of pulmonary involvement are pulmonary artery aneurysms with fatal outcomes. Involvement of the heart may lead to myocarditis, coronary arteritis, endocarditis and valvular disease.

The renal involvement vary from minimal change disease to proliferative glomerulonephritis and rapidly progressive crescentric glomerulonephritis.

HISTOPATHOLOGY

Histopathological examination of early aphthae or lesions of pustular vasculitis showed leukocytoclastic or a neutrophilic vascular reaction; however the late lesions showed mainly a lymphocytic reaction.

DIAGNOSIS

Recurrent and extensive oral aphthosis should raise the suspicion of the disease. In absence of pathognomonic laboratory test or histopathologic findings, clinical criteria are used. Patients must have oral aphthae plus at least two of the following clinical features:

- Genital aphthae,
- Synovitis,
- Posterior uveitis,
- Cutaneous pustular vasculitis
- Meningoencephalitis.

An international study group was formed with an objective to obtain an agreed set of diagnostic criteria for Behcet's disease as presented in **Table 26.11**.

DIFFERENTIAL DIAGNOSIS

Patients with complex aphthosis have recurrent oral and genital aphthae but have no other features of Behcet's disease.

Reiter's disease is characterized by an axial erosive arthritis and by psoriasiform muco cutaneous lesions but there is conspicuous absence of aphthae and pustular vasculitis.

Patients with inflammatory bowel disease have an increased incidence of oral aphthae and have a

TABLE 26.11: Diagnostic criteria for Behcet's disease

Criteria	Clinical feature	Characteristics
Major	Recurrent oral aphthae	Minor aphthous or herpetiform ulceration observed by physician or patient that recurred at least 3 times in a 12 month period.
Plus two of the following minor criteria	Recurrent genital ulceration	Aphthous ulceration or scarring observed by physician or patient.
	Eye Lesions	Anterior uveitis, posterior uveitis, cells in vitreous on slit lamp examination or retinal vasculitis observed by ophthalmologist.
	Skin Lesions	Erythema nodosum observed by physician or patient, pseudo folliculitis or papulo pustular lesions, acneiform nodules observed physician in post adolescent patients not on corticosteroid treatment
	Positive Pathergy Test	Read by physician after 24 hours

'Dermatosis – Arthritis syndrome' mimicking Behcet's Disease but eye involvement is generally absent.

Patients with isolated pustular vasculitis alone may have gonococcal or meningococcal sepsis or it may occur as an idiopathic syndrome.

TREATMENT

A wide array of therapeutic agents has been used for Behcet's disease, including systemic steroids, colchicine, chlorambucil, azathioprine, cyclosporine and thalidomide. Clinical indications of different drugs have been presented in **Table 26.12**.

Colchicine shows higher efficacy in children than in adults, especially for oral ulcers, skin rash, joint symptoms and occasionally eye disease. A placebo controlled study of 96 patients with Behcet's disease showed that thalidomide is effective for treating the oral and genital ulcers and follicular lesions of Behcet's disease. Uveitis, epidydimitis and arthritis may not respond to thalidomide. Recently anti-TNF antibody infliximab has been used with successful outcomes.

TABLE 26.12: Summary of treatment in Behcet's disease

Condition	Therapeutic agent
Palliative treatment of aphthae	Topical corticosteroids Intralesional corticosteroids Topical tacrolimus Topical viscous lidocaine
Mucocutaneous manifestations	Colchicine Dapsone Dapsone and colchicine
Systemic involvement	Systemic corticosteroids Immunosuppressive for most severe disease: • Azathioprine • Methotrexate • Ciclosporine

COURSE AND PROGNOSIS

Behcet's disease has a highly variable clinical course. Mucocutaneous and arthritic manifestations are the first to occur. Ophthalmic involvement is the leading cause of morbidity. Central nervous system, pulmonary and large vessel involvement as well as bowel perforation are the major life threatening complications.

Markers of poor prognosis are

- HLA-B51 positivity,
- Male gender
- Early development of systemic features.

Early onset of clinical features in childhood does not tantamount to poor prognosis. Spontaneous remissions occurs in certain or all manifestations of Behcet's disease.

GRAFT-VERSUS-HOST DISEASE

Dermatologists play an important role in the evaluation and management of patients at risk for or diagnosed with graft *vs.* host disease (GVHD). Of all organ dysfunctions associated with GVHD, the skin serves as the earliest and the most frequent target.

DEFINITION

GVHD develops when immunocompetent lymphoid cells, which are histoincompatible, are administered to an immunodeficient patient.

If the recipient is normal, donor lymphocytes would be destroyed, but if the recipient is immunodeficient, these proliferate and attack the host tissue producing a reaction involving skin, gastrointestinal tract and liver.

Prerequisites for GVHD to occur are:
- Graft should be immunocompetent
- Host should be immunodeficient
- Difference in histocompatibility is present.

Clinical manifestations, histopathology, pathogenesis and treatment of GVHD with emphasis on the skin manifestations are considered in the following section.

GVHD can be classified into acute and chronic:
Acute: Develops between 1 week to 3 months after transplantation
Chronic: Appears after 3 months of transplantation.

Clinical settings in which GVHD can occur:
- Allogenic marrow transplant
- Maternal fetal transfer of lymphocytes
- Blood transfusion
- Solid organ transplant, usually liver

ACUTE GVHD

Acute GVHD develops in 20-80% of patients, usually 10-30 days after bone marrow transfusion.

Clinical Features

The eruption usually begins with faint erythematous macules, usually on the palms, soles and pinna, but may occur on any skin surface. Edema and tenderness often accompanies the erythema regardless of cause. As GVHD evolves, the erythematous macules increase in size and distribution, and become confluent commonly over the upper back. Erythroderma may ensue. Development of bullae indicates poor prognosis. Bullae are usually subepidermal with necrotic roof. This progression usually takes over several weeks. An explosive variant has also been described, in which erythroderma develops rapidly and then evolves into lichen planus like eruption resembling chronic disease. **Tables 26.13 and 26.14** presents clinical staging and grading of the disease, respectively.

Prognostic Factors

1. Extent of skin involvement
2. Total bilirubin value
3. Stool output/day

Resolution occurs in the same pattern as its appearance. It resolves with desquamation and leaves behind a brown–grey discoloration of the skin .Significant blister formation results in widespread denudation with exposed dermis, placing the patient at greater risk of sepsis and fluid and electrolyte imbalance.

Pathogenesis

In acute GVHD, it is believed that preparative regimen before the infusion of the graft causes extensive tissue

TABLE 26.13: Clinical staging of GVHD

Stage	Skin; MP rash	Liver; Bilirubin	GIT; loose stools
+	<25% of BSA	2-3mg/dl	>500 ml/day
++	>25%-50% of BSA	3-6mg/dl	>1000 ml/day
+++	Generalized erythroderma	6-15mg/dl	>1500 ml/day
++++	Generalized erythroderma with bulla formation	>15mg/dl	Severe abdominal pain with or without paralytic ileus

TABLE 26.14: GVHD grading

GVHD grade	Skin stage	Liver	Intestinal Tract	Clinical response
I	+ to ++	0	0	None
II	+ to +++	+	+	Mild
III	++ to +++	++ to ++++	++ to +++	Marked
IV	++ to ++++	++ to ++++	++ to ++++	Extreme

damage, which releases inflammatory cytokines and expose recipient major histocompatibility complex antigens (MHC).Recognition of the host antigen by donor T cells, and activation and proliferation of them is crucial in the initial phase. The greater the disparity between donor and the recipient MHC, the higher is the T cell response. Infiltration of both CD4+ and CD8+ T cells or with either one of them predominating has been reported. B cells are not found. The inflammatory cytokines (interleukins, GM-CSF, TNF-α, IFN) are produced by activated T cells and by tissue damage during the preparative regimen. It activates mononuclear phagocytes and natural killer cells. Both apoptosis and perforin /granzyme-dependent killing are important in GVHD-induced damage. In skin, young rete ridge keratinocyte, follicular stem cells, and Langerhans cells are preferred targets. However, the exact mechanisms by which the skin, liver, and GIT are targeted are not clear. Expression of the cutaneous lymphocyte antigen by lymphocytes returning to the peripheral circulation after marrow transplant would explain homing to the skin.

Histopathology

The early changes in acute phase consist of focal basal vacuolation, superficial perivascular lymphocytic infiltrate with exocytosis of individual cells into the epidermis and follicular epithelium. The number of lymphocytes correlates positively with the probability of developing more severe acute GVHD.

Histologic grading scheme for the acute cutaneous GVHD

Grade	Description
0	Normal skin or changes not referable to GVHD
1	Basal cell vacuolization of the dermo-epidermal junction
2	Basal cell vacuolization, necrotic epidermal cells, lymphocytes in the dermis and/or epidermis
3	Subepidermal cleft formation plus grade 2 changes
4	Separation of epidermis from dermis plus grade 2 changes/ complete loss of epidermis

Minimal Criteria for the Diagnosis

- Infiltrate of lymphocytes in the dermis
- Basal cell vacuolar alteration
- Necrosis of epidermal cells at a frequency of at least 4/linear millimetre of epidermis

In grade 2, satellite cell necrosis is seen, which is described as direct apposition of a lymphocyte to a necrotic keratinocyte.

In accordance with the clinical observation that the acute cutaneous GVHD begins around the hair follicle, early histopathologic changes also begin in a perifollicular array. At the follicular epithelium, evidence of interface changes is observed with necrosis of follicular keratinocyte and extension of lymphocytes into the follicular epithelium. In association with the perivascular infiltrate, there is marked endothelial swelling and narrowing of the vascular lumen.

Diagnosis

Diagnosis of acute cutaneous GVHD rests on the combination of clinical findings, including the onset of variably distributed erythematous macules and papules at the time of peripheral lymphocyte recovery, and a minimum of grade 2 histopatholgic changes.

CHRONIC CUTANEOUS GVHD

Chronic GVHD presents between 3 to 14 months post hematopoietic stem cell transplant in approximately 20% of matched sibling transplants and 40% of matched unrelated donor recipients.

Chronic GVHD is divided into lichenoid and sclerodermoid forms. The lichenoid phase develops earlier than the sclerodermoid phase. Some patients may have both forms at the same time. Prior acute GVHD is the greatest predictor. The lichenoid form resembles lichen planus, with erythematous to violaceous polygonal papules, distributed over the flexors. Wart like lesions has also been described. Patients have typical oral involvement which resolves with postinflammatory pigmentation. The sclerodermoid form resembles scleroderma. Patients have thickened skin plaques, which are shiny, erythematous and atrophic with progressive loss of pilosebaceous unit. Some patients may go on to develop joint contractures, chronic cutaneous ischemia and erosions. Fascitis can occur. Sicca syndrome due to diminished lacrimal and salivary output is known to occur. Bacterial skin infections are quite common.

The two forms of the disease overlap in many patients.

Pathogenesis

Improper regulation of autoreactive elements of the immune system is proposed as an explanation for the development of different phases of cutaneous GVHD. Strong evidence links transforming growth factor beta to the development of skin and visceral changes in sclerodermoid GVHD with neutralizing antibodies capable of reversing the fibrosis in a mouse model. Cutaneous fibroblasts in sclerodermatous skin express MHC class II and make abnormally large amounts of type I collagen.

Histopathology

Overall picture resembles lichen planus with hyperkeratosis, hypergranulosis, acanthosis, apoptotic keratinocytes and a mononuclear cell infiltrate immediately below the epidermis with pigmentary incontinence. A rare manifestation is the 'columnar epidermal necrosis', characterized by small foci of total epidermal necrosis accompanied by a lichenoid tissue reaction.

In the late sclerodermoid phase, the epidermis is atrophic, with the keratinocytes being small, flattened and hyper pigmented. Basal layer vacuolization, inflammation and colloid body formation is rare or absent. Dermis is thickened, with sclerosis extending into subcutaneous tissue resulting in septal hyalinization. The adnexal structures are destroyed. Subepidermal bullae may be present.

Treatment

Treatment of established GVHD is difficult; hence success of bone marrow transplantation depends on prevention of GVHD. Prophylactic regimes include use of cyclosporine or tacrolimus with methotrexate and lymphocyte depletion using alemtuzumab, a humanized monoclonal antibody directed against lymphocyte CD52 antigen. A new approach in the prevention of acute GVHD involves use of genetically manipulated donor T cells expressing the herpes simplex virus thymidine kinase suicide gene.

Systemic steroids remain the standard therapy for acute GVHD.

When the condition worsens, patients may require secondary therapy with mycophenolate mofetil, sirolimus or monoclonal antibodies against cytokines or their receptors (infliximab, basiliximab, daclizumab, visilizumab and ABX-CBL). Tolerance induction agents such as cytotoxic T lymphocyte antigen (CTLA)-4 Ig and anti CD-40 ligand can also be used. Pentostatin may also be helpful. IL-18 has the capacity to modulate acute GVHD when administered to either the donor or to the recipient.

Therapy directed specifically at the skin includes topical glucocorticoids and UV radiation. Psoralen plus UVA (PUVA) produces clinical improvement in the cutaneous features of GVHD. Extracorporeal photopheresis has reported benefit in some acute phases, including steroid refractory GVHD, possibly by promoting a shift from a Th1 to Th2 lymphocyte distribution.

For chronic GVHD, oral immunosuppressives like steroids, cyclosporine and azathioprine are used in varying combinations. Thalidomide has received renewed interest as an immunomodulating agent due to its ability to ameliorate chronic GVHD.

The dermatologist is involved in treating chronic cutaneous infections, manifestations of lichenoid disease and sclerodermoid disease. Intermittent cultures for bacteria and fungi should be undertaken. For the lichenoid lesions, PUVA treatment is quite effective.

Etretinate has been tried in sclerodermoid phase. Halofuginone, an inhibitor of collagen type I synthesis, has been reported as beneficial.

PRURITUS IN CHILDREN

The word pruritus comes from latin word prurire which means to itch. Itching or pruritus is a predominant symptom of inflammatory skin disease.

Itch is an unpleasant sensation in the skin that provokes a desire to scratch.

Various peripheral mediators of itch are histamine, histamine liberators like morphine and codeine, serotonin, prostaglandins, platelet activating factor, kallikrein, interleukin 2, proteases, substance ρ, calcitonin gene related peptides, β-endorphins, leu enkephalin and met enkephalin.

Itching is almost universal in all dermatological as well as in some systemic disorders. Adult individuals can ignore the sensation, while it may be disturbing to the children. While more than one visit may be needed to identify the cause of pruritus, common conditions eventually respond to specific agents.

ETIOLOGY

While establishing the cause of a pruritic eruption in a child, the steps to follow are; identifying the primary lesion, recognizing the pattern of involvement, the location of the eruptions, and any secondary lesions. **Table 26.15**

TABLE 26.15: Common causes of pruritus in children

Pruritus associated with dermatoses	Scabies Dermatitis (endogenous & exogenous) Eczematised molluscum contagiosum Papular urticaria Urticaria Insect bites
Pruritus associated with systemic disorders	Cholestasis Chronic renal failure
Hematological disorders	Polycythemia vera Iron deficiency anemia Leukemias Lymphomas Plasma cell dyscrasias Mastocytosis (Urticaria pigmentosa)
Parasitosis*	Ankylostomiasis Ascariasis Trichinosis Giardiasis Weil's disease Onchocerciasis Gnathostomiasis
Neurological disorders**	Multiple Sclerosis Tumors Abscesses Neurofibromatosis
Endocrine disorders	Hyperparathyroidism Hypothyroidism Diabetes Mellitus Sipple's syndrome Carcinoid syndrome

*Mechanism is thought to be due to allergic sensitization of the host to the parasite. Treating the cause relieves pruritus.
** Can present with diffuse itching

shows the common conditions leading to pruritus in children.

Dermatological disorders giving rise to pruritus will be detailed in the respective sections. Characteristic clinical features of individual conditions clinch the diagnosis.

Scabies

The classic presentation of scabies includes small, symmetrical, pruritic, erythematous papules involving the hands (particularly the finger-web spaces), flexural aspects of wrists, anterior axillary folds, buttocks, and genitalia). Scalp, face and palms and soles are involved in infants. Pruritic, excoriated, penile papules in children are almost always scabetic in origin and may be the sole evidence of the disease. Diffuse excoriation and eczematization, sometimes with secondary infection may obscure the classic features of scabies. Nocturnal pruritus and history of involvement of other family members or playmates are characteristic. The classic burrow—a short, linear, and sometimes wavy lesion may be present on occasions.

The definitive diagnosis includes demonstration of burrows and microscopic identification of the mite, eggs, or feces. This is not an easy method and not always practical. Several lesions may have to be firmly scraped to get positive identification.

Treatment includes specific anti-scabies agents, topical and/or systemic. All family members and close contacts, whether symptomatic or not, should be treated.

Atopic Dermatitis

It is a highly pruritic skin condition that affects more than 10% of children. The patients have inherently dry skin.

Classically, the infants present with recurrent episodes of eczema on face, trunk and extensor extremities. In later childhood, the pattern is more flexural, involving antecubital and popliteal fossae and flexural aspects of the wrists. Pruritus is always worse at night. In atopics, a mere touch with clothings may cause a persistent itching, termed as 'alloknesis'. Family history of cutaneous atopy, asthma, and hay fever are common.

Management protocol of such children includes general measures like skin hydration, emollients, and therapy with mild to moderate topical steroids, topical calcineurin inhibitors and sedative antihistamines.

Papular Urticaria

Recurrent episodes of symmetrically distributed, erythematous papules with a central punctum are present predominantly over exposed body parts. These are caused by the bites of insects such as mosquitoes, fleas, and bed bugs and may be frequent in rainy season. Pruritus may be significant, especially at night and repeated scratching may produce thickened cutaneous nodules. Bed-bug bites may be localized and linear,referred to as the *breakfast-lunch-supper* pattern. Management includes protection from insects by use of nets or repellants, topical corticosteroids, and oral antihistamines.

PRURITUS DUE TO CHOLESTASIS

Intense generalized itching may occur in patients with cholestasis due to conjugated hyperbilirubinemia irrespective of the degree of hyperbilirubinemia. It may result from intra or extrahepatic cholestasis. Symptomatic relief of the pruritus may occur following administration of various therapeutic agents including bile acid binding agents such as cholestyramine, cholerectic agents such as phenobarbitone or ursodeoxycholic acid. Other agents used with variable success are opioid antagonists, antihistamines and antibiotics such as rifampicin. Surgical diversion of bile via a procedure called partial external biliary diversion has provided relief for medically refractory pruritus.

PRURITUS DUE TO CHRONIC RENAL FAILURE

Itching can occur in chronic renal failure, more so in patients on dialysis. Various probable mechanisms include xerosis, secondary hyperparathyroidism, metastatic calcification, cutaneous mast cell proliferation, deficient sweating, increased endogenous vitamin A and opioids and cutaneous nerve proliferation. Renal transplantation is thought to be the definitive therapy. UVB phototherapy, oral cholestyramine, oral charcoal and emollients have been tried.

PRURITUS DUE TO HEMATOLOGICAL DISORDERS

In childhood, lymphoma and leukemias may be associated with generalized pruritus. There is no primary cutaneous change, but excoriation marks may be observed. Patients with iron deficiency anemia may present with generalized pruritus and often respond to oral ferrous sulfate. Systemic mastocytosis may be the cause of itching without any skin lesions.

ANOGENITAL PRURITUS

Anogenital pruritus is usually multifactorial. In children, enterobiasis has to be ruled out. Mostly patients have perianal or perineal itching, especially at night. Chronic infestations are common because of autoinoculation. Treatment with albendazole gives a cure rate of 90-100%. Other causes include atopic diathesis, fecal contamination. In prepubertal and young girls, vulvovaginal candidiasis may be present.

It is not always easy to make a rapid and definitive diagnosis in a pruritic child. Common dermatological conditions at this age-group should be ruled out initially followed by detailed screening for systemic disorders.

BIBLIOGRAPHY

1. Abdelmalek NF, Gerber TL, Menter A. Cardiocutaneous syndromes and associations. J Am Acad Dermatol 2002;46:161-83.
2. Bem J, Bradley EL. Subcutaneous manifestations of severe acute pancreatitis. Pancreas 1998;16:551.
3. Bergassa NV, Link MJ, Keogh M et al. Pilot study of bright-light therapy reflected towards the eyes for the pruritus of chronic liver disease. Am J Gastroenterol 2001;96:1563-70.
4. Bernhard JD, Jorizzo JL, Callen JP. Pruritus. In: Callen JP .Jorizza JL, Eds. Dermatological signs of internal disease, 3rd edn.Philadelphia: Saunders, 2003:65-8.
5. Bork K, Barnstedt SE. Treatment of 193 episodes of laryngeal edema with C1 inhibitor concentrate in patients with hereditary angioedema. Arch Intern Med 2001;161:714
6. Brady RO, Schiffman R. Clinical features and recent advances in Fabry's disease. JAMA 2000;284:2771.
7. Braverman IM. Skin changes of systemic disease, 3rd edn. Philadelphia: Saunders, 1998:405-37.
8. Brik R, Shamali H, Bergman R. Successful Thalidomide treatment of Severe Infantile Behcet's disease. Pediatr

Dermatol 2001;18:143-5.
9. Costopanagiotou E, et al. An unusual cause of massive gastric bleeding in a young patient Am J Gastroenterol 2000;95:2400.
10. Dajani AS, Taubert KA, Gerber MA, et al. Diagnosis and therapy of Kawasaki disease in children. Circulation. 1993;87:1776 –1780.
11. Deaver C, Miltenberger RG, Stricker JM. Functional analysis and treatment of hair twirling in children. J Appl Behav Anal 2001;34:535-8.
12. Dinkel H-P, et al. Sonographic appearances of the abdominal manifestations of hereditary angioedema. Pediatr Radiol 2001;31:296.
13. Eng CM, Guffon N, Wilcox WR, et al. International collaborative Fabry group study group. Safety and efficacy of human recombinant alpha-galactosidase. A replacement therapy in Fabry's disease. N Engl J Med 2001;345:9-16.
14. Flynn JA, Provost TT. Rheumatic fever. In: Provost TT, .Flynn JA, eds. Cutaneous medicine: Cutaneous manifestation of systemic disease. Hamilton, Ontario: Decker, 2001;205-7.
15. Friedman S, et al. Intravenous cyclosporine in refractory pyoderma gangrenosum complicating inflammatory bowel disease. Inflammal Bowel Dis 2001;7:1.
16. George WM. Cutaneous findings related to cardiovascular disorders (review). Int JDermatol 1998;37:161-72.
17. Ghate JV, Jorizzo JL. Behcet's disease and complex apthosis. J Am Acad Dermatol1999;40:1-18.
18. Gorlin RJ et al. Syndromes of the head and neck, 4th ed. New York, Oxford University Press, 2001:1455-72
19. Grebe TA, Clericuzio C. Neurological and gastrointestinal dysfunction in cardio- facio-cutaneous syndrome, identification of a severe phenotype. Am J Med Gener 2000;95:135-143.
20. Happle R. Lyonization and the lines of Blaschko. Hum Genet 1985;70:200.
21. Jonelle K McDonnell. Cardiac disease and the skin. Dermatol Clin 2002;20:503-11.
22. Kone Paul et al. Clinical features of Behcet's disease in children: An international collaborative study of 86 cases. J Paediatr 1998;132:721.
23. Lahteenoja H, et al. Oral mucosa is frequently affected in patients with dermatitis herpetiformis. Arch Dermatol 1998;134:756.
24. Lankisch M R, et al. Acute abdominal pain for Degos disease (malignant atrophic papulosis). Am J Gastroenterol 1999;94:1098.
25. Lowitt M, Dover J. Necrobiosis lipoidica. J Am Acad Dermatol.1991;25:735-748.
26. Lucky AW, Biro FM, Huster GA, et al. Acne vulgaris in premenarchal girls. Arch Dermatol 1994;130:308-314.
27. Markinokovich MP. Update on inherited bullous dermatoses. Dermatol Clin 1999;17:473.
28. Miller AM, et al. Rapid response of severe refractory metastatic Crohn's disese to infliximab. J Gastroenterol Hepatol 2001;16:940.
29. Nanette B Silverberg, Anup Singh, Terestia A Laude. Cutaneous manifestations of chronic renal failure in children of color. Pediatric Dermatology 2001;18:199-204.
30. Oppenheimer E, Linder B, DiMartino-Nardi J. Decreased insulin sensitivity in pre-pubertal girls with premature adrenarche and acanthosis nigricans. J Clin Endocrinol Metab 1995. 80:614-618.
31. Pepin M, et al. Clinical and genetic features of Ehlers –Danlos syndrome type IV, the vascular type. N Engl J Med 2000;342:673.
32. Ratnaike RN. Whipple's disease. Postgrad Med J 2000;76:760-6.
33. Rogers M, Fairley M, Santhaman R. Artefactual skin disease in children and adolescents. Australas J Dermatol 2001;42:264-70.
34. Rucco V, Psilogenis M, Lo Schiavo A, et al. Dermatological manifestations of alcoholic cirrhosis. Clin Dermatol 1999;17:463-8.
35. Shah D, Goraya JS, Poddar B, Parmar VR: Acute infantile hemorrhagic edema and Henoch-Schonlein purpura overlap in a child. Pediatr Dermatol 2002;19:92-3
36. Shimuzu H. Darier's disease with oesophageal carcinoma. Eur J Dermatol 2000;10:470.
37. The International Incontinentia Pigmenti Consortium: Genomic Rearrangement in NEMO impairs NF-kappa-B activation and is a cause of incontinentia pigmenti. Nature 2000;405:466.
38. Tizard EJ. Henoch-Schonlein purpura. Arch Dis Child 1999;80:380.
39. Tsao H. Update on familial cancer syndrome and the skin . J Am Acad Dermatol 2000;42:939-69.
40. Victoria J, Trujillo R. Topical Ivermectin: A new successful treatment for scabies. Pediatr Dermatol 2001;18:63.
41. Vogelsang GB, Lee L,Bensen-Kennedy D. Pathogenesis and treatment of graft-versus-host disease after bone marrow transplant.Annu Rev Med 2003;54:29-52.

27

Infantile and Adolescent Acne

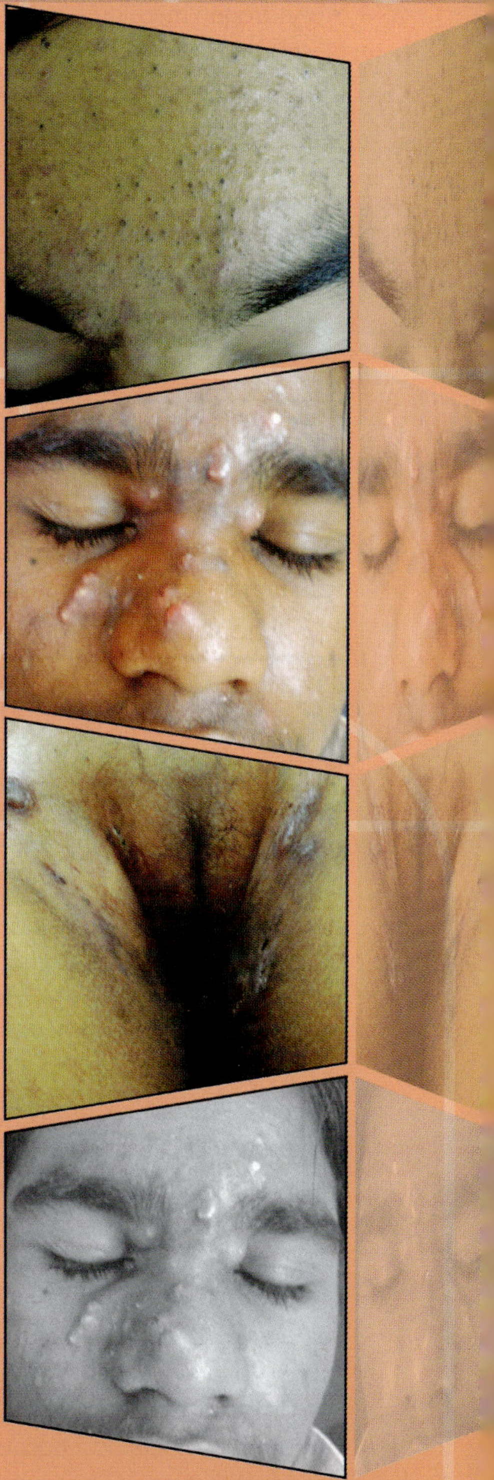

Shernaz Walton
Thomas Oliphant

SALIENT FEATURES

- Infantile acne is relatively uncommon compared to adolescent acne.
- Adrenal androgens are implicated in the etiology of infantile acne.
- Androgen mediation and polycystic ovarian syndrome should be considered in adolescents, especially when associated with hirsutism, obesity and menstrual dysfunction.
- Topical/systemic therapy is prescribed on the basis of severity of acne and should be tailored to the needs of the pediatric age-group.
- Physical methods and alternative medicine both have a place in treatment.

INTRODUCTION

Acne is a chronic inflammatory disease of the pilosebaceous units – characterized by seborrhea, comedones, papules, pustules and less frequently by nodules and cysts resulting in scarring.

EPIDEMIOLOGY AND NATURAL HISTORY

Acne usually starts in adolescence and frequently resolves in the twenties. In one study, prevalence of significant acne among adolescents (aged between14 and16 years) was 56% (boys) and 45% (girls). A peak in prevalence and severity occurs between 14 and 17 years in females, when 40% are affected and 16 and 19 years in males, when 35% are affected. A study from the USA indicated that the prevalence by the midteens was virtually 100%.

Acne develops earlier in females than in males, reflecting the earlier onset of puberty. Mild, comedonal acne can be the first sign of puberty. Significant comedones usually precede inflammatory lesions by 2–3 years. Some children show small non-inflamed lesions by the age of 8–9 years. After the age of 20 years, acne resolves slowly. However, in 7–17% of individuals, acne persists beyond the age of 25 years with physiological acne in females having a prevalence of 24%. Factors that underlie the resolution of acne or the relative persistence in females are poorly understood because improved treatment has modified the prevalence, severity and age of presentation to dermatology clinics.

ETIOLOGY

The etiology of acne is multifactorial and often due to the interaction of the following factors:

- Increased sebum production (seborrhea)
- Ductal colonization with *Propionibacterium acnes* (*P. acnes)*
- Keratinization of the pilosebaceous duct (comedogenesis)
- Production of inflammation.

HORMONAL FACTORS

Active sebaceous glands are a prerequisite for the development of acne. Acne patients excrete, on average, more sebum than normal subjects and the level of secretion correlates well with the acne severity. Androgens of gonadal or adrenal origin exert a major influence on sebum production. Serum dehydroepiandrosterone sulphate (DHEAS) levels are used to screen for an adrenal source of excess androgen production. Late-onset adrenal hyperplasia due to partial deficiency of 21-hydroxylase should be considered in patients with persistent acne.

An ovarian source of excess androgen can be suspected in cases where the serum total testosterone is elevated. The free androgen index (FAI), which is a ratio of total testosterone and sex hormone binding globulin (SHBG), is raised in patients with polycystic ovary syndrome. Greater elevations in serum testosterone may indicate an ovarian tumor.

There is general agreement that plasma testosterone levels are not abnormally high in males with acne. In females with acne, some investigators have found testosterone levels to be normal, while others have found testosterone levels to be raised. An enhanced peripheral response to androgens must therefore be considered as a probable factor in many subjects, hypothesizing the theory that certain follicles in acne-bearing areas are more prone to acne.

As per authors' experience in clinical practice and that of other acne centers, it is not usually necessary to investigate all patients for an associated endocrinopathy. An endocrine assessment may be indicated for adolescent and adult females, with a sudden onset of severe acne or with acne that has proven resistant to conventional therapy, especially when associated with hirsutism, irregular menstrual periods or signs of hyperandrogenism.

Polycystic ovary syndrome is the most frequently associated endocrinal disease. In most acne clinics, the majority of female patients with acne have no other clinical features of the syndrome, which consists of hirsutism, infertility or menstrual irregularities. Infantile acne results from transplacental stimulation of the adrenal gland, as most neonates have elevated plasma adrenal androgen levels. After three months of age, the sebaceous glands atrophy, seborrhea declines and the lesions disappear over a 2–3 months period. An associated virilizing tumor or underlying congenital adrenal hyperplasia is extremely rare.

GENETIC FACTORS

A genetic influence is confirmed by the very high concordance between monozygotic twins, in whom sebum excretion rate (SER) is virtually identical. Comedone numbers are also similar in identical twins but not in dizygotic twins, which suggest a genetic role in comedone formation.

Patients with persistent acne have a strong family history of severe acne, in contrast to patients with adolescent acne.

The association between acne and Apert's syndrome is linked to two genetic mutations in receptor 2 fibroblastic growth factor. These patients develop early epiphyseal closure, which, like acne, is an androgen mediated event. They have characteristic facial abnormalities which include hypertelorism, flattened occiput, proptosis, prognathism, parrot-beaked nose and fused shortened digits.

PATHOGENESIS

Androgens are responsible for increased sebum production, which occurs during adolescence. Adolescence and its attendant seborrhea are associated with a significant increase in *P. acnes* numbers.

Comedogenesis occurs due to ductal hypercornification and is manifested clinically as blackheads, whiteheads and macrocomedones. Comedones are due to abnormalities in the proliferation and differentiation of ductal keratinocytes and represent the retention of hyperproliferating ductal keratinocytes/corneocytes in the duct. Several factors have been implicated in the induction of keratinocyte hyperproliferation, and include sebaceous lipid composition, androgens, local cytokine production and bacteria.

The precise factors that induce inflammation in acne lesions are unknown. Micro-organisms, especially *P. acnes,* are an obvious source of antigenic stimulation; in particular, its cell wall fraction is a potent chemo attractant for polymorphonuclear and mononuclear cells. There is also evidence to support the involvement of toll-like receptors in acne inflammation. Toll receptors recognize 'abnormal' organisms; *P. acnes* are considered 'abnormal' as it is not often present in follicles from subjects without acne. The toll receptors in turn regulate the production of cytokines which contribute to acne inflammation. P. *acnes* also produce a prostaglandin-like substance which might also be involved. Cytokines are known to play a role in inflammatory acne.

PREDISPOSING/TRIGGERING/ EXACERBATING FACTORS

DIET

Acne is blamed on certain foods, in particular chocolate and oily foods, but scientific proof is lacking. A hypothesis that needs to be tested is that the 'Gujarati' diet, like the western diet, has a high glycemic index which in turn can trigger insulin and insulin-like growth factor that influence androgens and thereby may induce seborrhea, comedones and acne. The trend of increased weight among children and earlier puberty may be reflected in the early development of clinical acne.

PREMENSTRUAL FLARE

About 70% of girls experience a flare premenstrually but it is unlikely that a variation in sebum excretion occurs during the menstrual cycle.

ULTRAVIOLET RADIATION (UV)

Natural sunlight often improves acne, but scientific evidence is lacking. The cosmetic effect of tanning may be the explanation. Artificial UV radiation is less satisfactory than natural radiation, and psoralen and UVA (PUVA) have been reported to induce acne uncommonly.

DRUGS

Corticosteroids are the most common cause of iatrogenic acne. Oral and potent topical steroids can induce acne in a dose-dependant manner. Acne is not uncommonly seen in organ-transplant recipients.

Antiepileptic medications such as phenytoin and phenobarbitone are known to cause acne.

Less commonly, *isoniazid* and *rifampicin* have been reported to induce acne. Intravenous *Dactimomycin* used to treat pediatric malignancies may also precipitate acne, associated with elevated androgen levels.

COSMETICS

A few cosmetics are comedogenic. Acne is more commonly produced by cosmetics those contain lanolin, vegetable oils, fatty acid esters and waxes. The acne takes 6–8 weeks to improve once the products are discontinued.

STRESS

Appearance is an important factor in social and emotional interaction. A recent paper, in which acne severity was graded before and during examinations, suggested that stress can induce acne. In addition, acne itself induces stress, and the 'picking' of the lesions will aggravate the symptoms. This is particularly obvious in young females who present with acne excoriée.

Questionnaires that relate specifically to acne – the Acne Quality of Life Scale (Acne- QoL), when compared with other chronic illnesses have shown that the social, psychological and emotional disability levels of acne patients are similar to those reported by patients with 'more serious' diseases, such as asthma, epilepsy, diabetes or arthritis. Younger acne patients are subject to bullying, teasing and stigmatization from their peers.

CLINICAL FEATURES

Acne is a disease of the pilosebaceous follicles and therefore affects the face and upper trunk.

Physical signs of acne include:

- Seborrhea (oily skin)
- Non-inflamed lesions (whiteheads, blackheads)
- Superficial inflamed lesions (papules, superficial pustules)
- Deep inflamed lesions (nodules)
- Scarring
- Post-inflammatory hyperpigmentation

Seborrhea is due to excessive production of sebum by acne-prone follicles. It is manifested as obvious oiliness.

Blackheads or open comedones vary in size from microscopic to 2–3mm in diameter. The black tip of the comedone is not due to dirt but to oxidation of melanin **(Figure 27.1)**.

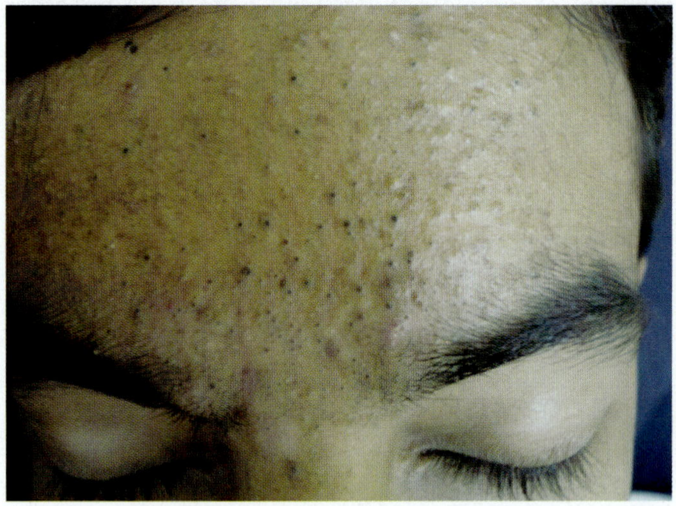

FIGURE 27.1: Blackheads over forehead

Whiteheads, or closed comedones, are very small, usually less than 1 mm, skin-colored, pink or white papule or macule, better visualized with a lens in good light. Comedones may be seen 2-3 years prior to the onset of significant inflammatory acne in adolescents and young adults.

Superficial inflamed lesions are easily recognized. These are usually papule and pustules (≤ 5 mm).

Deep inflamed lesions (nodules) refer to large inflammatory lesions ≥ 0.5 cm in diameter and may last

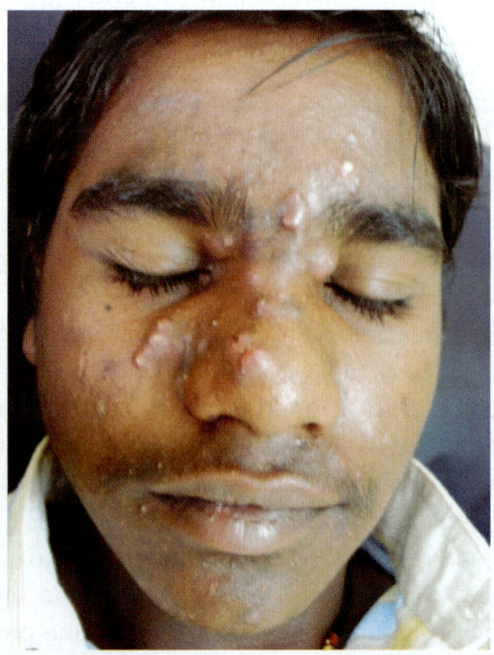

FIGURE 27.2: Deep inflammatory and pustular lesions

for many weeks to months. Sometimes pustulation occurs within the nodule and the lesion is referred to as a deep pustule, which can be mistaken for a boil **(Figure 27.2)**.

Scarring is not infrequent in pediatric patients with acne and can either be associated with loss or increase of collagen.

Persistent post-inflammatory hyperpigmentation is a common feature of Asian or Afro-Caribbean skin and may be more disfiguring than the original disease.

CLINICAL ACNE VARIANTS

HIDRADENITIS SUPPURATIVA AND DISSECTING FOLLICULITIS

Hidradenitis suppurativa **(Figure 27.3)** and dissecting folliculitis of the scalp may accompany acne and are classified as the follicular occlusion triad when accompanied by acne conglobata. All these conditions have in common a deep, recurrent, chronic folliculitis that results in abscess and sinus track formation and scarring. These, however, are uncommon in adolescents and predominantly occur in females.

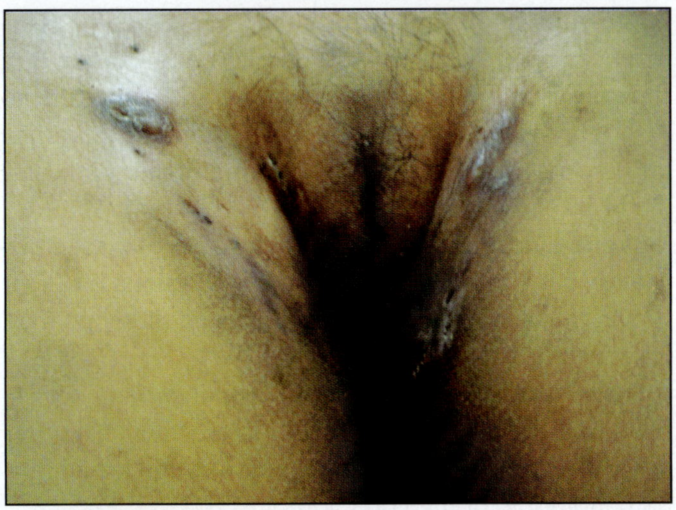

FIGURE 27.3: Hidradenitis suppurativa in a girl

ACNE FULMINANS

Acne fulminans is a rare ulcerative form of acne that most commonly affects adolescent boys. It has an acute onset and is associated with systemic symptoms such as fever, weight loss, arthralgia, mygalgia, erythema nodosum and hepatosplenomegaly. Etiology is uncertain but the presence of microscopic hematuria, erythema nodosum, increased response to *P. acnes* antigen in skin tests and depressed response to intradermal purified protein derivative are all pointers to an abnormal immunological response.

These patients require urgent dermatological review and may require admission to hospital. Treatment involves a combination of oral prednisolone and oral isotretinoin. Prednisolone is started immediately at an initial dosage of 0.5-1 mg/Kg/day, and continued for 4 to 8 weeks to prevent relapse. Oral isotretinoin is started after 4–6 weeks of steroid therapy and is given at a dose of 0.5-1mg/Kg/day for approximately 6 months. In patients with the severe form of the disease, a lower starting dose of isotretinoin (0.1-0.25 mg/Kg/day) is recommended.

ACNE EXCORIÉE

Acne excoriée is seen predominantly in females. Anxious patients may pick and scratch the existing lesions to produce this morphology. The importance of not picking the skin lesions must be emphasized to these patients. Systemic treatment is often required as they are often non-compliant with topical therapy.

GRAM-NEGATIVE FOLLICULITIS

Gram-negative folliculitis occurs as a complication of long-term antibiotic therapy. Clinical features consist of sudden onset of multiple pustules, frequently localized to the perioral and perinasal areas. Occasionally, the condition presents with nodular lesions or simply as a flare of 'ordinary' acne. The organisms isolated include *Escherichia coli, Proteus, Pseudomones* and *Klebsiella*. The ongoing antibiotic therapy has to be stopped. Trimethroprim 300 mg twice daily or oral isotretinoin is the usual treatments. As relapse is not uncommon when trimethroprim is stopped, isotretinoin is often the treatment of choice.

HYPERANDROGENISM

Hyperandrogenism should be considered in a young patient, between 18 months to 7 years of age, with acne associated with precocious puberty, hirsutism, menstrual dysfunction and obesity. The most common cause of hyperandrogenism presenting in a teenage girl is polycystic ovary syndrome. Plasma-free testosterone is a sensitive indicator of hyperandrogenism. The pattern of response of plasma-free testosterone, DHEAS and cortisol to dexamethasone suppression tests will allow the source of excess androgen to be identified.

NEONATAL, INFANTILE AND JUVENILE ACNE

Neonatal, infantile and juvenile acne; acne may rarely occur in neonates or during the first 18 months of life and often persists until the age of 3 or 4 years. Males are more frequently affected and the face is virtually always involved. Lesions rarely occur on the trunk. The infants are in good health, and endocrine investigations are only warranted in the presence of other features of androgen excess.

The sebaceous glands of neonates produce a considerable amount of sebum in the first few weeks of life due to the effect of maternal androgens. Many infants have tiny whitish yellow papules over the nose, forehead and cheeks as a result of the sebaceous hyperplasia. After three months of age, the glands atrophy, seborrhea declines and the lesions will disappear over a 2–3 month period. Sebum production is then hardly measurable until puberty. Quantified data on comedone formation in neonatal and infantile acne is lacking but *P. acnes* have been shown to colonize the skin surface and pilosebaceous ducts.

APERT'S SYNDROME

Apert's syndrome (acrophalasyndactyly) is thought to occur as a result of an androgen end-organ hypersensitivity response affecting the epiphyses and sebaceous glands. This produces early epiphyseal fusion, resulting in short stature, short and fused digits and acrocephaly. The characteristic facial features are distinctive. Most patients have subnormal intelligence. Occurrence is mainly sporadic but can be inherited as an autosomal dominant trait. The acne in Apert's syndrome is often extensive, severe and resistant to treatment and oral isotretinoin is often required.

DIFFERENTIAL DIAGNOSIS

Acne vulgaris is rarely misdiagnosed. Various conditions can look similar and need to be differentiated.

Rosacea occurs in older patients and lacks comedones, cysts, nodules and scarring. Facial flushing that is induced by heat, spicy food or alcohol is a pointer towards a diagnosis of rosacea. Patients with rosacea may also have ocular involvement.

Perioral dermatitis also presents in older patients. The skin is dry without comedones. Itching is a prominent symptom.

Milia may be confused with whiteheads (closed comedones). The lesions are often infraorbital in distribution and are whiter. They are very common and can occur in association with (although unrelated to) acne. In neonates, milia are common and would need to be differentiated from lesions of acne.

Folliculitis due to Gram-negative organisms can complicate acne therapy and the rare folliculitis due to *Candida* sp. may also present as multiple pustules, as may *S. epidermidis* folliculitis in immunocompromised individuals. Demodex folliculitis can present as non-responsive acne. It is difficult to diagnose since many individuals have this mite in their normal pilosebaceous follicles. The best diagnostic help is the therapeutic response to topical metronidazole or permethrin.

Pityrosporum folliculitis presents on the upper trunk as small scattered papules and pustules. It is likely, though unproven, to be a host reaction to a normal skin commensal *M. furfur*.

Plane warts, particularly on the face, may cause diagnostic confusion.

Zoophilic ringworm can cause localized pustular eruptions resulting in kerion formation.

Dermatitis herpetiformis may rarely present as an itchy vesicular, pustular facial eruption and **Linear IgA disease** can also present uncommonly as a papular facial rash without comedones. Biopsy, including immunofluorescence studies, is essential to confirm this particular diagnosis.

Acne agminata (granulomatous rosacea) presents as a facial rash in the older patient. The lesions are light brown in color (darker in Asian skin) and diascopy may reveal an apple-jelly color.

Tuberous sclerosis also presents with monomorphic, brownish papules on the face. There may be other associated features like periungual fibroma which are pathgnomonic of the condition.

Zinc deficiency can produce a severe papulo-pustular eruption, associated with a periorificeal rash and diarrhea. Several cases have also been reported after prolonged intravenous feeding without zinc supplementation.

LABORATORY INVESTIGATIONS

Most patients with acne do not need endocrine investigations.

However, underlying endocrine abnormalities are to be excluded if acne is part of SAHA syndrome (seborrhea, acne, hirsutism and alopecia) or associated with irregular menstruation suggestive of polycystic ovary syndrome (PCOS). In such cases, following investigations are indicated:

- Free androgen index – this is a ratio of total testosterone and steroid hormone binding globulin (SHBG) and it is raised. High elevation in serum testosterone may be indicative of an ovarian tumor.
- Ovarian ultrasonography –more than 10 follicles per ovary are suggestive of the diagnosis of PCOS.
- Luteinizing (LH) and follicle stimulating hormone (FSH) levels – reveal an elevated level of LH, often with an increased LH: FSH ratio.
- Fasting glucose and lipid profile as 50% of the PCOS patients have hyperinsulinemia.

Ovarian tumors are suspected if there is marked hirsutism and signs of systemic virilization (deep voice, cliteromegaly and a male muscular physique). The plasma-free testosterone level is double the upper limit of normal in such cases.

If an adrenal source of excess androgen production is suspected, following tests may be useful:

- Serum DHEAS level, which is markedly elevated (in contrast to modest elevation seen in PCOS).
- Serum 9.00 am cortisol and 17α-hydroxyprogesterone levels are raised in patients with congenital adrenal hyperplasia.

Baseline investigation to monitor drug therapy:

MINOCYCLINE

- Liver function tests
- Antinuclear antibody (ANA)
- Perinuclear antineutrophil cytoplasmic antibody (pANCA)

These should be done prior to starting treatment and repeated every 3 to 6 months whilst on therapy.

SPIRONOLACTONE

- Serum urea and electrolyte estimation at regular intervals.

ISOTRETINOIN

- Liver function tests
- Fasting lipid profile

Published evidence suggests that these tests need not be repeated except in groups at risk, such as diabetics and patients with known familial hypertriglyceridemia.

MANAGEMENT

GENERAL PRINCIPLES

The treatment of acne depends upon four factors:

- Type of lesion
- Acne severity
- Age-group affected
- Psychological impact of the disease

Type of Acne

Type of acne in a particular patient needs to be established. A good light is necessary for optimal assessment. Lesions can be predominantly comedonal, inflammatory or a combination of both. Blackheads, papules, pustules, deep pustules and nodules are easily recognized but whiteheads can be difficult to see. It may be necessary to stretch the skin gently and examine by shining a light at different angles to reveal the maximum number of whiteheads. This is particularly important in Asian patients, in whom whiteheads are even more difficult to appreciate. Determination of the type of acne lesions present is particularly relevant while deciding on the best topical therapy to use **(Table 27.1)**.

TABLE 27.1: Topical therapies for acne*

Anticomedonal therapy:
Adapalene
Tretinoin
Azelaic acid
Isotretinoin
Anti-inflammatory therapy:
Adapalene
Benzyoyl peroxide 2.5%, 4%, 5% and 10%
Clindamycin
Erythromycin
Tetracycline
Combined therapy:
Benzoyl peroxide and erythromycin
Isotretinoin and erythromycin
Zinc and erythromycin

*Reprinted with permission from Dermatology in Practice, S Walton et al.

Acne Severity

Acne severity depends on several factors that the clinician must take into account: the physical severity of the disease, the presence of or the risk of scarring, the psychological effects of the disease and the failure of previous treatments.

Grading scales can be developed by the clinician to suit the individual practice. Scarring has been described previously and must be included in the assessment of the severity. Post-inflammatory pigmentation also contributes to the severity, especially in dark-skinned patients.

Age-group

The **age-group** affected needs to be taken into consideration, especially before deciding on systemic treatment. In infants, the principles of treatment are the same as for adult patients with acne, except that the tetracycline group of drugs are avoided because of the risk of discoloration of permanent teeth. For mild disease, topical therapies such as topical retinoids, benzoyl peroxide, topical erythromycin or clindamycin are recommended—the preferred choice is a combination of a topical retinoid and a topical antimicrobial agent. For moderate disease, a topical retinoid and/or benzoyl peroxide combined with oral erythromycin (as ethyl succinate, 125 mg three times a day) for 6 months is essential until lesions have totally disappeared. Alternative is oral trimethoprim, 100 mg twice daily. Isotretinoin is rarely needed, and only for severe non-responding cases. Patients with infantile acne may develop significant acne as adolescents.

In adolescents, the same principles of treatment apply as in adults, provided there are sufficient clinical indications.

Psychological Impact

The psychological impact of acne may be significant. Several questionnaires are available to assess this, but one suitable for the adolescent age group has to be developed. Nevertheless, the existing ones are very helpful to monitor the progress of the psychosocial status of the disease and the effect of treatment and only take 1-2 minutes to complete.

TOPICAL TREATMENT

Topical therapy forms the mainstay of treatment in all grades of acne severity – it should be prescribed alone for mild acne, in conjunction with appropriate oral therapy for moderate acne and as maintenance therapy in severe acne after oral therapy has been stopped. Topical therapy may be necessary for several years and should be used regularly once or twice daily. It is necessary to apply the topical therapy not just to the spots, but to the whole of the acne-bearing skin on the face and trunk.

The most commonly used topical agents are benzoyl peroxide, retinoids, antibiotics and azelaic acid, either as monotherapy or in combinations.

Benzoyl Peroxide

Benzoyl peroxide is available in concentrations of 2.5%, 4%, 5% and 10% either alone or in combination with hydroxyquinolines, tretinoin, miconazole or antibiotics. The rationale for combining benzoyl peroxide and erythromycin is effective in reducing the number of pre-existing resistant organisms on the skin of acne patients.

Adapalene

Adapalene, a synthetic retinoid, is a relatively new topical agent that is effective in the treatment of mild to moderate acne. Available in gel and cream formulations, it appears to be significantly better tolerated than several tretinoin formulations. Although the structure of adapalene is unlike other retinoids, it has a retinoid function with respect to the antiproliferative effect on keratinocytes. It also has significant anti-inflammatory effects by inhibiting polymorphonuclear leukocyte chemotaxis, and, in contrast to tretinoin, it also inhibits the -5 and -15 lipoxygenase pathways of metabolism of arachidonic acid. Clinically, adapalene is a useful monotherapy in patients with mild disease and, after oral therapy has been discontinued, it can be used as a maintenance therapy. It can be safely combined with oral and topical antibiotics, as there is no risk of enhancing *P. acnes* resistance. Similarly, it can be used concomitantly with other topical antimicrobials such as benzoyl peroxide and azelaic acid.

Adapalene was introduced in India in 2001. A post-marketing survey was conducted to assess the safety and efficacy of 0.1% adapalene gel as monotherapy or in combination with other anti-acne agents in 571 Indian patients from 21 centers across India. An improvement of > 96% in patients with acne was observed. It was well tolerated with no serious adverse effects.

Tazarotene

A new third generation topical acetylenic retinoid has a significant effect on inflammatory lesions and has good efficacy and safety data on its use on Indian patients with acne.

Azelaic Acid

Azelaic acid is an endogenous C9-dicarboxylic acid synthesized by omega-oxidation from fatty acids and found physiologically in human urine. After topical application, about 3.6% is absorbed through the skin. It is metabolized via the β-oxidation pathway ending in the formation of malonyl-CoA or acetyl-CoA. It has two major effects in the pathogenesis of acne. It leads to normalization of the dysfunctional keratinocytes in the follicular infundibulum and it has a strong antimicrobial effect. The major advantage of azelaic acid is its lower irritant property compared with benzoyl peroxide and tretinoin. Also, it does not bleach clothes or bed linen – a common complaint against benzoyl peroxide. Azelaic acid does not produce resistance in *P. acnes* – an important consideration for long-term use.

Topical Antibiotics

Topical antibiotics include tetracycline, erythromycin and clindamycin. Lincomycin 2% gel has been used in India and has been found to be effective and safe in the treatment of mild and moderate acne. Combination antibiotics include erythromycin with zinc or with benzoyl peroxide and these are marginally better than used singly.

SYSTEMIC TREATMENT

Oral therapy for acne includes antibiotics, hormones, isotretinoin and occasionally steroids.

Oral antibiotics are the most widely prescribed oral therapy for acne worldwide.

Tetracyclines (oxytetracycline, doxycycline, lymecycline, minocycline and azithromycin) are the antibiotics of choice. Erythromycin is preferred in young females who may become pregnant. Trimethroprim (400-600 mg/day), which is similar in efficacy to tetracyclines, is often used as a third-line antibiotic in resistant cases complicated by Gram-negative folliculitis.

Patients who require antibiotics should be given 1g/day of tetracycline or erythromycin in divided doses. The major disadvantage of tetracycline (and less so of erythromycin) is the need to take the medication with water (not milk) half an hour before food to ensure adequate absorption. Thus, daily doxycycline (100 mg/day) or lymecycline (408 mg/day) or the more expensive minocycline (100 mg/day) which are better absorbed, may improve patient compliance. Minocycline, despite its widespread use, should not be the first-line drug for treatment of acne.

Oral therapy should be combined with topical therapy for a minimum of 6 months, for

- Patients with moderate to severe acne;
- Patients who are depressed and suffer from dysmorphophobia;
- Asian patients who are likely to develop post inflammatory hyperpigmentation;
- Patients prone to develop scarring.

Hormonal treatments are usually indicated when

- Standard antibiotic regimens have failed,
- Concomitant menstrual regularization or contraception and acne treatment are required
- Oral isotretinoin is inappropriate or unavailable.

The contraceptive pill, in the name **Dianette®** (35 mg of ethinylestradiol and 2 mg of the antiandrogen, cyproterone acetate) may occasionally be useful in younger adolescent female patients with menstrual problems and who may require oral contraception. **Yasmin®** (drospirinone 3 mg, ethinyloestradiol 30 mg) is an alternative for patients who are unable to tolerate Dianette. The clinical efficacy of this combination can be enhanced by giving an extra 50-100 mg of cyproterone acetate (CPA) from the 5th to 14th day of the cycle. At this dosage, the reduction in sebum production is 50-67%.

For how long CPA (2 mg) combined with ethinylo-estradiol (35 mg) can be administered safely is uncertain. Given recent evidence, it is prudent to change to a lower estrogen-containing pill once the acne is under control, to minimise the risk of thrombo-embolism.

Spironolactone is an effective treatment and is used for its antiandrogenic effects in reducing sebum production. It is useful in females who are at risk of thrombo-embolic disease from the estrogen content of the combined contraceptive pills.

Isotretinoin is the only treatment that has an effect on all the major etiological factors involved in acne. It significantly reduces elevated sebum production, comedogenesis and surface/ductal colonization with *P. acnes*; it also possesses anti-inflammatory action. It is a third-line systemic agent and reserved for severe forms of acne. Age should not be a barrier to the use of isotretinoin. A very small number of neonates and young acne patients who had not responded to all appropriate topical/oral therapy have been treated successfully with isotretinoin, the usual dose being 0.5 mg/Kg/day. Some pre-adolescent youngsters under the age of 10 years develop severe acne with scarring. Oral isotretinoin should be prescribed for pediatric patients with acne if there are sufficient clinical indications.

Table 27.2 summarizes the various treatment regimens in all severities of acne.

TABLE 27.2: Treatment regimens based on severity of acne

Physiological and mild acne	Topical therapy
Moderate acne	Topical therapy + Oral antibiotics or Hormonal regimen
Severe acne	Topical therapy + Hormonal regimen or Isotretinoin

SIDE EFFECTS

These are rarely severe enough requiring discontinuation of therapy.

Topical Therapies

All of these may produce a primary irritant dermatitis consisting of erythema and scaling at the site of application. This may reduce patient compliance and therefore it may be necessary to explain this common occurrence at the initial visit. Adapalene and the newer preparations are less irritant. A true allergic dermatitis is rare.

Oral Antibiotics

Side effects are not usually a major problem and consist mostly of gastrointestinal tract disturbance, such as nausea, abdominal colic and diarrhea. Vaginal candidiasis, which is common in adults, is extremely unusual in the pediatric population.

Rare side effects can also occur, especially with the tetracycline group of drugs. A photo-sensitive rash and photo-onycholysis may occur with tetracyclines, particularly doxycyline. Minocycline can induce pigmentation, not only at the site of acne scars, but also on the shin and mucous membranes. A diffuse gray pigmentation can also occur very rarely. Pigmentation resolves usually within 18 months of stopping therapy. Benign intracranial hypertension is also a very rare side effect of tetracyclines, especially minocycline. Patients present with a headache, nausea, blurred vision and, in extreme cases, impaired concentration and a confusional state. Minocycline may also very rarely produce hepatitis, pulmonary eosinophilia and a lupus erythematosus-like syndrome. Minocycline should not be given to patients with a personal or family history of lupus and screening/monitoring tests as mentioned in an earlier section are recommended.

Tetracyclines should be avoided in infants and young acne patients due to discoloration of teeth during dentition. Side effects of Dianette® are similar to those of other oral contraceptives.

Isotretinoin has many side effects but the more serious ones include teratogenicity, depression (particularly in adolescents) and benign intracranial hypertension. Most other side effects of oral isotretinoin are predictable and rarely require cessation of therapy. A flare of acne occurs in 6% cases and patients must be informed of this possible side effect. If severe, one may need to taper the dose of isotretinoin and treat with oral prednisolone (0.5-1mg/kg/day) for a 2-3 week period with a slow reduction in dosage over 6 weeks. The mucocutaneous side effects can be minimized by the regular use of moisturizers (except on areas with acne) and lip salves. Secondary impetiginization due to *S. aureus* may occasionally occur necessitating a combined intermediate strength steroid and antiseptic combination applied topically. In more severe cases, oral flucloxacillin and/or topical mupirocin (2%) ointment may be required.

TREATMENT OF RESISTANT/REFRACTORY CASES

There are several reasons why patients with acne do not respond to therapy. These include:

Poor Compliance

It is important to emphasize to patients that acne responds slowly to treatment and improvement may not occur for 4-6 weeks and that, it is necessary to apply topical treatment not just to the acne lesions but to the whole of the acne-prone skin. Education and time spent with patients, especially the adolescents, can improve compliance.

P. acnes Resistance

This is another reason for treatment failure. This should be suspected in:

- Patients, who are compliant to treatment, but fail to respond to adequate antibiotic dosage,

- Patients who relapse while on antibiotics,
- Patients who have been treated with multiple different topical and systemic antibiotics.

P. acnes resistance is more likely to develop during treatment with erythromycin (65%) and tetracyclines, including doxycycline (40%). It occurs less frequently with trimethoprim and rarely with minocycline. If *P. acnes* resistance to erythromycin is suspected, a combination of erythromycin and benzoyl peroxide has been shown to dramatically reduce the organism, both *in vivo* and *in vitro*. Patients receiving systemic antibiotics will require a change of antibiotic, one to which *P. acnes* is sensitive. Treatment with isotretinoin may also be required occasionally.

Cystic acne is a further cause of poor response. Acne cysts are not in fact true cysts as they are not lined by epithelium and are best referred to as large nodules. A recently developed large nodule should be treated with the topical application of a potent steroid such as clobetasol propionate cream, applied sparingly twice daily for 5 days, or by intralesional injection of triamcinolone. Sometimes, cryotherapy is the preferred treatment and patients can tolerate 20 seconds of freezing with little discomfort. The rationale of this treatment is to encourage polymorphonuclear leucocytes to enter the nodule, which is developing early fibrosis, and facilitate resolution.

Acne variants also respond poorly to conventional treatment. These include Gram-negative folliculitis, acne fulminans and acne conglobata and their management has already been discussed.

PHYSICAL MODALITIES

Physical modalities are used as an adjunct to treatment.

For active acne, the following have been used:

Comedone extraction, using a blackhead extractor or host compress is useful.

Light electrocautery after application of a local anesthetic cream has been shown to be helpful in patients with multiple 'macrocomedones' or whiteheads. The cautery should be used at a low setting so as to produce minimal discomfort. The aim is to produce very low-grade thermal damage so as to stimulate the body's own defence mechanisms to eradicate the comedones.

UV light (DermaLux lamp): Combination of blue UV light (peak at 415 nm) and mixed blue and red UV light (peaks at 415 and 660 nm) were investigated in 107 patients with mild to moderate acne. The light sources were portable and the treatment was performed daily for 15 minutes over a 12 week period. At 12 weeks, there was a mean improvement of 76% with blue-red light and was significantly superior to the improvement seen from blue light, benzoyl peroxide and the control white light.

Photodynamic therapy (PDT) using topical amino levulinic acid (ALA) plus broadband light (550-700 nm) has been shown to produce statistically significant clearance of inflammatory acne for at least 20 weeks after multiple treatments and 10 weeks after a single treatment. The therapy produced acute damage to the sebaceous glands, resulting in significant suppression of sebum production and a decrease in *P. acnes* for many weeks.

Laser therapy (N Lite laser), which emits light at 585 nm, has been reported to produce a 50% improvement in acne grade and lesion counts by 12 weeks following a single treatment.

TREATMENT OF ACNE SCARS

Dermabrasion and Laser Resurfacing

Atrophic scars are treated with these modalities. Laser resurfacing has gradually replaced dermabrasion in the past 5 years. An increasing array of lasers is being used for this purpose. Although scientific data on their benefit are limited, the future outlook may be promising.

Collagen Injections

Purified bovine dermal collagen is of limited benefit but has shown to help soft scars that are easily stretched. Deep ice-pick and fibrotic scars show little improvement. Hypersensitivity must be excluded and technical expertise is necessary.

Chemical Peeling

The chemical agents used include; hydroxy acids, glycolic acids and resorcinol. Chemical peels promote desquamation and may help to dislodge comedonal plugs. There is limited scientific evidence to support the use of chemical peels.

For treatment of hypertrophic scars and keloid, available options include steroids (either potent topical steroid creams or intralesional triamcinolone injections), excision, cryotherapy or topical application of silicon gels. There are several studies testifying the benefits and pitfalls of such therapies.

Cosmetic Camouflage

Cosmetic camouflage is necessary for patients with scars and post-inflammatory hyperpigmentation (seen in Asian skin). Patients should be advised to use light, non-greasy make-up.

ALTERNATIVE MEDICINE

Systemic and topical use of herbal extracts to treat acne have been developed and standardized. Herbal extracts derived from plants described in ayurvedic treatise like Bhavprakasha Nighantu and Charak Samhita, used in a Phase II clinical trial confirmed that the combination of systemic and topical preparation was more efficacious than the oral formulation alone. In another double-blind randomized placebo-controlled trial comparing four ayurvedic formulations, used orally, a significant reduction in lesion count was observed in patients receiving Sunder Vati when compared with placebo and the other ayurvedic formulations.

Further evidence of the effectiveness of herbal drugs comes from an open clinical trial where patients were treated with tablets containing multiple herbal drugs (Purim) and the application of a herbal cream (Clarina) for a four week period. This trial revealed good clinical responses in all grades of acne and the tablet (Purim) and cream (Clarina) were well tolerated.

Plant extracts from *Berberis aristata* (Berber-idaceae), *Pterocarpus santalinus* (Fabaceae) and *Bombax ceiba* (Bombacaceae) have been shown to possess antibacterial activity against *P. acnes* and form the essential ingredients of a 'herbal cream' developed for the treatment of acne.

Tea tree oil is in use both in Asia and Europe, mainly for its antiseptic qualities. In a randomized, double-blind placebo-controlled study, using 5% topical tea tree oil gel, a significant improvement in the acne severity index with a reduction in total lesion count was found in the active group compared to the placebo. It was well tolerated as in the placebo group.

BIBLIOGRAPHY

1. Altman RS, Altman LJ, Altman JS. A proposed set of new guidelines for routine blood tests during isotretinoin therapy for acne vulgaris. Dermatology 2002; 204: 232-5.
2. Chu A, Chon S Y, Kimball A B. The response of skin disease to stress: changes in the severity of acne vulgaris as affected by examination stress. Arch Dermatol 2003; 139: 897-900.
3. Cordain L, Lindeberg S, Hurtado M, et al. Acne vulgaris: a disease of western civilisation. Arch Dermatol 2002; 138: 584-90.
4. Cunliffe W J, Baron S E, Coulson I H. A clinical and therapeutic study of 29 patients with infantile acne. Br J Dermatol 2001; 145: 463-6.
5. Eushaich S, Jooya A, Siadat AH, et al. The efficacy of 5% topical tea tree oil gel in mild to moderate acne vulgaris: a randomized, double-blind placebo-controlled study. Indian J Dermatol Venereol Leprol 2007;73: 22-5.
6. Fernandez-Obregon A C. Azithromycin for the treatment of acne. Int J Dermatol 2000; 39: 45-50.
7. Gollnick H, Cunliffe W J, Berson D, et al. Management of acne. A report from a global alliance to improve outcomes in acne. J Am Acad Dermatol 2003; 49: S1-36.
8. Herane MI, Ando I. Acne in infancy and acne genetics. Dermatology 2003; 206: 24-8.
9. Hongcharu W, Taylor CR, Chang Y, et al. Topical ALA – photodynamic therapy for the treatment of acne vulgaris. J Invest Dermatol 2000; 142: 973-80.
10. Itoh Y, Ninomiya Y, Tajima S, et al. Photodynamic therapy of acne vulgaris with topical amino laevulinic acid and incoherent light in Japanese patients. Br J Dermatol 2001; 144: 575-9.
11. Janniger C K. Neonatal and infantile acne vulgaris. Cutis 1993; 52:16.
12. Jappe U, Ingham E, Henwood J, et al. Propionibacterium acnes and inflammation in acne; P. acnes has T-cell mitogenic activity. Br J Dermatol 2002;146:202-9.
13. Klasson AF, Newton JN, Mallon E. Measuring quality of life in people referred for specialist care of acne, comparing generic and disease no-specific measures. J Am Acad Dermatol 2003; 43:229-33.
14. Nigam PK, Anant S. An evaluation of the efficacy and safety of tazarotene (0.1%) cream in acne vulgaris. Indian J Dermatol Venereol Leprol 2005; 71:360-1.
15. O'Brien SC, Lewis JB, Cunliffe WJ. The Leeds revised acne grading system. J Dermatol Treatment 1998; 9: 215-20.
16. Papageorgiou P, Katsambas A, Chu AS. Phototherapy with blue and red light in the treatment of acne vulgaris. Br J Dermatol 2000; 142: 973-80.
17. Sachidanand YN, Anand Kumar BH. Treatment of acne vulgaris with new polyherbal formulations. Indian J Dermatol Venereol Leprol 2000;45:138-41.
18. Sanjana PH. Safety and efficacy of adapalene gel 0.1% in acne vulgaris : results of a post-marketing surveillance study. Indian J Dermatol Venereol Leprol 2003; 69: 277-80.
19. Saple DG, Torsekar RG, Pawanarkar V, et al. An open study to evaluate the efficacy and safety of tazarotene gel (0.1%) in acne vulgaris. Indian J Dermatol Venereol Leprol 2004; 70: 92-5.
20. Seaton E, Charikida A, Mouser PE, et al. Pulsed dye laser treatment for inflammatory acne vulgaris: a randomised controlled trial. Lancet 2003;362:1347-52.
21. Sharma AD, Gupta PD, Sundaram M, et al. Topical lincomycin gel in acne vulgaris: a multicentric placebo controlled study. Indian J Dermatol Venereol Leprol 2003; 69: 271-3.
22. Singhi MK, Ghiya BC, Dhabhai RK. Comparison of oral azithromycin pulse with daily doxycycline in the treatment of acne vulgaris. Indian J Dermatol Venereol Leprol 2003; 69: 274-6.
23. Smithard A, Glazebrook C, Williams H C. Acne prevalence, knowledge about acne and psychological morbidity in mid-adolescence: a community-based study. Br J Dermatol 2001; 145: 274-9.
24. Walton S, Gowda P. Topical treatment for acne – recent additions. Dermatology in Practice 2004; 10: 6-8.

28

Pediatric Dermatological Emergencies

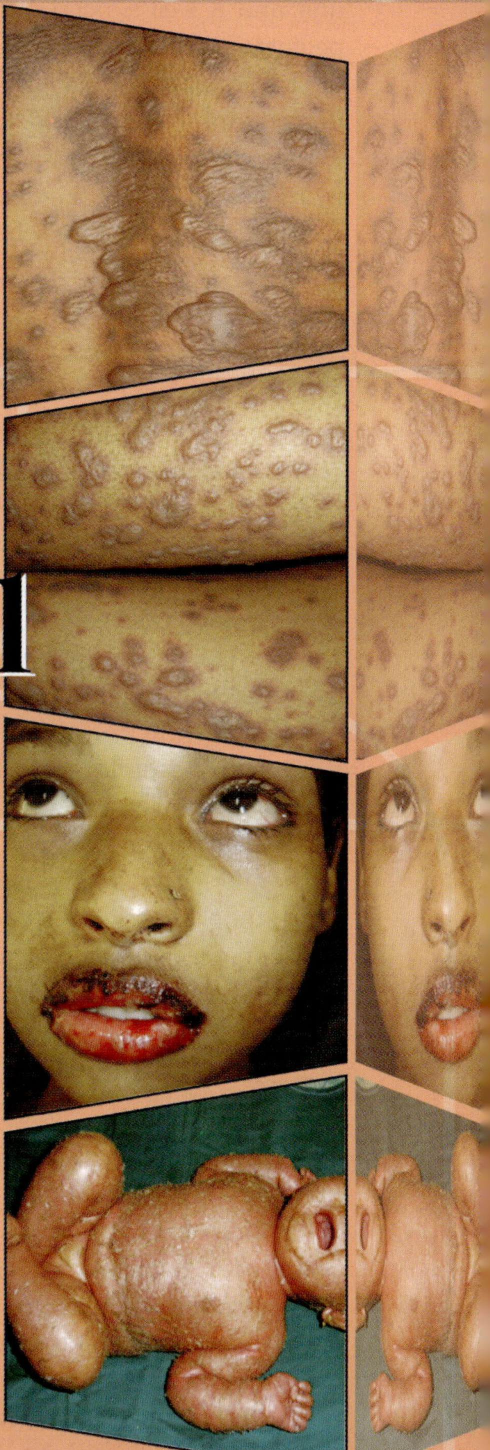

Arun C Inamadar
Ragunatha S

INTRODUCTION

Dermatological emergencies comprise of diseases that demand early diagnosis, hospitalization, careful monitoring and multidisciplinary intensive care to minimize the associated morbidity and mortality. An intensive care unit and a well synchronized team of dermatologist, pediatrician and devoted nursing staff are necessary for the management of patients. In this chapter, the clinical presentation that should alert the possibility of life threatening diseases, and emergency care of such patients is discussed. Details on etiology, pathophysiology and specific treatment of each disease are described in respective chapters.

EPIDEMIOLOGY

A wide range of dermatological conditions need intensive care in children. Some of these disorders, for e.g. epidermolysis bullosa (EB), ichthyoses, staphylococcal scalded skin syndrome (SSSS), Kawasaki disease, etc., are exclusively seen in children. The incidence and spectrum of dermatological emergencies differ in different pediatric age groups. In an Indian study, of total emergency dermatological referrals, 15.5% were neonates, 9.7% were infants, 36.9% were preschool and 37.2% were school going children. Genodermatoses like EB, Collodion baby and Harlequin ichthyosis (37.5%), and SSSS (31.7%) were common in neonates whereas severe atopic and seborrheic dermatitis were common in infants. In preschool and school going children, infections (42.1%) and cutaneous drug reactions (56.4%) respectively, formed majority of cases.

CLASSIFICATION

The presentations of dermatological emergencies vary from localized to extensive skin lesions. Any skin disease in children causes considerable anxiety in parents. Sometimes, relatively benign conditions like Pityriasis rosea, mild viral exanthemas, etc, are perceived by parents as emergencies. Therefore, categorization of diseases that really require emergency care is essential. Depending upon the extent of skin involvement and underlying systemic illness, the dermatological emergencies can be classified into three groups **(Box 28.1)**.

DISEASES CAUSING ACUTE SKIN FAILURE

The dermatological diseases with extensive skin lesions can result in total loss of skin function. In the absence of treatment, acute skin failure can lead to death like any other organ failure. The systemic complications are consequence of primary skin disease. Various vesiculobullous disorders and erythrodermas result in acute skin failure **(Figures 28.1 to 28.4)**. The knowledge of clinical clues and rapid diagnostic tests of these disorders is essential for arriving at the diagnosis and initiation of specific treatment immediately **(Table 28.1)**.

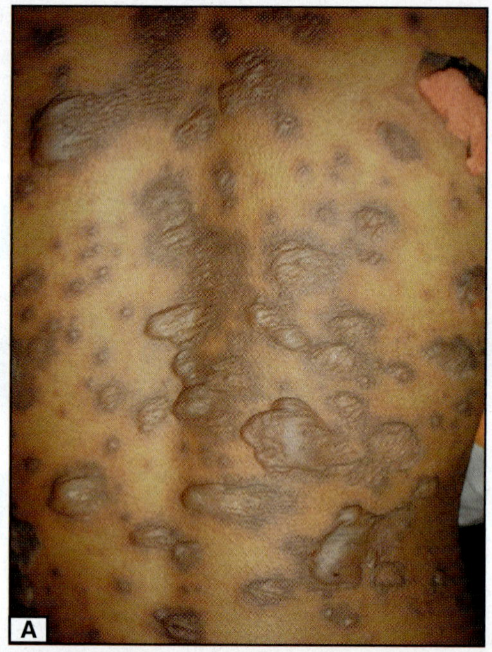

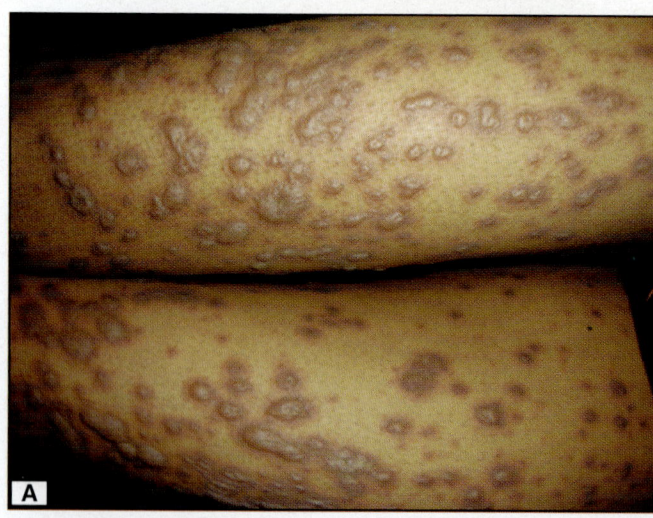

FIGURES 28.1A AND B: Stevens-Johnson syndrome

Box 28.1: Classification of dermatological emergencies

I. Diseases causing Acute Skin Failure
- A. Vesiculobullous and erosive disorders
  1. Mechanobullous diseases: Epidermolysis bullosa (EB)
  2. Staphylococcal scalded skin syndrome (SSSS)
  3. Immunobullous diseases:
     - a. Chronic bullous disorder of childhood
     - b. Pemphigus vulgaris (PV)
     - c. Childhood bullous pemphigoid (BP)
  4. Steven-Johnson syndrome (SJS)/ Toxic epidermal necrolysis (TEN)
- B. Erythroderma
  1. Ichthyoses
     - a. Harlequin Ichthyosis
     - b. Collodion baby
     - c. Bullous congenital ichthyosiform erythroderma (BCIE)
     - d. Non bullous congenital ichthyosiform erythroderma (NBCIE)
     - e. Netherton's syndrome
  2. Leiner's phenotype
  3. Eczemas
     - a. Atopic dermatitis
     - b. Seborrheic dermatitis
     - c. Contact dermatitis
  4. Psoriasis and pustular psoriasis

II. Diseases with or due to underlying severe systemic illness
- A. Kawasaki disease
- B. Purpura fulminans
- C. Urticaria and Angioedema
- D. Infections:
  1. Neonatal herpes simplex infection
  2. Kaposi's varicelliform eruption
  3. Neonatal Varicella
- E. Diffuse cutaneous mastocytosis
- F. Sclerema neonatorum

III. Localized diseases
- A. Subcutaneous infections
- B. Kasabach-Merritt phenomenon

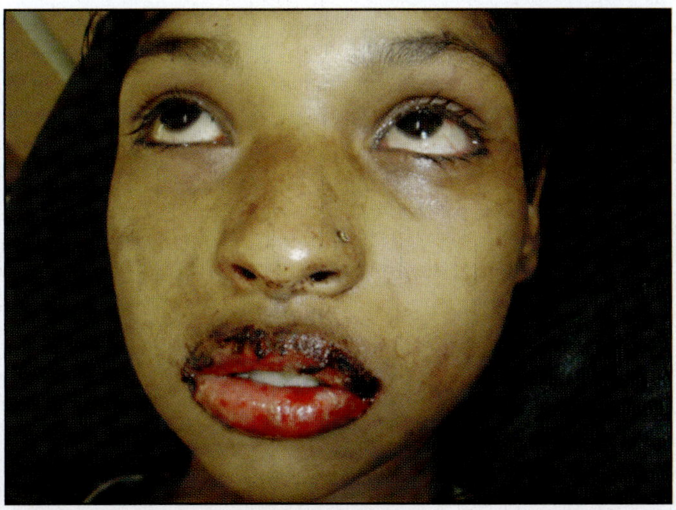

FIGURE 28.2: Hemorrhagic crust on lips and conjunctival congestion in Stevens-Johnson syndrome

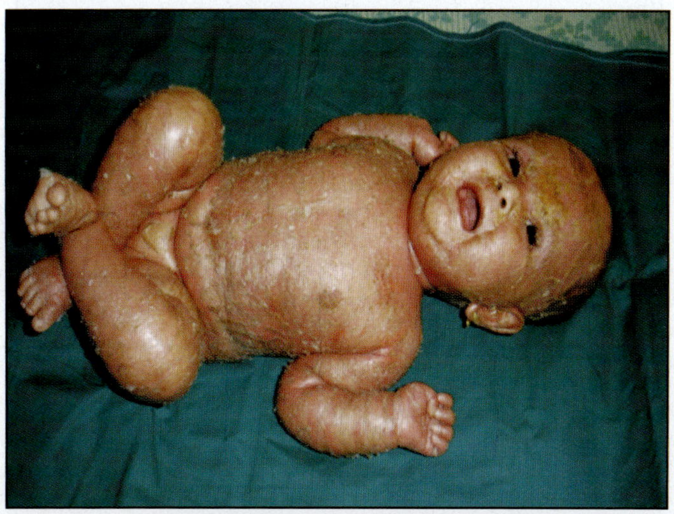

FIGURE 28.3: Infantile erythroderma

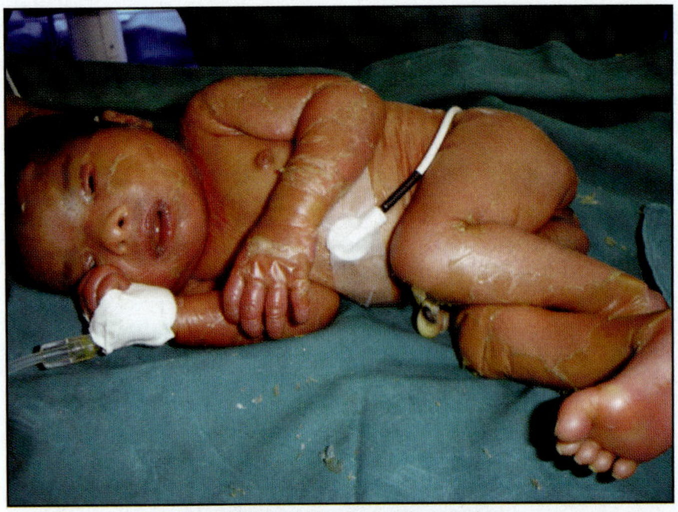

FIGURE 28.4: Collodion baby

ACUTE SKIN FAILURE

Acute skin failure is defined as loss of normal temperature control with inability to maintain the core temperature, and failure to prevent percutaneous loss of fluid, electrolyte and protein with resulting imbalance, and failure of the mechanical barrier to prevent penetration of foreign materials. As with other organ failures, patients with acute skin failure deserve special attention and management protocol.

Consequences of Acute Skin Failure

Fluid and electrolyte imbalance: The transepidermal water loss (TEWL) in erythroderma, and loss of fluid and electrolytes in blister fluid in vesiculobullous disorders result in hypovolemia, dehydration and decreased urinary

TABLE 28.1: Diagnostic clues and rapid diagnostic methods of vesiculobullous disorders causing acute skin failure

Disease/ age group	Diagnostic clues	MM	NS	Investigations	Specific therapy
Neonates					
JEB-H	Tense blisters over buttocks and ear pinnae. Exuberant granulation tissue over periorificial area and nape of neck	Present	-ve	IHC with GB3 (laminin5) antibody, Tzanck test negative	No specific therapy, supportive care
RDEB-HS	Generalized blistering, mitten hands, severe scarring, contractures and involvement of nails	Severe	-ve	IHC with LH7:2 (collagenVII), Tzanck test negative	No specific therapy, supportive care
SSSS	Generalized erythema with tenderness, periorificial and flexural involvement	Absent	+ve	Fried egg like cells with no PMNL on Tzanck test	Antistaphylococcal antibiotics
Preschool or school going					
CBDC	Pruritic tense bullae arranged in cluster jewels pattern predominantly over perineum and periorificial region	Present	-ve	Tzanck test negative, frozen section and IF	Dapsone/ prednisolone
SJS/ TEN	Target like lesions, large parchment like epidermal detachment, prior drug intake	Severe ≥2MM	+ve	Necrotic keratinocytes with PMNL on Tzanck test, frozen section	IV immunoglobulin 3 g/kg in divided doses over 2-3 days, systemic steroid is controversial
Juvenile BP	Pruritic tense bullae, urticarial plaques over inner aspect of thighs, forearms, lower abdomen and groin	Present	-ve	Tzanck test may show eosinophils, frozen section, IF	Prednisolone, 1-2 mg/kg/day
Pemphigus	Flaccid bullae, painful erosions and crusts with involvement of scalp	Severe	+ve	Acantholytic cells on Tzanck test, frozen section, IF	Prednisolone, 1-2 mg/kg/day

Note: BP—bullous pemphigoid, CBDC—chronic bullous disease of childhood, IF—immunofluorescence, IHC—immunohistochemistry, JEB-H—junctional epidermolysis bullosa- Herlitz type, MM—mucus membrane, NS- Nikolsky's sign, PMNL—polymorphonuclear leukocyte, SJS—Steven Johnson syndrome, SSSS—staphylococcal scalded skin syndrome, TEN—toxic epidermal necrolysis output. The blister fluid of autoimmune bullous disorders and TEN contains around 40 g/L of protein, 120-150 mmol/L of Na^+, 100 mmol/L of Cl^- and 5-10 mmol/L of K^+. The serum creatinine and urea nitrogen levels are also raised. If not corrected, hypovolemia may lead to hemodynamic changes, organic renal failure and increased risk of irreversible septic shock.

Protein and calorie loss: In erythroderma, the basal metabolic rate (BMR) may reach a maximum of 2 to 2.5 times to compensate for hypothermia induced by increased cutaneous blood flow. Energy expenditure occurs at the expense of catabolism of proteins as an energy source. This is because of abnormal glycogen regulation resulting from inhibition of insulin secretion and/or insulin resistant. Low environmental temperature also increases the energy expenditure. The dermatogenic enteropathy and decreased synthesis of albumin are other causes of protein loss. In blistering disorders, proteins are lost in the blister fluid.

Impaired thermoregulation: Both hypothermia and fever can occur in acute skin failure. The former is heat loss resulting from increased blood flow and the latter is mediated by interleukin-1 (IL-1) secreted by damaged keratinocytes. The failure of compensatory mechanisms, like increased BMR and shivering, results in poikilothermia (body temperature as that of environmental temperature). Every degree raise in temperature increases the energy loss by 12%. Therefore, any change in temperature worsens both protein and caloric loss, and also evaporative water loss.

Alteration in immunologic function and infection: Alterations in host defense mechanisms are mainly seen in extensive blistering disorders like TEN. IL-1 and tumor necrosis factor-α (TNF-α) released by keratinocytes are probably responsible for decreased immunity against infectious agents. In addition, damaged skin and exudates support the growth of wide spectrum of organisms. *Staphylococcus aureus* is the commonest cause of septicemia in these patients. The use of steroids and broad spectrum antibiotics, and invasive procedures may increase the risk of infection with candida and other unusual organisms.

Systemic Involvement

Pulmonary involvement may be a systemic manifestation and a dreaded complication of TEN. Pulmonary edema can occur as a complication of erythroderma or overzealous correction of hypovolemia.

Management of Acute Skin Failure

In addition to specific treatment, general measures; monitoring hemodynamic changes; fluid and electrolyte balance; nutritional and protein supplementation; prevention of complications; and topical therapy are the pillars of successful management.

General measures:

- Patients should be managed in an intensive care unit or burns unit.
- In infants and young children the body temperature is dependent on the environmental temperature. The temperature regulation is one of the important aspects of management (see above). Hence, the environmental temperature should be maintained at 30-32°C (e.g. using infrared lamp).
- Barrier nursing should be followed strictly in order to prevent the sepsis.
- Periodic examination of involved mucus membranes and their regular cleaning is mandatory to prevent stricture or synechiae formation.
- Once or twice daily bathing with lukewarm water (35-38°C) is recommended.
- Urinary catheter or condom drainage, intravenous line and nasogastric tube are mandatory in severely ill patients.
- In EB, care must be taken to avoid trauma by using protective pads and keeping the environmental temperature cool.

Monitoring hemodynamic changes: In acute skin failure, the body tends to maintain the hemodynamic status through various mechanisms (e.g. release of catecholamines). In the presence of complications such as sepsis and hypovolemia, the indicators of hemodynamic status should be interpreted carefully. The important indicators are pulse rate, urine osmolality and urine output. A drop in urine output is an early and sensitive marker of disturbed hemodynamics and/or of sepsis. Two other sensitive indicators are state of consciousness and respiratory rate. Anxiety, excitement or confusion is often the first symptoms of sepsis. Tachypnea indicates hypoxemia, metabolic acidosis or both. Tachycardia even in the presence of fever suggests hypovolemia. The variation in body weight, total amount

TABLE 28.2: Fluid and electrolyte therapy, and nutrition and protein supplementation in a severely ill child with acute skin failure

Phase	Fluid and Electrolytes	Nutrition*	Protein*
Initial phase (First 24 hrs)	2 ml/kg/%BSA of Ringers lactate plus maintenance fluid-first 10 kg-100 ml/kg second 10 kg-50 ml/kg above 20 kg- 20 ml/kg		
Second 24 hrs	0.25 ml/kg/% BSA 5% albumin in normal saline plus D5W to maintain urine output 1ml/kg/hr	60 kcal/kg + 35 kcal/ %BSA as enteral feeding in equal amount of fluid	3 mg/kg + 1 mg/% BSA
Maintenance phase** (EWL+MF)	[(%BSA + 35)× BSA× 24] / 2 + [1500× BSA (m^2)] of D5 half normal saline with potassium supplements†. (Gradually IV fluid is converted to oral fluids over next few days)		

Note: BSA—body surface area, D5W- 5% dextrose, EWL—evaporative water loss, IV—intravenous, MF—Management fluid. *similar to burns, **should be guided by clinical and laboratory assessment (Box 28.2), †potassium chloride 40mEq/L at a rate of 3 mEq/kg/24 hr

of fluid administered and urine output help in calculation of amount of fluid loss. The acute loss of body weight >1% suggests loss of body water.

Fluid and electrolyte replacement: The infants and younger children have a larger daily turnover of water relative to total body water and large extracellular fluid space, whereas the neonates have high body surface area to weight ratio and functionally immature kidneys. All these factors predispose the children with acute skin failure to a greater risk of fluid and electrolyte imbalance than adults. Though, acute skin failure secondary to vesiculobulous disorders is compared to burns, the fluid requirement is 2/3 to 3/4th of that of burns covering the same area. The fluid and electrolyte therapy in children include, restoration of losses that have already occurred, replacement of ongoing losses and maintenance fluid. During initial 24 hours Ringer's lactate is the fluid of choice. In infants and younger children who are more prone to hypernatremia and lactic acidosis, 0.33% normal saline is preferred instead of Ringer's lactate. The calculation of resuscitation fluid is similar to that of burns. However, in acute skin failure the loss of fluid and electrolytes is far less than what is seen in burns. Therefore, half of the resuscitation fluid calculated for burns is administered in order to avoid pulmonary edema due to fluid overload. These resuscitation formulas are only a rough guide for replacement of fluid and electrolytes, and frequent clinical and laboratory assessment of hydration is necessary **(Box 28.2)**. The main goal of fluid therapy is to maintain the urine output at 1 ml/kg/hr and urine specific gravity at <1.020. After first 24 hrs, the maintenance phase should include maintenance fluid and replacement of ongoing losses **(Table 28.2)**. The former depends on the energy expenditure of the patient and obligatory daily water loss. The latter depends on the composition of the fluid lost, usually evaporative water loss. The potassium should be supplemented only after the correction of urine output.

BOX 28.2: Non invasive guide to fluid resuscitation

1. **Vital signs**
   - Pulse rate
   - Respiratory rate
   - Temperature
   - Blood pressure
2. **Physical examination**
   - Sensorium
   - Body weight
   - Peripheral circulation (capillary filling)
   - Urine output
3. **Laboratory investigations**
   - Hematocrit
   - Blood urea nitrogen and serum creatinine
   - Serum electrolytes
   - Urine electrolytes and osmolality
   - Blood gases and pH
4. **Fluid losses**
   - Gastric
   - Urine
   - Stool

Nutrition and protein supplementation: Aggressive nutrition supplementation should be started preferably through enteral route to minimize the catabolism of proteins, and to provide proteins required for healing of skin lesions, and also for rapid growth of the child. Enteral feeding has the advantage of preserving gastrointestinal integrity and decreasing the incidence of bacterial transmigration across the gut. Severely ill patients may have impaired gastric emptying. Hence, the enteral feeding is initially started with 1/4th of the desired volume and the volume is gradually increased at a rate of 5 ml/hr. The residual gastric volume should be checked by periodic aspiration and feeding is stopped if it is more than 50 ml.

Prevention of sepsis: Hand washing and aseptic handling of the patients has the greatest impact in reducing the risk of infection. The invasive monitoring through contaminated skin can predispose the patient to septicemia and is better avoided. Bacteriology of the skin lesions or discharge or pus should be done at presentation and then on alternate days. The prophylactic antibiotic in the absence of infection is not recommended by many authors. However, antibiotics are indicated in a patient with altered sensorium, sudden hypothermia, high bacterial count from skin or catheter urine sample, and symptoms of systemic infection e.g. pneumonia or urinary tract infection.

Topical therapy: In TEN, the detachable epidermis is preferably left in place. Silver nitrate (0.5%) can be used as paints or dressings. Bland emollients like white petrolatum in vapor permeable dressings (gauze) can be used as epidermal barrier. These emollients prevent the damaged skin surface from sticking to the bed or the apparel. In many centers in India banana leaves are used as non sticky dressings. If available, the biological dressings like amnion and collagen-based skin substitutes, and newer wound dressings like cadaveric allograft, cultured human allogenic or autologous epidermal sheets, and human newborn fibroblasts cultured on a nylon mesh of Biobrane are used to cover the epidermal detachment.

DISEASES WITH OR DUE TO UNDERLYING SYSTEMIC ILLNESS

Certain dermatological diseases are associated with severe systemic involvement and some are manifestations of severe systemic disease. Unlike dermatoses causing acute skin failure, the skin lesions in these disorders per se do not cause any systemic complication. However, the associated mortality is due to underlying systemic disease. Many such cases may present first to the dermatologist or require emergency dermatological opinion. Therefore, these disorders are considered under dermatological emergencies.

KAWASAKI DISEASE

Kawasaki disease (KD) is a multisystem vasculitic syndrome mainly affecting infants and young children. It is an acute febrile illness presenting with characteristic skin and mucus membrane lesions, and lymphadenopathy. The morbidity and mortality is determined by underlying cardiac abnormality. Death can occur at any time during the disease due to acute myocarditis or coronary artery aneurysm. The former is frequently seen during the first week of illness and the latter starts 7 days after the onset of fever. The maximum numbers of deaths occur 3-4 weeks into the illness due to either rupture of coronary artery aneurysm, or myocardial insufficiency caused by coronary artery stenosis or myocarditis. The fatality rate has declined from 10% to 0.1-0.2%.

Diagnosis

The diagnosis of KD is based on fulfillment of five of six diagnostic clinical criterias. However, atypical KD (< 4 criterias) which occurs predominantly in infants is diagnosed when coronary artery abnormality is detected by two- dimensional echocardiography (2- DE). An infant with fever of more than 1 week duration should be investigated for atypical KD. The heart rate and gallop rhythm disproportionate to the degree of fever should also alert the possibility of KD. Once diagnosed, a baseline 2-DE should be done in all cases during the first week and repeated 3-5 weeks later. Coronary angiogram is considered when there is evidence of myocardial insufficiency or to distinguish between stenosis and obstruction which are common in giant aneurysms (>8 mm in diameter).

Management

The coronary artery aneurysm occurs in 25% of untreated patients. The aim of the therapy is to initiate intravenous immunoglobulin (IV Ig) within 10 days of illness, ideally within 7 days. IV Ig can be given even after 10 days if the patient is febrile and there is evidence of ongoing cardiac damage. The recommended therapy is a combination of single dose IV Ig 2 g/kg given as infusion over 8-12 hours and high dose aspirin (30-50 mg/kg/day) to be reduced to 3-5 mg/kg/day after defervescence. If fever recurs, IV Ig dose should be repeated. In the presence of myocardial infarction percutaneous transluminal coronary recanalization should be done within 6 hours. Intravenous urokinase, nitroglycerine, balloon angioplasty or coronary artery bypass grafts can also be considered. If angiography shows three vessel obstruction, severe left coronary artery occlusion or severe occlusion of both left anterior descending and right coronary artery, surgical treatment is indicated.

PURPURA FULMINANS

Purpura fulminans (PF) is a fatal complication of disseminated intravascular coagulation (DIC) that occurs during (acute infectious PF) or immediately after (post infectious PF) a variety of infections. It has been associated with varicella, scarlet fever, streptococcal and pneumococcal bacteremia, and meningococcemia. Neonatal PF can occur in the presence of congenital or acquired protein C and/ or protein S deficiency. During the course of infection or immediately after the child becomes febrile and toxic which heralds appearance of large, sharply demarcated ecchymoses with narrow zone of surrounding erythema. They are usually localized to extremities, though any part of the body may be involved. Hemorrhagic blebs, infarction and necrosis may develop at the site. The disorder is rapidly progressive with peripheral vasoconstriction and shock developing over 48-72 hours. The mortality rate may range from 20% to 30%.

Diagnosis

The characteristic skin lesion and laboratory evidence of DIC [prolonged prothrombin time (PT) and partial thromboplastin time (PTT); reduced fibrinogen levels and platelet count] will clinch the diagnosis of PF. Underlying infection and protein C activity is detected by relevant investigations.

Management

In acute infectious PF, the treatment should be aimed at septic shock. Administration of broad spectrum antibiotics, correction of hypovolemia and electrolyte imbalance is the mainstay of treatment. Fresh frozen plasma (FFP), 8-12 l/kg q 12 hours is given to reduce the risk of hemorrhage and to restore coagulation factors (protein C, protein S and antithrombin). In severe cases, protein C and antithrombin concentrates are given. Low dose heparin, 10 U/kg/hr infusion may be helpful in reducing DIC. In post infectious PF, immediate heparinization should be undertaken. The use of anticoagulants should outweigh the risk of hemorrhage into internal organs. Heparin is given as 100 U/kg IV bolus followed by continuous infusion of 25 U/kg/hr. FFP infusion helps in correction of coagulation factor deficiency (especially protein S). In patients with critical limb ischemia or impending gangrene low dose tissue plasminogen activator, 0.05-0.1 mg/kg/hr is administered carefully to avoid visceral hemorrhage. Surgical intervention is delayed because of severe coagulopathy and absence of clear demarcation between viable and dead tissue during acute phase. However, fasciotomy is necessary if there is evidence of compression of vessels by edematous tissue.

URTICARIA AND ANGIOEDEMA

Ordinary urticaria and angioedema rarely cause serious problems in children. However, they can occur in association with bronchospasm and circulatory collapse in anaphylaxis. Patients with anaphylaxis develop pruritus within seconds to minutes, immediately followed by urticaria and angioedema. Certain physical urticarias like cold induced and aquagenic urticaria (especially during swimming); food allergy and hymenoptera sting may cause anaphylactic reaction. Fatal laryngeal edema is always a manifestation of hereditary angioedema. It is usually associated with diffuse brawny swelling of limbs and abdominal pain. If untreated it may cause death in almost 30% of patients. Laryngeal edema is unlikely to develop if it does not occur during initial few hours of an episode of acute urticaria.

Diagnosis

The diagnosis of anaphylaxis is mainly clinical. Persistently low complement 4 (C4) level and functional assay of C1 esterase inhibitor helps in the diagnosis of hereditary angioedema.

Management

Anaphylaxis is a medical emergency. Venous access and endotracheal tube should be secured immediately. Subcutaneous epinephrine 0.01ml/kg is administered as soon as possible and repeated every 15-20 minutes if necessary. Intravenous or endotracheal administration of a more dilute epinephrine may be required in the presence of complete circulatory collapse. Supplemental therapy with IV fluids, intravenous aminophylline and bronchodilator inhalation is given to treat shock and bronchospasm. However, acute airway obstruction in hereditary angioedema does not respond to epinephrine, steroids or antihistamines. The acute attack is managed by IV fluids, airway maintenance and IV infusion of C1 esterase inhibitor concentrate. In children with increased risk of anaphylactic reaction, an epinephrine injection kit is prescribed, and both children and parents should be educated regarding the injection of epinephrine.

INFECTIONS

Neonatal Herpes Simplex Infection

Neonatal Herpes Simplex infection caused by Herpes Simplex virus-1 (HSV-1) may be localized or disseminated. The latter is life threatening presenting with pneumonia, hepatitis, coagulopathy and encephalitis with or without cutaneous involvement. If untreated the fatality rate of HSV infection and disseminated visceral herpes can be 60% and 90% respectively.

Diagnosis: Any newborn presenting with vesicles, bullae, vesiculopustules, erosions or ulcer should be evaluated for HSV infection. Demonstration of multinucleated giant cells in Tzanck smear is a simple and rapid method of diagnosis. For more quick results direct fluorescent antibody test, PCR and ELISA tests are used. Cerebrospinal fluid analysis is important in diagnosing necrotizing encephalitis. Computed tomography (CT) and magnetic resonance imaging (MRI) of brain are helpful in detecting central nervous system (CNS) inflammation. Electroencephalogram (EEG) may be positive before any imaging study if the infection involves temporal lobe.

Management: Intravenous acyclovir (30 mg/kg/day 8th hrly for 7-10 days) should be started as soon as possible before any systemic complication develops.

Kaposi's Varicelliform Eruption

Kaposi's varicelliform eruption (KVE) is a manifestation of primary HSV-1 or HSV-2 infection in a child with atopic dermatitis and other predisposing conditions like mycosis fungoides, Sézary syndrome, Darier's disease, ichthyosiform erythroderma, second or third degree burns etc. An abrupt onset of umbilicated vesicles predominantly over the area of active or recently healed dermatitis with disproportionately severe systemic symptoms (dehydration and shock) should give rise to the suspicion of KVE. The super infection caused by *Staph aureus, Streptococcus* or *Pseudomonas* and internal organ involvement may lead to death in 10% of patients.

Diagnosis: The laboratory diagnosis is similar to neonatal HSV infection (see above).

Management: Early treatment with intravenous acyclovir (10-15 mg/kg 8th hrly or 40-80 mg/kg/day in 3-4 divided doses for 14-21 days) along with adequate hydration and control of fever is life saving.

Neonatal Varicella

Fulminant neonatal varicella occurs if mother acquires the infection within 4 days prior to or within 2 days after delivery. Disseminated infection with pneumonia, hepatitis or meningoencephalitis is usually fatal. Death from severe pneumonitis and respiratory distress often occurs 4-6 days after the onset of lesions. In the absence of therapy, the mortality rate has been estimated to be 10-30%.

Diagnosis: Detection of viral DNA by PCR and ELISA, direct fluorescent antibody test and Tzanck tests aid in the rapid diagnosis of varicella.

Management: All high risk neonates should receive varicella zoster immunoglobulin (VZIG). In children with fulminant infection, intravenous acyclovir 20 mg/kg every 8 hours for minimum of 5 days and aggressive supportive therapy is required.

Diffuse Cutaneous Mastocytosis

Diffuse cutaneous mastocytosis (DCM) is a rare type of cutaneous mastocytosis characterized by diffuse infiltration of mast cells. Clinically, it presents as generalized thickening of skin with yellowish hue. Hemorrhagic bullae may be the first signs of the disease. Infants presenting with bullae are more likely to have systemic involment. The patients are usually at risk of massive degranulation of mast cells resulting in flushing, hypotension, dyspnea, hemorrhage or overt shock. Various drugs, physical and chemical agents and trauma may act as triggering factors. Unlike urticaria pigmentosa, the prognosis of DCM is guarded.

Diagnosis: DCM should be differentiated from SSSS. Tzanck test and diffuse infiltration of mast cells on histopathology help in correct diagnosis of DCM.

Management: The management of patients with hypotension and shock is similar to anaphylactic reactions. Subcutaneous epinephrine, IV fluids, pressor agents and antihistamines should be started immediately. For bullae and erosions, topical Mupirocin ointment is safe as other antibiotics may contain polymyxin B, a mast cell degranulator. The parents are given a list of triggering factors which should be avoided in order to prevent the massive degranulation of mast cells.

Sclerema Neonatorum

Sclerema neonatorum is a rare skin disease that occurs during first 1-2 weeks of life in severely debilitated term and preterm infants. It is characterized by sudden onset of diffuse hardening of skin appearing first over the lower limb and later spreading to thighs, buttocks, trunk and cheeks sparing palms, soles and genitalia. The involved skin is cold, smooth, hard and bound down. The infant is usually poorly nourished, dehydrated, hypotensive and hypothermic. Septicemia, necrotizing enterocolitis, pneumonia, intracranial hemorrhage, hypoglycemia or electrolyte disturbance is often associated with sclerema. It is regarded as end stage of severe systemic diseases and the death is likely in most of cases except for sepsis where the chance of survival may be 70%.

Diagnosis: The diagnosis is mainly clinical. The laboratory abnormalities may include hyperkalemia, hyponatremia, hypoglycemia and azotemia.

Management: Systemic corticosteroids with exchange transfusion and antibiotics improved the survival rate in infants with sepsis. Thermoregulation, fluid electrolyte balance and nutritional supplementation are also important in reducing the inevitable mortality.

LOCALIZED DISEASES

SUBCUTANEOUS INFECTIONS

Subcutaneous infections span wide spectrum of severity. Though localized, they can cause significant morbidity in the form of amputation of the affected limb. In the absence of signs and symptoms requiring immediate surgical intervention **(Box 28.3)**, relatively less severe infections like erysipelas and cellulitis can be treated conservatively with appropriate antibiotics. While on conservative management, extension of lesions beyond initial limits, fever lasting more than 2 days after antibiotic therapy and worsening of general status warrant emergency surgery. More invasive infections like necrotizing fascitis, gangrenous cellulitis and myonecrosis are considered as surgical emergencies. Excision of devitalized skin by an experienced surgeon will prevent the extension of the infection and compartmental syndrome.

BOX 28.3: Signs and symptoms requiring immediate surgical intervention

Local
- Skin anesthesia
- Skin necrosis
- Mottled or livedoid cyanosis
- Livid and cold extremity
- Crepitations
- Presence of gas on X- ray

Systemic
- Rapid respiration
- Altered consciousness
- oliguria

KASABACH-MERRITT PHENOMENON

Kasabach-Merritt phenomenon (KMP) is a localized variant of consumptive coagulopathy usually seen in infants younger than 3 months of age. It is caused by sequestration of platelets, accumulation of activated coagulation factors and local fibrinolysis in a congenital vascular tumor. Contrary to earlier belief that the tumor is a true hemangioma of infancy, the KMP occurs in infants with Kaposi's hemangioendothelioma (KHE) or tufted angioma. KHE is an aggressive, rapidly enlarging, deep red to violaceous indurated tumor with advancing ecchymotic ring. The rapidly enlarging tumor may compress the vital structures and the thrombocytopenia may cause acute hemorrhage in various internal organs. Visceral KMP such as cervicothoracic, abdominal, pelvic or intracranial is always life threatening. In an infant, any rapidly growing vascular tumor with or without ecchymosis should be evaluated for both cutaneous and visceral KMP. The presence of pallor, prolonged bleeding, spontaneous ecchymosis and petechiae, hematuria, and epitaxis indicate DIC. The disease causes mortality in 20-30% of patients.

Diagnosis

Laboratory evidence of consumptive coagulopathy (prolonged PT and PTT, reduced fibrinogen, and elevated D-dimer levels) and thrombocytopenia along with clinical course of the tumor confirm the diagnosis of KMP. Destructive vascular lesions on MRI aid in the diagnosis of visceral KMP.

Management

KMP is unique in that the manifestations of coagulopathy are localized to the vascular tumor itself. No single treatment modality is universally effective and hence combination therapy is necessary. Prednisolone 2-5 mg/kg/day have been effective in increasing platelet count and decreasing the size of tumor in some cases. Vincristine (1-1.5 mg/m^2 or 0.05-0.65 mg/kg weekly IV) has been found to be effective which can be used as first line of treatment. Controversies exist about transfusion of blood products in the presence of accelerated consumption of coagulation factors. However, supportive therapy with FFP and cryoprecipitate may be helpful. Platelet transfusion should be avoided unless there is significant bleeding. Surgical excision by an experienced vascular surgeon with prior transfusion of platelet is safe in well circumscribed, superficial vascular tumors with KMP. Other therapeutic options are interferon-α, ticlopidine plus aspirin, ε-aminocaproic acid, cyclophosphomide, and arterial embolization. Ionizing radiation (X-ray) is considered only if the condition is life threatening and the tumor is not responding to medical treatment.

REFERENCES

1. Beltrani VS. Urticaria and angioedema. Dermatol Clin 1996; 14(1):171-97.
2. Cohen PR. Tests for detecting herpes simplex virus and varicella- zoster virus infections. Dermatol Clin 1994; 12: 51-68.
3. Duarte AM, Pruksachatkunakorn C, Schachner LA. Life-threatening dermatoses in pediatric dermatology. Advances in dermatology 1995;10: 329-72.
4. Finkelstein JL, Schwartz SB, Madden MR, Marano MA, Goodwin CW. Pediatric burns. An overview. Pediatr Clin Nor Am 1992; 39(5): 1145-64.
5. Inamadar AC, Palit A. Acute skin failure: Concept, causes, consequences and care. Indian J Dermatol Venereol Leprol 2005; 71: 379-85.
6. Irvine C. "Skin failure"- a real entity: discussion paper. J R Soc Med 1991; 84: 412-13.
7. Kane TD, Warden GD. Pediatric burn injury. In: Rudolph AM, Hoffman JIE, Rudolph CD, eds. Rudolph's Pediatrics. 20th edn. London: Pentice Hall International Ltd, 1996; 861-7.
8. Kimberlin DW, Jacobs RF, Powell DA et al. The safety and efficacy of high dose acyclovir in neonatal herpes simplex virus infection. Pediatrics 2001; 108: 230-8.
9. Kwong KY, Maalouf N, Jones CA. Urticaria and angioedema: pathophysiology, diagnosis and treatment. Pediatr Annals 1998; 27: 719-24.
10. Levin M, Eley B. Purpura fulminans. In: Harper J, Oranje A, Prose N, eds. Textbook of pediatric dermatology. Blackwell Science 2006;1:1574-87.
11. Newburger JW, Takahashi M, Beiser AS et al. A single intravenous infusion of gamma globulin as compared with four infusions in the treatment of acute Kawasaki syndrome. New Eng J Med 1991;324:1633-9.
12. Roujeau JC, Revuz J. Intensive care in dermatology. In: Champion RH, Pye RJ, eds. Recent advances in dermatology. Edinburgh: Churchill Livinstone, 1990; 8:85-100.
13. Siegel NS, Lattazi WE. Fluid and electrolyte therapy in children. In: Arieff AI, DeFronzo RA, eds. Fluid, Electrolyte and Acid-Base disorders. New York: Churchill Livingstone, 1985;1:1211-30.
14. Whitney R, Arvin A, Prober C et al. Predictors of morbidity and mortality in neonates with herpes simplex virus infections. The National Institute of Allergy and Infectious Diseases Collaborative Antiviral Study Group. N Engl J Med 1991; 324:450-4.

29

Nutritional Deficiency Disorders

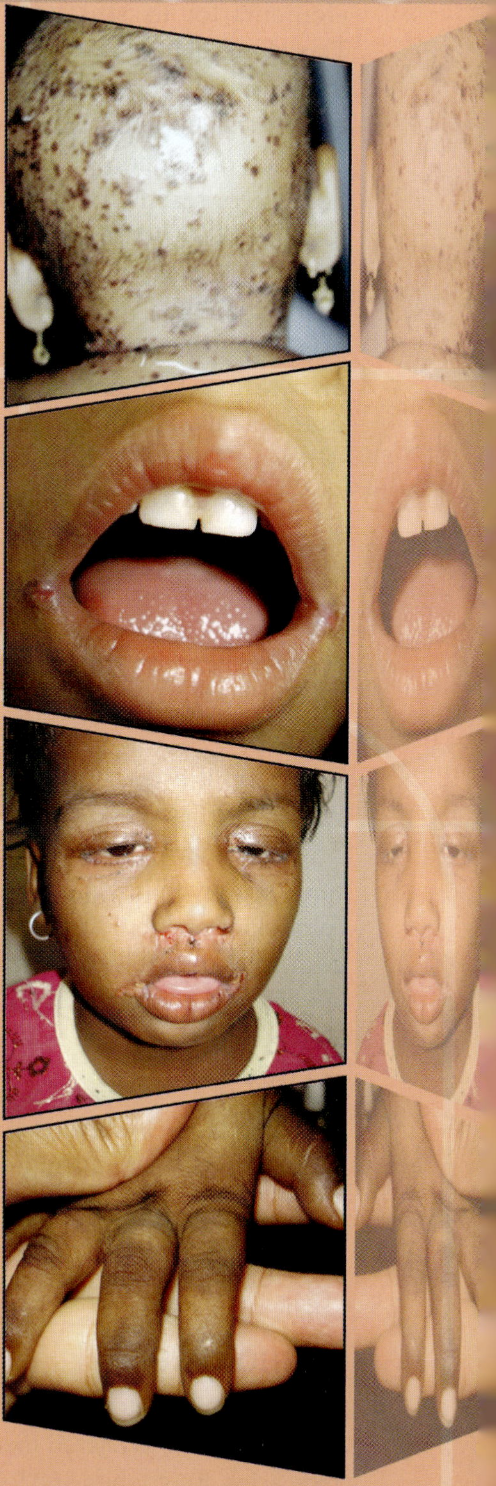

Aparna Palit
Ragunatha S

INTRODUCTION

Nutrition is necessary for growth of the body and maintenance of health. Like other organs of the body, skin is also dependent on various nutrients such as proteins, lipids, carbohydrates, vitamins and trace elements for its structural integrity and functions. Therefore, skin changes can develop if any of these nutrients are deficient. The infants, children and elderly are particularly susceptible to the risk of malnutrition. The disorders of nutrition are common in third world countries because of scarcity of food. Malabsorption syndromes, hepatic diseases, inborn errors of metabolism and intestinal surgeries may also result in malnutrition. Certain eating disorders like anorexia nervosa and bulimia nervosa can present with malnutrition. The biochemical pathways of pyridoxine, thiamine, riboflavin, niacin, zinc and essential fatty acids intersect with each other. Therefore, deficiency of multiple nutrients should be suspected if a child presents with a disorder of nutrition. In this chapter cutaneous manifestation of various nutrition deficiency disorders is discussed.

RIBOFLAVIN (VITAMIN B_2) DEFICIENCY

Riboflavin is a component of co-enzymes flavin mononucleotide (FMN) and flavin-adenine dinucleotide (FAD). These coenzymes are required for various metabolic and oxidative-phosphorylation pathways in the body. Pyridoxine metabolism also requires flavins. Once absorbed in the proximal small intestine by active transport, riboflavin is converted into FMN and then to FAD.

CAUSES

The clinical manifestations of riboflavin deficiency usually occur after 3-5 months of an inadequate diet. The riboflavin deficiency is seen in patients with hypothyroidism, acute boric acid poisoning, neonatal phototherapy for hyperbilirubinemia, and chlorpromazine ingestion.

PATHOGENESIS

The clinical manifestations seen in riboflavin deficiency are mainly due to altered metabolism of pyridoxine, free fatty acids, tryptophan and folic acid. Flavins are required for the metabolic pathway of these nutrients.

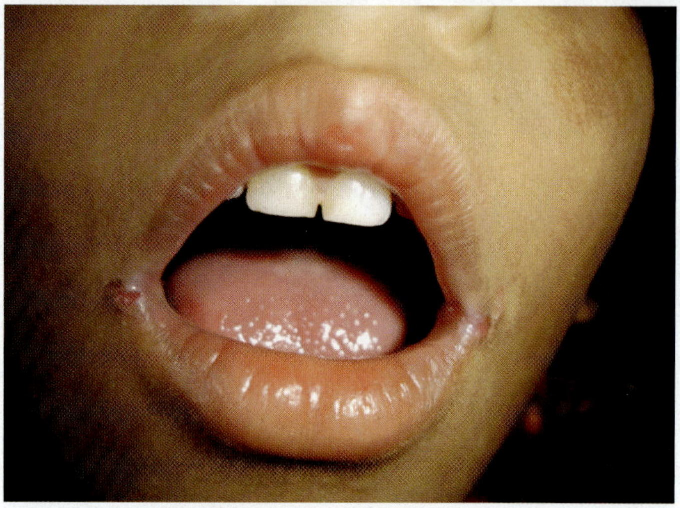

FIGURE 29.1: Angular cheilosis

CLINICAL MANIFESTATIONS

The characteristic cutaneous manifestations include stomatitis, angular cheilosis **(Figure 29.1)**, glossitis, and seborrheic dermatitis like lesions. Glossitis presents as magenta tongue with loss of filiform papillae. Scrotal dermatitis with sparing of median commisure is also seen in riboflavin deficiency.

Extracutaneous features include retarded intellectual development and electroencephalogram changes.

MANAGEMENT

Dietary supplementation rich in riboflavin such as milk, meat, fish and eggs is recommended. In deficient infants 1-3 mg/ day of riboflavin is indicated.

NIACIN (VITAMIN B_3) DEFICIENCY

Niacin (nicotinic acid) plays an important role in various metabolic pathways. The coenzymes synthesized from niacin, nicotinamide-adenine dinucleotide (NAD) and NAD phosphate (NADP) are involved in electron transport, respiratory chain, and fatty acid synthesis. Meat, poultry, fish, dry beans, nuts and eggs are rich sources of niacin. Trigonelline, an alkaloid present in coffee, can form nicotinic acid in the presence heat and acid. This reaction occurs during the roasting of coffee beans and increases the niacin content of the coffee by 30 folds.

CAUSES

Niacin deficiency occurs as a result of inadequate diet, malabsorption, or defects in the tryptophan-niacin pathway. The deficiency is endemic in certain areas where maize or jowar is the stapple diet. In maize, niacin is present in bound form which cannot be utilized in the body. The alkaline hydrolysis (washing corn with lime water) method releases niacin and thereby forestalls the deficiency. Jowar contains large quantities of leucin apart from adequate levels of niacin. Leucin interferes with the tryptophan and niacin pathway resulting in niacin deficiency.

Certain drugs such as isonoazid, 6-mercaptopurine and 5-fluorouracil have been found to cause niacin deficiency by interfering with the tryptophan-niacin pathway. Isoniazid impairs the function of pyridoxine which is a cofactor in the tryptophan-niacin pathway. 6-mercaptopurine inhibits the synthesis of NAD by interfering with NAD phophorylase.

Niacin deficiency is also seen in patients with carcinoid syndrome and Hartnup disease. In the former, tryptophan is utilized for the synthesis of excess of serotonin whereas in the latter, the absorption and reabsorption of tryptophan and other monoamine and monocarboxylic amino acids is impaired due to defect in the neutral brush border system throughout the body.

In the body every 60 mg excess of tryptophan is converted into 1mg of niacin. This conversion requires vitamin B_1 and vitamin B_6. Therefore, deficiency of one of these vitamins can also precipitate pellagra.

PATHOGENESIS

NAD and NADP are required for high energy transfer reactions in the body. Therefore, the organs with high energy requirement (brain) and high turnover rates (skin and gut) are predominantly affected by niacin deficiency. Impaired zinc or fatty acid metabolism may also contribute to the cutaneous manifestations.

Photosensitivity seen in pellagra has been postulated to occur as a result of deficiency of urocanic acid, a chromophore synthesized in the skin which absorbs ultraviolet-B rays. Similarly, accumulation of kynurenic acid in pellagra induces phototoxic changes when exposed to ultraviolet radiation. Ichthyotic skin changes are probably due to atrophy of sebaceous glands and decrease in wax ester content of sebum. The gastrointestinal symptoms are secondary to degenerative changes in dorsal vagal nuclei. Similarly, chromatolysis of cortical and brain stem nuclei result in neurological manifestations.

CLINICAL FEATURES

The disease caused by niacin deficiency is called as pellagra. The classical manifestations of pellagra are referred as 3 D's, dermatitis, diarrhea and dementia. Eventually 4th D, death, follows if the patient is not treated. The dermatitis component presents as painful, erythematous, well demarcated patches symmetrically distributed over sun-exposed areas of the body such as dorsal aspect of hands, extensor aspect of forearms, neck, face and upper part of the chest. There may be appearance of flaccid bullae. Eventually the lesions become well demarcated keratotic, hyperpigmented, ichthyotic plaques. The involvement of upper central portion of chest and neck resembles Casal's necklace. Other features like cheilosis, glossitis, angular stomatitis, and oral and perirectal ulcers are also seen.

Extracutaneous manifestations of pellagra include diarrhea, anorexia, and neuropsychiatric changes such as apathy, depression, psychosis, coma and encephalopathy.

MANAGEMENT

Fluorometric assay of urinary levels of N-methyl-nicotinamide (NMN) below 0.8 mg and ratio of urinary NMN to N-methyl-2-pyridone-5-carboxamide >2.0 are suggestive of niacin deficiency. Pellagra responds dramatically to treatment. Niacinamide is preferred to niacin because the former lacks vasomotor disturbances. Niacinamide is used in the dosage of 100-300 mg/ day in divided doses. Following initiation of treatment mental disturbances disappear within 24-48 hours but skin lesions may take 3-4 weeks.

PYRIDOXINE (VITAMINE B_6) DEFICIENCY

Pyridoxine exists in three biologically interchangeable forms, pyridoxine, pyridoxamine and pyridoxal. These undergo phosphorylation to become active coenzymes. Pyridoxal 5-phosphate (PDP) is an important coenzyme of pyridoxine which is essential for the metabolism of amino acids.

CAUSES

Pyridoxine deficiency can occur in patients taking isoniazid, hydralazine and penicillamine. These drugs increase excretion or decrease activity of PDP. A low level of pyridoxine has been reported in patients with uremia and cirrhosis.

PATHOGENESIS

The cutaneous changes that occur in pyridoxine may be due to its role in tryptophan-niacin pathway and essential fatty acid synthesis. Pyridoxine is required for kynurenase that converts 3-hydroxy kynurenine to 3-hydroxy anthranilic acid in tryptophan-niacin pathway. In pyridoxine deficiency, it has been shown that there is decreased synthesis of arachadonic acid and accumulation of essential fatty acids.

CLINICAL FEATURES

The cutaneous manifestation of pyridoxine deficiency resembles that of riboflavin and niacin deficiency. Seborrheic-like dermatitis, glossitis, angular stomatitis, cheilosis, conjunctivitis and intertrigo are the common cutaneous manifestations. Rarely, pellagra-like dermatitis can occur.

Extracutaneous manifestation mainly involves the nervous system. Somnolence and confusion are commonly seen in pyridoxine deficiency. Sensory neuritis presents as hyperesthesias, ascending parasthesias, altered vibration and position sense, and hypoactive deep tendon reflexes. Hematologic abnormalities like normocytic, normochromic anemia and absolute lymphopenia may also occur especially in patients taking deoxypyridoxine. In severe cutaneous involvement, eosinophilia has been reported.

MANAGEMENT

The plasma or serum level of pyridoxine-6-phosphate <20 ng/ ml indicates pyridoxine deficiency. Replacement of pyridoxine depends on the underlying cause of deficiency. The normalization of tryptophan metabolism induced by isoniazid and penicillamine requires 30 mg/ day and 100 mg/ day of pyridoxine respectively. Following replacement therapy the oral lesions resolve in days, skin and hematological changes in weeks and neurological changes in months.

VITAMIN B_{12} DEFICIENCY

Vitamin B_{12}, cyanocobalamine, is required for folate metabolism and synthesis of myelin. Following oral intake vitamin B_{12} is absorbed from the ileum. Intrinsic factor synthesized by the gastric mucosa is necessary for its absorption. A period of 3 to 6 years is required for deficiency states to manifest because of large body stores of vitamin B_{12} (4 mg).

CAUSES

Vitamin B_{12} deficiency occurs due to impaired absorption in the ileum and decreased synthesis of intrinsic factor by gastric mucosa. The former is caused by tropical sprue, regional enteritis, tuberculosis, Whipple's disease, postilectomy states, and Zollinger-Ellison syndrome, and the latter is caused by pernicious anemia and postgastrectomy states. Microbial competition for vitamin B_{12} in the gut because of bacterial overgrowth and Diphyllobothrium latum infection, can also lead to the deficiency.

PATHOGENESIS

The vitamin B_{12} deficiency indirectly affects synthesis of melanin resulting in hyperpigmentation. Normally, the reduced glutathione inhibits tyrosinase and vitamin B_{12} maintains the reduced form of glutathione. In vitamin B_{12} deficiency, the increased activity of glutathione results in hyperpigmentation. Similarly, biopterin which is required for hydroxylation of phenylalanine, a step in the melanogenesis, is increased as a result of altered folate metabolism. There is also impaired incorporation and redistribution of melanin in epidermis due to megablastic changes in keratinocytes.

The abnormal folate metabolism and myelin synthesis are responsible for hematological and neurological manifestations of vitamin B_{12} deficiency, respectively.

CLINICAL FEATURES

The clinical manifestations of vitamin B_{12} deficiency commonly involve blood and nervous system. The cutaneous changes are rare. The typical presentation is generalized hyperpigmentation with accentuation in flexures, palmar creases and knuckles **(Figure 29.2)**. The palms and soles show multiple, descrete, hyperpigmented macules. The nail changes include longitudinal melanonychia. Pigmentation of oral mucosa, an enlarged beefy red tongue and poliosis may also be seen.

The extracutaneous features include paresthesias, numbness of extremities, ataxia, abnormal reflexes, altered mental status and megaloblastic anemia.

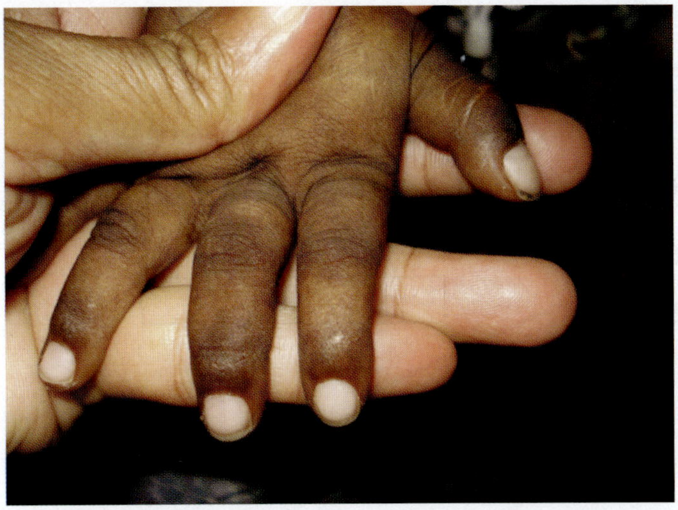

FIGURE 29.2: Knuckle pigmentation in vitamin B_{12} deficiency

MANAGEMENT

Vitamin B_{12} deficiency can be detected by microbiologic or radioassay of plasma or serum cyanocobalamine (<150 pg/ml). Vitamin B_{12} deficiency is treated with parenteral cyanocobalamin with initial dose of 1mg/ week for one month and thereafter, 1mg/ month. Following therapy, the weakness diminishes in days, hematocrit normalizes in weeks and cutaneous changes disappear in years. However, the neurologic manifestations may or may not resolve.

VITAMIN C (ASCORBIC ACID) DEFICIENCY

Vitamin C is a water soluble vitamin. Human body cannot synthesize vitamin C and hence it depends on exogenous dietary sources such as citrus fruits and vegetables. It is a potent reducing agent that is easily oxidized and destroyed by heating.

CAUSES

Chronic inadequate intake of dietary sources is the main cause of vitamin C deficiency. Inadequate intake may be due to anorexia nervosa, food faddism, restrictive diet imposed by food allergies, neurodevelopmental abnormalities compromising the oral intake of food and famines. The vitamin C requirement is increased by febrile illnesses, iron deficiency, cold exposure, or protein depletion. Vitamin C deficiency in mother may cause scurvy in her breast-fed infant.

PATHOGENESIS

Vitamin C is an important cofactor for enzymes involved in the synthesis of catecholamines, melanin, corticosteroids, carnitine, peptide hormones and collagen. Vitamin C also increases the intestinal absorption of iron. As a potent redox agent, vitamin C protects DNA, proteins, lipids, lipoproteins and vessel walls from free radical injury. Other functions of vitamin C include conversion of folate into active metabolites and formation of reduced disulfide bonds in hair follicles.

The major manifestations of vitamin C deficiency are due to defective synthesis of collagen. Therefore, the pathologic changes and respective clinical features are common in organs or tissues containing collagen such as skin, cartilage, bone, dentine and blood vessels **(Figure 29.3)**.

CLINICAL FEATURES

The clinical condition resulting from vitamin C deficiency is known as scurvy. It usually manifests after 1-3 months of inadequate intake of vitamin C. Scurvy is commonly seen in children between 6 months to 7 years of age. Majority of cases of infantile scurvy occur between 6-24 months of age. Development of scurvy during neonatal period is very rare.

In children, the organs or tissues in growth phase are predominantly affected. Therefore, characteristic manifestations of scurvy involve in musculoskeletal system, gums, and teeth **(see Figure 29.3)**. Cutaneous features such as perifollicular hemorrhages, perifollicular hyperkeratotic papules, and corkscrew hairs are rarely seen in infantile scurvy. Initially child presents with non-specific symptoms like irritability, lethargy, malaise, tachypnea, fever, diarrhea and poor weight gain.

The gum changes are seen only if teeth have erupted. The child assumes a frog like position due to severe tenderness. Scorbutic rosary, sharply angled beads at the costochondral junctions of ribs with depressed sternum is characteristic of scurvy. A Sjogren-like sicca syndrome characterized by xerostomia, keratoconjunctival sicca and enlargement of salivary glands has been reported.

MANAGEMENT

The diagnosis of scurvy is established by characteristic clinical features, radiological changes and history of

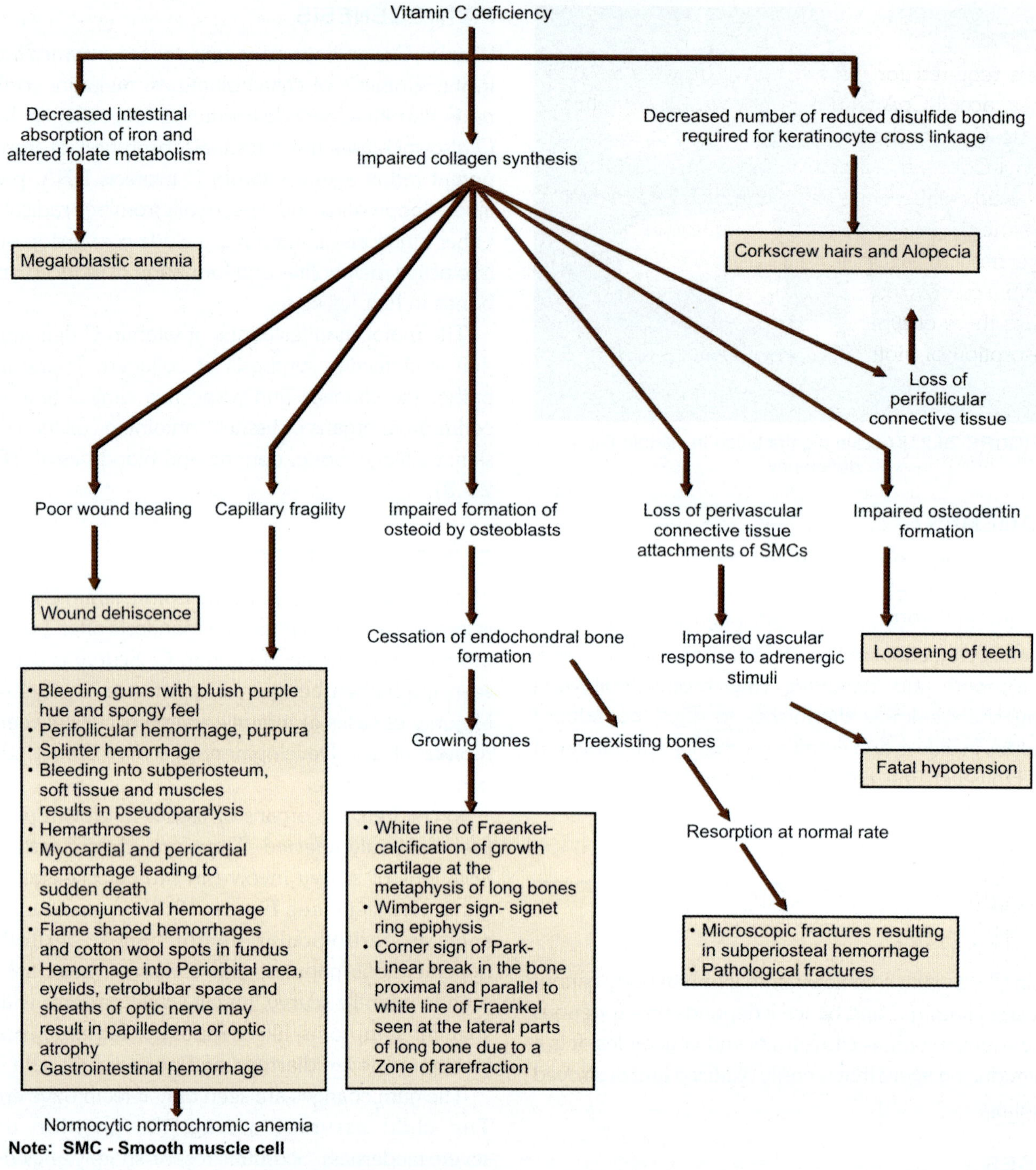

FIGURE 29.3: Clinicopathological correlation in scurvy

inadequate intake of vitamin C. Laboratory tests are usually not of much help in the diagnosis of scurvy. Though serum ascorbic acid levels <0.1 mg/dl suggest scurvy, this value may be affected by recent dietary intake of vitamin C. The more specific leukocyte ascorbic acid level is difficult to perform and is not available in all centers.

Vitamin C should be given in dosage of 25 mg orally every 6 hourly for 1 week and then recommended daily allowance is continued. Following initiation of therapy hypotension normalizes in 24 hours, spontaneous bleeding and gum changes resolve in 2-3 days, ecchymoses in 10-12 days, and anemia in 2-3 weeks.

BIOTIN (VITAMIN H) DEFICIENCY

Biotin is required for the function of four carboxylase enzymes, acetyl-CoA carboxylase (fatty acid synthesis); pyruvate-CoA carboxylase (gluconeogenesis); and propionyl-CoA and 3-methylcrotonyl-CoA carboxylases (amino acid catabolism). These enzymes become active when biotin is linked to inactive apocarboxylase by the enzyme holocarboxylase synthetase. The recycling of biotin from carboxylase is carried out by biotinidase which degrades these enzymes. Biotinidase is also responsible for absorption of biotin from the intestine.

CAUSES

Impaired absorption and bacterial synthesis of biotin in the intestine, deficiency of holocarboxylase synthetase and biotinidase enzymes can all lead to biotin deficiency. The first two causes are acquired and rare, whereas the last two are genetic.

The acquired form is rare and is usually due to excess intake of raw eggs. The avidin present in egg white binds tightly to biotin and impairs its absorption from the gut. Impaired absorption along with decreased bacterial synthesis of biotin can also occur in infants with short gut syndrome on broad spectrum antibiotics.

The genetic forms are inherited as autosomal recessive disorders. Holocarboxylase synthetase deficiency causes neonatal biotin deficiency which usually manifests during first 6 weeks of life. Biotinidase deficiency causes infantile biotin deficiency after first 3 months of life.

CLINICAL FEATURES

The biotin deficiency results in metabolic, neuropsychiatric, and cutaneous changes that resemble acrodermatitis enteropathica **(Figure 29.4)**. The severity of manifestations depends on the cause of biotin deficiency **(Table 29.1)**. Neonatal biotin deficiency is fatal if not treated or diagnosed early. The intercurrent illnesses may precipitate metabolic acidosis.

MANAGEMENT

In genetic forms, the diagnosis is established by estimation of urinary organic acid excretion. 3-hydroxyisovaleric acid is the major metabolite excreted in biotin deficiency. Low biotinidase level in serum is diagnostic of infantile biotin deficiency.

The signs and symptoms resolve completely following biotin therapy. The dosage of biotin and duration of therapy depends on the cause of biotin deficiency **(see**

TABLE 29.1: Clinical features of different forms of biotin deficiency

Characteristics	Acquired biotin deficiency	Genetic forms	
		Neonatal biotin deficiency	Infantile biotin deficiency
Cause	Excess intake of raw egg (avidin), impaired absorption, microbial production in gut	HCS deficiency (AR)	Biotidinase deficiency (AR)
Age of onset	Any	First 6 wks of life	After 3 months of life
Presentation	Xerosis, periorifial eczema, alopecia, atrophic tongue and pallor	Severe metabolic acidosis, organic aciduria, extensive dermatitis of intertrigenous area, universal alopecia	Metabolic acidosis, lactic academia, organic aciduria, less severe periorifial dermatitits, patchy alopecia
Other features	Anorexia, irritability, depression, myalgia, hyperesthesia, hypotonia	Seizures, abnormal muscle tone, athetosis, coma	Seizures, ataxia, optic nerve atrophy, neurosensory hearing loss Keratoconjunctivitis
Diagnosis	Clinical	Urinary organic acid excretion (3-HIVA)	Urinary organic acid excretion (3-HIVA), low biotidinase levels in serum
Treatment	150ìg/ day of biotin	10-40 mg/ day of biotin	5-10 mg/ day of biotin

Note: AR, Autosomal recessive; HCS, Holocarboxylase synthetase; 3-HIVA, Hydroxyisovaleric acid

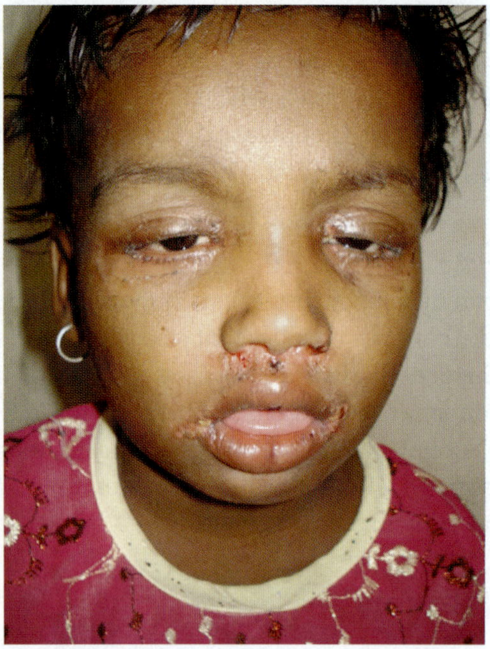

FIGURE 29.4: Periorificial dermatitis resembling acrodermatitis enteropathica in biotin deficiency

Table 29.1). In inherited forms, the biotin supplementation is life long.

VITAMIN A DEFICIENCY

Vitamin A is a fat soluble vitamin essential for normal functioning of eyes, gonads and skin. There are three physiologic forms of vitamin A, retinol, retinal and retinoic acid. Vitamin A presents in the animal sources as retinyl ester which is hydrolyzed to retinol before intestinal uptake. The vegetable sources (beta-carotene) contain retinal which is reduced to retinol in the villous cells.

CAUSES

Vitamin A deficiency commonly occurs following inadequate dietary intake. In developed countries it is associated with fat malabsorption and liver disease. Vitamin A deficiency occurring following small bowel bypass surgery has been reported.

CLINICAL FEATURES

Follicular hyperkeratosis presenting as asymptomatic, discrete, keratotic, acuminate and pigmented follicular papules with central keratinous plug **(Figure 29.5)** is the characteristic cutaneous manifestation of vitamin A deficiency. This condition is commonly refered as

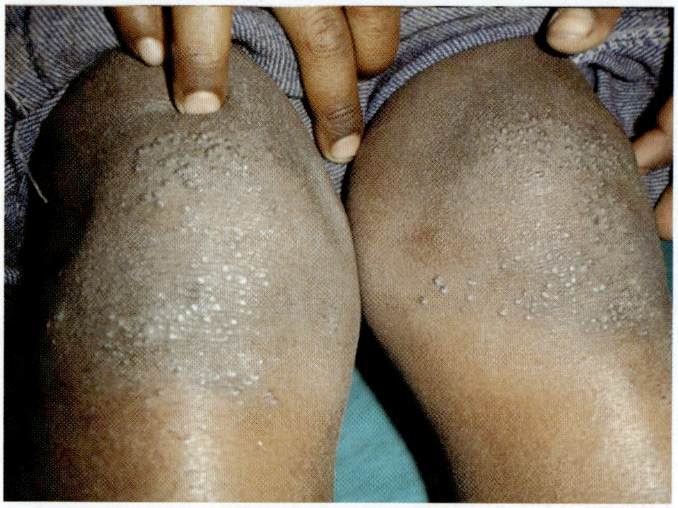

FIGURE 29.5: Phrynoderma

phrynoderma, meaning 'toad skin'. Generalized xerosis is usually seen in vitamin A deficiency.

Phrynoderma is a disorder of follicular keratinization commonly seen in children and adolescents. The exact etiology of phrynoderma is not yet clear. Deficiencies of various nutrients such as vitamin A, essential fatty acids, vitamin B complex, vitamin E, and vitamin C have been proposed. However, the evidences in favor of these nutrients as the sole cause of phynoderma are inconsistent.

Phrynoderma is common in children between 5-15 years of age. Clinically, the lesions (see above) are distributed symmetrically over areas of friction such as elbows, knees and buttocks. The lesions feel like nutmeg grater. The surrounding skin usually shows pigmentation and dryness. The lesions may be generalized involving face and trunk. Increased prevalence of phrynoderma during winter season has been reported.

The ocular manifestations of vitamin A deficiency are commonly seen in children less than 5 years of age. These include night blindness, Bitots spots, xerophthalmia, keratomalacia and blindness.

MANAGEMENT

The diagnosis of phrynoderma is mainly clinical. Low serum retinol, vitamin B complex, vitamin E or essential fatty acids levels have been reported. Similarly, all these nutrients have been used in the treatment of phrynoderma with variable success. Systemic vitamin A, vitamin B complex and essential fatty acids were found to be effective. Topical keratinolytics can also be used.

ESSENTIAL FATTY ACID DEFICIENCY

EFAs are unsaturated fatty acids with 18-, 20-, or 22-carbon chain length. There are three series of fatty acids exist (n-3, n-6, and n-9) each originating from a different 18-carbon chain EFAs. Linoleic acid, from which arachidonic acid is produced, belongs to n-6 series. Essential fatty acids (EFAs) cannot be synthesized in the human body and hence they must be derived from the diet. Inadequate linoleic acid intake results in increased levels of products (eicosatrienoic acid) of n-9 series. Therefore, high ratio (>0.4) of eicosatrienoic acid to arachidonic acid (tetraenoic acid) indicates essential fatty acid deficiency.

CAUSES

EFA deficiency can develop in low birth weight infants because of insufficient EFA stores. It can also occur in infants with gastrointestinal abnormalities, or inflammatory bowel disease. Feeding an infant with skimmed milk or total parenteral nutrition without lipid supplementation can result in EFA deficiency.

PATHOGENESIS

Linoleic acid is necessary for formation of lamellar granule in the epidermis which is responsible for prevention of loss of water from the skin. Deficiency of linoleic acid results in increased evaporative water loss by 10 folds. This leads to generalized xerosis and scaling. Eczematous changes have been attributed to impaired eicosanoid production.

CLINICAL FEATURES

Cutaneous manifestations of EFA deficiency include alopecia, generalized xerosis, and intertriginous erosions. Extracutaneous features include growth retardation, fatty liver, anemia, thrombocytopenia, poor wound healing and increased susceptibility to infections.

MANAGEMENT

Increased ratio of eicosatrienoic acid to arachidonic acid is diagnostic of EFA deficiency. The condition is treated with supplementation of linoleic acid in the diet. It should constitute 1-4% of total caloric intake.

PROTEIN-ENERGY MALNUTRITION

Protein-energy malnutrition is comprised of marasmus and kwashiorkor. The former is a state of total starvation and the latter is a result of protein deficiency with relative carbohydrate excess.

CAUSES

Marasmus is commonly seen in third world countries where there is a scarcity of food. Kwashiorkor occurs in a disposed baby who is fed on high starch diet during weaning.

PATHOGENESIS

Clinical manifestations of marasmus and kwashiorkor are mainly due to inadequate intake of essential nutrients. The skin ulceration has been attributed to low zinc levels.

CLINICAL FEATURES

Generalized wasting without peripheral edema is the prominent feature of marasmus. The child weighs less than 60% of expected body weight. The skin appears dry, wrinkled and loose. Loss of buccal pad of fat results in wizened "Monkey facies". Several hair abnormalities like, slow growth, thinning, easy shedding, and lanugo hairs on face and posterior aspect of neck have been reported. Nails may show fissures.

Kwashiorkor refers to a child with peripheral edema **(Figure 29.6A)** who weighs 60 to 80% of expected body weight. The skin and hair shows several characteristic changes **(Table 29.2)**.

The extracutaneous features include anorexia, irritability and apathy, diarrhea, bilateral parotitis, fatty liver, hypoalbuminemia and immunosuppression.

TABLE 29.2: Cutaneous manifestations of kwashiorkor

1. "Enamel paint spots": Sharply demarcated hyperpigmented plaques with a burnished surface and waxy feel seen over elbows, knees, ankles, and intertrigenous area (trauma prone areas).
2. "Flaky paint" or "Crazy paving" dermatosis: Extensive skin peeling with erosions and flexural fissuring (Figure 29.6B).
3. Mosaic pigmented pattern: Dry, glossy surface with cracks over extensor aspect of tibia.
4. Hypopigmented patches with bran like desquamation over edematous areas and around the mouth.
5. "Flag sign": Alternating bands of normal and hypopigmention on scalp hair.

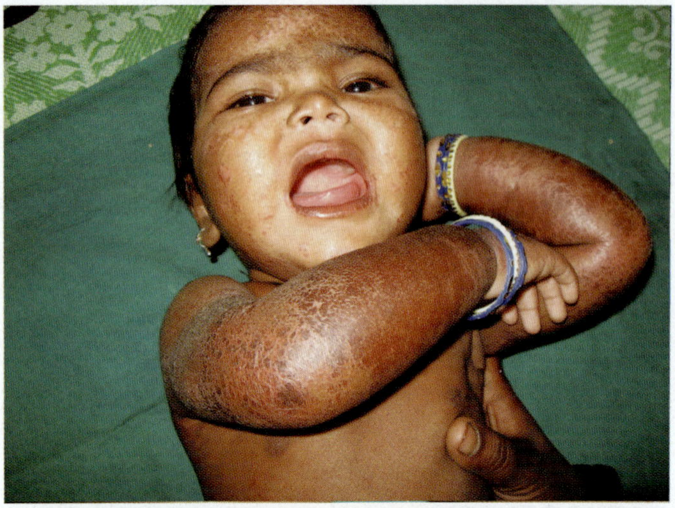

FIGURE 29.6A: Generalized edema with 'Moon facies'

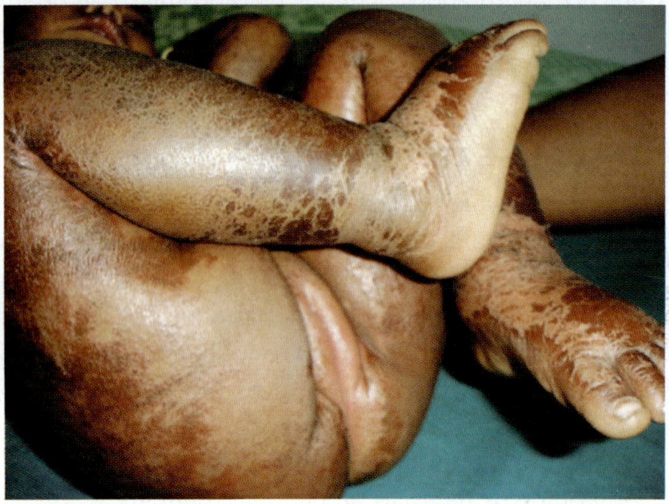

FIGURE 29.6B: Flaky paint dermatosis—Extensive skin peeling with erosions

MANAGEMENT

Treatment of protein-energy malnutrition includes adequate diet consisting of sufficient proteins, carbohydrates, lipids, vitamins, and minerals. Maintenance of electrolyte balance especially potassium is also important. A parkinsonian-like tremor known as kwashi shakes has been reported to develop during treatment. They usually resolve after 2 weeks.

ZINC DEFICIENCY

Zinc is an essential micronutrient of body. It is a component of many important metallo-enzymes (e.g. carbonic anhydrase, alkaline phosphatase, RNA & DNA polymerase, thymidine kinase, carboxypeptidases) involved in various metabolic pathways. Its main physiological functions include;

- Protein and nucleic acid synthesis
- Carbohydrate and vitamin A metabolism
- Immune function related to T cell, natural killer cell and neutrophils
- Wound healing and tissue repair

Zinc is absorbed in the small intestine from dietary sources. Maximum bioavailability is from foods of animal origin like meat, fish and shellfish; other vegetarian foods like legumes, whole grains and green leafy vegetables contribute to far lesser amount of the body requirement. In case of children, mother's milk contains very high concentration of zinc, the absorption of which is facilitated by the presence of a zinc binding ligand in it. However, zinc level of human breast milk gradually declines in later months of lactation. Formula milk, though may contain still higher concentration of zinc, bioavailability is inferior to mother's milk.

In the plasma, zinc is present in bound form with albumin (50%) and other proteins. Body storage sites for zinc are bone, muscle, prostate and skin; however, these do not contribute to the plasma pool of zinc. Hence, continuous dietary source is required to maintain body functions. Recommended daily intake of zinc in children is as follows:

- < 6 months: 3 mg
- > 6 months to 1 year: 5 mg
- 1-7 years: 10 mg
- 11 years/> : 16 mg

Dietary fibers, phytate and calcium containing foods may impair zinc absorption.

Zinc deficient state is of immense clinical importance as it gives rise to specific signs and symptoms and may turn fatal unless promptly diagnosed and treated. In children, zinc deficiency may be acquired or may be a heritable disorder, i.e. acrodermatitis enteropathica. Clinical features of acquired zinc deficiency are similar to that of heritable disorder, except that the onset is acute in the latter with a rapid, fatal course.

ACQUIRED ZINC DEFICIENCY

Zinc-deficient state may be acquired in children in the following situations:

- Premature infants, whose zinc requirement is higher to meet the need of rapid growth and the zinc content of mother's milk is insufficient for them. Moreover, intestinal zinc absorption is poor in such infants because of prematurity.

- Protein energy malnutrition
- Children on total parenteral nutrition without zinc supplementation, and cancer chemotherapy
- Endemic zinc deficiency has been reported from countries like Iran, Egypt and Turkey because of high dietary content of phytates.
- Chronic diseases like nephrotic syndrome, cystic fibrosis and inflammatory bowel syndrome.
- Full-term, breast-fed infants may develop zinc deficiency even before weaning, which may be attributable to lower zinc content of mother's milk. This may result from a zinc-deficient state in the mother or defective mammary gland secretion of zinc in the breast milk.

Acquired zinc deficiency should be treated with oral or parenteral supplementation with zinc sulphate as required. Prophylactic dose of zinc sulphate (0.1-0.3 mg /Kg /day) should be administered in premature infants and children on total parenteral nutrition.

HERITABLE DISORDER OF ZINC DEFICIENCY

Acrodermaitis Enteropathica

Acrodermatitis enteropathica (AE) is a rare autosomal recessive disorder resulting in clinical manifestations of zinc deficiency during weaning period in breast-fed infants and earlier in bottle-fed infants.

Pathogenesis: Pathogenesis of AE is not yet clearly understood. There is mutation of SLC39A gene, which encodes an endogenous zinc binding ligand (ZIP4 protein) produced by pancreas. This results in structural and functional, as well as quantitative defect in this ligand, resulting in poor intestinal absorption of zinc.

Clinical features: Clinical manifestations are multi-systemic, presenting with a triad of diarrhea, peri-orificial dermatitis and alopecia. In the acute stage, there is oozy dermatitis and vesiculo-bullous or pustular eruptions involving peri-oral, peri-nasal, peri-ocular **(Figure 29.7A)**, peri-anal and perineal locations **(Figure 29.7B)** as well as symmetrically on the distal extremities. Grayish, flat bullae surrounded by dull erythema are found on hands (finger flexion creases) and feet **(Figure 29.7C)**. Without treatment, peri-orificial lesions rapidly progresses to form areas of necrosis and eschar formation **(Figure 29.7D)**. There may be diffuse hair loss involving scalp

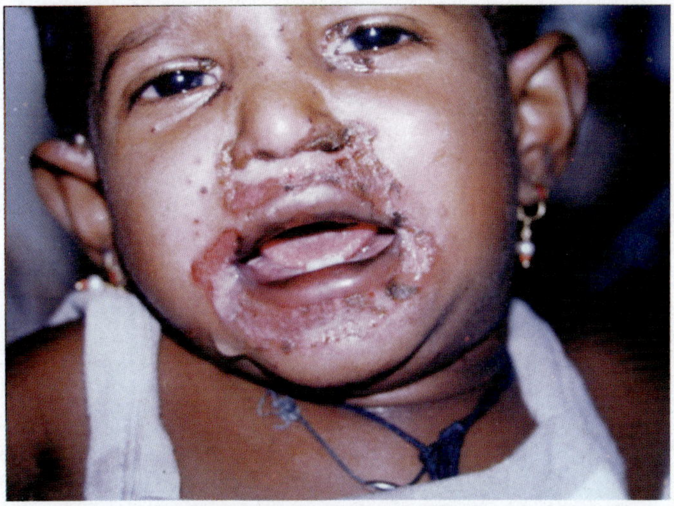

FIGURE 29.7A: Periocular and perioral dermatitis in acrodermatitis enteropathica

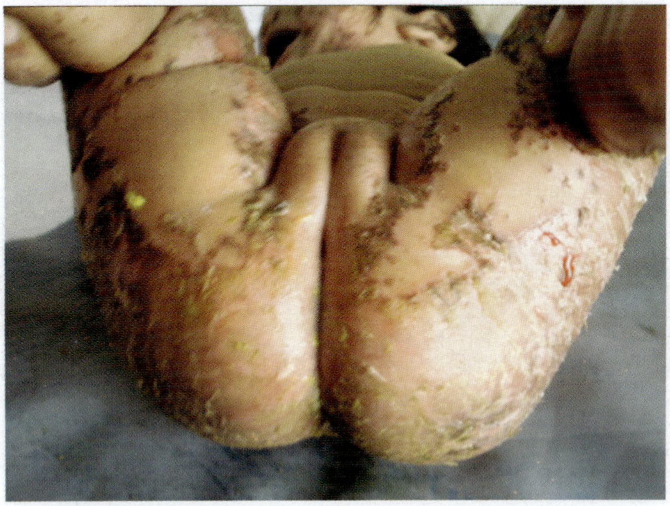

FIGURE 29.7B: Perianal and perineal dermatitis in acrodermatitis enteropathica

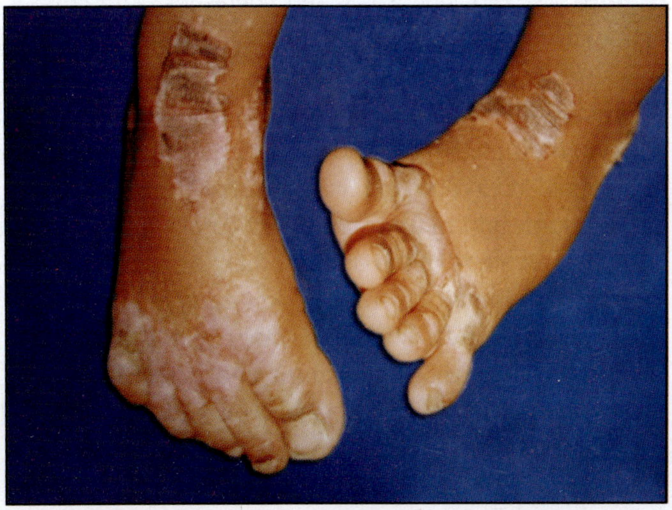

FIGURE 29.7C: Acral dermatitis in acrodermatitis enteropathica

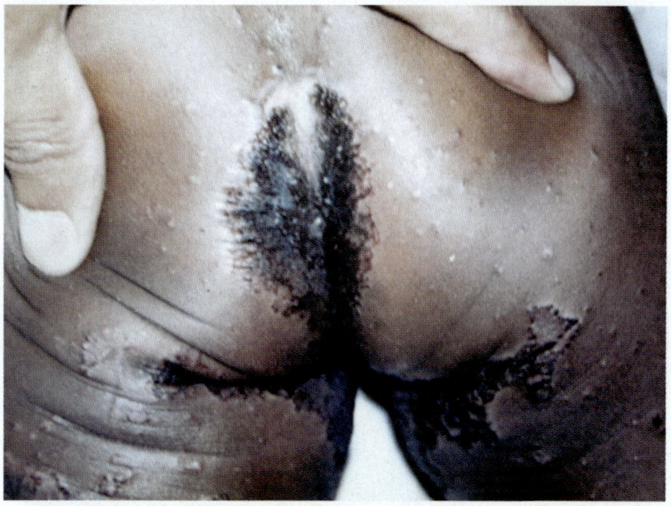

FIGURE 29.7D: Eschar formation in periorificial areas acrodermatitis enteropathica

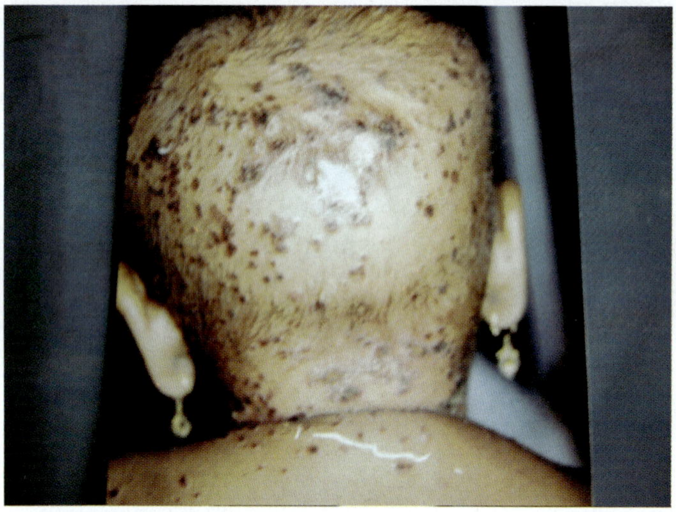

FIGURE 29.7E: Alopecia in acrodermatitis enteropathica

(Figure 29.7E), eyebrows and eyelashes. The child is extremely irritable with photophobia, refuses food and occasionally depressed. Voluminous, frothy, foul-smelling diarrhea is common in acute stage and may precede the cutaneous eruptions. Secondary bacterial (*Pseudomonas*) and fungal (*Candida sp.*) infections of the skin lesions are common and may result in septicemia.

In chronic stage of the disease, there are well-defined, lichenified eczematous eruptions on trauma-prone areas like knees, elbows, knuckles, malleoli and buttocks. Seborrheic dermatitis-like lesions and acral depigmentation simulating vitiligo has been reported. There is perleche and perioral eczema with sparing of the vermilion border. Stomatitis and glossitis may be associated. Hair is thin, sparse and lightly pigmented and there may be complete alopecia. Structural hair changes like bayonet-hairs, spearhead hair ends, split hair shaft, transverse bands, pseudomonilethrix may be present. Nails show Beau's lines once zinc supplementation is started. The affected children are often apathetic, depressed and anorexic.

Diagnosis: Diagnosis of AE is mostly clinical, confirmed by a low serum zinc level ($\geq$ 50 μg/dl). Simultaneous estimation of serum albumin is required as low albumin may falsely depict a lower serum zinc level. Estimation of serum alkaline phosphatase (ALP) level, a zinc dependent enzyme, may give an approximate idea of serum zinc status. It is low in zinc deficient state (normal reference range in children, 1-9 years; 145-420 U/L). There are reports of AE with normal serum zinc level, which may occur due to presence of a variant of the intestinal zinc-binding ligand. Such ligands allow intestinal zinc absorption leading to normal serum level but release at the cellular level is impaired giving rise to features of zinc deficiency. Estimation of ALP level is especially helpful in detecting such cases.

Histopathological examination from eczematous skin lesions show spongiosis and occasional suprabasal cleft. Epidermis is lost in ulcerative lesions, and psoriasiform in chronic lesions.

Treatment: Oral (2-5 mg/Kg/day in 2-3 divided dosage) or parenteral (0.2-0.3 mg/Kg/day) zinc-sulphate is the treatment of choice (a total dose of 50 mg/day in infants and 150-200 mg /day in children is recommended). Oral preparations should be administered before meals to avoid impaired absorption by food. Patients with established AE should receive life-long zinc supplementation at a minimum effective dosage.

Course and follow-up: Prompt diagnosis and early institution of therapy is mandatory for AE as delay may result in fatality. Earliest evidence of adequate therapy is subsidence of irritability and return of a normal mood within 24-48 hours. Skin lesions start healing by 2-3 days and clear completely in a week **(Figure 29.7F).** Diarrhea and anorexia improves in another few days. Re-growth of hair takes 2-3 weeks.

During follow-up, serum zinc level should be estimated at 6-monthly intervals. Estimation of serum ALP gives an approximate idea of serum zinc status as it rises and falls proportionate to zinc level.

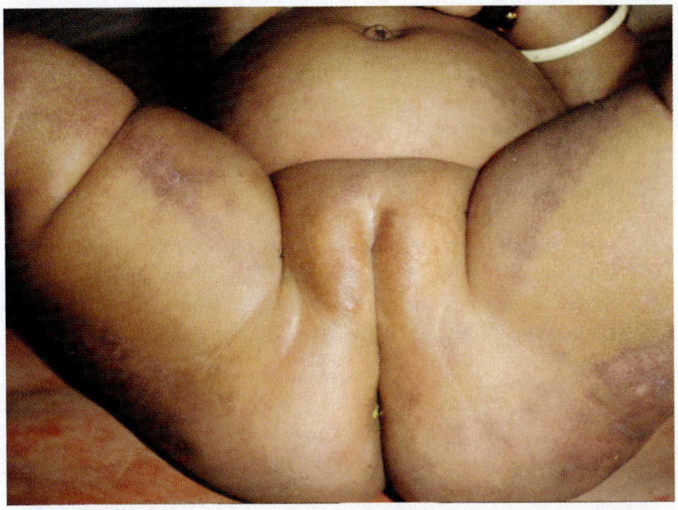

FIGURE 29.7F: Child in Figure 29.7B showing complete response to zinc therapy

Differential diagnosis: Conditions simulating AE are biotin deficiency and certain heritable organic acid related disorders like propionic acidemia, methylmalonic acidemia, maple syrup urine disease, citrullinemia and some other similar conditions. Periorificial skin lesions and hair changes in these conditions provide a look-alike of AE. In doubtful cases, therapeutic challenge with adequate dosage of zinc sulphate may be tried. Lack of clinical improvement in 3-4 days should dictate the clinician to rule out others causes than zinc deficiency.

COPPER DEFICIENCY

Copper is an important cofactor for functioning of various enzymes. The acquired copper deficiency seen in infants with severe protein-energy malnutrition or those on strict cow milk diet is rare. The cutaneous changes do not occur in acquired copper deficiency. However, characteristic hair changes are seen in X-linked recessive disorder of copper metabolism, Menke's kinky hair syndrome (See Chapter 13 for details). Repetitive twisting of hair (Pili torti) **(Figures 29.8A and B)** has been attributed to functional deficiency of amine oxidase activity which is required for disulfide bond formation within hairs. Other hair changes include trichorrhexis nodosa and monilethrix.

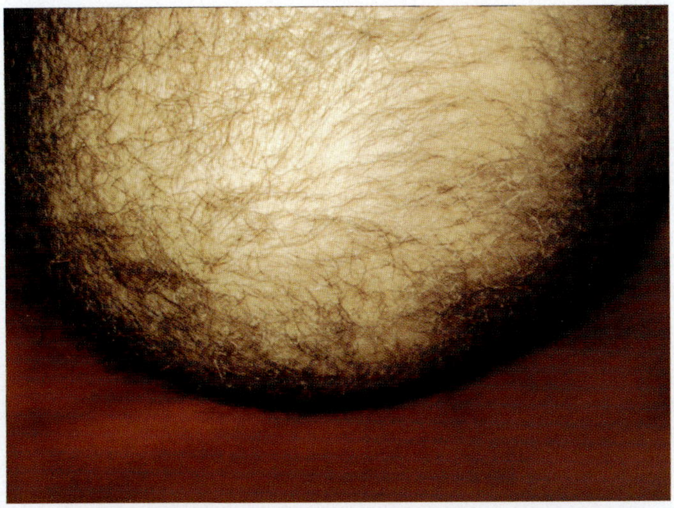

FIGURE 29.8A: Steel wool hairs Menke' syndrome

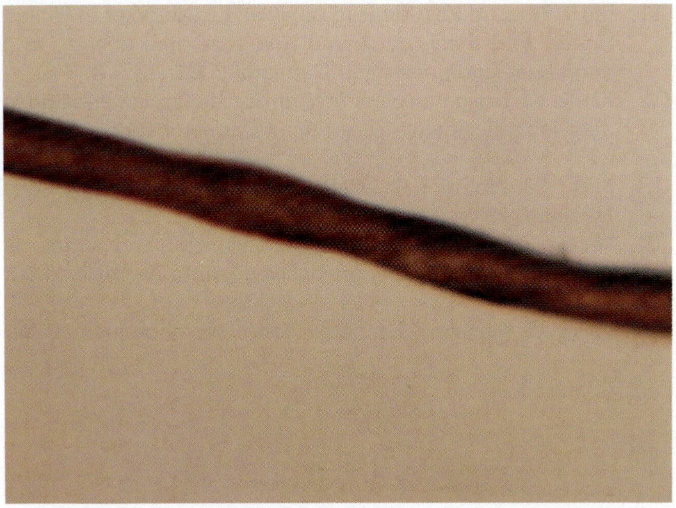

FIGURE 29.8B: Microscopic feature of pili torti (repetitive twisting of hair)

BIBLIOGRAPHY

1. Al-Rashid RA, Spangler J. Neonatal copper deficiency. N Engl J Med 1971; 285: 841-3.
2. Curran JS, Barness LA. Nutrition. In: Behrman RE, Kliegman RM, Jensen HB (Eds). Nelson Textbook of pediatric, 16th edn. Singapore: Harcourt Asia PTE, Ltd, 2000: 138-88.
3. Horrobin DF. Essential fatty acids in clinical dermatology. J Am Acad Dermatol 1989; 20: 1045-53.
4. Inamadar AC, Palit A. Acrodermatitis enteropathica with depigmented skin lesions simulating vitiligo. Pediatr Dermatol 2007; 24:668-9.
5. Jen M, Shah KN, Yan AC. Skin in nutritional, metabolic and heritable disease. In: Wolff K, Goldsmith LA, Katz SI, Gilchrist BA, Paller AS, Leffell DJ. Fitzpatrick's dermatology in general medicine, New York: McGraw Hill 2008;7(2):1201-18.
6. Karthikeyan K, Thappa DM. Pellagra and skin. Int J Dermatol 2002; 41: 476-81.
7. Koley SK, Sen MK, Panja RK. Phrynoderma-A review. Indian J Dermatol Venereol Leprol 1975; 41 (5): 171-5.
8. Kumaravel R. Scurvy. http://www.emedicine.com/ped/topic2073.htm (accessed on December 25, 2006).
9. Lakshmi AV. Riboflavin metabolism-relevance to human nutrition. Indian J Med Res 2000; 108: 182-90.
10. Latham MC. The dermatosis of kwashiorkor in young children. Semin Dermatol 1991; 10: 270-72.

11. Liu T, Howard RM, Mancini AJ, et al. Kwashiorkor in United States. Fad diets, perceived and true milk allergy, and nutritional ignorance. Arch Dermatol 2001; 137: 630-6.
12. Marks VJ, Briggman RA, Wheeler CE. Hyperpigmentation in megaloblastic anemia. J Am Acad Dermatol 1985; 12: 914-17.
13. Miller SJ. Nutritional deficiency and the skin. J Am Acad Dermatol 1989; 21: 1-30.
14. Navarro PC, Guerra A, Alvarez JG. Cutaneous and neurologic manifestations of biotinidase deficiency. Int J Dermatol 2000; 39: 363-5.
15. Paller AS, Mancini AJ. Inborn errors of metabolism. In: Paller AS, Mancini AJ (Eds). Hurwitz clinical pediatric dermatology, 3rd edn. Philadelphia: Elsevier Saunders 2006;631-49.
16. Perafán-Riveros C, Franca LFS, Alves ACF, Sanches Jr. JA. Acrodermatitis enteropathica: case report and review of literature. Pediatr Dermatol 2002;19:426-31.
17. Petit JHS. Phrynoderma. Int J Dermatol 1983; 22: 117-9.
18. Ragunatha S, Inamadar AC, Palit A, Sampagavi VV, Deshmukh NS. Diffuse nonscarring alopecia of scalp: An indicator of early infantile scurvy? Pediatr Dermatol 2008; 25: 644-6.
19. Seymons K, De Moor A, De Raeve H, Lambert J. Dermatologic signs of biotin deficiency leading to diagnosis of multiple carboxylase deficiency. Pediatr Dermatol 2004; 21: 231-5.

Index

A

B

E

F

G

I

J

K

L

M

N

R

S